# Intensity-Modulated Radiation Therapy

## The State Of The Art

Medical Physics Monograph No. 29

# Intensity-Modulated Radiation Therapy

## The State Of The Art

**Edited by**

**Jatinder R. Palta**
**T. Rockwell Mackie**

**American Association of Physicists in Medicine**
**2003 Summer School Proceedings**
**Colorado College**
**Colorado Springs, Colorado**
**June 22–26, 2003**

Published for the
American Association of Physicists in Medicine
by Medical Physics Publishing

To order American Association of Physicists in Medicine (AAPM) publications, contact:

Medical Physics Publishing
4513 Vernon Boulevard
Madison, WI 53705-4964
Phone: 1 (800) 442-5778 or (608) 262-4021
Fax: (608) 265-2121
E-mail: mpp@medicalphysics.org
Web: www.medicalphysics.org



Published by:
Medical Physics Publishing
Madison, Wisconsin

Published for:
American Association of Physicists in Medicine (AAPM)
One Physics Ellipse
College Park, MD 20740-3846
(301) 209-3350
Fax: (301) 209-0862

Library of Congress Catalog Card Number: 2003105917
ISBN 1-930524-16-1

Printed in the United States of America

# Contents

# Preface

The discipline of radiation oncology is reaching new heights with continued advancement in treatment planning, delivery, and treatment verification. These advances are attributed to newer innovations in several areas including volumetric imaging, optimized 3-D dose calculations and display, computer-controlled treatment delivery equipment, and on-line treatment verification. Volume imaging with advanced computed tomography and magnetic resonance imaging, functional imaging with positron emission tomography scanning, inter- and intra-image registration, and automatic image segmentation tools have enhanced our ability to define target volumes and critical structures with improved accuracy. Fast computers have made it possible to implement more rigorous and accurate model-based dose calculation and optimization algorithms for estimating dose distributions in three dimensions. Computer-controlled linear accelerators with multileaf collimators are capable of delivering highly complex radiation intensity patterns. Electronic portal imaging devices can provide real-time treatment verification. Such innovations have made it possible to plan and deliver radiation therapy treatments to patients that are highly conformal. Delivery of conformal therapy has traditionally been accomplished with radiation beams having a uniform radiation intensity across the field. More recently, conformal therapy is being implemented with radiation beams that have non-uniform radiation intensity across the field in two dimensions. This new type of conformal therapy is called intensity-modulated radiation therapy (IMRT). IMRT can achieve even greater conformity by optimally modulating the radiation fluence from the computer-controlled radiation delivery system. There are preliminary indications that this conformality leads to reduced early-onset of complications to normal tissues.

IMRT represents one of the most significant technical advances in radiation therapy since the advent of the medical linear accelerator. IMRT is not just an add on to the current radiation therapy process; it represents a new paradigm that requires knowledge of multimodality imaging, setup uncertainties and internal organ motion, tumor control probabilities, normal tissue complication probabilities, three-dimensional dose calculation and optimization, and dynamic beam delivery of non-uniform beam intensities. This new process of planning and treatment delivery shows significant potential for further improving the therapeutic ratio and reducing toxicity. There is a great push to make this technology available for all cancer patients, but it does not come without a price and a risk. The price lies in the fact that IMRT utilizes expensive hardware, complex and voluminous multimodality imaging and planning data, and significant personnel resources. The risk lies in the fact that complex radiation therapy techniques can be misunderstood and misapplied, possibly resulting in excess tumor recurrences or excess complications that will negate the potential benefits of these new technologies. Therefore, the task of safely implementing IMRT in radiation therapy clinics around the country will require innovative and efficient methodologies of quality assurance. Most IMRT planning and delivery systems are essentially first generation systems and are changing rapidly.

This book presents the proceedings of a comprehensive five-day program devoted to the state-of-the-art and future IMRT techniques presented at the 2003 American Association of Physicists in Medicine (AAPM) summer school in Colorado Springs, Colorado. The goal of the program is to present a snapshot of the current IMRT planning and delivery technology, to discuss issues that confront safe implementation of IMRT, and finally to encourage a reflection on the future of IMRT. The contributors to the proceedings of the AAPM summer school are among the foremost in the field. The result of their hard work is a textbook-quality handbook that will aid both experienced radiation oncology physicists and newcomers to the field in understanding the nuances of IMRT and its safe implementation in the clinics. The level of presentation was designed for practicing medical physicists who are not specialists in IMRT. IMRT is an emerging technology, which is still in its infancy. Therefore, some IMRT issues such as imaging and target delineation, quality assurance and its frequency, and achievable accuracy are discussed in multiple chapters and from differing points of view, reflecting the diversity of opinions in this rapidly evolving field.

The editors wish to thank all authors who took time from their extremely busy schedules to contribute quality material for this book. We would also like to acknowledge the local arrangement committee, headed by Jerry White, Chris Dennett, and Robin Miller, who arranged outstanding facilities and superbly organized the conference. The committee handled critical details that enabled the success of the 2003 AAPM summer school. We are most appreciative of the professional editing of this book done by Betsey Phelps of Medical Physics Publishing.

*T. Rockwell Mackie, Ph.D.*
*Jatinder R. Palta, Ph.D.*

Colorado Springs, Colorado
June 2003

# List of Contributors

John P. Balog, Ph.D.
TomoTherapy Inc.
1240 Deming Way
Madison, WI 53717-1954

James Balter, Ph.D.
Radiation Oncology Department
University of Michigan
1500 E. Medical Center Drive
B1F510B
Ann Arbor, MI 48109-0030

Jerry J. Battista, Ph.D.
Radiation Oncology Program
London Regional Cancer Centre
790 Commissioners Road East
London, ON N6A 4L6
Canada

Glenn S. Bauman, M.D.
London Regional Cancer Centre
790 Commissioners Road East
London, ON N6A 4L6
Canada

Angel I. Blanco, M.D.
Department of Radiation Oncology
Washington University
4511 Forest Park Blvd., Suite 200
St. Louis, MO 63108

Thomas R. Bortfeld, Ph.D.
Department of Radiation Oncology
Massachusetts General Hospital
30 Fruit Street
Boston, MA 02114

Lionel G. Bouchet, Ph.D.
ZMed Inc.
200 Butterfield Drive
Ashland, MA 01721

Francis J. Bova, Ph.D.
Department of Neurological Surgery
University of Florida
Box 100265 JHMHC
Gainesville, FL 32610

Arthur L. Boyer, Ph.D.
Department of Radiation Oncology
Stanford University
School of Medicine
300 Pasteur Drive
Stanford, CA 94305-5304

John M. Buatti, M.D.
University of Iowa
Department of Radiation Oncology
W189Z-GH
200 Hawkins Drive
Iowa City, IA 52242-1077

Yair Censor, D.Sc.
Department of Mathematics
University of Haifa
Mt. Carmel
Haifa 31905, Israel

K. S. Clifford Chao, M.D.
Department of Radiation Oncology
U.T. M.D. Anderson Cancer Center
1515 Holcombe Boulevard
Houston, TX 77030

Yan Chen, Ph.D.
Department of Radiation Oncology
Thomas Jefferson University Hospital
111 South 11th Street
Philadelphia, PA 19107

Zhe Chen, Ph.D.
Department of Radiation Oncology
Yale University School of Medicine
New Haven, CT 06510

Cynthia Chuang, Ph.D.
Department of Radiation Oncology
University of California
at San Francisco
1600 Divisadero Street, Suite H1031
San Francisco, CA 94115

Bruce H. Curran, M.E., M.S.
University of Michigan
Medical Center
1500 E. Medical Center Drive
UH-B2C438, Box 0010
Ann Arbor, MI 48109-0010

Matthew A. Earl, Ph.D.
Department of Radiation Oncology
University of Maryland School
of Medicine
22 Greene Street
Baltimore, MD 21201

Gary A. Ezzell, Ph.D.
Mayo Clinic Scottsdale
13400 E. Shea Blvd., Desk R
Scottsdale, AZ 85259

Lisa Forrest, V.M.D.
College of Veterinary Medicine
and Surgical Sciences
University of Wisconsin
Veterinary Medicine Building,
Room 2060
Madison, WI 53706

Kenneth M. Forster, Ph.D.
Department of Radiation Physics
U.T. M.D. Anderson Cancer Center
1515 Holcombe Boulevard
Houston, TX 77030

James M. Galvin, D.Sc.
Thomas Jefferson University Hospital
Jefferson Medical College
111 South 11th Street
Philadelphia, PA 19107-5097

Michael T. Gillin, Ph.D.
Department of Radiation Physics,
Box 94
U.T. M.D. Anderson Cancer Center
1515 Holcombe Boulevard
Houston, TX 77030-4009

Thomas Guerrero, M.D., Ph.D.
Department of Radiation Oncology
U.T. M.D. Anderson Cancer Center
1515 Holcombe Boulevard
Houston, TX 77030

Paul Harari, M.D.
Department of Human Oncology
University of Wisconsin
Medical School
K4/B100 Clinical Science Center
600 Highland Avenue
Madison, WI 53792

A. Curtis Hass, M.D.
University of Iowa
Department of Radiation Oncology
W189Z-GH
200 Hawkins Drive
Iowa City, IA 52242-1077

Susanta Hui, Ph.D.
Medical Physics Department
University of Wisconsin
1300 University Avenue
Madison, WI 53706

David A. Jaffray, Ph.D.
Department of Radiation Oncology
University of Toronto
University Health Network/
Princess Margaret Hospital
610 University Avenue, Rm. 1B-727
Toronto, ON M5G 2M9
Canada

Robert Jeraj, Ph.D.
Medical Physics Department
University of Wisconsin
1300 University Avenue
Madison, WI 53706

Jeffrey M. Kapatoes, Ph.D.
TomoTherapy Inc.
1240 Deming Way
Madison, WI 53717-1954

Paul Keall, Ph.D.
Department of Radiation Oncology
Virginia Commonwealth University
401 College Street
MVC Box 980058
Richmond, VA 23298

Jong Oh Kim, Ph.D.
Department of Radiation Oncology
Virginia Commonwealth University
401 College Street, B-129
MVC Box 980058
Richmond, VA 23298

Siyong Kim, Ph.D.
Department of Radiation Oncology
University of Florida
P.O. Box 100385
2000 SW Archer Road
Gainesville, FL 32610-0385

Michael Kissick, Ph.D.
Medical Physics Department
University of Wisconsin
1300 University Avenue
Madison, WI 53706

Mark Langer, M.D.
Department of Radiation Oncology
Indiana University
Indiana Cancer Pavilion
535 Barnhill Drive RT 041
Indianapolis, IN 46202-2486

Jonathan G. Li, Ph.D.
Department of Radiation Oncology
University of Florida
P.O. Box 100385
2000 SW Archer Road
Gainesville, FL 32610-0385

Chihray Liu, Ph.D.
Department of Radiation Oncology
University of Florida
Shands Cancer Center
2000 SW Archer Road
Gainesville, FL 32610-0385

Tony Lomax, Ph.D.
Paul Scherrer Institute
5232 Villigen-PSI
Switzerland

Thomas J. LoSasso, Ph.D.
Medical Physics Department
Memorial Sloan-Kettering
Cancer Center
1275 York Avenue
New York, NY 10021

Daniel A. Low, Ph.D.
Associate Professor
of Radiation Oncology
Washington University
School of Medicine
4921 Parkview Place
St. Louis, MO 63110

Gary Luxton, Ph.D.
Department of Radiation Oncology
Stanford University
School of Medicine
300 Pasteur Drive
Stanford, CA 94305-5304

T. Rockwell Mackie, Ph.D.
Medical Physics Department
University of Wisconsin
1300 University Avenue
Madison, WI 53706

Sanford L. Meeks, Ph.D.
University of Iowa
Department of Radiation Oncology
W189Z-GH
200 Hawkins Drive
Iowa City, IA 52242-1077

Minesh P. Mehta, M.D.
Department of Human Oncology
University of Wisconsin
Medical School
K4/B100 Clinical Science Center
600 Highland Avenue
Madison, WI 53792

Radhe Mohan, Ph.D.
Department of Radiation Physics
U.T. M.D. Anderson Cancer Center
Box 94
1515 Holcombe Boulevard
Houston, TX 77030

Jean M. Moran, Ph.D.
Department of Radiation Oncology
University of Michigan
Medical Center
UH-B2C438 Box 0010
1500 E. Medical Center Drive
Ann Arbor, MI 48109-0010

Gustavo H. Olivera, Ph.D.
Medical Physics Department
University of Wisconsin
1300 University Avenue
Madison, WI 53706

Jatinder R. Palta, Ph.D.
Department of Radiation Oncology
University of Florida
P.O. Box 100385
2000 SW Archer Road
Gainesville, FL 32610-0385

Charles A. Pelizzari, Ph.D.
Radiation and Cellular
Oncology Department
University of Chicago,
Chicago, Illinois
MC9006
5758 South Maryland Avenue
Chicago, IL 60637

Alan Pollack, M.D., Ph.D.
Department of Radiation Oncology
Fox Chase Cancer Center
7701 Burholme Avenue
Philadelphia, PA 19111

Robert A. Price, Ph.D.
Department of Radiation Oncology
Fox Chase Cancer Center
7701 Burholme Avenue
Philadelphia, PA 19111

Paul J. Reckwerdt, B.S.
TomoTherapy Inc.
1240 Deming Way
Madison, WI 53717-1954

Mark Ritter, M.D., Ph.D.
Department of Human Oncology
University of Wisconsin
Medical School
K4/B100 Clinical Science Center
600 Highland Avenue
Madison, WI 53792

Kenneth J. Ruchala, Ph.D.
TomoTherapy Inc.
1240 Deming Way
Madison, WI 53717-1954

Michael B. Sharpe, Ph.D., DABMP
Department of Radiation Oncology
Princess Margaret Hospital and
University of Toronto
610 University Avenue
Toronto, ON M5G 2M9
Canada

David M. Shepard, Ph.D.
Department of Radiation Oncology
University of Maryland
School of Medicine
22 Greene Street
Baltimore, MD 21201

Jeffrey V. Siebers, Ph.D.
Medical College of Virginia Hospitals
Virginia Commonwealth University
P.O. Box 980058
401 College Street
Richmond, VA 23298-0058

Y. Song, Ph.D.
Department of Radiation Oncology
Stanford University
School of Medicine
300 Pasteur Drive
Stanford, CA 94305-5304

Craig W. Stevens, M.D., Ph.D.
Department of Radiation Oncology
U.T. M.D. Anderson Cancer Center
1515 Holcombe Boulevard
Houston, TX 77030

Wolfgang A. Tomé, Ph.D.
Department of Human Oncology
University of Wisconsin
Medical School
K4/B100 Clinical Science Center
600 Highland Avenue
Madison, WI 53792

Timothy J. Waldron, M.S.
Department of Radiation Physics
U.T. M.D. Anderson Cancer Center
1515 Holcombe Boulevard, Unit 94
Houston, TX 77030-4095

Steve Webb, Ph.D., D.Sc.
The Institute of Cancer Research
Joint Department of Physics
The Royal Marsden NHS Trust
Downs Road
Sutton, Surrey SM2 5PT
United Kingdom

James S. Welsh, M.D.
Department of Human Oncology
University of Wisconsin
Medical School
K4/B100 Clinical Science Center
600 Highland Avenue
Madison, WI 53792

John Wong, Ph.D.
Radiation Oncology Department
William Beaumont Hospital
3601 W. Thirteen Mile Road
Royal Oak, MI 48073-6769

Chuan Wu, M.S.
Medical Physics Department
University of Wisconsin
1300 University Avenue
Madison, WI 53706

Qiuwen Wu, Ph.D.
Department of Radiation Oncology
Virginia Commonwealth University
401 College Street
MVC Box 980058
Richmond, VA 23298

Yan Wu, M.S.
Department of Radiation Oncology
Virginia Commonwealth University
401 College Street
Richmond, VA 23298

Ping Xia, Ph.D.
Department of Radiation Oncology
University of California
at San Francisco
P.O. Box 0226
San Francisco, CA 94143-0226

Ying Xiao, Ph.D.
Radiation Oncology/Medical Physics
Thomas Jefferson University Hospital
11th and Sansom
Philadelphia, PA 19107

Lei Xing, Ph.D.
Department of Radiation Oncology
Stanford University
School of Medicine
300 Pasteur Drive
Stanford, CA 94305-5304

Y. Yang, Ph.D.
Department of Radiation Oncology
Stanford University
School of Medicine
300 Pasteur Drive
Stanford, CA 94305-5304

Ellen D. Yorke, Ph.D.
Medical Physics Department
Memorial Sloan-Kettering
Cancer Center
1275 York Avenue
New York, NY 10021

Cedric X. Yu, D.Sc.
Department of Radiation Oncology
University of Maryland
School of Medicine
22 Greene Street
Baltimore, MD 21201

# Historical Perspective On IMRT

**Steve Webb, Ph.D., D.Sc.**
Joint Department of Physics
Institute of Cancer Research and Royal Marsden NHS Trust, London, UK



## Introduction

### My View Is Not The Only One

Historical records are rarely as objective as one might think they should be. At first sight history might seem to be just the requirement to get straight the past order of events and to string them together in some neat way to capture the attention of the reader. At rock bottom level this is indeed what we amateur-historian writers do.

However, historical writing is inevitably colored with the subjectivity of the writer and, had the AAPM chosen one of the other pioneers of IMRT to do the writing, the story may have come out differently. Hopefully the main landmarks, the stepping stones of progress, would have been the same but the detail and interpretation would inevitably have varied. The author wishes to add a note of introductory caution that the review is from his perspective and that others may view the history differently. It is also a "history" in the sense of an account written by one who worked right through the period, a professional physicist but effectively an amateur historian. A professionally trained historian might not write in this way.

## What Is History?

Then there is the issue of what constitutes history? A common understanding is that historians are interested in unraveling events from many years ago. The term "IMRT" was coined about 1996. We had been working on "beam modulation," "fluence structuring," and so on, but the acronym IMRT is less than a decade old and no one has come forward to claim they were first to say the words[1]. So the history of IMRT is a very recent history. Table 1 summarizes the main developments. In my opinion, everything significant in IMRT has transpired in the last 15 years (although I will point to some historical antecedents). This means that the vast majority of the IMRT pioneers are alive, indeed are still working. Indeed many are at this meeting and in this audience. The author considers it might be somewhat presumptuous to pick out key people in that those not mentioned may feel offended. He apologizes for this and hopes a generous spirit can allow the highlighting of some central figures. Amateur writers of history tread dangerously.

## Is IMRT "Completed"?

The next observation is to ask whether the desire to open this Summer School with a historical perspective is in itself a statement that there is some international consensus that the main issues in IMRT are all worked out and there is now less to do. Certainly it seems to me that, if I were writing a four-sentence history, I would say that in 1988 just one person (Anders Brahme) had suggested fluence modulation and inverse planning. Then, by 1995, the main planning and delivery techniques had been worked out (but with little commercial apparatus and almost no clinical implementation). Then, by 2000, all the major companies were offering IMRT planning and delivery; the first clinical deliveries were being made. By 2003 "everyone wants IMRT."

---

[1] Thomas Bortfeld, one of the pioneers of IMRT, told me a nice anecdote about another pioneer Art Boyer. Answering the same question one day Boyer had said "well it must have been me because: I aM aRT". It was undoubtedly tongue-in-cheek but it's a nice story.

**Table 1.** The Development of IMRT: the One-Page History

**IMRT is poised to make a major clinical impact.
How has the field reached the present position?**

| | |
|---|---|
| **1895** | The x ray was discovered on November 8th in Germany by Roentgen. |
| **1896** | Doctors understood the need to "concentrate radiation" at the target but had means to neither do this nor even to know where the target was precisely. |
| **1950s** | Takahashi first discussed conformation therapy. |
| **1959** | Invention and patenting of the first multileaf collimator. |
| **1960s** | Proimos developed gravity-oriented blocking and conformal field shaping. |
| **1970s** | The Royal Free Hospital built the "tracking cobalt unit" and MGH Boston did similarly. |
| **1982** | Brahme et al. discussed inverse-planning for a fairly special case of rotational symmetry. |
| **1984** | First commercial MLCs appeared. |
| **1988** | Brahme published first paper on algebraic inverse planning. |
| **1988** | Källman postulated dynamic therapy with moving jaws. |
| **1989** | Webb developed simulated annealing for inverse planning. So did Mageras and Mohan. |
| **1990** | Bortfeld developed algebraic/iterative inverse-planning, the precursor of the KONRAD treatment-planning system. |
| **1991** | Principle of segmented-field therapy developed (Boyer / Webb). |
| **1992** | Convery showed the DMLC technique was possible. |
| **1992** | Mark Carol first showed the NOMOS MIMiC® and associated PEACOCK-PLAN® planning system (now CORVUS). |
| **1993** | Tomotherapy (the Wisconsin machine) first described by Mackie. |
| **1994** | Stein, Svensson, and Spirou independently discovered the optimal DMLC trajectory equations. |
| **1994** | Bortfeld and Boyer conducted the first multiple-static-field (MSF) experiments. |
| **1999** | First discussion of possible robotic IMRT. |
| **2002** | Commercial tomotherapy began. |
| **2003** | Large number of competing IMRT planning systems and systems for delivery. IMRT is well established in several geographically distributed centers. |

I have heard some young people ask if there is any serious IMRT science left to do. I have had this question too from my hospital and university chiefs and I have implicitly heard it from grant review bodies. All my training as a physicist teaches me that just as one reaches such a period of questioning, the next avenue opens up. I personally believe that development in IMRT is anything but concluded and I expect this Summer School to reinforce this view. We are good at shaping a high-dose distribution to a stationary target ("dead patient") but we are still embryonic on solving the problem of irradiating the moving target. Image guidance-IM-radiotherapy (IG- IM-RT) will help us. Also some of us are developing simpler non-MLC (multileaf collimator) IMRT delivery techniques and IMRT with $^{60}$Co machines (see the later sections *Cobalt IMRT* and *Shuttling Multileaf Collimators And Jaws+Mask*). There is the whole issue of how to determine target volumes from more than anatomical tomographic data. Multimodality imaging is hardly applied yet to IMRT. Perhaps when molecular genetics moves from the lab to the clinic, there will be an enhanced response due to combination with radiation, which will be required to be selectively delivered to precise geometric sites. Despite the now 15-year history of effort in inverse planning for IMRT and 10-year history of effort in MLC delivery of IMRT there is still a flow of new papers in this area. Controversially, I wish to suggest that recently there has been some "wheel reinventing" and that research effort would more appropriately be directed at IG-IM-RT.

## Critics Of IMRT

A further observation is that, just as IMRT is becoming clinically widespread, there has started the flow of papers from those who question whether it is all going too fast and is on shaky premises. This is welcomed and, at least in the UK, multicentric randomized clinical trials are planned to determine whether IMRT is going to deliver on its expected promise. Certainly, there is huge manufacturer interest and pressure to purchase, and a doubter might say that the volume of IMRT clinical implementation has more to do with dollars than patient care. It is also gripped by fashion in radiotherapy and by an "if they've got it, then we too must have it" mentality (Schulz and Kagan 2002). All this is probably an unstoppable consequence of some basic human characteristics.

## Weightier Reviews Of IMRT

I have been in the enviable position of being a reviewer of conformal radiation therapy (CFRT) and IMRT since its inception and wrote a trilogy of books (Webb 1993, 1997, 2001c) in which aspects of this history have already appeared (for the most relevant one see figure 1). Others have since done similar jobs, which I welcome. Sternick (1997) produced the first book with IMRT in its title (figure 2). Particularly useful is the e-book from Schlegel and Mahr (2001). Van Dyk (1999) has produced a massive overview. Smith (1995) also reviewed CFRT and IMRT. There have been a number of Special Journal Supplements and issues. In fact, there is really no shortage at all of review material. I have produced three "lay" accounts (Webb 1998, 2000a, 2002c). The history of radiotherapy in general was reviewed in Webb (1993, 2002c).

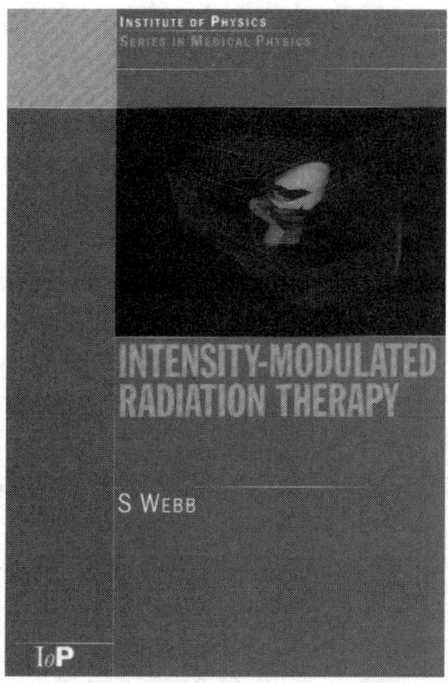

**Figure 1.** Cover of author's text on IMRT (November 2000) [Webb (2001c)].

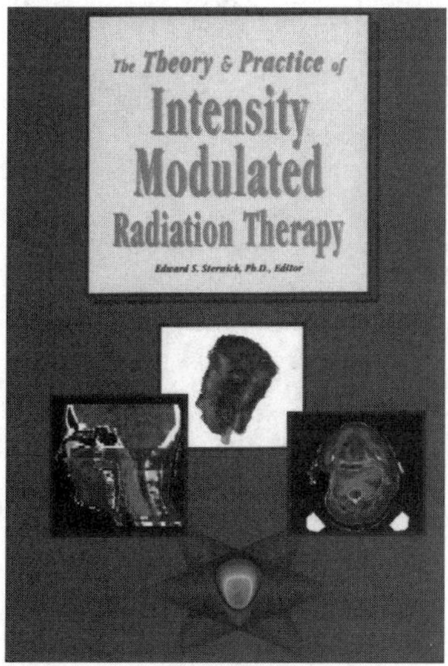

**Figure 2.** Cover of the first book with IMRT in its title (Summer 1997). [Sternick (1997)].

## Prehistory

The first paper showing how one could move from a dose prescription to a fluence modulation was by Brahme, Roos, and Lax (1982) (see figures 6 and 7) and the paper by Brahme (1988) followed up. But these did not just come from nowhere. It might be argued that there are precedents—let's call this prehistory and start with this.

## Birkhoff's Drawing Theory

George Birkhoff, an American mathematician, showed in 1940 that any grayscale drawing could be made up of a finite series of intersecting straight lines. A key proviso was that there needed to exist lines of negative blackness that could cancel out positive blackness in some areas. These he called "rectilinear erasures". They did not erase all in their path but simply added in some negative weight along their path. The overall drawing was the sum of the different positive and negative weights of blackness (Birkhoff 1940). In essence he had described the principle of IMRT since perfect pictures (dose distributions) would be made by adding lines (rays) of different blackness (intensity). However negative blackness was also needed (negative X-rays) and there the analogy with IMRT breaks down. It is a fanciful analogy because of course radiation physics was not in mind, but it is a neat analogy in retrospect. The exact mathematical equivalences are written down in appendix D of Webb (1997) and Birkhoff's example picture is shown in figure 3.

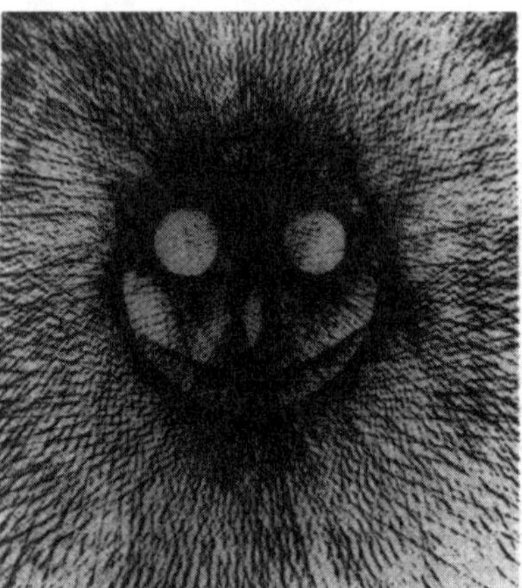

**Figure 3.** The diagram in the paper by Birkhoff showing how a black & white picture of a cat can be made up from a series of pencil lines of different thickness (density) provided these are both positive (normal pencil) and negative (unphysical erasure). [Reprinted from *Journal des Mathématiques Pures et Appliquées*, vol 19, G. D. Birkhoff, "On drawings composed of uniform straight lines," pp. 221–236. © 1940, Société de Periodiques Spécialisés.]

## Gravity Blocking

Several workers in the 1960s produced radiotherapy techniques that had the harshest modulation possible, i.e., binary radiation: on (open aperture) or off (shield). It was arranged that, as the gantry rotated about the patient, the shield changed its position with respect to the patient by hanging under gravity, in such a way that organs to be spared were always in the line-of-sight of the gravity block (Proimos 1960). An alternative realization arranged for the absorbers to co-rotate under chain drive (figure 4) as the gantry rotated, thus always aligning the long edge of the absorber with the line-of-sight into the tissue. Apart from some small transmission component these organs were thus spared primary radiation although they received scatter. Sometimes, at the same time, the open aperture also varied its shape in response to the beam's-eye view (BEV) of the target. The problems with these methods were several. Firstly, they inherently led to an inhomogeneous planning target volume (PTV) dose distribution especially when the PTV was abutting the spared organs. Secondly, the blocks had to be fabricated for each patient individually. Thirdly, the apparatus was inherently mechanical. Recall this was before the days of computer control. This idea has actually resurfaced comparatively recently from its original proposer. Webb (1993) has provided a lengthy review with pictures.

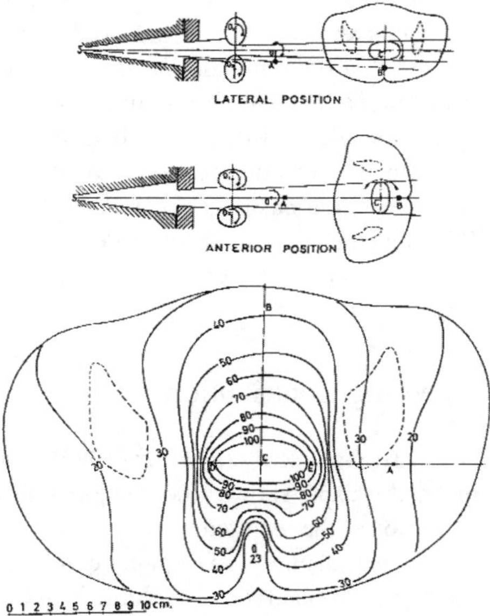


**Figure 4.** Treatment of an elliptical area in the pelvis by synchronous field shielding. Note that the circular absorber at A protects the spinal cord at B. The dose distribution obtained is shown below the irradiation arrangement. [Reprinted from *Radiology*, vol 77, B. S. Proimos, "Synchronous protection and field shaping in cyclotherapy," pp. 591–599. © 1961, with permission from Radiological Society of North America (RSNA).]

## Tracking $^{60}$Cobalt Unit

With hindsight early developments might be seen as antecedents to IMRT. For example, the tracking cobalt unit developed by Jennings and co-workers in the 1970s at London's Royal Free Hospital tracked target aiming to spare organs at risk (Jennings 1985).

## Blocks, Wedges, And Compensators

Finally, in a strict sense, the use of a block, a wedge, or a compensator modulates the intensity. But it is pushing too hard to claim these were also genuine historical antecedents to IMRT.

## **Modern IMRT History**

## What Exactly Is IMRT?

Let us agree that IMRT means the delivery of several fields in which the modulation is more complex than can be achieved with a block, wedge, or compensator. The modulation could be fine resolution in one or both of the spatial and fluence domains (see figure 5). If I had been writing this review 3 years ago, I would have categorically stated that a useful aid to definition is that such modulation should have been calculated by inverse-planning, i.e., the technique by which beam modulations are "automatically" deduced by computer from input desired dose distributions and input constraints. However, recently, there has been a considerable trend to adapt forward planning to multisegment beams so this definition has begun to fall over. Perhaps now the only surviving "label" for IMRT is that the modulation be moderately complex. If we accept this, then this creates clear blue water between those concepts from prehistory and IMRT as we know it today.

## Anders Brahme's Pioneering Contribution

The paper (figures 6 and 7) by Brahme, Roos, and Lax (1982) is generally regarded as the first paper on IMRT in that this paper shows how to begin with a desired dose distribution and arrive at a specification of the required fluence modulation to create it. Today we refer to this process as "inverse-planning". The paper considered what is generally believed to be the only problem that is analytically soluble, that of obtaining a uniform annulus of dose $D$ with outer radius $R$ surrounding a central circle of radius $r_0$ of zero primary dose (the problem was two-dimensional). It was shown that this would be achieved by a rotation technique in which the fluence was zero from the origin out to the inner radius $r_0$ of the annulus and which then rose suddenly (figure 7) to infinity (or in practice "large") followed by a falloff with distance $x > r_0$ according to:

$$F(x) = \exp\left[\mu(R^2 - x^2)^{0.5}\right] D \, x \, \cos\left[\mu\,(x^2 - r_0^2)^{0.5}\right] / (x^2 - r_0^2)^{0.5}$$

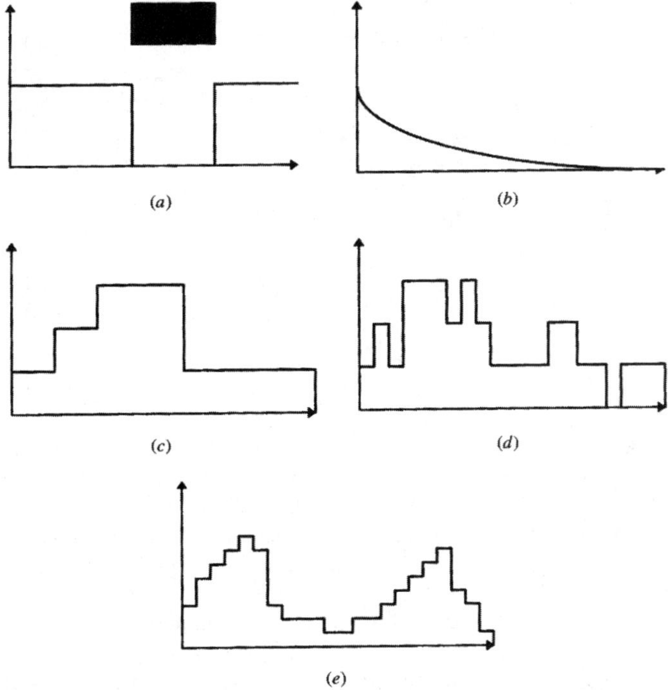

**Figure 5.** IMRT of varying complexity: (a) "binary on-off" (block); (b) wedge; (c) full modulation (coarse spatial and intensity scale); (d) full modulation (fine spatial, coarse intensity scale); (e) full modulation (fine spatial and intensity scale). The vertical axis in each case represents intensity or fluence and the horizontal axis represents distance. Here are presented just 1-D IMBs corresponding to one line of a 2-D modulation. [Reprinted from *Intensity-Modulated Radiation Therapy* by Steve Webb, Fig. 1.5, © 2001, with permission from IOP Publishing Limited.]

# Solution of an integral equation encountered in rotation therapy

A Brahme†, J-E Roos‡ and I Lax§

§ Department of Hospital Physics, Karolinska Sjukhuset, Box 60204, S-104 01 Stockholm, Sweden
‡ Department of Mathematics, University of Stockholm, Box 6701, S-113 85 Stockholm, Sweden
§ Department of Hospital Physics, Karolinska Sjukhuset, Box 60204, S-104 01 Stockholm, Sweden

Received 30 March 1981, in final form 4 December 1981

**Figure 6.** Title page of the pioneering paper by Brahme, Roos, and Lax (1982).

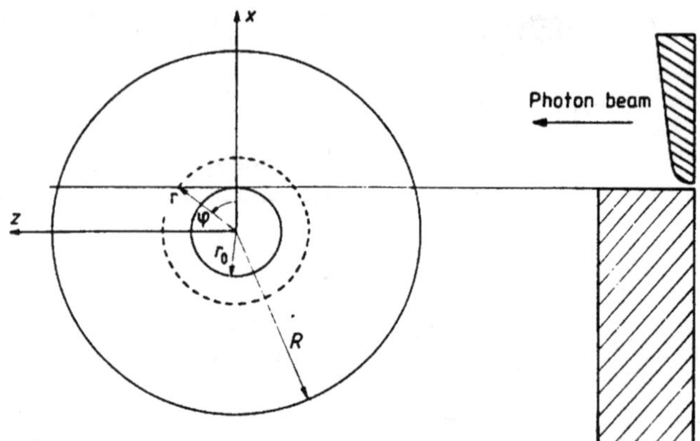


**Figure 7.** A diagram from the paper in figure 6 showing how a uniform annular dose distribution surrounding a circle of zero dose could be obtained by rotating an intensity-modulated beam. [Reprinted from *Physics in Medicine and Biology*, vol 19, A. Brahme, J. E. Roos, and I. Lax, "Solution of an integral equation encountered in rotation therapy," pp. 1221–1229. © 1982, with permission from Elsevier.]

where $\mu$ is the X-ray linear attenuation coefficient. Chapter 2 of Webb (1993) develops the algebra in detail and shows further extensions from this concept.

The next milestone in inverse planning was the paper by Brahme (1988) in which was explained the notion of creating fluence profiles from dose distributions by first inspecting the dose distribution in dosespace, then deconvolving the point-spread dose kernel from this to create the density of fluences required. The next step was to back-project the density of fluence back into fluence space to create the fluence profiles. Then, from the profiles so generated, the deliverable dose distributions could be formed by a process of projecting the fluence back into dosespace. The projection and back-projection processes both involved exponential (+/−) depth operations. However, projection and backprojection are not inverse processes and so the technique was only approximate. Also, the process could generate negative fluences and so required some form of truncation to zero or the addition of constant terms in fluence space. The work was a landmark because it established the idea of this kind of planning viewed as a form of inverse computed tomography, a term which actually was used for a while but later abandoned.


## Early Inverse Planning

The term "inverse planning" has however become well established. Several authors, notably Bortfeld et al. (1990), observed that this was a mirror of the CT process. In CT the known quantities are the projection data and one requires to reconstruct the image. In inverse planning for IMRT the known (or at least specified) quantities are the dose prescription distributions and constraints and the goal is to find the (back)projected fluence patterns that, when projected into dosespace, generate a realistic approximation to the desired dose prescription. Bortfeld et al. (1990) showed that by introducing filtering steps, and then in later work (Bortfeld et al. 1994a) iterative repeated forward and backprojection, the process of inverse planning could be fine-tuned. Just a little after, a similar CT-based algorithm was developed by Holmes and Mackie (1992).

## Simulated Annealing

At the same time Webb (1989) published the first of a suite of four papers (1989–1992) showing how IMRT could be planned via inverse-planning techniques using simulated annealing. He had been working on simulated annealing for reconstruction of gamma camera SPECT (single photon emission computed tomography) data, had heard of the mirror concept through Brahme's visit to the Royal Marsden Hospital in 1988 and saw the opportunity to switch the technique into a new field and create fluence profiles this way. The early papers considered firstly 2-D dosemaps from 1-D projections, with and without scatter and then subsequently went on to consider how to deliver modulations using the then quite new multileaf collimator (MLC). In fact, the third of the four papers introduced the idea of "two weights per field", one weight for that part of the BEV seeing just target and the other weight for that part of the BEV seeing target and under- or overlying organs at risk (OARs). This idea has been taken up in more recent years by many others and now is often referred to as segmental IMRT. Mageras and Mohan (1992) were performing quite similar work at Memorial Sloan-Kettering Hospital, New York. They too had developed simulated annealing and the concept of two-weights per field. Their paper is a little later but the dates on papers are never a perfect indicator of the time work was done and I have made it clear in many reviews in the past that these two projects may well have been taking place simultaneously. Certainly there is striking similarity between them although no collaboration as such (see chapter 2 of Webb 1997).

## Cone-Beam IMRT

Around 1991 Boyer generalized the inverse planning technique to cone-beam geometry and also described a "field-within-field" technique whereby modulated 2-D fields could be constructed by multiple applications of the MLC with different irregular field profiles. Boyer should be credited with the "invention" of the multiple-static-field (MSF) MLC technique for IMRT (Boyer, Desobry, and Wells 1991) (see also the later section *Multiple-Static-Field (MSF) MLC Technique*).

## NOMOS, The MIMiC®, PEACOCKPLAN®

Mark Carol, founder of NOMOS Corporation, presented a concept for delivering IMRT at his commercial exhibit at the 1992 AAPM meeting in Calgary. At the same meeting, Tim Holmes from the University of Wisconsin presented the first work on tomotherapy.

At the European Association of Radiology meeting in Geneva on October, 1992, Mark Carol showed slides of a device called the MIMiC®, then manufactured by the Medical Equipment Development Company Inc. (MEDCO), soon to be rebadged as the NOMOS Corporation. The audience was spellbound because he opened with words like "You have heard how we want to do it; now I shall show you apparatus that can do it". It was one of those moments one sensed would have long-term impact. If I recall correctly, Carol was encouraged to over-run well into a scheduled coffee break and then asked to return in the afternoon to an unscheduled session, so much interest was there in the new apparatus (Carol et al. 1993).

The MIMiC was extraordinary because it was not a product from one of the well-known accelerator manufacturers. It was a device capable of being mounted on any accelerator. It created two adjacent 1-D profiles, each with 20 bixels at any gantry angle chosen. By changing the dwell time of tungsten attenuators in these 40 bixels as a function of gantry rotation, and under electropneumatric control, the required 1-D intensity-modulated beams were created which, when delivered, yielded conformal dose distributions with invaginations. For the period 1992–1997 the use of the MIMiC dominated clinical IMRT practice and it continues to be the device which has delivered more IMRT worldwide than its rivals (see later). A prototype 2-D MIMiC comprising mercury-fillable balloons was also manufactured in the factory but never developed for sale. In the hands of its supporters, those trained to use the MIMiC and those with the wisdom to apply it to situations where tissue movement was not a major issue, the MIMiC became a front runner. It was coupled to a treatment-planning system initially called PEACOCKPLAN®, now CORVUS®, that was based on simulated annealing. Carol kindly acknowledged me as the source of these ideas although I want to make it clear that the development was entirely by NOMOS. My papers were in the public domain and rightly available for use. Later, CORVUS became a more versatile tool for planning MLC-based IMRT.

NOMOS hosted the first international conference on IMRT (figures 8 and 9) in the Strater hotel theatre in Durango, Colorado, filmed the whole proceedings, issued video sets, and published the first book with the words IMRT in the title (Sternick 1997) (figure 2).

The workings of the apparatus are so well known that this is not the place to repeat the description. A few further observations are made. Why was the MIMiC such a turning point? Probably the reason lay in the fact that it was not announced until it was ready for purchase. There were no advanced warning papers, modeling papers, proofs of principle, etc. One could simply hook up to the company and start IMRT. The company offered an integrated planning and delivery package and one could go for training. The equipment, like all radiotherapy equipment, was of course quite complex but the user had relatively simple tasks to just attach the MIMiC in the accelerator tray ring and perform well-documented commissioning tasks. NOMOS had also enlisted early clinical support, particularly from Baylor College of Medicine where the first clinical deliveries were made. In time the numbers of installations grew to the hundreds. Possibly the Achilles' heel of the MIMiC IMRT was the need for exquisite matchline accuracy, the subject of some criticism and many studies. To its credit the NOMOS Corporation diversified into planning for non-MIMiC IMRT and also became the first company to market ultrasound-guided therapy [the BAT® (B-mode acquisition and targeting system)] so taking seriously the issues of image-guided therapy which were beginning to emerge in the mid 1990's as the next focus for serious attention to improvement of the physics of conformal radiotherapy and IMRT.

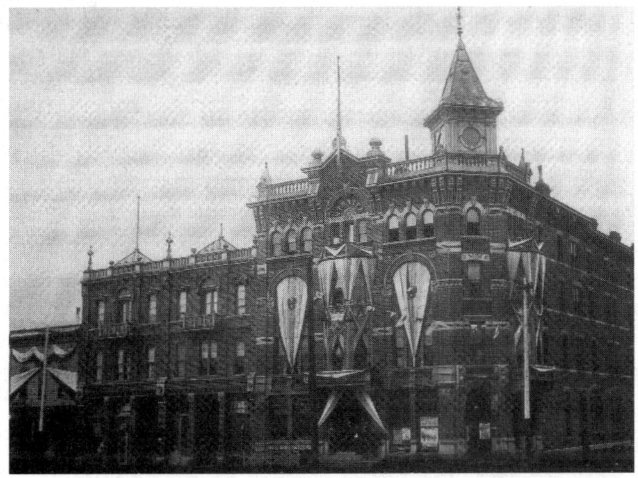

**Figure 8.** The location of the first ever conference on IMRT (May 1996).

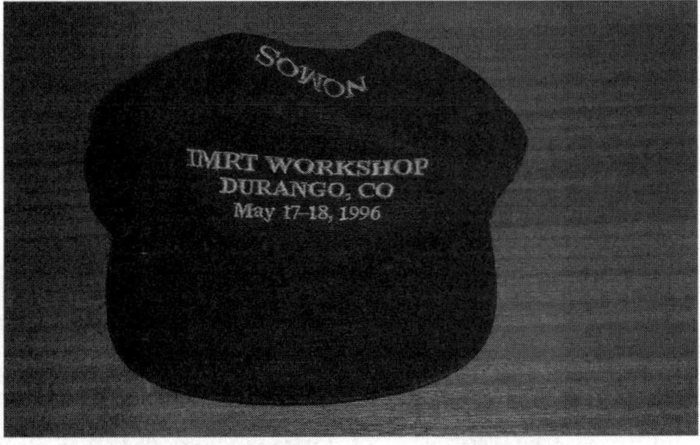


**Figure 9.** The first IMRT conference attendees wore these hats.

## Tomotherapy

In 1993 a seminal paper appeared from the University of Wisconsin describing what was then quite a futuristic concept for radiotherapy (Mackie et al. 1993). The concept was to abandon the conventional design of accelerator. Instead, an in-line short-length linear accelerator (linac) would be mounted on a continuously rotatable ring directed at its center. The linac would rotate in circles whilst the patient slowly translated through the ring. Thus a spiral of slit-field radiation was directed at the patient. The slit was to be modulated by a collimator identical in principle to the MIMiC. At the same time a megavoltage CT detector was to be mounted opposite the source for verification purposes and for creating transit dosimetry maps, sinograms, and a host of other dose-imaging tasks which could be fed back to correct for changes in patient anatomy and movement. At right angles to this a kilovoltage CT system would make conventional CT scans. The system was described as "radiotherapy in a box".

For the next nearly 10 years attendees at radiation oncology and medical physics conferences grew used to expecting the latest news in the development of this exciting concept. Many Ph.D. students worked on the project and a flood of papers appeared showing how the design could in principle overcome many of the concerns for conventional radiotherapy. The approach was quite different to that of the NOMOS Corporation because there was a 10-year period in which the community was tempted towards a then non-existent piece of apparatus. However, as we now know, the prototype tomotherapy equipment has treated its first patient, other machines are being commercially produced, and a company has now been formed to manufacture and distribute equipment.

In many reviews MIMiC slice-by-slice tomotherapy and helical tomotherapy are often considered together because indeed they share the concept of using a binary modulated slit aperture. In fact, the patents for the MIMiC were disclosed originally by Mackie and colleagues. I was told that the ideas (figure 10) originally came from a student of Mackie's called Stuart Swerdloff, the first name on the two patents for the equipment (Swerdloff, Mackie, and Holmes 1994a,b). The patents make very interesting reading and describe a variety of implementations including split-level shuttling vanes. Pictures are reproduced in chapter 2 of Webb (1997).

## Multiple-Static-Field (MSF) MLC Technique

In 1993 Thomas Bortfeld from DKFZ spent a sabbatical period in Houston, Texas, with Art Boyer. During that period they made the first ever IMRT delivery using a MLC and by the technique of multiple-static fields. A polystyrene multi-slice phantom was constructed based on the outlines of the CT data for a patient with prostate cancer for whom a high-dose volume was required to the prostate, sparing rectum and bladder as organs at risk. The phantom comprised nine slices, 1 cm thick with film sandwiched in-between. The treatment was delivered with a Varian accelerator fitted with a Varian MLC and a leaf-sweep method in which the leaves moved unidirectionally in creating the next shape in a sequence. The number of leaf settings per leaf pair varied between 21 and 30. The experiment took many hours to perform because the accelerator was under manual control. Art Boyer drew by hand neat 3-D pictures of the high dose wrapped around the prostate (Bortfeld et al. 1994b) (figure 11). These have been much reproduced since. Somehow they capture the pioneering nature of that experiment. This work was re-presented at the 11th ICCR (International Conference on the use of Computers in Radiation Therapy) in Manchester in 1994 and, appropriately for a groundbreaking landmark, won the prize for best paper (Bortfeld et al. 1994c).

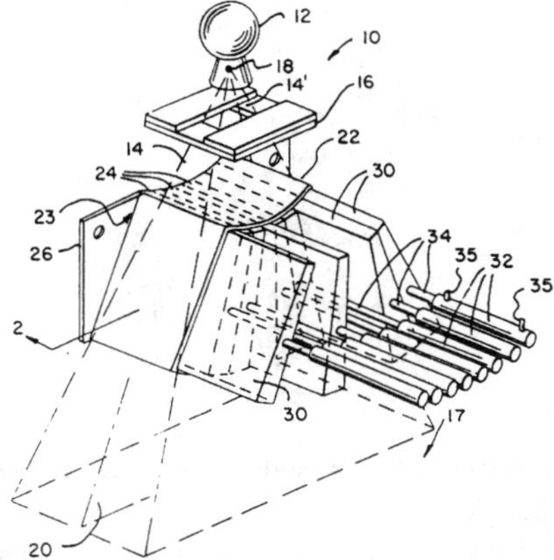

**Figure 10.** A general schematic diagram of the collimator proposed by Swerdloff et al. (1994a) for creating intensity-modulated fan-beams of radiation.
[From Swerdloff, Mackie, and Holmes 1994a.]

This experiment set the scene for the MSF-MLC technique that is now commercially available from Varian, Elekta, and Siemens. There have been tens of similar studies since and interestingly the experiment represents one of the main ways of verifying IMRT, that of replanning the patient fields on to a slice-phantom with films and comparing the digitized films with the predictions from a planning computer.

## The Dynamic MLC (DMLC) IMRT Technique

By sweeping the leaves of an MLC from one side to the other unidirectionally and at varying speeds, a 2-D fluence-modulated map can be created. To first order one can consider the delivery of 2-D fluence as a summation of the deliveries of 1-D fluence profiles, each created by the movement of just two opposing leaf pairs. The leading leaf starts to move and the trailing leaf follows. Depending on the velocity profiles of the two the primary radiation delivered to each point along the path can be made to vary. To first order this will be proportional to the time for which that point is open to the line-of-sight of the source. The principle is delightfully simple.

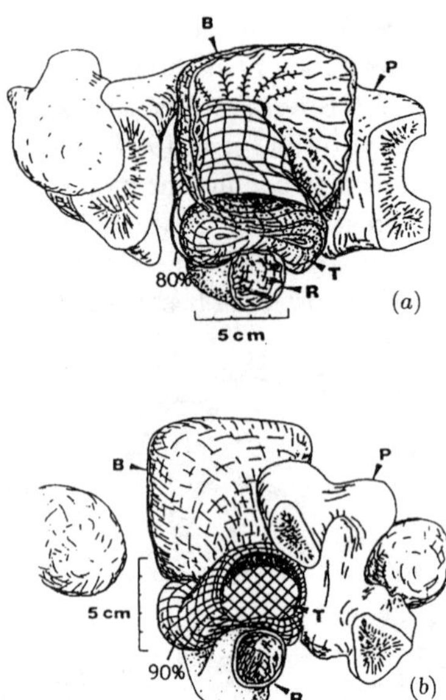

**Figure 11.** Three-dimensional display of isodose surfaces and the anatomical structures. R is the rectum, B is the bladder, P is the pelvis, and T is the target. (a) Direction of view: superior to inferior. The isodose value is 80% of the maximum dose. The dome of the bladder is shown cutaway for better appreciation of the isodose surface with the inner wall of the bladder. The seminal vesicles are enclosed in the invaginating target volume. (b) Visualization from inferior to superior, showing the 90% isodose. The pubis symphysis and right pelvic bones are removed to show the juxtaposition of the isodose surface between the bladder and the rectum. [Reprinted from *International Journal of Radiation Oncology Biology and Physics,* vol 30, T. Bortfeld, A. L. Boyer, W. Schlegel, D. L. Kahler, and T. J. Waldron, "Realisation and verification of multileaf modulated conformal radiotherapy with modulated fields," pp. 899–908. © 1994, with permission from Elsevier Science.]

Three groups were simultaneously working on this and three papers appeared in 1994 with the mathematics that described the optimum velocity profiles in terms of minimizing the treatment time (Stein et al. 1994; Spirou and Chui 1994; Svensson, Källmann, and Brahme 1994). The groups were in three different countries (Heidelberg, Germany; New York, USA, and Stockholm, Sweden). As far as I know they had no knowledge of each other's work and they came to effectively identical conclusions. What are sometimes now known as the "Stein equations" govern the motion. The algebra showing the equivalence of the approaches is reproduced in chapter 2 of Webb (1997). Art Boyer at the 12th ICCR in Salt Lake City produced a particularly nice graphical way of obtaining the same results, reproduced in Webb (2001c).

When creating 2-D modulations, it is not advisable to simply apply the equations to each of the MLC leaf tracks simultaneously because this may lead to situations in which the trailing leaf of one pair tries to overlap the leading leaf of another pair. Some accelerator MLCs forbid this interdigitation. There followed many attempts to build the MLC equipment limitations into the leaf motions. These inevitably led to less efficient but practical deliveries. Also, the simple description applies to only the primary fluence and many workers produced techniques to factor in the finite leaf transmission and also the varying head scatter. These became cyclic iterative methods in which the leaf motions were adjusted so the total fluence matched the planned fluence.

From about 1995 through to 1998-ish there was overconcern about what was known as the "tongue-and-groove effect." MLC leaf sides are like interlocking floor planks and for some of the motion the partial-depth leaf sides protrude into the open field creating potential underdoses. However this problem is entirely overcome by a method of leaf synchronization due to van Santvoort and Heijmen (1996). Others, including myself, provided more general formulations. The problem does *not* automatically go away with MSF-MLC deliveries and I showed in a pair of papers that in general the effect could not be removed. Coming right up to date, most workers believe that by using collimator rotations for different components and taking into account patient motion and electron transport the whole problem is something of a non-problem in practice. Perhaps we made too much of it at the time?

The dynamic MLC (DMLC) technique was first applied by a few research workers in university hospitals. At the midpoint of the 1990s just a handful of experiments had been made. However, there was a burgeoning development of quality assurance and at about this time the MLC became a much more standard tool to be had on a linac. Also the big electrotechnical companies were all putting resources into developing commercial packages for clinical MLC-based IMRT. Varian, Elekta, and Siemens were each offering equipment by about 1997. Some of these were so-called research releases but gradually the market shook down and now one can purchase almost plug-and-play systems from each. Not surprisingly they vie with each other for customers. The market is polarized. Varian has a lion's share in the USA, Elekta in the UK, and Siemens in Germany, but there are examples to be had in each country of all of them.

## Moving Jaw Therapy

The developments of the DMLC technique described above had some antecedents. Convery and Rosenbloom (1992) had studied how modulated fields could be created by moving accelerator jaws at different speeds. The bulk of their paper concerns jaw motion but they appended on the use of MLC leaves for 2-D modulation. Four years earlier Källman et al. (1988) had presented a theory for dynamic modulation using an MLC. However, the paper is somewhat theoretical and more concerned with how to calculate the opening density of the leaves than with practicalities. These were two important landmarks. However, in terms of presenting a thorough analysis of how to use MLC leaves, the three 1994 papers (Stein et al. 1994; Spirou and Chui 1994; Svensson, Källmann, and Brahme 1994) are often regarded as the most seminal. If one wanted to be specifically generous to some workers from far off days, one could acknowledge that Kijewski, Chin, and Bjärngard (1978) showed how to use moving jaws to make wedge distributions and of course Takahashi (1965) had described primitive MLCs for what he called conformation radiotherapy. By way of completeness we might note that the MLC was patented in 1959 by Gscheidlen (1959). Despite this Brahme (1985) also has a patent on the MLC, admittedly a more up-to-date computer-controlled model.

## Ultramodern IMRT History

Perhaps there is a thin line between a history and a review. The bulk of this paper was meant to be a history. However, as said at the outset, the history is very new. For this reason it seems logical to include the most recent proposals for IMRT.

## Robotic IMRT?

Levin (2001) has described in detail the scientific and business history of Accuray, the company which markets the CyberKnife®. The CyberKnife is a robotic device holding an X-band linac, which is capable of irradiating tumors stereotactically with feedback of organ motion to the robot. The initial vision of the person, John Adler, who started the development was that this would extend the concept of frame-based head-and-neck stereotactic radiotherapy and radiosurgery to frameless whole body radiotherapy and radiosurgery. Adler had worked with Lars Leksell in Sweden, the developer of the Gamma Knife (now manufactured by Sweden's Elekta AB Company). Adler first worked at the Harvard Medical School in Massachusetts General Hospital in Boston. He then left Harvard in 1990 to go to the Stanford University School of Medicine where he founded Sunnyvale, California-based Accuray with the goal of carrying Lars Leksell's vision from the brain to the rest of the body. The development is described as the third major step in radiotherapy technology this century (the first being the use of computed tomography data post 1972 to better define radiation shapes), the second being the development of non-robotic IMRT, and the third being the future of radiotherapy centered around the CyberKnife. The main thrust of the approach is to take account of patient movement, breathing, and other involuntary movements so that the exact location of where the tumor is at any one moment is tracked by the robotic linac. Adler's philosophy was that, because radiosurgery works so well in the brain, there was no biological reason why it should not have the same clinical application throughout the rest of the body.

The development of the CyberKnife became possible when one of Adler's patients introduced him to a small California-based company, Schoenberg Radiation, that made portable linear accelerators originally designed for industrial inspections, which could be carried on a person's back and therefore easily attachable to a robot.

The key feature described as the "crown jewels" of the CyberKnife system is its use of minimally invasive on-the-fly imaging to continually feed back the position of the tumor to the robot. Essentially, the procedure ensures that the tumor is in the same place with respect to the robot at the beginning, during, and at the end of the treatment. The robot "chases the tumor." The procedure is painless but can last anywhere from 30 to 90 minutes. Accuray received 510(k) approval for the Cyberknife for treatments of head and neck tumors in July 1999 and in 2001 lodged the application to the FDA (U.S. Federal Drug Administration) for approval to treat extracranial tumors such as those of the prostate, breast, and liver.

Can the CyberKnife be genuinely considered part of the IMRT story? Well, it can essentially place pencils of radiation of different intensities at different orientations with respect to the patient. So in this sense the answer is yes. It would be more useful if it were fitted with a small MLC and some of us are considering how that might be arranged.

## Cobalt IMRT

As evident, most IMRT has been built around delivery with a linear accelerator. However, many of the (so-called) less well-developed countries routinely use cobalt machines; some developed countries too. There have been attempts to perform IMRT with a cobalt source. Shreiner (2001) is building a slice-based tomotherapy machine on this principle. At present, a laboratory prototype is under construction. Warrington and Adams (2002) are developing an automatic compensator carousel for IMRT on a cobalt machine. Barthold (2002) at DKFZ is developing a machine called CORA using a scanned arc of multiple cobalt sources. At present, these do not rival linac IMRT.

## Shuttling Multileaf Collimators And Jaws+Mask

Webb (2000b, 2001b) has designed and modeled a new concept of using two banks of shuttling vanes to create IMRT with maximum monitor unit (MU) efficiency. Webb (2002a,b) has also proposed using a tertiary mask together with the jaws of an accelerator for performing IMRT without an MLC. The proof of principle of these options has been thoroughly modeled but no equipment yet built. Again, they do not rival linac IMRT.

## Other Forms Of IMRT

In the early 1990s the Racetrack Microtron was used to deliver IMRT. However, this has not developed widely. Another concept was the use of rotational techniques with the MLC continually changing shape as the gantry rotated. When this was geared to generating fluence modulation it was called intensity-modulated arc therapy (IMAT) and Cedric Yu (1995) was the inventor. Alternatively, the shape of the MLC was the projected view of the PTV and in this case the therapy was a form of dynamic therapy. Another concept was the scanning 1-D attenuating bar, developed in Milan.

## Clinical IMRT

No one has ever been treated with a concept, however smart. Hence it might be argued that this account should have only included those IMRT devices that have actually been used to treat patients. For two reasons I have not followed this path. The first is that, as a physicist, I am interested possibly more in the development of new tools than their use. I think the overall picture is clearer if one can see the ideas that existed in the dim past, even when they did not gain widespread use and also the same for the newest embryonic ideas that may be only at the modeling stage. Secondly, imagine the account had been written early last year and restricted to clinically implemented concepts. The Wisconsin tomotherapy machine would, for example, have been missed out and that clearly would have made no sense. So I hope my approach has been justified.

Moreover, of interest also is the history of clinical implementation. This is harder to track and I have avoided even starting on the lists of centers now known to be performing IMRT in one form or another. There are so many.

## Further Comments And Disclaimers

With respect to the topics in the previous sections (tomotherapy, robotic IMRT, cobalt IMRT, shuttling MLCs and jaws+mask, and other forms of IMRT) it may be commented that, given the very widespread use of (conventional) MLC-based IMRT delivery, competing technologies face a somewhat uphill battle to be fairly evaluated. Until there are an equivalently large number of installations, the data are hard to gather to assess their competitive value. This is the familiar "Catch-22."

We may also note that there is often a very long time period between proof of concept and widespread clinical use. Consider the MLC, first patented in 1959 (figure 12) but not used clinically until the late 1980's.

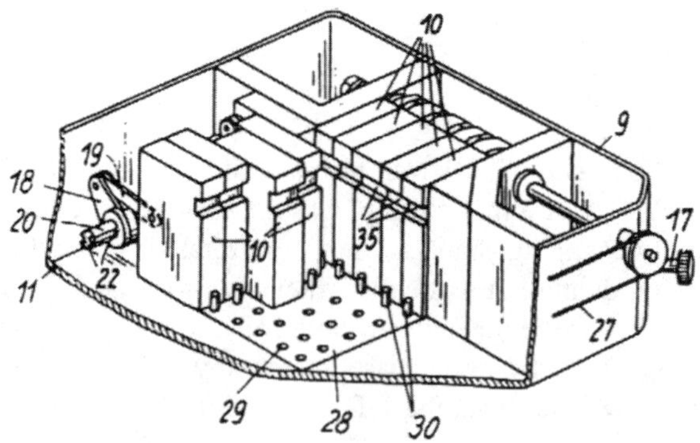


**Figure 12.** A schematic view of Gscheidlen's multileaf collimator patented in 1959, showing just two of the four sets of leaves. The actuating mechanism and the template for setting the field shape may be seen, as well as some of the guide bars. [From Gscheidlen (1959).]

IMRT has become a major research speciality. As such, there are so many aspects one could also consider in a historical review. Included could be: (1) capitalizing on multimodality imaging for IMRT optimization, (2) verification of IMRT, (3) image-guided IMRT, (4) IMRT planning optimisation, (5) the development of commercial inverse-planning systems, (6) the link of MLC design to IMRT, specifically the design of microMLCs, (7) transit and *in vivo* dosimetry. To start on this would however depart too much from history into review of state-of-the art and this is the role of the rest of this School.

# References[2]

Barthold, S. (2002). Private communication.

Birkhoff, G. D. (1940). "On drawings composed of uniform straight lines." *J. Math. Pures Appl.* 19:221–236.

Bortfeld, T., J. Burkelbach, R. Boesecke, and W. Schlegel. (1990). "Method of image reconstructions from projections applied to conformation therapy." *Phys. Med. Biol.* 35:1423–1434.

Bortfeld, T., D. L. Kahler, T. J. Waldron, and A. L. Boyer. (1994a). "X-ray field compensation with multileaf collimators." *Int. J. Radiat. Oncol. Biol. Med. Phys.* 28:723–730.

Bortfeld. T., A. L. Boyer, W. Schlegel, D. L. Kahler, and T. J. Waldron. (1994b). "Realisation and verification of three-dimensional conformal radiotherapy with modulated fields." *Int. J. Radiat. Oncol. Biol. Med. Phys.* 30:899–908.

Bortfeld, T., A. L. Boyer, W. Schlegel, D. L. Kahler, and T. J. Waldron. "Experimental Verification of Multileaf Modulated Conformal Radiotherapy" in *Proceedings of the XIth International Conference on the Use of Computers in Radiation Therapy.* A. R. Hounsell, J. M. Wilkinson, and P. C. Williams (Eds.). Manchester, UK, 20–24 March 1994. Manchester, UK: North Western Medical Physics Dept., Christie Hospital NHS Trust, pp. 180–181, 1994c.

Boyer, A. L., G. E. Desobry, and N. H. Wells. (1991). "Potential and limitations of invariant kernel conformal therapy." *Med. Phys.* 18:703–712.

Brahme, A. (1985). "Multileaf collimator." U.S. Patent 4672212.

Brahme, A. (1988). "Optimisation of stationary and moving beam radiation therapy techniques." *Radiother. Oncol.* 12:129–140.

Brahme, A., J. E. Roos, and I. Lax. (1982). "Solution of an integral equation encountered in rotation therapy." *Phys. Med. Biol.* 27:1221–1229.

Carol, M. P., H. Targovnik, C. Campbell, A. Bleier, J. Strait, B. Rosen, P. Miller, D. Scherch, R. Huber, B. Thibadeau, D. Dawson, and D. Ruff. "An Automatic 3D Treatment Planning and Implementation System for Optimised Conformal Therapy" in *Three-dimensional Treatment Planning.* P. Minet (ed.). Geneva: WHO, pp.173–187, 1993.

Convery, D. J., and M. E. Rosenbloom. (1992). "The generation of intensity-modulated fields for conformal therapy by dynamic collimation." *Phys. Med. Biol.* 37:1359–1374.

Gscheidlen, W. (1959). "Device for collimation of a ray beam." U.S. Patent 2904692.

---

[2] There are literally thousands of references to IMRT and hundreds of important ones. I have here been extremely selective. My books (see list) give comprehensive bibliographies up to 2000.

Holmes, T., and T. R. Mackie. (1992). "Simulation studies to characterize the search space of a radiotherapy optimization algorithm." Proceedings of the AAPM Conference, August 1992. *Med. Phys.* 19:842.

Jennings, W. A. "The tracking cobalt project: From moving beam therapy to three dimensional programmed irradiation" in *Progress in Medical Radiation Physics*: 2. C. Orton (Ed.). New York: Plenum Press, pp. 1–44, 1985.

Källman, P., B. Lind, A. Eklöf, and A. Brahme. (1988). "Shaping of arbitrary dose distributions by dynamic multileaf collimation." *Phys. Med. Biol.* 33:1291–1300.

Kijewski, P. K., L. M. Chin, and B. E. Bjärngard. (1978). "Wedge-shaped dose distributions by computer controlled collimator motion." *Med. Phys.* 5:426–429.

Levin, S. (2001). "Accuray: Tightly targeting tumours." *Windhover's In Vivo The Business and Medicine Report* 19(4):1–12.

Mackie, T. R., T. Holmes, S. Swerdloff, P. Reckwerdt, J. O. Deasy, J. Yang, B. Paliwal, and T. Kinsella. (1993). "Tomotherapy: A new concept for the delivery of dynamic conformal radiotherapy." *Med. Phys.* 20:1709–1719.

Mageras, G. S., and R. Mohan. (1992). "Application of fast simulated annealing to optimisation of conformal radiation treatments." *Med. Phys.* 20:639–647.

Proimos, B. S. (1960). "Synchronous protection and field shaping in rotational megavolt therapy." *Radiol.* 74: 753–757.

Proimos, B. S. (1961). "Synchronous protection and field shaping in cyclotherapy." *Radiol.* 77: 591–599.

Schlegel, W., and A. Mahr. *3D Conformal Radiation Therapy: Multimedia Introduction to Methods and Techniques*. Heidelberg: Springer (e-book), 2001.

Schreiner, L. J. (2001). "The potential for intensity modulated radiation therapy with cobalt 60." *NORDION Insights* 3(1):3.

Schulz, R. J., and A. R. Kagan. (2002). "On the role of intensity-modulated radiation therapy in radiation oncology." *Med. Phys.* 29:1473–1482.

Smith, A. *Radiation Therapy Physics*. Berlin: Springer, 1995.

Spirou, S. V., and C. S. Chui. (1994). "Generation of arbitrary intensity profiles by dynamic jaws or multileaf collimators." *Med. Phys.* 21:1031–1041.

Sternick, E. S. (ed.). *The Theory and Practice of Intensity Modulated Radiation Therapy*. Madison, WI: Advanced Medical Publishing, 1997.

Stein, J., T. Bortfeld, B. Dörschel and W. Schlegel. (1994). "Dynamic x-ray compensation for conformal radiotherapy by means of multileaf collimation." *Radiother. Oncol.* 32:163–173.

Svensson, R., P. Källmann, and A. Brahme. (1994). "Analytical solution for the dynamic control of multileaf collimators." *Phys. Med. Biol.* 39:37–61.

Swerdloff, S., T. R. Mackie, and T. Holmes. (1994a). "Method and apparatus for radiation therapy." U.S. Patent 5317616.

Swerdloff, S., T. R. Mackie, and T. Holmes. (1994b). "Multi-leaf radiation attenuator for radiation therapy." U.S. Patent 5351280.

Takahashi, S. (1965). "Conformation radiotherapy, rotation techniques as applied to radiography and radiotherapy." *Acta Radiol. Suppl.* 242.

Van Dyk, J. (ed.). *The Modern Technology of Radiation Oncology*. Madison, WI: Medical Physics Publishing, 1999.

van Santvoort, J. and B. Heijmen. (1996). "Dynamic multileaf collimation without "tongue-and-groove" underdose effects." *Phys. Med. Biol.* 41:2091–2105.

Warrington, A. P., and E. J. Adams. (2002). "Cobalt-60 Teletherapy for Cancer — a Revived Treatment Modality for the 21$^{st}$ Century." Proc. Sem. on appropriate medical technology for developing countries. Feb 6$^{th}$ 2002. IEE London, pp. 21.1–21.19.

Webb, S. (1989). "Optimisation of conformal dose distributions by simulated annealing." *Phys. Med. Biol.* 34:1349–1370.

Webb, S. (1991a). "Optimisation by simulated annealing of three-dimensional conformal treatment planning for radiation fields defined by a multileaf collimator." *Phys. Med. Biol.* 36:1201–1226.

Webb, S. (1991b). "Optimisation of conformal radiotherapy dose distributions by simulated annealing: 2-inclusion of scatter in the 2D technique." *Phys. Med. Biol.* 36:1227–1237.

Webb, S. (1992). "Optimisation by simulated annealing of three-dimensional, conformal treatment planning for radiation fields defined by a multileaf collimator: 2. Inclusion of two-dimensional modulation of the x-ray intensity." *Phys. Med. Biol.* 37:1689–1704.

Webb, S. *The Physics of Three Dimensional Radiation Therapy: Conformal Radiotherapy, Radiosurgery and Treatment Planning.* Bristol: IOP Publishing, 1993.

Webb, S. *The Physics of Conformal Radiotherapy: Advances in Technology.* Bristol: IOP Publishing, 1997.

Webb, S. (1998). "The physics of radiation treatment." *Physics World* November 1998:39–43.

Webb, S. (2000a). "Advances in three-dimensional conformal radiation therapy physics with intensity modulation." *The Lancet Oncology* 1:30–36.

Webb, S. (2000b). "A new concept of multileaf collimator (the shuttling MLC) – an interpreter for high-efficiency IMRT." *Phys. Med. Biol.* 45(11):3343–3358.

Webb, S. (2001a). "The future of photon external beam radiotherapy: The dream and the reality." *Physical Medica* 17:207–215.

Webb, S. (2001b). "Concepts for shuttling multileaf collimators for intensity-modulated radiation therapy" *Phys. Med. Biol.* 46:637–651.

Webb, S. *Intensity-Modulated Radiation Therapy.* Bristol: IOP Publishing, 2001c.

Webb, S. (2002a). "Intensity-modulated radiation therapy using only jaws and a mask." *Phys. Med. Biol.* 47:257–275.

Webb, S. (2002b). "Intensity-modulated radiation therapy using only jaws and a mask: A simplified concept of single bixel attenuators." *Phys. Med. Biol.* 47:1869-1879.

Webb, S. (2002c). "Some snapshots from the history of radiotherapy physics." *SCOPE* 11(1):8–12.

Yu, C. (1995). "Intensity modulated arc therapy with dynamic multileaf collimation: An alternative to tomotherapy." *Phys. Med. Biol.* 40:1435–1449.

# Mathematical Optimization For The Inverse Problem Of Intensity-Modulated Radiation Therapy

**Yair Censor, D.Sc.**
Department of Mathematics, University of Haifa
Haifa, Israel



## Introduction

We consider intensity-modulated radiation therapy (IMRT) where beams of penetrating radiation are directed at the lesion (tumor) from external sources. Based on understanding of the physics and biology of the situation, there are two principal aspects of radiation teletherapy that call for mathematical modeling. The first is the calculation of the *radiation dose*, which is a measure of the actual energy absorbed per unit mass everywhere in the irradiated tissue. In dose calculation the relevant physical, geometric and biological characteristics of the irradiated object and the relevant information about the radiation source (geometry, physical nature, intensity, etc.) serve as input data. The result of the calculation is a *dose function* (distribution) whose values are the dose absorbed as a function of location inside the irradiated body. This dose calculation is the *forward problem* of IMRT.

The second aspect is, mathematically speaking, the *inverse problem* of the first. In addition to the availability of the physical and biological parameters of the irradiated object we assume here that the relevant information about the capabilities and specifications of the available *treatment machine* (i.e., radiation source) is given. Based on medical diagnosis, knowledge, and experience, the physician prescribes a *desired* dose function to the case. The output of a solution method for the inverse problem should be a *radiation intensity function*, whose values are the radiation intensities at the sources as a function of source location, that would result in a dose function that is identical to the desired one. To be of practical value, this resulting radiation intensity function must be implementable, in a clinically acceptable form, on the available treatment machine.

Historically, working in two dimensions (2-D) where only a single plane through the center of the target is considered, the treatment planning was done (and is still frequently done) in a trial-and-error fashion. A machine setup that gives rise to a certain external radiation intensity field (function) is picked up and then, using a forward-problem-solver software package, the resulting dose function is determined. If the discrepancy between this dose function and the prescribed dose function is unacceptable, then some changes are made to the external radiation intensity field (i.e., the machine setup parameters) and the process is repeated until the physician and dosimetrist are satisfied with the resulting dose function. Only then is actual patient treatment performed.

Such 2D-RTTP (radiation therapy treatment planning) has achieved success due to accumulated experience and also because of the ever-increasing quality, sophistication, and speed of forward-problem-solvers. However, automated solution of the inverse problem of IMRT should be useful in handling difficult planning cases, particularly in three dimensions (3-D) (see figure 1). There, it would be much more difficult to reach an acceptable plan by trial-and-error because of the multitude of potential directions from which the 3-D object can be irradiated. Nonetheless, even a 2-D discussion, as given here, is enough to expose the nature of the dilemmas that we consider in the sequel.

In the next section we present the continuous forward and inverse problems and then we give their discretizations. The feasibility approach is formulated and optimization formulations are given in later sections. Finally, we very briefly discuss some of the methods and techniques that have been applied to the inverse problem of IMRT, namely, global optimization (including simulated annealing), multi-objective optimization, linear and mixed integer programming, and projection methods (including Cimmino's algorithm). This paper is written as a tutorial and there is neither an intention to present a full survey of optimization methods in RTTP, nor an attempt to properly cover the literature. We also admit a slight bias in space allocation below towards projection methods, which are our own main field of research.

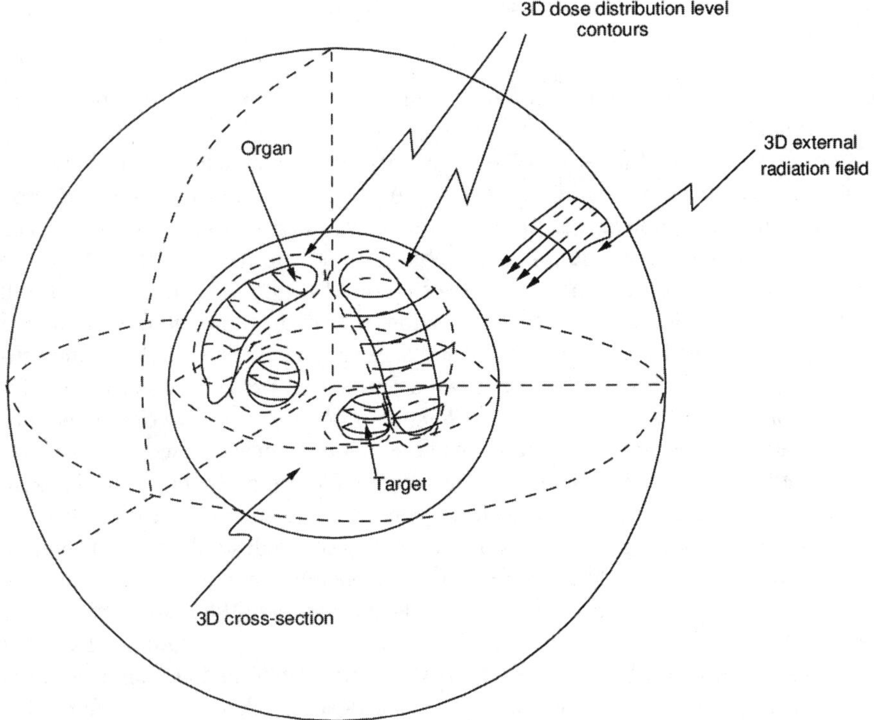


**Figure 1.** A 3-D cross-section, external radiation field, and dose distribution
for 3-D IMRT planning.

## Problem Definition And The Continuous Model

Let $D(r, \theta)$ be a real-valued nonnegative function, of the polar coordinates $r$ and $\theta$, whose value is the dose absorbed at a point in the patient's planar cross-section $\Omega$ coincident with the plane of the machine's gantry motion. This is the *dose function*, or dose distribution. A *ray* is a directed line along which radiated energy travels away from the *source* (the *teletherapy source* ). Rays are parametrized by variables $u$ and $w$ in some well-defined way and the real-valued nonnegative function $\rho(u, w)$ represents the *radiation intensity* along the ray $(u, w)$ due to a point source on the gantry circle, located at $(u, w)$.

**Problem 1**. *The continuous forward problem of IMRT. Assume that the cross-section $\Omega$ of the patient and its radiation absorption characteristics are known. Given an external radiation intensity function $\rho(u, w)$, for $0 \leq u < 2\pi$ and $-W \leq w \leq W$, find the dose function $D(r, \theta)$, for all $(r, \theta) \in \Omega$, from the formula*

$$D(r,\theta) = \mathfrak{D}\big[\rho(u,w)\big](r,\theta) \tag{1}$$

*where $\mathfrak{D}$ is the dose operator which relates the dose function to the radiation intensity function.*

In other words, the forward problem amounts to the calculation of the total dose absorbed at each point of a patient's cross-section when all parameters of all radiation beams are specified and the description of the patient's cross-section is known. The difficulties associated with the forward problem stem from the fact that to this date there exists no closed-form analytic representation of the dose operator $\mathfrak{D}$ that will enable us to use equation (1) for the calculation of $D(r, \theta)$. Although the interaction between radiation and tissue is measured and understood at the atomic level, the situation is so complex that, to solve the forward problem in practice, a state-of-the-art computer program, which represents a *computational approximation* of the operator $\mathfrak{D}$ and which enables reasonably good dose calculations, must be used.

By stating that "there exists no closed-form analytic representation of the dose operator $\mathfrak{D}$" we mean that only if drastically simplifying assumptions are made about the physics of the model as well as of the particulars of the desired dose distribution, then it is sometimes possible to express the dose operator in a closed-form analytic formula. This has been done first by Brahme, Roos, and Lax (1982) and extended by Cormack and co-workers; consult the review paper of Cormack and Quinto (1990) for further references. See also Brahme's review (Brahme 1995) and Goitein's editorial (Goitein 1990). In current practice of IMRT, when dose calculations are performed to verify the dose that will result from a proposed treatment plan, the goal is to obtain results that are as accurate as possible. To achieve this, various empirical data, which are often condensed in look-up tables, are incorporated into the forward calculation. Thus, the true forward calculation, or true dose operator, is not represented by a closed-form analytic relation between the radiation intensity function $\rho(u, w)$ and the dose function $D(r, \theta)$, but by a software package that calculates $D(r, \theta)$ from $\rho(u, w)$. We choose to adhere to the software representation of $\mathfrak{D}$ rather than to compromise by allowing simplifying assumptions that might lead to a closed-form analytic mathematical formula at the expense of the physical and biological reality of the forward calculation.

**Problem 2**. *The continuous inverse problem of IMRT. Assume that the cross-section $\Omega$ of the patient and its radiation absorption characteristics are known. Given a prescribed dose function $D(r, \theta)$, find a radiation intensity function $\rho(u, w)$ such that equation (1) holds, or, equivalently,*

$$\rho(u,w) = \mathfrak{D}^{-1}\big[D(r,\theta)\big], \tag{2}$$

*where $\mathfrak{D}^{-1}$ is the **inverse operator** of $\mathfrak{D}$.*

Solving problem 2 gives an external configuration and relative intensities of radiation sources (i.e., the radiation field) that will deliver the prescribed radiation dose distribution (or some acceptable approximation thereof). This inversion problem needs to be solved, in a computationally tractable way, although no closed-form analytic mathematical representation is available for the dose operator $\mathcal{D}$. Without such a mathematical representation of $\mathcal{D}$ it is impossible to employ mathematical methods for analytic inversion to find the inverse operator $\mathcal{D}^{-1}$. This is why full discretization of the problem has to be adopted, as we did in Altschuler and Censor (1984) and Censor, Altschuler, and Powlis (1988a).

The dose at $(r, \theta)$ is the sum of the dose contributions from the sources at all the different gantry angles. Thus,

$$D(r,\theta) = \sum_{s=1}^{s} y_s D_s(r,\theta) \tag{3}$$

where, for each $s = 1, 2, \ldots, S$, the value $D_s(r, \theta)$ is the dose deposited at point $(r, \theta)$ by a beam of unit intensity from the $s$th source, and $y_s$ is the time the $s$th beam is kept on. It will be assumed here that the dose $D_s(r, \theta)$ can be calculated accurately once the beam parameters and patient's cross-section information are specified. That is, we assume that we can solve the forward problem and calculate $D(r, \theta)$ accurately from (3). This assumption is confirmed by innumerable direct measurements in water and tissue-equivalent phantoms. Whereas a dose distribution that solves the forward problem is always obtained for a specified external radiation intensity field, the inverse problem may have no solution at all, since some prescribed dose functions may be unobtainable from any radiation field.

## Discretization Of The Problem

In the approach presented here, we adhere to the computational approximation of the dose operator $\mathcal{D}$. Full discretization of the problem at the outset is used to circumvent the difficulties associated with the analytic inversion of $\mathcal{D}$. We also neglect in the present description the effects of scattered radiation. The patient's cross-section $\Omega$ is discretized into a grid of points represented by the pairs$\{(r_j, \theta_j) \,|\, j = 1, 2, \ldots, J \}$. Define $\mathcal{D}_j[\rho]$ by

$$\mathcal{D}_j[\rho] := \big[\mathcal{D}\rho\big]\big(r_j,\theta_j\big) \tag{4}$$

and call $\mathcal{D}_j$ a *dose functional*, for every $j = 1, 2, \ldots, J$. Acting on a radiation intensity function $\rho(u, w)$, the functional $\mathcal{D}_j$ provides $\mathcal{D}_j[\rho]$, which is the dose absorbed at the $j$th grid point of the patient's cross-section $\Omega$ due to the radiation intensity field $\rho$. To continue the discretization process of the problem it is assumed that a set of *I basis radiation intensity fields* is fixed and that their nonnegative linear combinations can give adequate approximations to any radiation intensity field we wish to specify. This is done by discretizing the region $0 \le u < 2\pi$, $-W \le w \le W$ in the $(u, w)$-plane into a grid of points given by $\{(u_i, w_i) \mid i = 1, 2, \ldots, I\}$. A radiation intensity function

$$\sigma_i(u, w) := \begin{cases} 1, & \text{if } (u, w) = (u_i, w_i) \\ 0, & \text{otherwise,} \end{cases} \tag{5}$$

is a *unit intensity ray* (or *beamlet*) and serves as a member of the set of basis radiation intensity fields for $i = 1, 2, \ldots, I$. In this fully discretized model, a desired radiation intensity function $\rho$ that solves the inverse problem is always approximated by

$$\hat{\rho}(u, w) = \sum_{i=1}^{I} x_i \sigma_i(u, w) \tag{6}$$

where $x_i$ is the intensity of the $i$th ray and it is required to be nonnegative, i.e., $x_i \ge 0$ for all $i = 1, 2, \ldots, I$. Once the grid points are fixed, any radiation intensity function $\hat{\rho}$, that can be represented as a nonnegative linear combination of the rays, is uniquely determined by the intensity coefficients $x_i$. The latter form the components of the vector $x = (x_i)_{i=1}^{I} \in R^I$, in the $I$-dimensional Euclidean space, referred to as the *radiation intensity vector*.

Further, assume that the dose functionals $\mathcal{D}_j$ are linear and continuous. This assumption cannot be mathematically verified due to the absence of an analytic representation of either $\mathcal{D}$ or $\mathcal{D}_j$, but it is a reasonable assumption based on the empirical knowledge of $\mathcal{D}_j$. Using linearity and continuity of all $\mathcal{D}_j$'s, we can write

$$\mathcal{D}_j[\rho] \cong \mathcal{D}_j(\hat{\rho}) = \sum_{i=1}^{I} x_i \mathcal{D}_j[\sigma_i] \tag{7}$$

For $j = 1, 2, \ldots, J$, and $i = 1, 2, \ldots, I$, denote by

$$a_{ij} := \mathcal{D}_j[\sigma_i] \tag{8}$$

the dose deposited at the $j$th grid point $(r_j, \theta_j)$, in the patient's cross-section $\Omega$, due to a unit intensity ray $\sigma_i(u, w)$, and define vectors $a^j = (a_{ij})_{i=1}^{I} \in R^I$, for $j = 1, 2, \ldots, J$. Then the right-hand side of (7) becomes equal to the inner product $\langle a^j, x \rangle = \sum_{i=1}^{I} a_{ij} x_i$ in $R^I$. The desired dose functional is also discretized by defining

$$b_j := D(r_j, \theta_j), \text{ for all } j = 1, 2, \ldots, J. \tag{9}$$

**Problem 3**. *The fully discretized inverse problem of IMRT. Let $a_{ij}$ be as in (8) and let $b_j$ be the desired doses as in (9), for $j = 1, 2, \ldots, J$, and $i = 1, 2, \ldots, I$. Find a radiation intensity vector $x^* \in R^I$ such that*

$$\left\langle a^j, x^* \right\rangle = b_j, \; for \; j = 1, 2, \ldots, J, \tag{10}$$

$$and \; x_i^* \geq 0, \; for \; i = 1, 2, \ldots, I. \tag{11}$$

Defining the $J \times I$ matrix $A$ as the matrix whose transpose $A^T$ has $a^j$ in its $j$th column, and the $J$th dimensional vector $b = \left(b_j\right)_{j=1}^{J}$, the system (10)–(11) can be rewritten as

$$Ax^* = b \; and \; x^* \geq 0. \tag{12}$$

This fully discretized model calls for the quantities $a_{ij}$ which can be precalculated with any state-of-the-art forward-problem-solver. Numerous iterative techniques are available for the solution of (12), some of which are discussed in the sequel. The tendency to make the discretization finer results in very large values of $I$ and $J$. If the available treatment machine cannot deliver such finely discretized radiation intensity fields, by shooting energy along rays, we need an additional computational step after a solution vector $x^*$ (or an approximation thereof) of the system (12) has been obtained. This is a "consolidation" step in which a clinically acceptable machine setup, usually with few (up to 5 to 6) beam positions, is derived from the fully discretized solution vector $x^*$ by using the individual ray intensities to rank the prominence of beams; see, e.g., Censor, Altschuler, and Powlis (1988a). Modern computer-controlled *multileaf collimator* (MLC) technology, capable of generating arbitrary intensity modulation, fills in the gap that existed between the fully discretized beamlet-based solution of the inverse problem and the delivery capabilities; see, e.g., Cho and Marks (2000) and references therein. To sum up, the fully discretized model is not difficulties-free, but it offers a route of circumventing the inversion problem of the computational dose operator $\mathfrak{D}$ without compromising on any of the heuristics and empiricism involved in advanced dose calculations. Brahme (1995) reaches also a conclusion in favor of full discretization and says: "...In either case it is very useful to transform the relevant integral equation into an algebraic form by discretizing the transport quantities along the coordinates of the free variables."

## The Feasibility Approach

The feasibility formulation relaxes the equality in (1). Let $\overline{D} = \overline{D}(r,\theta)$ and $\underline{D} = \underline{D}(r,\theta)$ be two dose functions whose values represent upper and lower bounds, respectively, on the permitted and required dose inside the patient's cross-section.

    **Problem 4**. *The feasibility formulation for the continuous inverse problem of* **IMRT**. *Assume that the cross-section $\Omega$ of the patient and its radiation absorption characteristics are known. Given prescribed dose functions $\overline{D}(r,\theta)$, and $\underline{D}(r,\theta)$, find a radiation intensity function $\rho(u, w)$ such that*

$$\underline{D}(r,\theta) \leq \mathcal{D}[\rho(u,w)](r,\theta) \leq \overline{D}(r,\theta), \text{ for all } (r,\theta) \in \Omega, \tag{13}$$

*where $\mathcal{D}$ is the dose operator.*

    A radiation therapist defines $\overline{D}(r,\theta)$ and $\underline{D}(r,\theta)$ for each given case and will accept as a solution to the IMRT inverse problem any radiation intensity function $\rho(u, w)$ that satisfies (13). In target regions (tumors) the lower bound $\underline{D}$ is usually the important factor because the dose there should exceed that given value. In critical organs and other healthy tissues $\underline{D}(r,\theta) = 0$, and $\overline{D}(r,\theta)$ is the dose that cannot be exceeded. Any solution $\rho(u, w)$ that fulfills (13), for given $\overline{D}$ and $\underline{D}$, is a *feasible solution* to the IMRT continuous inverse problem 4. In order to discretize (13) we must specify the dose functions $\overline{D}$ and $\underline{D}$ at the grid points by giving, for all $j = 1, 2, \ldots, J$,

$$\overline{D}(r_j,\theta_j) = \overline{D}_j \text{ and } \underline{D}(r_j,\theta_j) = \underline{D}_j \tag{14}$$

thus, converting (13) into a finite system of *interval inequalities*

$$\underline{D}_j \leq \mathcal{D}_j[\rho] \leq \overline{D}_j, \quad j = 1, 2, \ldots, J. \tag{15}$$

Denoting hereafter by $\overline{D}$ ($\underline{D}$) the $J$-dimensional column vector whose $j$th component is $\overline{D}_j(\underline{D}_j)$, the inverse problem of IMRT can be restated as follows:

    **Problem 5**. *The feasibility formulation for the fully discretized inverse problem of* **IMRT**. *Assume that the cross-section $\Omega$ of the patient and its radiation absorption characteristics are known. Given vectors $\overline{D} = (\overline{D}_j)$ and $\underline{D} = (\underline{D}_j)$ of permitted and required doses, respectively, at J grid points in the patient's cross-section $\Omega$, find a radiation intensity vector $x \in R^I$ such that*

$$\underline{D}_j \leq \sum_{i=1}^{I} x_i a_{ij} \leq \overline{D}_j. \quad j = 1, 2, \ldots, J, \tag{16}$$

$$x_i \geq 0, \quad i = 1, 2, \ldots, I. \tag{17}$$

*where $a_{ij}$ are as in (8).*

Let the set of pixels in the discretized patient's cross-section be denoted by $N = \{1, 2, \ldots, J\}$, so that the $j$th pixel is identified with the $j$th grid point at $(r_j, \theta_j)$. Organs within the patient's cross-section are then defined as subsets of $N$. The subsets $B_l \subset N$, where $l = 1, 2, \ldots, L$, denote $L$ *critical organs* that have to be spared from excessive radiation. Let the values $b_l$ denote the corresponding upper bounds on the dose permitted in each critical organ. The subsets $T_q \subset N$, where $q = 1, 2, \ldots, Q$, denote $Q$ *target regions*. Let the values $t_q$ denote the corresponding prescribed lower bounds for the absorbed dose in each target organ. All the $B_l$ and $T_q$ are pairwise disjoint. The set of pixels inside the patient's cross-section that are not in any $B_l$ or $T_q$ are called the *complement*, denoted as the subset $C \subset N$, and $c$ is the upper bound for the permitted dose there. It is assumed that the definition of all subsets $B_l$ and $T_q$ and $C$ and the prescription of all $b_l$, $t_q$, and $c$ are given by the radiotherapist as input data for the treatment planning process. Problem (16)–(17) then becomes the following system of linear inequalities.

$$\sum_{i=1}^{I} a_{ij} x_i \leq b_l, \quad \text{for all } j \in B_l, l = 1, 2, \ldots, L, \tag{18}$$

$$t_q \leq \sum_{i=1}^{I} a_{ij} x_i, \quad \text{for all } j \in T_q, q = 1, 2, \ldots, Q, \tag{19}$$

$$\sum_{i=1}^{I} a_{ij} x_i \leq c, \quad \text{for all } j \in C \tag{20}$$

$$x_i \geq 0, \quad \text{for all } i = 1, 2, \ldots, I. \tag{21}$$

With $b_l$, $t_q$, and $c$ given and the $a_{ij}$'s pre-calculated from (8) with a forward problem solver, the mathematical question represented by the basic model (18)–(21) is to find a nonnegative solution vector $x^* = (x_i^*)$ for a system of linear inequalities. This fully discretized feasibility inverse problem appeared in Altschuler and Censor (1984) and Censor, Altschuler, and Powlis (1988a).

## Optimization Formulations

We use the term optimization as it is used in the field of *mathematical optimization,* namely to designate a situation where an *objective function* (also called: cost function or merit function) has to be optimized (i.e., minimized or maximized). This explains why the feasibility approach, discussed above, is not called optimization, although in the field of IMRT the term *optimization* is frequently used in a more general manner to refer to the process of treatment planning where the treatment has to be "optimized" even if the underlying mathematical model is a feasibility model where no objective function appears. When it comes to discussing an optimization approach to IMRT we must distinguish between two different kinds of optimization problems depending on the space in which they are formulated. One possibility is to define an objective function $f: R^I \rightarrow R$ over the space of radiation intensity vectors $x$ and use either the system (12) or the constraints (18)–(21) as the feasible set (i.e., the constraints set). For example, choosing $f(x) = (1/2) \| x \|^2$ (where $\| \cdot \|$ stands for the Euclidean norm) and solving a minimization problem

$$\min\left\{ (1/2) \| x \|^2 \mid (18) - (21) \text{ hold} \right\}, \tag{22}$$

leads to a minimum-norm solution vector $x^*$; i.e., a feasible vector closest to the origin so that the total radiation intensity is smallest possible in the Euclidean norm sense. This was recently studied via a special-purpose iterative minimization method in Xiao et al. (2003a).

Regardless of the specific choice of $f$, in this approach the *interval-constrained optimization* problem

$$\min\left\{ f(x) \mid \alpha \leq Ax \leq \beta, \ x \geq 0 \right\} \tag{23}$$

where $\alpha \leq Ax \leq \beta$ represents the system (18)–(20), with appropriately defined $\alpha, \beta \in R^I$, is still aiming at a solution of the fully discretized formulation of the inverse problem. A solution vector $x^*$ will represent a radiation field that will deliver a dose which is both feasible (i.e., adheres to the upper and lower dose bounds imposed by the physician) and is optimal in the sense that it minimizes the objective function $f$. This approach of optimization in the space of radiation intensity vectors is called *radiation intensity optimization.*

The second possibility for introducing an optimization problem in IMRT is to use (12) or (18)–(21) as constraints but choose an objective function $g : R^J \rightarrow R$ defined over the space of dose vectors. Such objective functions may be either *biological,* or *physical.* Biological objective functions represent knowledge (statistical or other) about various biological mechanisms that affect our ability to control the disease. An example is the conditional probability of having tumor control without severe injury, denoted in the literature by $P_+$. Physical objective functions aggregate physical features which are important for tumor control and prevention of normal tissue complications, such as dose variance over target volume or peak dose to organs at risk. A thorough discussion of biological and physical objective functions can be found in Brahme (1995), see also Alber and Nüsslin (1999). Let us call this kind of optimization, over the space of dose vectors, *dose optimization*.

Early work on dose optimization was not geared towards solving an optimization problem but rather towards *comparing rival plans*. In this mode, several treatment plans were compared, based on their score with respect to some pre-determined quality index. The treatment plans were all fixed prior to the comparison and, therefore, the selection of the plan of choice depended largely on the choice of the quality index. Various quality indices were proposed and advocated on different grounds; see, e.g., Wolbarst et al. (1980), Dritschilo et al. (1978) and Kartha et al. (1982). In general, the dose optimization approach leads to a problem of the form

$$\min \{g(y) \mid \alpha \le y \le \beta\}, \tag{24}$$

where $g : R^J \to R$ assigns real values to dose vectors $y = \left(y_j\right)_{j=1}^{J} \in R^J$ whose $j$th component $y_j$ is dose at pixel $j$. The question of feasibility versus optimization is not crucial if only radiation intensity optimization is considered because both the feasibility formulation and the optimization formulation [regardless of the particular choice of the objective function $f(x)$] occur in the same space (of radiation intensity vectors) and, thus, aim at a solution of the discretized inverse problem. Therefore, the difference between these two formulations is, from the mathematical point of view, only technical. Raphael (1992) studied the inverse problem of RTTP as constrained optimization in the $L^2$ Hilbert space. Recently, Cho et al. (1997) reported on the advantage of the feasibility approach over a global optimization model solved by simulated annealing; see also Cho et al. (1998). In case when the composite function $g(Ax)$ is simple enough the approach of (24) can still be efficiently used for solving directly the discretized inverse problem in its full generality. Otherwise, the inversion problem has to be abandoned and the optimization can be performed with respect to only few parameters of the external radiation field. See, for example, Gustafsson (1996) and Gustafsson, Lind, and Brahme (1994). This is done while other important parameters are left out of the optimization problem and must be given as input to the process; see also the discussion in Censor and Zenios (1997, section 11.7). The question whether to use biological or physical objective functions in the space of dose vectors (and thereby possibly compromise on the full generality of the inverse problem) remains unsettled.

## Mathematical Optimization Techniques

A variety of mathematical optimization techniques have been applied to the inverse problem of IMRT. Additional methods and approaches are being applied and tested as the collaboration between researchers in this field with experts in mathematical optimization and operations research surges in recent years. This trend is evident from the growing number of special issues devoted to the interface between optimization theory and radiation therapy, e.g., Lee and Sofer (2003), Holder and Newman (2003), and Ferris and Zhang (2003), and the recent dedicated site on the Internet (Holder 2003). In this section we briefly review the following methods and approaches that have been applied to solving the inverse problem of IMRT, with emphasis on more recent publications in each category: (1) Simulated annealing and global optimization, (2) Multi-objective optimization, (3) Linear optimization and mixed integer programming (MIP), and (4) Cimmino's algorithm and other projection methods.

Other optimization models and methods, not mentioned here, were also used in RTTP in recent years; see Shepard et al. (2000), Xing and Chen (1996), Bortfeld et al. (1990) and the gradient and gradient-like methods of Spirou and Chui (1998) and others.

## Simulated Annealing And Global Optimization

The NEOS (Network Enabled Optimization System) Guide Optimization Tree (at: http://www-fp.mcs.anl.gov/otc/Guide/OptWeb/index.html) uses, in its *Introduction to Global Optimization*, the following definition: "Global optimization is the task of finding the absolutely best set of admissible conditions to achieve your objective, formulated in mathematical terms. It is the hardest part of a subject called nonlinear programming (NLP)." It goes on to supply references and links to the field that are most useful to anyone who wishes to learn about it. A general mathematical optimization problem has the form

$$\min\{f(x) \mid x \in Q\}, \tag{25}$$

where

$$Q = \{x \in R^l \mid x \in \Gamma, g_j(x) \le 0, (j = 1, 2, \ldots, J), h_m(x) = 0, (m = 1, 2, \ldots, M)\} \tag{26}$$

is the feasible set of the problem, represented by a set-constraint $\Gamma$ and equality $h_m(x) = 0$ and inequality $g_j(x) \le 0$ constraints. A point $x^* \in Q$ is a global optimal solution (global minimizer) of (25) if

$$f(x^*) \le f(x), \text{ for all } x \in Q. \tag{27}$$

A point $\tilde{x} \in Q$ is a *local optimal solution* (local minimizer) of (25) if there exists a neighborhood $U \subset R^l$ of $\tilde{x}$ so that

$$f(\tilde{x}) \leq f(x), \quad \text{for all } x \in Q \cap U. \tag{28}$$

The problem (25) is *multi-extremal* if it has multiple local minimizers with different objective function values. The occurrence of multiple extrema makes problem solving in nonlinear optimization a hard task. Without supplying global information, which is usually unavailable, the search for a global optimizer is not simple. There are stochastic methods and deterministic methods for global optimization, but one can also classify different methods based on their underlying philosophy, as Rinnooy Kan and Timmer (1989) do, as follows. (a) *Partition and search*: the feasible set $Q$ is partitioned into successively smaller subregions among which the global minimum is sought. (b) *Approximation and search*: the objective function $f$ is replaced by an increasingly better approximation that is easier from a computational point of view. (c) *Global decrease*: in this class of methods the aim is for permanent improvement in the values of $f$, culminating in arrival at the global minimum. (d) *Improvement of local minima*: exploiting the availability of an efficient local search routine, these methods seek to generate a sequence of local minima of decreasing function values. (e) *Enumeration of local minima*: here one strives to reach a complete enumeration of all local minima or, at least, of a promising subset of them.

*Simulated annealing* (SA) is a global optimization method. Its fundamental idea appears in Metropolis et al. (1953) and was applied to optimization problems by Kirkpatrick, Gelatt, and Vecchi (1983). The underlying principle of SA is to simulate the cooling process of material in a heat bath and it uses this simulation to systematically search for feasible points in a way that makes the generated sequence converge to a global minimum. Webb first introduced the SA algorithm into the field of RTTP (Webb 1989); see also his book (Webb 2001). A concise description of Webb's application of SA appears in his book (Webb 1993, subsection 2.5.4).

Global optimization can be used also for the IMRT inverse problem when the trajectories of the leaves of the MLC are integrated into the model. This has been recently done by Trevo et al. (2003) who arrived at a very high-dimensional constrained nonlinear global optimization problem and solved it by a, commercially available, software package called LGO (Lipschitz (continuous) Global Optimizer).

## Multi-Objective Optimization

*Multi-objective* (also called *multicriteria*) *optimization* handles problems in which more then one objective function is defined over the feasible set. The standard form of such a problem is

$$\min\{F(x) \mid x \in Q\}, \tag{29}$$

where $F(x)$ is a vector of (objective) functions, i.e., for $S \geq 2$,

$$(F(x))^T = (f_1(x), f_2(x), \ldots, f_S(x)), \tag{30}$$

and for each $s = 1, 2, \ldots, S$, the function $f_s(x)$ maps $R^I \to R$. We denote by $Q \subset R^I$ the feasible set that may be defined by equality constraints, inequality constraints, set constraints, or any mixture of them, as in (26). An optimal point for problem (29) is a point that is feasible ($x \in Q$) and minimizes $F(x)$. But what does it mean to minimize a vector of functions? Moving from one point $x^1$ in $R^I$ to another point $x^2$ may cause some function values to decrease while others increase; so how should one decide if a move is acceptable? The situation thus differs from the case of *scalar optimization*, when $S = 1$, because the vector of functions $F(x)$ induces on the feasible set $Q$ a *partial order* and not a *linear order*, i.e., not every two points are ordered by their $F$ values. Therefore, the solution (or solutions) to problem (29) depends *a priori* on which *solution concept* is adopted for solving the problem; see, e.g., Censor (1977). One way to handle this is by employing *scalarization*. This refers to the conversion of the multi-objective problem into a family of scalar optimization problems. This family has the form

$$\min\left\{ \sum_{s=1}^{S} \gamma_s f_s(x) \mid x \in Q \right\}, \tag{31}$$

where $\gamma = \left(\gamma_s\right)_{s=1}^{S} \in R^S$ is a parameter vector whose components $\gamma_s$ are the weights of relative importance which combine all scalar functions $f_s(x)$ into the linear combination. The difficulty here is that one usually does not know how to choose appropriately a vector $\gamma$ by which a specific scalar optimization problem of the form (31) will be picked out of the family of all possible such problems. Obviously, this choice strongly affects the final outcome.

An alternative approach to multi-objective optimization is to preserve the multi-objective nature of the problem and use a solution concept that does not involve scalarization. A frequently used such concept is the *Pareto optimality*, also termed *Pareto efficiency*.

**Definition 6.** *A point* $x^* \in R^I$ *is called* **Pareto optimal** (**efficient**) *for problem* (29) *if* $x^* \in Q$ *and there is no other* $x \neq x^*$ *such that* $x \in Q$, *for which* $f_s(x) \leq f_s(x^*)$ *for all* $s = 1, 2, \ldots, S$, *with a strict inequality for at least one* $s$, $1 \leq s \leq S$.

This means that $x^*$ is Pareto efficient if it is impossible to decrease the value of any individual scalar objective function from its value at $x^*$ without increasing at least one other scalar objective function. See, e.g., Ehrgott's recent book (Ehrgott 2000). In a recent paper, Hamacher and Küfer (2002) propose and investigate a *linear multicriteria programming* (LMP) problem for the inverse problem in RTTP. The concept of multicriteria optimization without prior scalarization is indeed tempting to work with.

It has been utilized in a variety of real-world problems in other technological and scientific fields. In operations research and the management sciences, multiple criteria decision making has developed into a solid body of literature in the past 30 years. The International Society on Multiple Criteria Decision Making (MCDM) offers relevant software solutions (at: http://www.mit.jyu.fi/MCDM/soft.html). Further scientific research and evaluation are needed to gauge the usefulness of this methodology in the field of RTTP. Küfer et al. (2003) develop this approach further and find that they must use adaptive reduction by appropriate approximation schemes to cope with the large scale nature of the LMP problem.

## Linear Optimization And Mixed Integer Programming (MIP)

*Linear optimization* (traditionally called *linear programming*) is the field of study of optimization problems in which all constraints as well as the objective function are linear. The literature of this field is vast and the leading algorithms for solving such problems are the famous SIMPLEX method and primal-dual interior point methods. We direct the reader to Shepard et al. (1999, subsection 4.1) and to Holder (2003) for recent works that describe this approach and supply many useful references. An early application of linear optimization to radiotherapy treatment planning is Bahr et al. (1968) where the approach is used to optimize the treatment plan with respect to just a few setup parameters which are kept free after the plan has been obtained by the trial and error methods of those days. Rosen et al. (1991) critically compares linear optimization approaches, as used until 1990, with simulated annealing and with projection methods for the feasibility approach.

There are several ways to apply linear optimization to the IMRT inversion problem, depending mainly on the choice of the objective function. For example, if we choose to minimize the total dose to all pixels in the patient's cross-section while obeying the upper and lower bounds on organs we may consider the linear optimization problem

$$\min\left\{ \sum_{j=1}^{J} \sum_{i=1}^{I} a_{ij} x_i \mid (18)-(21) \text{ hold} \right\}. \tag{32}$$

Alternatively, one can use an organ-weighted total dose objective function of the form

$$\sum_{l=1}^{L} \beta_l \sum_{j \in B_l} \sum_{i=1}^{I} a_{ij} x_i + \sum_{q=1}^{Q} \theta_q \sum_{j \in T_q} \sum_{i=1}^{I} a_{ij} x_i + \gamma \sum_{j \in C} \sum_{i=1}^{I} a_{ij} x_i, \tag{33}$$

and minimize it over (18)–(21) after choosing user-specified weights of importance

$$\{\beta_l\}_{l=1}^{L}, \{\theta_q\}_{q=1}^{Q}$$

and $\gamma$. See, e.g., Shepard et al. (1999, subsection 4.1) for other formulations.

Mixed integer programming (MIP) occurs when some variables in an optimization problem are restricted to take only integer values. In the case of linear optimization, the MIP problem has the general form

$$\min\left\{\langle c, x\rangle \;\middle|\; Ax = b,\; l \le x \le u, \;\; \text{and some or all } x_i \text{ are integers}\right\}, \qquad (34)$$

where $c \in R^I$, the matrix $A$, and the vectors $b \in R^J, l, u, \in R^I$, are given, see, e.g., Bixby et al. (2000). In RTTP the need for this kind of optimization arises in a natural way when *dose-volume constraints* (also called *partial volume constraints*) are considered. Such constraints appear when the oncologist is willing to sacrifice a portion of a region at risk in order to improve the probability of curing the disease. In such a case, in addition to the upper and lower bounds on required and permitted radiation doses, as formulated in (18)–(21), he might state that "up to $\varphi\%$ of all pixels inside a certain organ $B_l$ in (18) might be allowed to exceed $b_l$ by $\psi\%$", without specifying *a priori* which of the pixels in $B_l$ will actually use this relaxed upper bound. The MIP formulation reached at in this way can be found in Langer et al. (1996) and also in Shepard et al. (1999, p. 737). Other applications of MIP in this field include Lee, Fox, and Crocker (2000) who used it for radiosurgery treatment planning, Boland, Hamacher, and Lenzen (2002) who employed a nonlinear MIP formulation to incorporate MLC settings within the treatment planning, and Bednarz et al. (2002) who compared MIP performance with that of Cimmino's algorithm. Ferris, Meyer, and D'Souza (2002) give details of the mathematical formulations and algorithmic approaches as well as pointers to supporting literature for MIP-based approaches to problems of RTTP. As Ferris, Meyer, and D'Souza correctly notice, the main difficulty associated with the MIP approach is that these formulations can become quickly impractical due to large numbers of voxels in the region of interest (i.e., the number $J$, above). These difficulties have then to be attacked by approximate techniques.

## Cimmino's Algorithm And Other Projection Methods

The *convex feasibility problem* is to find a (i.e., any) point in the nonempty intersection $C := \cap_{j=1}^{J} C_j \ne \emptyset$ of a family of closed convex subsets $C_j \subseteq R^I$, $1 \le j \le J$, of the $I$-dimensional Euclidean space. It is a fundamental problem in many areas of mathematics and the physical sciences, see, e.g., Combettes (1993, 1996) and references therein. It has been used to model significant real-world problems such as image reconstruction from projections [see, e.g., Herman (1980)] and crystallography [see Marks, Sinkler, and Landree (1999)] and has been used under additional names such as *set theoretic estimation* or the *feasible set approach*. A common approach to such problems is to use projection algorithms; see, e.g., Bauschke and Borwein (1996). *Projection algorithms* employ projections onto convex sets in various ways. They may use different kinds of projections and, sometimes, even use different projections within the same algorithm. They serve to solve a variety of problems, which are either of the feasibility or the optimization types. They have different algorithmic structures, of which some are particularly suitable for parallel computing, and they demonstrate nice convergence properties and/or good initial behavior patterns. This class of algorithms has witnessed great progress in recent years and its member algorithms have been applied with success to fully discretized models of problems in image reconstruction and image processing; see, e.g., Stark and Yang (1998), Censor and Zenios (1997).

Projection algorithms often employ *orthogonal projections* (i.e., nearest point mappings) onto the individual sets $C_j$. The orthogonal projection $P_\Omega(z)$ of a point $z \in R^l$ onto a closed convex set $\Omega \subseteq R^l$ is defined by

$$P_\Omega(z) := \arg\min\left\{ \| z - x \| \mid x \in \Omega \right\}. \tag{35}$$

Frequently a *relaxation parameter* is introduced so that

$$P_{\Omega,\lambda}(z) := (1 - \lambda)z + \lambda P_\Omega(z) \tag{36}$$

is the relaxed projection of $z$ onto $\Omega$ with relaxation $\lambda$. Another problem that is related to the convex feasibility problem is the *best approximation problem* of finding the projection of a given point $y \in R^l$ onto the nonempty intersection $C$ of a family of closed convex subsets $C_j \subseteq R^l$, $1 \leq j \leq J$; see, e.g., Deutsch's recent book (Deutsch 2001). In both problems the convex sets $\left\{ C_j \right\}_{j=1}^{J}$ represent mathematical constraints obtained from the modeling of the real-world problem, e.g., in IMRT, each constraint of (18)–(20) can be used to define a halfspace $C_j$. In the convex feasibility approach any point in the intersection is an acceptable solution to the real-world problem whereas the best approximation formulation is usually appropriate if some point $y \in R^l$ is given and one wishes to find the point in the intersection of the convex sets which is closest to the point $y$. Iterative projection algorithms for finding a projection of a point onto the intersection of sets are more complicated than algorithms for finding just any feasible point in the intersection. This is so because they must have, in their iterative steps, some built-in "memory" mechanism to remember the original point whose projection is sought after. The sequential or parallel algorithms of Dykstra [see, e.g., Bregman, Censor, and Reich (1999)], Haugazeau [see, e.g., Bauschke and Combettes (2001)], Bauschke (1996), and others and their modifications employ different such memory mechanisms.

Projection algorithmic schemes for the convex feasibility problem or for the best approximation problem are, in general, either *sequential* or *simultaneous* or *block-iterative* (see, e.g., Censor and Zenios (1997) for a classification of projection algorithms into such classes, and the review paper of Bauschke and Borwein (1996) for a variety of specific algorithms of these kinds). In what follows we explain and demonstrate these structures along with the recently proposed *string-averaging* structure. The philosophy behind these algorithms is that it is easier to calculate projections onto the individual sets $C_j$ than onto the whole intersection of sets. Thus, these algorithms call for projections onto individual sets as they proceed sequentially, simultaneously, or in the block-iterative or the string-averaging algorithmic modes.

*The String-Averaging Algorithmic Structure*

The *string-averaging* algorithmic scheme was proposed by Censor, Elfving, and Herman (2001). For $t = 1, 2, \ldots , M$, let the *string* $J_t$ be an ordered subset of $\{1, 2, \ldots , J\}$ of the form

$$J_t = \left( j_1^t, j_2^t, \ldots , j_{J(t)}^t \right). \tag{37}$$

with $J(t)$ denoting the number of elements in $J_t$. Suppose that there is a set $Q \subseteq R^l$ such that there are operators $R_1, R_2, \ldots , R_J$ mapping $Q$ into $Q$ and an operator $R$ which maps $Q^M = Q \times Q \times \cdots \times Q$ ($M$ times) into $Q$. Initializing the algorithm at an arbitrary $x^0 \in Q$, the iterative step of the string-averaging algorithmic scheme is as follows. Given the current iterate $x^k$, calculate, for all $t = 1, 2, \ldots , M$,

$$T_t\left( x^k \right) = R_{j_{J(t)}^t} \ldots R_{j_2^t} R_{j_1^t}\left( x^k \right) \tag{38}$$

and then calculate

$$x^{k+1} = R\left( T_1\left( x^k \right), T_2\left( x^k \right), \ldots , T_M\left( x^k \right) \right). \tag{39}$$

For every $t = 1, 2, \ldots , M$, this algorithmic scheme applies to $x^k$ successively the operators whose indices belong to the $t$th string. This can be done in parallel for all strings and then the operator $R$ maps all end-points onto the next iterate $x^{k+1}$. This is indeed an algorithm provided that the operators $\left\{ R_j \right\}_{j=1}^J$ and $R$ all have algorithmic implementations. In this framework we get a sequential algorithm by the choice $M = 1$ and $J_1 = (1, 2, \ldots , J)$. The well-known "Projections Onto Convex Sets" (POCS) algorithm for the convex feasibility problem is such a *sequential* projection algorithm; see Bregman (1965), Gubin, Polyak, and Raik (1967), Youla (1987), and the review papers by Combettes (1993, 1996). Starting from an arbitrary initial point $x^0 \in R^l$, the POCS algorithm's iterative step is

$$x^{k+1} = x^k + \lambda_k\left( P_{C_{j(k)}}\left( x^k \right) - x^k \right), \tag{40}$$

where $\{\lambda_k\}_{k\geq 0}$ are relaxation parameters and $\{j(k)\}_{k\geq 0}$ is a *control sequence*, $1 \leq j(k) \leq m$, for all $k \geq 0$, which determines the individual set $C_{j(k)}$ onto which the current iterate $x^k$ is projected. A commonly used control is the *cyclic control* in which $j(k) = k \bmod J + 1$, but other controls are also available (Censor and Zenios 1997). This algorithm was used in RTTP in Censor, Altschuler, and Powlis (1988b) and by Cho and Marks and co-workers in Cho et al. (1997, 1998) and Cho and Marks (2000). The celebrated ART (Algebraic Reconstruction Technique) of Gordon, Bender, and Herman (1970) [see also Herman (1980)], is equivalent to the application of POCS to a system of linear equations.

A *simultaneous* algorithm is obtained by the choice $M = J$ and $J_t = (t)$, $t = 1$, $2, \ldots, M$, and Cimmino's projections method is indeed such an algorithm. Using relaxation parameters $\{\lambda_k\}_{k\geq 0}$ and *weights of importance* $\left\{w_j\right\}_{j=1}^{J}$, such that $w_j > 0$ and $\sum_{j=1}^{J} w_j = 1$, the iterative step of Cimmino's algorithm for the derivation of the next iterate $x^{k+1}$ from the current one $x^k$ is

$$x^{k+1} = x^k + \lambda_k \left( \sum_{j=1}^{J} w_j P_{C_j}\left(x^k\right) - x^k \right). \tag{41}$$

For halfspaces as constraints sets, i.e.,

$$C_j = \left\{ x \in R^I \,\middle|\, \langle a^j, x \rangle \leq d_j \right\}, \quad \text{for all } j = 1, 2, \ldots, J, \tag{42}$$

the formula becomes:

$$x^{k+1} = x^k + \lambda_k \sum_{j=1}^{n} w_j c_j\left(x^k\right) a^j, \tag{43}$$

where

$$c_j\left(x^k\right) = \min\left( 0, \frac{d_j - \langle a^j, x^k \rangle}{\left\| a^j \right\|^2} \right). \tag{44}$$

String-averaging schemes offer a variety of options for steering the iterates towards a solution of the convex feasibility problem. It is an *inherently parallel* scheme in that its mathematical formulation is parallel (like the fully simultaneous method mentioned above). We use this term to contrast such algorithms with others that are sequential in their mathematical formulation but can, sometimes, be implemented in a parallel fashion based on appropriate model decomposition (i.e., depending on the structure of the underlying problem). Being inherently parallel, this algorithmic scheme enables flexibility in the actual manner of implementation on a parallel machine. At the extremes of the "spectrum" of possible specific algorithms, derivable from the string-averaging algorithmic scheme, are the generically sequential method, which uses one set at a time, and the fully simultaneous algorithm, which employs all sets at each iteration.

The *block-iterative projections* (BIP) scheme of Aharoni and Censor (1989) also has the sequential and the fully simultaneous methods as its extremes in terms of block structures, but the string-averaging algorithmic structure gives users further options to design new inherently parallel computational schemes. The behavior of the string-averaging algorithmic scheme in the inconsistent case when the intersection $C = \cap_{j=1}^{J} C_j$ is empty is not known at this time. For results on the behavior of the fully simultaneous algorithm with orthogonal projections in the inconsistent case see, e.g., Combettes (1994). We demonstrate some of the algorithmic possibilities offered by the general string-averaging method in figure 2. The constraints sets of the convex feasibility problem are assumed in this special case to be the six hyperplanes $H_1$, $H_2$, $H_3$, $H_4$, $H_5$, and $H_6$.

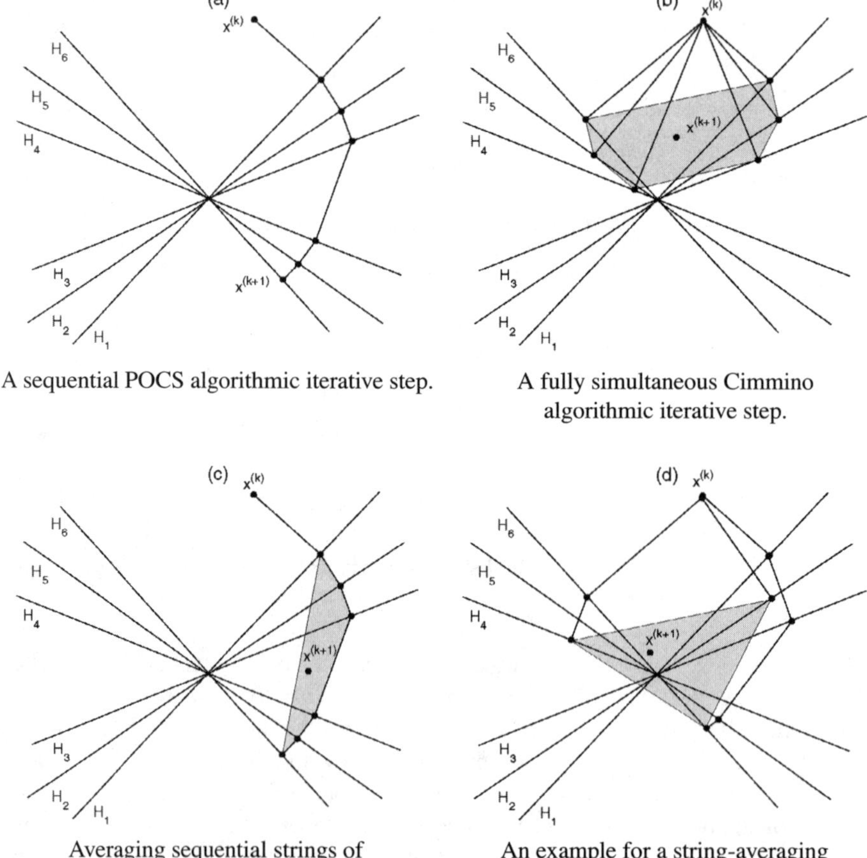



A sequential POCS algorithmic iterative step.

A fully simultaneous Cimmino algorithmic iterative step.

Averaging sequential strings of consecutive projections.

An example for a string-averaging algorithmic iterative step.

**Figure 2.** Some algorithmic possibilities offered by the string-averaging method.

The fully simultaneous Cimmino algorithm, applied to halfspaces, defined by the inequalities of the system (18)–(20), was first used in RTTP by Censor, Altschuler, and Powlis (1988a) [see also Powlis et al. (1989)]. There are several advantages of the simultaneous projections Cimmino algorithm over the sequential projections POCS algorithm for the linear feasibility problem arising from the fully discretized model of IMRT. When initialized at zero intensities it generates an approximate LIF (least-intensity feasible) solution; see Xiao et al. (2003a). It converges globally to a feasible solution, if such a solution exists, or to a minimal value of a proximity function in the inconsistent case; see Combettes (1994) and Byrne and Censor (2001). It is an inherently parallel iterative algorithm, thus, implementable on parallel computing equipment regardless of problem structure. It can be accelerated by using strong over-relaxation, see Höffner et al. (1996), or by using it with oblique projections (i.e., the CAV algorithm; see, e.g., [Xiao et al. (2203b), appendix] and references therein). It is a special case of more general algorithmic schemes, such as BIP and the string-averaging scheme, which allow processing of various sets of constraints instead of a single (POCS) or all (Cimmino) constraints, in each iterative step. It generates smoother intensity patterns; see Xiao et al. (2003b).

## Acknowledgments

The author gratefully acknowledges useful discussions with Martin Altschuler, Greg Bednarz, Christopher Börgers, Yan Chen, James Galvin, Chris Hauser, Gabor Herman, Darek Michalski, William Powlis and Ying Xiao. The support and hospitality and the inspiring research atmosphere at the Medical Physics Division (Prof. James Galvin, Director), Department of Radiation Oncology, Thomas Jefferson University, Philadelphia, PA, where some of the work reported here was done, are gratefully acknowledged. This work was partially supported by grant 592/00 of the Israeli Science Foundation, founded by The Israel Academy of Sciences and Humanities. Some material was adopted from Censor (1999) which appeared in the book: *Computational Radiology and Imaging: Therapy and Diagnosis*, C. Börgers and F. Natterer (eds.), The IMA Volumes in Mathematics and its Applications, Vol. 110, New York, NY: Springer-Verlag, copyright Springer-Verlag, with permission.

## References

Aharoni, R., and Y. Censor. (1989). "Block-iterative projection methods for parallel computation of solutions to convex feasibility problems." *Linear Algebra and Its Applications* 120:165–175.

Alber, M., and F. Nüsslin. (1999). "An objective function for radiation treatment optimization based on local biological measures." *Phys. Med. Biol.* 44:479–493.

Altschuler, M. D., and Y. Censor. "Feasibility Solutions in Radiation Therapy Treatment Planning" in *Proceedings of the Eighth International Conference on the Use of Computers in Radiation Therapy*. J.R. Cunningham, D. Ragan, and J. Van Dyk, (eds.), Silver Spring, MD, USA: IEEE Computer Society Press, pp. 220–224, 1984.

Bahr, G. K., J. G. Kereiakes, H. Horowitz, R. Finney, J. Galvin, and K. Goode. (1968). "The method of linear programming applied to radiation treatment planning." *Radiol.* 91:686–693.

Bauschke, H. H. (1996). "The approximation of fixed points of compositions of nonexpansive mappings in Hilbert space." *J. Math. Analys. Appl.* 202:150–159.

Bauschke, H. H., and J. M. Borwein. (1996). "On projection algorithms for solving convex feasibility problems." *SIAM Review* 38:367–426.

Bauschke, H. H., and P. L. Combettes. (2001). "A weak-to-strong convergence principle for Fejér-monotone methods in Hilbert spaces." *Math. Oper. Res.* 26:248–264.

Bednarz, G., D. Michalski, C. Hauser, M. S. Huq, Y. Xiao, P. R. Anne, and J. M. Galvin. (2002). "The use of mixed-integer programming for inverse treatment planning with pre-defined field segments." *Phys. Med. Biol.* 47:1–11.

Bixby, R. E., M. Fenelon, Z. Gu, E. Rothberg, and R. Wunderling. "MIP: Theory and Practice—Closing the Gap" in *System Modelling and Optimization: Methods, Theory and Applications*. M. J. D. Powell and S. Scholtes (eds.). Boston, MA: Kluwer Academic Publishers, 2000.

Boland, N., H. W. Hamacher, and F. Lenzen. "Minimizing beam on time in cancer radiation treatment using multileaf collimators." Technical report in Wirtschaftsmathematik Nr. 78/2002. Department of Mathematics, University of Kaiserslautern, Germany. 2002.

Bortfeld, T., J. Bürkelbach, R. Boesecke, and W. Schlegel. (1990). "Methods of image reconstruction from projections applied to conformation radiotherapy." *Phys. Med. Biol.* 35:1423–1434.

Brahme, A. "Treatment Optimization Using Physical and Radiological Objective Functions" in *Medical Radiology: Radiation Therapy Physics*. A.R. Smith (eds.), Berlin: Springer-Verlag, pp. 209–246, 1995.

Brahme, A., J.-E. Roos, and I. Lax. (1982). "Solution of an integral equation encountered in rotation therapy." *Phys. Med. Biol.* 27:1221–1229.

Bregman, L. M. (1965). "The method of successive projections for finding a common point of convex sets." *Soviet Mathematics Doklady* 6:688–692.

Bregman, L. M., Y. Censor, and S. Reich. (1999). "Dykstra's algorithm as the nonlinear extension of Bregman's optimization method." *J. Convex Analys.* 6:319–333.

Byrne, C., and Y. Censor. (2001). "Proximity function minimization using multiple Bregman projections, with applications to split feasibility and Kullback-Leibler distance minimization." *Ann. Oper. Res.* 105:77–98.

Censor, Y. (1977). "Pareto optimality in multiobjective problems." *Appl. Math. Optim.* 4:41–59.

Censor, Y. "Mathematical Aspects of Radiation Therapy Treatment Planning: Continuous Inversion Versus Full Discretization and Optimization Versus Feasibility" in *Computational Radiology and Imaging: Therapy and Diagnosis*, C. Börgers and F. Natterer (eds.). The IMA Volumes in Mathematics and its Applications, Vol. 110, New York: Springer-Verlag, pp. 101–112, 1999.

Censor, Y., and S. A. Zenios. *Parallel Optimization: Theory, Algorithms, and Applications*. New York: Oxford University Press, 1997.

Censor, Y., M. D. Altschuler, and W. D. Powlis. (1988a). "On the use of Cimmino's simultaneous projections method for computing a solution of the inverse problem in radiation therapy treatment planning." *Inverse Problems* 4:607–623.

Censor, Y., M. D. Altschuler, and W. D. Powlis. (1988b). "A computational solution of the inverse problem in radiation therapy treatment planning." *Appl. Math. Comput.* 25:57–87.

Censor, Y., T. Elfving, and G. T. Herman. "Averaging Strings of Sequential Iterations for Convex Feasibility Problems" in *Inherently Parallel Algorithms in Feasibility and Optimization and Their Applications.* D. Butnariu, Y. Censor, and S. Reich (eds.). Amsterdam: Elsevier Science Publishers, 2001, pp. 101–114, 2001.

Cho, P. S., and R. J. Marks II. (2000). "Hardware-sensitive optimization for intensity modulated radiotherapy." *Phys. Med. Biol.* 45:429–440.

Cho, P. S., S. Lee, R. J. Marks II, J. A. Redstone, and S. Oh. "Comparison of Algorithms for Intensity Modulated Beam Optimization: Projections onto Convex Sets and Simulated Annealing" in *Proceedings of the XII International Conference on the Use of Computers in Radiation Therapy.* May 27–30, 1997, Salt Lake City, Utah. D. D. Leavitt, and G. Starkschall (eds.). Madison, WI: Medical Physics Publishing, pp. 310–312, 1997.

Cho, P. S., S. Lee, R.J. Marks II, S. Oh, S. G. Sutlief, and M. H. Phillips. (1998). "Optimization of intensity modulated beams with volume constraints using two methods: Cost function minimization and projections onto convex sets." *Med. Phys.* 25:435–443.

Combettes, P. L. (1993). "The foundations of set-theoretic estimation." *Proc. IEEE* 81:182–208.

Combettes, P. L. (1994). "Inconsistent signal feasibility problems: Least squares solutions in a product space." *IEEE Trans. Sig. Proc.* 42:2955–2966.

Combettes, P. L. (1996). "The convex feasibility problem in image recovery." *Adv. Imag. Electron Phys.* 95:155–270.

Cormack, A. M., and E. T. Quinto. (1990). "The mathematics and physics of radiation dose planning using X-rays." *Contemp. Math.* 113:41–55.

Deutsch, F. *Best Approximation in Inner Product Spaces.* New York: Springer-Verlag, 2001.

Dritschilo, A., J. T. Chaffey, W. D. Bloomer, and A. Mark. (1978). "The complication probability factor: A method for selection of radiation treatment plans." *Br. J. Radiol.* 51:370–374.

Ehrgott, M. *Multicriteria Optimization.* Lecture Notes in Economics and Mathematical Systems. Vol. 491. Berlin: Springer-Verlag, 2000.

Ferris, M. C., and Y. Zhang (eds.). Special Issue on Mathematical Programming in Biology and Medicine. *Mathematical Programming Series B,* 2003. To appear.

Ferris, M. C., R. R. Meyer, and W. D'Souza. (2002). "Radiation treatment planning: Mixed integer programming formulations and approaches." Optimization Technical Report 02-08, Computer Science Department, University of Wisconsin, Madison, WI, October 2002.

Goitein, M. (1990). "The inverse problem." *Int. J. Radiat. Oncol. Biol. Phys.* 18:489–491.

Gordon, R., R. Bender, and G. T. Herman. (1970). "Algebraic reconstruction techniques (ART) for three-dimensional electron microscopy and X-ray photography." *J. Theoret. Biol.* 29:471–481.

Gubin, L., B. Polyak, and E. Raik. (1967). "The method of projections for finding the common point of convex sets." *USSR Computational Mathematics and Mathematical Physics* 7:1–24.

Gustafsson, A. (1996). Development of a Versatile Algorithm for Optimization Of Radiation Therapy. Ph.D. Thesis. Department of Medical Radiation Physics. University of Stockholm, Sweden.

Gustafsson, A., B. K. Lind, and A. Brahme. (1994). "A generalized pencil beam algorithm for optimization of radiation therapy." *Med. Phys.* 21:343–356.

Hamacher, H. W., and K.-H. Küfer. (2002). "Inverse radiation therapy planning—a multiple objective optimization approach." *Discrete Appl. Math.* 118:145–161.

Herman, G. T. *Image Reconstruction From Projections: The Fundamentals of Computerized Tomography*. New York: Academic Press, 1980.

Höffner, J., P. Decker, E. L. Schmidt, W. Herbig, J. Rittler, and P. Weiss. (1996). "Development of a fast optimization preview in radiation treatment planning." Strahlentherap. Onkol. 172:384–394.

Holder, A. (2003). "Radiotherapy Treatment Design and Linear Programming" in *The Handbook of Operations Research/Management Science Applications in Health Care*. M. Brandeau, F. Sainfort, M. Brandeau, and W. Pierskalla (eds.). New York: Kluwer Academic Press, 2003. In press.

Holder, A. (Internet site founder and maintainer). "Operations Research & Radiation Oncology." http://www.trinity.edu/aholder/HealthApp/oncology/.

Holder, A., and F. Newman (eds.). Special Issue on Radiation Oncology. Optimization and Engineering. In preparation. http://www.trinity.edu/aholder/research/CallForPapers.html.

Kartha, P. K. I., A. Pagnamenta, A. Chung-Bin, and F. R. Hendrickson. (1982). "Optimization of radiation treatment planning for the isocentric technique by use of a quality index." *Appl. Radiol.* 11:101–110.

Kirkpatrick, S., C. D. Gelatt, and M. P. Vecchi. (1983). "Optimization by simulated annealing." *Science* 220:671–680.

Küfer, K.-H., A. Scherrer, M. Monz, F. Alonso, H. Trinkaus, T. Bortfeld, and C. Thieke. (2003). "Intensity-modulated radiotherapy—A large scale multi-criteria programming problem." *OR Spectrum*. In press.

Langer, M., S. Morrill, R. Brown, O. Lee, and R. Lane. (1996). "A comparison of mixed integer programming and fast simulated annealing for optimizing beam weights in radiation therapy." *Med. Phys.* 23:957–964.

Lee, E. K., and A. Sofer (eds.). (2003). Special Issue on Optimization in Medicine. *Ann. Oper. Res.* 119.

Lee, E. K., T. Fox, and I. Crocker. (2000). "Optimization of radiosurgery treatment planning via mixed integer programming." *Med. Phys.* 27:995–1004.

Marks, L. D., W. Sinkler, and E. Landree. (1999). "A feasible set approach to the crystallographic phase problem." *Acta Crystallograph.* A55:601–612.

Metropolis, N., A. W. Rosenbluth, M. N. Rosenbluth, A. H. Teller, and E. R. Teller. (1953). "Equation of state calculation by fast computing machines." *J. Chem. Phys.* 21:1087–1091.

Powlis, W. D., M. D. Altschuler, Y. Censor, and E. L. Buhle Jr. (1989). "Semi-automatic radiotherapy treatment planning with a mathematical model to satisfy treatment goals." *Int. J. Radiat. Oncol. Biol. Phys.* 16:271–276.

Raphael, C. (1992). "Radiation therapy treatment planning: An $L^2$ approach." *Appl. Math. Computat.* 52:251–277.

Rinnooy Kan, A. H. G., and G. T. Timmer. (1989). "Global Optimization" in *Optimization. Handbooks in Operations Research and Management Science, Vol. 1*. G. L. Nemhauser, A. H. G. Rinnooy Kan, and M. J. Todd (eds.). Amsterdam: Elsevier Science Publishers B.V., pp. 631–662, 1989.

Rosen, I. I., R. G. Lane, S. M. Morrill, and J. A. Belli. (1991). "Treatment plan optimization using linear programming." *Med. Phys.* 18:141–152.

Shepard, D. M., M. C. Ferris, G. H. Olivera, and T. R. Mackie. (1999). "Optimizing the delivery of radiation therapy to cancer patients." *SIAM Review* 41:721–744.

Shepard, D. M., G. H. Olivera, P. J. Reckwerdt, and T. R. Mackie. (2000). "Iterative approaches to dose optimization in tomotherapy." *Phys. Med. Biol.* 45:69–90.

Spirou, S. V., and C.-S. Chui. (1998). "A gradient inverse planning algorithm with dose-volume constraints." *Med. Phys.* 25:321–333.

Stark, H., and Y. Yang. *Vector Space Projections: A Numerical Approach to Signal and Image Processing, Neural Nets, and Optics.* New York: John Wiley & Sons, 1998.

Trevo, J., P. Kolmonen, T. Lyyra-Laitinen. J. D. Pinter, and T. Lahtinen. (2003). "An optimization-based approach to the multiple static delivery technique in radiation therapy." *Ann. Oper. Res.* 119. In press.

Webb, S. (1989). "Optimisation of conformal radiotherapy dose distribution by simulated annealing." *Phys. Med. Biol.* 34:1349–1370.

Webb, S. *The Physics of Three-Dimensional Radiation Therapy.* Bristol, UK: Institute of Physics Publishing (IOP), 1993. Reprinted with corrections 2001.

Webb, S. *Intensity-Modulated Radiation Therapy.* Bristol, UK: Institute of Physics Publishing (IOP), 2001.

Wolbarst, A. B., E. S. Sternick, B. H. Curran, and A. Dritschilo. (1980). "Optimized treatment planning using the complication probability factor (CPF)." *Int. J. Radiat. Oncol. Biol. Phys.* 6:723–728.

Xiao, Y., Y. Censor, D. Michalski, and J. M. Galvin. (2003a). "The least intensity feasible solution for aperture-based inverse planning in radiation therapy." *Ann. Oper. Res.* 119:183–203.

Xiao, Y., Y. Censor, D. Michalski, and J. M. Galvin. (2003b). "Inherent smoothness of intensity patterns for intensity modulated radiation therapy generated by a simultaneous projection algorithm." Technical Report, May 19, 2002. Revised: January 21, 2003.

Xing, L., and G. T. Y. Chen. (1996). "Iterative methods for inverse treatment planning." *Phys. Med. Biol.* 41:2107–2123.

Youla, D.C. "Mathematical Theory of Image Restoration by the Method of Convex Projections" in *Image Recovery: Theory and Applications.* H. Stark, (ed.). Orlando, Florida: Academic Press, pp. 29–77, 1987.

# Physical Optimization

**Thomas R. Bortfeld, Ph.D.**
Department of Radiation Oncology
Massachusetts General Hospital, Boston, Massachusetts



Intensity-modulated radiation therapy (IMRT) provides the potential to yield better dose distributions than uniform beam therapy because of its much larger number of degrees of freedom. However, even with IMRT it is impossible to deliver the ideal dose distribution with 100% dose in the tumor and 0% in the relevant critical structures, i.e., true inverse dose planning is not feasible (Bortfeld 1999). We therefore want to find the best plan within the wider physical limits of IMRT, i.e., we are confronted with an optimization problem. Before trying to find solutions, we need to define the problem clearly. More specifically, clinically meaningful *objectives* and *constraints* of the treatment must be *quantitatively* defined. This may look like a simple task at first glance, but it is in fact one of the most critical and important tasks in radiotherapy planning. As of today, there are still strongly varying opinions concerning such optimization criteria.

Clinicians often find it difficult to formulate a complete, unique, optimization representation of radiotherapy planning, even though they feel capable of ranking individually prepared plans. This problem is not unique in radiotherapy planning but is commonly encountered by operations researchers (optimization experts) working in many diverse fields. It is one of the central questions in a collaborative effort between operations researchers, medical physicists, and clinicians (http://www.isye.gatech.edu/nci-nsf.orart.2002/). As a consequence of these difficulties, IMRT optimization and the evaluation of the optimized plans are usually separate procedures. If the evaluation based on dose-volume histogram (DVH) and visual isodose inspections reveals some problems with the plan, another optimization run is performed with adjusted optimization parameters. An important requirement on optimization criteria is therefore to allow for a high degree of steerability of the plan.

Basically the optimization objectives and constraints that have been proposed and implemented up to now can be classified into *physical criteria*, which we will concentrate on here, and *biological criteria*, which will be dealt with in the subsequent lecture. Naturally, combinations of criteria belonging to both types have also been suggested, cf., Niemierko (1992), Wang et al. (1995), and Fraass (2002). It is beyond the scope of this tutorial to discuss the pros and cons of the two approaches in any detail. The IMRT treatments that have been delivered so far have been optimized almost exclusively based on physical criteria.

First we discuss different physical optimization criteria. Next we learn how different criteria are combined to define the objective function. The next section describes which treatment variables are optimized. Finally, we study an illustrative example of an optimization algorithm based on a gradient technique. Because of the introductory nature of this presentation we recommend that the interested reader study the more detailed descriptions in IMRT Collaborative Working Group (2001), Bortfeld (1999), and especially the excellent overview in the book of Webb (2001), which contains a complete set of references.

## Physical Optimization Criteria

By physical optimization criteria we mean criteria that provide a *clinically* relevant characterization of radiotherapy dose distributions and that can be expressed in terms of well-defined and measurable physical quantities such as dose and volume. In addition, we will briefly discuss purely physical and technical criteria such as the non-negativity of intensities, and the deliverability of the intensity maps.

### Clinically Relevant Criteria

All the criteria discussed below can be used as either constraints or as objectives. In the constraint formulation one merely requests that the criteria should stay within certain limits. If they are defined as (part of) the objective function, the goal is to maximize or minimize these quantities.

*Deviation From Prescribed Dose*

An important criterion is that the prescribed dose in the target volume(s) should be reached as closely as possible. The sum of the quadratic deviation from the prescription dose taken over every volume element (voxel) in the target is often used as the optimization objective to be minimized. Because in the target volume underdosage is more critical than overdose, different weight factors (also called penalty factors or importance factors) can be used for underdose and overdose. The objective function for the target volume is then:

$$F_T(\vec{b}) = \sum_{i=1}^{N_T} \left( u\left[D_{\min} - d_i(\vec{b})\right]_+^2 + w\left[d_i(\vec{b}) - D_{\max}\right]_+^2 \right) \tag{1}$$

where $u$ and $w$ are the weight factors for under- and overdose, respectively. $d_i(\vec{b})$ is the dose at voxel $i$ as a function of the beam element (bixel) intensities $\vec{b}$. $D_{min}$ and $D_{max}$ are the *prescribed* minimum and maximum doses that should ideally not be exceeded. Note that $D_{min}$ and $D_{max}$ are *not* the minimum and maximum doses of the *actual* dose distribution $d_i(\vec{b})$. One often sets $D_{min} = D_{max} =$ prescribed dose in the target volume. $[x]_+$ stands for $x$ if $x > 0$ and 0 otherwise.

This quadratic approach has been criticized because it does not sufficiently penalize very low doses in the target volume. Even if the dose at one point becomes zero, $F_T$ may still be in an acceptable range, as long as most voxels receive the prescription dose. The global (i.e., over all voxels), as opposed to local, nature of this criterion may result in unacceptable doses in some areas that get compensated in the criterion value by values at other voxels. Higher order measures of the deviation (such as differences taken to the power of 4, 6, …) have been suggested (Fraass 2002) but are not common in clinical IMRT optimization.

*Target Dose Homogeneity Issues*

It is a common misconception that IMRT necessarily leads to a reduction of target dose homogeneity when compared to conventional uniform beam therapy. In fact, in complex cases, the only way to obtain a rather homogeneous target dose is through the use of IMRT. To understand this point it is instructive to take a closer look at the original IMRT work of Brahme (Brahme, Roos, and Lax (1982). The example presented therein can serve as a general motivation of the use of intensity-modulated fields. Consider the irradiation of a target volume that is ring-shaped in a transversal slice and that has a circular critical structure, i.e., organ at risk (OAR), at its center; see figure 1. At first glance, an obvious treatment technique for such a tumor would be a rotation technique with a central block as schematically shown in figure 1. Now, it is well known that this does *not* produce a uniform dose distribution in the ring-shaped target at all. In fact, the resulting dose profile through the center of the ring falls off gradually toward the OAR, where the dose is almost zero, as desired (solid line at the bottom of figure 1). The considerable target dose inhomogeneity resulting from blocking the central part of the beam can be understood with a simple geometrical argument: Consider point 1 at the boundary of the target. This point is connected with the source, i.e., within the unblocked region of the field, for a large range of gantry angles, such as for the angle shown in figure 1. Point 2 located just inside the target but close to the OAR, on the other side, is blocked for the most part like, for instance, for the angle shown. Consequently, point 2 receives significantly less dose than point 1. Another point of view is that the total dose distribution is in this case given by the dose from the rotated open field without block (thereby treating both the ring and the OAR) *minus* the dose resulting from treating the OAR alone. Then the tails of the latter distribution outside the OAR are responsible for the inhomogeneous dose distribution in the ring-shaped target.

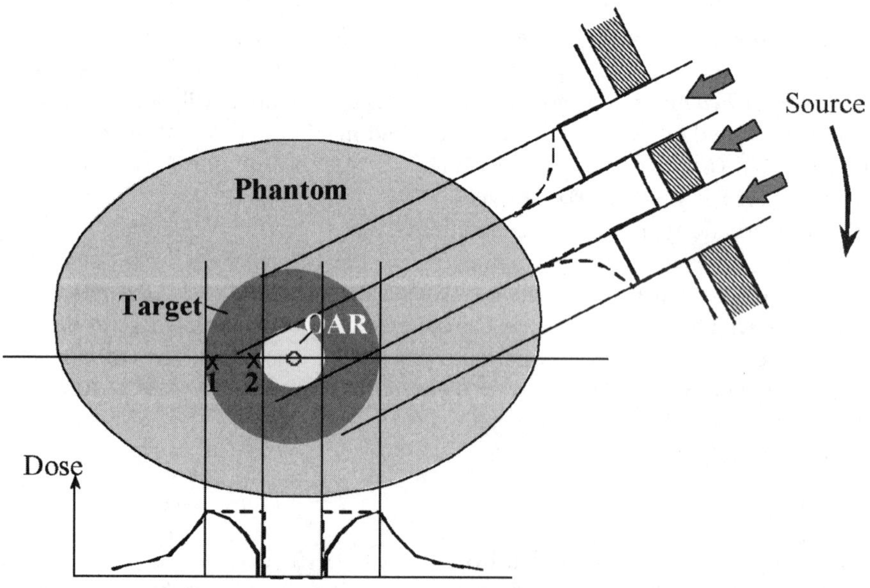


**Figure 1.** Target dose homogeneity issues: In complex cases one needs inhomogeneous beam intensity maps to deliver homogeneous target doses. The example shows the original example of Brahme (Brahme, Roos, and Lax 1982), which is an abstract case of a ring-shaped target volume around a critical structure (say, the spinal cord). The rotation with a centrally blocked beam produces an inhomogeneous dose distribution in the target. This can be seen from the solid line at the bottom, which is a dose profile through the isocenter. Only through a modulation of the intensity within the open part of the beam (dashed curve) can the missing dose be filled up (dashed curve at the bottom). [Reprinted from *Seminars in Radiation Oncology,* vol. 9, issue 1, T. Bortfeld, "Optimized planning using physical objectives and constraints," pp. 20–34. © 1999, with permission from Elsevier.]

The important idea is that the dose distribution in the target can be made *homogeneous* by applying an *inhomogeneous* beam intensity distribution (beam profile) in the unblocked part of the beam, as shown schematically by the dashed line in figure 1. In this way the missing dose in the target can be "filled up." In reality, the resulting dose distribution is of course not as ideal as the dashed line at the bottom of figure 1. There will be some scatter dose in the OAR, and the dose profile deviates somewhat from the rectangular shape due to penumbra. Nevertheless, IMRT allows pushing the dose conformation potential to the physical limits. This means in particular that the penumbra between the target and the OAR can be made as narrow or even somewhat narrower than the penumbra at the boundary of a single fixed beam.

In spite of these theoretical considerations it is true that in practice IMRT dose distributions are often less homogeneous than conventional dose distributions. Several reasons are responsible for this:

1. Margins: many IMRT optimization algorithms set the intensities of all pencil beams that do not directly hit the target volume to zero. This increases dose conformality but compromises target coverage.

2. Number of beams: The considerations above assumed an infinite number of beams. With a smaller finite number of beams, there is less potential to compensate dose inhomogeneities of one beam with other beams.

3. Trade-off with critical structures: If there is a nearby critical structure with low dose tolerance, the target dose will be compromised because even with IMRT the dose gradient is limited.

4. Objective function: As discussed above, the choice of the objective function has some influence on the target dose distribution.

However, as already said, the target dose inhomogeneities are not a necessary consequence of IMRT per se.

*Min/Max Dose*

One way to enforce dose homogeneity is to put hard constraints on the actual minimum and maximum dose in the target volume. For example, an optimization constraint might require keeping the target dose within −5% and +7% of the prescription dose, as recommended by the International Commission on Radiation Units and Measurements (ICRU) (1993). A possible optimization objective is to maximize the minimum dose value in the target volume (Langer et al. 1996). Maximum dose limitations (but, of course, not minimum dose limitations) make sense in critical structures as well. In structures with a serial organization, such as the spinal cord, the complication is correlated with the maximum dose. For example, in the spinal cord the maximum dose should be limited to, say, 45 Gy. Maximum dose constraints can also be formulated as objectives that require to minimize (to zero) the quadratic deviation of the actual dose distribution from the prescribed $D_{max}$, just like in *Deviation From Prescribed Dose* above with $u = 0$.

### Mean Dose

The mean dose is a useful descriptor of the dose effect in the target volume as long as deviations from the mean are not too big (Brahme 1984; Levegrun et al. 2001). The mean dose is also a useful clinical parameter in critical structures that are organized in parallel, such as the lung (Kwa et al. 1998). It should be noted, however, that different regions in the lung have different radiation sensitivities. The mean dose overall can therefore only be a very coarse predictor of side effects. It should also be emphasized that different kinds of complication can occur in the same organ, for example in the lung, such that different criteria may have to be used for one organ in the optimization.

### Dose-Volume Criteria

Another common method to represent dose effects in parallel critical structures is to use DVH constraints (Langer and Leong 1989; Langer et al. 1990; Niemierko 1992; Bortfeld, Stein, and Preiser 1997; Spirou and Chui 1998; Gustafsson and Langer 2000), which take into consideration the volume dependence to some degree. DVH constraints can be formulated as "no more than $V_{max}\%$ of the volume should receive more than a dose of $D_{max}$." They can be visualized as a barrier with a corner at the point $D_{max}$, $V_{max}$ in the DVH. See figure 2. The use of multiple DVH constraints may also be indicated in some cases (Carol et al. 1997), and DVH constraints can be used for the target volume as well.

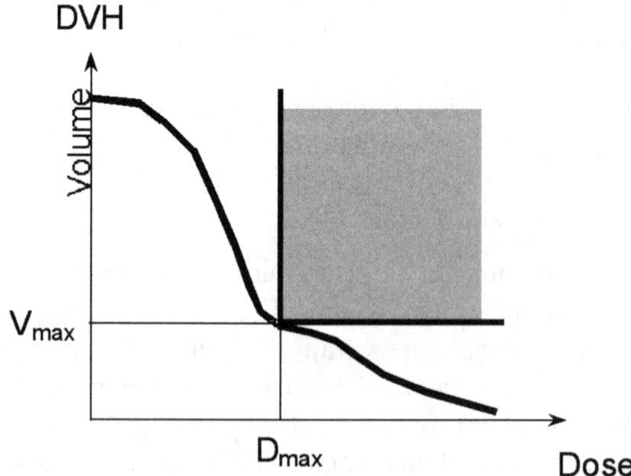


**Figure 2.** Structures with a large volume effect are appropriately spared through the application of DVH constraints. They prevent the DVH from going above the point $D_{max}$, $V_{max}$.

One general advantage of physical criteria is that, due to their clear and easy definition, they can be used easily in clinical protocols. It may be illustrative to look at a concrete example. In the Radiation Therapy Oncology Group (RTOG) protocol H022 for IMRT of oropharyngeal cancer the following physical dose specification is used:

<u>RTOG-022</u>

<u>Target dose prescription (homogeneity):</u>

No more than 1% of planning target volume (PTV) can receive less than 93% of prescription

No more than 20% of the PTV can receive greater than 110% of prescription

No more than 1% or 1 cc of tissue outside of PTVs will receive greater than 110% of prescription dose to primary PTV

<u>Critical Structures dose limits:</u>

Brainstem: 54 Gy

Cord (+ 5mm): 45 Gy

Mandible: 70 Gy

<u>Parotids (3 options):</u>

Mean dose to either parotid < 26 Gy or

At least 50% of either parotid gland < 30 Gy or

At least 20 cc of the combined parotid volume will receive < 20 Gy

A potential problem with dose-volume constraints is that they are non-convex (Deasy 1997). As a consequence of this, optimization based on DVH constraints may get trapped in local minima. However, it has been shown that this is mainly a theoretical problem, which is of little relevance in practical optimization (Wu and Mohan 2002).

*EUD*

The equivalent uniform dose (EUD) is defined as the uniform dose that would create the same biological effect in a specific organ as the actual non-uniform dose distribution (Brahme 1984; Niemierko 1997). Because it involves the biological effect, the EUD can be interpreted as a biological criterion. However, according to a more recent definition by Niemierko (1999) the EUD is simply the generalized mean (a norm) of the physical dose distribution:

$$\text{EUD} = \left( \sum_i v_i \cdot d_i^a \right)^{1/a} \tag{2}$$

where $v_i$ is the volume of voxel $i$ divided by the total volume of the organ. With this definition and with $a = 1$, the EUD is in fact the mean dose and with $a = \infty$, it equals the maximum dose. Of course, the value of $a$ is organ specific. Values between 1 and infinity represent organs with a mixture between parallel and serial structure. It is interesting to note that the value of $a$ can be derived from the well-known power-law relationship of the tolerance *TD* dose as a function of the relative treated volume $v$:

$$TD(v) = \frac{TD(1)}{v^n} \tag{3}$$

One finds that $a = 1/n$.

For target volumes, the value of $a$ is negative. The beauty of this approach is its simplicity and generality. All organs can be characterized by just one parameter. The EUD has recently been implemented into experimental IMRT optimization systems (Thieke, Bortfeld, and Niemierko 2002; Wu et al. 2002). A convenient feature of the EUD is that it is a convex function of the dose distribution, and therefore of the beam intensities, for $a \geq 1$ and $a \leq 0$, that is for almost all organs. This facilitates optimization and makes the use of projection onto convex sets (POCS) methods possible (Cho et al. 1998; Thieke, Bortfeld, and Niemierko 2002).

## Physical And Technical Criteria

### Non-Negativity Of Intensities

An obvious physical limitation is that the beam intensities must not be allowed to take negative values.

### Deliverability, Smoothness Of Intensity Maps

An important aspect of optimized treatment plans is that they have to be deliverable in an acceptable amount of time. Also, small errors in the delivery should not affect the resulting dose distribution too much, i.e., the plan should be robust. Both these requirements can be fulfilled with intensity maps that are smooth. If there are multiple solutions to the optimization problem, which is frequently the case, one should obviously choose the solution with the smoothest (easiest to deliver) intensity maps. If one has the choice between a highly conformal plan with extremely complex intensity maps, and a plan that is almost as good but much easier and safer to deliver, one would probably choose the latter plan. Basically, there are two ways to ensure smooth intensity maps. First, one can smoothen the maps using a filter. Median filters can be used for this purpose (Webb, Convery, and Evans 1998; Kessen, Grosser, and Bortfeld 2000). Secondly, one can add a smoothness term to the objective function (Alber and Nüsslin 2000).

## The Objective Function

As discussed in the lecture about mathematical optimization, the objective function is the function that needs to be minimized or maximized. Historically, many optimization techniques were developed with the goal to reduce the cost of, say, production processes. The objective function is therefore also called "cost function" and most often the minimization of the objective function is desired. In radiotherapy planning we consequently want to define the objective function such that its minimum corresponds with the optimum treatment.

## Combination Of Criteria (Costlets) Using Weights (Importance Factors)

The criteria (or "costlets") mentioned in the previous section must somehow be combined to form the total objective function. The most common approach to do this is simply by adding up the criteria using weight factors that reflect the importance of the different criteria. Multiplication of costlets has also been suggested (Fraass 2002). A typical approach is to add the deviations from the dose prescription (tumor) and maximum doses (critical structures) as defined previously using weight factors $w$. According to this definition the optimum treatment is the one with the smallest overall deviation from the prescription. Mathematically, the objective function is then defined as $F = F_T + w_{R1}F_{R1} + w_{R2}F_{R2} + w_{R3}F_{R3} + \ldots.$ For example, by using a large value for $w_{R1}$, more emphasis is put on sparing the first critical structure, $R1$. Figure 3 shows DVHs of optimized IMRT plans for the treatment of a head and neck tumor. Plan 1 was obtained with an equal weighting of the target and the spinal cord. *A priori* it is not clear by how much to change the weights to achieve the desired effect on the dose distribution. Suitable weight factors have to be determined by trial and error, which can be quite time-consuming. Plan 2 shows that, in order to reduce the dose in the spinal cord below 25 Gy, the weight had to be increased by 5 orders of magnitude. Some researchers argued that optimized "inverse" IMRT planning has just replaced the conventional manual trial and error search to find the best beam parameters by a manual trial and error search for suitable weight factors and constraints. While there may be some truth to this statement, it is also true that IMRT allows one to deliver highly conformal dose distributions that are impossible to achieve with conventional 3-D techniques.

## Constraints, Feasibility Search

Formulating the criteria as constraints provides more direct control and a higher degree of "steerability" of the treatment plan as discussed above. For example, by formulating the maximum dose in the spinal cord as a constraint, one can control it directly, not through the use of weight factors. Constraints are essential to take hard physical facts into consideration, such as the non-negativity of intensities. Typically, in constraint optimization one criterion (for one organ) is optimized while all others are kept within certain constraints. To give an example, the minimum dose value in the target volume is maximized while the doses in all critical structures are limited (Langer et al. 1996). A potential problem with constraint optimization is that there is no reward for reducing the dose in the critical structures below the constraint. Figure 4 shows a clinical head and neck example with two critical structures, one of which is dose limiting for the target volume, but the other one is not. In fact, it is possible to reduce the

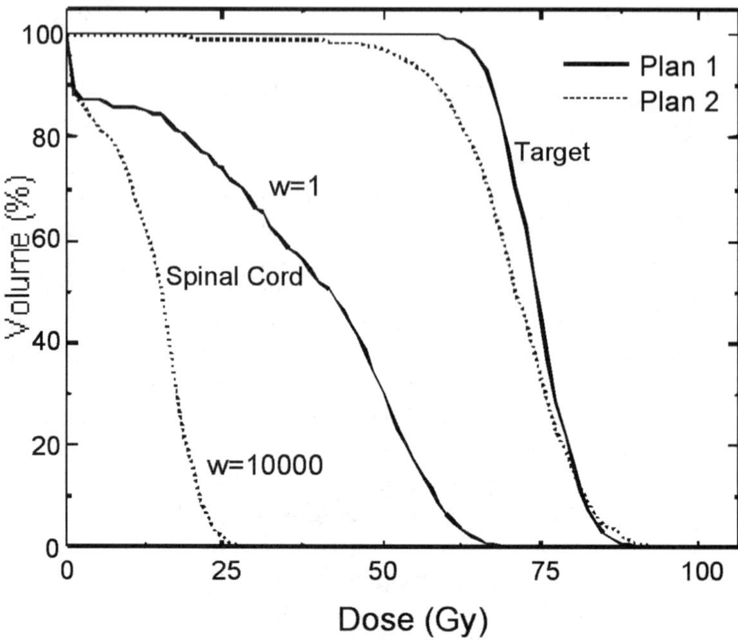



**Figure 3.** IMRT optimization for a head and neck tumor using a quadratic objective function with weight factors. Plan 1 is the optimization result with weight factors 1 for both target and spinal cord/brainstem, whereas plan 2 is the result with weightings 1 for target and 10,000 for spinal cord/brainstem. This shows that, to achieve a significant effect in the DVH, weight may have to be changed drastically, in this case by 5 orders of magnitude. Because weight factors have no obvious clinical interpretation, it is not *a priori* clear by how much to change the weight factors in order to achieve the desired effect in the DVH.

dose in the brainstem without compromising the dose in any of the other structures. Hence, although both plans in figure 4 are clinically acceptable, plan 2 is clearly better.

To facilitate optimization based on normal tissue dose constraints it is very helpful to know the sensitivity of the dose, say, in the target volume, to changing the dose constraints in one of the critical structures. This means, we want to know how much we have to pay in the target volume (in terms of reduction of the minimum target dose) if we reduce the dose in a critical structure by some amount, or vice versa. First approaches towards a sensitivity analysis along theses lines have been published (Alber, Birkner, and Nüsslin 2002).

An extreme case of a constraint "optimization" is one where there is no objective function at all, i.e., only constraints are used. This is called "feasibility search" (Censor, Altschuler, and Powlis 1988; Starkschall, Pollack, and Stevens 2000). The goal is to find a plan that "just" fulfills all constraints. This approach can be very useful if the constraints are carefully chosen: We do not want to make it too easy to fulfill the

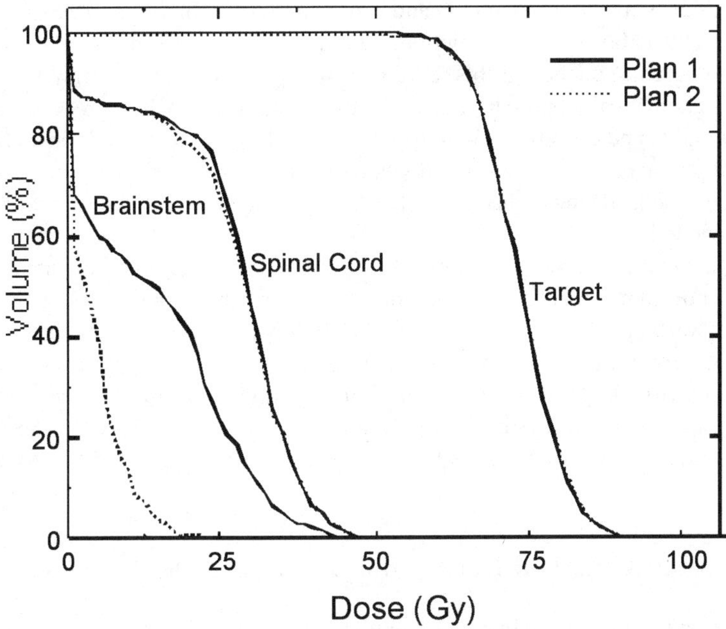


**Figure 4.** Same case as in figure 3. Here, constrained optimization was used. The dose constraints for the spinal cord and the brainstem were set to 37 Gy. According to these constraints, plan 1 is mathematically equivalent to plan 2. However, plan 2 is clearly better in terms of sparing the brainstem.

constraints because that may result in suboptimal plans. We also do not want to over-constrain the problem because then there will be no solution at all. The motivation of feasibility search comes from the fact that in practice it is often sufficient to find a suitable treatment plan, not necessarily the best plan. Feasibility search could be particularly successful for clinical cases that do not vary too much between individuals, such as prostate cancer. Here it is possible to find class solutions of constraints that will yield good treatment plans for most patients.

## Mono-Criteria Vs. Multi-Criteria Optimization

IMRT optimization is a typical multi-criteria or multi-objective optimization problem. As discussed above, optimality is difficult to define for this kind of problem. There are always trade-offs involved, and how well one can treat the target volume depends always on how much one is willing to "pay" in healthy organs. The basic problem is that something as complex as a radiation treatment plan can hardly be characterized by a single score, which is necessary in mono-criteria optimization. In most cases it is desirable to control multiple criteria and objectives (in the target volume(s) and in several critical structures) separately and simultaneously, which cannot easily be done with a single scalar objective function, even if it is the weighted sum of different costlets. As a consequence of this, current IMRT planning systems may yield plans that are mathematically optimal (maximal score) but not clinically appropriate. Adjusting the weights and constraints with trial and error leads to improved results, but the treatment planner never knows if and when the best clinical trade-off for the patient has been reached, and the trial and error has to be stopped when a time tolerance threshold is exceeded.

This issue was addressed in some detail at a National Cancer Institute/National Science Foundation (NCI/NSF) sponsored workshop in February of 2002 (http://www.isye.gatech.edu/nci-nsf.orart.2002/). It is perhaps surprising that, although multi-criteria optimization is a mature discipline of mathematical optimization (Steuer 1985; Conn, Gould, and Toint 1994; Gill, Murray, and Wright 1999; Miettinen 1999), it is only just beginning to surface in radiation therapy (Yu 1997; Küfer, Hamacher, and Bortfeld 2000; Cotrutz et al. 2001; Hamacher and Küfer 2002; Milickovic et al. 2002).

## A New Multi-Criteria IMRT Optimization Concept, Pareto Solutions

Here we want to briefly outline a new optimization concept that is being developed jointly by ITWM Kaiserslautern, Massachusetts General Hospital (MGH) Boston, and DKFZ Heidelberg with the goal to avoid some of the difficulties of current IMRT optimization. Instead of defining a single objective function as a measure of the quality of the treatment plan, the new approach is inherently multi-criterial. The dose distribution in each structure (critical structures and target) is characterized by its own, separate parameter. There are several options of what this parameter can be. One option is to use dose-volume parameters as described above. Perhaps the most promising parameter is the EUD. Using EUD, volume effects (e.g., in the lung and the kidneys) are "automatically" considered in the optimization process. The whole plan is characterized by the set of parameters (say, EUDs) in the different organs. What is sought is an optimal tradeoff between the target and the critical structures. Now, there is an infinite number of feasible combinations of those parameters. To make the search tractable, only so-called efficient (Pareto optimal) solutions are considered. These are defined as solutions that cannot be improved in the sense that an improvement in one organ will always lead to a worse result in at least one of the other organs. Figure 5 shows the Pareto frontier for a head and neck case as an example. The advantages of this concept are threefold:

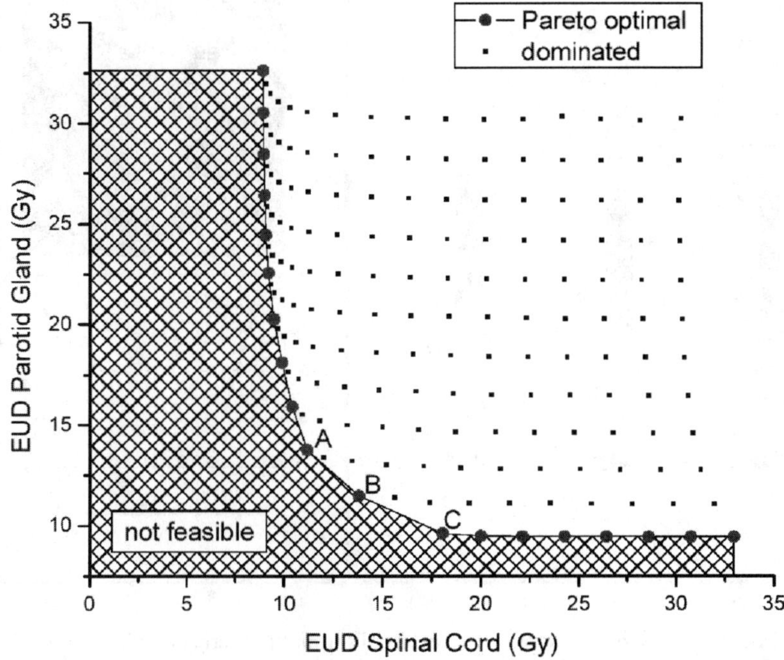


**Figure 5.** Exploration of the Pareto front for a head and neck case by brute force methods. Every black dot represents one treatment plan. A total of $16 \times 16 = 256$ plans was generated. The fat dots represent the Pareto front for this case, i.e., the set of "efficient" treatment plans.

1. Artificial weight factors, which have no clinical meaning, are avoided. The whole concept is based on dose-like values, which are amenable to a clinical interpretation.

2. Unnecessarily high doses in some of the critical structures, which can occur in constrained optimization (see above), are avoided by definition of the efficient (Pareto optimal) solution.

3. Plan tuning can be done interactively using "knobs" (figure 6) that have a clinical meaning. It is easy to do a sensitivity analysis and determine the dependency of, say, the target EUD on any of the critical structure EUDs.

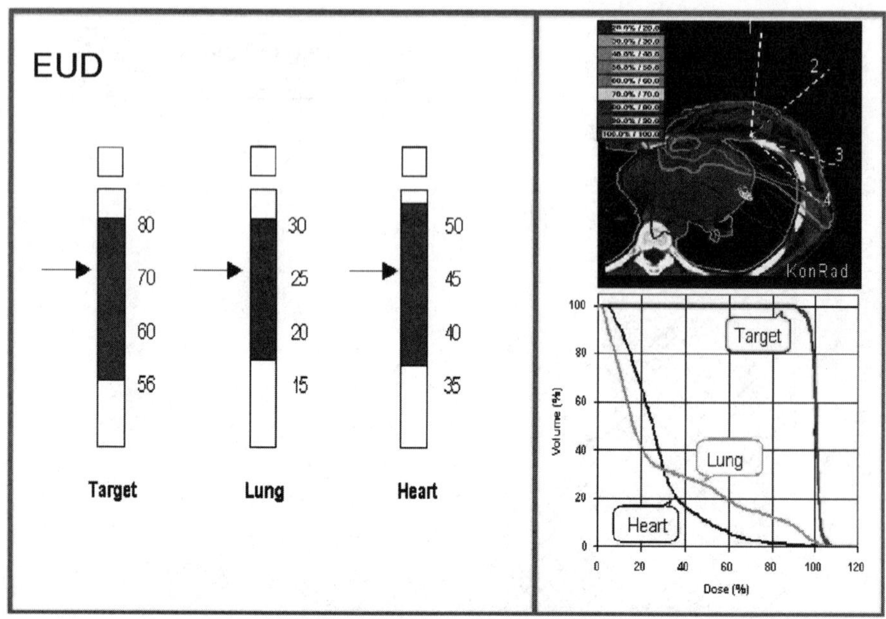


**Figure 6.** First prototype of an interactive search tool for multi-criteria optimization. In the left window, every structure is represented by a bar indicating the range of feasible organ parameters (e.g., EUD) and showing the actual value by an arrow. The dose distribution of the actual treatment plan is also visualized in the two windows to the right, in the upper one as isodoses and in the lower one as DVHs. The tool is fully interactive, i.e., by moving the EUD arrows one can immediately go to other solutions with the corresponding DVH and isodoses. [Reprinted from "New Approaches in Intensity-Modulated Radiotherapy" T. Bortfeld, C. Thieke, K.-H. Küfer, and H. Trinkaus in *Progress in Radio-Oncology* VII, H. D. Kogelnik, P. Lukas, F. Sedlmayer (eds.). © 2002, with permission from Monduzzi Editore, Bologna, Italy.]

The planning proceeds as follows: In a first step, the physician defines the prescribed dose in the target and the maximum tolerable doses for the normal structures. These data lead to an initial treatment plan that balances the consideration of all constraints to some degree. Based on the initial solution, the system generates a database of many alternative treatment plans. All these plans are efficient (Pareto optimal), and each of them represents a solution with a different emphasis on specific structures. For example, there will be a plan in which the target gets more dose than in the starting solution, but the dose in some normal structures will be higher as well. The following data is stored in each database entry:

- Treatment setup (beam directions and intensity matrices)

- Dose distribution with DVHs and isodoses

- The parameter set characterizing the doses in each structure

- The relation to the other database entries

The solutions are calculated and the database is filled overnight. It contains all treatment plans that lie in the area of clinical interest, whereby the definition of this area is very broad (a typical number of stored treatment plans is in the range 700 to 1000). One can see that in this concept the definition of the constraints is not critical. It is only used to generate an initial solution that lies somewhere in the area of clinically interesting solutions.

At the planning stage, the treatment planner and the physician can search the database interactively (see figure 6). At the beginning, the system suggests the plan of the initial solution. The dose distribution resulting from the plan is visualized in three ways: First, as the EUD values (or dose deviations as noted above) separately for each structure, second, as the DVH, and third, as isodoses.

If one or more aspects of the plan are not desirable (e.g., the EUD in one critical structure is too high), the planner can immediately go to another solution in which that specific criterion is fulfilled. This is done simply by dragging the EUD of the particular organ in the desired direction. Instantaneously, the system finds the corresponding solution in its database and updates the information for the other structures and in the DVH and isodose windows. This gives the planner immediate feedback about the sensitivity of the problem.

To give more control over the plan selection, it is possible to "lock" an organ by clicking on the box above the respective EUD bar. If an organ is "locked," all treatment plans with a worse EUD than the actual one are excluded from the further database exploration. In the future, for fine-tuning purposes it will be possible to find alternative plans not only by varying the organ parameter, but also by dragging the DVH and isodose curves.

The planner does not have to have a look at all the plans in the database. The interactive search tool allows him or her to find the most suitable trade-off in a few steps. Even the patient might be involved in this process at some point.

## Variables To Be Optimized

### Intensity Maps

In IMRT the main variables to be optimized are obviously the intensity maps for each beam. Each beam is typically subdivided into beam elements (bixels) of $5 \times 5$ to $10 \times 10$ mm$^2$. The intensity (fluence) for each of the bixels is optimized. The total number of bixels for all beams is typically in the order of 1000 to 10,000. Hence, IMRT optimization is a high-dimensional problem. Because there is no way to deliver intensity-modulated photon beams directly with a linear accelerator (linac), the intensity maps are then converted to a series of multileaf collimator (MLC) shapes (segments) in a second almost independent step, which is called "leaf sequencing." We say almost independent because there has to be some link between optimization and sequencing. For example, the optimizer must know the leaf width of the MLC and should use that as the bixel size in one dimension. More thorough approaches for the consideration of delivery constraints in intensity map optimization have also been suggested (Cho and Marks 2000; Alber and Nüsslin 2001).

## Direct Aperture Optimization

Besides the common two-step approach it has also been suggested to avoid the intermediate step of using intensity maps altogether and directly optimize MLC shapes (apertures) and their weights. This approach has been suggested by the group in Ghent (DeNeve et al. 1996) and at the Thomas Jefferson University hospital, among others. The MLC shapes can be determined manually based on the geometry (anatomy) of the problem, or they can be directly optimized together with the weights of the segments. The latter method has recently been published by Shepard et al. (2002). The direct optimization of MLC shapes and weights is mathematically a difficult, non-convex problem.

## Number Of Beams And Beam Angles

The question of how many intensity-modulated beams should be used is highly relevant for the practical delivery of IMRT. As a consequence of the analogy between image reconstruction in computed tomography (CT) and inverse radiotherapy planning, the early theoretical approaches to inverse planning assumed a very high number of coplanar beams (Brahme, Roos, and Lax 1982; Cormack and Cormack 1987). Later it was recognized that quite acceptable results can also be achieved with a moderate number of beams. In fact, some publications claim that one generally does not need more than three intensity-modulated beams to obtain results that can hardly be improved any more (Söderström and Brahme 1995). These issues have been discussed frequently in the literature (Brahme 1993, 1994; Mackie et al. 1994; Mohan and Ling 1995; Mohan and Wang 1996; Söderström and Brahme 1996).

In principle it is clear that the higher the number of beams, the higher is the dose conformation potential. However, the incremental improvement of the conformity of the total dose distribution diminishes as more and more beams are added. The real question about the "optimum" number of beams in IMRT is therefore: what is the number of beams beyond which one does not see any practically relevant improvement of the treatment plan? Several authors have found independently that it is hardly ever necessary to use much more than 10 intensity-modulated beams to achieve results that are close to optimum (Bortfeld et al. 1990; Webb 1992; Söderström and Brahme 1995; Stein et al. 1997).

On the other extreme, with a number of beams as small as 3 or 4, the conformity of the resulting dose distribution is considerably reduced when compared to a plan incorporating 10 beams. However, thanks to intensity modulation, it is still possible to imprint the desired shape on at least one isodose line, e.g., the 80% isodose. This finding is related to image reconstruction of homogeneous objects using only three or four projections (Natterer 1986). Hence, in cases where the tolerance of the critical structures is not too low as compared to the required target dose, one may get away with very few intensity-modulated beams (Söderström and Brahme 1995).

The question about the optimum beam angles is related to the number of beams. Clearly, if very many beams (>>10) are used, they can be placed at evenly spaced angular intervals and there will be no need to optimize beam orientations. Even with a moderate number of beams in the order of 7 or 9, one may often use evenly spaced beams without compromising the dose distribution (Bortfeld and Schlegel 1993). However, it has been shown that this is case dependent, and complex cases such as head and neck sometimes benefit from beam orientation optimization even for 9 or more beams (Pugachev et al. 2001). With very few beams, such as four or less, very careful and time-consuming optimization of beam orientations is always essential. Otherwise one will not be able to achieve acceptable results.

It should be noted that optimum orientations of intensity-modulated beams are generally different from those of uniform beams: in IMRT it is not generally necessary and often not even advantageous to avoid beam directions through organs at risk, because these can be spared by reducing the intensity for the corresponding rays (Stein et al. 1997). Also, for similar reasons, non-coplanar beams are rarely used in IMRT. Another point worth mentioning is that parallel- opposed beams should be avoided in IMRT, such that, for evenly spaced beams, the number of beams should be odd. The reason for that is that a parallel opposed beam adds much less beam shaping potential than a slightly angled beam. Clearly, if the attenuation were zero, parallel-opposed beams would be completely useless.

## Number Of Intensity Levels

Most IMRT planning methods assume a *continuous* modulation of the intensity. Several investigations have shown that promising results can be achieved with step-like beam profiles as well (Bortfeld et al. 1994; Gustafsson, Lind, and Brahme 1994; DeNeve et al. 1996). In fact, using a moderate number of stair-steps with 5 to 7 "intensity levels" in each beam profile, the results are almost as good as with continuous modulation (Keller-Reichenbecher et al. 1998). Consequently, it is not necessary to go to a fully dynamic treatment mode to perform IMRT with an MLC. IMRT can rather be realized in a "step-and-shoot" mode, i.e., by the successive delivery of a number of static MLC-shaped beam segments from each direction of incidence. The total number of beam segments or "subfields" to be delivered in this way is in the order of 100. Modern treatment machines can deliver such a sequence of subfields automatically and quickly. A comparison of the features of dynamic vs. step-and-shoot IMRT has been published by Chui et al. (2001). Both techniques will be discussed in subsequent chapters.

## Beam Energy

The choice of the beam energy is less critical in IMRT than in conventional radio-therapy. In fact, it was suggested that very low energies around 1 MeV or less suffice in IMRT. The reason is once again that in IMRT one tends to spread the beams more evenly around the patient, and the depth-dose fall-off is therefore not very relevant.

For IMRT with charged particles such as electrons or protons, on the other hand, the selection of the right energies is crucial. In practice, for electron or proton IMRT optimization, the energy is not optimized directly, but pencil beams with different energies are employed from each beam direction, and their weight is optimized pretty much as in photon IMRT. This optimization approach falls into the general framework of this chapter.

## Optimization Algorithm: An Illustrative Example

The past 10 to 15 years have witnessed exciting advances in the field of mathematical optimization and a large number of different optimization algorithms have been published. Many optimization algorithms that were developed for general optimization problems were applied to the radiation therapy problem. These approaches are too numerous to be described here in any detail. We therefore focus on one specific but rather typical and frequently used optimization technique, the gradient method. We study a very simple version of the gradient technique and apply it to a strongly simplified model problem. In spite of its simplicity, this example will give some insights into how IMRT optimization works in practice. For details about other optimization techniques the reader is referred to the works mentioned in the introduction.

Assume that our objective is to minimize the quadratic deviation of the actual dose $d_i$ from the dose prescription $P_i$ at every voxel $i$, similar to the model in *Deviation From Prescribed Dose*. We write the objective function $F$ in the form

$$F = \sum_{i=1}^{N} w_i \left[ d_i - P_i \right]^2. \tag{4}$$

The sum is taken over all $N$ voxels indexed by $i$. $P_i$ is the prescription dose if $i$ is a target voxel, and it is the tolerance dose if $i$ refers to a voxel in a critical structure. The weight factors $w_i$ are chosen such that in critical structures the weights are zero whenever the dose is below the tolerance dose, i.e., in critical structures we only penalize doses that are too high. The dose at any voxel $i$ depends on the beam element (bixel) intensities $\vec{b}$. Usually, the dependence is to a good approximation linear, i.e.:

$$d_i = d_i(\vec{b}) = \sum_j D_{ij} b_j, \tag{5}$$

where $D_{ij}$ is the dose contribution resulting due to a unit intensity from bixel $j$ to voxel $i$ and the sum is taken over all bixels. $D_{ij}$ can be calculated once before the optimization starts or it can be calculated online during the iterative optimization. These issues will be discussed in the chapter on (Monte Carlo) dose calculation for IMRT.

In employing the idea of the gradient technique we do an iterative optimization, and at every optimization step we correct the current $t$-th vector of bixel intensities $\vec{b}^1$ along the gradient (the slope) of the objective function with respect to $\vec{b}$. This is somewhat similar to a skier going downhill into the valley (of the objective function). Gradient techniques are therefore also called "downhill techniques."

The $j$-component of the gradient, i.e. the partial derivative of $F$ with respect to $b_j$, can easily be calculated as:

$$\frac{\delta F}{\delta b_j} = 2\sum_{i=1}^{N} w_i(d_i - P_i)D_{ij} \tag{6}$$

The gradient gives us the direction at every iteration step. We also need to know how far to move in this direction at each step. It is intuitively clear that the curvature of the objective function can provide some useful information here. If the curvature is large, we should be more careful and take smaller steps, and vice versa. The curvature is given by the second partial derivative, and in higher dimensions by the Hessian matrix consisting of all the (mixed) second partial derivatives. For quadratic objective functions it can be shown that one can reach the optimum (minimal value of $F$) by taking a single step that equals the product of the gradient and the inverse Hessian matrix. The technique works well in general because many objective functions can be locally approximated by a quadratic function. It is the basis of a large class of optimization methods called "Newton" or "quasi-Newton" methods. Because the calculation of the inverse Hessian matrix is often too difficult and time-consuming, approximations are generally used. Even the simple inverse of the second derivative

$$\frac{\delta^2 F}{\delta b_j^2} = 2\sum_{i=1}^{N} w_i D_{ij}^2 \tag{7}$$

can be quite useful.

With these prerequisites we can now formulate the simple gradient optimization algorithm as:

$$b_j^{t+1} = \left[ b_j^t - \alpha \, \frac{\frac{\delta F}{\delta b_j}}{\frac{\delta^2 F}{\delta b_j^2}} \right]_+ = \left[ b_j^t - \alpha \, \frac{\sum\limits_{i=1}^{N} w_i (d_i - P_i) D_{ij}}{\sum\limits_{i=1}^{N} w_i D_{ij}^2} \right]_+ \tag{8}$$

where $\alpha$ is a constant "damping factor" that has to be determined experimentally. One way to do this is by requiring that after the first iteration the mean dose in the target volume should equal the prescribed dose. Sometimes a value of $\alpha = 1/N_B$ has been used, where $N_B$ is the number of beam orientations. The + sign at the lower right side of the bracket indicates that only the positive part of the term in brackets is used. Negative values are cut off, i.e., set to zero. This is, of course, to avoid negative intensities. It is important to realize that the cutting off of negative values does not affect the convergence of the algorithm. The mathematical reason is that the set of non-negative numbers is convex.

We now take a look at the specific example in figure 7. The goal is to deliver a dose value of 1 unit to the C-shaped target volume, which wraps around a critical structure consisting of two voxels. The dose in the critical structure should not exceed 0.5 units. No other structures will be considered. For those voxels that belong neither to the target nor to the critical structure, we set $w_i = 0$. To keep it as simple as possible, we will use only two beams (see figure 7a). Furthermore, we assume that unit intensity from every bixel $j$ contributes the dose of $D_{ij} = 1$ unit to all voxels $i$ along the ray $j$, and no dose to the side, i.e., the depth dose is constant and there is no side scatter.

We begin by setting all bixel intensities $b_j^0 = 0$, which results in a dose distribution $d_i = 0$ in all voxels. To calculate the next approximation of the bixel intensities, $b_j^1$, for all $j$, we follow the recipe of equation (8). First we calculate the gradient in the numerator. Here we simply have to take the sum of the differences between actual and prescribed doses along ray $j$. Because the actual dose is still zero, this is simply the projection of the target volume along each beam.

Next we normalize (scale) the gradient with the second derivative in the numerator of equation (8). Due to our definition of $w_i$ and $D_{ij}$, this is again the projection of the target volume, such that the ratio becomes 1 in the target volume. The value of $\alpha$ is 1/2 in this case. That means, we obtain $b_j^1 = 1/2$ for all $j$ inside the projection of the target volume, and 0 outside. This yields, as a first step toward intensity modulation, the field shape of the treatment beams, similar to those used in conformal radiotherapy.

Due to our definition of $D_{ij}$, the dose distribution $\vec{d}^1$ for intensities $\vec{b}^1$ is a back-projection of the bixel intensities along the rays. The total dose distribution as a sum of both beams is shown in the lower right of figure 7a.

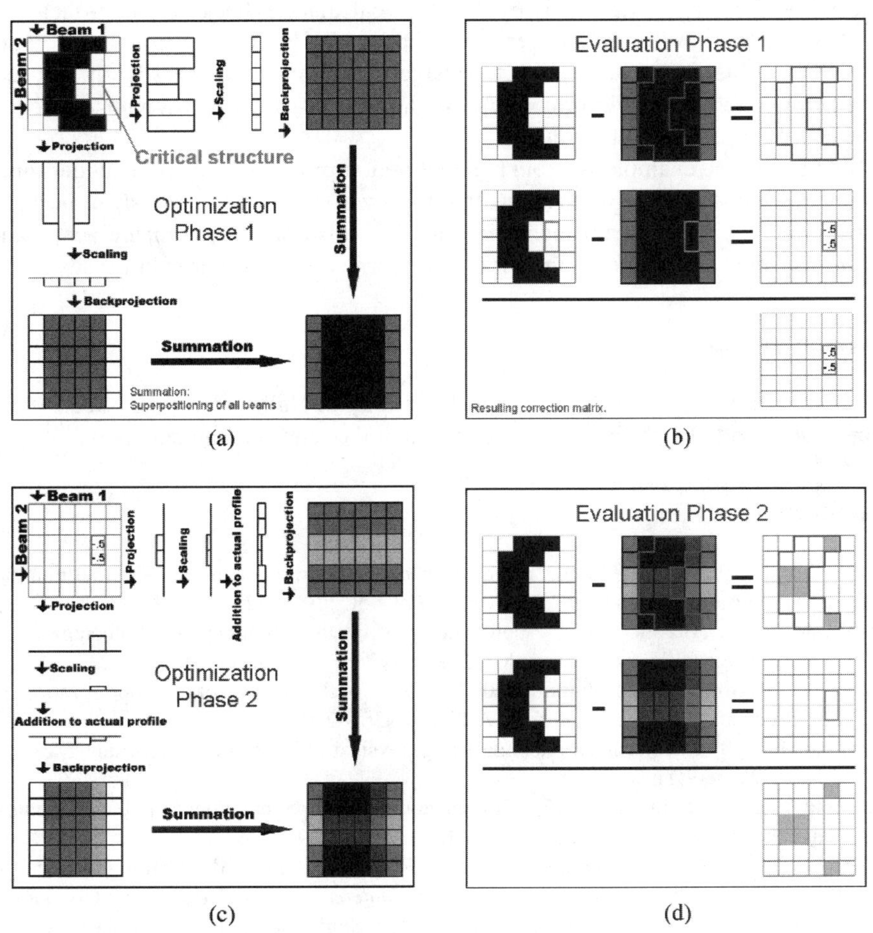









**Figure 7.** A graphical illustration of a gradient optimization algorithm. See the text for details.

For the next iteration, we start again by calculating the gradient in the numerator of equation (8). First we take the difference between prescribed and actual dose in the relevant voxels (target and critical structure, figure 7b) to calculate a correction matrix. Because the dose in the target volume is all 1, as it should be, the difference is 0. However, in the critical structure the dose is also 1 unit, i.e., it is too high by 0.5 units. Hence, the difference is –0.5. The correction matrix has to be summed along rays, which yields the projection of the correction along the two beams. This ends the calculation of the gradient. Note that in this case the projection has a negative sign (figure 7c). Scaling with the inverse of the second derivative and with $\alpha$ reduces the height of the projection. The scaled projection is then added to the previous bixel intensities (actual profile), $b_j^1$, which yields $b_j^2$. The dose calculation (back-projection) leads to $\vec{d}^2$. As can be seen from the lower right of figure 7c, the critical structure is better spared after this second iteration, but the target dose homogeneity is slightly reduced. Further iteration steps will further improve the dose distribution, but with two beams one cannot expect perfect results.

Although the example is strongly simplified, it provides some basic understanding of how most IMRT optimization algorithms work: They continuously project and back-project between beam intensities and dose distributions, compare actual and prescribed dose distributions, and apply some correction to the current intensity maps.

## Acknowledgment

I am grateful to Professor Yair Censor (University of Haifa) and to Drs. John Wolfgang and David Gierga (MGH Boston) for their thoughtful comments.

## References

Alber, M., and F. Nüsslin. (2000). "Intensity modulated photon beams subject to a minimal surface smoothing constraint." *Phys. Med. Biol.* 45(5):N49–52.

Alber, M., and F. Nüsslin. (2001). "Optimization of intensity modulated radiotherapy under constraints for static and dynamic MLC delivery." *Phys. Med. Biol.* 46(12):3229–3239.

Alber, M., M. Birkner, and F. Nüsslin. (2002). "Tools for the analysis of dose optimization: II. Sensitivity analysis." *Phys. Med. Biol.* 47(19):N265–270.

Bortfeld, T. (1999). "Optimized planning using physical objectives and constraints." *Semin. Radiat. Oncol.* 9(1):20–34.

Bortfeld, T., and W. Schlegel. (1993). "Optimization of beam orientations in radiation therapy: Some theoretical considerations." *Phys. Med. Biol.* 38:291–304.

Bortfeld, T., J. Stein, and K. Preiser. "Clinically Relevant Intensity Modulation Optimization Using Physical Criteria" in *XIIth International Conference on the Use of Computers in Radiation Therapy.* (XII ICCR). D. D. Leavitt and G. Starkschall (eds.). Salt Lake City, May 27–30, 1997. Madison, WI: Medical Physics Publishing, pp. 1–4, 1997.

Bortfeld, T., J. Bürkelbach, R. Boesecke and W. Schlegel. (1990). "Methods of image reconstruction from projections applied to conformation radiotherapy." *Phys. Med. Biol.* 35:1423–1434.

Bortfeld, T., A. L. Boyer, W. Schlegel, D. L. Kahler, and T. J. Waldron. (1994). "Realization and verification of three-dimensional conformal radiotherapy with modulated fields." *Int. J. Radiat. Oncol. Biol. Phys.* 30(4):899–908.

Brahme, A. (1984). "Dosimetric precision requirements in radiation therapy." *Acta Radiol. Oncol.* 23(5):379–391.

Brahme, A. (1993). "Optimization of radiation therapy and the development of multileaf collimation." *Int. J. Radiat. Oncol. Biol. Phys.* 25(2):373–375.

Brahme, A. (1994). "Optimization of radiation therapy." *Int. J. Radiat. Oncol. Biol. Phys.* 28(3):785–787.

Brahme, A., J. E. Roos, and I. Lax. (1982). "Solution of an integral equation encountered in rotation therapy." *Phys. Med. Biol.* 27:1221–1229.

Carol, M. P., R. V. Nash, R. C. Campbell, R. Huber, and E. Sternick. "The Development of a Clinically Intuitive Approach To Inverse Treatment Planning: Partial Volume Prescription and Area Cost Function" in *XIIth International Conference on the Use of Computers in Radiation Therapy*. (XII ICCR). D. D. Leavitt and G. Starkschall (eds.). Salt Lake City, May 27–30, 1997. Madison, WI: Medical Physics Publishing, pp. 317–319, 1997.

Censor, Y., M. D. Altschuler, and W. D. Powlis. (1988). "A computational solution of the inverse problem in radiation-therapy treatment planning." *Appl. Math. Comput.* 25:57–87.

Cho, P. S., S. Lee, R.J. Marks II, S. Oh, S. G. Sutlief, and M. H. Phillips. (1998). "Optimization of intensity modulated beams with volume constraints using two methods: Cost function minimization and projections onto convex sets." *Med. Phys.* 25:435–443.

Cho, P. S., and R. J. Marks II. (2000). "Hardware-sensitive optimization for intensity modulated radiotherapy." *Phys. Med. Biol.* 45:429–440.

Chui, C. S., M. F. Chan, E. Yorke, S. Spirou, and C. C. Ling. (2001). "Delivery of intensity-modulated radiation therapy with a conventional multileaf collimator: Comparison of dynamic and segmental methods." *Med. Phys.* 28:2441–2449.

Conn, A., N. Gould, and P. Toint. *Large-Scale Nonlinear Constrained Optimization: A Current Survey*. Dordrecht: Kluwer Academic Publishers, 1994.

Cormack, A. M., and R. A. Cormack. (1987). "A problem in rotation therapy with x-rays: Dose distributions with an axis of symmetry." *Int. J. Radiat. Oncol. Biol. Phys.* 13:1921–1925.

Cotrutz, C., M. Lahanas, C. Kappas, and D. Baltas. (2001). "A multiobjective gradient-based dose optimization algorithm for external beam conformal radiotherapy." *Phys. Med. Biol.* 46(8):2161–75.

Deasy, J. O. (1997). "Multiple local minima in radiotherapy optimization problems with dose-volume constraints." *Med. Phys.* 24:1157–1161.

DeNeve, W., C. DeWagter, K. DeJaeger, M. Thienpont, C. Colle, S. Derycke, and J. Schelfhout (1996). "Planning and delivering high doses to targets surrounding the spinal cord at the lower neck and upper mediastinal levels: static beam-segmentation technique executed with a multileaf collimator." *Radiother. Oncol.* 40(3): 271–279.

Fraass, B. (2002). "Differences between plan evaluation and the optimization problem statement, and the difference it makes." http://www.isye.gatech.edu/nci-nsf.orart.2002/talks.php.

Gill, P., W. Murray, and M. Wright. *Practical Optimization*. San Diego: Academic Press, 1999.

Gustafsson, A., and M. Langer. "Dose-Volume Constrained Radiotherapy Optimization for a Clinical Treatment Planning System" in *XIII International Conference on the Use of Computers in Radiation Therapy*. (XIII ICCR). W. Schlegel and T. Bortfeld (eds.). Heidelberg, Germany. Heidelberg: Springer Verlag, 2000.

Gustafsson, A., B. K. Lind. and A. Brahme. (1994). "A generalized pencil beam algorithm for optimization of radiation therapy." *Med. Phys.* 21(3):343–356.

Hamacher, H. W., and K.-H. Küfer. (2002). "Inverse radiation therapy planning-A multiple objective optimization approach." *Discrete Appl. Math.* 118:145–161.

International Commission on Radiation Units and Measurements (ICRU) Report 50. "Prescribing, Recording, and Reporting Photon Beam Therapy." Bethesda, MD: International Commission on Radiation Units and Measurements, 1993.

IMRTCWG (Intensity Modulated Radiation Therapy Collaborative Working Group). (2001). "Intensity-modulated radiotherapy: Current status and issues of interest." *Int. J. Radiat. Oncol. Biol. Phys.* 51(4):880–914.

Keller-Reichenbecher, M. A., T. Bortfeld, S. Levegrun, J. Stein, K. Prieser, and W. Schlegel. (1999). "Intensity modulation with the 'step and shoot' technique using a commercial MLC: A planning study. Multileaf collimator." *Int. J. Radiat. Oncol. Biol. Phys.* 45:1315–1324.

Kessen, A., K.-H. Grosser, and T. Bortfeld. "Simplification of IMRT Intensity Maps by Means of 1-D and 2-D Median-Filtering During the Iterative Calculation " in *XIII International Conference on the Use of Computers in Radiation Therapy.* (XIII ICCR). W. Schlegel and T. Bortfeld (eds.). Heidelberg, Germany. Heidelberg: Springer Verlag, 2000.

Küfer, K.-H., H. W. Hamacher. and T. R. Bortfeld (2000). "A Multicriteria Optimization Approach for Inverse Radiotherapy Planning " in *XIII International Conference on the Use of Computers in Radiation Therapy.* (XIII ICCR). W. Schlegel and T. Bortfeld (eds.). Heidelberg, Germany. Heidelberg: Springer Verlag, pp. 26–29, 2000.

Kwa, S. L., J. V. Lebesque, J. C. Theuws, L. B. Marks, M. T. Munley, G. Bentel, D. Oetzel, U. Spahn, M. V. Graham, R. E. Drzymala, J. A. Purdy, and A. S. Lichter. (1998). "Radiation pneumonitis as a function of mean lung dose: An analysis of pooled data of 540 patients." *Int. J. Radiat. Oncol. Biol. Phys.* 42:1–9.

Langer, M., and J. Leong. (1987). "Optimization of beam weights under dose-volume restrictions." *Int. J. Radiat. Oncol. Biol. Phys.* 13:1255–1260.

Langer, M., R. Brown, M. Urie, J. Leong, M. Stracher, and J. Shapiro. (1990). "Large scale optimization of beam weights under dose-volume restrictions." *Int. J. Radiat. Oncol. Biol. Phys.* 18:887–893.

Langer, M., S. Morrill, R. Brown, O. Lee, and R. Lane. (1996). "A comparison of mixed integer programming and fast simulated annealing for optimizing beam weights in radiation therapy." *Med. Phys.* 23:957–964.

Levegrun, S., A. Jackson, M. J. Zelefsky, M. W. Skwarchuk, E. S. Venkatraman, W. Schlegel, Z. Fuks, S. A. Leibel, and C. C. Ling. (2001). "Fitting tumor control probability models to biopsy outcome after three-dimensional conformal radiation therapy of prostate cancer: Pitfalls in deducing radiobiological parameters for tumors from clinical data." *Int. J. Radiat. Oncol. Biol. Phys.* 51(4):1064–1080.

Mackie, R., J. Deasy, T. Holmes, and J. Fowler (1994). "Optimization of radiation therapy and the development of multileaf collimation." *Int. J. Radiat. Oncol. Biol. Phys.* 28(3):784–785.

Miettinen, K. *Nonlinear Multiobjective Optimization.* Norwell. MA: Kluwer Academic Publishers, 1999.

Milickovic, N., M. Lahanas, M. Papagiannopoulo, N. Zamboglou, and D. Baltas. (2002). "Multiobjective anatomy-based dose optimization for HDR-brachytherapy with constraint free deterministic algorithms." *Phys. Med. Biol.* 47(13):2263–2280.

Mohan, R., and C. C. Ling. (1995). "When becometh less more?" *Int. J. Radiat. Oncol. Biol. Phys.* 33:235–237.

Mohan, R., and X. H. Wang. (1996). "Physical vs. biological objectives for treatment plan optimization." *Radiother. Oncol.* 40:186–187.

Natterer, F. *The Mathematics of Computerized Tomography.* Stuttgart: Teubner, 1986.

Niemierko, A. (1992). "Random search algorithm (RONSC) for the optimization of radiation therapy with both physical and biological endpoints and constraints." *Int. J. Radiat. Oncol. Biol. Phys.* 23:89–98.

Niemierko, A. (1997). "Reporting and analyzing dose distributions: A concept of equivalent uniform dose." *Med. Phys.* 24(1):103–110.

Niemierko, A. (1999). "A generalized concept of equivalent uniform dose (EUD)." *Med. Phys.* 26(6):1100.

Pugachev, A., J. G. Li, A. L. Boyer, S. L. Hancock, Q. T. Le, S. S. Donaldson, and L. Xing. (2001). "Role of beam orientation optimization in intensity-modulated radiation therapy." *Int. J. Radiat. Oncol. Biol. Phys.* 50(2):551–560.

Radiation Therapy Oncology Group (RTOG) H-0022. Phase I/II Study of Conformal and Intensity Modulated Irradiation for Oropharyngeal Cancer, Feb 2001 (Rev. 1-2, Jan 15, 2002). Available at rtog.org.

Shepard, D. M., M. A. Earl, X. A. Li, S. Naqvi, and C. Yu. (2002). "Direct aperture optimization: A turnkey solution for step-and-shoot IMRT." *Med. Phys.* 29(6):1007–1018.

Söderström, S., and A. Brahme (1995). "What is the most suitable number of photon beam portals in coplanar radiation therapy." *Int. J. Radiat. Oncol. Biol. Phys.* 33:151–159.

Söderström, S. and A. Brahme (1996). "Small is beautiful-and often enough." *Int. J. Radiat. Oncol. Biol. Phys.* 34(3):757–758.

Spirou, S. V., and C.-S. Chui. (1998). "A gradient inverse planning algorithm with dose-volume constraints." *Med. Phys.* 25:321–333.

Starkschall, G., A. Pollack, and C. W. Stevens. "Using a Dose-Volume Feasibility Search Algorithm for Radiation Treatment Planning" *XIII International Conference on the Use of Computers in Radiation Therapy.* (XIII ICCR). W. Schlegel and T. Bortfeld (eds.). Heidelberg, Germany. Heidelberg: Springer Verlag, 2000.

Stein, J., R. Mohan, X. H. Wang, T. Bortfeld, Q. Wu, K. Preiser, C. C. Ling, and W. Schlegel (1997). "Number and orientation of beams in intensity-modulated radiation treatments." *Med. Phys.* 24(2):149–160.

Steuer, R. *Multicriteria Optimization: Theory, Computation and Applications.* New York: Wiley, 1985.

Thieke, C. Multicriteria Optimization in Inverse Radiotherapy Planning. University of Heidelberg, 2003.

Thieke, C., T. Bortfeld, and A. Niemierko. (2002). "Direct consideration of EUD constraints in IMRT optimization." *Med. Phys.* 29(6):1283.

Wang, X. H., R. Mohan, A. Jackson, S. A. Leibel, Z. Fuks, and C. C. Ling. (1995). "Optimization of intensity-modulated 3D conformal treatment plans based on biological indices." *Radiother. Oncol.* 37:140–152.

Webb, S. (1992). "Optimisation by simulated annealing of three-dimensional, conformal treatment planning for radiation fields defined by a multileaf collimator: 2. Inclusion of two-dimensional modulation of the x-ray intensity." *Phys. Med. Biol.* 37:1689–1704.

Webb, S. (2001). *Intensity-Modulated Radiation Therapy.* Bristol: Institute of Physics (IOP) Publishing, 2001.

Webb, S., D. J. Convery, and P. M. Evans. (1998). "Inverse planning with constraints to generate smoothed intensity-modulated beams." *Phys. Med. Biol.* 43(10):2785–2794.

Wu, Q., and R. Mohan. (2002). "Multiple local minima in IMRT optimization based on dose-volume criteria." *Med. Phys.* 29:1514–1527.

Wu, Q., R. Mohan, A. Niemierko, and R. Schmidt-Ullrich. (2002). "Optimization of intensity-modulated radiotherapy plans based on the equivalent uniform dose." *Int. J. Radiat. Oncol. Biol. Phys.* 52:224–235.

Yu, Y. (1997). "Multiobjective decision theory for computational optimization in radiation therapy." *Med. Phys.* 24(9):1445–1454.

# Biological Indices For Evaluation
# And Optimization Of IMRT


**Ellen D. Yorke, Ph.D.**
Memorial Sloan-Kettering Cancer Center
New York, New York




## Introduction

The mantra of conformal radiation therapy is "high dose to the tumor and low or no dose to normal tissue." Dose is a surrogate for the two desired biological endpoints — high probability of local tumor control (TCP) and acceptably low probability of normal tissue complications (NTCP). For conventional treatment, standard beam arrangements (four-field box), simple rules of thumb ("maximum cord dose <45 Gy"), and clinical intuition based on experience within this framework are an adequate guide for designing and evaluating treatment plans. With the advent of advanced methods to design and deliver novel computer-sculpted intensity-modulated radiation therapy (IMRT) dose distributions based on multi-modality patient images, physicists and physicians must make more use of clinical outcomes data as well as participate directly in studies that add to the knowledge base. Biological criteria are increasingly used to evaluate dose distributions and decide total treatment dose. There are also hopes that directly integrating such criteria into the IMRT optimization process will improve the dose distributions or at least increase planning efficiency.

This chapter aims to provide information to assist physicists involved in these endeavors. Since radiation-induced cell death or loss of cellular reproductive capacity is responsible for both good and bad radiation therapy outcomes, this chapter reviews the widely-used linear-quadratic (LQ) model, the status of TCP models, and NTCP data of particular interest for IMRT and some of the models which summarize these data. The material in the sections on Tumor Control Probability (TCP) Models and Normal Tissue Complications is relevant to both plan evaluation and plan optimization and also indicate how far we are from the ambitious goal of "reliable" data and models. The last section reviews efforts to directly integrate biological indices into optimization algorithms. This field is in its infancy and it is not yet known whether better IMRT dose distributions than those obtained with dose and dose-volume based score functions will result. Three books (Thames and Hendry 1987, Hall 1994, Steel 1997) provide detailed information and primary literature references for many topics covered below.

## The Linear-Quadratic (LQ) Model

### The LQ Equation

Numerous dose-response experiments have been performed for well-defined *in vitro* and animal models to understand the ability of cells to survive and reproduce following irradiation, a quantity often called "the surviving fraction." $SF_d$ is the surviving fraction survival following a single dose $d$. Semi-log plots ($\log(SF_d)$ vs. dose) have general shapes shown in figure 1. For low-LET (linear energy transfer) radiation, there is usually a shoulder at low dose while for high-LET radiation, $\log(SF_d)$ decreases linearly with dose. Both logarithm curves are well described by an LQ function

$$Ln\ (SF_d) = -\alpha d - \beta d^2 \tag{1a}$$

so that

$$(SF_d) = \exp(-\alpha d - \beta d^2). \tag{1b}$$

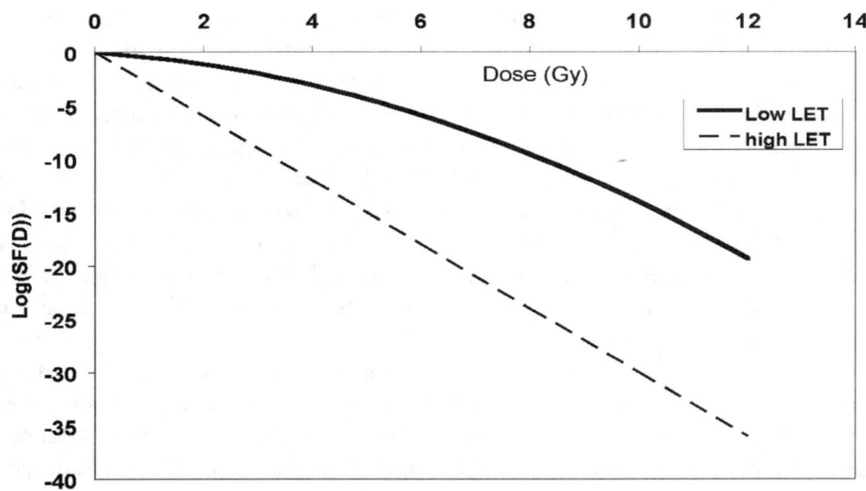


**Figure 1.** Typical curves of the log of the surviving cell fraction vs. a single dose of low and high LET radiation.

Here $\alpha$ and $\beta$ are experimentally determined and depend on many factors including the cell strains, environmental conditions (e.g., oxygen tension), dose rate, and the type of ionizing radiation (e.g. for high-LET radiation, $\beta/\alpha$ is approximately zero while for low LET, it ranges from 0 to ~0.5 Gy$^{-1}$). The linear term ($\alpha$) is attributed to non-repairable DNA lesions and the quadratic term (potentially lethal or sublethal damage) is often described as two repairable lesions that interact to kill the cell if they are sufficiently close together. According to this interpretation, $\beta/\alpha$ is zero for high-LET radiation because the dense ionization tracks produce only non-repairable lesions and $\beta/\alpha$ is reduced for low dose rate, low-LET radiation when the time scales of sublethal damage creation and repair are comparable. Whether or not these mechanistic explanations are completely correct, the LQ model is a good phenomenological description of measured cell survival curves for clinically relevant doses and dose rates.

For fractionated delivery of total dose $D$ in $n$ equal fractions of dose $d$ (so $D = nd$), the surviving cell fraction, $SF(D,d)$ in the absence of damage repair or cell proliferation, is given by

$$SF(D,d) = (\exp(-\alpha d - \beta d^2))^n \qquad (2a)$$

or

$$SF(D,d) = \exp(-\alpha\,(1 + d\,/[\alpha/\beta]) \qquad (2b)$$

These equations are easily generalized to unequal doses per fraction.

Determining $\alpha$ *in vivo* is difficult because cell survival depends on uncontrollable environmental factors and, furthermore, a tumor or normal tissue is a mixture of cells with differing radiosensitivities. However, from *in vitro* measurements, $\alpha$ for low-LET radiation is between 0.1 $Gy^{-1}$ (very radioresistant) and 2 $Gy^{-1}$ (very radiosensitive). *In vivo* determination of $\alpha/\beta$ is easier, as it involve the efficacy of different dose fractionation schedules at creating radiation damage. Damage to a tissue with a large value of $\alpha/\beta$ (>10 Gy) depends on total dose but is insensitive to the dose per fraction; damage to a tissue with a small value (<5 Gy) is strongly affected by both total dose and fractionation. The three books mentioned in the Introduction have tables of LQ parameters and Deschavanne and Fertil (1996) lists *in vitro* values of $SF_2$ for almost 700 human tumor and normal cells.

A relationship between $\alpha/\beta$ and the time post-irradiation for a radiation-induced tissue effect to occur is experimentally and clinically observed (though not completely understood). Early-responding tissues are affected during or shortly after a treatment course and are functionally dependent on rapidly dividing cells. They include skin, mucosa, and many tumors. They also have large values of $\alpha/\beta$; for model calculations, $\alpha/\beta$ is often estimated to be 10 Gy for tumors. Recent evidence indicates that slow-growing prostate cancers are an exception and have low $\alpha/\beta$ (~1.5 to 3 Gy) (Fowler, Chappell, and Ritter 2002; Brenner et al. 2002). Late-responding tissues express radiation damage months to years after the end of treatment, perhaps because they contain critical cells with low proliferation rates. These tissues, which can suffer the most feared radiation complications, have small values of $\alpha/\beta$ (~1 to 4 Gy); they include spinal cord, kidneys, and liver. Tabulations of $\alpha/\beta$ are found in Thames and Hendry (1987, Tables 3.1 and 3.2) and in Joiner and van der Kogel (1997).

Late and early normal tissue complications have different consequences for radiation therapy. Early complications occur during treatment, are often non-lethal, and can be handled by treatment breaks. Many of the lethal or serious complications are late effects. Since they occur after the end of treatment, their probability of occurrence must be estimated "up front" and limited by changing the dose distribution or reducing the total dose. Radiation pneumonitis occurs during or within the first 6 months after treatment, but it is handled like a late effect for planning purposes and also has a low $\alpha/\beta$ (~3 to 4 Gy).

Some authors prefer to specify cellular radiosensitivity directly in terms of $SF_d$. The surviving fraction after a single 2 Gy dose, $SF2$, is particularly convenient because 2 Gy per fraction is a common schedule. Equation (2) can be recast as

$$SF(D,2) = (SF2)^{D/2} \qquad\qquad (3)$$

For most tumors, $SF2$ is between 0.1 and 0.8 (Deschavanne and Fertil 1996).

## The LQ Model And Dose Fractionation Schedules

Because of its mathematical simplicity and the relationship between $\alpha/\beta$ and late vs. early normal tissue reactions, the LQ model is very successful in designing dose fractionation schedules. Both dose and fractionation effects are summarized in the "biological effective dose" (BED), which is defined as

$$BED = D(1 + d/(\alpha/\beta)) \tag{4}$$

The poorly known quantity $\alpha$ drops out of BED, which depends only on the better-known $\alpha/\beta$. For a single tissue, the LQ equations show that fractionation schedules with the same BED result in the same surviving cell fraction and therefore produce the same TCP or NTCP. However, late-and early-responding tissues that receive the same dose have different BEDs. A rationale for hyperfractionation schedules based on BED arguments is given below.

*A treatment plan is given according to a standard treatment schedule of a total dose $D_{std}$ in 2 Gy fractions, once daily. The isodose distribution is such that the late-responding normal tissue dose is $\leq$ the tumor dose. Let the tumor $\alpha/\beta$ be 10 Gy and the late-responding normal tissue $\alpha/\beta$ be 3 Gy. For the same relative dose distribution, find the hyperfractionated (HF) treatment dose, $D_{HF}$, given at 1.2 Gy/fraction, twice daily (b.i.d) which produces the same late normal tissue effect and assess the advantages of hyperfractionation for tumor control.*

***Iso-late-complications require equal normal tissue BEDs. Using equation (4) with $\alpha/\beta = 3$ Gy***

$$1.4 D_{HF} = (1.667) D_{std} \text{ or } D_{HF} = 1.19\, D_{std}.$$

***At total dose $D_{HF}$ , the ratio of tumor BEDs is***

$$BED_{tum,HF}/BED_{tum,std} = 1.19\, D_{std}\, (1.12)/1.2\, D_{std} = 1.11.$$

***The hyperfractionated schedule has an 11% increase in tumor BED with no cost to late-responding tissues. Of course, acutely responding tissues (e.g., mucosa), with large $\alpha/\beta$, also experience increased BED and might suffer more severe reactions.***

For classical examples of the power of the LQ model for comparing treatment schedules, see Hall (1994), Fowler (1989, 1992), and Joiner and van der Kogel (1997). There is current interest, sparked by evidence of low $\alpha/\beta$ for prostate cancer, in finding hypofractionation schedule (lower total dose in fewer, but larger fractions) that could improve tumor BED while not increasing normal tissue complications (Fowler, Chappell, and Ritter 2002).

For non-uniform dose distributions, dose-per-fraction effects are different in different parts of a tissue. Dose-volume histograms (DVHs) can be directly converted to BED-VHs providing that the dose per fraction for each volume element is known (straightforward for a single-phase treatment course). Fractionation effects for non-uniform dose distributions are more readily appreciated if the LQ model is used to convert the dose in each dose bin to its biological equivalent at standard fractionation (Fowler 1989; Wheldon et al. 1998). A common equivalence is to the BED for dose in 2 Gy fractions, LQED2, where

$$LQED2 = BED/(1 + 2/(\alpha/\beta)). \tag{5}$$

This conversion is useful for TCP and NTCP calculations because most model parameters are determined at standard fractionation. The lung and spinal cord DVHs in figure 2 are compared with LQED2-VHs for a treatment of 70 Gy to the 100% isodose line (at 2 Gy/fraction), assuming $\alpha/\beta$ = 3 Gy for both organs. Above 70 Gy, the dose per fraction exceeds 2 Gy and LQED2 is greater than the physical dose (region 2); in region 1, total dose <70 Gy, dose per fraction <2 Gy, and LQED2 is lower than the physical dose.

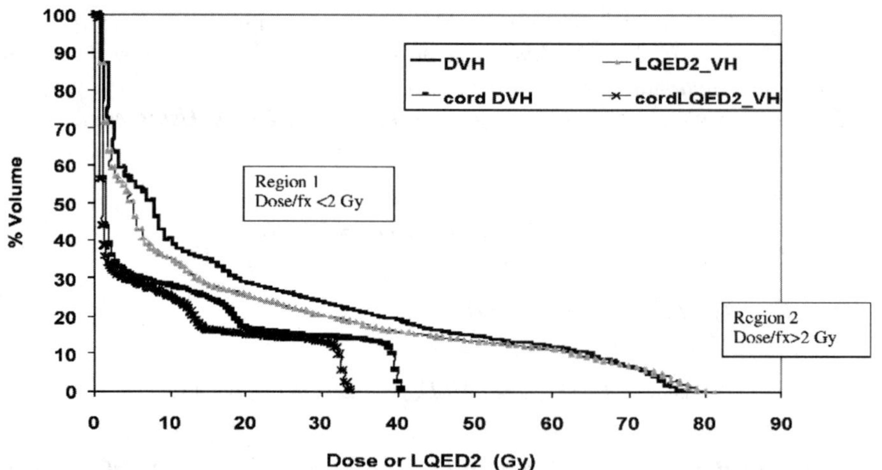


**Figure 2.** Lung and cord DVHs and LQED2-VHs. The prescription dose is 70 Gy in 2 Gy fractions and $\alpha/\beta$ = 3 Gy for both organs.

## Time-Dependent Effects

The LQ model has been generalized to include two important time-dependent effects—sublethal damage repair and proliferation. Repair causes the coefficient of the quadratic term to depend on the dose rate, including the time between treatments for fractionated external beam therapy. Experimental evidence for sublethal damage repair is provided by split dose and low dose rate experiments (Thames and Hendry 1987; Hall 1994, Ch 7; Joiner and van der Kogel 1997; Brenner, Huang, and Hall 1991). The simple approximation assumes exponential decay of the number of sublethal lesions with half time $T_{1/2}$ or repair constant $\mu = Ln2/T_{1/2}$. Repair effects are expressed as $g(\mu t)$, a multiplicative correction factor to $\beta$. Measured values of $T_{1/2}$ range between 0.2 and 2 hours, depending on the tissue (table 3.6 in Thames and Hendry, table 13.3 in Joiner and van der Kogel). A general expression for $g(\mu t)$ is given in Brenner, Huang, and Hall (1991) while special cases of equally spaced acute dose fractions and constant dose-rate radiation are in Thames and Hendry (1987, Ch 7) and continuous constant and exponentially decaying radiation in Dale (1985). If $\beta_\infty$ is the quadratic term coefficient with complete repair following a single acute dose fraction, then for two such fractions, $d$, separated by time $t$, the effective value of $\beta$ varies as

$$\beta_{eff} = \beta_\infty (1 + \exp(-\mu t)). \tag{6}$$

As the interfraction interval increases from $t\sim0$ (no repair) to $t\gg T_{1/2}$ (complete repair), $\beta_{eff}$ decreases by a factor of two (Thames and Hendry 1987, Ch 7). The clinical rule of thumb, "at least 6 (or 8) hours between fractions" for twice daily treatments comes from data showing that these intervals are long enough for substantial repair of normal tissues.

The low dose-rate expression was motivated by brachytherapy applications but it may be relevant to slow IMRT delivery techniques. The solid curves in figure 3 are the ratio of BED with and without repair vs. delivery time (units of $T_{1/2}$) for a single 2 Gy dose given at a continuous dose rate. The upper curve is for an early responding tissue (acute dose $\alpha/\beta$ is 10 Gy) and the lower for a late responder ($\alpha/\beta = 2$ Gy). To reduce BED by $\sim$10%, $\alpha/\beta$ should be small and the delivery time at least 50% of $T_{1/2}$ (thus >6 minutes for very short $T_{1/2}$ of 0.2 hours). Fair comparison with "historical" data should include inter-beam delays due to room entry to change blocks and/or wedges. The dotted curves in figure 3 shows similar BED ratios for a 2 Gy fraction delivered as four acute 0.5 Gy subdoses (four fields with blocks) vs. the time interval between the sub-doses. Clinically typical time intervals of 1 to 2 minutes are unlikely to seriously degrade BED.

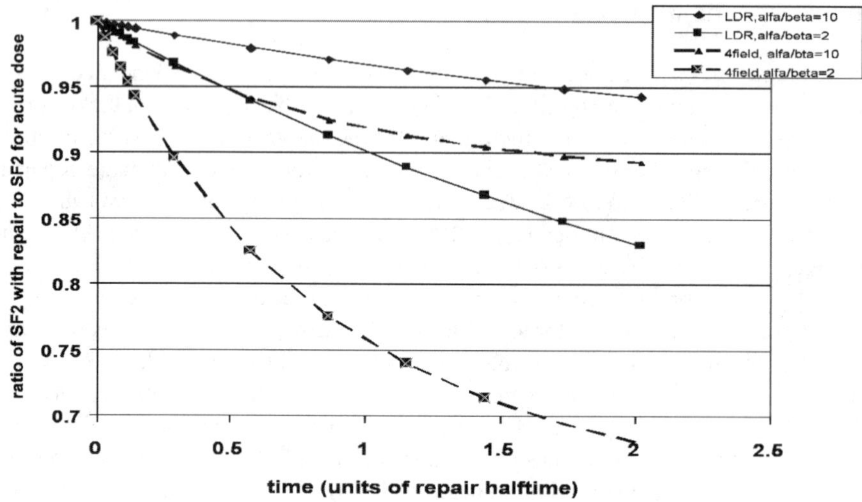


**Figure 3.** Effect of exponential sublethal damage repair on the BED for a single 2 Gy fraction. The solid curves are the ratio (BED for dose given as continuous dose rate radiation) to (BED for acute dose) vs. delivery time (units of $T_{1/2}$). The dots are a similar ratio for four acute 0.5 Gy sub-fractions vs. the time between the subfractions (units of $T_{1/2}$).

Cell proliferation or "repopulation" during treatment is also very relevant to tumor control and recovery of some normal tissues (especially early responders). Proliferation *in vitro* is often exponential with a doubling time of $T_{pot}$. *In vivo* tumor doubling times, $T_{eff}$, are usually longer than $T_{pot}$ due to cell cycle effects and cell loss from the tumor (Hall 1994, Ch 12). Measured tumor $T_{eff}$'s depend on the clinical or experimental situation and there are large uncertainties in knowledge of this parameter in a clinical setting. Reported values vary from approximately 2 to 100 days (Hall 1994; Mackillop et al. 1996). "Accelerated repopulation" ($T_{eff}$ decreases part way through the treatment course) is sometimes observed (Fowler 1989; Hall 1994, Ch 13). The effect of exponential doubling throughout a fractionated treatment course which takes time $T$ is estimated by multiplying the surviving cell fraction by the factor exp($Ln2$ $T/T_{eff}$) while accelerated repopulation is represented as exponential growth which kicks in after a lag time, $T_0$. In general, delay or break in treatment for a proliferating tumor increases the surviving fractions (reduces cell kill). Short treatment schedules ("accelerated hyperfractionation") have been proposed to reduce the resulting loss of tumor control (Joiner 1997). The loss of TCP due to delay in start of treatment was modeled by (Mackillop et al. 1996) for tumors with rather long mean doubling times (>50 days) who found that delays over ~2 weeks can seriously decrease the calculated TCP.

## Tumor Control Probability (TCP) Models

*In vitro* experiments, animal studies and clinical experience show that TCP for a uniformly irradiated tumor increases sigmoidally from zero at low dose to near unity (100%) at high dose with a generic shape illustrated in figure 4. Two parameters—$D_{50}$ (or $TCD_{50}$) and $\gamma_{50}$—determine the curve's location and slope. $D_{50}$ is the dose for 50% TCP and $\gamma_{50}$ is the change in TCP (expressed as %) per percent change in dose at $D_{50}$ and is proportional to the slope at $D_{50}$ (the tangent line in the figure). Clinical estimates for radiocurable tumors place $D_{50}$ is in the range 40-70 Gy and $\gamma_{50}$ in the range 1–3.

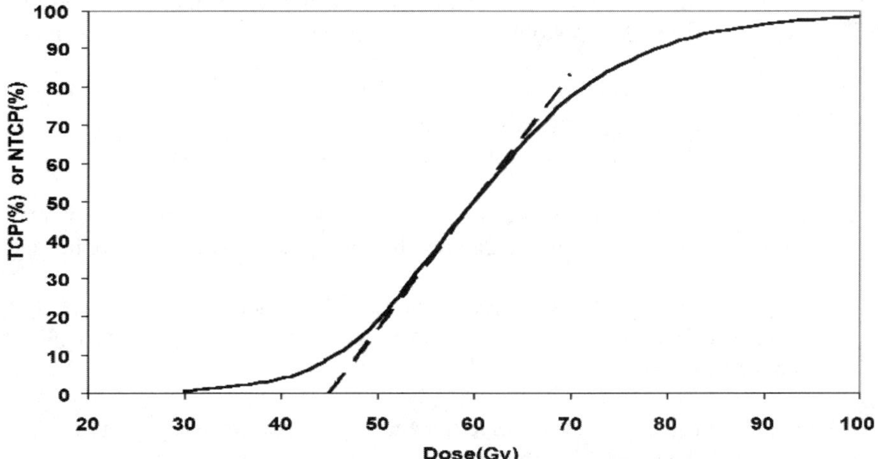


**Figure 4.** The sigmoidal shape of a TCP vs. dose curve and the tangent line with the same slope passing through the midpoint. For TCP, $D_{50}$ (here 60 Gy) is the dose at which TCP is 50% and $\gamma_{50}$ is proportional to the slope at this point. The same general shape also describes NTCP vs. dose; the "tolerance dose" at which NTCP reaches 50% is called "$TD_{50}$."

Changes in TCP due to dose changes near $D_{50}$ can be estimated by approximating TCP curve by the tangent line through the point ($D_{50}$, 50%) that has slope 100 $\gamma_{50}/D_{50}$. The change in TCP due to dose change $\Delta D$ is approximately 100 $\gamma_{50}\,\Delta D/D_{50}$. For example, in figure 4, $D_{50}$ is 60 Gy and $\gamma_{50}$ is 2.0. A 10% dose increase (dose- > 66 Gy) increases TCP to ~70% and a 10% dose decrease ( dose- >54 Gy ) decreases TCP to ~30%.

Simple phenomenological functions of prescription dose D, such as a logistic function

$$TCP(D) = 1/(1 + (D_{50}/D)^{4\,\gamma_{50}})$$

$$(6)$$

are convenient for quick calculations. However, the logistic is rather insensitive to cold spots (Deasy 1998). Further, it is hoped that radiobiology-based TCP models will provide better guides for treatment planning, extrapolation to novel dose distributions, and outcome analysis. Unfortunately, developing reliable TCP models has proven difficult for reasons including those listed below.

1.  Scarce data relating local control to details of dose distributions in tumors.

2.  Soft-tissue tumors contain approximately $10^9$ cells per cc, but not all these cells are clonogenic cells, whose growth causes tumor recurrence. Discriminating clonogenic from non-clonogenic cells *in vivo* is an unsolved problem so data relating dose distributions to their spatial distribution are almost nonexistent.

3.  The delivered dose (setup error, organ motion, etc.) is seldom known although TCP is determined by the delivered—rather than the planned—dose.

4.  Scoring *local* failure as opposed to nearby recurrence is difficult, especially for sites such as lung where detailed follow-up imaging studies are needed.

5.  The structure of otherwise reasonable models is such that they can easily be parameterized to agree for uniform dose distributions but differ drastically for non-uniform ones.

While these problems are unresolved, the use of TCP in treatment plan design or evaluation should be taken with a grain of salt.

## Poisson–LQ Models Of TCP

Most mechanistic TCP models start with the hypothesis (Munro and Gilbert 1961) that local control is achieved if and only if all the clonogenic cells are destroyed and that, if the average surviving fraction for a population of identically irradiated N-clonogen tumors is *SF*, TCP is given by Poisson statistics.

$$TCP = \exp(-N\,SF). \tag{7}$$

At zero dose, *SF* is unity so that for large *N*, *TCP* is approximately zero and at high dose, *SF*<<*N* and *TCP* approaches 1.0. Combining the LQ model and equation (7), *TCP* for uniform tumor irradiation is given by

$$TCP = \exp(-N\exp[-\alpha D(1 + d/(\alpha/\beta))]) \tag{7a}$$

or

$$TCP = \exp(-N\,(SF2)^{D/2}). \qquad (7b)$$

Equations (7a) or (7b) are easily generalized to include intra-tumor radiobiological heterogeneity; if a fraction $f_i$ of clonogens in each tumor have surviving fraction $SF_i$, then

$$TCP = \exp(-N\Sigma_i f_i\, SF_i) \qquad (7c)$$

Repair of sublethal damage can be included by modifying $\beta$ by $g(\mu t)$ as discussed previously. Repopulation is more problematic, but for large $N$ and tumors with a slow repopulation rate relative to the dose delivery, Poisson statistics is believed to be a good approximation (Tucker, Thames, and Taylor 1990).

$D_{50}$ and $\gamma_{50}$ can be calculated from equations (7). For example, from equation (7b)

$$D_{50} = 2 \ln (\ln 2/N)/\ln (SF2) \qquad (8a)$$

and

$$\gamma_{50} = (\ln 2/2) \ln (N/\ln 2). \qquad (8b)$$

Note that $\gamma_{50}$ depends *only* on the number of clonogens. If the clonogen density is approximately equal to $10^8$ to $10^9$ per cc, the cell density in soft tissue, $\gamma_{50}$ is predicted to rise logarithmically with tumor volume, starting at ~8 for a 10 cc tumor. However, according to clinical data, $\gamma_{50}{\approx}2$, corresponding to N~200—a very small fraction of the total number of cells in a detectable soft-tissue tumor. Further, these clonogens must be quite radioresistant: if $D_{50}$ of 60 to 70 Gy and $N = 200$, equation (8a) predicts $SF2$~0.83 or $\alpha$<0.1 Gy$^{-1}$. Many authors believe that TCP is determined by a small number of radioresistant clonogens and that the vast majority of cells in a tumor are either not clonogenic or are radiosensitive and killed by doses well below $D_{50}$ [see, for example, Brenner (1993) and Zaider and Minerbo (2000)]. It is easy to choose LQ parameters that illustrate this point. The solid curves in figure 5 are TCP for two "pure" tumors—one with $10^7$ radiosensitive clonogens (SF2 = 0.5, $D_{50}$~47.5 Gy) and the with 200 radioresistant clonogens ($SF2 = 0.8$, $D_{50}$~50.8 Gy). The dotted TCP curve is for a tumor which is a mixture of $10^7$ radiosensitive clonogens with $SF2 = 0.5$ and 200 radioresistant clonogens with $SF2 = 0.8$. By 50 Gy, most of the radiosensitive cells are killed, leaving the tiny radioresistant fraction to dominate TCP. If the radiosensitive cells had slightly smaller $SF2$ (<0.45), the effect would be even more pronounced and the TCP curves of the mixture and the radioresistant tumor would be almost identical. In any case, *in vitro* experiments using cells from the mixture would be dominated by the far more numerous radiosensitive clonogens.

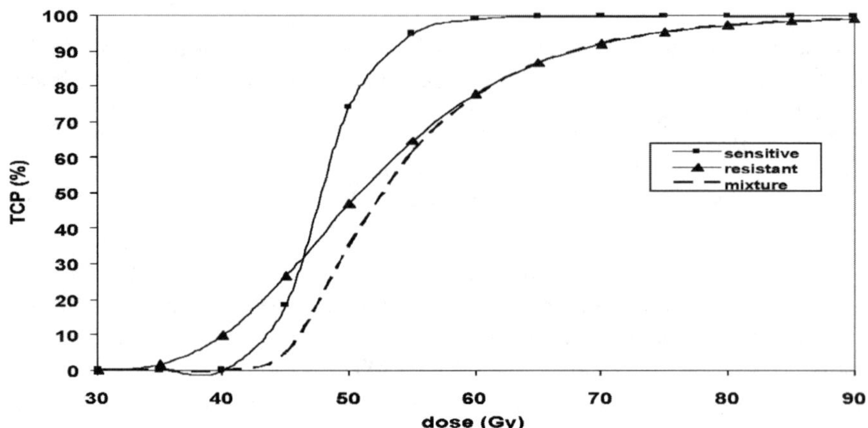


**Figure 5.** Simple example of the domination of TCP by radioresistant cells in a tumor that is a mixture of a large number ($10^7$) cells and a much smaller number (200) of radioresistant cells.

However, Goitein (1987) pointed out that if a very few clonogens control TCP and their number increases proportional to tumor volume, equation (8a) predicts overly strong dependence of $D_{50}$ on tumor size. A modification which also agrees with the observed low $\gamma_{50}$'s is based on the fact that TCP is a statistical concept which is observed for a population (an individual either fails or is controlled) (Goitein 1987; Zagars, Schultheiss, and Peters 1987; Suit 1992). Even if a population is stratified as to disease, stage, etc., there is *inter*-tumor variability such that tumors of different individuals differ in radiobiological characteristics (e.g., *SF*2 or $\alpha$, $\beta$, and *N*) and the observed *TCP* is an average over the population. Figure 6 is a simple illustration of reduction of $\gamma_{50}$ by population averaging. The "patient population" consists of three equal size groups—one slightly radiosensitive (*SF*2 = 0.55), one intermediate (*SF*2 = 0.6) and one slightly radioresistant (*SF*2 = 0.65). For each group, the number of clonogens is $10^7$. For the individual TCP curves, $\gamma_{50}$ is ~5.7, but $\gamma_{50}$ of the average curve for the population (dotted) is ~2.0.

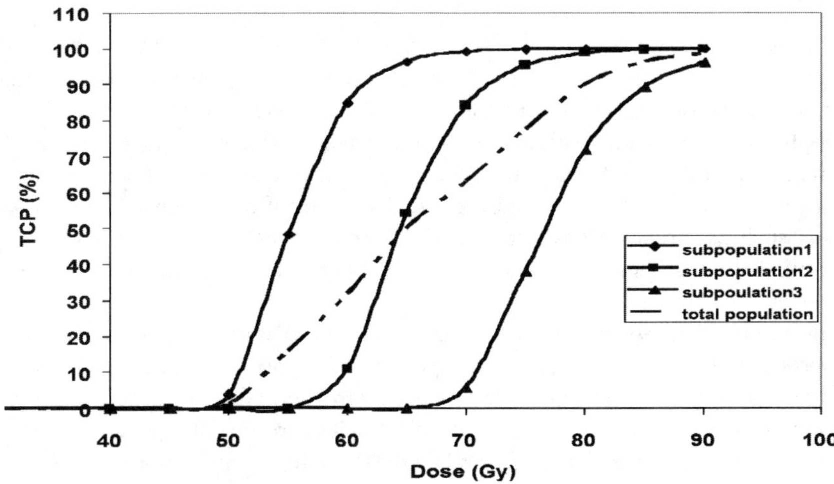


**Figure 6.** Simple example of how population averaging of three equal sized subpopulations (solid curves) reduces the $\gamma_{50}$ observed for the entire population.

In reality, both intra-tumor and inter-patient variation of all the radiobiological parameters, including clonogen density, probably exist. Several authors [Niemierko and Goitein (1993a), Roberts and Hendry (1998), and Webb (1994)] have fit clinical tumor control data to normal or log normal distributions of inter-patient and intra-tumor radiobiological parameters and obtained values of $\gamma_{50}$ in agreement with data together with high clonogen densities. However, these methods do not uniquely determine the number (or density) of clonogens, so the question of few vs. many remains unresolved. For example, in Webb (1994), data sets for control of four types of cancer are fit by population averaging models with clonogen densities ranging over 7 orders of magnitude. This great uncertainty in key TCP model parameters has implications for application of TCP to non-uniform dose distributions.

## TCP For Non-Uniform Dose Distributions

To calculate TCP for a non-uniform dose distribution, the tumor is divided into small subvolumes or "tumorlets" (Goitein 1987) in each of which the dose is approximately uniform. Each tumorlet is assumed to respond to radiation independently of its neighbors. If $V_i$, $\rho_i$, and $n_i$ ($= \rho_i\, V_i$) are, respectively, the volume, clonogen density, the number of clonogens in the $i$th clonogen and $D_i$ and $d_i$ the dose and dose per fraction it receives, then the probability (without population averaging), then if $TCP$ is the probability that no clonogens survive anywhere in the tumor

$$TCP = \prod_i \{\exp(-n_i\, SF\, (D_i\, ,\, d_i)\}. \tag{9}$$

$D_i$ and $V_i$ are given by the tumor DVH. The equation can also be written in terms of tumorlet volume fractions, $v_i$, where $v_i = V_i/\Sigma_i(V_i)$ . Each factor in equation (9) is Poissonian, even if $n_i$ is small. For population-averaged models, equation (9) is averaged over the population distribution of radiobiological parameters. A similar formalism can be applied to other mathematical representations of TCP (e.g., logistic functions). It is straightforward to accommodate spatial variations of clonogen density such as low clonogen density in regions of microscopic disease or of other radiobiological parameters such as larger $SF2$ where functional imaging indicates "aggressive" cells. Unfortunately, the parameters associated with such spatial variations are generally unknown.

From equation (9), it is obvious that a "sufficiently deep" cold spot seriously compromises TCP. In the limit of a complete miss of part of the tumor, some clonogens receive zero dose, a factor in the product is zero, and TCP falls to zero (signifying local failure). But what is "sufficiently deep"? For less drastic cold spots, the predicted decrease of TCP is model dependent and models with few clonogens and simple logistic functions are less sensitive to cold spots. As an extreme example, figure 7 compares two models. Model A is a population averaged model with parameters from (Webb 1994) for a 100 cc squamous tumor with clonogen density of $10^7$ cells/cc and model B is a few-clonogen model, with TCP controlled by 90 radioresistant clonogens ($SF2$ = 0.846) which are equally likely to be anywhere in the tumor. These parameters give almost identical TCP curves for uniform irradiation (figure 7a) but dramatically different predictions for the impact of a very small cold spot (1% of the volume) as shown in figure 7b, where 99% of the tumor is irradiated to 70 Gy and the x-axis is the percent of underdose in the cold spot. A plan evaluation or optimization scheme using model A would discriminate much more strongly against cold spots than one using model B. Furthermore, 1% of the volume is *small*—if distributed as a shell at the periphery of a 100 cc sphere, it would be approximately 0.01 cm thick! Such a tiny cold spot has negligible effect on global aspects of the DVH that are often used for plan evaluation. A 1 cc cold spot of 50% in an otherwise uniformly irradiated 100 cc tumor does not change the dose to 95% of the tumor ($D_{95}\%$), reduces the volume within the 95% isodose line ($V_{95}\%$) by 1% and reduces the mean dose by only 0.5%, yet model A predicts a TCP which is so low that the treatment would be considered a failure. Discussions of geometric aspects of small-volume dose inhomogeneities are given by Withers (2000) and Tomé and Fowler (2002).

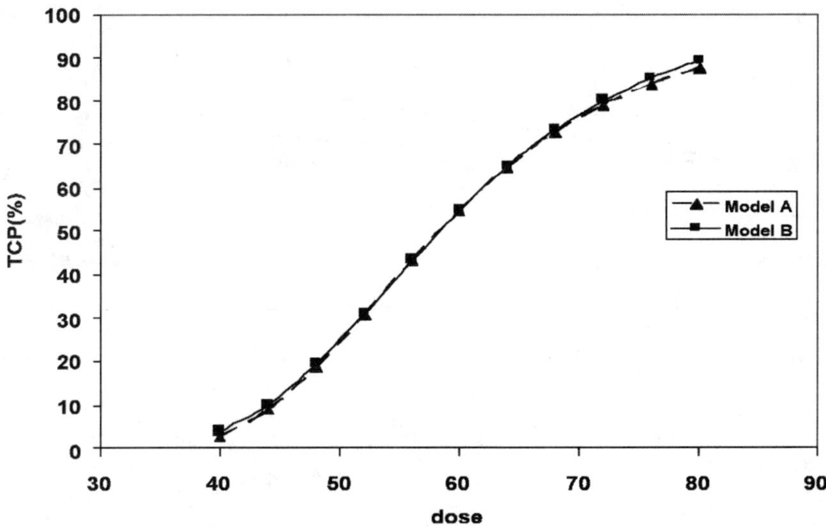

**Figure 7a.** Model A, a population averaged model ($10^7$ clonogens) and model B, with 90 clonogens, have almost identical TCP curves for uniform tumor irradiation. The models are described in more detail in the text.

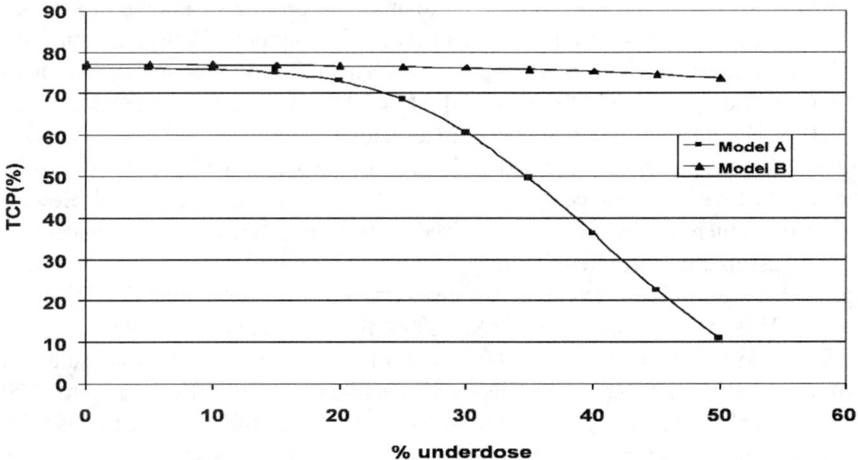

**Figure 7b.** A cold spot comprising 1% of the tumor model degrades TCP much more for model A than for model B. The dose to the bulk of the tumor is 70 Gy and the x axis is the % underdose (10% corresponds to a dose in the cold spot of 63 Gy).

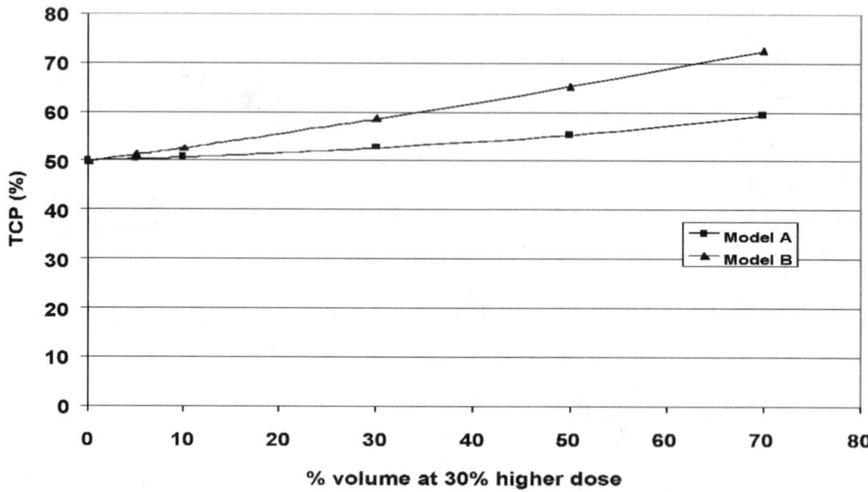


**Figure 7c.** Increase in TCP for 30% higher dose for models A and B vs. percent volume at high dose. The remaining volume is at $D_{50}$.

It is important to stress that figure 7, like many other examples [Withers (2000), Tomé and Fowler (2002)], assumes uniform clonogen density over the entire target region. If low dose regions occur in a "good" treatment plan, they are at the edge of the planning target volume (PTV) rather than within regions of known or suspected microscopic disease. Such cold spots are likely to be in regions of low clonogen density so that they cause minimal reduction in *observed* TCP (no reduction if there are no clonogens). Levegrun et al. (2000 and 2001) looked for dosimetric correlates of biopsy-proven local control of prostate cancer in a data set where the cold spots in the PTV almost always fell outside the gland as defined on the planning CT scan. They did not find significant correlation between minimum PTV dose and local control. However, for tumors which are less clearly localized than encapsulated prostate cancers, it is safest to assume uniform density or to "dose paint" by increasing dose where imaging or other studies indicate aggressive disease rather than decreasing dose elsewhere in the PTV [see Goitein and Niemierko (1996) for cautionary warnings].

IMRT dose distributions in the target are sometimes less uniform than static field conformal distributions, though this is by no means a necessity (Chui and Spirou 2001; Vineberg et al. 2002). The predicted ability of hot spots to substantially increase TCP is qualitatively insensitive to the model. To improve TCP, high dose regions must either occupy a large fraction of the tumor or be targeted to an area of known aggressive disease — in either case be a boost rather than a hot spot. For smaller high dose regions, the bulk of the tumor acts as a huge cold spot. Figure 7c illustrates the effect of a hot spot on predictions of models A and B described above. Here, the bulk of the tumor receives approximately $D_{50}$ (58.2 Gy), the hot spot dose is 30% higher and the hot spot volume is varied. Withers (2000) and Tomé and Fowler (2000) provide many TCP model calculations for simple non-uniform dose distributions.

## Equivalent Uniform Dose (EUD)

Niemierko (1997) defined the equivalent uniform dose (EUD) as the dose which, "when distributed uniformly across the target volume, causes the survival of the same number of clonogens" as the true dose distribution. He suggested that EUD has advantages over TCP for evaluating tumor dose distributions and derived some of its general properties. If the clonogen density and $SF2$ are uniform throughout the tumor and $\beta/\alpha{\sim}0$, the $EUD$ (Gy) of a dose distribution where volume fraction $v_i$ receives dose $D_i$ is

$$EUD = 2 \ln (\Sigma v_i\, (SF2)^{Di/2})/(\ln SF2) \tag{10}$$

While calculation of $EUD$ from the tumor DVH requires radiobiological parameters, it does not involve the number or density of clonogens. $EUD$ is bounded above by the mean dose and below by the minimum dose in the tumor (or structure whose DVH is used in the calculation). It is insensitive to $\beta/\alpha$ and to population averaging; the population averaged $EUD$ is well approximated by using the population mean value of $SF2$ or $\alpha$. While $EUD$ is model dependent, it is less so than TCP. Figure 8a shows the $EUD$ for models A and B and the same small cold-spot dose distribution as used for figure 7b. Figure 8b illustrates the relative model sensitivity of EUD and TCP for this dose/TCP model example. Equation (10) has also been generalized to include dose per fraction effects, spatial variation of relative clonogen density, and population averaging of radiobiological parameters (Niemierko 1997).

## Tumor Proliferation Or Repopulation

In the presence of tumor proliferation Tucker, Thames, and Taylor (1990) and Zaider and Minerbo (2000) showed that Poisson statistics do not describe the probability distribution of surviving clonogens. Nonetheless, Poisson-based expressions with SF multiplied by $\exp($ (Ln 2) $T/T_{eff}$, are almost always used for TCP calculations applied to inhomogeneous dose distributions. A more accurate formalism was derived by Zaider and Minerbo (2000), who gave examples of parameter choices for which the exact and Poisson expressions predict quite different TCPs, with the Poisson model always predicting lower TCP. To my knowledge, there are no systematic explorations of the effects of repopulation on plan evaluation and/or design. It is also of interest that several studies (Wilner et al. 2002) use local control at different times after treatment as endpoints and find fewer recurrences shortly after treatment than later, as surviving clonogens repopulate the site of the original tumor. Mechanistic models that deal with such endpoints will have to include the number distribution of surviving clonogens and their post-treatment tumor growth.

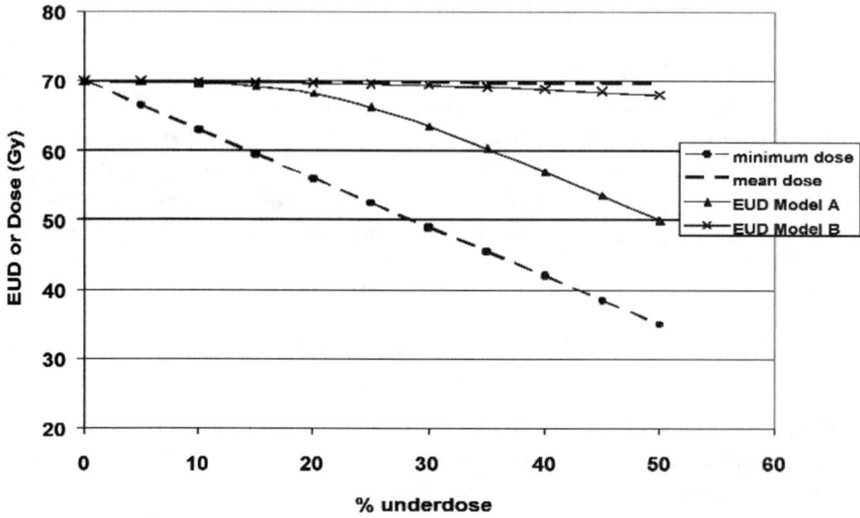

**Figure 8a.** EUD vs. percent underdose in a 1 cc volume (remaining 99 cc getting 70 Gy) for the tumor models A and B described in reference to figures 7. EUD is bounded above by the mean dose and below by the minimum dose.

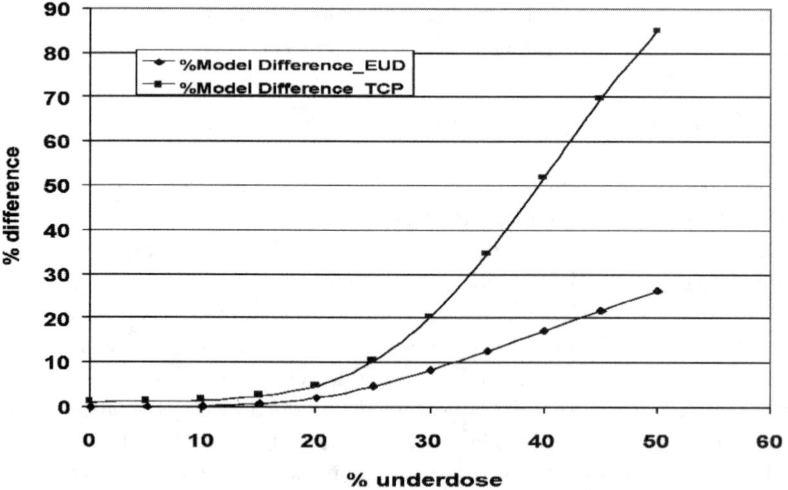

**Figure 8b.** Percent difference between models B and A for EUD (defined as 100(EUD_B − EUD_A)/EUD_B) and TCP (100 (TCP_B-TCP_A)/TCP_B) for the dose distribution of figures 7b and 8a. EUD is model dependent but less so than TCP.

## Normal Tissue Complications

### Some General Problems

If TCP were the only concern, it would be sufficient to treat the tumor to high dose with a few large fields. But the NTCP for most tissues increases with dose, often following a sigmoidal curve similar to TCP (e.g., figure 4), where NTCP reaches 50% at the tolerance dose, $TD_{50}$. Treatment planning thus requires consideration of normal tissues as well as tumor coverage. As with TCP, accurate prediction of NTCP, especially for unconventional dose distributions and dose escalation situations is a difficult problem. Some of the issues are listed below.

1. Data based on accurately known dose distributions are scarce. The widely used 1991 compilation (Emami et al. 1991) is based on many studies that predate the CT-planning era. Data from "delivered" dose distribution (setup error, organ motion, etc.) is almost non-existent.

2. Most NTCP data are at the low complications (<25%) end of the dose-response curve, and were acquired at low (<70 Gy) total treatment doses.

3. Many organs suffer several types of complication, each with a different time of onset and dosimetric correlates.

4. Different classification criteria are used in different studies and by different institutions (e.g., (Yorke et al. 2002) use Radiation Therapy Oncology Group (RTOG) grade 3 pneumonitis as an endpoint, while (Kwa et al. 1998) use Southwest Oncology Group (SWOG) grade 2 pneumonitis—both endpoints include prescription of steroids but they are not identical).

5. Factors other than radiation such as pre-existing medical conditions or chemotherapy change normal tissue responses.

### Features Of Available NTCP Data

Despite these problems, a fair amount of normal tissue complications information is available and used. The main source of information is still the 1991 compilation of tolerance doses for 50% and 5% complication probability within five years ($TD_{50/5}$ and $TD_{5/5}$) and associated volume effects for serious complications in 28 dose-limiting organs (Emami et al. 1991). "Standard fractionation" (1.8 to 2 Gy per daily treatment) is assumed. Below, we drop the time-scale from the notation and refer to $TD_{50}$, etc.

For many normal organs, the tolerance dose for a given probability of a complication varies inversely with the irradiated volume. This volume effect is often approximated by a power law, which is defined for the condition of "partial organ irradiation" in which a volume fraction $v$ receives a uniform dose while the remainder of the organ receives zero dose. If $TD_{c(v)}$ is the dose required for complication probability $c\%$ for partial organ irradiation of volume fraction $v$ and $TD_{c(1)}$ is the tolerance dose for the same complication probability with uniform whole organ irradiation then

$$TD_{c(v)} = TD_{c(1)}/v^n \tag{11}$$

because of the inverse relationship, $n \geq 0$, and it is usually assumed that $n \leq 1$. The power law is computationally simple and approximates dose-volume effects, but it has no underlying radiobiological rationale.

Complications for which $n \ll 1$ depend weakly on the irradiated volume fraction. For plan evaluation or optimization, even small volumes of the organ with dose should be kept below tolerance, but low doses to large fractions of the organ are acceptable. The best dose distributions for these complications give "a little to a lot" (Zaider and Amols 1998). Plan evaluators look at the maximum organ dose or a related DVH parameter and dose-based optimization score functions penalize exceeding a maximum dose. Examples of such complications include radiation myelitis, brainstem necrosis, and bowel perforation. It is also prudent to limit the maximum dose to small normal structures (e.g., optic chiasm, cochlea) that occupy only a few voxels.

Complications for which $n$ is close to 1 have strong volume dependence, are insensitive to small hot spots, and depend on the organ's entire DVH. Mean dose has been found to correlate well with the incidence of these complications. The best dose distributions for these complications give "a lot to a little" (Zaider and Amols 1998). Plan evaluators might look at the mean organ dose or points at the middle of the DVH (the volume receiving more than a critical dose, such as $V_{20}$ or $V_{30}$). To deal with these complications, optimization score functions based on physical dose criteria should include dose-volume or mean dose constraints. Severe radiation pneumonitis, radiation induced liver disease (RILD), and xerostomia have strong volume dependence, with $n \sim 1$ and NTCP depending approximately on the mean organ dose.

In a companion paper Burman et al. (1991) tabulated values of $n$ consistent with the data in Emami et al. (1991) and volume effects have been actively investigated ever since. Volume 31 Issue 5 (1995) of the "Red Journal" (*International Journal of Radiation Oncology, Biology, Physics*) and the July 2001 issue of *Seminars in Radiation Oncology* are excellent sources of more current information. Since IMRT improves dose distributions for curative or aggressive palliative treatment of recurrent disease, re-treatment tolerances of normal tissues are of interest and are reviewed by Stewart (1997) and Nieder, Milas, and Ang (2000). Below, we briefly and selectively and summarize some NTCP data updates with particular relevance to IMRT. Since changes are always "in the works", it is worthwhile to check primary references and keep up with developments.

## Updates For Some Dose-Limiting Complications

### Radiation Myelitis/Spinal Cord

In the 1991 compilations, $TD_5$ and $TD_{50}$ for myelitis at standard fractionation are 47 to 50 Gy and 70 Gy, respectively. The weak volume dependence (n = 0.05 in Burman et al. (1991) is confirmed in more recent studies. Myelitis is a late complication (6 months to 7 years) and tolerance doses are dependent on dose fractionation. A thorough review (Schultheiss et al. 1995) summarizes evidence that $TD_5$ is substantially above 50 Gy and volume dependence is small. However, myelitis is so serious that most planners aim to keep complication probability well below 5%. For this reason, when the maximum cord dose comes close to the local standard for tolerance, it is advisable to include the effects of setup error in the evaluation process. The spinal cord is often a concern in re-treatment and there is evidence in the above-cited reviews and in Grosu et al. (2002) that it recovers some tolerance 4 to 6 months after initial treatment.

### Radiation Pneumonitis: Lung

Probability up to 25% of pneumonitis requiring steroids or other prescription medication is often considered clinically acceptable for curative radiation treatment of lung cancer. The parameters in the 1991 compilations, ($TD_{50(1)}$ = 24.5 Gy, $n = 0.87$), have held up well although Martel et al. (1994) find that a higher tolerance dose ($TD_{50(1)}$ = 28 Gy) and $n = 1$ were better fits to their data where dose calculations with lung density corrections. Many recent studies agree that mean lung dose is a good predictor of pneumonitis. For an overview see Marks (2002) and for more detail, Seppenwoolde and Lebesque (2001). Other DVH features that correlate with pneumonitis include the volume fraction above a cutoff dose. For example, in a study of non-small-cell lung cancer patients treated with 3DCRT, Graham et al. (1999) saw no severe pneumonitis providing $V_{20} < 32\%$. $V_{30}$ has also been found to correlate with pneumonitis (Hernando et al. 2001). Clinically validated correlation of complications with such model-independent indices as mean dose and $V_{20}$ is useful, as they are obtained directly from the DVH and can be implemented in physical dose-based optimization algorithms without extra radiobiological parameters.

### Rectal Bleeding

IMRT has enabled striking dose escalation for prostate cancer without concurrent increase in normal tissue complications (Zelefsky et al. 2002) and severe rectal bleeding, requiring medical intervention, is a major dose-limiting complication for radiation therapy of prostate and other pelvic tumors. According to the 1991 compilations, $TD_5$ and $TD_{50}$ are 60 Gy and 80 Gy, respectively, and there is little volume dependence ($n = 0.12$). Recent analyses of CT-based conformal radiation therapy to high treatment doses find a more complicated volume dependence, indicating a need for both dose-volume and maximum dose considerations in score functions and plan evaluation. Jackson (2001) thoroughly reviews these studies. There is a volume effect relating to the fraction of rectal wall (on the planning scan) exposed to doses above 75 Gy and also to the wall fraction exposed to doses in the intermediate range of 40 to 50 Gy (Jackson et al. 2001). Memorial Sloan-Kettering Cancer Center's (MSKCC's) evaluation requirements for high dose prostate plans incorporates these findings and allows no more than 30% of the rectal wall volume to exceed 75 Gy. Also, when possible without compromising target coverage, at most ~50% of the wall is taken to doses above 47 Gy. For IMRT prostate treatments to prescription doses of 81 Gy and 86.4 Gy, these dose-volume constraints are consistent with both acceptably uniform doses in the gland and very low (<5%) rectal bleeding rates (Zelefsky et al. 2002). These clinical rectal bleeding data are acquired at standard fractionation and should not be applied to hypofractionation schedules which aim to exploit prostate cancer's possible low $\alpha/\beta$ ratio without further studies.

It is of interest that CT-based studies since 1991 show severe esophagitis also has mixed maximum dose, dose-volume, and dose-circumference correlates (Maguire et al. 1999), though the 1991 compilations assigns it $n = 0.06$.

*Xerostomia/Parotids*

Head and neck cancers are another disease where IMRT improves dose distributions. Xerostomia adversely affects quality of life but is not lethal, so higher complication rates are permitted. For unilateral tumors, judicious beam selection can spare one parotid and for bilateral disease, IMRT treatments can often improve parotid sparing without compromising target coverage. According to the 1991 compilation, $TD_{5(1)}$ and $TD_{50(1)}$ are 32 and 46 Gy, respectively, and there is fairly strong volume dependence ($n = 0.7$). Recent studies of patients treated with CT-based conformal therapy suggest stronger volume effect ($n = 1$) and find correlation between the mean dose and saliva flow preservation in an individual gland. Several studies find a threshold mean dose for suppression of saliva flow without recovery at $\leq 1$ year [24 to 26 Gy mean dose threshold by Eisbruch et al. (1999), 32 Gy by Chao et al. (2001)] while Roesink et al. (2001) find no threshold but agree that $n = 1$ and that the $TD_{50}$ mean dose for flow recovery increases with time from $TD_{50}$ is 31 Gy at 6 weeks to 39 Gy at 1 year post therapy. Parotid complications studies are reviewed by Eisbruch et al. (2001).

*Radiation-Induced Liver Disease (RILD)*

RILD is potentially lethal and is a major dose-limiting complication in radiation treatment of primary liver tumors and liver metastases. According to the 1991 compilation, $TD_{5(1)}$ and $TD_{50(1)}$ are 30 Gy and 40 Gy respectively and there is moderate volume dependence ($n = 0.32$). These parameters have changed, due largely to an NTCP model-based dose escalation protocol in progress since 1987 at the University of Michigan. Treatments are at with CT based conformal radiation therapy, 1.5 Gy, twice daily, with concurrent chemotherapy (FUdR or BUdR). An overall review of RILD data is given in Dawson, Ten Haken, and Lawrence (2001) and complications outcomes for 203 patients in the trial were recently been reported (Dawson et al. 2002). The reference volume evaluated was the normal liver [gross tumor volume (GTV) not included]. A strong volume effect was found ($n = 0.94$) such that RILD correlated with mean dose and no RILD was seen for mean normal liver dose below 30 Gy. $TD_{50(1)}$ was higher for patients with liver metastases (45.8 Gy) than those with primary hepato-biliary cancer ($TD_{50(1)} = 39.8$ Gy).

## NTCP Models

NTCP models provide mathematical expressions that summarize data and compress an entire dose distribution into a single number that can be used for plan evaluation or optimization. There are both phenomenological and mechanistic models, but all have free parameters which are adjusted to fit clinical data. Current models are simplistic, and should not be lightly extrapolated to novel dose distributions, fractionation schemes, or high dose levels. A model validated for dose distributions that resemble partial organ irradiation should be applied cautiously to very different distributions. Most models were fit to data at standard fractionation (1.8 to 2 Gy per daily fraction) at which it is reasonable to use DVHs or substitute LQED2-VHs (Martel et al. 1998), but new parameters might be needed for drastically different schedules (e.g., extreme hypofractionation). With these warnings, some common models are described in the next subsections.

### The Lyman Model

The Lyman model (Lyman 1985) is widely used in North American radiation oncology. It is a combination of the probability integral to describe the sigmoidal curve, the power law for volume effects, and a "histogram reduction" scheme for general dose distributions. It is applied to different complications by changing four parameters. One parameter is a reference volume (usually whole organ), and the other three are fit to clinical data. They are $TD_{50}$, the volume effect exponent $n$ and a parameter $m$ that determines the mid-point slope or the $\gamma_{50}$ of the NTCP curve. For partial organ irradiation of volume fraction $v$ to dose $D$, NTCP is given by

$$NTCP(D) = 1/\sqrt{(2\pi)} \int_{-\infty}^{\left(D-TD_{50(v)}\right)/\left(mTD_{50(v)}\right)} \exp\left(-t^2/2\right) dt \tag{12}$$

For general dose distributions, the Lyman model is supplemented by a "histogram reduction" algorithm. This is a systematic method that converts a general DVH to a simple one with the same NTCP—either an equivalent uniform whole organ dose ($D_{\text{eff}}$) or partial irradiation of an effective volume, $V_{\text{eff}}$, to a representative dose (e.g., maximum dose, $D_{\text{max}}$). Equation (12) is then applied to the reduced DVH. There are at least two histogram reduction algorithms [Lyman and Wolbarst (1989) and Kutcher and Burman (1991)] and there is no biological reason to prefer one over the other. Both obey common-sense limits (Kutcher and Burman 1991) including consistency with equation (11) for partial organ irradiation, prediction that NTCP increases (decreases) for small hot (cold) spots and correct volume dependence for small $n$ and $n = 1$. The reduction algorithms predict similar but not identical NTCP for the same DVH (Moiseenko, Battista, and Van Dyk 2000). The Kutcher-Burman reduction scheme, which is widely implemented in treatment planning, reduces the DVH (volume fraction $v_i$ in dose bin centered at $D_i$) to either an equivalent uniform whole-organ dose, $D_{eff}$, given by

$$D_{eff} = (\Sigma \, v_i \, (D_i)^{1/n})^n \tag{13a}$$

or an equivalent partial irradiation of a volume fraction $v_{eff}$ to $D_{max}$,

$$v_{eff} = \Sigma \, v_i \, (D_i/D_{max})^{1/n}. \tag{13b}$$

These equations are equivalent and both reduce to equation (11) for partial organ irradiation. When $n = 1$, $D_{eff}$ is the mean dose and for small $n$, $D_{eff}$ approaches $D_{max}$.

Burman et al. (1991) found Lyman model parameters that fit the data of Emami et al. (1991) and updated values are given in some of the work referenced previously in the section **Updates For Some Dose Limiting Complications**. Since NTCP vs. dose curve is steep ($\gamma_{50}$~2 or 3), Lyman model estimates of NTCP are sensitive to $TD_{50}$. For example, the 1991 estimate of $TD_{50(1)}$ for radiation pneumonitis was 24.5 Gy, but Martel et al. (1994) found a better fit with $TD_{50(1)} = 28$ Gy and $m$ approximately the same. If the calculated $D_{eff}$ for a dose distribution is 24.5 Gy, an evaluation according to the 1991 parameters predicts pneumonitis probability of 50%, while using the 1994 parameters predicts approximately 25%. Given the evolving state of outcomes analysis, some studies rely on the monotonic relationship of NTCP and $D_{eff}$ or $V_{eff}$, calibrate these quantities against complications data (e.g., an acceptable complications level is found in a patient group if $D_{eff}$ <22 Gy) and then use $D_{eff}$ or $V_{eff}$ for plan comparison or evaluation. This approach has been applied very effectively to dose escalation protocols by the University of Michigan (Martel et al. 1994; Dawson et al. 2002). It is similar in spirit to using EUD as a surrogate for TCP and a generalization of EUD to include normal tissues was proposed by Niemierko (see the section *EUD*).

Fractionation can be included in the Lyman model by reducing the DVH to an equivalent BED-VH at standard fractionation (e.g., LQED2-VH) and keeping the model parameters unchanged. If the DVH represents a small-n tissue and $D_{max}$ is delivered at dose/fraction>prescription (e.g., $D_{max}$ in region 2 of figure 2), $D_{eff}$ corrected for fractionation is higher than that calculated from the physical DVH while if $D_{max}$ is in region 1 (as with the cord DVH in figure 2), the LQ-corrected $D_{eff}$ is lower than that calculated from the physical DVH. Similarly, for tissues with n~1 if most of the DVH is in region 1 (lung DVH in figure 2) the fractionation corrected $D_{eff}$ is reduced. When comparing NTCP studies, one should be aware of how fractionation effects were handled.

While not based on cellular radiobiology, the Lyman model is easy to use. With parameter updates, it summarizes clinical observations well enough to justify its wide application in plan evaluation, analyzing clinical outcomes and deciding treatment doses, especially when deviations from traditional doses and distributions are approached cautiously.

*Tissue Architecture Models*

NTCP models based upon radiation biology and organ physiology were developed that might be better than phenomenological expressions for predicting normal tissue response to new treatment regimes. Withers, Taylor, and Maciejewski (1988) set out a conceptual framework for a class of such models. They hypothesized that normal organs are composed of multicellular "functional subunits" or FSUs. The radiation response of an individual FSU depends on the radiosensitivity and regenerative properties of its component cells, but an NTCP dose-response depends on the general arrangement (tissue architecture) of the FSUs and how they carry out organ function. Although this suggestion is almost 15 years old, there is no organ-complication pair for which the FSU has been unambiguously identified. Candidate structures include the nephron in kidney and the alveolus in lung but in a recent *Medical Physics* "Point-Counterpoint," it was argued that NTCP dose and volume dependence is due to microvascular architecture (Hendee, Hopewell, and Withers 1998).

Three types of response models were proposed: serial (critical element model), parallel (critical volume model), and graded response. Serial and parallel models reduce NTCP evaluation to a binary choice—only events above a chosen endpoint (e.g., grade 2 pneumonitis) are rated as complications. Graded response models apply to complications caused by the same underlying mechanisms but covering a continuum of severity. There are few graded response models; recently one was applied to salivary flow reduction in parotid irradiation (Chao et al. 2001). Current tissue architecture models include a common set of simplifying assumptions including: (1) an FSU is either incapacitated by radiation or remains completely functional; (2) the probability of destroying an FSU is independent of the condition of the other FSUs; (3) dose gradients across a single FSU are negligible. With these assumptions, it is straightforward to make model NTCP calculations for inhomogeneous dose distributions. Although there is no definitive evidence that tissue architecture models agree better with clinical outcomes than the Lyman model, we discuss serial and parallel models for completeness.

**The serial architecture or critical element model**. In the serial architecture model, the FSUs are arranged in series, like a string of Christmas tree lights. The complication occurs if even a single FSU is destroyed (Schultheiss, Orton, and Peck 1983; Withers, Taylor, and Maciejewski 1988; Niemierko and Goitein 1991) so that NTCP is the probability of destroying at least one FSU. This linear picture suggests applying the serial model to long, thin organs (cord, rectum, esophagus), but experimental and clinical data show this is an oversimplification (Jackson 2001; Maguire et al. 1999).

A unified formalism for applying the serial model to general DVHs was developed by Niemierko and Goitein (1991). If $p(D)$ is the probability of destroying an FSU with dose $D$ and the organ is composed of $N$ FSUs, then NTCP for uniform irradiation of the whole organ to dose $D$ is

$$NTCP(D) = 1 - (1 - p(D))^N. \tag{14a}$$

Finding $p(D)$ requires no additional assumptions about individual FSUs, as it is derived from the whole organ NTCP by inverting equation (14a):

$$p(D) = 1 - (1 - NTCP(D))^{1/N} \tag{14b}$$

For a general dose-distribution where $n_i$ FSUs receive dose $D_i$, NTCP is given by

$$NTCP(\{n_i, D_i\}) = 1 - \prod_i (1 - p(D_i))^{n_i} \tag{14c}$$

where the product is over all the dose bins of the DVH. Dose per fraction effects can be handled similarly to the Lyman model.

At low complication probabilities, the predictions of the serial model predictions and the Lyman model with $n = 0.1$ are similar but for simple DVHs with small hot spots, the Lyman model predicts higher NTCP (Niemierko and Goitein 1991). Despite different predictions, the Lyman model with small $n$ is more widely used, perhaps because it covers NTCP for many tissues with the same equation.

**The parallel architecture or critical volume model.** The FSUs of a parallel architecture organ work "in parallel" and some FSUs can be destroyed without causing complication. Only when more than a critical number of FSUs are destroyed does the complication occur. If too few FSUs are damaged—for example, by irradiating a sufficiently small volume, even to a high dose—one might observe local damage such as radiological changes but not observe "the complication" (Yorke et al. 1993). The ultimate parallel model is TCP, where the "FSU" is the clonogenic cell and the critical number is all clonogens (Kallman, Agren, and Brahme 1992; Jackson, Kutcher, and Yorke 1993). The parallel model might apply to complications with strong volume dependence such as radiation pneumonitis, radiation nephritis, radiation hepatitis, and severe xerostomia (Withers, Taylor, and Maciejewski 1988). Some of the "parallel" organs may also suffer complications which are not described by the parallel model (e.g., clinical lung fibrosis or changes in local pulmonary function).

Features of the parallel model were elucidated by Niemierko and Goitein (1993b), Yorke et al. (1993), and Jackson, Kutcher, and Yorke (1993). NTCP calculations require at least four parameters, two of which determine the slope and radiosensitivity of p(D). A logistic function (Jackson et al. 1995) or a Poisson-LQ model resembling a tumor control probability model (Niemierko and Goitein 1993b) have been used. If there are many FSUs, NTCP is determined by the fraction, rather than the absolute number, of FSUs destroyed and the critical fraction for producing the complication is called the "functional reserve." NTCP is determined by the average fraction of destroyed FSUs (mean or fractional damage or $f_{dam}$) relative to the functional reserve. For a general dose distribution, $f_{dam}$ is calculated from p(D) and the organ's DVH, or LQED2_VH as

$$f_{dam} = \Sigma_i p(D_i) v_i \ . \tag{15}$$

Equation (15) can be generalized to handle FSU densities or radiosensitivities that vary within the organ (Yorke 2001).

If there are many FSUs and the functional reserve is not too close to 1 or 0, the model predicts an unrealistically steep dependence of NTCP on dose. As with TCP models, averaging over a population distribution of FSU radiobiological parameters and critical reserve flattens the slope and brings the NTCP curve into agreement with clinical observation. The distribution of functional reserves has been shown to have the greatest effect on the NTCP curve, and the mean and standard deviation of this distribution are the other two model parameters. The parallel model was fit to clinical data for RILD (Jackson et al. 1995), updated by Dawson, Ten Haken, and Lawrence (2001) and for radiation pneumonitis (Ten Haken, personal communication) using a logistic function for $p(D)$ and a Gaussian distribution of functional reserves.

Since NTCP increases monotonically with $f_{dam}$, it rather than NTCP can be used in plan evaluation or optimization (similarly to using $EUD$, $D_{eff}$, or $V_{eff}$). This requires only two parameters and is computationally simpler than population averaging. It is easy to design simple dose distributions for which the parallel model and the Lyman model with $n\sim1$ give different plan rankings. One such example, due to Jackson, is shown in Yorke et al. (2000) and Yorke (2001). For clinical dose distributions, the two models are strongly correlated, but at least for conformal plans for lung cancer, the parallel model is more forgiving at high doses ($>>$ the FSU $D_{50}$) because $f_{dam}$ saturates while $D_{eff}$ can increase without bound. According to recent analysis, the two models are equivalently significant predictors of severe pneumonitis (Yorke et al. 2002) and the parallel model is still under consideration for RILD (Dawson, Ten Haken, and Lawrence, 2001).

**Kallman's "relative seriality" or "s" model**. In the "Kallman s-model" or "relative seriality model" (Kallman, Agren, and Brahme 1992), which is often used in European studies, the organ is thought of as an assembly of FSUs. It requires at least four parameters, one of which is a reference volume. Two other parameters—$TD_{50}$ and the slope of the sigmoidal whole organ NTCP vs. dose curve—are determined from clinical data and the s-model shares with the serial architecture model the convenient feature of not requiring extra parameters to describe an individual FSU response. The fourth parameter, also fit from data, is the "relative seriality", $s$, which can be any positive number. If $s$ is small (<<1.0), the complication has strong volume dependence, if $s = 1.0$, the model reduces to the serial architecture model, and $s$ can exceed 1.0. For a general dose distribution, NTCP is given by

$$NTCP = (1 - \prod_i (1 - p(D_i)^s)^{1/v_i})^{1/s} \tag{16}$$

where $p(D)$ is found by inverting equation (16) for uniform whole organ irradiation. The s-model was fit to the data of Emami et al. (1991) for seven complications (Kallman, Agren, and Brahme 1992) and it was recently used to analyze late cardiac (Gagliardi et al. 1996) and rectal (MacKay et al. 1997) complications.

## EUD

Niemierko (1999) generalized the concept of EUD to NTCP and suggested a phenomenological expression to calculate EUD from a DVH:

$$EUD = \left(\left[\sum_i v_i D_i^a\right]\right)^{1/a} \tag{17}$$

where the sum is over all the dose bins. Only one complication-specific parameter, $a$, needs to be fit from data and it can range over all real numbers ($-\alpha < a < \alpha$). The EUD equation has the same form and the same interpretation for normal tissues as the Lyman model $D_{\text{eff}}$, with $1/n = a$. Complications with a small volume dependence have large values of $a$ and those which depend on the mean dose have $a = 1$. If $a$ tends to $-\infty$, $EUD$ tends to the minimum dose, so that tumor $EUD$ can be modeled with large negative values of a. Since $EUD$ and the Lyman $D_{\text{eff}}$ are mathematically identical, $EUD$ has the same strengths and weaknesses as the Lyman model relative to correlation with clinical NTCP data. However, it has the advantage of placing TCP and NTCP in the same computational framework. This makes it attractive to use EUD rather than more complex models in optimization algorithms (Wu et al. 2002; Jones and Hoban 2002).

## Summary

There is no doubt that there is frequent clinical use of NTCP-related features of dose distributions and NTCP models, both for plan evaluation and to set dose and dose-volume constraints in optimization. Data from follow-up of patients treated with 3DCRT feed back to improve understanding of dosimetric correlates of complications and this, in turn, changes treatment of future patients. Fortunately, many complications correlate with quantities such as maximum dose, mean dose, or percent volume above a critical dose level, which are easily extracted from DVHs and used as constraints in existing optimization algorithms. As better clinical data become available, the process of plan design and evaluation becomes more rational and informed.

There are several NTCP models but all are rather simple descriptions of clinical data sets so it is not surprising that different models can lead to different conclusions about a specific treatment plan. As a simple example, the patient whose treatment plan produced the dose distribution from which the DVH of figure 2 was obtained was enrolled in a lung cancer dose escalation protocol at MSKCC. In the initial years of the protocol, a patient could be treated at the highest permitted dose level provided that the Lyman model lung NTCP [parameters from Burman et al. (1991)] was $\leq$25%. Subsequently, the protocol was amended to replace the Lyman model with the parallel model (parameters by Ten Haken) with $f_{dam}$ held to $\leq$0.28. Both of these criteria were consistent with an acceptable level of radiation pneumonitis. The Lyman model criterion would limit the total dose for this particular treatment plan to 75 Gy while the parallel model would allow the same plan to go to 84 Gy (where dose constraints to other normal tissues were still met). For this patient, the NTCP model in force in the protocol determines the total treatment dose. For interesting discussion of how NTCP model affects the ranking of rival treatment plans (with the model parameters adjusted to fit the same clinical data) see Moiseenko, Battista, and Van Dyk (2000).

Given the current status of NTCP models and the lack of definitive evidence for which is more "correct," perhaps it is most practical for a department to choose one well-documented set of criteria (models or DVH features) per complication and to calibrate the choice with local clinical outcomes and a large scoop of common sense. Simultaneously, one should expect and keep up with new understanding of treatment outcomes.

## Direct Use Of Biological Indices In IMRT Plan Design

The title of this section is *not* "biological indices in treatment plan optimization" because the "optimal" plan, which is lethal dose to every tumor cell and dose nowhere else, is physically unattainable. Even if our understanding of the connections between dose distributions and radiation-induced complications and TCP were superior to the present day level, there would remain a large subjective component in what an individual physician, physicist, or even a patient would consider "the best plan available." Provocative examples are given by Amols and Zaider (1997) and Lind et al. (1999).

To my knowledge, optimization score functions in commercial North American treatment planning systems are based on dose and/or dose-volume constraints (although at least one implements biological indices in a pre-release version). Few commercial systems include TCP or NTCP model calculations for plan evaluation. Thus, much work remains to determine if and when direct use of biological indices in optimization is advantageous. Clinical users of IMRT have invested a great deal of effort to find combinations of beams, constraints, and penalties that work for them so that, in a reasonable time frame, they can design deliverable IMRT plans which are superior to conventional plans in comparisons based on dose-volume and biological criteria and clinical judgment. To conduct fair comparisons between dose-based and biology-based optimization algorithms, investigators will have to climb a learning curve with the biology-based system. It has been argued that score functions based on biological indices explore a wider range of dose distributions than those which overtly constrain the DVH (Wu et al. 2002). But because few comparisons appear in the literature, the benefits of "biology-based optimization" are still unclear.

The remaining sections are not an exhaustive review, but only describe some studies' score functions that directly incorporate biological indices. Three of these also include terms to help strike a balance between tumor control and normal tissue complications of different severity to make the resulting dose distribution clinically acceptable. A background normal tissue is often added to prevent overly high doses in or near the target.

## Uncomplicated Control

Uncomplicated control is the probability of local tumor control without normal tissue complications. If $P_B$ is the probability of benefit (i.e., TCP), $P_I$ the probability of injury and $\delta$ the fraction of patients for whom benefit and injury are statistically independent, then Agren, Brahme, and Turesson (1990) show that uncomplicated control, $P_+$, is given by

$$P_+ = P_B - P_I + \delta\, P_I\, (1 - P_B) \tag{18}$$

$P_I$ is obtained from the NTCPs of concern. If $c$ independent complications are considered (e.g., $c = 3$, corresponding to myelitis, pneumonitis, and esophagitis) and the $j$th complication probability is $NTCP_j$

$$P_I = 1 - \prod_j (1 - NTCP_j) \tag{19}$$

where the product runs from 1 to $c$. In addition to "real" critical organ complications, an NTCP term can be introduced to limit hotspots in the target. Optimization with $P_+$ as the score function is discussed by Södertsröm and Brahme (1993) while Lind et al. (1999) describe the use of $P_+$ in choosing the treatment dose for plans designed by other means.

Goitein (1992) pointed out that if $P_+$ is the score or ranking function it does not discriminate serious from tolerable adverse outcomes and also "…implies that a 6% increase in TCP would outweigh a 5% chance of a cord transection." The three score functions discussed below address this deficiency by including factors that weight TCP and NTCP according to clinical judgment.

## TCP And NTCP With Prioritization

Wang et al. (1995) implemented a score function that utilized TCP and NTCP models but allowed prioritization of the desired biological outcomes. The $i$th normal tissue complication was represented by subscore, $s_i$, which was a piecewise continuous function of NTCP. The user controlled the importance of the complication through three numbers—the maximum value of $s_i$, the NTCP at which $s_i$ begins to drop sharply and the NTCP at which $s_i$ reaches zero (thereafter staying zero). For example, by choice of these numbers, the user could allow the xerostomia NTCP to go to 30% without much penalty but force the risk of myelitis to be <1%. The overall score function to be maximized was

$$S = TCP \prod_i s_i \tag{20}$$

where the product is over all the normal tissue complications of interest. Dose distributions obtained through optimization with this score function were compared with results using a quadratic score function with maximum and minimum dose (but not dose-volume) constraints for a six-field prostate plan and a nine-field lung plan. Both methods gave acceptable distributions for the prostate plan, but for the lung plan, the biologically optimized plan was clearly superior. Whether that would still be true if dose-volume constraints had been used was not explored, though such constraints would be needed for a fair comparison of optimizations including complications with a strong volume effect.

## EUD

At least two groups have investigated the use of score functions based on the generalized EUD. Wu et al. (2002) maximized the product of subscores, $f_i$, each of which was a logistic function of EUD calculated with equation (17). The tumor subscore was

$$f_{\text{tum}} = 1/(1 + (EUD_0/EUD)^n) \tag{20a}$$

and the subscore for the $i$th normal tissue complication was

$$f_{\text{N,I}} = 1/(1 + (EUD/EUD_{0,\text{N,i}})^{n'}) \tag{20b}$$

The $EUD_0$'s are the desired target dose for the tumor or are related to the maximum allowed normal tissue EUD. The exponents, $n$, determine how rapidly the score function changes when the constraint EUD is violated. The user controls the allowed levels of complications through the $EUD_0$'s (taken from NTCP data) and their relative importance through the choice of $n$'s. A background normal tissue was introduced to limit hot spots within the tumor. The study compared prostate and head-and-neck plans optimized with the EUD-based score function to plans optimized with dose and dose-volume constraints. The EUD method achieved better normal tissue sparing (better even than the score function requirements) with equivalent target coverage and required less tweaking of constraints by the planner.

Optimization with a quadratic dose/dose-volume based score function was also compared with optimization using a quadratic EUD and integral BED-based score function for a phantom geometry of a concave-tumor partly surrounding a critical organ (Jones and Hoban 2002). They also investigated effects of changing the tumor and normal tissue $\alpha/\beta$. Again, a mock normal tissue had to be added to prevent excessive hot spots in the target volume. They found only minor differences between the dose-based and biology-based optimizations and suggested that biological indices were better used for plan ranking than optimization.

## Summary

### LQ Model

The LQ model is well supported by decades of experiment and clinical observation. It is mathematically simple, good for "back of the envelope" calculations, very useful for comparing dose fractionation schedules and thoroughly covered by accessible radiation oncology literature. It should be part of the knowledge base of all clinical physics staff involved in treatment plan design or evaluation.

### TCP

Although there are well-developed TCP calculation models, key parameters governing their sensitivity to dose inhomogeneities have not yet been extracted from experiments or clinical data. But two robust conclusions of TCP models agree qualitatively with clinical common-sense: cold spots in the GTV or CTV (clinical target volume) should be avoided and small hot spots in the target are of little benefit. However, estimates of the extent of TCP degradation or improvement are highly model dependent. While these problems are being resolved, prescription dose, target coverage, and perhaps EUD are practical and prudent surrogates for TCP.

### NTCP

Many clinical studies reveal simple features of dose distributions (DVHs) that correlate with normal tissue complications. These are model-independent and very helpful for setting dose and dose-volume constraints and for plan evaluation of all forms of conformal radiation therapy.

NTCP models are sometimes included in the clinical decision process. However, different models (and different parameters in the same model) lead to different conclusions. Interpretation of NTCP numbers calculated with a chosen model can be evaluated by retrospective study for later application to the local patient population and treatment plan types.

## IMRT

Direct use of biological indices to design IMRT intensity patterns is still in a research phase. It is not known whether such methods will improve the quality of IMRT dose distributions or the efficiency of IMRT treatment planning. Given the difficulties of developing reliable TCP/NTCP models, intermediate quantities such as EUD might be preferable and a cautious approach is justified.

## General

Outcomes analysis is an active subfield of radiation oncology. Physicists should remain alert to progress, maintain dialog with physician colleagues and work toward using the new information for better patient treatment.

## References

Agren, A., A. Brahme, and I. Turesson. (1990)."Optimization of uncomplicated control for head and neck tumors." *Int. J. Radiat. Oncol. Biol. Phys.* 19:1077–1085.

Amols, H. I., M. Zaider, M. K.Hayes, and P. B. Schiff. (1997). "Physician/patient driven risk assignment in radiation oncology: Reality or fancy?" *Int. J. Radiat. Oncol. Biol. Phys.* 38:455–461.

Brenner, D. J. (1993). "Dose, volume and tumor control predictions in radiotherapy." *Int. J. Radiat. Oncol. Biol. Phys.* 26:171–179.

Brenner, D. J., Y. Huang, and E. J. Hall. (1991). "Fractionated high dose-rate versus low dose-rate regimens for intracavitary brachytherapy of the cervix, equivalent regimens for combined brachytherapy and external irradiation." *Int. J. Radiat. Oncol. Biol. Phys.* 21:1415–1423.

Brenner, D. J., A. A. Martinez, G. K. Edmundson, C. Mitchel, H. D. Thames, and E. P. Armour. (2002). "Direct evidence that prostate tumors show high sensitivity to fractionation (low $\alpha/\beta$ ratio) similar to late-responding normal tissue." *Int. J. Radiat. Oncol. Biol. Phys.* 52:6–13.

Burman, C., G. J. Kutcher, B. Emami, and M. Goitein. (1991). "Fitting of normal tissue tolerance data to an analytic function." *Int. J. Radiat. Oncol. Biol. Phys.* 21:123–135.

Chao, K. S., J. O. Deasy, J. Markman, J.Hayne, C. A. Perez, J. A. Purdy, and D. A. Low. (2001). "A prospective study of salivary function sparing in patients with head-and-neck cancers receiving intensity-modulated or three-dimensional radiation therapy: initial results." *Int. J. Radiat. Oncol. Biol. Phys.* 49:907–916.

Chui, C. S., and S. V. Spirou. (2001). "Inverse planning algorithms for external beam radiotherapy." *Med. Dosim.* 26:189–197.

Dale, R. G. (1985). "The application of the linear-quadratic dose-effect equation to fractionated and protracted radiotherapy." *Br. J. Radiol.* 58:515–528.

Dawson, L. A., R. K. Ten Haken, and T. S. Lawrence. (2001). "Partial irradiation of the liver." *Semin. Radiat. Oncol.* 11:240–246.

Dawson, L. A., D. Normolle, J. M. Balter, C. J. McGinn, T. S. Lawrence, and R. K. Ten Haken. (2002). "Analysis of radiation-induced liver disease using the Lyman NTCP model." *Int. J. Radiat. Oncol. Biol. Phys.* 53:810–821.

Deasy, J. "Tumor Control Probability Models for Nonuniform Dose Distributions" in *Volume & Kinetics in Tumor Control & Normal Tissue Complications*. B. R. Paliwal, J. F. Fowler, D. E. Herbert, and M. P. Mehta (eds.). Madison WI: Medical Physics Publishing, pp. 65–85, 1998.

Deschavanne, P. J., and B. Fertil. (1996). "A review of human cell radiosensitivity in vitro." *Int. J. Radiat. Oncol. Biol. Phys.* 34:251–266.

Eisbruch, A., R. K. Ten Haken, H. M. Kim, L. H. Marsh, and J. A. Ship. (1999). "Dose, volume and function relationships in parotid salivary glands following conformal and intensity-modulated irradiation of head and neck cancer." *Int. J. Radiat. Oncol. Biol. Phys.* 45:577–587.

Eisbruch, A., J. A. Ship, H. M. Kim, and R. K. Ten Haken. ( 2001). "Partial irradiation of the parotid gland." *Semin. Radiat. Oncol.* 11:234–239.

Emami, B., J. Lyman, A. Brown, L. Coia, M. Goitein, J. E. Munzenrider, B. Shank, L. J. Solin, and M. Wesson. (1991). "Tolerance of normal tissue to therapeutic irradiation." *Int. J. Radiat. Oncol. Biol. Phys.* 21:109–122.

Fowler, J. F. (1989). "The linear-quadratic formula and progress in fractionated radiotherapy." *Br. J. Radiol.* 62:679–694.

Fowler, J. F. (1992*).* "Brief summary of radiobiological principles in fractionated radiotherapy." *Semin. Radiat. Oncol.* 2:16–21.

Fowler, J., R. Chappell, and M. Ritter. (2002). "The prospects for new treatments for prostate cancer (editorial)." *Int. J. Radiat. Oncol. Biol. Phys.* 52:3–5.

Gagliardi, G., I. Lax, A. Ottolenghi, and L. E. Rutqvist. (1996). "Long-term cardiac mortality after radiotherapy of breast cancer—application of the relative seriality model." *Br. J. Radiol.* 69:839–846.

Goitein, M. "The Probability of Controlling an Inhomogeneously Irradiated Tumor" in *Report of the Working Group on the Evaluation of Treatment Planning for Particle Beam Radiotherapy*. S. Zink (ed.). Bethesda, MD: National Cancer Institute, 1987,

Goitein, M. (1992). "The comparison of treatment plans." *Semin. Radiat. Oncol.* 2:246–256.

Goitein, M., and A. Niemierko. (1996). "Intensity modulated therapy and inhomogeneous dose to the tumor: A note of caution." *Int. J. Radiat. Oncol. Biol. Phys.* 36:519–522.

Graham, M. V., J. A. Purdy, B. Emami, W. Harms , W. Bosch, M. A. Lockett, and C. A. Perez. (1999). "Clinical dose-volume histogram analysis for pneumonitis after 3D treatment for non-small cell lung cancer (NSCLC)." *Int. J. Radiat. Oncol. Biol. Phys.* 45:323–329.

Grosu, A., N. Andratschke, C. Nieder, and M. Molls. (2002). "Retreatment of the spinal cord with palliative radiotherapy." *Int. J. Radiat. Oncol. Biol. Phys.* 52:1288–1292.

Hall, E. J. *Radiobiology for the Radiologist, 4th Edition*. Philadelphia: J. B. Lippincott, 1994.

Hendee, W. R., J. Hopewell, and H.R.Withers. (1998). "Point/Counterpoint Proposition: Long-term changes in irradiated tissues are due principally to vascular damage in the tissues." *Med. Phys.* 25:2265–2268.

Hernando, M. L., L. B. Marks, G. C. Bentel, S.-M. Zhou, D. Hollis, S. K. Das, M. Fan, M. T. Munley, T. D. Shafman, M. S. Anscher, and P. A. Lind. (2001). "Radiation-induced pulmonary toxicity: a dose-volume histogram analysis in 201 patients with lung cancer." *Int. J. Radiat. Oncol. Biol. Phys.* 51:650–659.

Jackson, A. (2001)."Partial irradiation of the rectum." *Semin. Radiat. Oncol.* 11:215–223.

Jackson, A., G. J. Kutcher, and E. D.Yorke. (1993). "Probability of radiation-induced complications for normal tissues with parallel architecture subject to non-uniform irradiation." *Med. Phys.* 20:613–625.

Jackson, A., R. K. Ten Haken, J. M. Robertson, M. L. Kessler, G. J. Kutcher, T. S. Lawrence. (1995). "Analysis of clinical complication data for radiation hepatitis using a parallel architecture model." *Int. J. Radiat. Oncol. Biol. Phys.* 31:883–891.

Jackson, A., M. W. Skwarchuk, M. J. Zelefsky, D. M. Cowen, E. S. Venkatraman, S. Levegrun, C. M. Burman, G. J. Kutcher, Z. Fuks, S. A. Leibel, and C. C. Ling. (2001). "Late rectal bleeding after conformal radiotherapy of prostate cancer (II): volume effects and dose-volume histograms." *Int. J. Radiat. Oncol. Biol. Phys.* 49:685–698.

Joiner, M. C., and A. J. van der Kogel. "The Linear-Quadratic Approach to Fractionation and Calculation of Isoeffect Relationships" in *Basic Clinical Radiobiology, 2ⁿᵈ Edition*. G. G. Steel (ed.). New York: Oxford University Press Inc., pp. 106–121, 1997.

Joiner, M. C. (1997). "Hyperfractionation and Accelerated Radiotherapy" in *Basic Clinical Radiobiology, 2ⁿᵈ Edition*. G. G. Steel (ed.). New York: Oxford University Press Inc., pp. 123–131.

Jones, L., and P. Hoban. (2002). "A comparison of physically and radiobiologically based optimization for IMRT." *Med. Phys.* 29:1447–1455.

Kallman, P., A. Agren, and A. Brahme. (1992). "Tumor and normal tissue responses to fractionated non uniform dose delivery." *Int. J. Radiat. Biol.* 62:249–262.

Kutcher, G. J., and C. Burman. (1991). "Calculation of complication probability factors for nonuniform normal tissue irradiation: the effective volume method." *Int. J. Radiat. Oncol. Biol. Phys.* 21:123–135.

Kwa, S. L. S., J. V. Lebesque, J. C. M. Theuws, L. B. Marks, M. T. Munley, G. Bentel, D. Oetzel, U. Spahn, M. V. Graham, R. E. Drzymala, J. A. Purdy, A. S. Lichter, M. K. Martel, and R. K. Ten Haken. (1998). "Radiation pneumonitis as a function of mean lung dose: An analysis of pooled data from 540 patients." *Int. J. Radiat. Oncol. Biol. Phys.* 42:1–9.

Levegrun, S., A. Jackson, M. J. Zelefsky, E. S. Venkatraman, M. W. Skwarchuk, W. Schlegel, Z. Fuks, S. A. Leibel, and C. C. Ling. (2000). "Analysis of biopsy outcome after three-dimensional conformal radiation therapy of prostate cancer using dose distribution variables and tumor control probability models." *Int. J. Radiat. Oncol. Biol. Phys.* 47:1245–1260.

Levegrun, S., A. Jackson, M. J. Zelefsky, M. W. Skwarchuk, E. S. Venkatraman, W. Schlegel, Z. Fuks, S. A. Leibel, and C. C. Ling. (2001). "Fitting tumor control probability models to biopsy outcome after three-dimensional conformal radiation therapy of prostate cancer: Pitfalls in deducing radiobiologic parameters for tumors from clinical data." *Int. J. Radiat. Oncol. Biol. Phys.* 51:1064–1080.

Lind, B. K., P. Mavroidis, S. Hyodynmaa, and C. Kappas. (1999). "Optimization of the dose level for a given treatment plan to maximize the complication-free tumor cure." *Acta Oncol.* 38:787–798.

Lyman, J. T. (1985). "Complication probability as assessed from dose-volume histograms." *Radiat. Res.* 104:S13–S19.

Lyman, J. T., and A. B. Wolbarst. (1989). "Optimization of radiation therapy IV: A dose-volume histogram reduction algorithm." *Int. J. Radiat. Oncol. Biol. Phys.* 17:433–436.

MacKay, R. I., J. H. Hendry, C. J. Moore, P. C. Williams, and G. Read. (1997). "Predicting late rectal complications following prostate conformal radiotherapy using biologically effective doses and normalized dose-surface histograms." *Br. J. Radiol.* 70:517–526.

MacKillop, W. J., J. H. T. Bates, B. O'Sullivan, and H. R. Withers. (1996). "The effect of delay in treatment on local control by radiotherapy." *Int. J. Radiat. Oncol. Biol. Phys.* 34:243–250.

Maguire, P. D., G. S. Sibley, S.-M. Zhou, T. A. Jamieson, K. L. Light, P. A. Antoine, J. E. Herndon, M. S. Anscher, and L. B. Marks. (1999). "Clinical and dosimetric predictors of radiation-induced esophageal toxicity." *Int. J. Radiat. Oncol. Biol. Phys.* 45:97–103.

Marks, L. B. (2002). "Dosimetric predictors of radiation-induced lung injury." *Int. J. Radiat. Oncol. Biol. Phys.* 54:313–316.

Martel, M. K., R. K. Ten Haken, M. B. Hazuk, A. T. Turrisi, B. A. Fraass, and A. S. Lichter. (1994). "Dose-volume histogram and 3-D treatment planning evaluation of patients with pneumonitis." *Int. J. Radiat. Oncol. Biol. Phys.* 28:575–581.

Martel, M. K., W. M. Sahudak, R. K. Ten Haken, M. L. Kessler, and A. T. Turrisi. (1998). "Fraction size and dose parameters related to the incidence of pericardial effusion." *Int. J. Radiat. Oncol. Biol. Phys.* 40:155–161.

Moiseenko, V., J. Battista, and J. Van Dyk. (2000)."Normal tissue complication probabilities: Dependence on choice of biological model and dose-volume histogram reduction scheme." *Int. J. Radiat. Oncol. Biol. Phys.* 46:983–993.

Munro, T. R., and C. W. Gilbert. (1961). "The relation between tumor lethal doses and radiosensitivity of tumor cells." *Br. J. Radiol.* 34:246–251.

Nieder, C., L. Milas, and K. K. Ang. (2000). "Tissue tolerance to reirradiation." *Semin. Radiat. Oncol.* 10:200–209.

Niemierko, A. (1997). "Reporting and analyzing dose distributions: A concept of equivalent uniform dose." *Med. Phys.* 24:103–110.

Niemierko, A. (1999). "A generalized concept of equivalent uniform dose (EUD)" (Abstract), *Med. Phys.* 26:1100.

Niemierko, A., and M. Goitein. (1991). "Calculation of normal tissue complication probability and dose-volume histogram reduction schemes for tissues with a critical element architecture." *Radiother. Oncol.* 20:166–176.

Niemierko, A., and M. Goitein. (1993a). "Implementation of a model for estimating tumor control probability for an inhomogeneously irradiated tumor." *Radiother. Oncol.* 29:140–147.

Niemierko, A., and M. Goitein. (1993b). "Modeling of normal tissue response to radiation: The critical volume model." *Int. J. Radiat. Oncol. Biol. Phys.* 25:135–145.

Roberts, S. A., and J. H. Hendry. (1998). "A realistic closed-form radiobiological model of clinical tumor-control data incorporating intertumor heterogeneity." *Int. J. Radiat. Oncol. Biol. Phys.* 41: 689–699.

Roesink, J. M., M. A. Moerland, J. J. Battermann, G. J. Horduk, and C. H. J. Terhaard. (2001). "Quantitative dose-volume response analysis of changes in parotid gland function after radiotherapy in the head-and-neck region." *Int. J. Radiat. Oncol. Biol. Phys.* 51:938–946.

Schultheiss, T. E., C. G. Orton, and R. A. Peck. (1983). "Models in radiotherapy: Volume effects." *Med. Phys.* 10:410–415.

Schultheiss, T. E., L. E. Kun, K. K. Ang, and L. C. Stephens. (1995). "Radiation response of the central nervous system." *Int. J. Radiat. Oncol. Biol. Phys.* 31:1093–1112.

Seppenwoolde, Y., and J. V. Lebesque. (2001). "Partial irradiation of the lung." *Semin. Radiat. Oncol.* 11:247–258.

Södertröm, S., and A. Brahme. (1993). "Optimization of the dose delivery in a few field techniques using radiobiological objective functions." *Med. Phys.* 20:1201–1210.

Steel, G. G. (ed.). *Basic Clinical Radiobiology, 2ⁿᵈ Edition.* New York: Oxford University Press Inc., 1997.

Stewart, F. A. "Re-treatment Tolerance of Normal Tissues" in *Basic Clinical Radiobiology, 2nd Edition*. G. G. Steel (ed.). New York: Oxford University Press Inc., pp. 203–211, 1997.

Suit, H., S. Skates, A. Tahian, P. Okunieff, and J. T. Effird. (1992). "Clinical implications of heterogeneity of tumor response to radiation therapy." *Radiother. Oncol.* 25:251–260.

Ten Haken, R. (2003). Personal communication.

Thames, H. D., and J. H. Hendry. *Fractionation in Radiotherapy*. New York: Taylor and Francis, 1987.

Tomé, W. A., and J. F. Fowler. (2000). "Selective boosting of tumor subvolumes." *Int. J. Radiat. Oncol. Biol. Phys.* 48:593–599.

Tomé, W. A., and J. F. Fowler. (2002). "On cold spots in tumor subvolumes." *Med. Phys.* 29:1590–1598.

Tucker, S. L., H. D. Thames, and J. M. G. Taylor. (1990). "How well is the probability of tumor cure after fractionated irradiation described by Poisson statistics?" *Radiat. Res.* 124:273–282.

Vineberg, K. A., A. Eisbruch, M. M.Coselmon, D. L. McShan, M. L. Kessler, and B. A. Fraass. (2002). "Is uniform target dose possible in imrt plans in the head and neck?" *Int. J. Radiat. Oncol. Biol. Phys.* 52:1159–1172.

Wang, X.-H., R. Mohan, A. Jackson, S. A. Leibel, Z. Fuks, and C. C. Ling. (1995). "Optimization of intensity-modulated 3D conformal treatment plans based on biological indices." *Radiother. Oncol.* 37:140–152.

Webb, S. (1994). "Optimum parameters in a model for tumor control probability including interpatient heterogeneity." *Phys. Med. Biol.* 39:1895–1914.

Wheldon, T. E., C. Deehan, E. G. Wheldon, and A. Barrett. (1998). "The linear-quadratic transformation of dose-volume histograms in fractionated radiotherapy." *Radiother. Oncol.* 46:285–295.

Wilner, J., K. Baier, E. Caragiani, A. Tschammler, and M. Flentje. (2002). "Dose, volume and tumor control predictions in primary radiotherapy of non-small-cell lung cancer." *Int. J. Radiat. Oncol. Biol. Phys.* 52:382–389.

Withers, H. R. (2000). "Biological Aspects of Conformal Therapy." *Acta Oncol.* 39:569–577.

Withers, H. R., J. M. G. Taylor, and B. Maciejewski. (1988). "Treatment volume and tissue tolerance." *Int. J. Radiat. Oncol. Biol. Phys.* 15:751–759.

Wu, Q., R. Mohan, A. Niemierko, and R. Schmidt-Ullrich. (2002). "Optimization of intensity-modulated radiotherapy plans based on the equivalent uniform dose." *Int. J. Radiat. Oncol. Biol. Phys.* 52:224–235.

Yorke, E. D. (2001). "Modeling the effects of inhomogeneous dose distributions in normal tissues." *Semin. Radiat. Oncol.* 11:197–209.

Yorke, E. D., G. J. Kutcher, A. Jackson, and C. C. Ling. (1993). "Probability of radiation-induced complications in normal tissues with parallel architecture under conditions of uniform whole or partial organ irradiation." *Radiother. Oncol.* 26:226–237.

Yorke, E., A. Jackson, K. Rosenzweig, and C. C. Ling. (2000). "The Lyman and a current parallel model: are they equivalent in predicting radiation induced lung toxicity." CD-ROM Proceedings of the World Congress on Medical Physics and Biomedical Engineering, July 23–28, 2000, Chicago, IL.

Yorke, E. D., A. Jackson, K. E. Rosenzweig, S. A. Merrick, D. Gabrys, E. S. Venkatraman, C. M. Burman, S. A. Leibel, and C. C. Ling. (2002). "Dose-volume factors contributing to the incidence of radiation pneumonitis in non-small-cell lung cancer patients treated with three-dimensional conformal radiation therapy." *Int. J. Radiat. Oncol. Biol. Phys.* 54:329–339.

Zagars, G., T. E. Schultheiss, and L. J. Peters. (1987). "Inter-tumor heterogeneity and radiation dose-control curves." *Radiother. Oncol.* 8:353–362.

Zaider, M., and H. I. Amols. (1998). "A little to a lot or a lot to a little: Is NTCP always minimized in multiport therapy." *Int. J. Radiat. Oncol. Biol. Phys.* 41:945–950.

Zaider, M., and G. N. Minerbo. (2000). "Tumor control probability: A formulation applicable to any temporal protocol of dose delivery." *Phys. Med. Biol.* 45:279–293.

Zelefsky, M. J., Z. Fuks, M. Hunt, Y. Yamada, C. Marion, C. C. Ling, H. Amols, E. S. Venkatraman, and S. A. Leibel. (2002). "High-dose intensity modulated radiation therapy for prostate cancer: Early toxicity and biochemical outcome in 772 patients." *Int. J. Radiat. Oncol. Biol. Phys.* 53:1111–1116.

# Aperture-Based Inverse Planning

**D. M. Shepard, Ph.D.[1], M. A. Earl, Ph.D.[1], C. X. Yu, D.Sc.[1], Y. Xiao, Ph.D.[2]**
[1]University of Maryland School of Medicine, Baltimore, Maryland
[2]Thomas Jefferson University, Philadelphia, Pennsylvania



## Introduction

The full benefits of intensity modulated radiation therapy (IMRT) can only be realized through the application of inverse planning techniques. With inverse planning, the desired dose distribution or the desired biological end points are used to specify the goals of the treatment. An optimization algorithm determines the plan parameters that best reflect the treatment goals.

In this review, inverse planning techniques are divided into two distinct categories:

1. Beamlet-based inverse planning.

2. Aperture-based inverse planning.

This distinction is based on the treatment parameters that are optimized. In beamlet-based inverse planning, each field is divided into a grid of beamlets (pencil beams) and the weights of these beamlets are optimized. The optimization provides a distribution of the beamlet weights, also called a beam intensity distribution or an intensity map. After the optimization is complete, each intensity map is sequenced into a set of deliverable aperture shapes. In aperture-based inverse planning, a set of deliverable apertures is included in the optimization, and the optimization parameters include aperture shapes, weights, or both. The optimized treatment plan does not require sequencing, and it is ready to deliver.

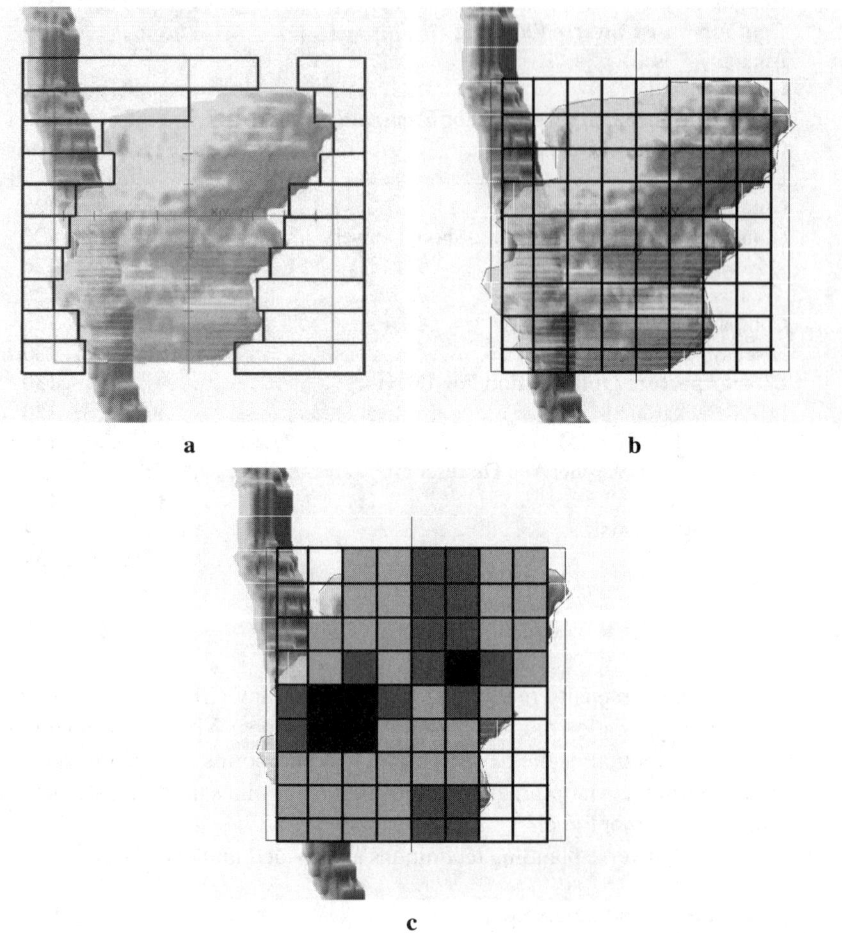

Figure 1. An illustration of the conventional inverse planning approach. (a) The leaves of the MLC are shaped to match the beam's eye view (BEV) of the tumor volume. (b) The BEV of the tumor is divided into a series of finite size pencil beams, and the corresponding pencil beam dose distributions are computed. (c) The pencil beam intensities are optimized and the result is an optimized intensity map. The three shades in the map represent three different intensity levels. Before delivery, this intensity map must be translated into deliverable shapes.

Current inverse-planning methods for IMRT (Bortfeld et al. 1994; Chui, LoSasso, and Spirou 1994; Galvin, Chen, and Smith 1993; Webb 1994, 1998a,b) are typically beamlet-based. They begin by dividing the beam's eye view (BEV) of the tumor into a series of finite-sized pencil beams or beamlets. The corresponding dose distribution for each pencil beam is then calculated. Next, a two-step approach is applied to produce an optimized treatment plan that is ready for delivery. In the first step, the pencil beam intensities are optimized (see figure 1). During the optimization, the quality of the treatment plan is scored using an objective function that reduces the entire treatment plan into a single numerical value. In the second step, a leaf-sequencing algorithm is applied that translates each optimized intensity pattern into a set of deliverable beam apertures (Xia and Verhey 1998; Crooks et al. 2002; Langer, Thai, and Papiez 2002; Saw et al. 2001; Convery and Webb 1998) (see figure 2). The goal of the leaf sequencing step is to determine a set of apertures that when combined will deliver the optimized map.

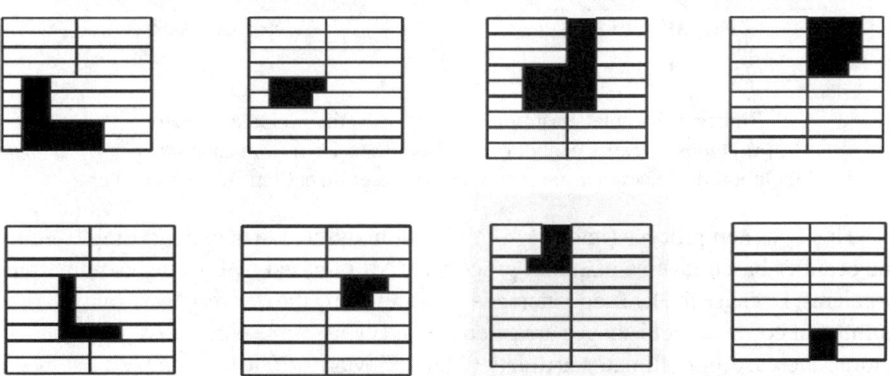

**Figure 2.** A leaf sequencing algorithm was applied to the intensity map in figure 1c. The leaf sequencer determined that the optimized intensity pattern with three intensity levels can be delivered with these eight apertures.

The multileaf collimator (MLC) design of each manufacturer imposes restrictions on the possible aperture shapes. Figure 3 illustrates sample constraints applicable to the Elekta SL20 MLC. For example, a minimum separation of 0.8 cm is enforced between each leaf and its opposing leaf. The separation requirement applies to each leaf and the leaves adjacent to its opposing leaf (MLC Manual 1993; Bortfeld, Stein, and Preiser 1997), thus making interdigitation impossible. The leaves also have a limit of travel across the central axis of 12.5 cm. With the two-step inverse planning approach, these constraints are accounted for in the leaf sequencing after the optimization is complete. Due to the separation of intensity optimization and leaf sequencing, a large number of apertures are typically required for recreating the optimized beam intensities. Each MLC constraint results in further increases of the required number of beam apertures.

The pencil beam intensities are often considered as continuous non-negative variables during the optimization process. Before the leaf-sequencing step some implementations of IMRT convert each optimized intensity map into a series of discrete levels. This introduces quantization errors and may result in a loss in some treatment plan quality. Further degradation can occur due to aperture-specific effects such as tongue-and-groove and leakage that are not considered during the optimization.

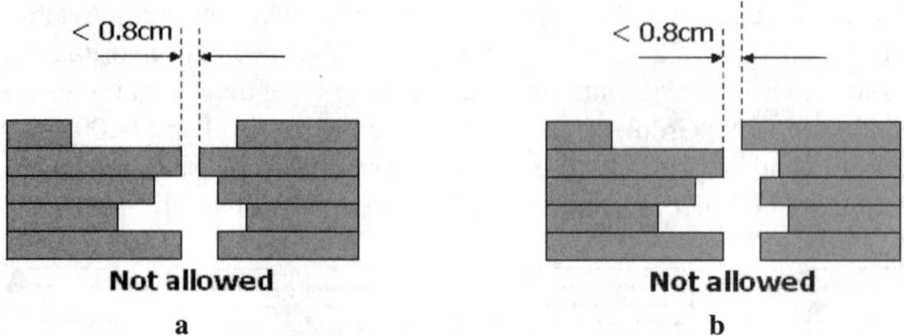


**Figure 3.** Sample constraints applicable to the Elekta collimator.
(a) Opposed leaves cannot come closer than 1 cm from each other.
(b) Opposed adjacent leaves cannot come closer than 1 cm from each other.

This two-step process (intensity optimization and leaf sequencing) employed in the beamlet-based inverse planning process for MLC-based IMRT creates numerous problems. Because the leaf sequencing is constrained by the delivery hardware, a large number of complex field shapes are often needed. This can lead to a loss in efficiency and an increase in collimator artifacts (Cho and Marks 2000). Attempts have been made to simplify the delivery by either grouping the intensity levels (Bar, Alber, and Nüsslin 2001) or smoothing the intensity distributions (Alber and Nüsslin 2000; Spirou et al. 2001). However, such attempts are always accompanied by a loss in treatment plan quality. Moreover, since the leaf sequencing process is often outside the optimization loop, the MLC specific effects such as leakage, the tongue-and-groove design, and head scatter variations are excluded from the optimization process. As the result, the highly conformal dose distributions of the "optimal" plan as shown on the computer cannot be realized in the patient (Cho and Marks 2000). Efforts to include these delivery-related effects in the leaf-sequencing process always increase the number of beam segments and decrease delivery efficiency (van Santvoort and Heijmen 1996; Webb et al. 1997). When a large number of segments are used, there are typically segments requiring a low number of monitor units (MUs) along with small off-axis fields. These segments introduce new challenges for accurate dose calculation and unrealistic requirements for geometric accuracy of the MLC and dosimetric accuracy of the linear accelerator (Budgell et al. 2000; LoSasso, Chui, and Ling 1998). As the result, QA efforts must be intensified in order to achieve the well-established safety and accuracy standards (LoSasso, Chui, and Ling 1998).

Aperture optimization is an inverse planning technique designed to reduce the complexity of IMRT treatment plans. With aperture optimization, each aperture considered by the optimizer is guaranteed to satisfy the delivery constraints. Hence, no leaf sequencing is required, and there is no need to divide the final intensity maps into discrete intensity levels. Current aperture optimization techniques can be subdivided into two approaches:

1.　Contour-based treatment planning, and

2.　Direct aperture optimization (DAO).

The details of these approaches are described separately in the following sections.

## Contour-Based Inverse Planning

### Anatomy-Based

One approach to aperture optimization is to predefine the aperture shapes (before the optimization) based upon the patient's anatomy (Xiao et al. 2000, 2003; Bednarz et al. 2002; Chen et al. 2002). For each beam angle, aperture shapes are constructed using the BEV of the target and the organs at risk (OARs). The first aperture is chosen to conform to the BEV of the target plus an appropriate margin. Additional apertures are added to protect any OAR that is exposed within the BEV of the target. For example, in treatment planning for a prostate patient, one might seek adequate tumor coverage while sparing the rectum and bladder. Thus, the following apertures could be created for each beam angle (see figure 4):

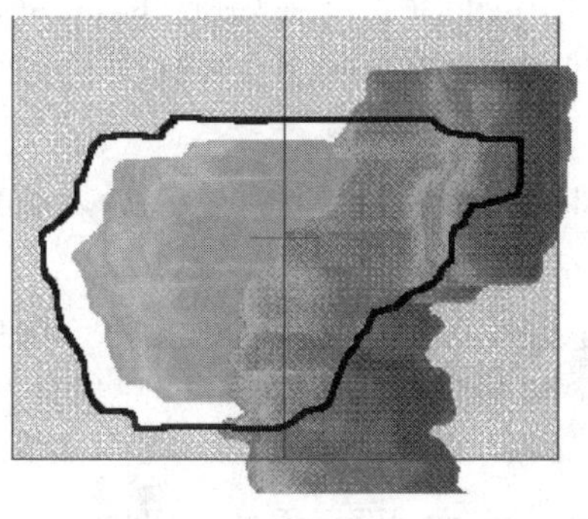
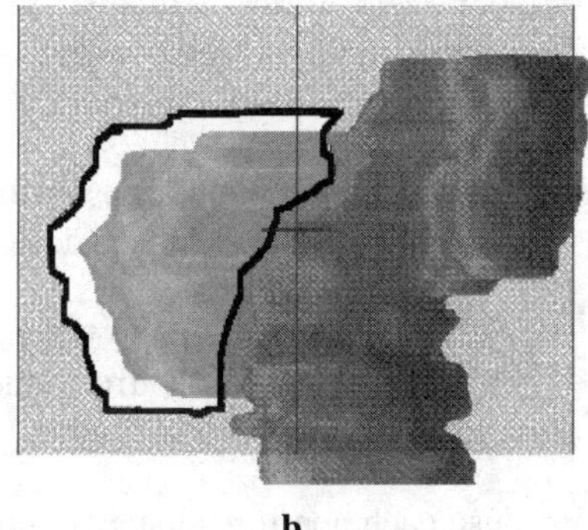

a　　　　　　　　　　　　　　　　b

**Figure 4.** (a) An aperture conforming to the prostate plus a margin.
(b) An additional portal aperture with the rectum blocked.

1.  An aperture shaped to match the BEV of the planning target volume (PTV).

2.  An aperture shaped to match the BEV of the PTV minus the BEV of the rectum.

3.  An aperture shaped to match the BEV of the PTV minus the BEV of the bladder.

4.  An aperture shaped to match the BEV of the PTV minus the BEV of the bladder and rectum.

If a particular OAR cuts through the center of the BEV of the target, two separate apertures are created to block the OAR and treat the uncovered region of the PTV.

In the implementation of Xiao et al. (2000, 2003), the apertures are created using the following steps:

1.  Select a field that conforms to the combined outline of all targets projected back to the radiation point source, and repeat for all orientations of the treatment unit.

2.  Select a field that conforms to the projection of the boost volume back to the radiation point source, and repeat for all orientations of the treatment unit. The boost volume is the portion of the target that is to receive a higher dose compared to regions of the target taken to the lowest dose.

3.  If there are other targets at different dose levels, repeat step 2 for regions of the target that are to receive the next higher level of dose.

4.  For every critical structure lying in the path of the conformal beam of the complete target, select a field segment that conforms to the target but fully shields the critical structure.

5.  Repeat the previous step for the field segments that encompass each of the volumes receiving higher dose.

6.  Select, for the complete target, extra segments to adjust for the dose inhomogeneity that results from shielding critical structures that do not run along the whole length of the target.

Because each aperture shape is known, aperture specific effects such as tongue-and-groove and leakage can be incorporated into the dose calculation. The aperture weights are optimized after the dose calculation. In the work of Xiao et al. (2000), the aperture weight optimization has been performed using a simultaneous projection algorithm (Cimmino's algorithm), mixed integer programming (Bednarz et al. 2002), and an iterative least-square algorithm (Chen et al. 2002). Figure 5 shows an optimized result produced by applying this technique to a prostate patient.

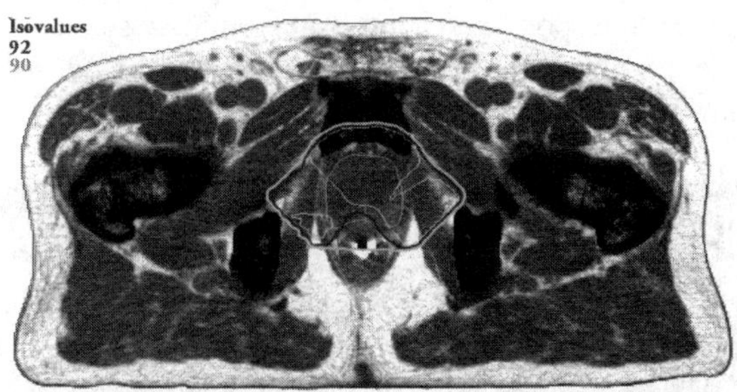


**Figure 5.** The 92% isodose line is pulled away from the rectum when an aperture is added with rectal blocking for all six beam angles (45°, 90°, 135°, 225°, 270°, 315°) treating the prostate.

An anatomy-based segmentation tool (ABST) has been developed by DeGersem (DeGersem et al. 2001a). ABST applies a series of rules that produce apertures in addition to those shaped to match either the BEV of the target or the BEV of the target minus one or more sensitive structures. For example, the ABST algorithm creates segments close to and conformally avoiding the organs at risk. These segments are designed based upon the following observation: If multiple beams are used to irradiate the PTV but the overlap of the PTV with critical organs is blocked, then an underdosage can be expected in the regions of the PTV that are close to the OARs. Additional segments are designed to boost these underdosed regions. A more detailed list of the rules applied in ABST was provided in DeGersem et al. (2001a,b).

## Isodose-Based

Through an iterative approach, isodose curves can be used to guide a contour-based approach to IMRT treatment planning. This technique has been employed at William Beaumont Hospital to improve dose uniformity with tangential breast radiotherapy (Kestin et al. 2000; Remouchamps et al. 2003). The inverse planning begins by computing the three-dimensional (3-D) dose distribution for equally weighted, open tangential fields (i.e., no blocks, no wedges). Separate MLC segments are then constructed to conform to the BEV projections of the 3-D isodose surfaces in 5% increments, ranging from the 120% to 100% isodose surface (see figure 6). Additional medial and lateral MLC segments are produced that conform to the lung tissue in the fields. Finally, the aperture weights are optimized to produce the IMRT treatment plan.

For ten early-stage breast cancer patients, researchers produced a conventional treatment plan (using wedges) and an IMRT plan (using the contour-based inverse planning) (Kestin et al. 2000). Between six and eight segments typically were employed, and the open segments delivered a majority of the dose (median of 78%). Because of the modest number of segments, treatment delivery was maintained to less than 10 minutes. In addition, the results demonstrated that the contour-based optimized plans result in smaller "hot spots" and a lower maximum dose while maintaining similar coverage of the treatment volume. Figure 7 shows an isodose comparison for a breast-patient optimized using this technique.

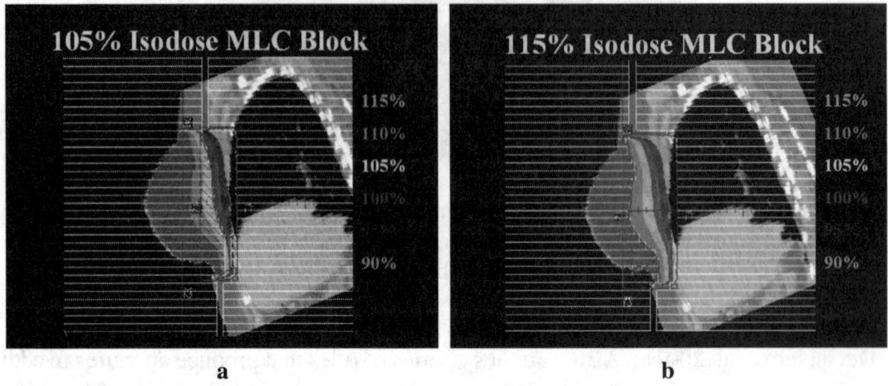


**Figures 6.** Aperture shapes are created to match the isodose curves for the open tangents.
(a) An aperture shaped to match the 105% isodose line.
(b) An aperture shaped to match the 115% isodose line.

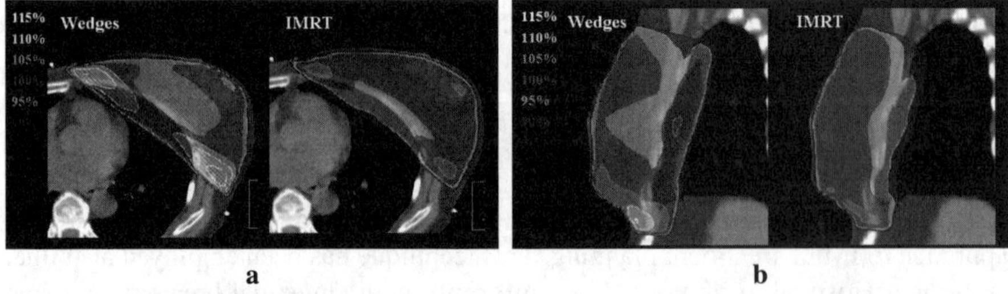


**Figure 7.** The aperture-based IMRT treatment plan as compared with the conventional plan.
Note the improved uniformity of dose in the breast with the aperture-based IMRT plan.
(a) Axial comparison. (b) Sagittal comparison.

## Direct Aperture Optimization For Step-And-Shoot IMRT

## Overall Scheme

Direct aperture optimization (DAO) (Shepard et al. 2002) is an inverse planning technique where the aperture shapes and aperture weights are optimized simultaneously. The beam angles and number of apertures per angle are both specified in the prescription. Unlike the contour-based planning methods described above, DAO includes the aperture shape as a parameter in the optimization. The optimization only considers aperture shapes that satisfy the constraints imposed by the MLC. Additional delivery considerations, such as the minimum aperture size and minimum number of MUs, can also be included in the optimization. At the end of the optimization, the treatment plan is ready for delivery.

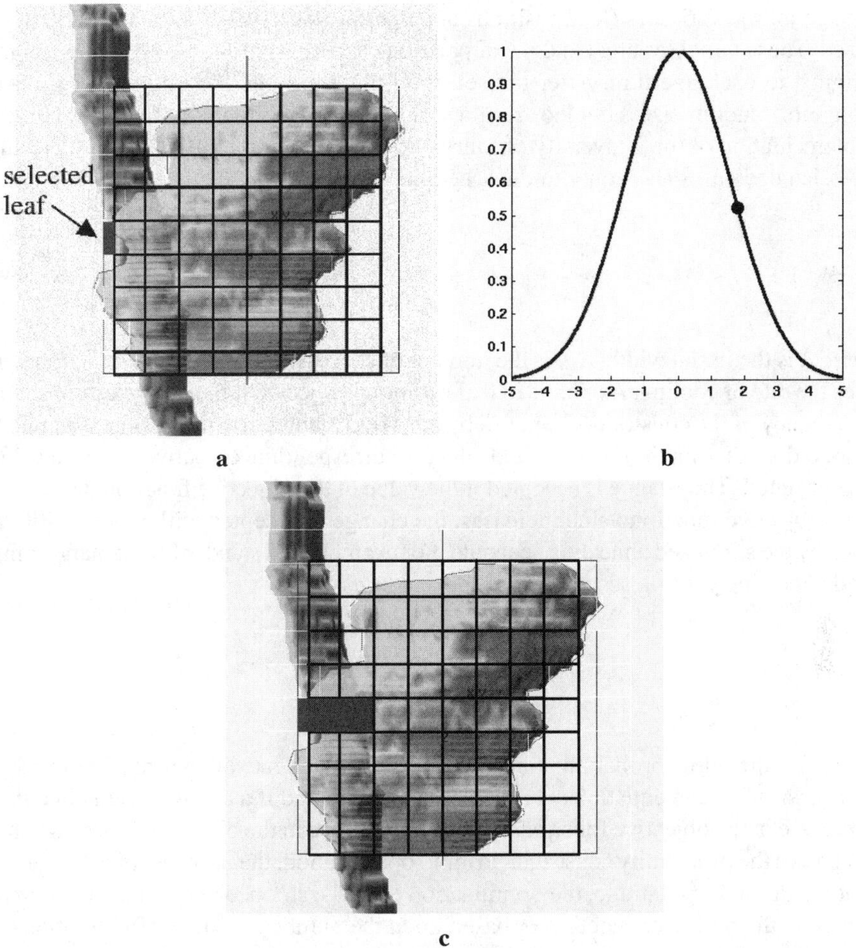


**Figure 8.** The DAO routine randomly selects a leaf position for modification. (a) The highlighted leaf has been chosen by the optimizer. (b) A random number is selected on a Gaussian scale to determine the size and direction of the change in leaf position. In this case, the leaf will move into the field by 2 units (2 pencil beam widths). (c) The modified aperture shape.

124                           **D. M. Shepard et al.**

A simulated annealing algorithm (Kirkpatrick, Gelatt, and Vecchi 1983; Geman and Geman 1984; Pincus 1970; Cerny 1982; Binder and Stauffer 1985) has been applied to perform the DAO optimization. The DAO algorithm takes as input the: (1) beam angles, (2) beam energies, and (3) number of apertures per beam angle. Each aperture is initialized to the BEV of the target. The optimization begins by computing the objective function for the initial beam configuration. The algorithm then cycles through all the variables (leaf positions and aperture weights), which are to be optimized. These variables are: (1) the leaf positions for each aperture, and (2) the weight assigned to each aperture. After the selection of a variable, the optimizer makes a change of random size sampled from a Gaussian distribution (see figure 8). In the implementation of the University of Maryland (Shepard et al. 2002), the width of the Gaussian decreases according to the schedule,

$$\sigma = 1 + (A - 1)e^{-\frac{\log(n_{succ} + 1)}{T_0^{step}}} \tag{1}$$

where $A$ is the initial width, $n_{succ}$ is the number of successful iterations, and $T_0^{step}$ quantifies the rate of cooling. A change in leaf position is rejected if the new aperture shape violates any of the constraints imposed by the MLC. Otherwise, the change is applied, the new dose distribution is computed, and the corresponding objective function value is determined. The change is accepted if the value of the objective function decreases. If the objective function value increases, the change is accepted with a probability $P$ given by the simulated annealing schedule. For example, if a standard Boltzmann simulated annealing cooling schedule is used:

$$P = 2B \frac{1}{1 + e^{\frac{\log(n_{succ} + 1)}{T_0^{prob}}}} \tag{2}$$

where $B$ is the initial probability and $T_0^{prob}$ quantifies the rate of cooling. The number of successes, $n_{succ}$, in equations (1) and (2) is incremented if a change results in either a decrease in the objective function value or an increase in the objective function value that passes the probability constraint. Prior to optimization, the user specifies the termination criteria. For example, the optimization could be stopped based upon the rate of change in the objective function or based upon the number of successful iterations.

Prior to evaluation of the objective function, each new aperture shape is tested for deliverability to ensure that the MLC constraints are satisfied. In addition, each aperture shape is checked to ensure that delivery restrictions specific to the intended machine are maintained. Hence, the resulting plan is ready for delivery and no additional step is required.

## Dose Calculation

DAO uses precomputed pencil beam dose distributions to increase the speed of the optimization algorithm. For each beam angle, the pencil beam dose distributions are computed before the optimization using a rectangular MLC shape large enough to cover the BEV of the target plus a margin.

A Monte Carlo-based dose engine (Rogers et al. 1995) was used to compute the pencil beams for the DAO results included in this chapter. The details of the Monte Carlo engine used are provided elsewhere (Naqvi, Earl, and Shepard 2003). The total dose from each aperture is computed as a sum of the unblocked pencil beams.

Each field shape undergoes hundreds of modifications during the optimization. After a change in leaf position, the affected pencil beams are simply added or subtracted from the total dose distribution. The dose calculation at each step in optimization can therefore be performed very rapidly. At the end of the optimization, a final dose calculation is performed using the optimized aperture shapes and aperture weights.

## Number Of Intensity Levels

With DAO, the intensity of each aperture is allowed to vary continuously. (This stands in contrast to the two-step approach where the intensity maps are binned into discrete levels before leaf sequencing.) In combination, these apertures produce complex intensity maps. The relationship between the number of intensity levels per beam direction and the number of apertures per beam direction can be expressed as:

$$N_n = 2^n - 1 \tag{3}$$

where $n$ is the number of apertures and $N$ is the possible number of intensity levels. For example, it is possible to produce seven intensity levels when just three apertures are used. This is illustrated with an optimized set of apertures from a DAO plan shown in figure 9. With five apertures, the number of possible intensity level jumps is 31. Sixty-three intensity levels are possible when six apertures are used. Consequently, highly modulated intensity patterns can be produced using a relatively small number of apertures per beam direction. This offers a significant advantage over the traditional two-step process where the number of apertures is typically two to three times the number of intensity levels (Xia and Verhey 1998). For instance, for 15 intensity levels, DAO requires 4 apertures as compared to the 30 to 45 apertures required by traditional algorithms.

                    **D. M. Shepard et al.**

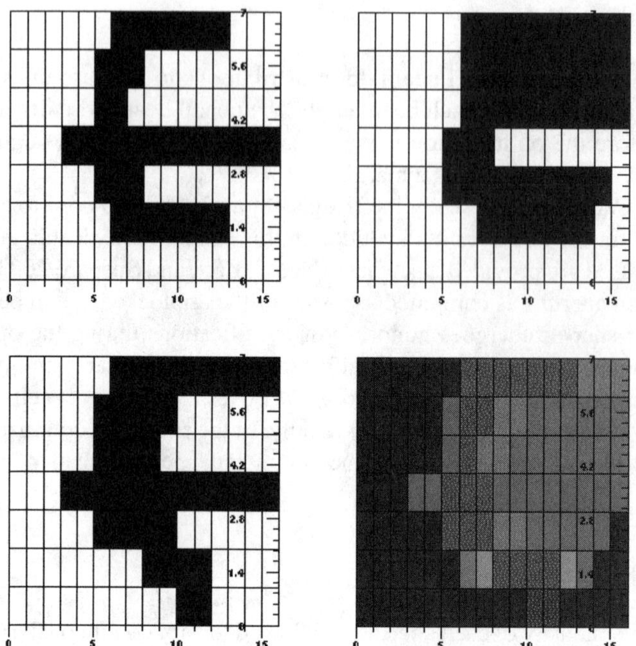

**Figure 9.** The three aperture shapes and corresponding intensity map for one beam direction from an optimized DAO plan. Here, three apertures result in seven intensity levels.

## Clinical Results Using Step-And-Shoot Delivery

### Head And Neck Patient

In figure 10, results are shown for a head and neck patient planned using nine beam angles with five apertures per angle. In the optimization 6390 voxels were included in the objective function with a grid size of $4 \times 4 \times 3$ mm$^3$. Because this patient had previously received radiation, spinal cord sparing was essential. The treatment plan also sought to spare the mandible. Note that the optimized plan maintained all of the spinal cord below 20% of the prescription.

### Pancreas Patient

Figure 11 show results from a DAO optimization for a pancreas patient. Seven beam angles were used with five apertures delivered from each. In the optimization 19,622 voxels were scored in the objective function, and a grid size of $4 \times 4 \times 3$ mm$^3$ was used. The goal was to obtain adequate tumor coverage while sparing the spinal cord, left kidney, right kidney, and liver.

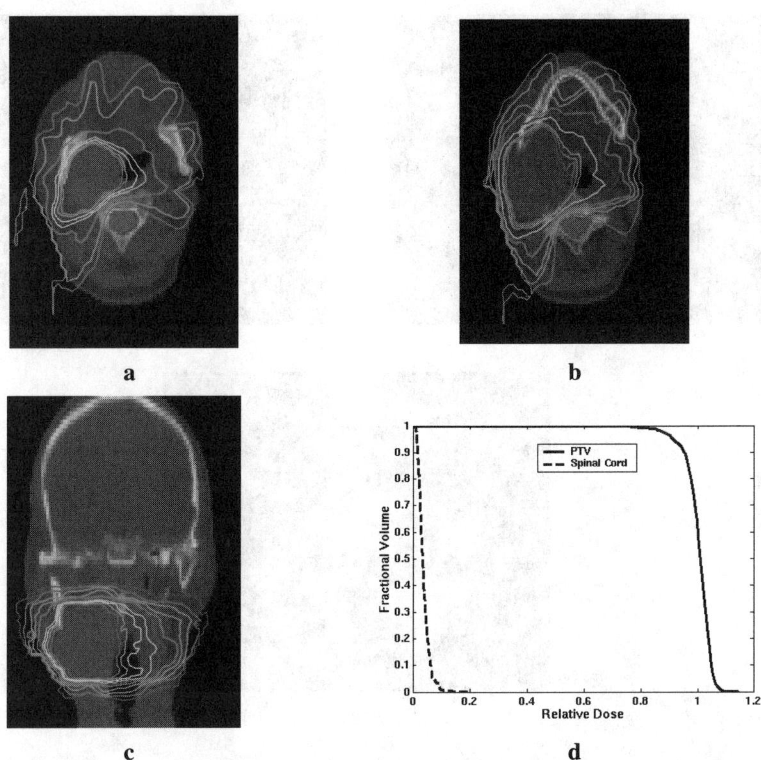



**Figure 10.** Optimized results using direct aperture optimization for a head and neck patient. The isodose lines plotted are 95%, 90%, 80%, 70%, 50%, 30%, and 20%. (a) An axial image; (b) a second axial image; (c) a coronal image; and (d) a cumulative dose volume histogram.

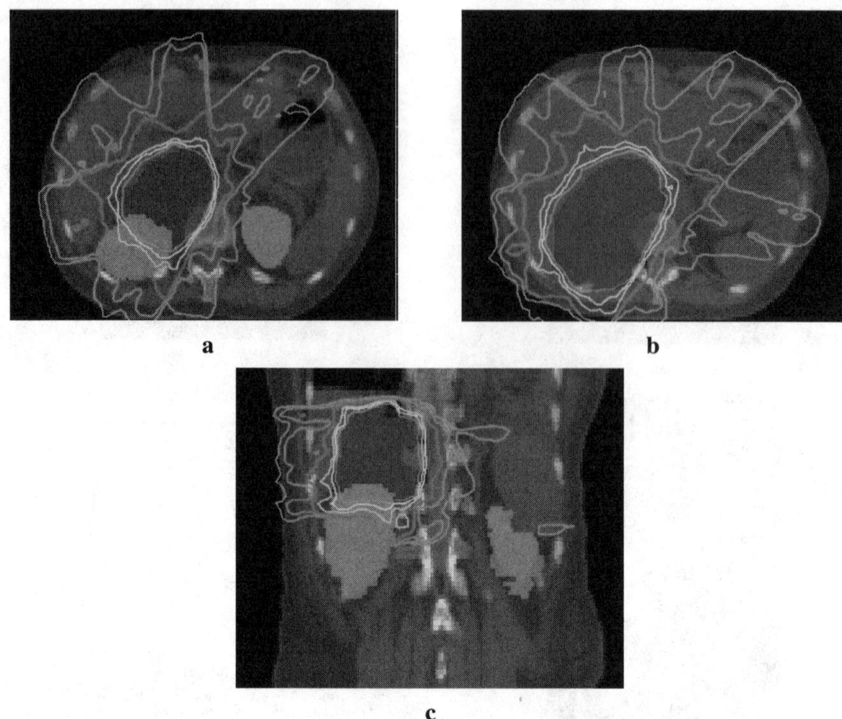

**Figure 11.** Optimized results using direct aperture optimization for a pancreas patient.
The isodose lines plotted are 90%, 80%, 70%, 50%, 40%, and 30%. (a) An axial image;
(b) a second axial image; and (c) a coronal image

## Comparison With CORVUS®

Treatment plans for four treatment sites (head and neck, lung, prostate, and pancreas)
were produced using the two-step approach as implemented in a commercial planning
system (CORVUS®). The same patients were planned using DAO. The prescription
parameters were adjusted so that both plans were judged by a clinician to be of comparable clinical value. The resulting plans were then compared in terms of efficiency.

Table 1 provides a comparison in terms of the number of segments and the total
number of monitor units.

**Table 1**

| Treatment Site | CORVUS No. of Segments | CORVUS No. of MU | DAO No. of Segments | DAO No. of MU |
|---|---|---|---|---|
| Head and Neck | 190 | 1094 | 20 | 283 |
| Lung | 576 | 2100 | 21 | 340 |
| Prostate | 251 | 1095 | 21 | 346 |
| Pancreas | 556 | 2187 | 21 | 330 |

Note that the DAO results provide a 75% reduction in the number of MUs and a 94% reduction in the number of segments.

It should be emphasized that these results are specific to the use of CORVUS in conjunction with an Elekta MLC. It is possible that with improved leaf sequencing (Langer, Thai, and Papiez 2001; Dai and Zhu 2001; Crooks et al. 2002) or smoothing of the intensity maps (Spirou et al. 2001; Webb, Convery, and Evans 1998), one could reduce the number of segments associated with the conventional two-step approach.

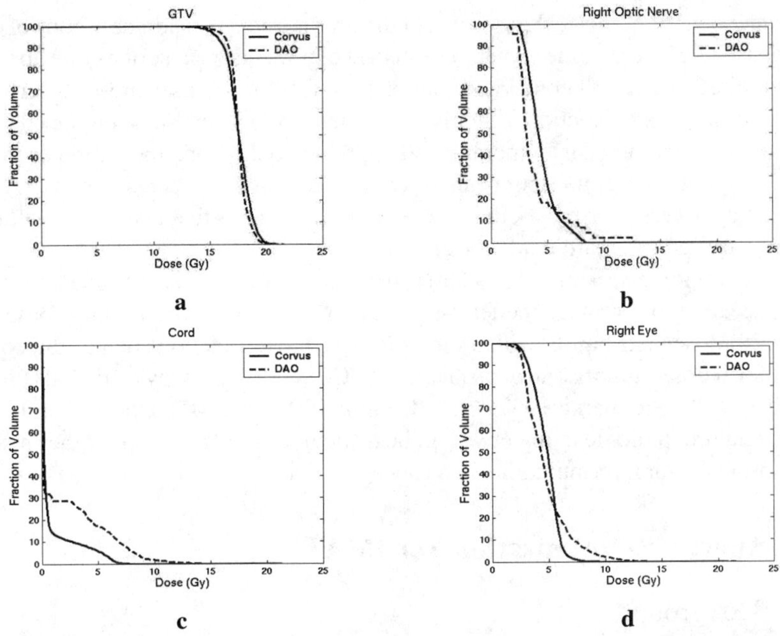

**Figure 12.** A DVH comparison with CORVUS® for a head and neck patient.

In figure 12 a dose-volume histogram (DVH) comparison is provided between DAO and CORVUS for the head and neck patient presented in table 1. This patient had previously been treated in our clinic using the CORVUS plan. The same seven beam angles were used in each case. In comparing the DVHs, it can be seen that the plan produced using DAO provided improved tumor dose homogeneity as compared with CORVUS. The CORVUS plan, however, provided improved sparing of the critical structures. By adjusting the relative weights assigned to the treatment goals, it may be possible to further reduce the differences between these two plans.

## Discussion

As compared with conventional IMRT planning techniques, DAO is able to produce comparable dose conformity with more efficient treatment deliveries. The reduction in the number of beam segments not only improves delivery efficiency, it also makes it easier to perform the required QA procedures. Concerns regarding the dosimetric effects associated with current IMRT delivery, such as the use of small MUs, tongue-and-groove effects, and head scatter uncertainties for very small off-axis fields are greatly reduced. As compared with contour-based inverse planning, the fact that the DAO does not pre-determine the aperture shapes not only saves the aperture definition step but also has the theoretical advantage of not confining the search space of the optimization.

Another benefit of this technique is that the user is given considerable control over the complexity of the treatment plan. For instance, if the user prescribes one aperture per beam direction, a 3-D conformal plan is produced; if the user prescribes five or six apertures per beam direction, a highly modulated IMRT plan can be produced. With this technique, one can take an incremental approach to the implementation of IMRT by starting with two apertures per beam direction and gradually increasing to a greater number of apertures. For most clinical cases, no more than five apertures per beam angle are required (Shepard et al. 2002).

Another important feature of this tool is the flexibility of simulated annealing algorithm. One can easily replace the least-squares objective function, which is based on the physical dose distribution with a biological objective function such as the equivalent uniform dose, tumor control probability (TCP), or P+ (Stavrev et al. 2001; Jones and Hoban 2000; Niemierko 1997, 1998; Brahme 1999a,b, 2001). Due to their highly nonlinear nature, biological objective can be difficult to implement into other mathematical programming formulations in a robust fashion.

## Direct Aperture Optimization For IMAT

### IMAT Background

Intensity-modulated arc therapy (IMAT) (Yu 1995; Yu et al. 2002; Earl et al. 2001, 2003; Li et al. 2001) is a rotational approach to IMRT that serves as an alternative to tomotherapy (Mackie et al. 1993, 1995; Olivera et al. 1999; Carol, Dawson, and Spied 1997). With tomotherapy, a binary MLC is used to modulate the intensity of radiation as the source rotates about the patient. In contrast, IMAT can be delivered on a conventional linear accelerator with a conventional MLC. Simultaneous MLC and gantry motion are incorporated into IMAT delivery. The treatment is composed of a series of arcs, and the MLC field shape changes continuously during gantry rotation from the beginning to the end of each arc. Overlapping arcs can be used to modulate the intensity of radiation delivered from each beam angle. With an appropriate number of arcs, IMAT plans can be delivered with an efficiency approaching that of conventional radiotherapy.

For IMAT treatment planning, each arc is approximated as a series of equi-spaced beams. Linear interpolation is used to determine the MLC shape at each point between adjacent beams. Consequently, an important link exists between adjacent shapes, and large changes in the aperture shape from one beam angle to the next will result in a degradation in the quality of the dose distribution.

The interconnectedness of shapes within each arc significantly complicates the leaf-sequencing step and makes production of IMAT treatment plans using this conventional two-step approach extremely cumbersome. Generally, 8 to 10 arcs are required to achieve three intensity levels (Yu 1995). IMAT is therefore not amenable to the traditional two-step inverse planning technique.

## Theory Of DAO For IMAT

For IMAT treatment planning, the optimizer takes as input: (1) the number arcs, (2) the angular range of the each, and (3) the beam energies (Earl et al. 2003). The optimization process is very similar to that used for creating step-and-shoot treatment plans for DAO. The parameters in the optimization are the leaf positions and the arc weights. If the gantry speed or dose rate is allowed to vary within an individual arc, a separate beam weight is assigned at each angle. Otherwise, a single weight is assigned to each arc.

Each MLC shape is initiated to conform to the BEV of the tumor. At each iteration in the optimization, a parameter is selected randomly. The parameter is then changed by an amount sampled from a Gaussian distribution whose width decreases with iteration number according to the simulated annealing schedule outline previously.

After each change in leaf position, the new aperture shape is checked to determine if it satisfies the delivery constraints. The delivery constraints are divided into two categories: MLC constraints and IMAT constraints. The MLC-based constraints are the same as those encountered in static beam delivery (see the previous section). IMAT constraints are based upon the leaf-travel speed and the gantry rotation speed. Leaves between adjacent angles within an arc are constrained so that their distance of travel does not exceed $d$ where $d$ can be computed using:

$$d = \frac{v_l \Delta \theta}{\omega} \qquad (4)$$

Here, $v_l$ is the leaf travel, $w$ is the gantry angular rotation speed, and $\Delta\theta$ is the angular separation between adjacent angles, typically 10°. Due to the interpolation that occurs between adjacent angles, there can be discrepancies between the calculated and delivered dose distributions. The degradation in the quality of the plan is minimal if a maximum leaf step size is set equal to 3 cm every 10° (Yu et al. 2002).

Some treatment machines require a constant dose rate and a constant gantry rotation speed in the delivery of IMAT plans. This constraint is imposed in the optimization by requiring that all angles composing an arc have the same relative weight. However, the full potential of IMAT can be better realized if either the dose rate or the gantry rotation speed can be varied during delivery.

During the optimization, a change in leaf position is rejected if any of the MLC constraints are violated. For a change that satisfies the delivery constraints, the new dose distribution and corresponding objective function are calculated. The change is accepted or rejected based on the rules outlined in the previous section, and the optimization terminates when the specified number of successful iterations has been reached.

## DAO For IMAT: Results And Discussion

Figure 13 shows the results of a DAO applied to an IMAT case. Six coplanar arcs were used to treat a tumor volume adjacent to the spinal cord. An IMAT treatment plan was also produced for a C-shape target located in a cylindrical phantom. The arc configuration is shown in figure 14. The IMAT treatment was then delivered on an Elekta SL20 linear accelerator. A comparison between the optimized dose distribution and the delivered dose as measured by film is shown in figure 15. DAO can also be used for IMAT treatment planning.

DAO serves as the first efficient inverse planning technique for IMAT. Because the number of arcs is specified in the prescription, the user has complete control over the complexity of the delivery.

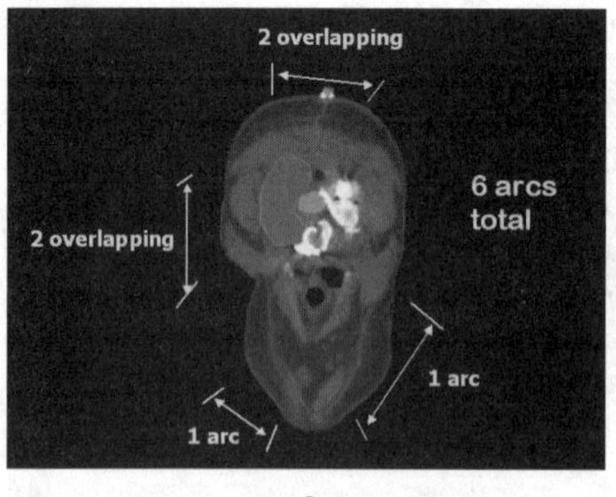


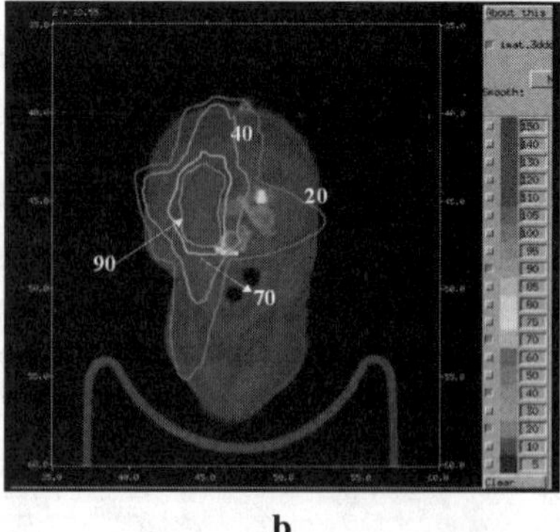


**Figure 13.** (a) The arc configuration for a patient with a tumor adjacent to the spinal cord. (b) The optimized IMAT dose distribution.

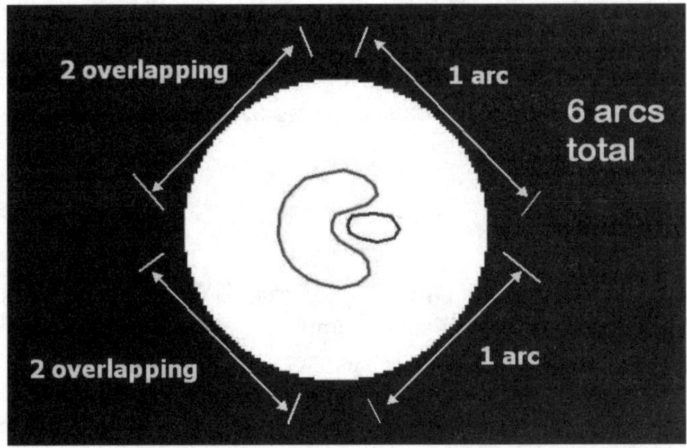



**Figure 14.** The arc configuration for a C-shaped target.

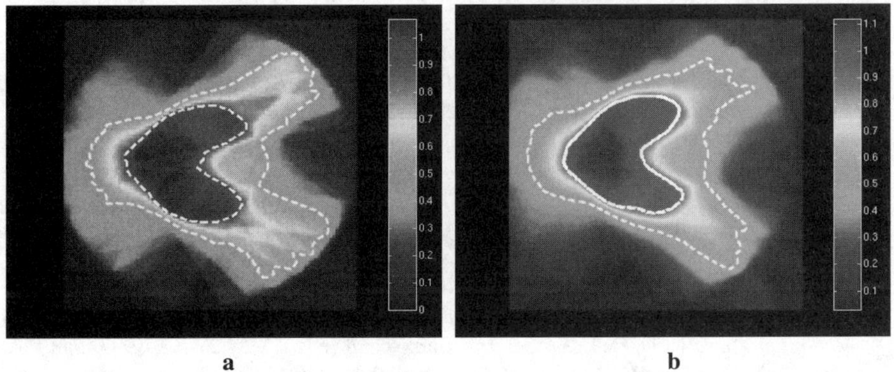

a  b

**Figure 15.** (a) The planned IMAT dose distribution. (b) The delivered dose distribution as measured by film. In both cases, the 90% and 20% isodose lines are shown.

## Summary

Aperture optimization is an inverse planning technique that eliminates the need for leaf sequencing in IMRT treatment planning. There are two main approaches to aperture optimization. The first, contour-based treatment planning, defines the aperture shapes based upon either: (1) the patient's geometry or (2) iteratively matching isodose curves. The second approach to aperture optimization is direct aperture optimization (DAO). This technique simultaneously optimizes the leaf positions and aperture weights. With DAO, the number of apertures per beam angle is specified in the prescription. High-quality IMRT treatment plans can be produced using five or fewer apertures per beam direction.

A key advantage of aperture optimization is that treatment plans are significantly simplified as compared to those produced using the traditional two-step approach to inverse planning.

## Acknowledgments

The authors would like to thank Di Yan, M. Sharpe, J. Wong, and F. Vicini for providing breast IMRT results from William Beaumont Hospital. We would also like to thank Shahid Naqvi and Allen Li for their assistance.

## References

Alber, M., and F. Nüsslin. (2000). "Intensity modulated photon beams subject to minimal surface smoothing constraint." *Phys. Med. Biol.* 45(5):N49–52.

Bar, W., M. Alber, and F. Nüsslin. (2001). "A variable fluence step clustering and segmentation algorithm for step and shoot IMRT." *Phys. Med. Biol.* 46(7):1997–2007.

Bednarz, G., D. Michalski, C. Houser, M. S. Huq, Y. Xiao, P. R. Anne, and J. Galvin. (2002). "The use of mixed-integer programming for inverse treatment planning with pre-defined field segments." *Phys. Med. Biol.* 47(13):2235–2245.

Binder, K., and D. Stauffer. "A Simple Introduction to Monte Carlo Simulations and Some Specialized Topics " in *Statistical Physics*. K. Binder (ed.). Berlin: Springer-Verlag, pp. 1–36, 1985.

Bortfeld, T., D. L. Haler, T. J. Waldron, and A. L. Boyer. (1994). "X-ray compensation with multileaf collimators." *Int. J. Radiat. Oncol. Biol. Phys.* 28:723–739.

Bortfeld, T., J. Stein, and K. Preiser. "Clinically Relevant Intensity Modulation Optimization Using Physical Criteria" in *XII International Conference on the Use of Computers in Radiation Therapy*. D. D. Leavitt and G. Starkschall (eds.). May 27–30, 1997, Salt Lake City, Utah. Madison, WI: Medical Physics Publishing, pp. 1–4, 1997.

Bortfeld, T., D. L. Kahler, T. J. Waldron, and A. L. Boyer. (1994). "X-ray compensation with multileaf collimators." *Int. J. Radiat. Oncol. Biol. Phys.* 28:723–730.

Brahme, A. (1999a). "Biologically based treatment planning." *Acta Oncol.* 38:61–68.

Brahme, A. (1999b). "Optimized radiation therapy based on radiobiological objectives." *Semin. Radiat. Oncol.* 9(1):35–47.

Brahme, A. (2001). "Individualizing cancer treatment: Biological optimization models in treatment planning and delivery." *Int. J. Radiat. Oncol. Biol. Phys.* 49(2):327–337.

Budgell, G. J., J. H. L. Mott, P. C. Williams, and K. J. Brown. (2000). "Requirements for leaf position accuracy for dynamic multileaf collimation." *Phys. Med. Biol.* 45:1211–1227.

Carol, M., D. Dawson, and R. Spied. (1997). "A binary volume delivery system temporal-based intensity modulation radiation therapy." *Med. Phys.* 24:996–997.

Cerny, V. (1982). A Thermodynamic Approach to the Traveling Salesman Problem: An Efficient Simulation Algorithm. Report, Comenius University, Bratislava, Czechoslovakia.

Chen, Y., D. Michalski, Y. Xiao, and J. M. Galvin. (2001). "Automatic aperture selection and IMRT plan optimization by beam weight renormalization." *Int. J. Radiat. Oncol. Biol. Phys.* 51(3): Suppl.1:74.

Chen, Y., D. Michalski, C. Houser, and J. Galvin. (2002). "A deterministic iterative least-squares algorithm for beam weight optimization in conformal radiotherapy." *Phys. Med. Biol.* 47(10):1647–1658.

Cho, P. S., and R. J. Marks II. (2000). "Hardware-sensitive optimization for intensity modulated radiotherapy." *Phys. Med. Biol.* 45(2):429–440.

Chui, C. S., T. LoSasso, and S. Spirou. (1994). "Dose calculation for photon beams with intensity modulation generated by dynamic jaw or multileaf collimations." *Med. Phys.* 21:1237–1244.

Convery, D. J., and S. Webb. (1998). "Generation of discrete beam-intensity modulation by dynamic multileaf collimation under minimum leaf separation constraints." *Phys. Med. Biol.* 43:2521–2538.

Crooks, S.M., L. F. McAven, D. F. Robinson, and L. Xing. (2002). "Minimizing delivery time and monitor units in static IMRT by leaf-sequencing." *Phys. Med. Biol.* 47(17):3105–3116.

Dai, J., and Y. Zhu. (2001). "Minimizing the number of segments in a delivery sequence for intensity-modulated radiation therapy with a multileaf collimator." *Med. Phys.* 28(10):2113–2120.

DeGersem, W., F. Claus, C. DeWagter, and W. DeNeve. (2001a). "An anatomy-based beam segmentation tool for intensity modulated radiation therapy and its application to head-and-neck cancer." *Int. J. Radiat. Oncol. Biol. Phys.* 51(3): 849–859.

DeGersem, W., F. Claus, C. DeWagter, B. VanDuyse, and W. DeNeve. (2001b). "Leaf position optimization for step-and-shoot IMRT." *Int. J. Radiat. Oncol. Biol. Phys.* 51(5):1371–1388.

Earl, M. A., D. M. Shepard, X. A. Li, and C. X. Yu. (2001). "Inverse planning for intensity modulated arc therapy using direct aperture optimization." *Int. J. Rad. Oncol. Biol. Phys.* 51(3):Suppl. 1:404.

Earl, M. A., D. M. Shepard, S. Naqvi, X. A. Li, C. X. Yu. (2003). "Inverse planning for intensity modulated arc therapy using direct aperture optimization" *Phys. Med. Biol.* Accepted for publication.

Followill, D., P. Geis, and A. Boyer. (1997). "Estimates of whole-body dose equivalent produced by beam intensity modulation conformal therapy." *Int. J. Radiat. Oncol. Biol. Phys.* 38:667–672.

Galvin, J. M., X. G. Chen, and R. M. Smith. (1993). "Combining multileaf fields to modulate fluence distributions." *Int. J. Radiat. Oncol. Biol. Phys.* 27:697–705.

Geman, S., and D. Geman. (1984). "Stochastic relaxation, Gibbs distribution and the Bayesian restoration in images." *IEEE Trans. PAMI* 6(6):731–741.

Jones, L. C., and P. W. Hoban. (2000). "Treatment plan comparison using equivalent uniform biologically effective dose (EUBED)." *Phys. Med. Biol.* 45(1):159–170.

Jordan, T. J., and P. C. Williams. (1994). "The design and performance characteristics of a multileaf collimator." *Phys. Med. Biol.* 39:231–251.

Kestin, L. L., M. B. Sharpe, R. C. Frazier, F. A. Vicini, D. Yan, R. C. Matter, A. A. Martinez, and J. W. Wong. (2000). "Intensity modulation to improve dose uniformity with tangential breast radiotherapy: Initial clinical experience." *Int. J. Radiat. Oncol. Biol. Phys.* 48:1559–1568.

Kirkpatrick S., C. D. Gelatt, Jr., M. P. Vecchi. (1983). "Optimization by simulated annealing." *Science* 220(4598):671–680.

Langer. M., V. Thai, and L. Papiez. (2001). "Improved leaf sequencing reduces segments or monitor units needed to deliver IMRT using multileaf collimators." *Med. Phys.* 28(12):2450–2458.

Li, X. A., L. Ma, S. Naqvi, R. Shih, and C. Yu. (2001). "Monte Carlo dose verification for intensity modulated arc therapy." *Phys. Med. Biol.* 46(9):2269–2282.

LoSasso T., C.-S. Chui, and C. C. Ling. (1998). "Physical and dosimetric aspects of a multileaf collimation system used in the dynamic mode for implementing intensity modulated radiotherapy." *Med. Phys.* 25:1919–1927.

Mackie, T. R., T. Holmes, S. Swerdloff, P. Reckwerdt, J. O. Deasy, J. Yang, B. Paliwal, and T. Kinsella. (1993). "Tomotherapy: A new concept for the delivery of dynamic conformal radiotherapy." *Med. Phys.* 20:1709–1719.

Mackie, T. R., J. Balog, K. J. Ruchala, D. M. Shepard, J. S. Aldridge, E. E. Fitchard, P. J. Reckwerd, G. H. Olivera, T. R. McNutt, and M. Mehta. (1995). "Tomotherapy." *Semin. Radiat. Oncol.* 32(4):1215–1225.

*Multileaf Collimator (MLC) Operator's Manual for MLC SA1.* Philips Medical Systems Document No. 4522 984 40891/764, Appendix C, 1993.

Naqvi, S. A., M. A. Earl, and D. M. Shepard. (2003). "Convolution/superposition using the Monte Carlo method." *Med. Phys.* Submitted.

Niemierko, A. (1997). "Reporting and analyzing dose distributions: a concept of equivalent uniform dose." *Med. Phys.* 24(1):103–110.

Niemierko, A. (1998). "Radiobiological models of tissue response to radiation in treatment planning systems." *Tumori.* 84(2):140–143.

Olivera, G. H., D. M. Shepard, K. Ruchala, J. S. Aldridge, J. Kapatoes, E. E. Fitchard, P. J. Reckwerdt, G. Fang, J. Balog, J. Zachman, and T. R. Mackie. "Tomotherapy" in *The Modern Technology of Radiation Oncology. A Compendium for Medical Physicists and Radiation Oncologists.* J. Van Dyk (ed.). Madison, WI: Medical Physics Publishing, pp. 521–587, 1999.

Pincus, M. (1970). "A Monte Carlo method for the approximate calculation of certain types of constrained optimization problems." *Oper. Res.* 18:1225–1228.

Rardin, R. *Optimization in Operations Research.* Upper Saddle River, NJ: Prentice Hall, 1998.

Remouchamps, V. M., F. A. Vicini, M. B. Sharpe, L. L. Kestin, A. A. Martinez, and J. W. Wong. (2003). "Significant reductions in heart and lung doses using deep inspiration breath hold with active breathing control and intensity-modulated radiation therapy for patients treated with locoregional breast irradiation." *Int. J. Radiat. Oncol. Biol. Phys.* 55(2):392–406.

Rogers, D. W. O., B. A. Faddegon, G. X. Ding, C.-M. Ma, J. We, and T. R. Mackie. (1995). "BEAM: A Monte Carlo code to simulate radiotherapy treatment unit." *Med. Phys.* 22:503–524.

Saw, C. B., R. C. Siochi, K. M. Ayyangar, W. Zhen, and C. A. Enke. (2001). "Leaf sequencing techniques for MLC-based IMRT." *Med. Dosim.* 26(2):199–204.

Shepard, D. M., G. H. Olivera, P. J. Reckwerdt, and T.R. Mackie. (1999)."Iterative approaches to dose optimization." *Phys. Med. Biol.* 45(1):69–90 .

Shepard, D. M., M. A. Earl, X. A. Li, S. Naqvi, and C. Yu. (2002). "Direct aperture optimization: A turnkey solution for step-and-shoot IMRT." *Med. Phys.* 29(6):1007–1018.

Spirou, S. V., N. Fournier-Bidoz, J. Yang, C. S. Chui, and C. C. Ling. (2001). "Smoothing intensity-modulated beam profiles to improve the efficiency of delivery." *Med. Phys.* 28:2105–2112.

Stavrev, P., N. Stavreva, A. Niemierko, and M. Goitein. (2001). "Generalization of a model of tissue response to radiation based on the idea of functional subunits and binomial statistics." *Phys. Med. Biol.* 46(5):1501–1518.

Tervo, J., and P. Kolmonen. (2000). "A model for the control of a multileaf collimator in radiation therapy treatment planning." *Inv. Problems* 16:1875–1895.

van Santvoort, J. P. C., and B. J. M. Heijmen. (1996). "Dynamic multileaf collimation without 'tongue and groove' underdosage effects." *Phys. Med. Biol.* 41:2091–2105.

Webb, S. (1994). "Optimizing the planning of intensity-modulated radiotherapy." *Phys. Med. Biol.* 39(12):2229–2246.

Webb, S. (1998a). "Configuration options for intensity-modulated radiation therapy using multiple static fields shaped by a multileaf collimator." *Phys. Med. Biol.* 43(2):241–260.

Webb, S. (1998). "Configuration options for intensity-modulated radiation therapy using multiple static fields shaped by a multileaf collimator. II: Constraints and limitations on 2D modulation." *Phys. Med. Biol.* 43(6):1481–1495.

Webb, S., D. J. Convery, and P. M. Evans. (1998). "Inverse planning with constraints to generate smoothed intensity-modulated beams." *Phys. Med. Biol.* 43(10):2785–2794.

Webb, S., T. Bortfeld, J. Stein, and D. Convery. (1997). "The effect of stair-step leaf transmission on the 'tongue-and-groove problem' in dynamic radiotherapy with multileaf collimator." *Phys. Med. Biol.* 42:595–602.

Wu, Y., D. Yan, M. B. Sharpe, B. Miller, J. W. Wong. (2001). "Implementing multiple static field delivery for intensity modulated beams." *Med. Phys.* 28(11):2188–2197.

Xia, P., and L. J. Verhey. (1998). "Multileaf collimator leaf sequencing algorithm for intensity modulated beams with multiple static segments." *Med. Phys.* 25:1424–1434.

Xiao, Y., J. Galvin, M. Hossain, and R. Valenti. (2000)."An optimized forward-planning technique for intensity modulated radiation therapy." *Med. Phys.* 9:2093–2099.

Xiao, Y., Y. Censor, D. Michalski, and J. Galvin. (2003). "The least-intensity feasible solution for aperture-based inverse planning in radiation therapy." *Ann. Oper. Res.* 119:183–203.

Yu, C. X. (1995). "Intensity-modulated arc therapy with dynamic multileaf collimation: An alternative to tomotherapy." *Phys. Med. Biol.* 40:1435–1449.

Yu, C. X., and J. Li. (2001). "Angular cost: A new concept for broad-scope planning optimization." *Int. J. Radiat. Oncol. Biol. Phys.* 51(3):Suppl. 1:406.

Yu, C. X., X. A. Li, L. Ma, D. Chen, S. Naqvi, D. Shepard, M. Sarfaraz, T. W. Holmes, M. Suntharalingam, and C. M. Mansfield. (2002). "Clinical implementation of intensity-modulated arc therapy." *Int. J. Radiat. Oncol. Biol. Phys.* 53(2):453–463.

# Medical Imaging In IMRT Planning


**Charles A. Pelizzari, Ph.D.**
Radiation and Cellular Oncology Department
University of Chicago, Chicago, Illinois

## Introduction: Rationale For Use Of Image Information In Radiation Treatment Planning, Delivery, And Followup

Over the past 25 years, dramatic improvements in multiple medical imaging technologies have been key enabling factors in fueling the development of the technology-intensive, image-guided modality that we recognize as modern radiotherapy. As new medical imaging modalities have become clinically available, their incorporation into various aspects of radiation treatment planning (RTP), delivery, assessment, and followup has typically been rapid. Frequently, developments in the technology of radiotherapy, notably intensity-modulated radiation therapy (IMRT) delivery systems, have opened new avenues for incorporation of imaging information of new types, such as use of biological information from various physiologic imaging modalities in the treatment planning process. Additionally, each technological advance leading to potential improvement in precision of dose delivery has necessitated the addition and/or improved utilization of information from imaging studies to the treatment planning process, in order to ensure these potential gains in precision might be translated to corresponding gains in treatment accuracy.

Radiation therapy was perhaps the original example of what has come to be called "image-guided therapy," and certainly one of the first areas in which use of three-dimensional (3-D) patient information from computed tomography (CT) was applied to clinical problems. In some of the earliest reported work, the group at Rhode Island Hospital developed CT-based treatment planning systems utilizing patient surface and internal structure contours on multiple slices which were digitized from films and plotted on a monochrome video monitor or on paper, as viewed from the perspective of candidate beam directions (Reinstein et al. 1978). Hardcopy perspective plots from each beam's point of view were used for design of field apertures and blocks. Subsequently, use of an interactive color graphics system replaced monochrome plots, and coupled with a calculation of dose on multiple planes, allowed interactive display of dose on arbitrarily oriented sections through the patient (McShan et al. 1979). Since no CT information in digital form was used, only contours from films, the 3-D display was limited to wireframe models. It is interesting to note that a feature of these early systems which was quickly recognized as extremely beneficial was the ability to visualize anatomical relationships from the perspective of the radiation source for any beam orientation. This allowed choosing beam orientations to best irradiate the target while sparing organs at risk.

Notwithstanding the considerable difficulties associated with getting 3-D information from CT scanners of the day into the planning process, the potential gain in incorporating this information into radiation treatment design was clearly recognized as being so great that treatment planning systems were designed whose capabilities (use of more than 50 CT slices in a study, interactive 3-D visualization of patient anatomy, calculation of computed radiographs for comparison with setup films) strained the capabilities of existing imaging systems, as well as data transmission, computer processing, hardcopy printing, and data storage technologies. Goitein and colleagues (Goitein and Abrams 1983; Goitein et al. 1983) described a 3-D treatment planning system used for both proton and photon planning, which incorporated a number of capabilities that have since become accepted as standards. Delineation of structures directly from CT image data using interactive graphic displays was supported, with sagittal and coronal reformatted images displayed along with the transverse slices to assist in the appreciation of anatomy. The display of structures or digitally reconstructed radiographs (DRRs) from the perspective of the radiation source was given the name "beam's-eye view." The advantage of using such views was stressed:

> The source of radiation is a very natural viewpoint from which to gauge anatomic relationships. If the user's eye is hypothetically placed at that point and directed along the central axis of a hypothetical radiation beam, the relative disposition of structures is readily apparent and judgments as to what would and would not be included in the beam can readily be made. If the user is able interactively to move his eye around to all locations accessible to a radiation source, he can explore which directions provide the greatest separation between, say, the target volume and critical normal structures. Beam-shaping apertures can be designed from these vantage points. These advantages have, of course, been appreciated by others.
>
> (Goitein et al. 1983)

The rationale for use of D image information in RTP has always been to improve the accuracy with which both the target to be irradiated, and the organs at risk to be spared, may be defined. The incorporation of information from multiple imaging modalities has proven useful in a number of ways in furthering this aim. In many situations, magnetic resonance imaging (MRI) provides superior visualization of both tumor and normal tissue regions, and inclusion of 3-D anatomical information from MR images into the planning process may thus allow more accurate definition of both regions to be irradiated, and regions to be avoided. Information from serial imaging datasets, for example pre-operative CT or MR in addition to postoperative treatment planning CT, can aid in definition of clinical target volumes (CTVs) including tumor margins at risk for microscopic disease. With the continuously improving potential offered today by IMRT planning systems to optimize a 3-D dose distribution using goals aimed at both adequate irradiation of the target and desired sparing of regions at risk, and of IMRT delivery systems to actually administer the optimized dose distribution to the patient, the ability to define all these regions accurately and in as much detail as possible takes on ever more significance. Furthermore, the continuing development of functional imaging modalities, providing an ever-expanding variety of information about the 3-D distribution of various physiologic processes, allows the incorporation of functional criteria into the definition of both target volumes and regions to be spared.

The treatment design task embodied in RTP is not the only stage of the overall radiation therapy process in which image information is valuable. To ensure that the treatment as planned on the "virtual patient," i.e., the image-based patient model including all relevant anatomic and functional information, is accurately delivered to the real patient, and that the patient's anatomy is treated consistently and correctly on a day-to-day basis throughout an extended course of fractionated radiotherapy, imaging provides key information. Historically, comparison of diagnostic quality simulation films with megavoltage radiographs taken on the treatment machine has been a critical step in quality assurance of treatment delivery. With the current availability of electronic portal imaging devices (EPIDs), such comparisons can be made electronically with either digital versions of simulation films, or with DRRs. Rapid analysis of patient positioning errors can thus be made, allowing either immediate corrections or periodic modification of patient position and/or field shape to ensure proper irradiation of the target volume and sparing of regions at risk. Numerous techniques have been developed for analysis of setup errors from electronic portal images. Significant difficulties exist in inferring 3-D differences in position from 2-D radiographs, and considerable research has been devoted to the development of methods to address this problem. Some of these methods can utilize information from multiple image modalities. For example, one may compare portal images with the 3-D virtual patient model from CT to verify the 3-D patient pose.

Imaging is also extensively used in patient followup and evaluation of treatment effect, in the assessment of both tumor response and potential radiation-associated complications. Both anatomic and functional modalities are useful in this regard, and fusion of functional with anatomic information, or of multiple functional images with one another, may prove valuable, for example in the differential diagnosis of tumor recurrence vs. radiation-induced necrosis.

## Sources Of Image Information: Image Modalities

### Anatomic Modalities

Fundamental to the process of RTP is the construction of an accurate and complete 3-D patient model which can be used for the computer-aided design of an optimized configuration of beams and IMRT beam intensities that satisfies as fully as possible an appropriate set of goals. These goals may include some or all of the following, alone or in combination: irradiation of at least a specified fraction of the target volume to a prescribed dose level; limitation of dose heterogeneity in the target volume to a specified range; limitation of dose to an entire organ at risk, or to one or more specified fractional volumes, to no more than a specified dose; maximization or minimization of biologically related indices such as tumor control probability (TCP) and normal tissue complication probability (NTCP) for target and organs at risk respectively. With the availability of IMRT delivery systems which can "sculpt" a 3-D dose distribution with a considerable degree of precision, it is a natural inclination to design dose distributions that conform ever more closely to target volumes, and which elegantly avoid ever more complex regions at risk. This places a premium on accurate definition of all the relevant volumes. Combining information from multiple modalities, each of which may have an advantage in defining a particular aspect of a structure, is often very helpful in this regard.

*CT*

Since the late 1970's, by far the most commonly used anatomical modality in RTP has been X-ray CT. CT offers a number of advantages, some of which are briefly summarized here. Unlike MRI, where magnetic field inhomogeneities and other physical effects, some of which can be changed by the patient, can lead to image distortions, a well-calibrated CT scanner produces images with consistent and reliable 3-D spatial coordinates. Thus, CT remains the "gold standard" for spatial fidelity in construction of a 3-D patient model. CT numbers are proportional to X-ray attenuation coefficient at each point, according to the relation

$$CT(x, y) = \frac{\mu(x, y) - \mu_{water}}{\mu_{water}} \times 1000$$

where $\mu(x,y)$ is the attenuation coefficient appropriate to the X-ray spectrum used in the scanner. Typical CT numbers for several tissue types are shown in table 1.

**Table 1.** CT Numbers for Several Materials

| Material | CT Number (Range) |
| --- | --- |
| Air | $-1000$ |
| Lung | $(-500,-200)$ |
| Fat | $(-200,-50)$ |
| Water | 0 |
| Blood | 25 |
| Muscle | $(25,40)$ |
| Bone | $(>200)$ |

Bones of course appear very bright in CT. Radiographs computed from CT can thus show bony anatomy with high contrast, and can be made to look like ordinary X-rays. Thus, these DRRs can be directly compared with actual radiographs such as simulation or verification films, or electronic portal images. It is fairly straightforward to derive from a set of CT images a 3-D map of Compton interaction coefficients that can be used in a dose calculation for photon beams (McCullough and Holmes 1985) or to produce megavoltage DRRs (Sherouse, Novins, and Chaney 1990). CT scanners are typically less expensive than MR units, and they can readily be installed in rooms originally designed for radiation therapy simulators. Thus, many radiation therapy clinics have their own dedicated CT scanners.

A number of operational characteristics of CT scanners affect their suitability for RTP purposes. Spiral data acquisition, in which the gantry rotates continuously while the patient couch moves through the aperture, allows collection of the complete projection dataset in a shorter time compared to axial mode, where the couch stops and the gantry makes a complete rotation at each slice position. This is useful in helping to minimize respiratory motion artifacts, if the projection dataset can be acquired during one or more patient breath holds in a reproducible state of inspiration. Multislice scanners that have multiple rows of detectors can acquire projections for several (e.g., 4, 8, 16) slices simultaneously, further reducing the time required to scan. Many scanners also allow gated imaging, where projection data are only acquired when a gating signal is within a certain range. This signal might be derived from a respiratory monitoring system, in which case only projections within a certain range around some point in the breathing cycle would be used to reconstruct the image. The image would then represent a "snapshot" of the patient's anatomy at that point in the cycle. Gated or breath-hold image acquisition must be done in a way that is appropriate to the way in which the treatment will be delivered. Slice thickness (the axial extent of the patient over which the slice is averaged) and index (the separation between slice centers along the direction of couch motion) for RTP applications can vary over a wide range of values, from 1 mm or less for high precision intracranial plans up to 5 mm or even 10 mm for thoracic or pelvic scans. It is noteworthy that to produce the highest quality DRRs, a small slice spacing is important. In fact, a scan with small slice separation and low X-ray tube current can produce better quality DRRs than a less noisy scan with larger slice separation (Balter and Lam 2001). Compared to diagnostic applications, the degree to which identification of extremely fine detail in CT images is needed in RTP is somewhat less. Thus spatial resolution of most modern CT scanners is more than adequate for RTP purposes. One interesting development that has occurred in the past several years is the introduction of a CT scanner (AcQSim CT, Philips Medical Systems) designed specifically for the RTP application. The major distinguishing feature of this scanner is its increased aperture—an opening of 85 cm, which allows scanning large patients and those immobilized or positioned in a way that would prevent their fitting through the smaller bore of conventional scanners. This is useful, for example, for patients to be treated with one or both arms above the head, as for many breast treatments.

CT scans for RTP are frequently done with continuous injection of iodinated contrast during image acquisition. This typically improves the visualization of vessels, certain glands, and lymph nodes, which are often important in defining the clinical target volume; and areas of increased vascularity or vascular leakage, which may be associated with tumor. A CT slice through the abdomen of a patient being planned for IMRT for an abdominal wall cancer, with several normal structures and tumor volumes outlined, is shown in figure 1.

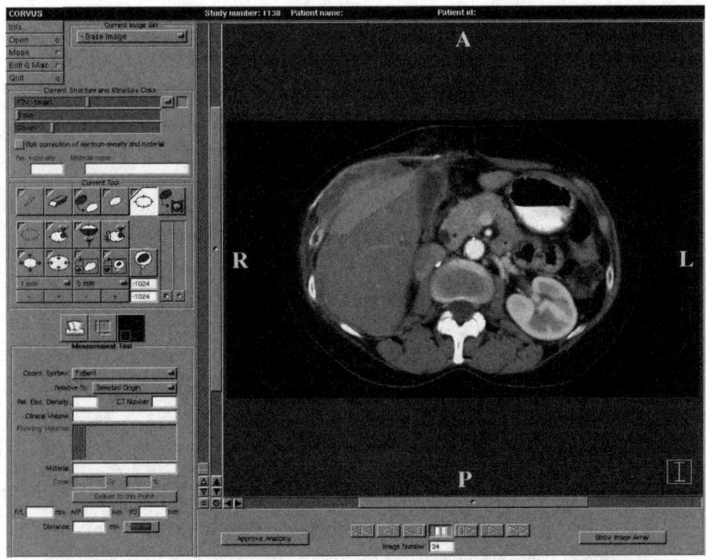

**Figure 1.** CORVUS® Anatomy module screen showing CT slice from abdominal wall IMRT plan with target and normal structures being defined.

A number of tumor types are well visualized on CT. For example, primary and metastatic tumors in the liver frequently appear with lower intensity than the surrounding parenchyma, as seen in figure 2. It is still often the case, however, that CT images cannot provide adequate discrimination of adjacent soft tissue structures, or of tumor from surrounding tissue. In these cases, the inclusion of MRI into the process of anatomy definition is frequently useful. For example, figure 3 shows CT and $T_1$-weighted MRI slices through the prostate. On CT, it is somewhat difficult to differentiate between the prostate gland and the surrounding musculature, while on MRI the boundary of the prostate can be clearly identified. Note that as mentioned earlier, due to the use of intravenous contrast, blood vessels, and lymph nodes in the anterior subcutaneous fat are clearly visible in CT. Merging information from these two studies requires image registration and fusion techniques, discussed in a later section. Note that the patient couch for CT is flat, and for MRI is curved. The distortion of the patient anatomy due to this difference complicates the image fusion process.

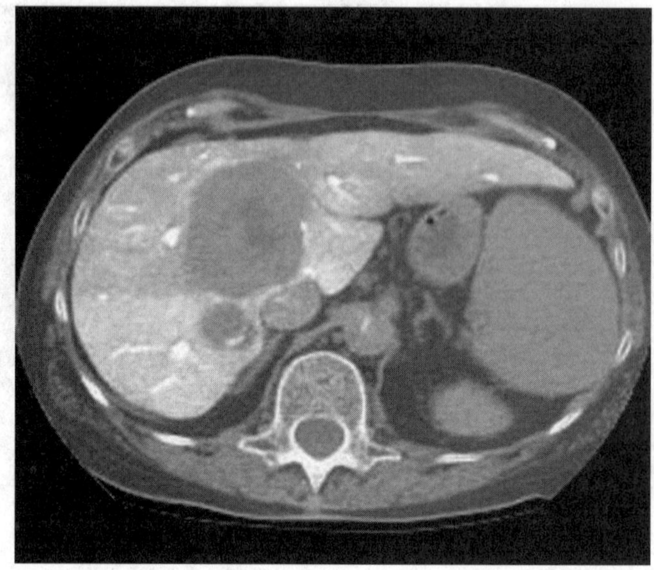

**Figure 2.** CT slice through liver with clear visualization of hypo-intense tumors.

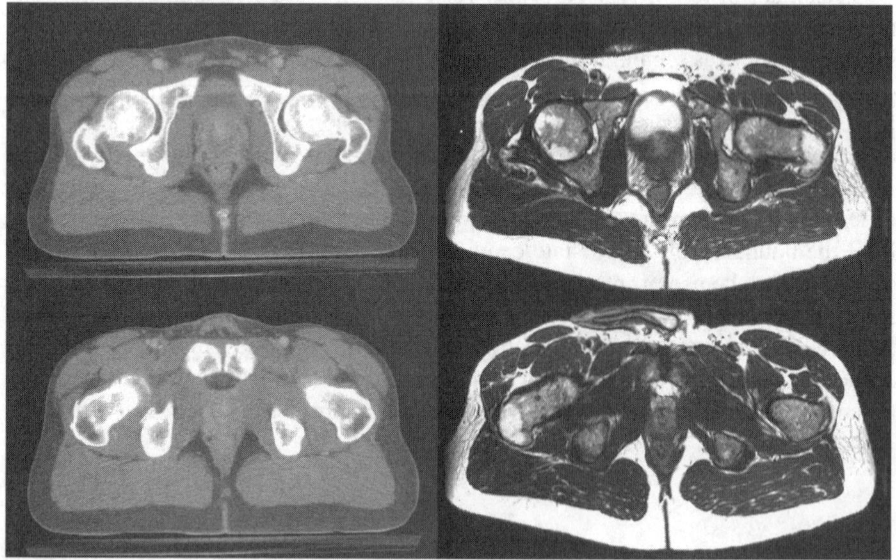

**Figure 3.** CT (left) and MR slices through approximately corresponding sections near the middle (above) and apex (below) of the prostate. Image parameters: CT, 5 mm slice thickness, single-slice axial acquisition mode, 0.78 mm pixel size; MR, 4.5 mm slice thickness, 0.74 mm pixel size.

*MRI*

The MR image signal is generated by precessing proton spins, as nuclear magnetization induced by an initial radio frequency (RF) pulse decays due to interactions of the polarized spins with their environment. Two characteristic decay times determine the time dependence of the signal: $T_1$, which characterizes the overall decay of the initially perturbed spin system to its equilibrium state; and $T_2$, which characterizes the loss of coherence of the originally polarized spins in the transverse plane due to various dephasing processes. In addition, the signal intensity depends directly on the local proton spin density. The relaxation times depend on physical and chemical properties of the local environment, including among others water content, viscosity, and diffusion coefficient. Local variations in magnetic field due to the presence of paramagnetic species or other effects also lead to dephasing of the transverse magnetization. The overall effective transverse decay time due to both the intrinsic $T_2$ and these other effects is called $T_2^*$. Using spin-echo techniques, the $T_2$ and $T_2^*$ effects can be separated. $T_2^*$-weighted images are useful in functional imaging, discussed later. Values of parameters for several tissue types of interest in brain imaging are shown in table 2.

**Table 2.** $T_1$ and $T_2$ Values for Several Tissue Types [Data from Hornak (2002)]

|  | $T_1$ (ms) | $T_2$ (ms) | $\rho^*$ |
|---|---|---|---|
| Cerebrospinal fluid | 800–2000 | 110–2000 | 70–230 |
| White | 760–1080 | 61–100 | 70–90 |
| Gray | 1090–2150 | 61–109 | 85–125 |
| Meninges | 500–2200 | 50–165 | 5–44 |
| Muscle | 950–1820 | 20–67 | 45–90 |
| Adipose | 200–750 | 53–94 | 50–100 |

*spin density relative to a standard calibration solution

As an example of the effects of the relaxation parameters on image contrast, the signal intensity vs. time for a repeated spin echo image sequence can be written as follows:

$$S(t) \propto \rho\left[1 - e^{-TR/T_1}\right] \times e^{-TE/T_2}$$

where *TR* is the repetition time between sequences, and *TE* is the echo time. Figure 4 shows S(t) for two tissues differing only in $T_1$, one with $T_1 = 500$ ms and one with $T_1 = 800$ ms. Figure 5 shows S(t) for two tissues differing only in $T_2$, one with $T_2 = 50$ ms and one with $T_2 = 80$ ms. In figure 4, if TR is chosen in the range 500 to 1000 ms, then the signal amplitude from the tissue with the shorter $T_1$ is approximately 20% greater, all other parameters being equal. In figure 5, if TE is chosen around 100 ms, signal from the tissue with the longer $T_2$ is approximately double that with the shorter $T_2$. Image contrast between tissues with different $T_1$ and $T_2$ values can thus be achieved by varying TR and TE. If TE is short relative to $T_2$, then image contrast will not be strongly affected by $T_2$ variation. If TR is comparable to $T_1$, then $T_1$ variation will affect image contrast. If TR is relatively long and TE is comparable to $T_2$, image contrast will be mainly due to $T_2$ variations. This is summarized in tables 3 and 4.

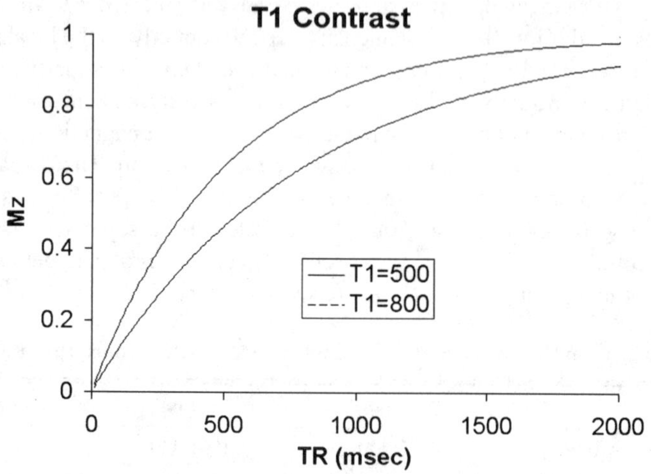


**Figure 4.** Signal intensity vs. TR for two values of $T_1$.

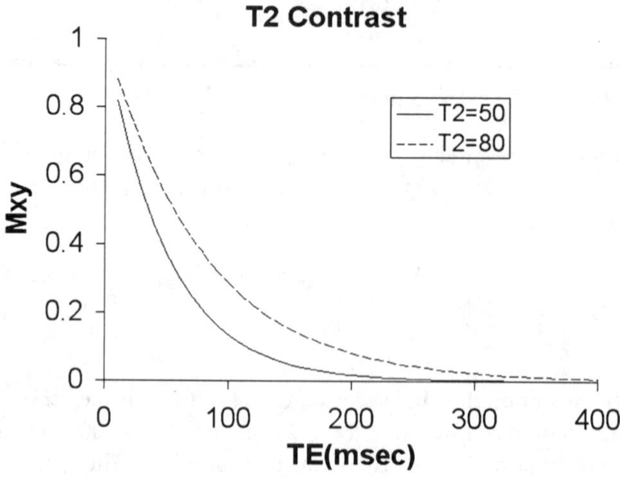


**Figure 5.** Signal intensity vs. TE for two values of $T_2$.

**Table 3.** MR Spin Echo Image Weighting [Data from Li and Bluemke (2001)]

| TR(ms) | TE(ms) | Image Type | Fat Intensity | Water Intensity |
|---|---|---|---|---|
| 400–800 | <30 | $T_1$ weighted | High | Low |
| 400–800 | >90 | Proton density | Intermediate | Intermediate |
| >1500 | <30 | Proton density | Intermediate | Intermediate |
| >1500 | >90 | $T_2$ weighted | Intermediate to low | High |

**Table 4.** Relative Intensity (1 = darkest, 5 = brightest) of Several Tissues in $T_1$- and $T_2$-Weighted MR Images [Data from Li and Bluemke (2001)]

| | Image Weighting | |
|---|---|---|
| **Tissue** | $T_1$ | $T_2$ |
| Adrenal | 3 | 4 |
| Cervix | 2 | 2 |
| Brain | | |
|   CSF | 2 | 5 |
|   Gray | 2–3 | 3–4 |
|   White | 4 | 2–3 |
| Cortical bone | 1 | 1 |
| Water | 2 | 4 |
| Fat | 4 | 2–3 |
| Muscle | 2 | 2 |
| Lung | 1 | 1 |
| Liver | 3–4 | 2–3 |
| Pancreas | 3–4 | 2–3 |
| Prostate | 3 | 4 |
| Spleen | 3 | 4 |

Due to the generally superior visualization of soft tissues and tumors in MRI, a considerable amount of effort has been directed toward inclusion of information from MRI into the treatment planning process. One of the original motivations for the development of image registration and fusion methods, discussed later, was to allow importing MRI-defined tumor volumes into an overall CT-based treatment planning process (Kessler et al. 1991; Thornton et al. 1992). However, entirely MRI-based treatment planning has not become widespread due to several of the desirable characteristics of CT mentioned earlier. Recently, commercial "MR simulation" systems analogous to CT simulation systems have been introduced. Several of the perceived drawbacks of MR in treatment planning have been addressed, for example in the Philips MR simulation product, which uses a low-field open MRI system, shown in figure 6. The low-field magnet is relatively inexpensive, so the overall system cost is comparable to a CT simulator. The relatively small aperture of most closed MRI systems would present a problem with scanning many patients immobilized in treatment position, and this problem is certainly less severe with the open system. Considerable effort has been expended in correcting distortions to address the problem of lower spatial accuracy which has traditionally been associated with MRI in treatment planning (Mah et al. 2002; Shukla, Vaisanen, and Steckner 2002). Data processing procedures have also been developed to allow the production of DRRs from MRI. An example of an image from the Philips system is shown in figure 7. Whether the use of dedicated MR simulation systems in radiation therapy departments will become widespread remains to be seen.

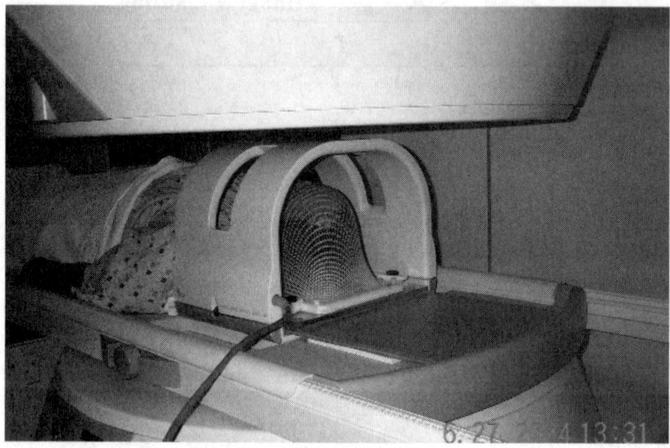

**Figure 6.** RT patient immobilized for planning scan in low field open MR imager. [Image courtesy of Philips Medical Systems]

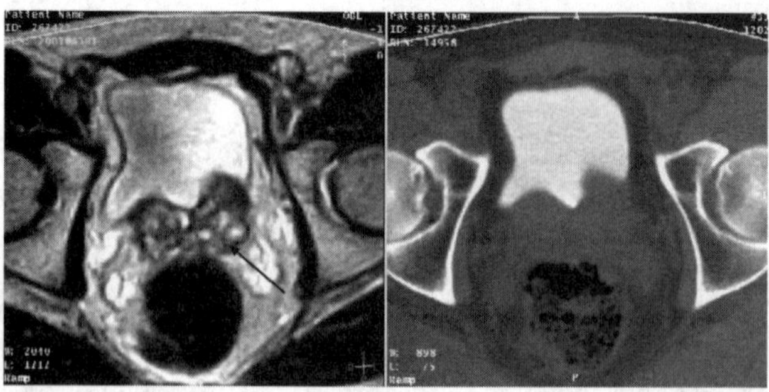

**Figure 7.** Comparison of MRI (left) with CT (right). The seminal vesicles are clearly contrasted with the extra-capsular extension (arrow). The CT does not readily distinguish between the two structures. [Image courtesy of Philips Medical Systems]

Frequently, MR contrast agents containing gadolinium, a paramagnet, are utilized. At relatively low concentrations, Gd shortens $T_1$, thus regions of contrast uptake appear brighter on $T_1$ weighted images, as seen in figure 8. As in the case of CT contrast, this improves visualization of regions of blood-brain barrier disruption, increased vascular permeability, and other effects that may reflect the presence of tumor. However, even with contrast, specificity of MR imaging alone in identifying tumor is less than ideal, and it is frequently difficult, for example, to differentiate image changes due to necrosis from tumor recurrence. Additional information from functional imaging is valuable in such cases, as discussed below. A bolus of paramagnetic contrast in relatively high concentration may decrease the image signal, and this effect may be used as the basis of flow sensitive imaging techniques.

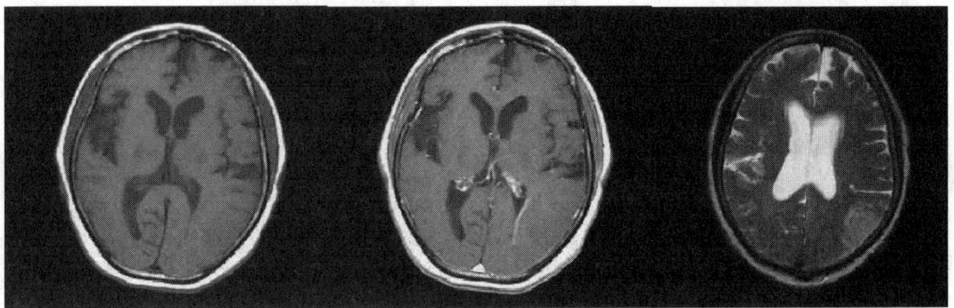

**Figure 8.** $T_1$ weighted pre (left) and post (center) contrast, and $T_2$-weighted (right) images showing tumor. Note regions of contrast enhancement in center image. [Image courtesy of P. MacEneaney, M.D., University of Chicago]

*Ultrasound*

Ultrasound imaging has typically not been used in the treatment planning phase of external beam radiation therapy, due to the lack of a well-defined 3-D image coordinate system, limited scan volume and problematic image quality. However, ultrasound-aided patient setup has been shown to be useful for some treatment sites, and commercial systems are available incorporating tracked ultrasound probes which can aid in locating the target region within the patient on a daily basis relative to the treatment machine (Lattanzi et al. 1999). Ultrasound is also widely used for radioactive seed implantation in image-guided interstitial brachytherapy of the prostate.

## Functional Modalities

Frequently it is difficult to identify tumor volumes with as much specificity and sensitivity as one would wish based on anatomic images alone. Furthermore, the CTV in concept is intended to include microscopic extensions of disease beyond the gross tumor visible on anatomic images. Inclusion of information from functional imaging modalities shows promise to aid in defining these volumes. In addition, the potential for IMRT to produce 3-D dose distributions with controlled inhomogeneities to both irradiate and avoid complicated 3-D regions raises the possibility of tailoring a dose distribution to place more dose where tumor burden is higher and vice versa. Regions to be avoided might also be better defined with the addition of information on the location of important functional regions, as in the brain, or of the level of function of different regions of an organ, as in the lung. The inclusion of functional imaging modalities into the treatment planning and assessment process, with the definition of a "biological target volume" (BTV) to which dose can be tailored, potentially with different doses delivered to more or less malignant or radioresistant regions, seems highly promising in moving toward these goals (Ling et al. 2000; Tepper 2000). Here we describe several well-established functional imaging modalities, and mention some others which are currently under development that may become useful in RTP in the near future.

### Nuclear Medicine: PET And SPECT

Emission tomography provides information on the 3-D distribution of a radiolabeled substance in the body. In positron emission tomography (PET) the isotopic label is a positron-emitting nucleus such as $^{18}$F, $^{15}$O, or $^{11}$C. When the positron annihilates with an electron, two 511 keV photons are emitted traveling in nearly opposite directions. The signature of these events is detection by two detectors nearly simultaneously, providing an "electronic collimation" that helps to discriminate true events from random counts or scattered photons. In addition, the total energy of the two photons depends not on the depth of the event in the patient, but on the line integral of photon attenuation coefficient through the patient, along the ray connecting the two detectors. Thus, an accurate attenuation correction can be made based on a separate measurement of these line integrals for each detector pair, which is typically made using an external source of 511 keV photons in a transmission geometry. For this reason, information from PET images is usually considered to have more quantitative potential than from single photon emission computed tomography (SPECT), in which radioisotopes are used that decay by photon rather than positron emission. On the other hand, the variety of tracers available for SPECT is larger and SPECT scanners are more widely available, so inclusion of functional information from SPECT into RTP is of considerable interest as well.

A few PET isotopes and tracers relevant to oncologic imaging are listed in table 5.

Two radioisotopes dominate clinical uses of SPECT: $^{99}$Tc and $^{111}$In. Technetium is the more commonly used of the two, since many pharmaceuticals can be labeled with generator-produced Tc in the nuclear medicine department using commercially available kits. A selection of tracers which have proven useful in oncologic imaging with SPECT is listed in table 6.

**Table 5.** Some PET Tracers Useful in Oncologic Imaging

| Isotope | Tracer | Physiology |
|---------|--------|------------|
| $^{15}$O | water, $CO_2$ | blood flow |
| $^{15}$O | $O_2$ | necrosis |
| $^{13}$N | ammonia | blood flow |
| $^{11}$C | acetate | oxidative metabolism |
| $^{11}$C | methionine, leucine | protein synthesis (tumor viability) |
| $^{18}$F | F$^-$ | osteoblastic activity (bone scan) |
| $^{18}$F | fluorodeoxyglucose (FDG) | glucose metabolism (tumor activity) |
| $^{64}$Cu | ASTM | Hypoxia |

**Table 6.** Some SPECT Tracers Used in Radiotherapy Planning and Evaluation

| Isotope | Tracer | Application |
|---------|--------|-------------|
| $^{111}$In | somatostatin receptor binding agents (octreotide, pentreotide) | lung, neuroendocrine tumors |
| $^{111}$In | OncoScint | colorectal, ovarian cancer |
| $^{111}$In | ProstaScint | prostate cancer |
| $^{99}$Tc | Macro aggregated albumen (MAA) | lung perfusion |
| $^{99}$Tc | antiCEA | colorectal cancer |
| $^{99}$Tc | DTPA | lung ventilation |
| $^{99}$Tc | MDP | bone metastases |
| $^{99}$Tc | HMPAO | brain perfusion |
| $^{99}$Tc | sulfur colloid | bone marrow activity |
| $^{67}$Ga | Gallium citrate | lymphoma |
| $^{123}$I | IMP | cerebral blood flow |
| $^{201}$Tl | thallium chloride | tumor detection- brain, head and neck |

A particularly successful application of SPECT imaging in radiation oncology has been the identification of regions of healthy and damaged lung, both for assessment of radiation induced lung complications and for adjusting treatment plans in an attempt to spare healthy lung regions (Boersma et al. 1993; Marks et al. 1993, 1997).

Application of nuclear medicine images in RTP requires registration and fusion of the functional information with CT and/or MR images, since the anatomical location of each functional region is critical to beam targeting. Examples of applications of the use of SPECT imaging in RTP for prostate and gynecologic cancers are discussed in the Image Registration section below.

### *fMRI*

In several situations, with appropriate analysis dynamic changes in MR images can yield qualitative or quantitative information concerning aspects of physiology. The most commonly used forms of functional MRI (fMRI) are blood oxygen level dependent (BOLD) contrast, which yields information concerning local oxygen concentration and/or oxygen utilization, and perfusion imaging, which yields information such as regional blood volume and blood flow, tissue perfusion or diffusion.

The BOLD effect is due to differences in the magnetic properties of oxygenated and deoxygenated hemoglobin. Deoxyhemoglobin is paramagnetic, and its presence in tissue leads to dephasing of precessing proton spins in the transverse plane and shortening of the effective transverse relaxation time $T_2^*$. Thus regions with higher levels of deoxyhemoglobin show decreased intensity on appropriately weighted MR images. BOLD signal intensities can thus be directly interpreted in terms of local tissue oxygenation, although only qualitatively. In turn, differences in $T_2^*$ sensitive images in two conditions can be used to identify regions in which oxygenation changes, for example between a resting and a task state (Belliveau et al. 1991). Such difference images can thus yield information as to which brain regions are involved in a specific activity. Hamilton et al. (1997) described the potential for including important functional brain regions as avoidance structures in planning for stereotactic radiosurgery.

Perfusion-weighted imaging is based on the analysis of time dependence of image intensity changes following the introduction of a contrast agent. The contrast agent may be endogenous, for example, saturated spins in flowing blood, or exogenous, such as a gadolinium-containing material. In the most basic technique, multiple $T_1$-weighted images are acquired in rapid succession following a bolus injection of Gd contrast. Analysis of the time dependence of image intensity at a particular voxel can yield measurements of blood volume, blood-brain barrier integrity, diffusion, perfusion, blood flow, and other parameters. Incorporation of perfusion maps from dynamic imaging has been reported to improve specificity in identification of active tumor areas in brain lesions, for example, in the differentiation of tumor from necrosis (Cha et al. 2002). Information on local diffusion coefficients from MR images has also been reported to be useful in identifying active regions in brain tumors (Tien et al. 1994). Such information may be useful in the definition of a BTV.

*MR Spectroscopic Imaging (MRSI)*

The actual magnetic field experienced by each proton in an MR imaging study is influenced by the electrons in the molecule of which the proton is a part. Different molecules introduce different degrees of shielding of the applied field, leading to a *chemical shift* in the proton resonance frequency for the various molecules—water, fat, etc. Analysis of the spectrum of resonant frequencies thus can yield information concerning the relative abundance of the different molecules. This in turn can be interpreted in terms of physiological processes that may be associated with the presence of some molecule in greater or lesser abundance relative to that observed in normal tissue. For example, choline, a metabolite which is associated with cell membrane turnover, has been observed to have higher abundance in malignant prostate tissue, compared to either normal or benign hypertrophic prostate (Scheidler et al. 1999). MRSI can map the location of tissue with high choline, and this spatial information can be used in definition of a BTV, with higher doses being delivered to regions that are spectroscopically more likely to be malignant. Spectroscopic information can also be used to identify active tumor regions in the brain. Figure 9 shows the same $T_2$-weighted brain slice as in figure 8, with spectra from normal (left) and tumor (right) regions. The relative heights of several peaks on the left increase approximately linearly. These peaks are associated with choline, creatine, glutamates, and N-acetylaspartate (NAA). Their linear relationship, shown with a dashed line in figure 9, is known as "Hunter's angle" and is a signature of normally functioning brain tissue. In the tumor region on the right, the spectrum is considerably altered, with the relative intensities of the choline and creatine peaks reversed. High levels of lactate observed in MRSI may also be used to identify hypoxic tumor regions, which may be useful in designing a BTV.

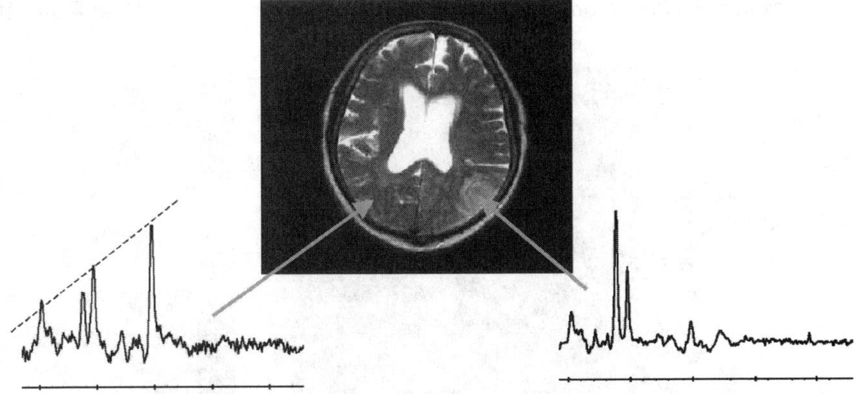

**Figure 9.** $T_2$-weighted brain image with spectra from normal and tumor regions. The normal linearly increasing relationship between several spectral peaks on the left is absent on the right, indicative of tumor. [Image courtesy of P. MacEneaney, M.D., University of Chicago]

*Other Modalities: Molecular Imaging, EPR Oxygen Imaging*

Recently there has been a rapid expansion of techniques aimed at imaging function at the molecular level. One approach to such imaging is to tag a radioisotope onto a substance that would be trapped due to chemical interactions in a particular physiologic process. Strategies have also been developed in which tracer molecules are targeted to specific cell-surface receptors, as in the case of several SPECT tracers mentioned earlier. Nuclear magnetic resonance (NMR) contrast generating tracers can also be targeted in this way. Contrast agents that are shielded within larger molecules, which can be cleaved by enzymatic activity specific to a physiologic process of interest, have also been demonstrated. For example, Meade and coworkers described the use of a molecular cage to shield paramagnetic gadolinium. When the cage was cleaved by a particular enzyme, MRI contrast was developed that indicated the distribution of cells producing the enzyme (Louie et al. 2000). Reporter molecules carrying radioisotopes that concentrate in regions where a particular gene is expressed have also been developed. This allows SPECT or PET imaging of regions of elevated expression of the targeted genes (Gambhir et al. 1999).

Spin resonance imaging utilizing electron rather than nuclear spins, known as EPRI, can also be used to produce 3-D maps of functional parameters. Using suitably designed contrast agents, the spectral line width in an EPR image can be converted to absolute values of tissue oxygen concentration (Halpern et al. 1994). Parameters of the microscopic tissue environment such as viscosity and pH can also be inferred using this technique. A capability for quantitative mapping of oxygen concentration with spatial resolution of ~1 mm and oxygen tension resolution of ~2 torr in small animals has been demonstrated (Elas et al. 2003). Regions of hypoxia that may require additional attention in treatment planning may be identified from such maps, and as such may play a role in BTV design. An example of an EPR oxygen image showing normoxic and hypoxic regions in an experimental tumor model is shown in figure 10.

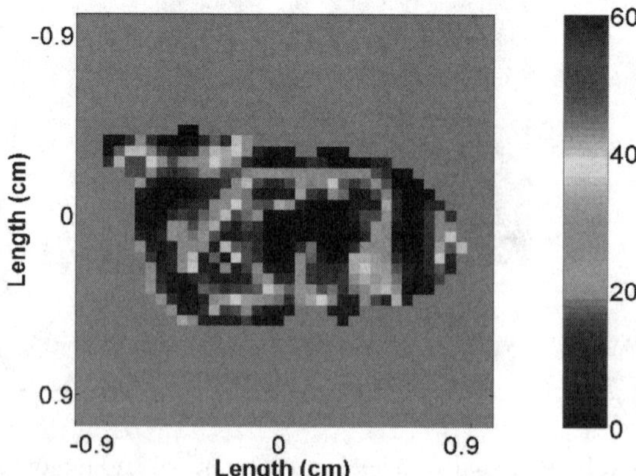


**Figure 10.** Coronal section from a 3-D tissue oxygen concentration map from EPR imaging of a rodent hind limb. Colorbar labeled in oxygen partial pressure (torr). [Image courtesy of H. Halpern, M.D., Ph.D., University of Chicago]

# Image Import Into RTP Systems" DICOM®[1] And DICOM-RT

In the early days of 3-D medical imaging modalities, each vendor developed unique data storage formats with features deemed desirable for their particular needs; for example, lossless data compression to minimize storage capacity requirements (recall that in the early 1980's, the cost of disk storage was in the range of $40 per megabyte, and not until the late 1980's were tapes and optical disks with capacity much beyond a few hundred megabytes available). CT and MRI storage formats even for a single vendor were typically different, reflecting their development by engineering groups with different priorities on what information needed to be accommodated in the archived files. For a treatment planning system to import data from any given scanner, custom software was required specific to the peculiar format of files from that modality and vendor. Furthermore, some scanners archived data onto reels of 1/2-inch tape, some onto tape cartridges, some onto floppy disks, some onto optical disks, so an RTP system might need several different storage devices to read all the required media. Different vendors' scanners used different computer hardware and operating systems, so their archived media might not be compatible with the hardware and software of any given RTP system. Network connectivity to scanners, even when it became available in the middle to late 1980's, was not intended to support transfer of data except between operating consoles and auxiliary viewing workstations produced by the same vendor.

One of the key technologies which has led to the ubiquitous use of image datasets in RTP is the industry standard Digital Imaging and Communications in Medicine, or DICOM, protocol. DICOM provides a consistent format and a set of protocols by which images may be communicated between computers and applications, and stored. Beginning in 1983, the American College of Radiology (ACR) and the National Electrical Manufacturers Association (NEMA) developed DICOM in order to facilitate standardized image communication, which was clearly required in order that picture archiving and communication systems (PACS) would ever move beyond single-vendor closed systems. Several versions of the basic standard were developed in the late 1980's (ACR-NEMA 1985, 1988) and development has continued since, with the current version of the standard, version 3.1, released in 2001. Initially DICOM was conceived in terms of communication over point-to-point links between computers, but later versions provide support for communication over local and wide-area networks, and for file storage on magnetic and optical media. DICOM is based on a number of key notions, of which a few will be described here. Quoted definitions are from the draft standards documents (ACR-NEMA 2001).

An *Information Object* is "an abstraction of a real information entity (e.g., CT Image, Study, etc.) which is acted upon by one or more DICOM Commands." An *Information Object Instance* is "a representation of an occurrence of an real-world

---

[1] DICOM is the registered trademark of the National Electrical Manufacturers Association for its standards publications relating to digital communications of medical information.

entity, which includes values for the attributes of the Information Object Class to which the entity belongs" (e.g., a specific CT image).

An *Information Object Definition* (*IOD*) is "an object-oriented abstract data model used to specify information about Real-World Objects. An IOD provides communicating Application Entities with a common view of the information to be exchanged."

IODs are thus a common language by which different computers and programs may "read" and "write" images. IODs must exist for each type of image (or non-image) dataset which is to be communicated using DICOM. IODs are defined in the 2001 standard for CT, Computed Radiography (CR), Nuclear Medicine, MR, PET, US, Secondary Capture (SC, e.g., digitized film, screen dump), Overlay, Curve, X-ray Angiography, X-ray Radiography/Fluoroscopy, RT Image, RT Dose, RT Structure Set, RT Plan, Digital Mammography, Digital Oral X-ray, RT Beams Treatment Record, RT Brachy Treatment Record, Visible Light Image, Waveform, and others.

A *Service Class* is "a structured description of a service which is supported by cooperating DICOM Application Entities using specific DICOM commands acting on a specific class of Information Object." Examples include storage, query, retrieval, and print service classes.

A *Service-Object Pair* (*SOP*) Class is "the union of a specific set of...Services and one related Information Object Definition (as specified by a Service Class Definition) which completely defines a precise context for communication." For example, CT Image (the object) Storage (the service) is a Service-Object Pair.

A *Service Class User* (*SCU*) is "the role played by a DICOM Application Entity...which invokes operations and performs notifications on a specific Association."

A *Service Class Provider* (*SCP*) is "the role played by a DICOM Application Entity...which performs operations and invokes notifications on a specific Association."

As an example, consider the frequently occurring "push" transfer of CT images from a scanner console to an RTP system. In this case, the scanner is actually requesting that the RTP system act as a Service Class Provider of CT Image Storage, for which the scanner console will be the Service Class User. On the other hand, if the RTP system queries the scanner console to find a particular study and then "pulls" the study from the console, the RTP system is a Service Class User of first the CT Image Query and then CT Image Retrieve services, provided by the scanner console.

The IOD for a particular Information Object defines a set of data elements which make up the object. Each element has a unique *Tag*, which is a pair of four-digit hexadecimal numbers of the form (gggg,eeee) where gggg is a *group number* and eeee is an *element number*. For example, the tag (0010,0010) corresponds to the patient's name, and (0010,0020) to the patient ID. For each tag there is a definition in the DICOM *data dictionary*, which defines the attributes of the data item corresponding to that tag (for example, patient name is a character string, possibly with certain length restrictions; CT matrix size is an integer; MR slice spacing is a real number). For a particular IOD, some data elements are mandatory, some are conditional (required if certain conditions exist) and some are optional. DICOM communication involves some initial negotiation between service class user and provider, followed by a stream of messages containing a tag, (sometimes) the number of bytes of data to be transmitted, (sometimes) information about how the data is represented, and finally the data corresponding to the current tag's data element. DICOM data are stored on disk in either this stream format, or in the file format defined in Part 10 of the standard, the so-called "Part 10" format. Most RTP systems today can import images directly from a scanner or PACS system via DICOM query and retrieve, or by reading either raw or Part 10 DICOM files received by a local storage server.

Of particular importance in RTP are the so-called "DICOM-RT" extensions to the original standard, developed in the 1990's and now part of the base standard. These include the IODs for *RT Image* (a simulator image, portal image or DRR, with optional curve overlays for collimator jaws, beam apertures, etc.); *RT Structure Set* (any number of 3-D structures, defined as multiple contours); *RT Dose* (dose information, expressed as lists of point doses, 2-D or 3-D dose grids, isodose curves, or dose-volume histograms), and *RT Plan* (beam definitions, fractionation information, brachytherapy application information, MLC control information, etc.). These are the information objects which are usually used, for example, to transmit structures contoured on a CT simulation workstation to an RTP system, an MLC sequence from an IMRT planning system to an RT information system, or a DRR to a portal image processing workstation. In the case of structures, another mechanism for transfer is also available. Image information objects in DICOM may also include data elements called *curves*, which can be used to store contours of structures or regions, among other uses. CT and MR IODs include curve modules for this purpose. Images transferred from a CT simulation workstation to an RTP system may include these curves for contours that have been defined on each image. If they do, the planning system may support extracting the curves associated with each image slice and using them to create 3-D planning structures. The PlanUNC RTP system developed at the University of North Carolina and used in numerous academic radiation oncology departments, for example, has the capability to convert DICOM curve data elements into the "anastruct" format used in that system to contain 3-D anatomical structures.

Quite a number of commercial or freeware programs are available for viewing images contained in DICOM files, for running a storage server on an RTP workstation or a personal computer, converting DICOM to popular image formats such as TIFF and JPEG, and so forth. An extensive list of available DICOM software is online at http://www.psychology.nottingham.ac.uk/staff/cr1/dicom.html.

## Image Registration And Fusion

In some instances, visual inspection of multiple image datasets is sufficient for their profitable use. This is particularly true in a diagnostic radiology setting. When multiple image datasets are utilized in therapy planning, it is typically desirable to include information from the several sources into a single geometric framework—for example, to include both CT and MRI-defined volumes of interest in a single beam's-eye view planning display, or to evaluate dose-volume statistics for MRI-defined volumes when a dose calculation has been done in a coordinate system defined with respect to CT images. Furthermore, it is frequently desirable to have an accurate estimate of how the *actual* patient, being treated or simulated, matches the planned position of the *virtual* patient model for which the treatment plan was designed.

## Rationale For Use Of Multimodality Imaging In RTP

Incorporation of information from more than one image study into RTP is motivated by the desire to use the most complete information available on each anatomical or functional region that affects the plan. In many instances this involves combination of anatomical information from multiple modalities. In other instances, combinations of anatomical and functional information can serve to improve the definition of a target or avoidance region.

### Multiple Anatomical Modalities

The earliest applications of multimodality fusion in RTP addressed the problem of locating brain lesions which were better visualized in MRI, in the coordinates of CT scans being used for planning (Kessler et al. 1991; Phillips et al. 1991). This continues to be the dominant application of this technology today. An example from a prostate planning case is shown in figure 11. It is also frequently useful to merge multiple scans of the same modality, e.g., treatment planning CT with diagnostic CT of the preoperative or prechemotherapy patient, to allow inclusion of suspected microscopic disease extension around a no longer visible tumor to be included in the CTV (Sailer et al. 1996). Fusion of serial imaging studies is also useful in assessment of tumor response to therapy, and for analysis of organ motion and patient setup uncertainties.

### Combination Of Anatomic And Functional Modalities

Fusion of PET and SPECT images with CT and MR was developed initially for the purpose of allowing more accurate analysis of the functional images, and to facilitate anatomically based interpretation, diagnosis, and surgery planning (Maguire et al. 1986; Pelizzari et al. 1987; Pelizzari 1989; Schad et al. 1987; Levin et al. 1989; Kovacic et al. 1989). The potential for using a set of anatomical images as a reference coordinate frame in which multiple functional images could be combined was also recognized useful early on, for example combining images reflecting metabolic, blood flow and blood-brain barrier breakdown status to assist in the differential diagnosis of recurrence vs. necrosis (Hollman et al. 1991). Fusion of functional lung images with CT, and also analysis of temporal changes in fused serial lung images, have been useful in analysis and in attempts to limit lung toxicity, as mentioned earlier. In addition, registration of SPECT images with CT was proposed for use in planning for radioimmunotherapy (Roeske et al. 1992).

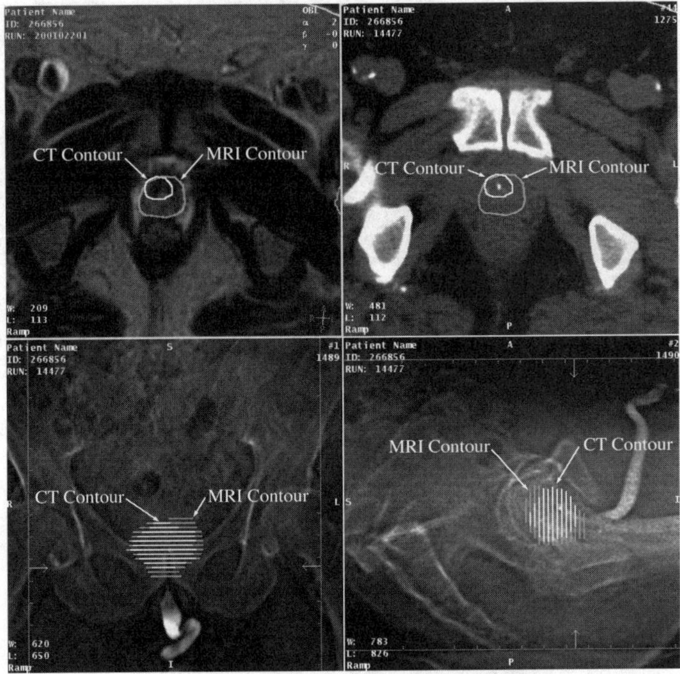


**Figure 11.** Image capture from a Philips AcQPlan workstation. The change in volume is seen on the digitally constructed radiographs below, with the MRI in the lighter shade and the CT in the brighter. [Image courtesy of Philips Medical Systems]

Inclusion of functional imaging in IMRT planning may allow optimization of dose distributions to minimize irradiation of identified functional regions. One such application is briefly described here. Originally, intensity-modulated whole pelvic radiotherapy (IM-WPRT) was developed in order to limit small bowel irradiation when treating whole pelvic fields in gynecologic cases (Roeske et al. 2000; Mundt et al. 2002). Recent work has investigated means to reduce hematologic toxicity due to irradiation of bone marrow in the pelvis (Brixey et al. 2002). Active bone marrow regions can be identified on nuclear medicine images, and the location of these regions can be transformed into the CT scan coordinate system used for IMRT planning. These functional bone marrow regions can then be used as avoidance structures in IMRT optimization. Figure 12 shows overlaid CT and $^{99}$Tc sulfur-colloid SPECT images, where the high intensity regions in SPECT correspond to active bone marrow. These images were merged using the multimodality registration capabilities of the Philips AcQSim software, by matching surfaces of marrow spaces contoured on CT with the boundaries of high-intensity regions contoured in SPECT (see below for discussion of surface matching). As shown in figure 13, dose to active bone marrow is significantly reduced when these functional regions are used as constraints in IMRT planning.

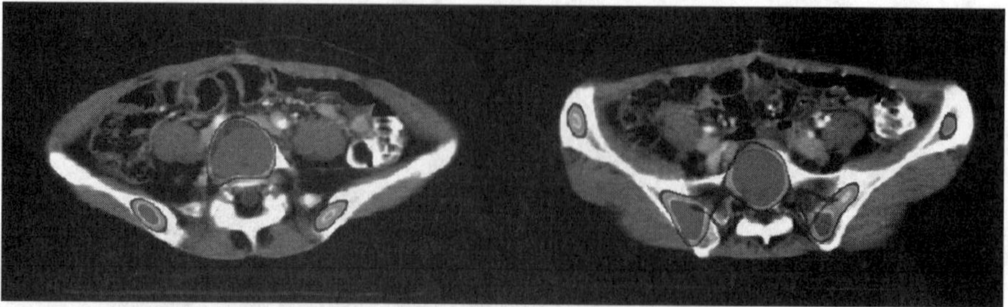

**Figure 12.** Fused ⁹⁹Tc sulfur colloid SPECT and CT images showing active bone marrow regions for IMRT planning. [Image courtesy of J. Roeske, Ph.D., University of Chicago]

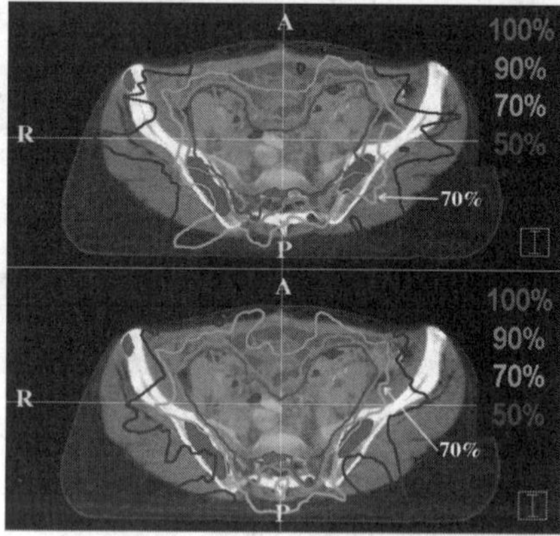

**Figure 13.** Example dose from bone-marrow sparing plan (bottom) showing avoidance of marrow regions (solid dark gray) by 70% isodose line. [Image courtesy of J. Roeske, Ph.D., University of Chicago]

## Methods Of Multimodality Fusion

*Registration And Fusion*

Several terms which are frequently used interchangeably, but which in fact have distinct meanings, are useful in this discussion. The combination of multiple images, or more generally the transfer of information from one image study to another, is referred to as *image fusion*. Taking the example of multiple tomographic image studies of a single patient, accurate image fusion clearly requires a knowledge of how the patient is oriented with respect to the image planes of the two studies. The process of establishing a coordinate transformation between the inherent coordinate spaces of two (or more) image studies, such that homologous points in the two spaces are mapped accurately onto each other, is termed *image registration*. Not surprisingly, interest in image registration and fusion is not limited to medical applications. Multispectral satellite imaging, astronomical imaging at widely varying wavelengths, robot vision, fingerprint analysis, and guidance of "smart" weapons are only a few examples of problems where accurate alignment of multiple images of the same scene, or of an image and a model of the scene, is useful. Several of the registration tools that are now applied routinely in medical imaging applications have their origins in one of these apparently unrelated fields. Several review articles have surveyed the field of medical image registration (Mauer and Fitzpatrick 1993; van den Elsen, Pol, and Viergever 1993; Maintz and Viergever 1998). Once the interscan coordinate transformation is known, it may be used to transfer any information from either scan to the other, which is the process of data fusion. For example, if a tumor volume has been identified on MRI sometime before the day of a stereotactic procedure, that volume may be transformed into the coordinate system of a stereotactic planning CT and used for beam planning. This is the sort of capability that is provided by the image fusion tools in the Radionics XKnife system, among others. Given the availability of image registration based on patient-intrinsic information, it has been suggested (Kooy et al. 1994) that use of MRI compatible stereotactic localizers is unnecessary, and in fact it may be the case that use of an intrinsic image registration method is a way of avoiding possible errors due to MRI localization uncertainties as discussed above (Alexander et al. 1995).

*Coordinate Transformations*

An important distinction between registration methods involves the class of coordinate transformations they are capable of utilizing in matching one dataset onto another. The simplest transformation is the *rigid body* transformation, which permits only translation and scaling in the mapping between the two coordinate spaces. Clearly such simple transformations are limited in their applicability, since few parts of any patient's anatomy actually move as rigid bodies. As might be expected, considerable success has been achieved in registration of brain images using rigid body transformations, and less so in other areas of the body. A slightly more complex transformation is the *affine* or general linear transformation, which includes anisotropic scaling and shearing. Progressively more complex, and with correspondingly more ability to model distortion of anatomy between two sets of images are *polynomial warping, elastic warping* [of which a particularly widely used variant is *thin plate spline warping* (Bookstein 1991)] and *viscous fluid deformation*. Each of these warping techniques allows every image voxel to effectively have its own coordinate transformation, slightly different from its neighbors. This allows the accommodation of continuous shape changes of tissues between scans, as would be caused by patient positioning on a flat instead of a curved couch, or of internal organ shape changes such as bladder and rectal filling or even tumor growth or resection. Additionally, coordinate transformations may be either *global* (i.e., a single transformation is applied to every voxel in the image spaces) or *local* (i.e., a different coordinate transformation may apply at different locations in the image spaces). Local transformations can be used to account for differences in the motions or distortions of different organs, for example.

A particularly promising approach to specifying coordinate transformations in image registration is the use of a biomechanical model of the underlying anatomy to control the mapping of one set of image data onto another. In this framework, it is possible to include realistic mechanical properties of multiple tissues, so that interorgan motions and deformations of individual tissue types between scans may be accurately modeled (Bharatha et al. 2001).

*Feature-Based Registration*

Since image registration requires the knowledge of a coordinate transformation between the two image studies, which relates the patient position in each of them, it is necessary to be able to learn the orientation of the slices of each study with respect to some coordinate system fixed to the patient. The basis of this coordinate system can be intrinsic to the patient, meaning defined by some aspect of the patient's anatomy, or it can be extrinsic, meaning added to the patient. The stereotactic localizer frame generally used in planning radiosurgery is a classic example of an extrinsic coordinate basis. To be useful in image registration, of course, the frame must be visible in all image sets of interest; frames have been designed over the years that are compatible with CT, MRI, angiography, and nuclear medicine images (Schad et al. 1987). Other extrinsic bases use point fiducial markers rather than a full coordinate frame. In either case, the positions in the image slices of the coordinate apparatus are used to solve for the orientation of the image coordinate system relative to the extrinsic frame. This idea is of course very familiar to those involved in stereotactic radiosurgery or radiotherapy planning. In principle, if the extrinsic apparatus is visible in each of two or more modalities, and its coordinate system remains fixed relative to the patient for the two image studies, then the orientation of the native coordinate system of each separate modality can be found *relative to the frame*. The relationship of the two relative orientations then defines the interscan coordinate transformation required for image registration.

The use of extrinsic registration methods with CT and MRI-compatible frames or fiducials requires either elimination of or correction for distortions which may be present in MR images (Schad et al 1987a; Dong, Fitzpatrick, and Maciunas 1992). It has been argued that under certain circumstances, errors of several millimeters may be inherent in uncorrected MR images (Sumanaweera et al. 1995); and that even when corrections are made, registration based on an external stereotactic frame in MRI may still be subject to errors on the order of millimeters (Kooy et al. 1994). The problem, in essence, is that the magnetic field experienced by the frame is different from that experienced by the head, due to susceptibility differences, so that a measurement of coordinates of the frame is no longer necessarily accurate with respect to patient anatomy. One approach to addressing this problem is to use an *intrinsic* rather than an extrinsic registration basis; that is, to use the patient's anatomy as the basis of registration.

Many registration methods using patient-intrinsic information as their basis have been developed, differing in one or more of several key areas. Most methods identify anatomical homologies between the two image studies and attempt to find an interscan coordinate transformation that matches the homologous structures. The characteristics of the structures used, and the particular mathematical algorithms used to maximize the interscan homology are the factors that generally differentiate one method from another. The structure to be matched may be 3-D "point" landmarks, either manually or in some cases automatically identified. Pointlike landmarks might include the crossing of two vessels; for example, the tips of bony prominences or the extrema of one soft tissue structure or another. Alternatively, "curve" landmarks such as the 3-D trajectory of vessels may be used. "Plane" landmarks are not frequently used, but the interhemispheric plane in the brain has indeed been used as a constraint in several registration methods. The use of all or portions of 3-D surfaces, such as the surface of the brain, as elements to be matched is also common.

An illustrative example of a surface-based registration method is the "chamfer matching" method developed by van Herk and Kooy (van Herk et al. 1992; Kooy et al. 1994) and integrated into the Radionics "XKnife" planning system. Chamfer matching is a calculational technique for minimizing the average distance between two models of the same surface, where one model for example might be the surface of the brain as defined from CT and another the same surface as defined from MRI. In each of the two scans, let us suppose the "native" coordinate system will have its x-y plane aligned with the transverse image slices and its z-axis normal to those planes. In case sagittal or coronal MR slices are used, the image planes might be x-z or y-z planes instead of x-y planes, but the procedure is the same. Assuming the brain has been contoured on some or all the slices, the x-y pixel coordinates along the contours on each plane together with their z coordinates define a 3-D locus of points that are on the surface of the brain in the scan coordinate system. All the contours together define a 3-D model of the brain surface. Contouring in both studies, then, results in two models of the brain surface, one in CT coordinates and one in MRI coordinates. In fact, identification of the surfaces to be matched may be done semiautomatically or even fully automatically, depending on the particular registration method. It is not even necessary to uniquely identify the 3-D objects of which the surfaces are to be matched—one may simply locate the positions of high gradients, intensity ridges, points of maximum curvature, or other mathematically defined features in the two scans, and use those features for registration. The object of image registration is of course to find the transformation between these two coordinate systems which when applied to one of the models (the MRI brain model, say) matches it most closely with the other (CT) model. Conceptually, one can think of interactively adjusting the interscan coordinate transformation to reorient the MRI model to bring it into coincidence with the CT model, while watching the two models on a display. Again, numerous methods for characterizing how well the two models fit together, and for finding the transformation that optimizes the match, have been developed. Chamfer matching involves precalculation of a 3-D distance field, which defines for each point (in CT space, say) the distance from that point in space to the nearest point which is on the brain surface. If the surface were an electrostatically charged object, the distance field would be analogous to a potential. Once having the distance field, the evaluation of the goodness of fit of the MRI model with the CT model consists simply of adding up the value of the distance field at each point on the MRI model. The procedure then consists of iteratively moving the MRI model around in CT space, evaluating the distance sum at each reorientation, and using some search procedure to find the reorientation of the MRI model which results in the minimum distance sum. This reorientation then represents an estimate of the interscan coordinate transformation—if the structure chosen for matching (the brain surface in this example) is an appropriate one, then the same transformation which matches the surface should also match the image data from which the surface was extracted, and should also match any other structures which are defined in either of the two scans. In fact, many matching procedures allow the definition of multiple homologous structures in the two scans, which are all used simultaneously in the matching process.

*Intensity-Based Registration*

A final step up in the complexity of features to be matched involves registration methods in which the entire volume of image data, that is, the intensities of the image voxels themselves, are utilized for matching. Understanding such methods is simplest in the context of single-modality registration. Consider the simple case of a single CT scan of a head, and a copy of the same dataset that has been translated and rotated. To register these two datasets, the second (transformed) dataset must be translated and rotated in an attempt to match it with the first (original). When the datasets are perfectly registered, every voxel of the second dataset, which is just the original dataset transformed away and then transformed back, should map onto an original voxel of exactly the same intensity. Thus a potential registration strategy might be to attempt to maximize the correlation in intensities between the original and the transformed datasets. Interestingly, the same type of strategy is useful for multimodality registration, even including functional images. This is true because although anatomical regions may appear with different relative intensities in different image modalities, their intensities are still highly correlated. Consider for example CT and MRI images in the head, and focus on three voxel classes: air is very dark in both CT and MRI; bone is bright in CT and dark in MRI, though not as dark as air; brain is intermediate in intensity in both modalities but with a considerable range of intensities in MRI. Let the intensities of air, tissue, and bone in CT and MRI be {Ac, Tc, Bc} and {Am, Tm, Bm}, for the moment taking a single value for brain in MRI. If the entire image volumes are perfectly registered with each other, then there is a high probability that bright CT voxels of intensity Bc will map onto dark MRI voxels of intensity Bm; and tissue CT voxels of intensity Tc will likewise have a high probability of mapping onto brain MRI voxels of intensity Tm. If the volumes are less than perfectly registered, some bright CT bone voxels may map onto MRI brain voxels and some dark MRI bone voxels onto CT brain voxels, and bone or tissue voxels in either scan may map onto air voxels in the other. Mathematically, we can say that when the registration is best, the joint distribution of intensity pairings in the overlapped volumes is most highly ordered. This is illustrated in figures 14 and 15.

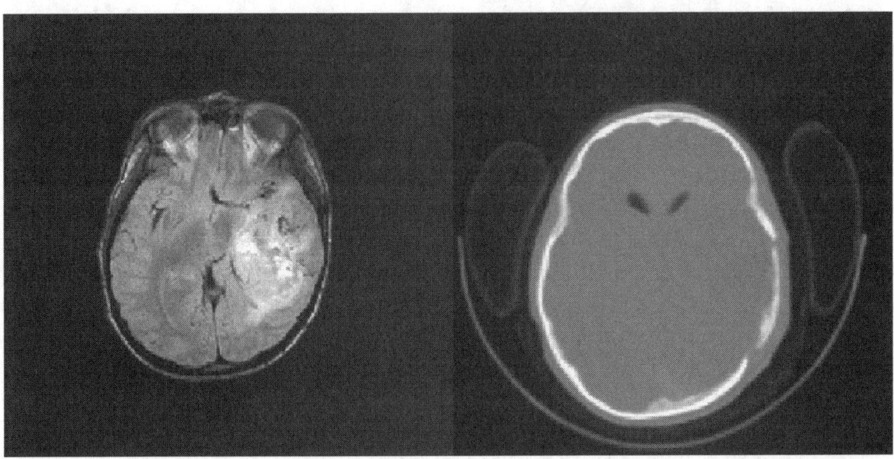

**Figure 14.** Principle of intensity correlation-based registration. Shown are MR and CT slices from the same patient, misregistered in 3-D. If perfectly registered, dark MRI bone voxels should have a high probability of mapping onto bright CT bone voxels. Very dark CT air voxels should map onto very dark MRI air voxels. Intermediate and bright MRI brain voxels should map onto intermediate CT brain voxels. This should hold true throughout the 3-D volume.

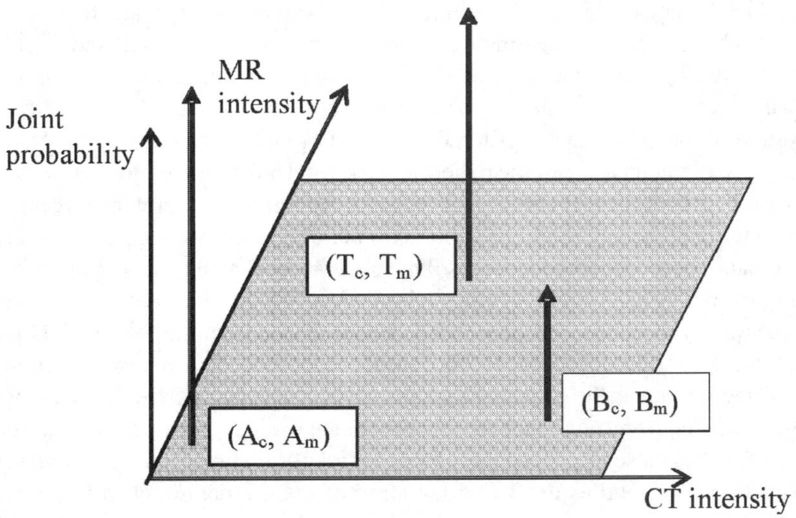


**Figure 15.** The joint intensity histogram plots probability of occurrence of CT and MRI intensity pairs. When the two spaces are properly aligned, strong peaks should occur for intensity pairs corresponding to the registered tissue types.

A useful information theoretic concept that quantifies the extent to which intensities are correlated, as evidenced in properties of the joint histogram, is mutual information (MI). Formally, MI expresses the extent to which knowledge of the value of one random variable allows prediction of the value of another. In our registration example, when the volumes are perfectly registered, then knowing that a CT voxel has bone intensity should mean there is a high probability that the corresponding MRI voxel also has bone intensity, and likewise for tissue and air voxels. Registration methods based on maximization of MI in the registered datasets have proven useful for a wide range of single- and multimodality problems, including both anatomic and functional images, in 2-D and in 3-D (Viola 1995; Wells, Viola, and Kikinis 1995). Several commercial image registration software systems provide MI-based registration capability, and the use of MI based registration on a routine basis in RTP has been reported (Kessler et al. 2002).

It has also been found useful in clinical practice to use an interactive intensity-based registration tool, where the operator manipulates the interscan coordinate transformation and is immediately presented with overlaid slices from the two registered datasets.

*2-D/3-D Registration*

A very important class of registration problems in radiation therapy planning and delivery involves the registration of a 3-D dataset such as a CT-based model of the patient's anatomy, with a 2-D dataset such as a simulation film or a megavoltage radiograph. Such 2-D/3-D registration would be utilized, for example, to evaluate the pose of the patient on the simulator or treatment machine in terms of the position and orientation of the CT-based patient model, since we know what the orientation of the model relative to the beam should be when the patient is perfectly positioned. Thus the difference in position of the 3-D model registered to the radiographs, compared to the "correct" position, is a direct measure of the patient setup error. Unfortunately, the 2-D/3-D registration problem is quite difficult. Using only one radiograph, positioning errors normal to the imaging plane and rotations about axes parallel to the imaging plane (so-called "out of plane rotations") cannot be resolved accurately, if at all, using straightforward techniques. By using two radiographs (simulation or portal images) to solve for the 3-D orientation of the patient model, it is possible to determine the full 3-D patient positioning error (Gilhuijs et al. 1996; Bansal et al. 1999). One important problem in 2-D/3-D registration is the choice of features which are to be matched between the 2-D and 3-D datasets. Bony edges are an obvious choice when registering CT datasets with radiographs, but these edges typically must be identified both in the 3-D dataset and in the radiographs, and as the 3-D orientation of the CT dataset changes, the set of image voxels that map onto the bony edges in the radiograph also changes. Effectively one wishes to map the "shadow" of the entire set of bony voxels in the CT, onto the bony region of the radiograph. Gilhuijs used a chamfer matching technique, as described above for 3-D surface matching, to register reconstructed radiographs from CT with the experimental radiographs, while varying the orientation of the CT dataset, to find the best agreement of the bony edges. Another interesting approach was taken by Bansal et al. (1999), who utilized an algorithm which simultaneously labeled and registered the bony voxels in both the CT and the radiographs. Excellent results were obtained when using two radiographs, and encouraging results were also obtained when using only a single radiograph.

## Patient-Image Registration

It is useful to note that although we typically speak of "image registration," there is also a very important application for registration of *image* space to *physical* space. This is, of course, the very purpose of stereotactic imaging—to impose a coordinate system on the patient that can be used to relate an image-identified coordinate with an actual location in the patient. It is also worth noting that the entire concept of virtual simulation rests on the assumption that the virtual patient (i.e., the images) and the real patient are registered, so a beam planned on the virtual patient will actually be delivered accurately to the real patient. So too, does any form of image-guided therapy, whether radiation therapy, focused ultrasound tissue ablation, cryosurgery, stereotactic neurosurgery, or any other modality. There has also been considerable work in the field of image-guided surgery on what has sometimes been called "frameless stereotaxy" and which is essentially the use of methods similar to those of image registration to determine a coordinate transformation between the image space of a virtual patient model, and the physical space of an actual procedure.

## Image Segmentation

An essential step in the use of image information to create the "virtual patient" model used in RTP is image segmentation, which is the process of identification and localization of each region of interest, both target and nontarget, that is to be considered in the treatment planning process. As discussed earlier, regions of interest may be either anatomic or functional, and may need to be identified and located in any number of image modalities. Techniques for performing these segmentation tasks have been the topic of intensive research for decades, and a complete, satisfactory set of methods for use in RTP still does not exist. The situation is much the same in other areas of medicine where quantitative use is made of image data for modeling or analysis, such as surgical planning.

## Requirements On Image Segmentation For RTP

Not very much attention has been devoted to formally characterizing the performance requirements for segmentation in RTP in terms such as specificity and sensitivity, which are widely used to evaluate image-processing algorithms used in diagnostic radiology. As pointed out by Jolesz (2002), "Diagnosis needs specificity, but it is less

**Charles A. Pelizzari**

susceptible to accuracy of localization. For therapy, sensitivity should be a fundamental feature." One may question to what extent the importance of sensitivity should be stressed at the extent of specificity, but certainly it is intuitive that if we desire to identify a target volume, it is necessary to identify all the image voxels that correspond to tumor, avoiding the possibility of leaving tumor cells inadequately treated, and perhaps less important not to include some non-tumor voxels in the target. Analogously, if we are identifying an organ at risk, we might prefer to use a technique that errs in the direction of more generous definition rather than missing some voxels at risk, which might then not be accorded all the dose sparing we had wished. In any given treatment situation, there will be some trade-off between the desires for complete identification of all the voxels that belong in a particular structure, and for leaving out voxels which are not in fact part of the structures. This of course applies to the imaging modalities used in RTP, as well as to the segmentation methods used to process them. There may also inevitably be ambiguities as to which region (target or organ at risk) certain voxels belong to. Another point of view concerning accuracy requirements for segmentation is that such requirements are context dependent, varying from one anatomical site or treatment technique to another. If uncertainties due to segmentation are insignificant compared to expected physiologic motion or patient setup uncertainty, then the segmentation may be "good enough," while for radiosurgery with rigid immobilization and minimal margins, more accuracy may be required of segmentation.

It is interesting to classify segmentation techniques according to what type of knowledge they use and what type of image features they operate on. One such classification, similar to that suggested by Udupa (2000) is shown in table 7. Methods are initially divided as to whether they identify regions by "delineation," that is, by identifying portions of the image with some specified properties (intensity, texture, gradient) and calling those the segmented objects, or by "recognition," that is, by looking for patterns or shapes known to be associated with the desired objects in the image. Delineation is by nature a more low-level, image processing-oriented approach. Recognition is a more high-level, computer vision-oriented approach.

**Table 7.** Outline of Semiautomatic and Automatic Segmentation Methods<br>[After Udupa (2000)]

<u>**Delineation**</u>
- **Boundary based (e.g., edge detection)**
- **Region based (e.g., region growing)**

<u>**Recognition**</u>
- **Automatic**
  - **Knowledge based**
- **Operator assisted**
  - **Specification of seed point**
  - **Specification of search region**
  - **Accept or reject delineated objects**

## Manual And Semiautomated Methods

The majority of image segmentation for radiation treatment planning continues to be done using manual or semiautomated software tools for structure delineation. Direct tracing of contours on an image display workstation remains by far the most common technique. A selection of flexible tools for freehand drawing, editing, copying from slice to slice, etc., is included in nearly every RTP system. The CORVUS® screen shown in figure 1 provides an example. A number of enhancements to the basic slice-by-slice contouring technique have been introduced in recent years. Several systems, for example the GE Advantage Sim, permit contouring on multiple planes, i.e., sagittal and coronal as well as transaxial, and visualizing the intersection of each contour with the other planes. This provides valuable context for the operator in identifying extrema of structures, such as the apex of the prostate. Interpolation of structures between planes is also supported by many systems. Most systems include some form of semiautomatic structure delineation. As indicated in table 7, such methods may be contour based, as in the case of isodensity threshold or edge following beginning near a point indicated by the operator, or region based, as in the case of region growing around a seed point indicated by the operator. In some cases these tools are able to propagate the identified region from slice to slice, allowing rapid definition of an entire 3-D region. Combination of 2-D and 3-D semiautomated tools to improve the efficiency of segmentation was the thrust of the Medical Anatomy Segmentation Kit (MASK) project at the University of North Carolina in the early 1990's (Tracton et al. 1994). Less commonly used in RTP, but quite popular in other areas of medical image analysis, are parametrically deformable or active contour models which can be initialized in the region where a structure is to be segmented, and allowed to find the contour or 3-D surface location which minimizes some combination of "image energy" having to do with image intensity, gradient, or texture properties, and "shape energy" having to do with shape descriptors such as curvature, size, and smoothness (Kass, Witkin, and Terzopoulos 1988; Staib and Duncan 1992; Cootes et al. 1993; Székely et al. 1996).

## Knowledge-Based Methods

A particularly promising class of segmentation methods includes those which use an "atlas" containing a statistical description of the shape, location, and image properties of tissues to be segmented, and attempts to "recognize" or "find" instances of these structures in the image data space (Bae et al. 1993; Boes et al. 1994). These methods have proven quite successful in brain image segmentation (Collins et al. 1995; Andreasen et al. 1996; Davatzikos 1996; Aboutanos and Dawant 1997; Thompson and Toga 1997). Ultimately, one may hope that such knowledge-based methods will allow nearly automated segmentation of an extensive set of normal tissues, and even perhaps of tissues which are severely distorted by tumors or surgery (by implication, possibly also labeling tumor voxels) (Dawant et al. 2002). Recently, the University of North Carolina group has presented a method based on a deformable multiscale medial shape descriptor which incorporates statistical shape variability explicitly in a user-guided segmentation method (Fletcher et al. 2002; Joshi et al. 2002), which has shown good agreement with segmentation by human experts, and with improved reproducibility (Chen et al. 2002).

A number of modality-specific methods for automatically segmenting high-contrast surfaces in CT by isosurfacing e.g., Lorenson and Cline (1987), or for brain structure segmentation in MRI using multispectral feature space discrimination and connected component analysis, e.g., Cline et al. (1990), have been successfully used in diagnostic and 3-D display applications. Considerable progress has been made in automated segmentation of a number of normal and pathologic structures in the brain from MRI, e.g., Ashton et al. (2003), and the atlas-based approaches discussed earlier. A recent review of segmentation methods by Pham (Pham, Xu, and Prince 2000) provides an introduction to a large number of methods. Since RTP demands that a number of different types of structures must be segmented from several different modalities, no single technique or tool is adequate to the entire task.

## Segmentation Of Planning Target Volumes

Unfortunately, even if all tumor and normal structures are correctly labeled in the image datasets, the segmentation task in RTP still requires the addition of margins to account for subclinical disease (clinical target volume, CTV) and positioning uncertainty (planning target volume, PTV). Usually, the PTV is developed via simple expansion, either isotropic or anisotropic, of the CTV using suitably chosen margins for a given treatment type. Automation of the process of identifying these volumes is also the subject of research. At the University of Washington, knowledge-based tools have been developed to create PTVs based on identified tumor location, using a rule-based system (Austin-Seymour et al. 1995) and compared with PTVs developed by humans using semiautomated tools (simple expansions) (Ketting et al. 1997). Another important application of knowledge-based systems in this area is in the prediction of disease spread for particular anatomical sites (Kalet et al. 2002), which may ultimately aid in CTV definition.

## Imaging For Targeting Verification: Electronic Portal Imaging

For many years, radiographs of the patient made with treatment beams have been compared with simulation films and more recently with DRRs to estimate the accuracy of beam delivery to the actual patient, relative to the simulated treatment (simulator films) or the virtual treatment (DRRs). The development of electronic portal imaging devices (EPIDs) since the early 1990's has revolutionized this application of imaging in radiation therapy. The ability to view images with no delay for film processing, and to electronically compare a just-acquired MV image with a reference DRR or electronically stored simulation image, allows the possibility of evaluating patient positioning errors as soon as the portal image is acquired, so that a correction may in fact be made on the spot, before the daily fraction is delivered. A great deal of work has gone into the development of both software tools and strategies to optimize the use of this critical information in ensuring the most accurate delivery of the planned doses to target and sparing of normal tissues.

## EPID Technology

Early EPID systems were based on a variety of technologies, with the dominant products using either a segmented liquid ion chamber that could be read out sequentially in a raster scanned mode, or a combination of fluorescent screen, mirror, and video camera. Currently, EPIDs are almost exclusively based on solid-state detector arrays, which differ widely in technologies of photon detection (conversion to charged particles, direct detection vs. fluorescence). With the EPID mounted on a robotic arm on the linear accelerator (linac) gantry, images can be acquired with minimal inconvenience, and both radiographic and fluoroscopic modes are available. Dose required to produce a useful image is continually decreasing with technological development, and is currently in the range of a few centiGray or less, with promise to be well under 1 cGy in the near future. In fluoroscopic "cine" mode, intratreatment motion of patient anatomy can be documented and studied.

## Detection Of Patient Positioning Errors

The basic technique for detection of patient positioning errors from portal images rests on image registration, as discussed earlier. At its simplest, portal image registration is a 2-D/2-D problem of matching the anatomy and the radiation portal as seen in a newly acquired image, to the anatomy and the desired portal outline in the simulation film or DRR. Prior to the era of electronic imaging, positioning errors were detected by physically overlaying port films with simulation films, aligning the field outline and beam axis fiducial markers, and evaluating the relative position of the anatomy. Given the poor contrast and noise characteristics of megavoltage radiographs, this process was less than satisfactory. With electronic imaging, contrast adjustment can be performed to highlight structures in both the reference image and the portal image, to aid in the task of matching. An early system for registration of radiographs was developed by Balter (Balter, Pelizzari, and Chen 1992). This method utilized matching of bony edges, which were identified by an operator as curve segments. The total area between portions of corresponding segments that overlapped was minimized by transforming one set of curves relative to the other, allowing both rotation and translation in the plane of the image. An example is shown in figure 16.

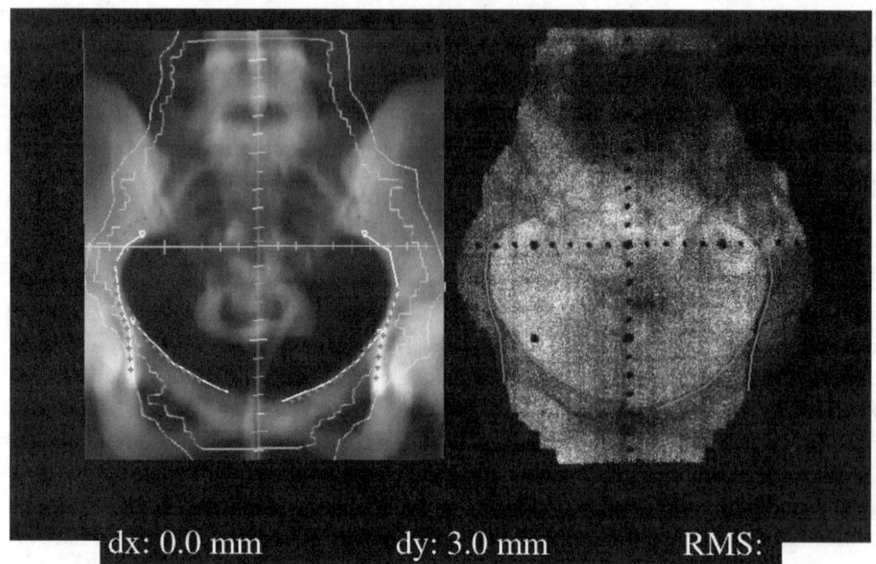



**Figure 16.** Example of matching DRR (left) and portal image using the method of Balter (Balter, Pelizzari, and Chen 1992). Overlap of curves drawn on the two images is maximized to define the inter-image coordinate transformation. [Image courtesy of A. Lujan, Ph.D., University of Chicago]

Many other methods have been developed for matching portal and DRR or simulation images. The Netherlands Cancer Institute (NKI) group utilized chamfer matching as described earlier for 3-D image registration, to match automatically detected edges in portal and reference images (Gilhuijs and van Herk 1993). As mentioned earlier, the matching of multiple portal images with the patient's full CT dataset to derive accurate estimates of the full 3-D patient positioning error has also been demonstrated (Gilhuijs et al. 1996; Gilhuijs, van de Ven, and van Herk 1996; Bansal et al. 1999). A number of image registration techniques described earlier in the context of 3-D image registration have been applied to this problem, including mutual information (Hadley et al. 1997; Kim et al. 2001).

*Adaptive Image Guidance Strategies*

Given an estimate of variation in the positions of target and/or organs at risk from imaging on a daily basis, a natural question how to make optimal use of this information to improve the quality of the treatment delivered (Balter et al. 1993). Clearly, there is a trade-off involved in making corrections to either the patient position or the radiation beams (moving the beams by adjusting MLCs may be viewed as an alternative to repositioning the patient), in that uncertainty in the estimates makes position corrections below some threshold likely to introduce as much or more error than they correct. It is important to analyze position deviations as measured by imaging techniques, whether EPI, serial CT, ultrasound or whatever, in order to understand the statistical distribution of positioning errors for each patient, and to utilize these measurements with proper consideration of the uncertainties in the measurements themselves. Yan and colleagues at William Beaumont Hospital have developed the concept of adaptive radiation therapy (ART) (Yan et al. 1997), where daily imaging is used to build a probability distribution of patient positioning errors, which can be used to predict the effect of making a setup correction (or moving fields) on the subsequent days. After four to nine daily images, more than 95% of patient specific setup margins could be predicted within 1 mm in a prospective study (Yan et al. 1998). Other schemes for making optimized use of image information to correct positioning errors have been published, including a recent scheme for making an optimized unconditional correction after a given number of fractions, with and without consideration of measurement error (Bortfeld, van Herk, and Jiang 2002).

## Conclusion

Radiation therapy planning has been at the forefront in using quantitative information from numerous imaging modalities for many years, and this trend is certain to continue as new imaging technologies become available. From early use of only a few CT slices per plan to today's availability of hundreds of slices from CT and MRI, along with multiple functional image modalities to aid in definition of both tumor and tissues at risk, imaging is at the heart of RTP in general and certainly for IMRT planning. In addition, imaging is critical in quality assurance of therapy delivery, adaptation of therapy to patient positioning and organ motion errors, evaluation of therapy effect and patient followup.

## Acknowledgments

The author is grateful to Himanshu Shukla of Philips Medical Systems, and Peter MacEneaney (Radiology), John Roeske, Howard Halpern, and Anthony Lujan (Radiation Oncology), all of The University of Chicago, for providing images. EPR imaging is supported by NCI/NCRR grant 1P41 RR12257 and DOD grant DAMD17-02-1-0034.

## References

Aboutanos, G., and B. Dawant. (1997). "Automatic brain segmentation and validation: Image-based versus atlas-based deformable models." *SPIE Proc. Med. Imaging* 3034:299–310.

ACR-NEMA. Digital Imaging and Communications in Medicine (DICOM), version 1.0: ACR-NEMA Standards Publication No. 300-1985. Reston, VA: American College of Radiology, 1985.

ACR-NEMA. Digital Imaging and Communications in Medicine (DICOM), version 2.0: ACR-NEMA Standards Publication No. 300-1988. Reston, VA: American College of Radiology, 1988.

ACR-NEMA. Digital Imaging and Communications in Medicine (DICOM). Reston, VA: American College of Radiology, 2001.

Alexander, E., H. Kooy, M. van Herk, M. Schwartz, P. Barnes, N. Tarbell, R. Mulkern, E. Holupka, and J. Loeffler. (1995). "Magnetic resonance image-directed stereotactic neurosurgery: use of image fusion with computerized tomography to enhance spatial accuracy." *J. Neurosurg.* 83(2):271–276.

Andreasen, N., R. Rajarethinam, T. Cizadlo, S. Arndt, V. N. Swayze, L. Flashman, D. O'Leary, J. Ehrhardt, and W. Yuh. (1996). "Automatic atlas-based volume estimation of human brain regions from MR images." *J. Comput. Assist. Tomogr.* 20(1):98–106.

Ashton, E., C. Takahashi, M. Berg, A. Goodman, S. Totterman, and S. Ekholm. (2003). "Accuracy and reproducibility of manual and semiautomated quantification of MS lesions by MRI." *J. Magn. Reson. Imaging* 17(3):300–308.

Austin-Seymour, M., I. Kalet, J. McDonald, S. Kromhout-Schiro, J. Jacky, S. Hummel, and J. Unger. (1995). "Three dimensional planning target volumes: A model and a software tool." *Int. J. Radiat. Oncol. Biol. Phys.* 33(5):1073–1080.

Bae, K., M. Giger, C. Chen, and C. J. Kahn. (1993). "Automatic segmentation of liver structure in CT images." *Med. Phys.* 20(1):71–78.

Balter, J., G. Chen, C. Pelizzari, S. Krishnasamy, S. Rubin, and S. Vijayakumar. (1993). "Online repositioning during treatment of the prostate: A study of potential limits and gains." *Int. J. Radiat. Oncol. Biol. Phys.* 27(1):137–143.

Balter, J., and K. Lam. (2001). "Technical note: Acquisition of CT models for radiotherapy applications with reduced tube heating." *Med. Phys.* 28: 590–592.

Balter, J., C. A. Pelizzari, and G. T. Y. Chen. (1992). "Correlation of projection radiographs in radiation therapy using open curve segments and points." *Med. Phys.* 19:329–334.

Bansal, R., L. Staib, Z. Chen, A. Rangarajan, J. Knisely, R. Nath, and J. Duncan. (1999). "Entropy-Based, Multiple-Portal-To-3-DCT Registration for Prostate Radiotherapy Using Iteratively Estimated Segmentation." Medical Image Computing and Computer Assisted Intervention-MICCAI 99, Cambridge, UK.

Belliveau, J., D. Kennedy Jr., R. McKinstry, B. Buchbinder, R. Weisskoff, M. Cohen, J. Vevea, T. Brady, and B. Rosen. (1991). "Functional mapping of the human visual cortex by magnetic resonance imaging." *Science* 254:716–719.

Bharatha, A., M. Hirose, N. Hata, S. Warfield, M. Ferrant, K. Zou, E. Suarez-Santana, J. Ruiz-Alzola, A. D'Amico, R. Cormack, R. Kikinis, F. Jolesz, and C. Tempany. (2001). "Evaluation of three-dimensional finite element-based deformable registration of pre- and intraoperative prostate imaging." *Med. Phys.* 28(12):2551–2560.

Boersma, L., E. Damen, R. de Boer, S. Muller, R. Valdes Olmos, C. Hoefnagel, C. Roos, N. van Zandwijk, and J. Lebesque. (1993). "A new method to determine dose-effect relations for local lung-function changes using correlated SPECT and CT data." *Radiother. Oncol.* 29(2):110–116.

Boes, J., P. Bland, T. Weymouth, L. Quint, F. Bookstein, and C. Meyer. (1994). "Generating a normalized geometric liver model using warping." *Invest. Radiol.* 29(3):281–286.

Bookstein, F. L. *Thin-Plate Splines and the Atlas Problem for Biomedical Images. Information Processing in Medical Imaging.* Wye, U.K. Berlin: Springer, 1991.

Bortfeld, T., M. van Herk, and S. Jiang. (2002). "When should systematic patient positioning errors in radiotherapy be corrected?" *Phys. Med. Biol.* 47(23):N297–302.

Brixey, C., J. Roeske, A. Lujan, S. Yamada, J. Rotmensch, and A. Mundt. (2002). "Impact of intensity-modulated radiotherapy on acute hematologic toxicity in women with gynecologic malignancies." *Int. J. Radiat. Oncol. Biol. Phys.* 54(5):1388–1396.

Cha, S., E. Knopp, G. Johnson, S. Wetzel, A. Litt, and D. Zagzag. (2002). "Intracranial mass lesions: Dynamic contrast-enhanced susceptibility-weighted echo-planar perfusion MR imaging." *Radiol.* 223:11–29.

Chen, J., G. Tracton, M. Rao, S. Joshi, E. Chaney, and S. Pizer. (2002). "Comparison of automatic and human segmentation of kidneys from CT images." *Int. J. Radiat. Oncol. Biol. Phys.* 54:82.

Cline, H. E., W. E. Lorensen, R. Kikinis, and F. Jolesz. (1990). "Three-dimensional segmentation of MR images of the head using probability and connectivity." *J. Comput. Assist. Tomogr.* 14:1037–1045.

Collins, D., C. Holmes, T. Peters, and A. Evans. (1995). "Automatic 3-D model-based neuroanatomical segmentation." *Human Brain Mapping* 3:190–208.

Cootes, T., A. Hill, C. Taylor, and J. Haslam. "The Use of Active Shape Models for Locating Structures in Medical Images" in *Information Processing in Medical Imaging*. H. Barrett and A. Gmitro (eds.). Berlin: Springer-Verlag, pp. 33–47, 1993.

Davatzikos, C. (1996). "Spatial normalization of 3-D brain images using deformable models." *J. Comput. Assist. Tomogr.* 20(4):656–665.

Dawant, B., S. Hartmann, S. Pan, and S. Gadamsetty. (2002). "Brain atlas deformation in the presence of small and large space-occupying tumors." *Comput. Aided Surg.* 7(1):1–10.

Dong, S., J. Fitzpatrick, and R. Maciunas. (1992). "Rectification of Distortion in MRI for Stereotaxy." Fifth IEEE Symposium on Computer-Based Medical Systems, Durham, NC, IEEE.

Elas, M., B. Williams, A. Parasca, C. Mailer, C. Pelizzari, M. Lewis, J. River, G. Karczmar, E. Barth, and H. Halpern. (2003). "Quantitative tumor oxymetric images from 4D electron paramagnetic resonance imaging (EPRI): Methodology and comparison with blood oxygen level-dependent (BOLD) MRI." *Magn. Reson. Med.* 49: In press.

Fletcher, P., S. Joshi, A. Gash, A. Thall, G. Tracton, S. Pizer, and E. Chaney. (2002). "Pablo: Clinical prototype software for automatic image segmentation of normal anatomical structures using medially based deformable models." *Int. J. Radiat. Oncol. Biol. Phys.* 54:81.

Gambhir, S., J. Barrio, M. Phelps, M. Iyer, M. Namavari, N. Satyamurthy, L. Wu, L. Green, E. Bauer, D. MacLaren, K. Nguyen, A. Berk, S. Cherry, and H. Herschman. (1999). "Imaging adenoviral-directed reporter gene expression in living animals with positron emission tomography." *Proc. Nat. Acad. Sci. USA* 96:2333–2338.

Gilhuijs, K., and M. van Herk. (1993). "Automatic on-line inspection of patient setup in radiation therapy using digital portal images." *Med. Phys.* 20(3):667–677.

Gilhuijs, K., P. van de Ven, and M. van Herk. (1996). "Automatic three-dimensional inspection of patient setup in radiation therapy using portal images, simulator images, and computed tomography data." *Med. Phys.* 23(3):389–399.

Gilhuijs, K., K. Drukker, A. Touw, P. van de Ven, and M. van Herk. (1996). "Interactive three dimensional inspection of patient setup in radiation therapy using digital portal images and computed tomography data." *Int. J. Radiat. Oncol. Biol. Phys.* 34(4):873–885.

Goitein, M., and M. Abrams. (1983). "Multidimensional treatment planning: I. Delineation of anatomy." *Int. J. Radiat. Oncol. Biol. Phys.* 9:777–787.

Goitein, M., M. Abrams, D. Rowell, H. Pollari, and J. Wiles. (1983). "Multidimensional treatment planning: II. Beam's eye view, back projection, and projection through CT sections." *Int. J. Radiat. Oncol. Biol. Phys.* 9:789–797.

Hadley, S. W., C. A. Pelizzari, L. S. Johnson, and G. T. Y. Chen. "Automatic Registration of Portal and Simulation Films by Mutual Information" in *XII International Conference on the Use of Computers in Radiation Therapy* (XII ICCR). Madison, WI: Medical Physics Publishing, pp. 243–244, 1997.

Halpern, H. J., C. Yu, M. Peric, E. Barth, D. J. Grdina, and B. A. Teicher. (1994). "Oxymetry deep in tissues with low-frequency electron paramagnetic resonance." *Proceedings of the National Academy of Sciences of the United States of America* 91(26):13047–13051.

Hamilton, R. J., P. J. Sweeney, C. A. Pelizzari, F. Z. Yetkin, B. L. Holman, B. Garada, R. R. Weichselbaum, and G. T. Chen. (1997). "Functional imaging in treatment planning of brain lesions." *Int. J. Radiat. Oncol. Biol. Phys.* 37(1):181–188.

Holman, B. L., R. E. Zimmerman, P. A. Carvalho, R. B. Schwartz, J. S. Loeffler, E. Alexander, C. A. Pelizzari, and G. T. Y. Chen. (1991). "Computer-assisted superimposition of magnetic resonance and high resolution Tc-99m HMPAO and TL-201 SPECT images of the brain." *J. Nucl. Med.* 32:1478–1484.

Hornak, J. (2002). *The Basics of MRI.* http://www.cis.rit.edu/htbooks/mri/inside.htm.

Jolesz, F. "Image-Guided Tumor Targeting for Diagnosis and Therapy in Oncology" in *Oncologic Imaging.* D. Bragg, P. Rubin, and H. Hricak (eds.). Philadelphia: W.B. Saunders, pp. 55–68, 2002.

Joshi, S, S. Pizer, P. T. Fletcher, P. Yushkevich, A. Thall, and J. S. Marron. (2002). "Multiscale deformable model segmentation and statistical shape analysis using medial descriptions." *IEEE Trans. Med. Imaging* 21(5):538–550.

Kalet, I., M. Whipple, S. Pessah, J. Barker, M. Austin-Seymour, and L. Shapiro. (2002). "A Rule-based Model for Local and Regional Tumor Spread." *Proc. AMIA Symposium*, pp. 360–364.

Kass, M., A. Witkin, and D. Terzopoulos. (1988). "Snakes: Active contour models." *Int. J. Comput. Vision* 1(4):321–331.

Kessler, M. L., S. Pitluck, P. Petti, and J. R. Castro. (1991). "Integration of multimodality imaging data for radiotherapy treatment planning." *Int. J. Radiat. Oncol. Biol. Phys.* 21:1653–1667.

Kessler, M., P. Archer, C. Meyer, S. Narayan, A. Eisbruch, H. Sandler, and T. Lawrence. (2002). "Routine clinical use of mutual information for automated 3-D registration of anatomic and functional image data." *Int. J. Radiat. Oncol. Biol. Phys.* 54(2):84.

Ketting, C., M. Austin-Seymour, I. Kalet, J. Jacky, S. Kromhout-Schiro, S. Hummel, J. Unger, L. Fagan, and T. Griffin. (1997). "Automated planning target volume generation: An evaluation pitting a computer-based tool against human experts." *Int. J. Radiat. Oncol. Biol. Phys.* 37(3):697–704.

Kim, J., J. Fessler, K. Lam, J. Balter, and R. Ten Haken. (2001). "A feasibility study of mutual information based setup error estimation for radiotherapy." *Med. Phys.* 28(12):2507–2517.

Kooy, H., M. van Herk, P. Barnes, E. Alexander, S. Dunbar, N. Tarbell, R. Mulkern, E. Holupka, and J. Loeffler. (1994). "Image fusion for stereotactic radiotherapy and radiosurgery treatment planning." *Int. J. Radiat. Oncol. Biol. Phys.* 30(5):1229–1234.

Kovacic, S., J. C. Gee, S. L. Ching, M. Reivich, and R. Bajcsy. "Three-dimensional Registration of PET and CT Images." IEEE Engineering in Medicine and Biology Society 11th International Conference, 1989.

Lattanzi, J., S. McNeeley, W. Pinover, E. Howritz, I. Das, T. Schultheiss, and G. Hanks. (1999). "A comparison of daily CT localization do a daily ultrasound-based system in prostate cancer." *Int. J. Radiat. Oncol. Biol. Phys.* 43(4):719–725.

Levin, D. N., X. P. Hu, K. K. Tan, S. Galhotra, C. A. Pelizzari, G. T. Chen, R. N. Beck, C. T. Chen, M. D. Cooper, J. F. Mullan, et al. (1989). "The brain: Integrated three-dimensional display of MR and PET images." *Radiol.* 172(3):783–789.

Li, A., and D. Bluemke. "Cancer Diagnosis: Imaging-Magnetic Resonance Imaging" in *Cancer: Principles and Practice of Oncology, 6th Edition.* V. DeVita, S. Hellman, and S. Rosenberg (eds.). Philadelphia: Lippincott Williams and Williams, 2001.

Ling, C., J. Humm, S. Larson, H. Amols, Z. Fuks, S. Leibel, and J. Koutcher. (2000). "Towards multidimensional radiotherapy (MD-CRT): Biological imaging and biological conformality." *Int. J. Radiat. Oncol. Biol. Phys.* 47(3):551–560.

Lorensen, W., and H. Cline. (1987). "Marching cubes: A high resolution 3-D surface reconstruction algorithm." *Computer Graphics* (SIGGRAPH '87) 21:163–169.

Louie, A., M. Huber, E. Ahrens, U. Rothbacker, R. Moats, R. Jacobs, S. Fraser, and T. Meade. (2000). "In vivo visualization of gene expression using magnetic resonance imaging." *Nature Biotech.* 18:321–325.

Maguire, G. Q. Jr., M. E. Noz, E. M. Lee, and J. H. Schimpf. "Correlation Methods for Tomographic Images Using Two and Three Dimensional Techniques" in *Information Processing in Medical Imaging*. S. L. Bacharach (ed.). Boston: Martinus Nijhoff, pp. 266–279, 1986.

Mah, D., M. Steckner, E. Palacio, R. Mitra, T. Richardson, and G. Hanks. (2002). "Characteristics and quality assurance of a dedicated open 0.23 T MRI for radiation therapy simulation." *Med. Phys.* 29:2541–2547.

Maintz, J., and M. Viergever. (1998). "A survey of medical image registration." *Med. Image Analysis* 2:1–36.

Marks, L., D. Spencer, G. Bentel, S. Ray, G. Sherouse, M. Sontag, R. Coleman, R. Jaszczak, T. Turkington, and V. Tapson et al. (1993). "The utility of SPECT lung perfusion scans in minimizing and assessing the physiologic consequences of thoracic irradiation." *Int. J. Radiat. Oncol. Biol. Phys.* 26(4):659–668.

Marks, L., M. Munley, D. Spencer, G. Sherouse, G. Bentel, J. Hoppenworth, M. Chew, R. Jaszczak, R. Coleman, and L. Prosnitz. (1997). "Quantification of radiation-induced regional lung injury with perfusion imaging." *Int. J. Radiat. Oncol. Biol. Phys.* 38(2):399–409.

Maurer, C., and J. Fitzpatrick. "A Review of Medical Image Registration" in *Interactive Image-Guided Neurosurgery*. R. J. Maciunas (ed.). Park Ridge, IL: American Association of Neurosurgeons, pp. 17–44, 1993.

McCullough, E., and T. Holmes. (1985). "Acceptance testing computerized radiation therapy treatment planning systems: Direct utilization of CT scan data." *Med. Phys.* 12(2):237–242.

McShan, D. L., A. Silverman, D. M. Lanza, L. E. Reinstein, and A. S. Glicksman. (1979). "A computerized three-dimensional treatment planning system utilizing interactive colour graphics." *Br. J. Radiol.* 52:478–481.

Mundt, A., A. Lujan, J. Rotmensch, S. Waggoner, S. Yamada, G. Fleming, and J. Roeske. (2002). "Intensity-modulated whole pelvic radiotherapy in women with gynecologic malignancies." *Int. J. Radiat. Oncol. Biol. Phys.* 52(5):1330–1337.

Pelizzari, C. A., G. T. Y. Chen, H. Halpern, C. T. Chen, and M. D. Cooper. (1987). "Three dimensional correlation of PET, CT and MRI images." *J. Nucl. Med.* 28(4):683.

Pelizzari, C. A., G. T. Y. Chen, D. R. Spelbring, R. R. Weichselbaum, and C. T. Chen. (1989). "Accurate three-dimensional registration of PET, CT and MR images of the brain." *J. Comput. Assist. Tomogr.* 13:20–27.

Pham, D., C. Xu, and J. Prince. (2000). "Current methods in medical image segmentation." *Ann. Rev. Biomed. Engr.* 2:315–337.

Phillips, M. H., M. L. Kessler, F. Y. S. Chuang, K. A. Frankel, J. T. Lyman, J. I. Fabrikant, and R. P. Levy. (1991). "Image correlation of MRI and CT in treatment planning for radiosurgery of intracranial vascular malformations." *Int. J. Radiat. Oncol. Biol. Phys.* 20:881–889.

Reinstein, L. E., D. L. McShan, B. M. Webber, and A. S. Glicksman. (1978). "A computer-assisted three-dimensional treatment planning system." *Radiol.* 1217:259–264.

Roeske, J. C., C. A. Pelizzari, G. T. Y. Chen, and M. J. Blend. (1992). "Image Registration of SPECT and CT Images for Radiolabeled Antibody Biodistribution Analysis and Dosimetry." Society of Nuclear Medicine Central Chapter 1992 Spring Meeting, Chicago.

Roeske, J., A. Lujan, J. Rotmensch, S. Waggoner, D. Yamada, and A. Mundt. (2000). "Intensity-modulated whole pelvic radiation therapy in patients with gynecologic malignancies." *Int. J. Radiat. Oncol. Biol. Phys.* 48(5):1613–1621.

Sailer, S., J. Rosenman, M. Soltys, T. Cullip, and J. Chen. (1996). "Improving treatment planning accuracy through multimodality imaging." *Int. J. Radiat. Oncol. Biol. Phys.* 35(1):117–124.

Schad, L. R., S. Lott, F. Schmitt, V. Sturm, and W. J. Lorenz. (1987a). "Correction of spatial distortion in MR imaging: A prerequisite for accurate stereotaxy." *J. Comput. Assist. Tomogr.* 11:499–505.

Schad, L. R., R. Boesecke, W. Schlegel, G. H. Hartmann, V. Sturm, L. G. Strauss, and W. J. Lorenz. (1987b). "Three dimensional image correlation of CT, MR, and PET studies in radiotherapy treatment planning of brain tumors." *J. Comput. Assist. Tomogr.* 11(6):948–954.

Scheidler, J., H. Hricak, D. Vigneron, K. Yu, D. Sokolov, L. Huang, C. Zaloudek, S. Nelson, P. Carroll, and J. Kurhanewicz. (1999). "Prostate cancer: Localization with three-dimensional proton MR spectroscopic imaging—clinicopathologic study." *Radiol.* 213(2):473–480.

Sherouse, G., K. Novins, and E. Chaney. (1990). "Computation of digitally reconstructed radiographs for use in radiotherapy treatment design." *Int. J. Radiat. Oncol. Biol. Phys.* 18(3):651–658.

Shukla, H., P. Vaisanen, and M. Steckner. (2002). "Distortion corrected MRI for radiotherapy." *Int. J. Radiat. Oncol. Biol. Phys.* 54:83–84.

Staib, L., and J. Duncan. (1992). "Boundary finding with parametrically deformable models." *IEEE Trans PAMI* 14(11):1061–1075.

Sumanaweera, T., G. Glover, P. Hemler, P. van den Elsen, D. Martin, J. Adler, and S. Napel. (1995). "MR geometric distortion correction for improved frame-based stereotaxic target localization accuracy." *Magn. Reson. Med.* 34(1):106–113.

Székely, G., A. Kelemen, C. Brechbühler, and G. Gerig. (1996). "Segmentation of 2-D and 3-D objects from MRI volume data using constrained elastic deformations of flexible Fourier contour and surface models." *Med. Image Analysis* 1(1):19–34.

Tepper, J. (2000). "Form and function: The integration of physics and biology." *Int. J. Radiat. Oncol. Biol. Phys.* 47(3):547–548.

Thompson, P., and A. Toga. (1997). "Detection, visualization and animation of abnormal anatomic structure with a deformable probabilistic brain atlas based on random vector field transformations." *Med. Image Analysis* 1(4):271–294.

Thornton, A. F., H. M. Sandler, R. K. Ten Haken, D. L. McShan, B. A. Fraass, M. L. LaVigne, and B. R. Yanke. (1992). "The clinical utility of magnetic resonance imaging in 3-dimensional treatment planning of brain neoplasms." *Int. J. Radiat. Oncol. Biol. Phys.* 24:767–775.

Tien, R., G. Felsberg, H. Friedman, M. Brown, and J. MacFall. (1994). "MR imaging of high-grade gliomas: value of diffusion-weighted echoplanar pulse sequences." *Am. J. Roentgenol.* 162:671–677.

Tracton, G. S., E. L. Chaney, J. G. Rosenman, and S. M. Pizer. (1994). "Medical anatomy segmentation kit: Combining 2D and 3-D segmentation methods to enhance functionality." *SPIE Math. Meth. Med. Imaging,* no vol, no page numbers.

Udupa, J. "3-D Imaging: Principles and Approaches" in *3-D Imaging in Medicine*. J. Udupa and G. Herman (eds.). Boca Raton, FL: CRC Press, pp. 1–73, 2000.

van den Elsen, P., E. Pol, and M. Viergever. (1993). "Medical image matching-a review with classification." *IEEE Engr. Med. Biol.* 12:26–39.

van Herk, M., K. Gilhuis, E. Holupka, and H. Kooy. (1992). "A new method for automatic three-dimensional image correlation." *Med. Phys.* 19(4):1134.

Viola, P. D. (1995). Alignment by Maximization of Mutual Information. Technical Report 1548. Artificial Intelligence Laboratory. Cambridge, MA: Massachussetts Institute of Technology.

Wells, W. M., P. Viola, and R. Kikinis. "Multi-Modal Volume Registration by Maximization of Mutual Information." Second Annual International Symposium on Medical Robotics and Computer Assisted Surgery. New York: John Wiley & Sons, 1995.

Yan, D., F. Vicini, J. Wong, and A. Martinez. (1997). "Adaptive radiation therapy." *Phys. Med. Biol.* 42(1):123–132.

Yan, D., E. Ziaja, D. Jaffray, J. Wong, D. Brabbins, F. Vicini, and A. Martinez. (1998). "The use of adaptive radiation therapy to reduce setup error: A prospective clinical study." *Int. J. Radiat. Oncol. Biol. Phys.* 41(3):7150–720.

# Target and Critical Structure Definitions, Dose Prescription, and Reporting for IMRT


**James Balter, Ph.D.**
Radiation Oncology Department
University of Michigan
Ann Arbor, Michigan




## Introduction

The safe and effective implementation of intensity-modulated radiation therapy (IMRT) invites a well-prepared radiotherapy department to re-visit the overall process of treatment planning. While the general concepts are comparable to those necessary for forward-planned, three-dimensional (3-D) conformal radiotherapy, the presence of steeper dose gradients, possible tighter margins, and differences in delivery techniques require further thought about all steps to be considered in developing and implementing a treatment plan. This chapter deals primarily with concepts related to target and critical structure definitions, as well as prescribing and reporting dose. The majority of information in this chapter is related to concepts presented in International commission on Radiation Units and Measurements (ICRU) report 62, and readers are strongly encouraged to obtain and read a copy of this reference when considering implementation of IMRT or other forms of conformal therapy.

## The Process Of Radiotherapy

Figure 1 describes the overall process of radiotherapy planning and treatment. The major processes involve: (1) establishing a model of the patient that includes appropriate definitions of target and critical structures; (2) defining objectives for an optimal plan; (3) developing a plan to attempt to meet those objectives; (4) translating this plan information to the treatment unit; and (5) verification and feedback to ensure proper accuracy of plan implementation. This chapter deals primarily with items 1, 4, and 5, although some concepts presented here influence items 2 and 3.

**James Balter**

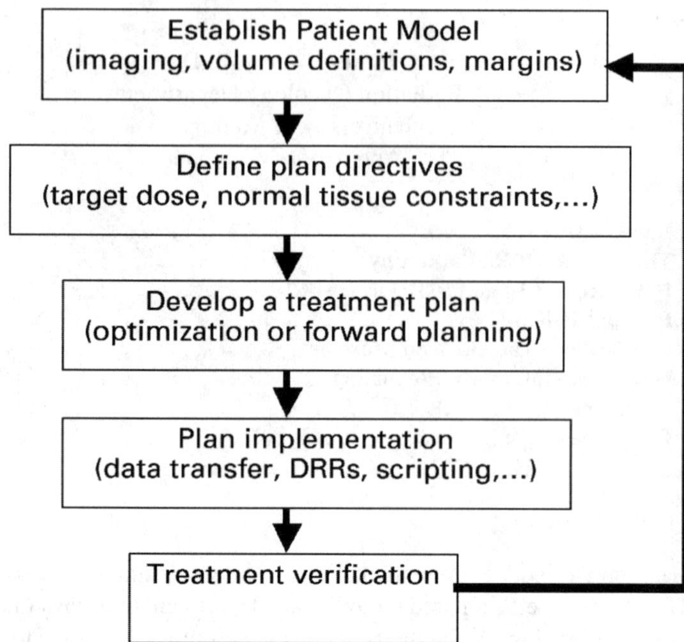



**Figure 1.** Overview of the radiotherapy process.

## ICRU Report 50 And ICRU Report 62

To help ensure accuracy and consistency in dose prescriptions, the ICRU has recommended a convention for dose reporting. The original form of these recommendations for external beam radiotherapy was ICRU report 50 (ICRU 50, 1993). The key concepts presented in ICRU report 50 are illustrated in figure 2.

The gross tumor volume (GTV) indicates the physician's observation of the tumor based on the imaging data available. In order to account for the likelihood of clonogenic tumor outside of the visualized GTV boundary, the clinical target volume (CTV), an expansion of the GTV, is created. The further uncertainty in tumor location due to setup error and/or internal organ movement and anatomic changes are considered in the planning target volume (PTV), and expansion of the CTV. Significant research has been applied recently in order to estimate necessary PTV expansions for different body regions.

While the constructs presented in ICRU report 50 provide the potential for ensuring adequate dose to tumor in most instances, there are a few limitations for treatment planning that remain to be addressed. ICRU report 62 (ICRU 62, 1999) deals with some of these issues. The additional constructs are described in figure 3.

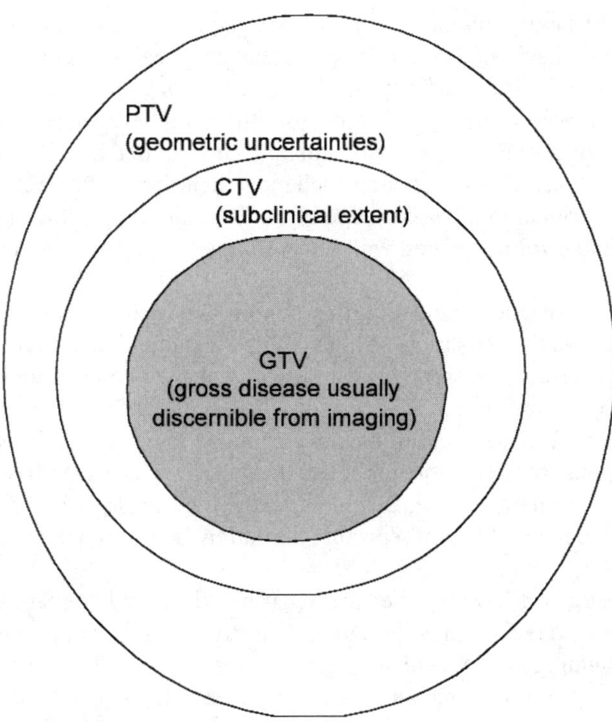


**Figure 2.** The GTV, CTV, and PTV concepts from ICRU report 50.

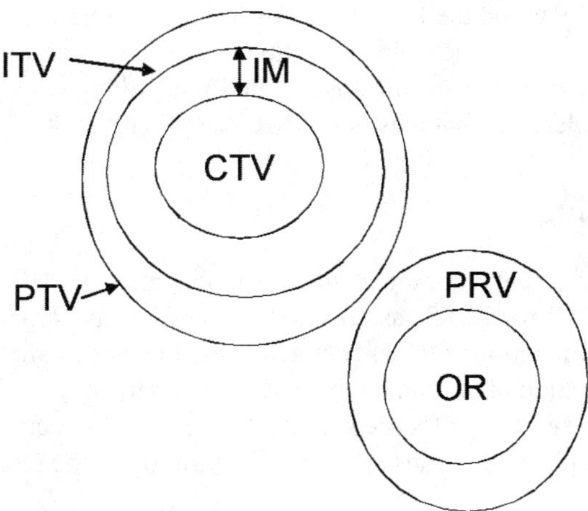


**Figure 3.** The internal margin (IM), internal target volume (ITV), organ at risk (OR), and planning organ at risk volume (PRV) concepts from ICRU report 62.

The internal target volume (ITV) was designed to account for practical issues related to patient treatment. It was considered that intratreatment physiological movement would be difficult to eliminate and, thus, the rules associated with margins for such movement may in fact be different from those for setup variation. The ITV is created by placing an anisotropic internal margin (IM) around the CTV to account for, e.g., breathing movement. Whether all such movements are in fact not manageable is not necessarily critical to the acceptance of the IM and ITV, as this margin can also consider residual error associated with interventions (e.g., gating) to reduce internal movement.

Improved understanding and reporting of normal tissue dosimetry is addressed in ICRU report 62 via the constructs of organ at risk and planning organ at risk volume (PRV). The OR represents some internal organ that may be dose limiting and thus needs to be considered in planning and dose reporting. The PRV incorporates and expansion of the OR to account for its movement and setup-induced position change. This construct may be acceptable for absolute assurance that a (serial) organ receives no more than a given point dose. Beyond this, the PRV presents a difficulty that can be generalized to the problem of reporting normal tissue doses, and will be discussed further below.

Some investigators have reported that the use of the PRV has enabled IMRT planning with improved reduction of dose to critical structures. It is important to note that most IMRT planning is done with a single representation of the patient, and thus the presence of the PRV may force an unnecessary trade-off. Figure 4 shows two possible treatment plan geometries. In figure 4a the expanded region of the PRV is distal from the high-dose region around the PTV, and thus the space of the PRV around the OR can be used to force lower doses to the region of anatomy near the OR during planning with less impact on the PTV dose distribution. In figure 4b, however, the expansions of the PRV and the PTV would overlap without modification of the PTV volume. Although it is possible in this scenario that the actual OR and CTV never reach such proximity, the demands of low dose to the PRV and high dose to the PTV force a trade-off during planning that may not be necessary in reality (Vineberg et al. 2002).

## Patient Modeling

The first step in treatment planning involves establishing a model of the patient. This step is highly critical for IMRT, as all information (density, structures) relevant for treatment plan optimization will be generated from this model, and as this model will reflect the configuration of the patient that any setup verification will attempt to reproduce. Significant research has focused on the differences between treatment planning computed tomography (CT) scans and the configuration of the patient at treatment.

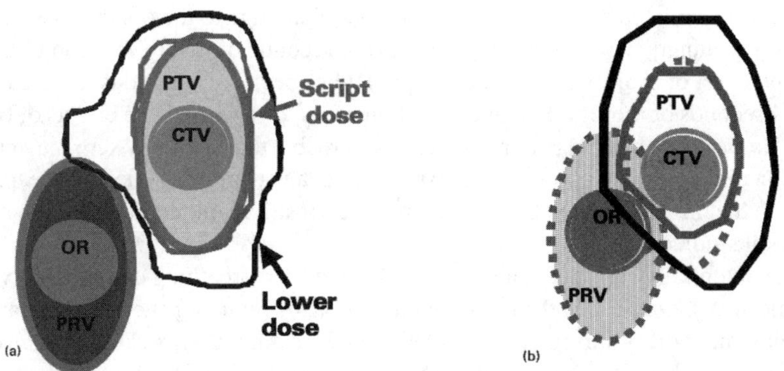


**Figure 4.** Dose coverage for a PTV and PRV in situations with (a) sufficient distance and (b) close proximity between the target and organ at risk.

One initial concern is to minimize the potential for artifacts to influence structure definition. Prior reports have described the effects of metal prostheses and other high-density implants on CT images. Of greater concern are artifacts associated with short-term movement of either the whole patient, or more likely internal anatomy of the patient due to normal physiologic processes. It is important to consider momentarily the nature of data collection for image reconstruction in CT. The general design of a CT scanner involves a rotating source that generates projections on either a large fixed (fourth generation) or a reduced traveling (third generation) array of detectors. In either instance, a complete set of projections is acquired over a source travel span of approximately 180° (plus travel to span the projection width). Maximum tube rotation speeds on modern CT scanners are on the order of 0.5 to 1.0 second, meaning that the data acquired per "slice" occurs over a time span of 0.3 to 0.6 seconds. The advent of multiple slice detector arrays improves this speed somewhat (Yamada et al. 2002), but nevertheless a helical scan of a typical thorax or abdomen can take up to 50 seconds depending on specific scanner hardware. During this time, it is expected that, even in an immobile patient, processes such as breathing, heartbeat, and peristalsis occur, leading to local movement and potential deformation of the patient. Such movements result in changes that impact subsets of the CT projections, resulting in a reconstructed model of the patient that does not in fact represent the true patient at any instance in time. The movement associated with patient breathing has been studied extensively (Henkelman et al. 1982; Ten Haken et al. 1996; Balter et al. 1996; Wong et al. 1999; Seppenwoolde et al. 2000; Shimizu et al. 2000a,b), and it is apparent that strategies to control breathing during CT scanning can reduce the magnitude of movement-related artifacts for targets in the thorax and abdomen (Wagman et al. 2003; Balter et al. 1998). It should also be noted that breathing-related movement has also been observed as in structures more distal to the thorax, such as the prostate in prone patients (Malone et al. 2000; Dawson et al. 2000).

Breathing-related movement also presents a challenge to the optimal use of cone-beam CT scanners, which may require over 30 seconds of gantry rotation to acquire a complete set of projections. One concept that has been considered is the use of very slow (4 seconds or more) CT scanner rotation times to "average" the effects of breathing by producing a blurred patient model. It is possible that such a system may provide a reasonable low-cost approach to establishing an average model of the patient, although the influence of such slow scans on the sensitivity of target definition has not been well studied.

The potentially significant artifacts associated with breathing can be dealt with in multiple ways. One method involves eliminating or reducing the allowed range of breathing movement during both simulation and treatment. This can be achieved via voluntary breath hold. Deep inspiration breath hold (DIBH) (Hanley et al. 1999; Remouchamps et al. 2003; Yorke et al. 2002) has been widely investigated, and has the further potential of both decreasing the regional volume of lung tissue in proximity to some lesions, as well as potentially reducing the volume of critical structures such as heart in breast cancer treatment. A more technically demanding method involves the use of either gated or actively breath-held CT scanning. All these mechanisms have to be evaluated prior to implementation, to establish the long- and short-term reproducibility of the breathing states attained. Coached shallow breathing and mechanically restricted shallow breathing are also viable options for reducing the magnitude of ventilatory movement.

Given that some patients will not be eligible for restricted breathing, or that gated breathing systems are not viable or available, other strategies to ensure proper treatment planning models involve acquiring one or more CT scans at controlled states of breathing. One example is the acquisitions of exhale breath-held CT scans. The exhale state has been shown to be the most geometrically reproducible over short time periods, and occupies a significant fraction of the breathing cycle in a typical patient. As such, CT scanning at exhale with margins to account for the motion towards inhale may be a feasible mechanism for creating a treatment planning model of the patient with density and position information that, while not completely modeling the variations during breathing, present a more reliable state than the artifact-prone free-breathing CT.

Another more challenging technique involves the acquisition of multiple CT scans at different phases of the breathing cycle. It is conceivable to use these multiple scans to map out the path that the CTV may move through during breathing. This concept has been described using CT scans at the inhale and exhale states. The recent development of "4-D" CT scans that sample a limited region of anatomy over multiple phases of the breathing cycle promises to improve the amount of information available for such modeling (Vedam et al. 2003), but will also present a challenge in optimally using this information, which inherently contains local deformation of anatomy. Some recent research into the development of deformable models of anatomy for radiotherapy may eventually aid in the utilization of 4-D CT (Brock et al. 2002). Another major concern in the development of such dynamic models for the construction of targets and guidance of treatment planning is developing a paradigm to consider potential variations in breathing cycles over the course of treatment.

The influence of cardiac movement on CT scans is known but less widely studied than that of breathing. Perhaps the best data on the magnitude of motion related to heartbeat come from fluoroscopic studies of patients with implanted radio-opaque markers for lung tumors. Shirato and colleagues (2000) performed a study of fluoroscopic tracking for radiotherapy of lung tumors. Their data, further analyzed by Seppenwoolde (Seppenwoolde et al. 2000), show movement of structures near the mediastinum of distances of several millimeters. By frequency analysis, the component of movement due to breathing is removed, and the higher temporal frequency component of cardiac movement is seen. It is perhaps most difficult to come to grips with this type of movement for routine planning of treatment, as modern CT scanning is not amenable to cardiac gating.

Issues of movement are one component in the overall for establishing a patient model that can be made to reasonably reflect the state of the patient during treatment. The presumably simpler problem of establishing a position and overall configuration of the patient that can be reproduced is also worthy of some forethought. As will be discussed in detail in the following sections, the random nature of immobilization and repositioning infer that the average position of the patient is unknown at the time of simulation, and can only be elucidated through observation during multiple sessions of positioning of the patient (typically during the delivery of treatment). It is critical to consider the immobilization employed, and the extent to which it will be able to repeat patient configurations through multiple uses over the course of up to 2 months of treatment.

## Positioning Strategies And Margins

The previous section of this chapter hinted somewhat at the geometric variability of the patient that may be expected during treatment. This section explores this concept further, and mentions some strategies for dealing with such variability during treatment planning and delivery.

Patient position is generally assumed to be random, with an average position of the patient that can be observed after multiple repeat positioning and a random variation about this average (figure 5a). It is the goal of patient positioning strategies to relate the position of the patient at treatment as closely as possible to the model acquired at simulation for the purposes of treatment planning.

The systematic component of setup variation has previously been classified as an error with potential sources related to differences between simulation and treatment equipment (e.g., laser calibration, table position calibration, table sag, patient comfort differences, etc.). Given the random nature of patient position, however, it is easy to speculate that "systematic" variations in position will exist even if no such differences occur. The simulation of the patient involves a session of positioning, which represents the average position of the patient plus a sample of the random distribution. This means that the likelihood of observing the true average position of the patient at the time of CT scanning is small and related directly to the magnitude of random variation in position. On the first day of treatment, the average position of the patient is again offset by a second sample of the random variation. The combination of these two random samples introduces a major component of the "systematic" error seen when establishing patient position on the first day of treatment. It is also important to reflect that, even if effort is taken on the first day of treatment to adjust patient position to exactly match that from CT [e.g., by alignment of portal images to digitally reconstructed radiographs (DRRs)], this correction further assumes that the first treatment fraction represents the average position of the patient. Any errors introduced by this assumption are thus propagated in the patient position until another correction is made.

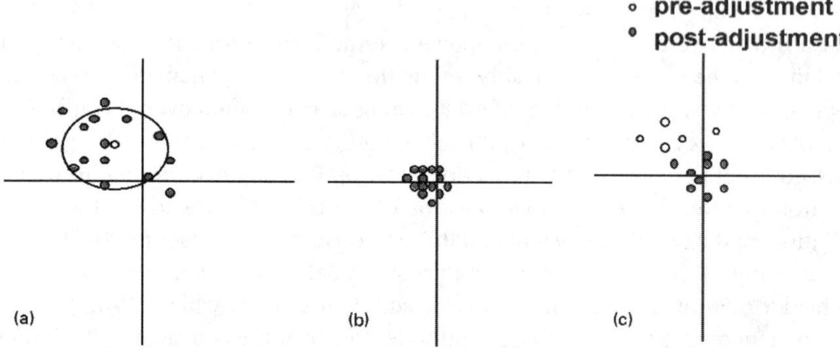


**Figure 5.** Position distributions. The initial setup position of a patient shown in (a) has an average "systematic" offset (clear point), and a random variation about this average (large circle represents 1 standard deviation). On-line setup adjustment shown in (b) reduces errors but does not eliminate them, and off-line protocols in (c) reduce the systematic error after a few early observations (clear points), but do not impact random variations.

The standard of practice for patient positioning recently has involved the acquisition of weekly portal films or digital portal images, with correction applied either immediately or on the fraction following observation of setup error. Given the nature of patient position, it is important to consider the benefit of such strategies. Figure 6 shows actual data of daily position variation of a patient treated using daily imaging and on-line setup correction. The data shown represent position variation in the inferior-superior axis. A simulation is shown of the impact of weekly setup adjustment with "perfect" correction. Perfect correction is simulated by taking the error seen on the days of imaging (every 5th fraction), and applying that correction on all subsequent fractions until the next imaging session. It can be seen that no significant improvement is made to patient position by weekly adjustment, and in fact the potential remains to increase setup error over doing nothing at all.

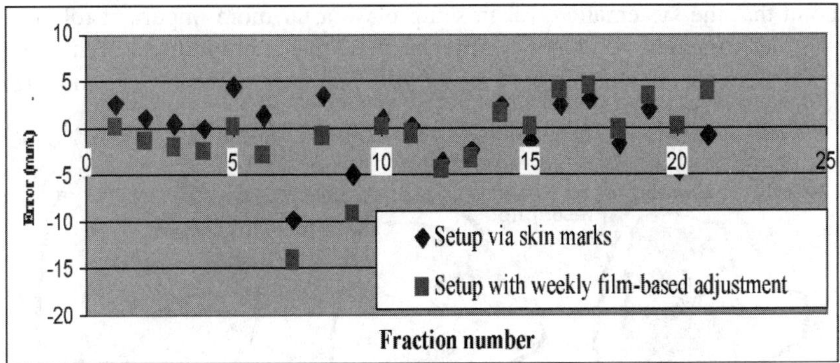


**Figure 6.** Actual measured position offsets of an abdominal setup in the inferior-superior direction (diamonds) and a simulation of offsets expected via exact implementation of weekly portal films and pre-treatment correction (squares).

A wealth of information has been gained recently on other potential strategies for patient setup correction. The simplest method to consider is on-line setup correction (Balter et al. 2002; Alasti et al. 2001; Pisani et al. 2000; Van de Steene et al. 1998; Brock, McShan, and Balter 2002; Gilhuijs and van Herk 1993; Jaffray, Yan, and Wong 1999). In this method (figure 5b), setup measurement is performed prior to treatment for each fraction, and all setup errors greater than a threshold level are corrected. This technique removes all considerations of systematic error, and furthermore dramatically reduces random variation in position. Some residual random variation remains, due to limits of accuracy of the mechanisms used to both measure and correct position. Application of a threshold for correction on the order of these residual uncertainties reduces the workload for setup adjustment dramatically. Nevertheless, on-line adjustment in its current form is both technically and time demanding.

In considering other strategies for setup adjustment, it is important to consider the impact of setup variations on target dose and margins for treatment. Figure 7 describes a general view of the impact of systematic and random variations on dose. To first order [ignoring effects of changing source-to-surface distances (SSDs) and depths], systematic errors will tend to shift the entire dose distribution, while random errors will tend to blur the dose distribution, reducing the volumes of high dose and increasing the volumes of low dose. Ignoring dose-per-fraction effects, it is possible to define a criterion for CTV dose coverage (e.g., 95% minimum dose) and to determine a PTV expansion necessary to ensure such coverage at an acceptable probability of success. Van Herk and others explored this concept in detail, and established the following formula for PTV margin (van Herk, Remeijer, and Lebesque 2002):

$$\text{PTV margin} = 2.5\Sigma + 0.7\sigma$$

Where $\Sigma$ represents the population standard deviation for systematic error, and $\sigma$ is the population averages random variation standard deviation. This formula emphasizes the point that the systematic error in setup plays a far more important role in dose coverage and margins than random variations, and that attempts to reduce the magnitude of systematic variation achieve most of the benefit possible in positioning for the majority of patients.

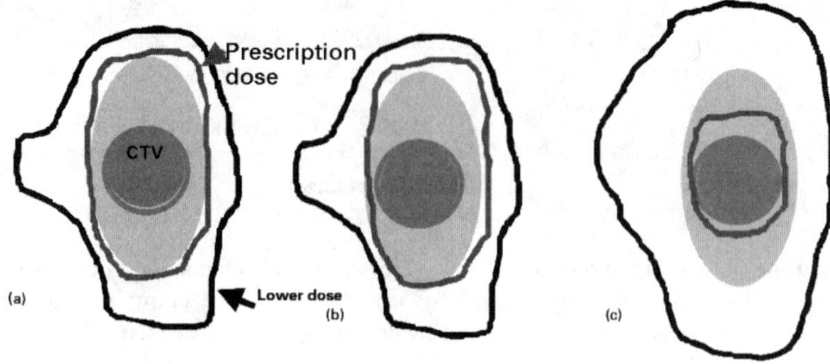


**Figure 7.** A dose distribution designed cover a PTV in (a) is, to first order, shifted by systematic error in (b) and blurred by random setup variation in (c).

Given that reduction of systematic offset is generally most critical, it is useful to consider other strategies for patient positioning that are beneficial at a reasonable cost of effort and technology. An off-line setup adjustment strategy (figure 5b) involves acquisition of patient setup position data (portal images, CT scans, etc.) over multiple positionings of the patient. Setup variation is generally measured retrospectively, and a prediction is made of the systematic offset. This offset is then corrected for subsequent treatment fractions, with periodic verification. Off-line techniques have many forms. Their major advantage over on-line adjustment lies in efficiency (no need to verify position prior to each treatment fraction, and added efficiency from retrospective off-line analysis of multiple images in one session). The major disadvantage is that margins are still required to account for the random variation of the patient, thus potentially limiting the utility of this technique for cases where the random variation of the patient's position is sufficiently large to introduce concerns of target miss (e.g., obese patients) or higher doses to organs at risk.

There are many strategies that primarily operate from this off-line measurement concept. The first concept is the no action level (NAL) protocol (deBoer and Heijmen 2001). This procedure generally involves observing setup over a small number (3 to 5) of fractions, followed by adjustment equal to the average position observed over these fractions. Research by a number of investigators indicate that a reasonable trade-off of effort versus accuracy in predicting systematic offsets via this approach results in observing three to four positionings of the patient. The first treatment fraction has recently been considered an outlying observation, and ignoring this measurement may in fact improve prediction of systematic offset. It is relatively easy to implement this protocol in a busy department with electronic portal imaging. Table 1 shows the magnitude of setup errors found and removed via this protocol during initial implementation at the University of Michigan.

**Table 1.** Systematic Errors Measured via a 4-Fraction Off-Line Setup Adjustment Protocol

| Site | Average (Maximum) "Systematic" Error Observed | | |
| --- | --- | --- | --- |
| | Lateral (mm) | Anterior-Posterior (mm) | Cranial-Caudal (mm) |
| Pelvis | 3.0 (8.3) | 2.3 (3.3) | 1.8 (8.0) |
| Chest | 2.3 (7.8) | 3.3 (10.3) | 3.1 (9.1) |
| Abdomen | 2.1 (5.4) | 2.4 (5.8) | 3.0 (5.8) |
| Head & Neck | 1.9 (4.5) | 1.9 (5.6) | 2.4 (5.0) |

A corollary to the NAL protocol is the shrinking action level (SAL) protocol (van Lin et al. 2001; Erridge et al. 2003). Also reasonable to implement, this protocol involves a larger tolerance for setup errors at the initiation of treatment, followed by a reduction in the threshold for adjustment as treatment fractions progress.

These strategies are reasonable cost-effective means to estimate systematic offset. They are simplifications of a strategy called adaptive radiotherapy (ART). Initially described by Yan (Yan et al. 1997), this statistical approach is designed to maximize the utility of prior knowledge combined with new measurements of patient position. Again an off-line or retrospective analysis technique, the ART process involves initiating treatment planning and delivery using a population model of setup variations as a guide for margins. Frequent observations are made of patient position at the initiation of treatment. Each new observation is used to adjust the probability model closer to the individual patient position model. After a small number of measurements, both the systematic and random variations of the individual patient are estimated, and corrections, including margin adjustment, can be made. Further observation can refine these estimates, and outlying observations trigger increased frequency of measurement and margin adjustment until statistical confidence is regained. Concepts of ART have been applied using both portal imaging as well as multiple CT scans early in treatment. This type of strategy is highly amenable to treatment validation concepts that acquire frequent 3-D patient models [e.g., cone-beam CT mounted on a gantry (Jaffray et al. 2000), tomotherapy (Mackie et al. 1993)]. The wealth of such data is currently prohibitive to most cases of on-line targeting and tracking, yet the wealth of data presented make such systems ideal candidates for adaptive strategies, especially those tied to treatment plan modification.

The nature of IMRT dose distributions (very steep dose gradients at interfaces between targets and organs at risk) place high demands on treatment precision. It is important to consider the accuracy required when establishing margins for treatment. Furthermore, the trade-offs required when a PRV overlaps a PTV, as mentioned earlier, may further dictate treatment strategies to ensure proper target dose. One concept that may be found in future IMRT systems is robust treatment planning. By considering multiple possible patient geometries at the time of optimization, IMRT planning systems could attempt to make plans that are robust in the face of expected motions and setup uncertainties.

## Dose Prescription And Reporting

IMRT presents a significant challenge in prescribing and reporting dose. This is due to the nature of delivered fluence distributions and the resulting 3-D dose distributions. Rapidly changing dose gradients may potentially obviate the presence of a reasonable reference point for dose prescription. A reference point should be within the target, in a region of minimal gradient, and surrounded by a sufficiently homogeneous region of dose to permit verification via measurement in a phantom. Furthermore, many current IMRT systems create dose distributions across targets (especially those in close proximity to organs at risk) with significantly larger heterogeneity than the 5% typically seen via conventional 3-D planning. Although improvements are being seen with advances in optimization strategies, dose heterogeneities of 10% to 20% may be possible within the target. These concepts will be explained in detail in later chapters.

One further difficulty with the PRV concept relates to the reporting of dose. A dose-volume histogram (DVH) for a PTV is, to first order, a reasonable estimate of the dose to a CTV given that the PTV was appropriately constructed. The veracity of this relationship relies in the fact that the dose to the PTV is inherently designed to be relatively homogeneous, and that an ideal plan will have minimal dose gradients within the resulting PTV. The dose distribution around the PRV, however, may be rapidly changing, and will most likely also show further changes when considering effects such as random setup variation (figure 6). It is very likely that the dose distributions planned to the PRV and delivered to the organ at risk will be significantly different, and it remains to be seen how strong a predictor of complications the PRV DVH will be for organs that exhibit a volume effect. For serial organs, the PRV maximum dose should be close to a reasonable estimate of the worst-case point dose to the organ at risk and may thus be a reasonable predictor.

## Summary

The implementation of IMRT involves, with any high-precision treatment planning concept, careful considerations of patient modeling. It is critical to understand generation of a model of the patient that will properly allow delineation of target volumes and volumes of organs at risk, and to understand their true range of movement in order to develop a safe and effective treatment plan. The decision on margins is closely linked to strategies for position verification, for which dramatic changes have occurred recently. It is worthwhile for a department considering implementation of an IMRT program to strongly consider all factors in the process in a prospective fashion to ensure safe and effective implementation of IMRT at the necessary accuracy.

# References


Alasti, H., M. Petric, C. N. Catton, and P. R. Warde. (2001). "Portal imaging for evaluation of daily on-line setup errors and off-line organ motion during conformal irradiation of carcinoma of the prostate." *Int. J. Radiat. Oncol. Biol. Phys.* 49(3):869–884.

Balter, J. M., R. K. Ten Haken, T. S. Lawrence, K. L. Lam, and J. M. Robertson. (1996). "Uncertainties in CT-based radiation therapy treatment planning associated with patient breathing." *Int. J. Radiat. Oncol. Biol. Phys.* 36:167–174.

Balter, J. M., K. L. Lam, C. J. McGinn, T. S. Lawrence, and R. K. Ten Haken. (1998). "Improvement of CT-based treatment-planning models of abdominal targets using static exhale imaging." *Int. J. Radiat. Oncol. Biol. Phys.* 41:939–943.

Balter, J. M., K. K. Brock, D. W. Litzenberg, D. L. McShan, T. S. Lawrence, R. Ten Haken, C. J. McGinn, K. L. Lam, and L. A. Dawson. (2002). "Daily targeting of intrahepatic tumors for radiotherapy." *Int. J. Radiat. Oncol. Biol. Phys.* 52(1):266–271.

Brock, K. K., D. L. McShan, and J. M. Balter. (2002). "A comparison of computer-controlled versus manual on-line patient setup adjustment." *J. Appl. Clin. Med. Phys.* 3(3):241–247.

Brock, K. K., S. J. Hollister, L. A. Dawson, and J. M. Balter. (2000). "Technical note: Creating a four-dimensional model of the liver using finite element analysis." *Med. Phys.* 29(7):1403–1405.

Dawson, L. A., D. W. Litzenberg, K. K. Brock, M. Sanda, M. Sullivan, H. M. Sandler, and J. M. Balter. (2000). "A comparison of ventilatory prostate movement in four treatment positions." *Int. J. Radiat. Oncol. Biol. Phys.* 48(2):319–323.

de Boer, H. C., and B. J. Heijmen. (2001). "A protocol for the reduction of systematic patient setup errors with minimal portal imaging workload." *Int. J. Radiat. Oncol. Biol. Phys.* 50(5):1350–1365.

Erridge, S. C., Y. Seppenwoolde, S. H. Muller, M. van Herk, K. De Jaeger, J. S. Belderbos, I. J. Boersma, and J. V. Lebesque. (2003). "Portal imaging to assess set-up errors, tumor motion and tumor shrinkage during conformal radiotherapy of non-small cell lung cancer." *Radiother. Oncol.* 66(1):75–85.

Gilhuijs, K. G., and M. van Herk. (1993). "Automatic on-line inspection of patient setup in radiation therapy using digital portal images." *Med. Phys.* 20(3):667–677.

Hanley, J., M. Debois, D. Mah, G. S. Mageras, A. Raben, K. Rosenzweig, B. Michalczak, L. H. Schwartz, P. J. Gloeggler, W. Lutz, C. C. Ling, S. A. Leibel, Z. Fuks, and G. J. Kutcher. (1999). "Deep inspiration breath-hold technique for lung tumors: The potential value of target immobilization and reduced lung density in dose escalation." *Int. J. Radiat. Oncol. Biol. Phys.* 45:603–611.

Henkelman, R. M., and K. Mah. (1982). "How important is breathing in radiation therapy of the thorax?" *Int. J. Radiat. Oncol. Biol. Phys.* 8(11):2005–2010.

ICRU Report 50. Prescribing, Recording and Reporting Photon Beam Therapy. Washington, DC: International Commission on Radiation Units and Measurements, 1993.

ICRU Report 62. Prescribing, Recording and Reporting Photon Beam Therapy. Supplement to ICRU Report 50. Washington, DC: International Commission on Radiation Units and Measurements, 1999.

Jaffray, D. A., D. Yan, and J. W. Wong. (1999)."Managing geometric uncertainty in conformal intensity-modulated radiation therapy." *Semin. Radiat. Oncol.* 9(1):4–19.

Jaffray, D. A., J. H. Siewerdsen, J. W. Wong, and A. A. Martinez. (2002). "Flat-panel cone-beam computed tomography for image-guided radiation therapy." *Int. J. Radiat. Oncol. Biol. Phys.* 53:1337–1349.

Mackie, T. R., T. Holmes, S. Swerdloff, P. Reckwerdt, J. O. Deasy, J. Yang, B. Paliwal, and T. Kinsella. (1993). "Tomotherapy: A new concept for the delivery of dynamic conformal radiotherapy." *Med. Phys.* 20:1709–1719.

Malone, S., J. M. Crook, W. S. Kendal, and J. Szanto. (2000). "Respiratory-induced prostate motion: Quantification and characterization." *Int. J. Radiat. Oncol. Biol. Phys.* 48(1):105–109.

Pisani, L., D. Lockman, D. Jaffray, D. Yan, A. Martinez, and J. Wong. (2000). "Setup error in radiotherapy: On-line correction using electronic kilovoltage and megavoltage radiographs." *Int. J. Radiat. Oncol. Biol. Phys.* 47:825–839.

Remouchamps, V. M., F. A. Vicini, M. B. Sharpe, L. L. Kestin, A. A. Martinez, and J. W. Wong. (2003). "Significant reductions in heart and lung doses using deep inspiration breath hold with active breathing control and intensity-modulated radiation therapy for patients treated with locoregional breast irradiation." *Int. J. Radiat. Oncol. Biol. Phys.* 55(2):392–406.

Seppenwoolde, Y., S. H. Muller, J. C. Theuws, P. Baas, J. S. Belderbos, L. J. Boersma, and J. V. Lebesque. (2000). "Radiation dose-effect relations and local recovery in perfusion for patients with non-small-cell lung cancer." *Int. J. Radiat. Oncol. Biol. Phys.* 47(3):681–690.

Shimizu, S., H. Shirato, H. Aoyama, S. Hashimoto, T. Nishioka, A. Yamazaki, K. Kagei, and M. Miyasaka. (2000a). "High-speed magnetic resonance imaging for four-dimensional treatment planning of conformal radiotherapy of moving body tumors." *Int. J. Radiat. Oncol. Biol. Phys.* 48(2):471–474.

Shimizu, S., H. Shirato, K. Kagei, T. Nishioka, X. Bo, H. Dosaka-Akita, S. Hashimoto, H. Aoyama, K. Tsuchiya, and M. Miyasaka. (2000b). "Impact of respiratory movement on the computed tomographic images of small lung tumors in three-dimensional (3D) radio-therapy." *Int. J. Radiat. Oncol. Biol. Phys.* 46(5):1127–1133.

Shirato, H., S, Shimizu, K. Kitamura, T. Nishioka, K. Kagei, S. Hashimoto, A. Aoyama, T. Kuneida, N. Shinohara, H. Dosaka-Akita, and K. Miyasaka. (2000). "Four-dimensional treatment planning and fluoroscopic real-time tumor tracking radiotherapy for moving tumor." *Int. J. Radiat. Oncol. Biol. Phys.* 48(2):435–442.

Ten Haken, R. K., J. M. Balter, M. K. Martel, and B. A. Fraass. (1996). "Tissue inhomogeneity in the thorax: Implications for 3-D treatment planning." *Front. Radiat. Ther. Oncol.* 29:180–187.

Van de Steene, J., F. Van den Heuvel, A. Bel, D. Verellen, J. de Mey, M. Noppen, M. De Beukeleer, and G. Storme. (1998). "Electronic portal imaging with on-line correction of setup error in thoracic irradiation: Clinical evaluation." *Int. J. Radiat. Oncol. Biol. Phys.* 40(4):967–976.

van Herk, M., P. Remeijer, and J. V. Lebesque. (2002). "Inclusion of geometric uncertainties in treatment plan evaluation." *Int. J. Radiat. Oncol. Biol. Phys.* 52(5):1407–1422.

van Lin, E. N., E. Nijenhuis, H. Huizenga, L. van der Vight, and A. Visser. (2001). "Effective-ness of couch height-based patient set-up and an off-line correction protocol in prostate cancer radiotherapy." *Int. J. Radiat. Oncol. Biol. Phys.* 50(2):569–577.

Vedam, S. S., P. J. Keall, V. R. Kini, H. Mostafavi, H. P. Shukla, and R. Mohan. (2003). "Acquiring a four-dimensional computed tomography dataset using an external respiratory signal." *Phys. Med. Biol.* 48(1):45–62.

Vineberg, K., et al. (2002). "IMRT plans robust to setup error and motion: Explicit incorporation of clinical setup data using the multiple instance of geometry approximation (MIGA)." *Int. J. Radiat. Oncol. Biol. Phys.* 54(2S):255.

Wagman, R., E. Yorke, E. Ford, P. Giraud, G. Mageras, B. Minsky, and K. Rosenzweig. (2003). "Respiratory gating for liver tumors: use in dose escalation." *Int. J. Radiat. Oncol. Biol. Phys.* 55(3):659–668.

Wong, J. W., M. B. Sharpe, D. A. Jaffray, V. R. Kini, J. M. Robertson, J. S. Stromberg, and A. A. Martinez. (1999. "The use of active breathing control (ABC) to reduce margin for breathing motion." *Int. J. Radiat. Oncol. Biol. Phys.* 44:911–919.

Yamada, K., T. Soejima, E. Yoden, T. Maruta, T. Okayama, and K. Sugimura. (2002) "Improvement of three-dimensional treatment planning models of small lung targets using high-speed multi-slice computed tomographic imaging." *Int. J. Radiat. Oncol. Biol. Phys.* 54(4):1210–1216.

Yan, D., F. Vicini, J. Wong, and A. Martinez. (1997). "Adaptive radiation therapy." *Phys. Med. Biol.* 42(1):123–132.

Yorke, E. D., L. Wang, K. E. Rosenzweig, D. Mah, J. B. Paoli, and C.-S. Chui. (2002). "Evaluation of deep inspiration breath-hold lung treatment plans with Monte Carlo dose calculation." *Int. J. Radiat. Oncol. Biol. Phys.* 53(4):1058–1070.

# What Is Different About IMRT?

**Mark Langer, M.D.**
Indiana University Medical School
Indianapolis, Indiana



What is different about IMRT? Medicine shares with physics the view that a new model should replace an old one only when it is shown to be superior. Clinical medicine does not lightly let go of the vast experience accumulated with standard drugs, techniques, and algorithms. The notion of a "standard" approach is enshrined in insurance, accreditation, legal and regulatory language, and is an integral part of the science of medical evaluation. A phase III randomized study is designed to demonstrate the clinical superiority of a new agent tested against a standard control. New drugs, at least, are expected to pass this hurdle before being accepted into the approved pharmaceutical formulary.

It is fair to ask in what ways can intensity-modulated radiation therapy (IMRT) be described as being different from radiotherapy practiced without this technique. What characteristics distinguish the distribution of dose given by one method from that given by another? Absent rigorous clinical trials, are the characteristics of the dose distribution planned by the new method unequivocally better than the old? Is their realization in delivery at least as free of error? If instead there are trade-offs between the methods, what procedures are available to choose between them?

These questions concern the practicing physicist and physician. Indeed, they must be able to pose these questions and formulate answers that can be agreed upon for each individual case. The dialogue that engages the physicist and physician in search of a solution can be a source of stimulation, excitement, and satisfaction but also lead to unending trials, anxiety, and frustration. Unanchored to the sheltered harbor of familiar practice, the practitioner of IMRT can discover new routes for more effective treatment, but must avoid foundering on the shoals of inexperience and surprise.

## Historical Experience

### 2-D Era

Historically, the radiation oncologist (then known as the radiation therapist) who used external beams treated with a limited number of fields, arranged in simple ways that could be regularly repeated from case to case. Surface anatomy had to be relied upon in earliest times, but once radiographic simulations became available, bony anatomy provided surer and more reproducible guides. Contrast provided by air or an administered agent (such as dye placed into the bladder) offered additional detail.

The utility of plain radiographic guides should not be lightly dismissed. Many normal tissues, for example, brain stem and spinal cord, are fairly well located by their surrounding bony anatomy. Other tissues, such as kidneys and small bowel, can be visualized once a suitable contrast agent is administered.

Soft tissue compartments enveloping a presumed tumor target, such as the tonsillar fossa or the prostate gland, often bear a fixed relation to the surrounding bony anatomy. The projection of these targets onto plain films oriented in familiar directions [e.g., anteroposterior (AP) or lateral] using known anatomic relations proved itself to the practicing physician over scores of successfully treated cases. Even when checked against the seemingly stricter standards of computed tomography (CT) or magnetic resonance imaging (MRI), fields constructed using these projections will be found to cover the intended target in most cases that have a reasonable probability of cure. The relation between an imaging irregularity and tumor invasion is ill defined and founded on little empiric data; abnormalities can be due to inflammation or edema and seemingly normal tissue elements may harbor neoplastic cells. In those cases where the gross target volume has escaped its assumed anatomic relations, the local clonigenic burden and expectation of metastases are both raised and the likelihood of cure with any field size may be remote.

Standardization of target projections lends itself to standardization of field design. The application of reproducible fields facilitated over many years the iterative adjustment to field borders needed to make isolated marginal failures a vanishingly rare occurrence for treatable conditions. The observations that directed refinements to treatment were seldom the conclusive results of controlled trials, but were nevertheless grounded in the reality of experience that formed the basis of retrospective reports in the scientific literature. There is inevitably a selection bias to such reports, but the adoption of reproducible fields across the community lends itself to successive processes of error finding and adjustment. In the language of physics, such a system might be termed "self-correcting."

The steps that were taken to make isolated marginal recurrence for head and neck cancer an uncommon event are illustrative of this process. Historically, such recurrence was related to disease insidiously spreading across the mucosa or infiltrating below the surface. Such disease still is sometimes better recognized as a subtle redness or a barely perceptible firmness on clinical examination than anatomic distortion on imaging. By understanding the sites of recurrence in light of the standardized field design, it was possible to make progressive corrections that greatly reduced the incidence of isolated marginal recurrence. The expansion of the anterior boundary of the standard lateral fields employed to treat upper head and neck cancers in the face of anteriorly sited recurrences provides one such example (Fletcher 1980).

Field design in the 2-D era was also made robust to set up inaccuracies. In their simplest form, they were based on elementary expansions of the smallest circle that enclosed the projection of the target onto the beam, or polygons that circumscribed this circle (figure 1). Such fields are robust to error: they will tend to be insensitive to rotational changes either in the plane of the beam or in a plane orthogonal to the beam. Straight edges or circular fields registered against lines templated on the patient's skin or overlying mask provided a means to detect and correct alignment errors at each treatment session, an early, simple but surprisingly robust form of adaptive radiotherapy.

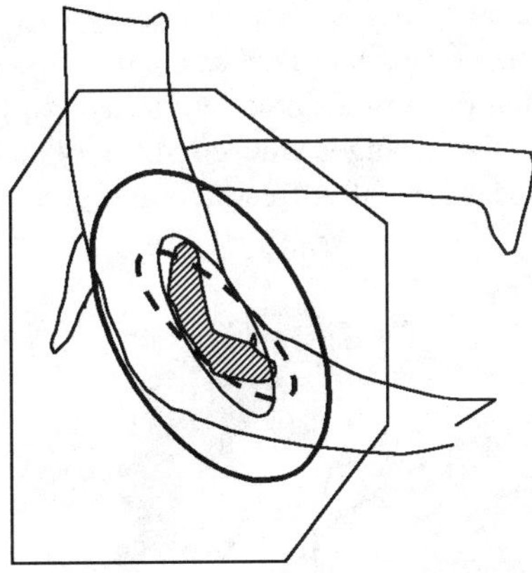

**Figure 1.** Field outlines devised for a hypothetical tonsillar fossa tumor using 2-D tools. The tumor (hatched lines) is concave shaped, but a convex envelope (small oval) has been drawn around it and expanded (dark oval) to form a beam "target". Straight blocks are used to form a polygonal-shaped field about the target. The convex shape of the target allows for avoidance of geographic miss of the tumor in the event of small rotational errors (dotted lines).

Even before the 3-D era dawned, the dangers of accepting untested innovations based only on a presumption of benefit from physical changes in the dose distribution appeared. Not infrequently one hears the argument that clinical trials of devices that "clearly improve" the dose distribution are unwarranted; there is no reason to delay their introduction by the long and tedious process of protocol writing, patient accrual, and results reporting. The story of how unexpected toxicity followed the introduction of flattening filters to improve the homogeneity of orthovoltage radiotherapy belies this assertion. In the post WWII period, flattening filters were devised to reduce the inhomogeneity across the orthovoltage fields then available. They were soon applied to the whole abdominal fields then prescribed for the treatment of many conditions (primarily seminomas) in the period prior to the availability of effective chemotherapy regimens. Some time after the introduction of the flattening filters, a complication that had been unexpected with whole abdominal treatment emerged with alarming frequency: nephritis and chronic renal damage (Luxton and Kunkler 1964). Upon inspection of the isodose plots (figure 2), it was discovered that the inhomogeneous dose distributions created without the flattening filters resulted in an underdosing at the field margin that had acted unintentionally to spare the upper pole of the kidneys. By applying an estimate, presumably extracted from the surgical experience, of the fraction of the renal parenchyma that must be spared to maintain physiologic function (about 1/3) to isodose plots on which the kidney outlines were superimposed, an estimate of the dose level corresponding to the threshold of renal tolerance was derived that is still in use today. Because the radiation damage did not appear until long after treatment, the warnings of renal toxicity came too late for many injured patients. The experience teaches that new methods of radiotherapy delivery that make a change assumed to be desirable in one characteristic of the dose distribution, whether that be homogeneity, conformality, or normal tissue complication probability (NTCP) may produce at the same time other changes whose risks may go unappreciated until their adverse consequences appear long after treatment has ended.

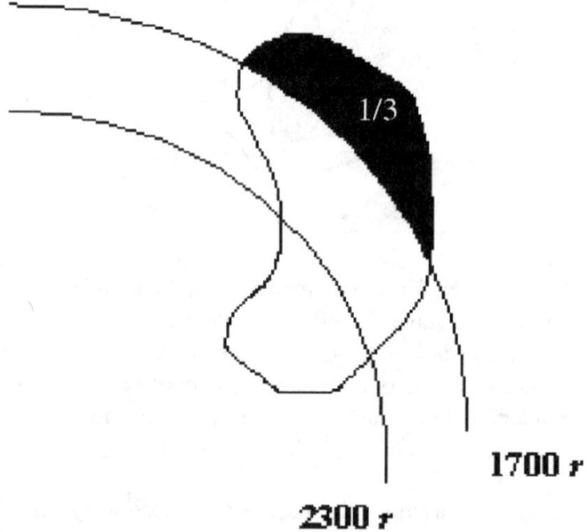


**Figure 2.** Early dose-volume analysis suggested by Luxton and Kunkler (1964). The investigators believed that 1/3 of the renal parenchyma was sufficient for renal reserve. Flattening filters that were later introduced removed the homogeneity that incidently spared the upper 1/3 of the kidney, here illustrated. Their introduction was followed by the later development of renal complications. By examining the isodose line that crossed the upper 1/3 of the kidney outline, Luxton and Kunker could estimate a threshold dose for renal tolerance. The actual dose levels they examined differed across a number of techniques that had been used prior to the introduction of the filters.

The simplified nature of 2-D therapy helped also to bring into stark contrast the economic trade-offs that appear when the resources commanded by a new technology intended to help one patient restricts access to medical care by other patients. Solzhenitsyn (1980) in his book *Cancer Ward* relates the fictionalized story of a physician who must balance the benefits to one patient of adding a hardening filter to a beam to improve its depth dose profile with the cost of the reduced dose rate that accompanies its use. The lengthened treatment time necessitated by the reduced dose rate worsened clinic throughput and diminished access to the therapy machine for other patients. The simplified structure of 2-D therapy helped to make such trade-offs recognizable to the practitioners of the day, to the author, and through his words, the public. The difficulty in tracing these connections through the complexities of modern medical technology and the health care delivery systems that support it represents a loss of information from the 2-D era whose importance can be underappreciated. In the present world of IMRT, a disproportionate share of personnel is consumed by the IMRT patients.

## 3-D Conformal Radiotherapy

The transition from 2-D to 3-D radiotherapy techniques provides a good model of how the benefits and drawbacks of new technology are absorbed in the radiotherapy community. Especially because adverse events in radiation oncology—whether tumor recurrence or normal tissue injury—emerge long after treatment is completed, the differences among techniques and their consequences may only be gradually perceived.

The introduction of 3-D techniques made it far easier to individualize the selection of beam direction to tumor geometry. Multiple coplanar and even non-coplanar orientations could be introduced. The imaging technology provided assurance to the oncologist that beams set in unfamiliar directions would nevertheless cover the required target and block out normal structures that were to be protected. By allowing multiple beams to be introduced, sharper margins around the target could be created because the penumbra of one beam could be placed in the interior of another. The arrangement opened up the possibility of reducing the risk of a marginal miss of target located in close proximity to normal structures.

The strong geometric arguments to employ 3-D technology ultimately proved persuasive to payors and the radiotherapy community and led to its widespread adoption in practice. The medical community at large will ask what is the quality of the evidence to support a gain? Because complications and recurrences may take years to appear after treatment ends, clinical evidence of improvement is expected to lag dosimetric gain. Absent such evidence, the physician community will look to the dose distributions to judge whether one technique provides superior results to another.

Rigorous planning studies of alternative techniques have been prepared. The results seldom establish an unequivocal benefit of one method over another. Instead, *trade-offs* among measures of the dose distribution tend to be found. A comparative planning study for lung cancer failed to substantiate the hypothesis that unrestricted beam arrangements (which this experiment took to be non-coplanar fields) could raise target dose over levels achieved with routine beam placement without at the same time increasing the dose delivered to some critical normal organ volume (Graham et al. 1994). Indeed, in most of the cases examined, standard beam arrangements for treating the target volume to a prescribed dose of 80 Gy had a smaller volume of contralateral lung exceed the critical threshold dose of 20 Gy than did the conformal non-coplanar fields. On the other hand, the volume of heart treated beyond a threshold dose of 40 Gy was higher with the standard field arrangements. In such situations, in which the dose distribution is improved in one structure but degraded in another, the value of one method over another is subject to judgment. In this instance, it was argued that the differences in lung volumes treated were small while the differences in heart volumes treated were substantial, and so the trade-offs favored the adoption of the non-coplanar 3-D approaches.

Judgments of this kind, weighing a favorable change in one tissue against an unfavorable change in another, will be on surer ground if the weighting rules are prospectively drawn. Otherwise, the comparisons may be subject to error. One source of error is that the weightings of the trade-offs may be biased by the results obtained. Another is that even if the weightings are deemed true, posing the evaluation rules after the plans are drawn forms a test of plan quality but not of the techniques used to generate them. A robust and effective technique will be able to produce treatment that is superior against the stated constraints and objective of the planning problem, but this treatment need not be best relative to conditions introduced after the planning exercise is completed.

Study of how the elements of 3-D technology affect the dose distribution showed that even small changes in the objective or constraints of the planning problem can produce large effects on the generated plan. The ability to employ treatment techniques that individualize planning to specifics of the treatment geometry and the prescribed rules for safe treatment would be expected to magnify this effect. Relaxation as small as 3% to 7% in a strict limit on dose homogeneity permitted tumor dose to rise by >20 Gy in a study of lung cancer cases in which the off cord boost angle was allowed to vary along the length of the patient (Langer et al. 1991). The strong sensitivity of tumor dose to the setting of the constraints was a finding made possible by the planning tools introduced by 3-D technology. In the 2-D era, the machinery to exhaust treatment constraints and check whether they were satisfied was much more limited.

Because small changes in the constraints can induce large changes in the dose distribution, the apparent advantage of one technique in raising tumor dose may be due to a failure to strictly meet a constraint rather than to an inherently superior method of treatment delivery. Other techniques may be more successful in meeting the constraints, but as a consequence may not achieve as high a tumor dose. Unless a plan scores worse by every criterion that is specified, it will always be possible to construct a set of weightings for the trade-offs so that a given plan will score best against them. Despite a maturation of 3-D technology, and investigation of its role, there remains a dearth of studies to show the advantage of 3-D technology over simpler methods using rules stated in advance of trial performance.

An additional source of error that can enter into comparison studies is that the advantage of one technique over another may hold only for a narrow range of settings for the prescription rules, and this range may differ from case to case. If the process of imposing the prescription requirements, such as dose, dose-volume, or homogeneity limits, is not blinded to the selection of cases, trials over the sample cases may be constructed, even inadvertently, to be systematically biased towards one technique or another. Such bias can be severe when the number of cases studied is small, or not representative of the population to which the conclusions are applied. This source of error has been exposed by an analysis of technique that the new methods of 3-D technology has helped excite (Ha, Kijewski, and Langer 1993). It was found that the advantage of varying along the length of the patient the angle at which the off cord boost for lung cancer was directed depended on the treatment geometry and the choice of dose limits. When strict limits were imposed on dose homogeneity, on spinal cord dose, and on the volume of contralateral lung that could exceed a threshold dose of 20 Gy, no advantage to varying the boost field angle along the patient length was found in three of six cases. In the remaining instances, the advantage held for only a narrow range of the volume of lung allowed more than 20 Gy, termed "V20". The range of V20 limits over which the new method proved better was not the same from one case to the next, and did not overlap among all three cases that showed a benefit for some choice of limits. In one case, only if the V20 was set to between 20% to 21% was an advantage found for the more sophisticated technique. At settings of the partial volume limit above this range, either boost method could deliver >80 Gy to the target without exceeding the tolerance constraints, while at settings below the range neither method achieved a significant tumor dose. Unless the requirements are chosen in advance of trial performance, the results may be subject to the selection bias of choosing conditions that appear to favor one technique over another for the patient series described. Such selection bias is the bane of all retrospective studies, but may be harder to discern in dosimetric studies where the endpoints are not as clearly established as those reported more generally in medicine, including death, failure, and toxicity.

While analysis of the gains achievable with new technology is subject to potential sources of error that review of the 3-D experience exposes, one must accept that comparisons not subject to any such error may be difficult to achieve. There may be too many conditions that govern safety for all to be specified in advance. Instead, shortfalls may only be recognized once they appear on isodose plots or dose-volume histograms, and their importance must be judged *ad hoc*. Indeed, it is possible to bury or miss undesirable properties in the dose distribution, if plans are described only in terms of a limited number of dose and volume combinations. Designers of 3-D technology responded to this need by inventing new displays that allowed the physician to rapidly inspect the dose distribution. These included color washes, dose-clouds, and multiplanar isodose plots. The practicing physician has learned to review one or more of these displays before electing a particular plan. In the medical literature, a variety of images are used to illustrate the differences in plans given by one technique over another to allow the reader the greatest freedom possible in judging plan quality.

Through such a process, a consensus governing the role of new technology may emerge, but one must beware the forces that can seek to manipulate the consensus building. While it may not be possible to base the judgments on rigorous scientific tests, the consensus may be sufficient to establish new standards, rules or practice guidelines that meet the expectations of physicians, regulators, and the public.

By probing for the advantage of 3-D technology across patient cases, the physician community has discovered unexpected connections among the different objectives of treatment, and forced a reconsideration of what the planning targets should be. Both clinical experience and planning studies have led to the realization that elective nodal irradiation in lung cancer enlists the inclusion of so much normal lung within the fields as to prohibit the safe escalation of dose to the gross target (Rosenzweig et al. 2001; Hayman et al. 2001; Senan et al. 2002). With only 2-D technology, dose escalation to the gross target is seldom feasible without violating standard limits on the dose delivered to the unaffected lung whether or not regional nodes are electively irradiated. When 3-D technology is introduced, dose escalation was found possible provided that elective irradiation of regional nodes was abandoned (McGibney et al. 1999). Here, 3-D technology did not provide improved treatment against the old dosimetric rules, but forced a rethinking of the rules that allowed new treatment strategies to be investigated.

The fact that new technology may bear hidden costs has also emerged as 3-D methods have become more widely implemented. These costs, not merely economic, can interfere with the theoretic gains otherwise expected. One is that the favored patient position may need to be revised to accommodate entry into the scanner; maintenance of arm position for the breast patient is one example. Another is that trial and error repositioning of the patient to create a preferred separation of target and normal tissue may be impaired by the cumbersome apparatus of the CT scanner. For example, certain decubitus positions designed to move the small bowel away from the right or left pelvic sidewall may be hard to achieve and evaluate using many kinds of scanning systems. Visualization of surface details may also be difficult, especially if available markers produce CT artifacts. Changes in patient contours over the course of treatment (e.g., due to weight change) may render planning based on pretreatment scanning of little worth or even dangerous. Because 3-D technology exploits individual differences in geometry, it is not robust to undetected errors in position or measurement. Using a pretreatment CT scan to estimate depth to spinal cord in a patient likely to have a much thinner neck by the time an electron boost is delivered presents a risk that demands special care to appreciate. So too, would building a custom compensator for a head and neck patient whose shoulder overlying the spine may rise or fall to different levels from simulation to treatment. Evaluation of motion over the treatment session ("intrafraction motion") is also more difficult with CT-based planning than with traditional fluoroscopic tools. While some of these problems may have work-arounds, complete remedies may not be available, and problem discovery and solution development are not always correctly amortized into calculations of the costs of changing the clinical environment.

The effect of patient motion on the quality of the delivered treatment is another problem that is difficult to measure. The concept of field margins essential to 2-D treatment design has been replaced by the construction of margins around clinical and planning target volumes (PTVs). However, because the falloff in the dose distributions may differ between 2-D and 3-D plans, uncertainty in treatment geometry may have different consequences. A small error may result in a more precipitous drop in dose using the sharper distributions available with 3-D treatment. The margins developed in the 2-D era, which may have allowed for an effective dose to be delivered in the event of a small positional error may not longer be effective. While it may be possible to use clinical experience to ultimately derive suitable margins for 3-D treatment, the required information is rarely available from pretreatment measurements. An iterative process of failure and response may need to be replayed to establish the margins appropriate for the new technology.

## IMRT: New Elements Of Treatment Construction

IMRT has changed the process of treatment construction from the design of fields to the design of dose distributions. As a result, the experience that has been learned in the process of designing treatment fields must be translated into the vocabulary of dose distributions. One no longer can speak of head and neck fields that cover boundaries marked by air cavities or cartilagineous projections, as in the 2-D era, or of fields that cover the projections of drawn targets, as with 3-D technology. Instead, the goal is to create dose distributions that meet the stated goals of therapy.

The problems are to determine what are the goals of therapy and what is to be done when the stated goals are not met. Deriving dosimetric goals from the experience of 2-D and conformal therapy is not simple, since the object of adopting new technology is not to merely replicate the old distributions but to change them.

Fundamental to the IMRT method is the ability to vary the radiation intensity across the face of the beam. Conventional therapy employs beams whose intensity is either uniform, or changes uniformly, such as by the addition of a wedge filter. The intensity profile of the IMRT technique need not observe such a restriction. This freedom means that features of the dose distribution that one has come to expect from conventional therapy need no longer be preserved but new features may be created. The ability to generate high dose volumes that are concave in shape is one advantage of the IMRT method. At the same time, other desirable properties may be lacking.

Homogeneity of dose across the target volume is one goal of conventional therapy that IMRT does not necessarily match. When fields of uniform or uniformly changing intensity were set to cover projections of the target volume, dose homogeneity was a realizable goal. The entire target volume was irradiated by each beam, and the dose delivered by that beam changed by a graded amount that could be adjusted by change of a wedge angle. Treatments could be expected to meet protocol prescriptions calling for dose homogeneity levels of ±5% to 10%, or the International Commission on Radiation Units and Measurements (ICRU) reports 50/62 recommendations of –5% to +7%. Of course, checks of these goals were sometimes done on only one or several planes taken through the target volume; the homogeneity of dose across the entire volume achieved in practice was likely worse. Nevertheless, these numbers gave guidelines around which treatment strategies could be built. IMRT has engendered a weakening of the homogeneity restrictions. Thus, one reads "The use of inhomogeneous dose distributions provides higher doses to the tumor without increasing normal tissue doses. For that reason, an IMRT technique was developed in our department" (DeMeerleer et al. 2000).

One difference from conventional therapy is that the sources of the described inhomogeneity are not necessarily known. As a result, a process to redesign treatment so as to eliminate the stated inhomogeneity is not established. It was primarily an unfavorable treatment geometry (e.g., tumor wrapped around spinal cord) that forbade simultaneous achievement of both an adequate tumor dose and the desired level of dose homogeneity with conventional treatment. Either the projection of the target over the critical normal tissue had to be blocked at the tolerance dose of the critical structure, in which case homogeneity was not achieved, or the entire treatment had to be terminated at this dose level, in which case tumor dose was inadequate.

The sources of the stated inhomogeneity with IMRT are more complex. First, it is possible that the cause still remains unfavorable treatment geometry. The desired level of homogeneity may not be realizable with any available method of delivery. Abutment of tumor against a critical organ structure on which an absolute dose limit has been placed will create this situation. Second, it is possible that a more homogeneous solution is feasible, but the method of planning has not discovered it. A trade-off between desired conformality and homogeneity has been surmised, and accepted in the IMRT environment. For example, one read: "Although with conventional therapy dose is usually prescribed to 100% of target volume, for the purpose of this study we chose a typical IMRT scenario where some of the target is allowed to be underdosed, thus giving the optimizer room to achieve a plan as conformal as possible" (Pirzkall et al. 2002). Recently, it has been shown that an entire range of homogeneity levels for a plan can be achieved, depending on which planning method is used and what parameters are chosen for it (Vineberg et al. 2002). Finally, it is possible that the stated homogeneity in the produced plan is wrong. The quoted level of homogeneity is only an approximation to the actual homogeneity achieved. The desired level of homogeneity may remain within an accepted range of error around the stated value. In the presence of error in determining homogeneity and other dose or dose-volume parameters, values for the 5th and 95th percentile doses in critical structures are now reported as surrogates for the maximum and minimum doses respectively (Hunt et al. 2001). The Radiation Therapy Oncology Group (RTOG) has imposed a minimum dose requirement on 99% of the planning target volume in its recent head and neck IMRT protocol, but none on 100% of the volume (RTOG H-0022).

Differences in the ability to develop the cause of failure to meet a treatment condition distinguish IMRT from conventional 2-D or conformal therapy. Because conventional therapy is simpler to plan, the possible changes to the dose distribution are limited. A new practice risk is created with IMRT by the possibility that the unmet conditions will be satisfied by a better plan produced after treatment has ended. It has been shown that an inverse plan routine may return a result that is inferior to one that can be produced by hand, both with respect to tumor and normal tissue (Mohan et al. 1994). Available planning routines do not disclose the quality of their solutions. It is possible to check whether a constraint is satisfied, but not whether a list of unmet conditions is feasible. Nor do the routines disclose by how much an objective can be raised under the constraints. An additional risk is that employing alternative methods of plan evaluation will expose shortfalls in the dose distribution that went unrecognized at the time of treatment delivery. Underdosing gross tumor in the face of a 1% short-fall in the PTV treated to a tumoricidal dose is one such risk. The shortfall may not occur along the periphery of the PTV, but in the interior deep within the gross target. Even a volume shortfall of only 1% within a $5 \times 5 \times 5$ cm$^3$ tumor can represent a signif-icant volume of disease (>1 cm$^3$) for which traditionally large doses of radiation must be employed to ensure sterilization. The risk of misinterpreting summaries of the deliv-ered treatment demands the physician rely on multiple illustrations of the dose distribution, complicating the process of plan generation and acceptance.

Clinicians, physicists, and physicians need to be alert to the fact that the tools for treatment display may not carry information regarding the delivered dose per fraction. The traditional use of successive cone-down fields with 2-D or 3-D treatment implied that the target was treated at a known dose per fraction. The dose per fraction deliv-ered to normal tissue took greater effort to estimate, but still could be adequately judged using information on prescription depth, field arrangement and energy in the 2-D era, or simple review of the different course plans in the 3-D era. With IMRT treatment, the planner must deliberately check not only that limits on total dose are satisfied, but that the dose per fraction lies within a range established to be safe and effective. With some systems, deliberate care must be exercised to acquire this information, depend-ing on the facility to combine or separate plans. Checks need to be performed separately not only on the gross and microscopic target volumes (which can show dose inhomogeneity) but also on normal tissues, which may unexpectedly lie within a high dose region.

The planner must also account for all tissue strata that can be affected by radia-tion within the treatment volume. Because the dose distributions created with IMRT can be unusual, the "treatment volume" which carries clinically significant dose may need to be redefined. Examination of integral dose, and of the dose carried by some sensitive structures that may lie distant from the target (e.g., contralateral lung in a breast case) is required. Structures that may have been unaffected by the homogeneous dose distributions delivered with conformal therapy may be placed at risk if they fall within high-dose regions lying in structures simply labeled as target. A widely accepted example is the urethra lying within the PTV of a prostate treatment plan. Another example less widely discussed is the tissue matrix comprising a "nasopharynx" target which may include mixtures of cartilage and soft tissue elements that can be injured at sufficiently high dose. High doses delivered to small points along bronchi lying within the PTV of a lung cancer target may evolve over time to produce a catastrophic or even fatal fistula connecting the bronchi with the parenchyma of the lung.

## Plan Evaluation

The process of generating dose distributions through IMRT creates uncertainties in the available tools of plan evaluation that challenge the physicist and physician developing treatment for the individual patient. One lies in the dose-volume histogram. Typically, sample points are generated within a volume of interest, and the dose at these sample points determined from interpolation on a fine dose grid that has been calculated. The intensity map of a conventional beam is convex—the intensity along a line connecting two points will be a weighted average of the values at the end points. By and large, the image of the dose distribution conserves this property, although it can deviate from it in the presence of large changes in the external surface, air cavities, and like disturbances to smoothness. On the other hand, the ability to create isodose maps that are concave is a critical property of the IMRT method. As a result, the dose along a line connecting two points may not be an average of the values of the endpoints, and interpolation ceases to be valid. Special care must be exercised in interpreting dose volume histograms constructed from such interpolations. It is conjectured that smoothness in the isodose lines (or in the difference between isodose lines and the target boundary) may be used instead to verify coverage of the target, but no formal method for establishing coverage is available.

The new kinds of dose distributions that can be created with IMRT have prompted a revisit to some of the traditional rules for plan acceptance and evaluation. The application of minimum dose requirements to less than 100% of the planning target volume is one example of such a revision. More broadly, NTCP and TCP (tumor control probability) indices have been applied to IMRT treatment design and evaluations in ways untried in conformal therapy. For example, the number of beams used and the choice of plans has been based on use of a P+ statistic, the probability of uncomplicated tumor control (Söderström and Brahme 1995). The choice to use three modulated beams for prostate cancer treatment has been adopted in one European center based on an assumed lack of clinical gain with more. The arguments that defend the use of biologic indices, whose values carry great uncertainty, can often be traced back to a statement of the national Cancer Institute (NCI) Photon Therapy Collaborative Working Group (NCI 1991), which noted that "Tumor control probabilities may be calculated to predict the likelihood of local control...Similarly, normal tissue complication probabilities may be calculated. While absolute probabilities are not yet attainable, relative probabilities may be used to rank treatment plans."

This statement was shown to be not true if score functions based on biologic indices, such as P+, are used to rank treatment plans (Langer 1998). The ranking is found to depend on the absolute probabilities, and cannot be determined from the relative probabilities alone. Nevertheless, score functions continue to be used to develop

IMRT treatment strategies, in ways that are foreign to the practitioner of conformal and 3-D therapy.

## Plan Acceptance

Criteria for plan acceptance may also be different. Uncertainty in the presented measures of the dose distribution (such as the dose-volume histogram) makes it difficult to gauge whether the prescribed conditions have been met, and there are no certain rules to decide how much additional effort should be expended to try to meet the conditions or improve the objective. While a similar problem can be stated for 2-D or 3-D treatment, the limited number of parameters that can be changed with the simpler technology seems to make a search over the feasible space a practical possibility. This is no longer the case with IMRT, for which the search can depend not only on the performance of the optimization engine with respect to its mathematical objective, but on how the parameters are set by the clinician to represent the clinical problem. A nasopharynx planning problem that carried maximum dose limits on critical structures, a prescribed dose for the target, and a dose homogeneity limit for target could not be represented as such for optimization. Instead, the stark clinical criteria had to be modified to form a "constraint template" on which the optimization engine operated (Hunt et al. 2001). The template required the assignment of "penalty factors" to each condition, and in order to produce useful results, artificial values for the constraint bounds had to be surmised and substituted for the clinically prescribed ones. For example, the clinically prescribed criteria were that the target receive a certain prescribed dose and the cord receive less than 40 Gy. In order to drive the engine to produce an acceptable solution, the max dose value allowed the spinal cord was set at 35 Gy rather than the 45 Gy specified in the clinical criteria, and penalty factors of 100 for spinal cord and 25 for target were chosen that were not part of the original problem statement. Such a process cannot be expected to maximize a dose objective subject to the clinically prescribed criteria, nor is it guaranteed to find a feasible solution if one exists.

An interesting perspective on the choice of penalty factors is given by linear programming. Under the typical convention that dose at a point is linear in the beam element intensities, the problem of developing a plan that meets the specified limits on absolute maximum and minimum doses, and on dose homogeneity can be represented as a linear program. The problem of choosing optimum values for the variables of a linear program that will maximize an objective subject to constraints is equivalent to finding a particular set of weights for the objective and constraints so that their weighted sum will be maximized at the optimum values of the variables (Dantzig 1963). The two problems are termed "duals" of one another. Choosing penalty factors is a task that goes to the heart of solving the optimization problem. When dose bounds are placed on tissue points, a particular set of penalty factors will correspond to the problem of maximizing a dose objective subject to these dose bounds. Finding these penalty factors is equivalent to solving the optimization problem. In practice, planning systems restrict the penalty set to classes of tissues, rather than placing them on individual points. The restriction means that fewer penalty factors have to be chosen. However, forcing all points in tissue to observe the same penalty rule is restrictive, and superior solutions may be eliminated by this artifice.

The apparent complexity of the planning problem has prompted the introduction of approximations to simplify the processes. These include stopping after a given number of iterations, accepting a solution that converges to a possibly local minimum, or developing an optimization solution based on setting the scatter dose component to zero beyond a selected distance from the central beamlet ray. In choosing fluences, the perturbations caused by collimator effects and discretization of intensity levels are not included. The validity of all these approximations remains unestablished by theory or experiment. In part, establishing the loss induced by these approximations means finding a solution that lies within a defined distance of the true optimum, a task that remains to be generally accomplished.

Because the methods of IMRT treatment delivery distort the delivered dose distribution from that planned, physicist and physician must exert care to review and either accept or reject the dose distribution that will actually be delivered. Sources of distortion include reduction of the continuous intensity maps to a limited number of discrete intensity levels to facilitate the leaf sequencing algorithms, and perturbation to the fluence caused by the construction of the collimator leaves (through leakage and tongue-and-groove effects). Measurements are also indicated, using routines that are distinct from those employed with conventional delivery apparatus.

## Robustness To Uncertainty

Robustness to uncertainty is different for IMRT than for conventional treatment. Unlike the change from 2-D to 3-D treatment, the effect of small movements is not due primarily to increased sharpness in the penumbra. Rather it is due to the inherent quality of IMRT in being able to produce high isodose lines that can follow the concave outlines of a tumor boundary. Because traditional treatment tends to produce a high isodose region that forms a convex envelope about the target, the results are relatively insensitive to rotational uncertainties—much like enclosing a shell within a ball that can be freely rotated within the conical margins of a beam (figure 3). IMRT tailors concave isodose regions to concave-shaped targets. Such shapes remain the quintessential targets for IMRT treatments (prostate indented by bladder or rectum, nasopharynx looped around the clivus, or cervical nodes curving around the parotid). Small rotational displacement in these concave targets can cut through critical isodose lines and produce substantial underdosing in the target (figure 4).

Simpler 2-D and 3-D technology allowed concave dose distributions to be created but mainly in a plane parallel to that of the beam front. The concavities simply followed the outline of the drawn blocks. These custom blocks, too, were less robust to rotational error than straight edged blocks that formed a convex polygon around the target (figure 3). Historically, physicians intuitively created blocks that took setup error into account by either forming a convex envelope around the target or allowing extra margin around boundary segments with increased curvature. Such rules were not necessarily followed when "automargins" that formed a fixed margin around the boundary were introduced. The circumspect physician learned to recognize the situation and override the routine when necessary (Ketting et al. 1997). Even when a tight margin around a concave boundary was required, rotational errors in the plane of a concavity could be detected on port films because the outlines to be observed lay parallel to the beam face and could be imaged. This is not the case for concavities in the isodose lines produced by IMRT, which lie in planes that are perpendicular to the beam face. New methods of CT guidance do allow visualization in planes perpendicular to the beam, and can capture rotational error within these planes. On-line correction are even possible to increase certainty beyond that achievable with current methods (Pisani et al. 2000). Until such imaging methods become widely established in the field, positional errors such as those related to patient rotation may jeopardize the clinical gains that could otherwise result from the novel dose distributions.

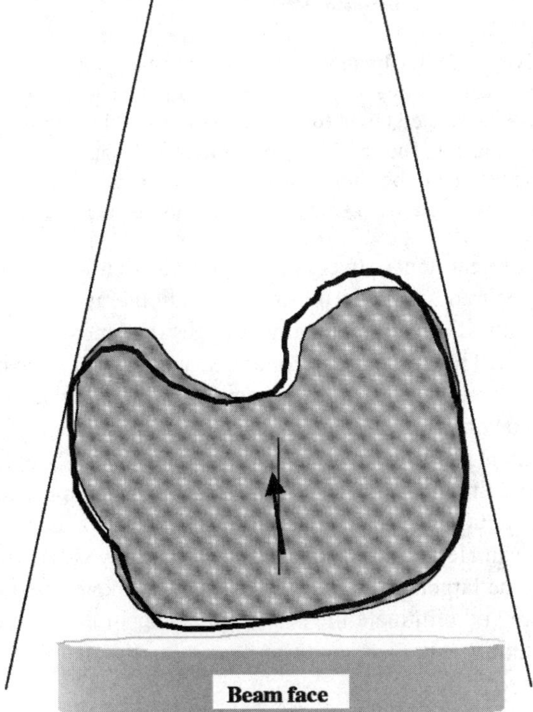



**Figure 3.** Conventional beams follow the projection of the target. The treatment volume forms a convex envelope around the target (shaded region) in the plane orthogonal to the beam face (shown here). Because the beam edges tangent the convex treatment volume, small rotational changes (arrow) retain the rotated target (dark boundary) within the treatment volume between the beam edges.

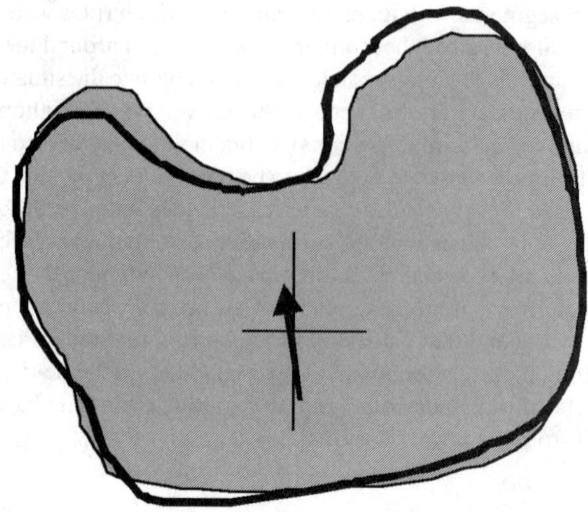

**Figure 4.** Sensitivity of IMRT treatment to rotational change. An IMRT dose distribution
forms a concave boundary outline around a concave target (shaded). A small rotational error
(arrow) will cause the rotated target (dark line) to now cut through the gray isodose line
intended to cover the target. The sensitivity of "conformal"-shaped fields to rotational error
in the plane of the beam will be similar, while the polygonal-shaped fields placed around
the target used in 2-D therapy will be insensitive to this error.

Each new era of treatment delivery has refocused attention on the problem of positional error and secured solutions of value to radiotherapy in general, such as the
positioning cases introduced about the time that the demands of 3-D conformal radiotherapy became felt. The process has continued with IMRT, whose introduction has
been accompanied by a plethora of inventions to stabilize the patient, to follow internal motions, and to correct or "adapt" to detected displacements. In general, creating
more secure treatment positions to allow reduced margins has both improved the accuracy of delivery and limited injury to normal structures. An approach of great interest
is the division of motional displacements into systematic and random error components (McKenzie, van Herk, and Mijnheer 2000). In many cases, the systematic error
has been found to be larger, a finding which suggest a new schedule for film review
in order to capture and eliminate the systematic error in the treatment course at the
earliest possible time.

## Predicting Outcomes

The changes to the dose distribution induced by IMRT include effects on the low-dose
regions whose clinical consequences may take a long time to register. Within IMRT,
variations in beam number or beam energy create ripple effects on the lower dose (e.g.,
70% to 80% regions), even when they are judged to hardly perturb target coverage by

the high isodose lines (Pirzkall et al. 2002). The clinical effects of changes to the lower regions may take time to discern. The Memorial Sloan-Kettering group, continuously reviewing outcomes in prostate cancer patients treated to high dose, has found a low dose criterion for avoiding rectal injury that is to be used in addition to a high dose criterion previously established (Jackson et al. 2001). Expanding the volume of soft tissue treated to even lower dose, or simply increasing integral dose may produce other, ill-defined aging affects, whose appearance may take years to recognize and discover.

At the same time, the shift in dose distributions created first by 3-D therapy and now more dramatically by IMRT has propelled a new look at traditional predictors of outcome. One is the use of mean dose to predict outcome. Mean tumor dose is more regularly increased by IMRT plans than minimum dose which is still constrained by the juxtaposition of tumor and normal tissues. The greater inhomogeneity seen with IMRT plans is associated with greater separation between minimum and mean dose, prompting a revisit of the question of what is the best dosimetric predictor of outcome using accumulated data. Mean dose has been found to be the best predictor of persistent tumor found on biopsy of previously irradiated prostate cancer patients (Levegrun et al. 2000). Whether the sampling results reflect the overall likelihood of persistent tumor within the treatment volume, or are biased by an inability to capture disease at the peripheral margin remains unanswered. The very area most likely to be excluded from biopsy because reasons of safety and geometric uncertainty (i.e., the peripheral margin closest to the rectal wall) is the one that for the same reasons is most likely to lie in the region receiving the lowest dose. Mean dose has also been found to be a suitable predictor of pulmonary complications in lung cancer treatment, offering the promise of a surrogate that is much easier to manipulate in optimization routines than dose-volume limits (Kwa et al. 2001). Caution needs to be taken in adopting these surrogate predictors for the purpose of steering optimization routines using new methods of treatment delivery. Predictors developed on the basis on correlations found with one kind of dose distributions (e.g., those given with 3-D treatment) may fail when a new kind of dose distribution is introduced, because a correlation with a more fundamental quantity affecting outcome (perhaps a dose-volume limit) may now be disturbed. A predictor that emerges when patients are treated by anteroposterior lung fields for a first course followed by off cord fields for a boost may no longer work when the technique is changed to alter the kinds of dose distributions that are produced. Changing the dose distribution may sever the connection between the predictor and some unknown set of dose-volume indices that actually affect the biology of the patient.

## IMRT Restrictions

IMRT, at least as defined for payment recognition, introduces new restrictions that may burden delivery, or constrain the dose distribution that can be produced. Increased numbers of monitor units may magnify issues of photon-neutron contamination from high-energy beams and limit their use. Patient motion may be exaggerated if treatment times are lengthened by the demands of increased monitor units or segments. An IMRT billing condition that at least four segments on average be used per field (Anon. 2001) may discourage techniques that use more efficient leaf sequencing, or rely on more beam angles. One study showed that by adopting an improved leaf sequencing strategy, the number of segments for a demonstrated prostate case could be reduced to 4.2, close to the lower limit below which IMRT billing is not allowed (Langer, Thai, and Papiez 2001). The billing rules must be regularly surveyed to avoid promoting inefficiencies in delivery. The absence of compensator or custom-based intensity modulation from the allowed billing definition of IMRT has been widely recognized. The distortions due to discretization, dose approximations during planning, incomplete optimization, leakage and tongue-and-groove effects in delivery, and limits on the segments or monitor units used all combine to limit the gains that might otherwise be achieved, and can produce results inferior to that given by simpler methods. For some sites for which IMRT has been examined, e.g., post lumpectomy whole breast treatment administered using an opposed pair of tangential fields, there was greater dose inhomogeneity and a more assured minimum tumor dose using conventional planning than realized with full modulation by IMRT (Fogliata, Bolsi, and Cozzi 2002). While it is sometimes thought that IMRT simply expands the degrees of freedom in treatment, these result underscore the truism that having more choices may make finding a good one that much harder.

## IMRT Advantages

Although the practitioner must be aware of the limitations, risks, and differences of IMRT from historic experience, it would be a mistake to dismiss the potential advantages of the technique. Coverage of structures at some small but not zero distance from critical normal structures have proved to be advantageously treated using the new technology. Examples include tumors of the sinus or nasopharynx partly eroding the clivus (Meeks et al. 1998), and the ease of creating dose distributions that cover cervical nodes while sparing sufficient parotid to preserve salivary function (Chao 2002). IMRT also offers the promise of limiting rectal irradiation in prostate cancer patients with the appropriate geometries (Mohan et al. 1994). The role of IMRT in other sites, such as post mastectomy irradiation of the chest wall and the regional lymphatics including the internal mammary nodes (Cho et al. 2002), and irradiation of the pelvis and/or para-aortic chain in gynecologic malignancy is undergoing investigation (Mundt et al. 2002).

Properly versed in how IMRT may differ from conventional or conformal therapy, and apprised of the sources of risk as well the benefits that are possible, the physician has the opportunity to improve patient care by the selective and considered use of this new tool.

# References


Anonymous. Summary of ACR/ASTRO Joint Economics Committee. *ASTRO News*. Jul–Aug 2001:15.

Chao, K. S. (2002). "Protection of salivary function by intensity-modulated radiation therapy in patients with head and neck cancer." *Semin. Radiat. Oncol.* 12(1 Suppl 1):20–25 (2002).

Cho, B. C., E. Hurkmans, E. M. Damen, I. J. Zijp, and B. J. Mijnheer. (2002). "Intensity modulated versus non-intensity modulated radiotherapy in the treatment of the left breast and upper internal mammary lymph node chain: a comparative planning study." *Radiat. Oncol.* 62:127–136.

Dantzig, G. B. "Basic Theorems on Duality" (ch. 6-4 ) and "Lagrange Multipliers" (ch. 6-5) in *Linear Programming and Extensions*. Princeton, NJ: Princeton University Press, 1963.

De Meerleer, G. O, L. A. Vakaet, W. R. De Gersem, C. De Wagter, B. De Naeyer, and W. De Neve. (2000). "Radiotherapy of prostate cancer with or without intensity modulated beams: A planning comparison." *Int. J. Radiat. Oncol. Biol. Phys.* 47:639–648.

Fletcher, G. "Head and Neck" (ch. 3). *Textbook of Radiotherapy*. 3rd ed. Philadelphia: Lea and Febiger, 1980.

Fogliata, A., A. Bolsi, and L. Cozzi. (2002). "Critical appraisal of treatment techniques based on conventional photon beams, intensity modulated photon beams and proton beams for therapy of intact breast." *Radiat. Oncol.* 62:137–145.

Graham, M. V., J. W. Matthews, W. B. Harms Sr., B. Emami, H. S. Glazer, and J.A. Purdy. (1994). "Three-dimensional radiation treatment planning study for patients with carcinoma of the lung." *Int. J. Radiat. Oncol. Biol. Phys.* 29:1105–1117.

Ha, C., P. Kijewski, and M. P. Langer. (1993). "Gain in target dose from using computer controlled radiation therapy (CCRT) in the treatment of non-small cell lung cancer." *Int. J. Radiat. Oncol. Biol. Phys.* 26:335–339.

Hayman, J. A., M. K. Martel, R. K. Ten Haken, D. P. Normolle, R. F. Todd 3rd, J. F. Littles, M. A. Sullivan, P. W. Possert, A. T. Turrisi, and A. S. Lichter. (2001). "Dose escalation in non-small-cell lung cancer using three-dimensional conformal radiation therapy: Update of a phase I trial." *J. Clin. Oncol.* 19:127–36.

Hunt, M. A., M. J. Zelefsky, S. Wolden, C. S. Chui, T. LoSasso, K. Rosenzweig, L. Chong, S. V. Spirou, L. Fromme, M. Lumley, H. A. Amols, C. C. Ling. (2001). "Treatment planning and delivery of intensity-modulated radiation therapy for primary nasopharynx cancer." *Int. J. Radiat. Oncol. Biol. Phys.* 49:623–632.

Jackson, A., M. W. Skwarchuk, M. J. Zelefsky, D. M. Cowen, E. S. Venkatraman, S. Levegrun, C. M. burman, G. J. Kutcher, Z. Fuks, S. A. leibel, and c. C. Ling. (2001). "Late rectal bleeding after conformal radiotherapy of prostate cancer. II. Volume effects and dose-volume histograms." *Int. J. Radiat. Oncol. Biol. Phys.* 49: 685–698 (2001).

Ketting, C. H., M. Austin-Seymour, I. Kalet, J. Jacky, S. Kromhout-Schiro, S. Hummel, J. Unger, L. M. Fagen, and T. Griffin. (1997). "Automated planning target volume generation: An evaluation pitting a computer-based tool against human experts." *Int. J. Radiat. Oncol. Biol. Phys.* 37:697–704.

Kwa, S. L., J. V. Lebesque, J. C. Theuws, L. B. Marks, M. T. Munley, G. Bentel, D. Oetzel, U. Spahn, M. V. Graham, R. E. Drzymala, J. A. Purdy, and A. S. Lichter. (1998). "Radiation pneumonitis as a function of mean lung dose: An analysis of pooled data of 540 patients." *Int. J. Radiat. Oncol. Biol. Phys.* 42:1–9.

Langer, M. (1998). "A test of the claim that plan rankings are determined by relative complication and tumor-control probabilities." *Int. J. Radiat. Oncol. Biol. Phys.* 41:451–457.

Langer, M., V. Thai, and L. Papiez. (2001). "Improved leaf sequencing reduces segments or monitor units needed to deliver IMRT using multileaf collimators." *Med. Phys.* 28:2450–2458.

Langer, M., P. Kijewski, R. Brown, and C. Ha. (1991). "The effect on minimum tumor dose of restricting target dose inhomogeneity in optimized 3-dimensional treatment of lung cancer." *Radiother. Oncol.* 21:245–256.

Levegrun, S., A. Jackson, M. J. Zelefsky, E. S. Venkatraman, M. W. Skwarchuk, W. Schlegel, Z. Fuks, S. A. Leibel, and C. C. Ling. "Analysis of biopsy outcome after three-dimensional conformal radiation therapy of prostate cancer using dose-distribution variables and tumor control probability models." *Int. J. Radiat. Oncol. Biol. Phys.* 47:1245–1260.

Luxton, R. W., and P. B. Kunkler. (1964). "Radiation nephritis." *Acta Radiol. Ther. Phys. Biol.* 2:169–178.

McGibney, C., O. Holmberg, B. McClean, C. Williams, P. McCrea, P. Sutton, and J. Armstrong. (1999). "Dose escalation of CHART in non-small cell lung cancer: Is three-dimensional conformal radiation therapy really necessary?" *Int. J. Radiat. Oncol. Biol. Phys.* 45:339–350.

McKenzie, A. L., M. van Herk, and B. Mijnheer. (2000). "The width of margins in radiotherapy treatment plans." *Phys. Med. Biol.* 45:3331–3342.

Meeks, S., J. M. Buatti, F. J. Bova, W. A. Friedman, W. M. Mendenhall, and R. A. Zlotecki. (1998). "Potential clinical efficacy of intensity-modulated conformal therapy." *Int. J. Radiat. Oncol. Biol. Phys.* 40: 483–495.

Mohan, R., X. Wang, A. Jackson, T. Bortfeld, A. T. Boyer, G. Kutcher, S. A. Leibel, Z. Fuks, and C. C. Ling. (1994). "The potential and limitations of the inverse radiotherapy technique." *Radiother. Oncol.* 32:232–248.

Mundt, A. J., A. E. Lujan, J. Rotmensch, S. E. Waggoner, S. D. Yamada, G. Fleming, and J. C. Roeske. (2002). "Intensity-modulated whole pelvic radiotherapy in women with gynecologic malignancies." *Int. J. Radiat. Oncol. Biol. Phys.* 5:1330–1337.

National Cancer Institute (NCI) Photon Treatment Planning Collaborative Working Group. (1991). "State-of-the-art of external photon beam radiation treatment planning." *Int. J. Radiat. Oncol. Biol. Phys.* 21:9–23.

Pirzkall, A., M. P. Carol, B. Pickett, P. Xia, M. Roach 3rd, and L. J. Verhey. (2002). "The effect of beam energy and number of fields on photon-based IMRT for deep-seated targets." *Int. J. Radiat. Oncol. Biol. Phys.* 53:434–442.

Pisani, L., D. Lockman, D. Jaffray, D. Yan, A. Martinez, and J. Wong. (2000). "Setup error in radiotherapy: On-line correction using electronic kilovoltage and megavoltage radiographs." *Int. J. Radiat. Oncol. Biol. Phys.* 47:825–839.

Radiation Therapy Oncology Group (RTOG) H-0022. Phase I/II Study of Conformal and Intensity Modulated Irradiation for Oropharyngeal Cancer, Feb 2001 (Rev. 1-2, Jan 15, 2002). Available at rtog.org.

Rosenzweig, K. E., S. E. Sim, B. Mychalczak, L. E. Braban, R. Schindelheim, and S. A. Leibel. (2001). "Elective nodal irradiation in the treatment of non-small-cell lung cancer with three-dimensional conformal radiation therapy." *Int. J. Radiat. Oncol. Biol. Phys.* 50:681–685.

Senan, S., S. Burgers, M. J. Samson, R. J. van Klaveren, S. S. Oei, J. van Sornsen de Koste, P. W. Voet, F. J. Lagerwaard, J. Marten van Haarst, J. G. Aerts, J. P. van Meerbeeck. (2002). "Can elective nodal irradiation be omitted in stage III non-small-cell lung cancer? Analysis of recurrences in a phase II study of induction chemotherapy and involved-field radiotherapy." *Int. J. Radiat. Oncol. Biol. Phys.* 54:999–1006.

Söderström, S. M., and A. Brahme. (1995). "What is the most suitable number of photon beam portals in coplanar radiation therapy." *Int. J. Radiat. Oncol. Biol. Phys.* 33:151–159.

Solzhenitsyn, A. *Cancer Ward*, N. Bethell and D. Burg (Translators). New York: Bantam Books, 1980.

Vineberg, K. A., A. Eisbruch, M. M. Coselmon, D. L. McShan, M. L. Kessler, and B. A. Fraass. (2002). "Is uniform target dose possible in IMRT plans in the head and neck?" *Int. J. Radiat. Oncol. Biol. Phys.* 52:1159–1172.

# IMRT Delivery Using Serial Tomotherapy

**Bruce Curran, M.E., M.S.**
University of Michigan Medical Center
Ann Arbor, Michigan



## Introduction

The era of modern intensity-modulated radiation therapy (IMRT) could be considered to have started with the papers by Brahme and Bortfeld at the end of the 1980's (Brahme 1988; Bortfeld et al. 1990). In those papers the concept of IMRT using modern, temporally varying delivery techniques was theorized, along with methods for the calculation of a fluence pattern starting from the desired dose distribution. As part of the discussion in these papers, a delivery device capable of producing a set of modulated pencil beams projected in a fan-beam orientation was imagined.

Following from this development, a number of researchers began to explore methods for the practical implementation of IMRT, including delivery devices and optimization/planning methods. This has been well reviewed and summarized by Webb, and more information can be found in his paper as part of this book and an earlier reference (Webb 1997, 2003).

One such group at the University of Wisconsin pursued the concept of delivering fan beams in a continuous, helical fashion (Holmes 1993; Mackie et al. 1993). As this concept (now known as "helical tomotherapy") is the subject of a later chapter in this book, readers are referred there for additional information (see *Helical Tomotherapy* by Mackie et al.)

Working at roughly the same time as the Wisconsin group, Mark Carol and associates at NOMOS Corporation (Cranberry Township, PA) developed a similar treatment procedure, now known as "serial tomotherapy" (Carol 1994, 1995). This technique delivers radiation using a rotational, modulated, slit beam aperture, similarly to the Wisconsin research. However, in the NOMOS technique the treatment couch does not move during irradiation. Thus, the total treatment is given as a series of arcs, each delivering dose to a narrow slice of the patient. The NOMOS product, known as the PEACOCK® system, consists of a serial tomotherapy collimator, computer controller, immobilization and couch positioning system, and a planning system for constructing the delivery patterns. This system is discussed in much greater detail in the section herein on implementation.

The first serial tomotherapy patient (and the first modern IMRT patient) was treated at The Methodist Hospital/Baylor School of Medicine, Houston, TX, in 1994 by Drs. Butler, Grant, and associates (Woo et al. 1994). Initial patients were predominantly brain and head and neck tumors, although some extra-cranial applications were done. They were followed in 1995 by Western Pennsylvania Hospital, Pittsburgh, PA; New England Medical Center, Boston, MA (Wazer et al. 1997); and Mercy Hospital, Oklahoma City, OK (Turner and Wizenberg 1997). In all these centers, the focus was on the treatment of cranial lesions, where good immobilization and minimal organ motion existed. By the end of 1996, approximately 30 centers had begun programs in IMRT using the NOMOS delivery system, extending the use of the system to target volumes throughout the body. Today, there are approximately 100 PEACOCK systems in use throughout the world.

## Characteristics of Serial Tomotherapy

A simple model of serial tomotherapy is shown in figures 1 and 2. The technique typically uses an arc of 270° to 340° for radiation delivery. Figure 1 shows such delivery of a single slice of radiation, conforming to the target volume and avoiding nearby critical structures (Note: this figure is animated on the CD). In order to treat the entire target volume, the patient is moved between successive arcs, as shown in figure 2. This movement is generally only along the longitudinal direction of the treatment couch, producing a series of treatment slices parallel to the patient's transverse plane. However, numerous researchers have used multiple couch angles to improve the conformity of the treatment for difficult lesions (Lam, Rogers, and Wichman 2001; Salter 2001).

There are several characteristics that distinguish serial tomotherapy from other IMRT techniques. In particular, three aspects of the method will be discussed: rotational delivery, table indexing, and delivery efficiency. Tomotherapy, in general, provides superior target conformity and organ-at-risk sparing compared to multileaf collimator (MLC)-based techniques (Xia et al. 2000). Some of the advantages/ disadvantages of serial tomotherapy, however, are related to the specific implementation of serial tomotherapy, and will be covered in more detail in the implementation section.

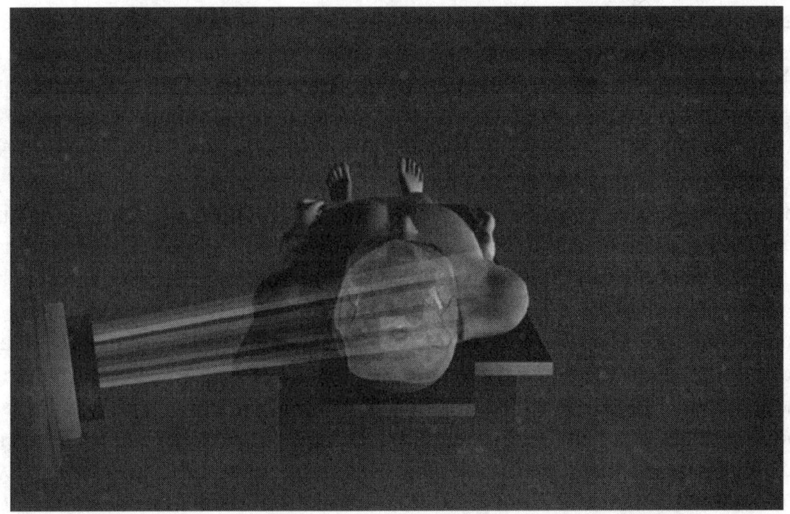

**Figure 1.** Animation showing delivery of an IMRT slice.
[Courtesy of NOMOS Corporation]

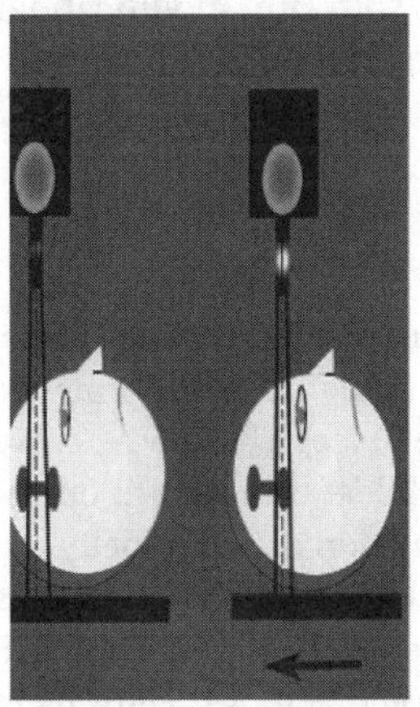 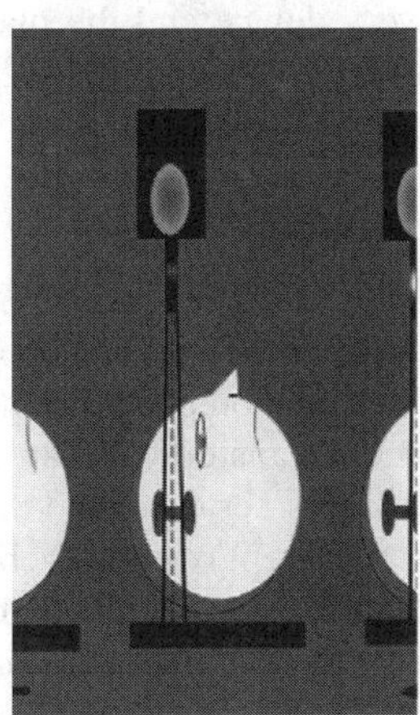 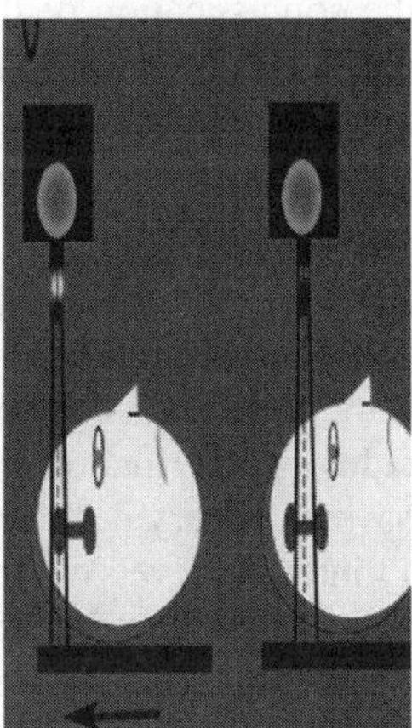

**Figure 2.** Cartoon showing the delivery of three slices of serial tomotherapy, each treating a different region of the target volume. [Courtesy of NOMOS Corporation]

Although other configurations may be possible, tomotherapy is generally conceived of as radiation delivery using a row of binary leaves oriented along the plane of rotation. These leaves, or vanes, open for various periods during the rotation to produce the desired delivery pattern. The width of each leaf, the number of leaves in a row, and the length of the opening are variables to be defined by specific implementations. Adding more leaves to a row increases the size of the target volume to be treated and the amount of modulation possible in a specific slice of the patient. However, more leaves results in increased weight for the collimator, as a result of the additional leaves and mechanics necessary to control them. This added weight may exceed the ability of individuals to easily position the device on the accelerator or the allowable weight of the mount or gantry motor of an accelerator. Thus, beyond a certain size, a specialized tomotherapy machine would be required.

In conventional external beam radiation therapy, rotational delivery is calculated by modeling the delivery as a series of static beams, evenly spaced along the path of the arc. A similar methodology can be used for tomotherapy. As with external beam, the rotation is modeled as a series of static beams, each with a modulation period, perhaps 5° to 10°. The planning system calculates an intensity pattern for each of these periods. From these intensity patterns, the rotational delivery is constructed, opening each leaf proportionally to its level of modulation. For example, let us assume a modulation period of 10° and modulation using 10% steps (0–100%). If the intensity pattern requires that a particular pencil beam open for 10%, the delivery system would open that leaf for 1° during the 10° modulation period, thus allowing 10% of the total radiation during that 10° period to be delivered, assuming a constant rotation speed and uniform dose rate. Similarly, a pencil beam open for 100% would open for all 10° of the modulation period. This allows standard, well understood, dose calculation algorithms to be used in tomotherapy dose calculations. Depending upon the sophistication of the delivery device and the planning software, modifications could also be made in the delivery to account for such perturbations as MLC transmission, mechanical delay, etc.

## Rotational Delivery

There are a number of advantages to the rotational delivery used in tomotherapy. First is the large number of potential irradiation positions that are available for tailoring the radiation distribution to the patient's anatomy. As an example, let us assume that we have a delivery device with 20 leaves per slice, and that each leaf can open to one of 11 intensity levels (0–100% by 10% steps) during each modulation period. Finally, we will assume that the modulation period is 5°, and that the modulation period centers are spread along an arc of 270° (these are the standard parameters for the NOMOS Peacock system, the only current implementation of serial tomotherapy). Thus, there are 1,100 potential pencil beams for each rotational slice ($55 \times 20$), nearly 8,000 pencil beams to treat a 7 cm lesion (assuming a pencil beam length of 1 cm). Using combinatorics, one can calculate that each slice has $(1{,}100)^{11}$ different treatment options, or approximately $2.85 \times 10^{33}$ potential pencil beam combinations for each slice. Of course, this will vary according to the implementation used, but clearly there are an enormous number of options that can be considered in finding the optimal treatment strategy.

A second advantage of rotational delivery is the reduced dependency of the delivery on such parameters as tissue heterogeneity and beam energy. It has long been understood that conventional arc treatments are not as sensitive to either of the above parameters as fixed-field deliveries (for a small number of fixed fields). This means that simpler dose calculation methods could be used to calculate the dose distribution, speeding up the calculation process, and allowing more options to be considered in an inverse planning scenario.

The disadvantages of a slice-by-slice rotational delivery center on divergence effects and the potential of added leakage radiation from the linear accelerator. Using a slice-by-slice delivery paradigm, precise table positioning must be achieved in order to maintain a homogeneous dose distribution. Incorrect or inconsistent spacing will result in hot and cold spots at these slice abutment regions. (A more detailed discussion of this issue can be found in the section *Implementation Of Serial Tomotherapy.*) Depending upon the target volume position and the organs-at-risk, there may be long areas of arc where no radiation is desired. However, conventional accelerators will continue to produce radiation during these periods, even though the tomotherapy collimator leaves are closed. This will result in increased radiation dose delivered through the tomotherapy leaves, and increased whole body dose as a result of overall accelerator leakage radiation.

Two additional aspects of rotational delivery should also be mentioned. The first of these is clearance. Current serial tomotherapy delivery devices are add-on, tertiary collimators. As such, the distance between the bottom face of the collimator and the patient/table is significantly reduced. For target volumes that are not centrally located, not all gantry angles may be possible. This is often not detectable until the patient is actually set up for treatment. The second issue is accelerator performance. Some accelerators are not designed for extensive rotational delivery, particularly with the added weight of a tertiary collimator. As a result, there may be an increase in needed repairs, particularly in the gantry bearings and motors. Such wear may also reduce the accuracy of tomotherapy delivery by introducing wobble in the gantry rotation bearing.

## Table Indexation

As mentioned above, serial tomotherapy is delivered as a set of arcs, each one treating a narrow slice of the patient. Matching of each slice (or set of slices, if more than one is delivered per arc) leads to two significant issues, accurate positioning/field matching and field divergence.

The sharp fall-off associated with linear accelerator delivery (and highly desirable for IMRT delivery as well) requires precise positioning of the patient between arc deliveries to accurately match the dose delivered from each arc, preventing hot and cold spots in this abutment region. The precision required, typically on the order of 0.1 to 0.3 mm, is much higher than conventional delivery, and thus requires special equipment and extra effort on the part of the radiation therapist. A more specific discussion of this issue is given in the section on implementation.

Also associated with field matching is the issue of divergence. Assuming one could, at a single distance, exactly match two adjacent arcs, there would still be under-lap/overlap at distances less than/greater than the match distance due to the divergence of the radiation field. Ideally, the divergence is compensated for by the opposing portion of the arc delivery. This compensation is reduced, however, by two factors. First is the total length of the arc. Due to table effects, collision issues, etc., the tomotherapy arc may not be a full 360°. This means that not all rotation positions have an opposing beam for compensation. Second, two opposing beams may not have the same intensity, resulting in an incomplete balancing of the divergence effect.

## Delivery Efficiency

The major issues associated with serial tomotherapy delivery are those of delivery efficiency. Although serial tomotherapy does not pay a penalty for the complexity of the intensity map to be delivered [which does occur with static and dynamic MLC-based deliveries and intensity-modulated arc therapy (IMAT)], its slice-by-slice delivery usually requires longer treatment times and longer beam-on times than other IMRT techniques. Some of the added time is implementation-specific, but most of it is inherent in the treatment technique.

*Treatment Time*

The delivery paradigm for serial tomotherapy is to treat each slice of a patient independently (or set of slices, if more than one slice is treated in a single arc). This requires one complete arc for each thickness of target volume to be treated. For example, a target volume of 7 cm would require seven arcs to be delivered, assuming a 1 cm slice thickness. Between each arc, the patient would need to be moved to a new position, typically by incrementing the table by the slice thickness. Using a conventional accelerator, the total treatment time [excluding patient setup and exit] would be on the order of 20 minutes (seven arcs, each requiring ~2 minutes, and six table motions, each requiring ~1 minute). These numbers could be improved by a number of methods, including auto-incrementing of the patient position, higher dose rates, and faster arc rotation. The treatment time is also directly proportional to the number of arcs used for treatment, and could be reduced by using a larger slice thickness for treatment. For example, prostate treatment may be delivered faster than other delivery methods of IMRT. However, using current treatment techniques and equipment, as was the basis for the estimates above, a 30 to 40 minute treatment slot is generally required, and can be longer for larger lesions. This time compares favorably to stereotactic treatment techniques, which often run 60 to 120 minutes, but is longer than conventional deliveries, which generally required 10 to 15 minutes for treatment, including setup and exit times.

*Monitor Unit Efficiency And Whole Body Dose*

In conventional external beam radiation therapy (excluding wedged treatments), the number of monitor units (MU) is approximately equal to the dose (in cGy) delivered to the center of the target volume. 3-D conformal techniques reduce this efficiency slightly, requiring approximately 1.5 MU/cGy delivered. Serial tomotherapy, however, due to the small fields used and the rotational technique (which may include dead periods) typically requires 2.5 to 3.0 MU/cGy for each arc. Coupled with the need to deliver multiple arcs in order to cover the entire volume, the overall number of monitor units (MUs) required to treat a target volume can approach 8 to 15 times the target dose. While this factor has some concern with regard to the wear on accelerator components, the primary concern is the additional whole body dose delivered as a result of leakage through the MLC and the accelerator itself.

The implications of these large MU deliveries has been studied by a number of researchers. Followill et al. published a theoretical study (Followill, Geis, and Boyer 1997) using three arcs per treatment volume. They estimated the MU/cGy factor to be 9.7, thus increasing the accelerator leakage dose by roughly a factor of 10 to approximately 543 mSv for a 70 Gy treatment using 6 MV photons. Mutic (Mutic and Low 1998) experimentally measured the dose at distance from the treatment region for serial tomotherapy deliveries. They estimated, for an average delivery (five arcs), that approximately 300 mSv would be received at a distance of 40 cm from the field, considerably less than the theoretical study, and significantly reducing the risk of an induced cancer from the whole body dose. Verellen (Verellen and Vanhavere 1999) also looked at the whole body dose from serial tomotherapy compared to conventional delivery. While the ratios of dose (~8) were similar to the previous studies, they estimated the total dose to be ~2,000 mSv. However, Verellen's dosimeters were placed at the skin surface, rather than in phantom, and therefore contained a greater amount of low-energy scattered radiation than Mutic's measurements.

The conclusions of these papers predicted a increase (1% to 3%) in the risk of induced cancers as a result of the use of IMRT and tomotherapy over conventional treatments. While significant, this increase will be difficult to verify without careful study of a large patient population. None of the papers attempted to compare this risk with the potential benefits of improved cures or decreased complications associated with IMRT.

*Collimator Transmission*

In addition to the increased whole body dose associated with serial tomotherapy, the increased number of MU require that the beam-shaping device designers pay more attention to transmission of radiation through its leaves than in conventional therapy. Most MLCs today have an average transmission of 2.0%. Should the tomotherapy collimator have similar characteristics, the transmitted radiation through the collimator could approach 10% to 20% of the delivered dose, thus significantly reducing any gain that might be achieved by IMRT delivery. Serial tomotherapy collimators need average transmissions to be on the order of 0.5% or less, so that the extra-target doses due to transmission through the collimator are less than 5.0%.

*Patient Positioning And Motion*

The extended treatment times associated with serial tomotherapy necessitate that consideration be given to the issues of patient motion and positioning. When delivering a precise treatment that could extend over 30 to 45 minutes, particularly a treatment requiring precise junctions, small movements of the patient during this process could result in significant dose errors. Patients need to be positioned in a comfortable and reproducible manner so that they will remain stable during the treatment. Xia and her colleagues at University of California San Francisco (UCSF) have looked at this problem for their treatment setup (Xia 2000). In this study, patients were positioned on a radiotherapy simulator table as if set up for IMRT treatment, and orthogonal fluoroscopy/radiographs done at regular intervals to check on patient position compared to the accelerator isocenter. They found that, using their setup, patient were able to maintain a consistent position for at least 30 minutes, the longest period examined. This can be seen in figures 3 and 4, showing a set of orthogonal radiographs taken at 0, 15, and 30 minutes for one of the patients studied.

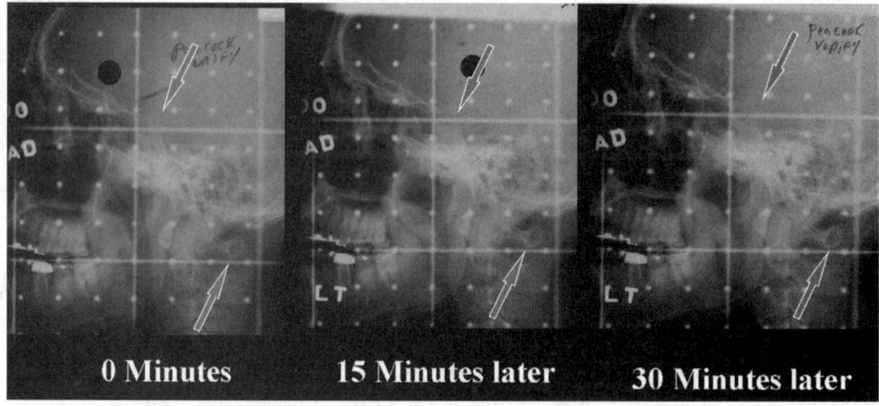


**Figure 3.** Lateral radiographs of patient. Arrows indicate points used for detection of patient shift during the 30-minute procedure. [Courtesy of Ping Xia, UCSF]

It may be, however, that a small amount of patient setup error/motion may be beneficial to the overall treatment. Small indexing errors are likely to occur, and, if done systematically, could result in an underdose/overdose for the perfectly positioned patient. A small amount of motion would result in a blurring of this underdose/overdose region, reducing the effect of any systematic treatment errors. This has been shown to be true for tongue-and-groove errors during MLC delivery of IMRT, a very similar situation to the abutment case of serial tomotherapy (Deng et al. 2001).

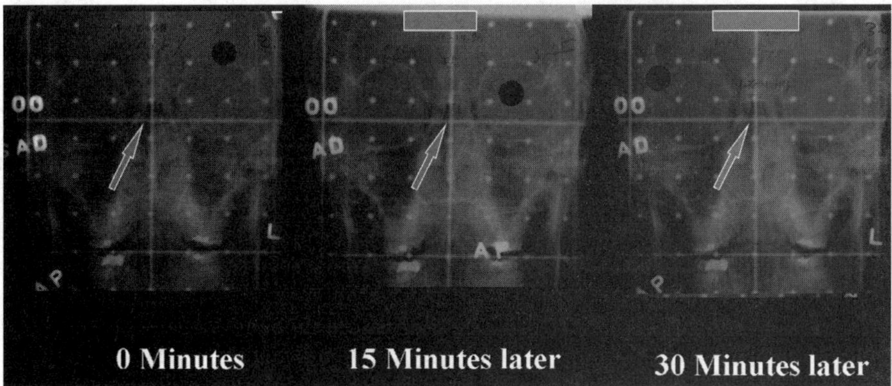


**Figure 4.** AP radiographs of patient. Arrows indicate points used for detection of patient shift during the 30-minute procedure. [Courtesy of Ping Xia, UCSF]

## Implementation Of Serial Tomotherapy

As only a single manufacturer has produced a serial tomotherapy product (NOMOS Corporation, Cranberry Township, PA) a description of how serial tomotherapy has been implemented can be quite specific. In this section, the general procedure for installing, commissioning, and use of the NOMOS product, known as the PEACOCK system is described. Acceptance tests and quality assurance (QA) procedures, both equipment and patient specific are also discussed. Finally, some typical clinical cases and their results are shown.

## Installation And Acceptance Testing

The delivery hardware used in the PEACOCK system is called the Multileaf Intensity Modulating Collimator (MIMiC®) and shown in figure 5. Designed specifically for IMRT delivery, it consists of two rows of 20 binary vanes, allowing two slices of the patient to be treated in a single arc (see figure 6). During an arc, each vane opens to produce a pencil beam aperture of nominal width 1 cm and length of 0.4 cm, 1.0 cm, or 2.0 cm. (As implemented by NOMOS, only a single length is used for a treatment.) Vanes open and close by an air pressure/solenoid system, having a typical transition time of 100 to 150 ms. Vanes are 8 cm of tungsten, double focused, and stepped to reduce interleaf leakage.

### *Typical Installation*

Depending upon the accelerator manufacturer and model, MIMiC is installed into or in place of the blocking tray. In either case, alignment pins are used to allow accurate and reproducible placement of the MIMiC on the accelerator. Thus the MIMiC can be installed as a removable collimator, allowing patients to be intermixed between tomotherapy and conventional deliveries.

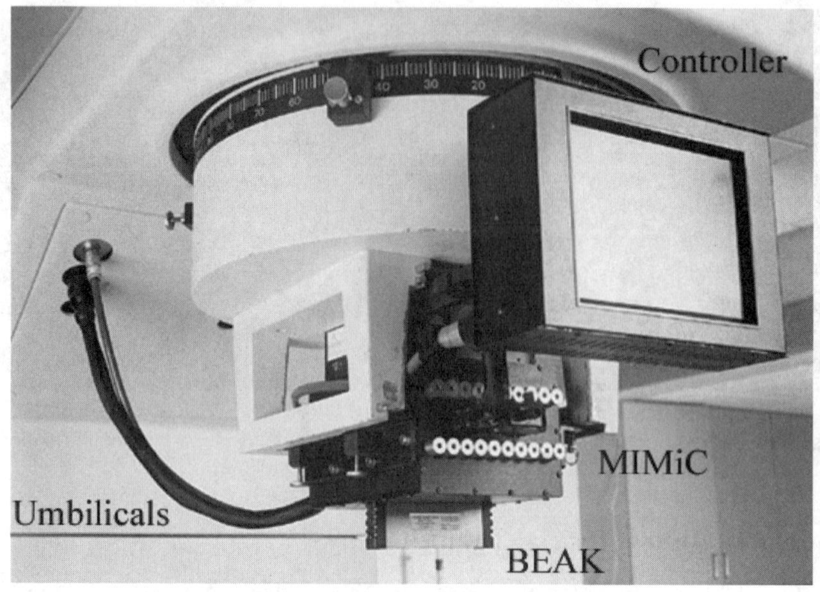



**Figure 5.** MIMiC mounted on a Siemens accelerator with the controller and the BEAK installed below it. [Courtesy of NOMOS Corporation]

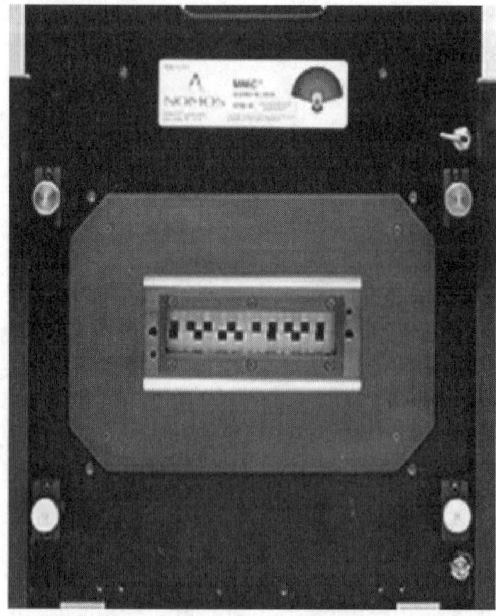

**Figure 6.** Patient's eye view of the MIMiC, showing the two rows of vanes, each of which creates a tomotherapy delivery slice. [Courtesy of NOMOS Corporation]

To supply the necessary power and air to the MIMiC, two supply lines, known as umbilicals, are run through the accelerator gantry and stand during installation. At the back of the accelerator, these lines lead to NOMOS-supplied air and power supplies, typically located on a small rack to one side of the accelerator stand. On the collimator side, the two umbilicals terminate in a pair of connectors located close to the collimator. Once place on the accelerator, the MIMiC and its associated controller are connected using a short pair of umbilicals. The installation of the MIMiC and umbilicals typically requires 1 to 2 evenings and can be done without interfering with normal operation of the accelerator during the day.

The MIMiC, its mount, and the controller have a total weight of approximately 40 kg. For some accelerators, this weight can alter the balance of the gantry and reduce the evenness of rotation. To offset this, a removable counterweight is also installed at the base end of the gantry. The counterweight is then adjusted to restore gantry balance when the MIMiC is installed.

The MIMiC controller interacts with the therapists via a touch-screen interface. This interface is calibrated, along with the redundant gantry angle sensors built into the controller.

Once installed, the MIMiC must be aligned to the center of the radiation field. Opposing pairs of alignment screws are provided on the MIMiC mount to accomplish this. Alignment is done in two steps. First, in-plane alignment is done using a film placed sagittally on the accelerator table and offset from the isocentric plane by approximately 20 cm. All MIMiC leaves are opened, and the film irradiated using lateral opposed beams. This produces a "box within a box" film (see figure 7) and the in-plane alignment screws adjusted until the boxes are well centered and the vertical edges parallel. Crossplane alignment is then accomplished by placing a film vertically at the isocentric plane and adjusting the MIMiC leaves to form a checkerboard pattern. Opposing lateral irradiations are once again done and the cross-plane alignment screws adjusted until a well-centered checkerboard is constructed from the opposing irradiations. Figure 8 shows the results of such an alignment.

**Figure 7.** MIMiC inplane alignment film. The film is placed vertically on the table, offset from isocenter ~20 cm, and then exposed from 90° and 270°. [Courtesy of Ping Xia, UCSF]

**Figure 8.** MIMiC crossplane alignment film. The film is placed vertically on the table at isocenter, the leaves opened in a checkerboard pattern, and the film then exposed at 90° and 270°. [Courtesy of Ping Xia, UCSF]

*Accelerator Issues*

The MIMiC alignment films shown above were taken after installation on a well-maintained accelerator. There are a number of issues associated with accelerator performance that will interfere with the quality of the MIMiC alignment that can be achieved, and thus the accuracy of delivery.

On many early MIMiC installations, a noticeable shift was detected in collimator rotation when the opposing lateral alignment films were taken. It was discovered that, for older accelerators in particular, the chains used to rotate the collimator would stretch, allowing a rotation of up to 1.0° for offset loads on the collimator. Due to the position of the MIMiC controller, such an offset load is present with the MIMiC. In later installations, collimator rotation was tested during installation and a collimator brake added if necessary.

Although alignment pins are used to ensure the reproducibility of MIMiC placement for those centers that do not mount the MIMiC permanently, the weight of the MIMiC can result in small, but noticeable, displacements of the MIMiC if not placed consistently. Sites are encouraged to develop a consistent method of placing the MIMiC on the accelerator, so that alignment will be consistent and accurate.

During radiation delivery, the MIMiC attempts to predict the delay time associated with the mechanical motion of vanes, and to initiate open and close commands slightly in advance of the desired transition. This delay time is calculated during the initial 5° to 10° of gantry rotation, with some allowance for initial start-up transients. Should the accelerator rotation fail to be relatively constant, this delay time can be misapplied, resulting in slight imperfections in the radiation delivery. The MIMiC controller checks for such rotation speed errors, and will shut down treatment delivery if the rotation speed exceeds a certain window. This window is quite wide, but the slight delivery errors that may occur within the window have not been shown to be of clinical significance.

As discussed previously, serial tomotherapy requires high precision in the incrementing of the table position, in order to precisely match adjacent treatment arcs. Current accelerator tables, with a precision of +/−1.0 mm, do not meet these criteria. The PEACOCK system includes a table positioning system (figure 9), allowing precise table motions on the order of 0.2 mm (Salter et al. 2001a). The dosimetric error associated with such precision has been investigated by several authors (Carol et al. 1996; Low et al. 1999) and will be discussed later in the commissioning section.

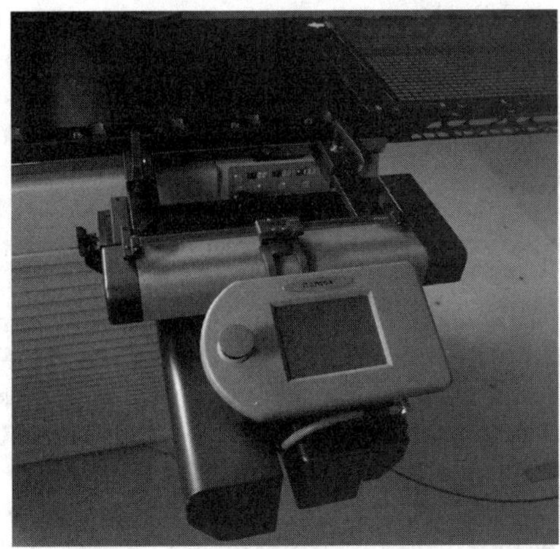

**Figure 9.** NOMOS Autocranea placed on treatment couch to allow unassisted, precise couch positioning between serial tomotherapy slices. [Courtesy of NOMOS Corporation]

Finally, similar to stereotactic radiotherapy (SRT) and stereotactic radiosurgery (SRS) systems, a stable and precise gantry isocenter is important for accurate tomotherapy delivery. Linear accelerators used for serial tomotherapy should meet the isocenter requirements discussed in AAPM Report 54 (AAPM 1995). Fortunately, most accelerators have a consistent isocenter pattern, or precession, as they rotate. This means that adjacent tomotherapy arcs do not overlap, but that nominally opposing pencil beams will have a slight offset, usually less than 1.0 mm, during radiation delivery.

*Commissioning*

In commissioning the PEACOCK system, one cannot completely separate the dosimetric issues of serial tomotherapy from those of the CORVUS® treatment planning system (NOMOS Corporation, Cranberry Township, PA), particularly since CORVUS is the only planning system supporting serial tomotherapy delivery. As such, this section will present a brief overview of the complete commissioning process, with specific emphasis on those issues that are uniquely associated with tomotherapy delivery.

The CORVUS planning system utilizes a finite-size pencil beam (FSPB) model for the calculation of dose in IMRT delivery (Bourland and Chaney 1992; Ostapiak, Zhu, and Van Dyk 1997) and has been described elsewhere (Kania et al. 1997; Nizin, Kania, and Ayyangar 2001). An idealized pencil beam is formed by extracting primary and scatter dose information from a series of percent depth dose (PDD) or tissue-maximum ratio (TMR) measurements along with the corresponding output factor measurements. The primary profile of the FSPB is derived from measurements of the in-plane and cross-plane profiles of a small field (central eight vanes open) and includes both vane shape parameters as well as an electron transport factor. A key parameter in this determination is the actual size of the pencil beam in the in-plane direction, as this will determine the match distance for adjacent arc deliveries.

The result of a typical procedure for measurement of the in-plane pencil beam size is shown in figure 10. Placing a film horizontally at the isocentric plane with appropriate build-up, a series of exposures is made with all vanes of the MIMiC open. Different increments are done for each static anterior-posterior (AP)-exposure and the match lines between the exposures are examined. The increment resulting in the most uniform exposure between adjacent arcs is selected as the *Table Index* value. Approximate values of this index are 8.0 mm for the BEAK® radiosurgical collimator, 16.5 mm for 1.0 cm mode, and 33.7 mm for 2.0 cm mode. Because the MIMiC beam is divergent, this increment assures only a correct match at the isocentric plane, with an underdose region above the isocenter and an overdose region below the isocenter, as one would expect from a conventional gap calculation. However, the rotational delivery of tomotherapy reduces the magnitude of these regions, dependent upon the total rotation used during treatment. Most serial tomotherapy deliveries use at least 270° of rotation, thus removing most of the underdose/overdose region resulting from the divergence.

**Figure 10.** MIMiC index test. Using a horizontal film and buildup material, successive AP irradiations are done with different spacings to determine the optimal slice index. [Courtesy of Ping Xia, UCSF]

At this point it is useful to look at the errors that might be introduced through incorrect indexing of the table between adjacent arcs. Several groups have looked at the dosimetry in this abutment region, both for shortened arcs and for errors in table indexing (Low and Mutic 1997; Low et al. 1999; Carol et al. 1996; Leybovich et al. 2000). Low and colleagues estimated that errors accumulated at a rate of 2.5% per 0.1mm of error. Thus a positioning device with a reproducibility of +/–0.2 mm could result in a dosimetric error in the abutment region of +/–5.0% (Low et al. 1999). This error would be further blurred by patient setup inaccuracies, typically no less than 1 to 2 mm.

In addition to the measurements of the standard beam profiles, CORVUS also requires an estimate of the radial fluence variation across the accelerator field. This information is acquired by averaging diagonal beam measurements taken at the same time as the PDD or TMR measurements are done. IMRT has the advantage of being able to compensate for non-uniform fluence sources (see the later paper in this proceedings on helical tomotherapy by Mackie et al.). Since the PEACOCK system is designed to work with a conventional accelerator, the fluence non-uniformity is small, but taken into account.

The final measurement required for initial beam entry is an estimate of the MIMiC vane transmission. CORVUS compensates, where possible, for the dose delivered through closed vanes in determining the duration of the opening of vanes for a particular pencil beam (Holmes et al. 1997). This value is typically measured at the center of the MIMiC opening, using the ratio of doses with all MIMiC vanes open to all vanes closed. A typical measured value is ~0.3%, considerably less than the nominal 1.0% specification.

The final step in commissioning a PEACOCK system for serial tomotherapy is the determination of the system calibration factor (CF). This factor adjusts the monitor unit (MU) calculation of CORVUS to agree with measurements. It accounts for small errors in the dose algorithm as well as some of the more sensitive measurements (for example, the measurement of the primary profile is sensitive to the detector volume). The CF is set by delivering a series of patient plans to phantom and adjusting the CF until the dose error is minimized for the set of plans. Typically, the CF is within 2% of unity and results in a dose accuracy for the system of +/–3%.

*Daily Setup And Use*

Converting an accelerator from conventional use to serial tomotherapy typically takes therapists 5 to 10 minutes. The blocking tray, if removable, is taken off and the MIMiC mount placed on the collimator, aligned, and fastened down. If used, the collimator brake is tightened. The controller is then attached to the MIMiC mount, and the electronic and air umbilicals attached. A switch located near the gantry stand is moved to the PEACOCK position, connecting the system to the accelerator (allows PEACOCK errors to interlock the accelerator). The MIMiC power supply is turned on and the system allowed to boot up. The recommended field size, typically 5 cm by 21 cm is set on the accelerator. While this is happening, the table positioning device is moved into position and attached and the MIMiC counterweight is attached.

Once the MIMiC controller has booted, the two computers inside perform a series of checks on the system and the MIMiC. The therapist adjusts the stops for the mode (1 cm or 2 cm) of the first patient, and positions any immobilization equipment needed.

Quality assurance for daily setup is fairly simple. Most institutions do a quick check of the delivery system alignment by rotating the gantry to a lateral position and viewing the intersection of the lateral laser with the closed vanes of the collimator. The table rotation angle may be checked, as well as the coincidence of the MIMiC gantry angle indicator with the accelerator. Most institutions develop a simple checklist so that the overall process becomes routine (Saw et al. 2001).

## Patient Setup And QA

For the most part, patient setup and QA for serial tomotherapy is no different from other forms of IMRT, and begins well before the actual treatment starts. The patient position must be well established and all setup accessories ready at the time of the patient's imaging studies, typically one week before the start of treatment. As previously discussed, the setup and immobilization must be designed to assist the patient in maintaining the desired reproducibility for the extended duration of most tomotherapy treatments. These materials should be checked regularly for defects or other variances that would reduce the accuracy and precision of patient placement (Saw et al. 2001).

Dosimetric QA starts with the generation of a "hybrid plan" (also called a phantom plan). This technique recalculates the patient treatment for delivery to a known phantom that has been previously scanned and aligned (Low et al. 1998). The plan is then delivered and the measured dose compared to the calculated one. While this does not completely check the actual patient dose, it provides a check on the accuracy of the delivery as calculated and transferred to the tomotherapy system. Figures 11 and 12 show typical results from dosimetry done using film and the hybrid plan option.

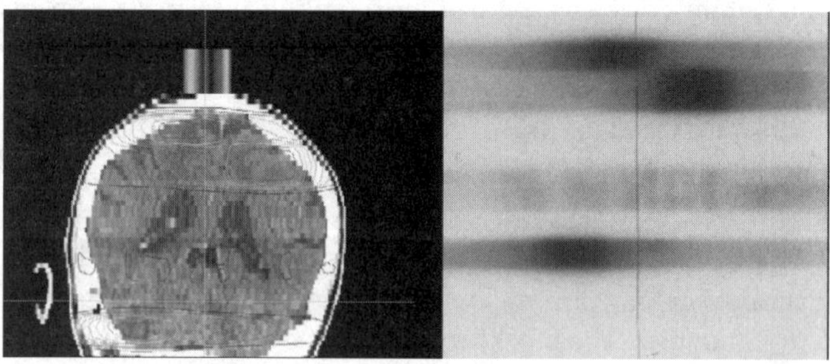

**Figure 11.** Coronal QA film for a multiple target IMRT plan.
[Courtesy of Walter Grant III, The Methodist Hospital, Houston, TX]

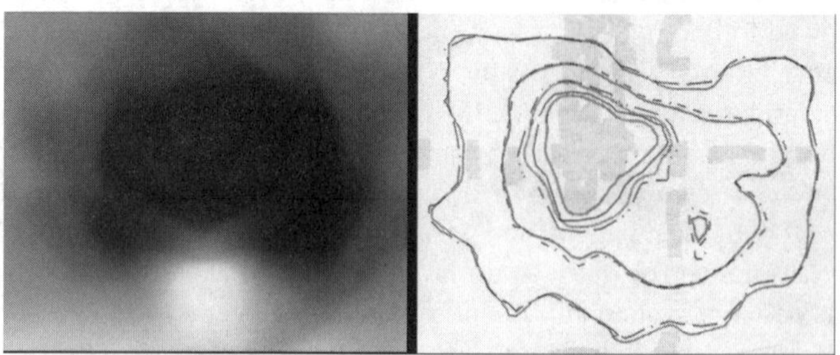

**Figure 12.** Axial QA film delivered to phantom and then compared with calculations.
[Courtesy of Ping Xia, UCSF]

## Clinical Examples

The first example of serial tomotherapy delivery is the fractionated treatment of an acoustic neuroma (Fuss et al. 2002; Salter 2001). The patient was immobilized using a high-precision, implanted head immobilization device capable of being used in fractionated treatment (Salter et al. 2001b). Computed tomography (CT) and magnetic resonance (MR) images were used to delineate the anatomy and target volumes, as seen in figure 13. Figure 14 shows the prescription for this target volume, delivering 54 Gy in 2 Gy fractions. The treatment was given using two couch angles (nominal and at one right angle) using a nominal 4 mm treatment slice. The 54 Gy (96% of maximum dose) line is shown in figure 15 for the central orthogonal cuts through the target volume. The statistics, also in figure 15, show that nearly 99.9% of the clinical target volume (CTV) is treated at the prescription dose, while all structures except the right lens are well below their prescription limits. Figure 16 shows the cumulative dose-volume histogram (DVH) for this plan, and figure 17 shows the fluence pattern for the first arc, as well as the MU for the four arcs used in the treatment. The treatment required nearly 1400 MU in order to deliver the daily fraction dose of 2 Gy.

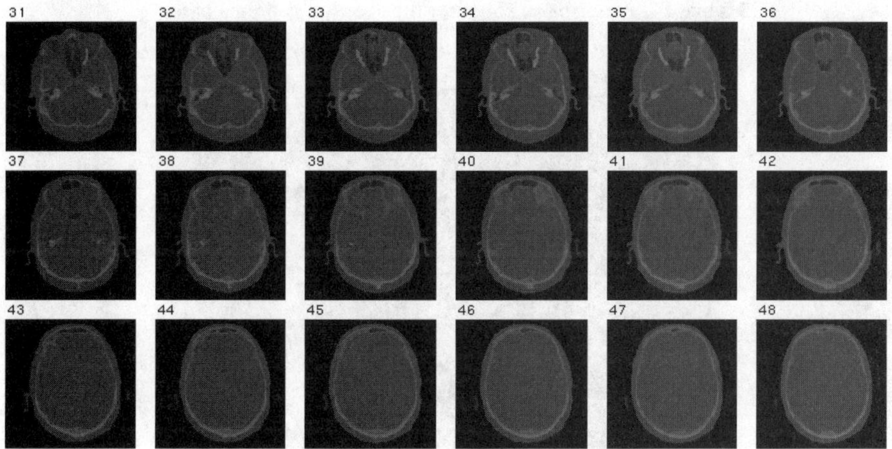

**Figure 13.** CT axial images showing the delineation of an acoustic neuroma. MR imaging was also used to identify target and sensitive volumes.

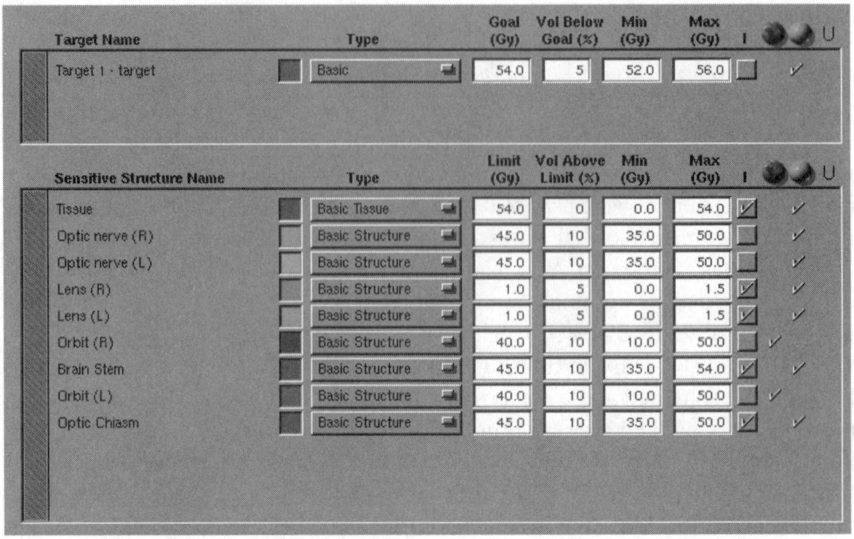

| Target Name | Type | Goal (Gy) | Vol Below Goal (%) | Min (Gy) | Max (Gy) |
|---|---|---|---|---|---|
| Target 1 - target | Basic | 54.0 | 5 | 52.0 | 56.0 |

| Sensitive Structure Name | Type | Limit (Gy) | Vol Above Limit (%) | Min (Gy) | Max (Gy) |
|---|---|---|---|---|---|
| Tissue | Basic Tissue | 54.0 | 0 | 0.0 | 54.0 |
| Optic nerve (R) | Basic Structure | 45.0 | 10 | 35.0 | 50.0 |
| Optic nerve (L) | Basic Structure | 45.0 | 10 | 35.0 | 50.0 |
| Lens (R) | Basic Structure | 1.0 | 5 | 0.0 | 1.5 |
| Lens (L) | Basic Structure | 1.0 | 5 | 0.0 | 1.5 |
| Orbit (R) | Basic Structure | 40.0 | 10 | 10.0 | 50.0 |
| Brain Stem | Basic Structure | 45.0 | 10 | 35.0 | 54.0 |
| Orbit (L) | Basic Structure | 40.0 | 10 | 10.0 | 50.0 |
| Optic Chiasm | Basic Structure | 45.0 | 10 | 35.0 | 50.0 |

**Figure 14.** Prescription panel for the acoustic neuroma case.

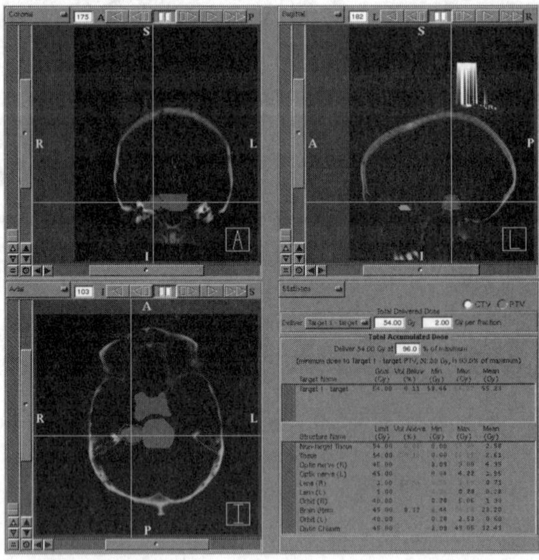

**Figure 15.** Results panel for a two table angle, serial tomotherapy plan showing the 96% isodose line (54 Gy) and statistics for the targets and organs-at-risk.

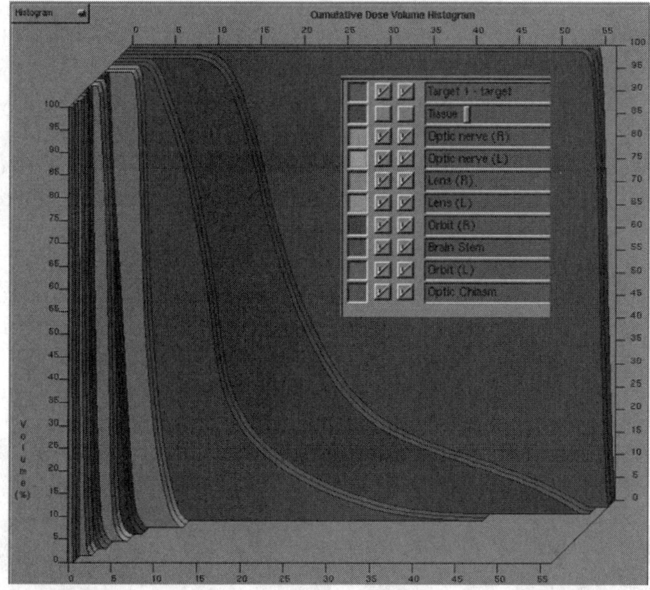

**Figure 16.** Acoustic neuroma dose volume histogram

**Figure 17.** QA report showing the fluence modulation for the first arc, the total number of arcs, and the MU required for each arc delivery.

The second clinical example of the use of serial tomotherapy is for treatment of prostate cancer (Xia et al. 2001; Teh et al. 2002). The patient was immobilized in an thermoplastic cast, and the CTV enlarged uniformly by 5 mm to form the planning target volume (PTV). CT images were used for delineation of the anatomy, as shown in figure 18. The prescription is shown in figure 19. Figures 20–22 show the results in a similar fashion to the first example. The prostate is well treated, with only 5% of the PTV receiving less than the prescription dose. However, the dose heterogeneity is high, resulting in the prostate and seminal vesicle mean doses being over 77 Gy and 69 Gy, respectively. In addition, the MU required to deliver 2 Gy exceed 3800. This very low efficiency in Dose/MU is a result of the low energy (6 MV) used for the treatment and the high modulation required due to the complex fluence pattern. The latter is a function of the planning system, and can be reduced by better optimization and fluence map control. The energy could potentially be raised to 10 MV, which would help to reduce the number of MU required, but cannot be raised further without significantly increasing the whole body dose from neutrons.

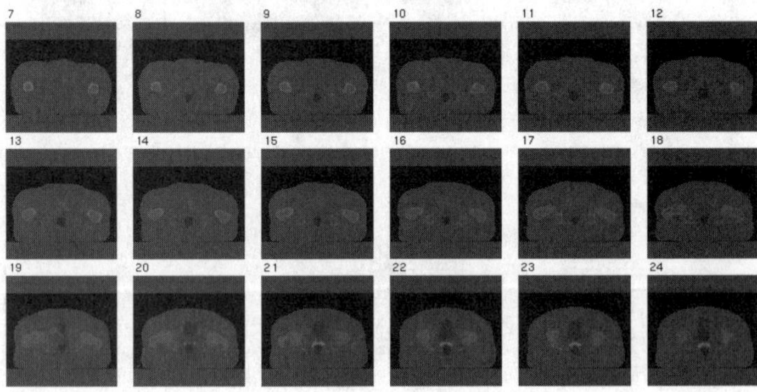

**Figure 18.** Prostate anatomy for case #2, showing delineation of the prostate, seminal vesicles, rectum, bladder, and femoral heads.

| Target Name | Type | Goal Dose (Gy) | Vol Below Goal (%) | Min (Gy) | Max (Gy) |
|---|---|---|---|---|---|
| Target1 - target | Basic | 72.0 | 6 | 69.0 | 78.0 |
| Seminal Vesicles - target | Basic | 60.0 | 20 | 57.0 | 72.0 |

| Sensitive Structure Name | Type | Limit (Gy) | Vol Above Limit (%) | Min (Gy) | Max (Gy) |
|---|---|---|---|---|---|
| Tissue | Basic Tissue | 72.0 | 0 | 0.0 | 72.0 |
| Bladder | Basic Structure | 60.0 | 30 | 30.0 | 72.0 |
| Femoral Heads | Reference | 45.0 | 30 | 30.0 | 50.0 |
| Rectum | Basic Structure | 50.0 | 30 | 30.0 | 72.0 |

**Figure 19.** Prostate prescription, showing prescribed doses to prostate (Target 1), seminal vesicles, and dose limits to non-target tissue, bladder, and rectum.

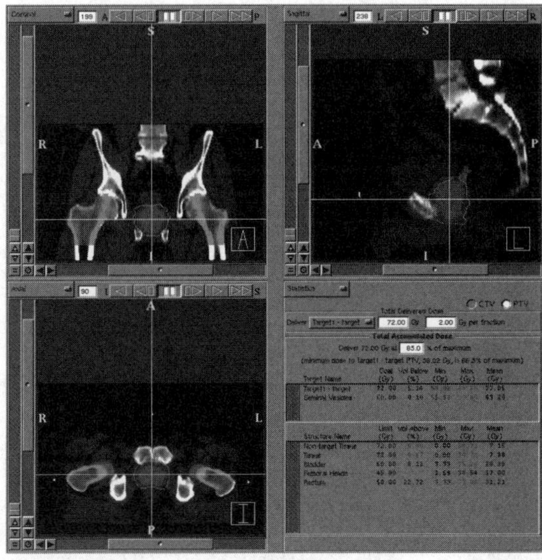

**Figure 20.** Results for prostate plan, showing mean dose to the prostate of 77 Gy and 69 Gy to the seminal vesicles. Although the max dose is higher than requested, the volume of rectum above 50 Gy is less than allowed.

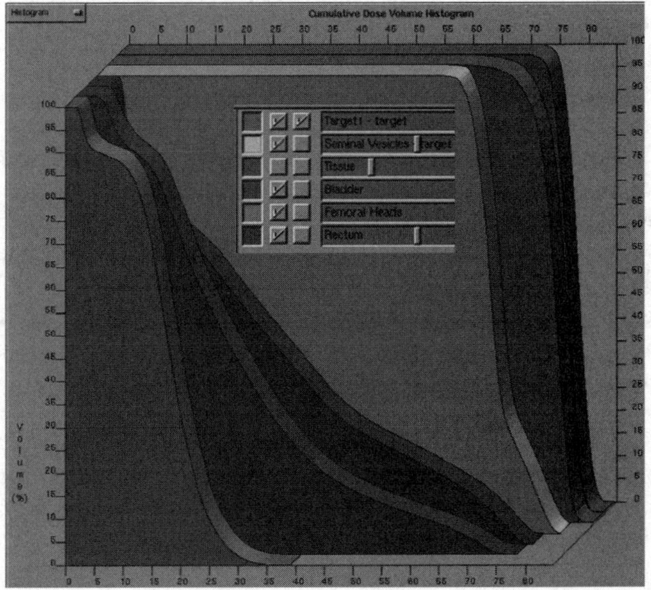


**Figure 21.** Prostate cumulative DVHs.

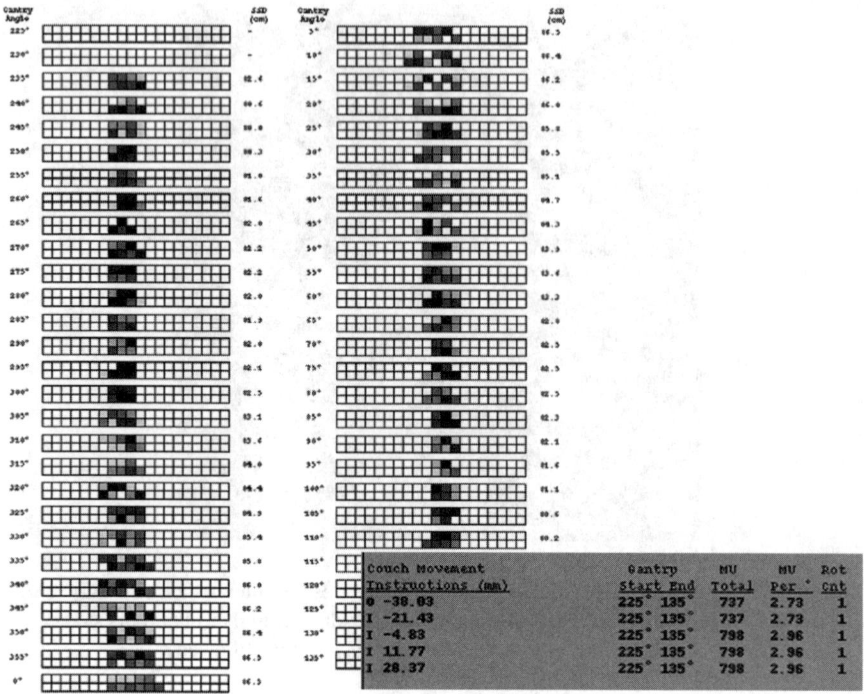

**Figure 22.** Prostate fluence pattern for the first arc and total MU.

## Conclusions

This paper has provided a short history of the development of serial tomotherapy, its clinical application, and some of the advantages and disadvantages regarding its use for IMRT treatments. Since only one commercial implementation of the technique is currently available, that system has been described in detail, from installation to patient treatment and quality assurance. Two clinical examples were given, one showing the advantages of tomotherapy in the treatment of a small lesion in the brain, a second showing some of the disadvantages of the technique in the treatment of a prostate lesion. It should be noted, however, that neither example should be taken as indicative of the overall applicability of serial tomotherapy to that class of lesions. A review of the references will show that serial tomotherapy has been used to significant advantage in the treatment of a wide variety of lesions of the brain, head and neck, thorax, abdomen, pelvis, and the extremeties.

## Acknowledgments

I would like to acknowledge several groups who have contributed to the development of this paper. Ping Xia and her colleagues at UCSF provided a number of images, as did Ron Lalonde and Dan Pavord of the Western Pennsylvania Hospital. Tim Biertempfel and NOMOS Corporation have also provided a number of images. Finally, I thank my former colleagues at NOMOS, with whom I worked for over 7 years, and whose knowledge and assistance over those years has contributed greatly to this work. In particular, Mark Carol, Ned Sternick, Tim Holmes, and Rob Hill, with whom I have spent many long evenings and weekends, have influenced more than a few of the brain cells that still function.

## References

American Association of Physicists in Medicine (AAPM). AAPM Report 54. Stereotactic Radiosurgery. Report of Task Group 42, Radiation Therapy Committee. Woodbury, NY: American Institute of Physics, 1995.

Bourland, J. D., and E. L. Chaney. (1992). "A finite-size pencil beam model for photon dose calculations in three dimensions." *Med. Phys.* 19(6):1401–1412.

Bortfeld, T. R., J. Burkelbach, R. Boesecke, and W. Schlegel. (1990). "Methods of image reconstruction from projections applied to conformation therapy." *Phys. Med. Biol.* 35:1423–1434.

Brahme, A. (1988). "Optimization of stationary and moving beam radiation therapy techniques." *Radiother. Oncol.* 12:129–140.

Carol, M. P. "Integrated 3-D conformal multivane intensity modulation delivery system for radiotherapy" in *XIth International Conference on the Use of Computers in Radiation Therapy*. A. R. Hounsell, J. M. Wilkinson, and P. C. Williams (eds.). Mar 20–24, 1994. Manchester, UK. Manchester: Christie Hospital NHS Trust, pp. 226–227, 1994.

Carol, M. P. (1995). "A system for planning and rotational delivery of intensity-modulated fields." *Int. J. Imaging Sys. Tech.* 6:56–61.

Carol, M. P., W.H. Grant, A. R. Bleier, A. A. Kania, H. Targovnik, B. Butler, and S. Woo (1996). "The field matching problem as it applies to the PEACOCK three dimensional conformal system for intensity modulation." *Int. J. Radiat. Oncol. Biol. Phys.* 34(1):183–187.

Curran, B. H. "Conformal radiation therapy using a multileaf intensity modulation collimator" in *The Theory and Practice of Intensity Modulated Radiation Therapy*. E. S. Sternick (ed.). Madison, WI: Advanced Medical Publishing, pp. 75–90, 1997.

Deng, J., T. Pawlicki, Y. Chen, J. Li, S. B. Jiang, and C.-M. Ma (2001). "The MLC tongue-and-groove effect on IMRT dose distributions." *Phys. Med. Biol.* 46(4):1039–1060.

Followill, D., P. Geis, and A. Boyer. (1997). "Estimates of whole-body dose equivalent produced by beam intensity modulated conformal therapy." *Int. J. Radiat. Oncol. Biol. Phys.* 38(3):667–672.

Fuss, M., B. J. Salter, A. Sadeghi, D. G. Vollmer, J. M. Hevezi, and T. S. Herman (2002). "Fractionated stereotactic intensity-modulated radiotherapy (FS-IMRT) for small acoustic neuromas." *Med. Dosim.* 27(2):147–154.

Holmes, T. W. (1993). A Model for the Physical Optimization of External Beam Therapy. Dept. of Medical Physics, University of Wisconsin, Madison.

Holmes, T. W., A. R. Bleier, M. P. Carol, B. H. Curran, A. A. Kania, R. J. Lalonde, L. S. Larson, and E. S. Sternick. "The Effect of MLC Leakage on the Calculation and Delivery of Intensity Modulated Radiation Therapy" in *XII International Conference on the Use of Computers in Radiation Therapy.* D. Leavitt and G. Starkschall (eds.). May 27–30, 1997, Salt Lake City, Utah. Madison, WI: Medical Physics Publishing, pp. 346–349, 1997.

Kania, A. A., A. R. Bleier, M. P. Carol, B. H. Curran, T. W. Holmes, R. J. Lalonde, L. S. Larson, C. E. Rasmussen, and E. S. Sternick. "Computational Beam Model for Narrow Field Photon Radiation Delivery" in *XII International Conference on the Use of Computers in Radiation Therapy.* D. Leavitt and G. Starkschall (eds.). May 27–30, 1997, Salt Lake City, Utah. Madison, WI: Medical Physics Publishing, pp. 95–98, 1997.

Lam, S., L. Rogers, and B. Wichman. (2001). "Non-coplanar inverse planning IMRT using the MIMiC system: Clinical significance in choice of 2-cm/1-cm mode and single couch vs. multiple couch angles." *Med. Dosim.* 26(1):11–16.

Leybovich, L. B., N. Dogan, A. Sethi, M. J. Krasin, and B. Emami. (2000). "Improvement of tomographic intensity modulated radiotherapy dose distributions using periodic shifting of arc abutment regions." *Med. Phys.* 27(27):1610–1616.

Low, D. A., and S. Mutic. (1997). "Abutment region dosimetry for sequential arc IMRT delivery." *Phys. Med. Biol.* 42:1465–1470.

Low, D. A., K. S. C. Chao, S. Mutic, R. L. Gerber, C. A. Perez, and J. A. Purdy (1998). "Quality assurance of serial tomotherapy for head and neck patient treatments." *Int. J. Radiat. Oncol. Biol. Phys.* 42(3):681–692.

Low, D. A., S. Mutic, J. F. Dempsey, J. Markham, S. M. Goddu, and J. A. Purdy (1999). "Abutment region dosimetry for serial tomotherapy." *Int. J. Radiat. Oncol. Biol. Phys.* 45(1):415–425.

Mackie, T. R., T. W. Holmes, S. Swerdloff, P. Reckwerdt, J. O. Deasy, J. Yang, B. Paliwal, and T. Kinsella. (1993). "Tomotherapy: A new concept for the delivery of conformal radiotherapy using dynamic collimation." *Med. Phys.* 20:1709–1719.

Mackie, T. R., G. Olivera, J. Kapatoes, K. Ruchala, J. Balog, W. Tomé, S. Hui, M. Kissick, C. Wu, R. Jeraj, P. Reckwerdt, P. Harari, M. Ritter, L. Forrest, J. Welsh, and M. Mehta. "Helical Tomotherapy" in *Intensity-Modulated Radiation Therapy: The State of the Art.* T. R. Mackie and J. Palta (eds.). Proceedings of the AAPM 2003 Summer School. Madison, WI: Medical Physics Publishing, pp. ###-###, 2003.

Mutic, S., and D. A. Low. (1998). "Whole-body dose from tomotherapy delivery." *Int. J. Radiat. Oncol. Biol. Phys.* 42(1):229–232.

Nizin, P. S., A. A. Kania, and K. M. Ayyangar. (2001). "Basic concepts of CORVUS dose model." *Med. Dosim.* 26(1):65–70.

Ostapiak, O. Z., Y. Zhu, and J. Van Dyk. (1997). "Refinements of the finite-size pencil beam model of three-dimensional photon dose calculation." *Med. Phys.* 24(5):743–750.

Salter, B. J. (2001). "NOMOS Peacock IMRT utilizing the BEAKa post collimation device." *Med. Dosim.* 26(1):37–46.

Salter, B. J., J. M. Hevezi, A. Sadeghi, and T. S. Herman. (2001a) "An oblique arc capable patient positioning system for sequential tomotherapy." *Med. Phys.* 28(12):2475–2488.

Salter, B. J., M. Fuss, D. G. Vollmer, A. Sadeghi, C. A. Bogaev, D. A. Cheek, T. S. Herman, and J. M. Hevezi. (2001b). "The TALON removable head frame system for stereotactic radiosurgery/radiotherapy: measurement of the repositioning accuracy." *Int. J. Radiat. Oncol. Biol. Phys.* 51(2):555–562.

Saw, C. B., K. M. Ayyangar, W. Zhen, R. B. Thompson, and C. A. Enke. (2001). "Quality assurance procedures for the PEACOCK system." *Med. Dosim.* 26(1):83–90.

Teh, B. S., S. Y. Woo, W.-Y. Mai, J. E. McGary, S. Carpenter, H. H. Lu, J. K. Chiu, M. T. Vlachaki, W. H. Grant III, and E. B. Butler. (2002). "Clinical experience with intensity-modulated radiation therapy (IMRT) for prostate cancer with the use of rectal balloon for prostate immobilization." *Med. Dosim.* 27(2):105–113.

Turner, A. P., and M. J. Wizenberg. "Resource Planning for IMRT" in *The Theory and Practice of Intensity Modulated Radiation Therapy.* E. S. Sternick (ed.). Madison, WI: Advanced Medical Publishing, pp. 229–242, 1997.

Verellen, D., and F. Vanahavere. (1999). "Risk assessment of radiation-induced malignancies based on whole-body equivalent dose estimates for IMRT treatment in the head and neck region." *Radiother. Oncol.* 53(3):199–203.

Wazer, D. E., M. Ling, B. Kramer, J. Wu, M. Engler, J.-S. Tsai, and M. Fagundes. "Clinical Applications of IMRT for Malignant Tumors of the CNS" in *The Theory and Practice of Intensity Modulated Radiation Therapy.* E. S. Sternick (ed.). Madison, WI: Advanced Medical Publishing, pp. 177–194, 1997.

Webb, S. (1997). "Inverse Planning for IMRT: The Role of Simulated Annealing" in *The Theory and Practice of Intensity Modulated Radiation Therapy.* E. S. Sternick (ed.). Madison, WI: Advanced Medical Publishing, pp. 51–74, 1997.

Webb, S. (2003). "Historical Perspective on IMRT" in *Intensity-Modulated Radiation Therapy: The State of the Art.* T. R. Mackie and J. Palta (eds.). Proceedings of the AAPM 2003 Summer School. Madison, WI: Medical Physics Publishing, pp. 1–23, 2003.

Woo, S. Y., M. Sanders, W. Grant, and B. Butler. (1994). "Does the Peacock have anything to do with radiotherapy." *Int. J. Radiat. Oncol. Biol. Phys.* 29:213–214.

Xia, P. (2000). "MIMiC vs MLC IMRT." Presented at the Stanford IMRT Course, Stanford, CA, July, 2000.

Xia, P., K. K. Fu, C. W. Wong, C. Akazawa, and L. J. Verhey. (2000). "Comparison of treatment plans involving intensity-modulated radiotherapy for nasopharyngeal carcinoma." *Int. J. Radiat. Oncol. Biol. Phys.* 48(2):329–337.

Xia, P., B. Pickett, E. Vigneault, L. J. Verhey, and M. Roach 3rd (2001). "Forward or inversely planned segmental multileaf collimator IMRT and sequential tomotherapy to treat dominant intraprostatic lesions of prostate cancer to 90 Gy." *Int. J. Radiat. Oncol. Biol. Phys.* 51(1):244–254.

# Helical Tomotherapy


T. Rockwell Mackie, Ph.D.[1,2,3], Gustavo H. Olivera, Ph.D.[1,3],
Jeffrey M. Kapatoes, Ph.D.[3], Kenneth J. Ruchala, Ph.D.[3],
John P. Balog, Ph.D.[3], Wolfgang A. Tomé, Ph.D.[2], Susanta Hui, Ph.D.[2],
Michael Kissick, Ph.D.[1], Chuan Wu, M.S.[1], Robert Jeraj, Ph.D.[1],
Paul J. Reckwerdt, B.S.[3], Paul Harari, M.D.[2], Mark Ritter, M.D., Ph.D.[2],
Lisa Forrest, V.M.D.[4], James S. Welsh, M.D.[2], and Minesh P. Mehta, M.D.[2]

[1]Medical Physics Department, University of Wisconsin, Madison, Wisconsin
[2]Department of Human Oncology, University of Wisconsin, Madison, Wisconsin
[3]TomoTherapy Inc., Madison, Wisconsin
[4]College of Veterinary Medicine and Surgical Sciences,
University of Wisconsin, Madison, Wisconsin

# Introduction

Tomotherapy literally means "slice therapy." The term was coined to describe the use of an intensity-modulated rotation therapy using a fan beam (Mackie et al. 1993). Serial (or sequential) tomotherapy refers to rotate-then-translate delivery using the fan beam and was the first form of intensity-modulated radiation therapy (IMRT) to treat patients (Carol et al. 1993). The gantry and couch motions are similar to those of a serial (or sequential) computed tomography (CT) scanner. Helical tomotherapy refers to the continuous gantry and couch motion, which from the patient's reference view, describes the helical trajectory of the radiation source. Helical tomotherapy has gantry and couch motions similar to a helical CT scanner. Both forms of tomotherapy utilize binary multileaf collimators (MLCs) that quickly move between the retracted (or open) position and the closed position, which blocks a portion of the slit field. Housed in a continuously rotating ring gantry, the helical tomotherapy unit is the first integrated CT-guided radiotherapy system.

## History Of Helical Tomotherapy

The concept of tomotherapy arose in the late 1980's well before the word "IMRT" was coined, as part of the fulfillment of a one-credit Special Topics course at the University of Wisconsin (UW). Under the supervision of Rock Mackie, Stuart Swerdloff, a doctoral student in nuclear medicine medical physics investigated potential methods to deliver the non-uniform optimized beams of radiation predicted by Anders Brahme (Brahme 1988). The methods investigated included forming a slit beam using the collimator jaws of a conventional linear accelerator (linac), translating it by moving the jaws and then rotating the collimator jaws to form a radon-transform-like delivery of one non-uniform intensity field. This method was abandoned because it would also require conventional field blocking to achieve regions of zero intensity. Another method was to deliver multiple shaped fields that defined the contour lines of equal intensity. This method would be later called "step-and-shoot IMRT" or "static MLC." The method that appealed to Swerdloff and Mackie was to use a slit field and to modulate the slit using a bank of parallel fast-moving collimator leaves, which came to be called a "binary MLC."

Paul Reckwerdt and Tim Holmes joined Mackie's group in 1988 and 1989 respectively and the basic properties of the collimator motion, geometrical configuration of the delivery system, and optimization system were developed. Holmes realized that a CT ring gantry would be ideal for tomotherapy, and with the inclusion of a detector system, it would also give the unit the ability to form CT scans of the patient. However, the idea was nearly abandoned because of a flaw that the group perceived. Multiple rotationally delivered slit fields would require extraordinary precision in the couch translation to avoid severe hot or cold spots along the junction of the fields. In 1991, Mackie was given the task to prepare specifications for a new CT scanner in the UW Radiation Therapy Clinic. In his investigation of CT, he became aware of the new developments in helical CT. It became clear to him that helical delivery would greatly reduce the potential for hot and cold junction artifacts. The first patent was filed in the spring of 1992 and the first talks given shortly thereafter.

At nearly the same time, Medco, a company formed by neurosurgeon Mark Carol began developing the serial tomotherapy concept. Their first presentation was in 1992 (Carol et al. 1993) and their first patient was treated with tomotherapy in 1994. The company changed its name to NOMOS Corporation and received FDA (510k) clearance to market the PEACOCK® IMRT product in 1996. NOMOS licensed the binary MLC patent, which they called the MIMiC®, from the UW's intellectual property agent, the Wisconsin Alumni Research Foundation.

Meanwhile Mackie's group began receiving research support from General Electric Medical System (GEMS) in 1994. This funding support included a benchtop tomotherapy unit employing a GEMS Orion 4 MV linac and the gantry and couch system from a HiSpeed Advantage CT scanner to build a clinical prototype. In 1997, GEMS sold its radiotherapy business to Varian. Mackie and Reckwerdt formed TomoTherapy Inc., to continue development of the clinical helical tomotherapy prototype and to commercialize the concept. The UW unit was completed in 2001 and following a long software integration and validation process, the first human patient was treated at the University of Wisconsin in August 2002 following FDA (510k) clearance.

## Redesign Of Radiotherapy Equipment And Processes For Image-Guided IMRT

Helical tomotherapy is designed for image-guided IMRT (Mackie et al. 1993, 1995, 1999; Yang et al. 1997; Olivera et al. 1999). Intensity-modulated delivery is characterized by high gradients between tumor volumes and sensitive structures (IMRTCWG 2001). In general, the more sensitive the structure is to radiation, the higher the necessary gradient. Small deviations in setup of the patient or internal shifts in the location of the regions of interest within the patient could move the high-dose region out of the target and into the sensitive structure. IMRT requires a higher standard for image guidance than conventional radiotherapy.

Image-guided IMRT is required for conformal avoidance radiotherapy (Mackie et al. 1995, 1999; Aldridge 1999). Conformal avoidance is the complement to conformal radiotherapy, which concentrates on the assured avoidance of sensitive structures. Conformal avoidance is ideal when the target volume is uncertain but the location of sensitive structures is well known. Image-guidance is required in order to verify the avoidance of sensitive structures.

Rotation therapy is relatively insensitive to the energy of the beam (Johns and Cunningham 1983). Before megavoltage beams were developed, rotation therapy was used to deliver x-radiation deep within the body. The lower exit dose of orthovoltage photon beams approximately compensated for the high entrance dose. With the advent of megavoltage beams, rotational delivery fell into disfavor because skin-sparing could be achieved even for single fields of radiation. There has to be a sufficiently high energy to produce reasonable beam intensities. Energies below 6 MV are insufficient. Modulation is achieved with IMRT by using the steep lateral fall-off at the edges of leaves or fields. A high-energy beam has a larger penumbra due to electron transport than a lower energy beam and so the degree of modulation used to avoid normal tissues is diminished. This effect is exaggerated in low-density structures. Shielding becomes heavier and more complex at high energies because the linacs become proportionately longer and there are increased concerns over the production of neutrons. The bremsstrahlung x-ray production probability becomes more and more forward directed at high energies and so it becomes more difficult to treat wider fields. These concerns grow at energies above 10 MV. The first helical tomotherapy unit chose 6 MV because such accelerators were in common usage but the ideal energy is likely around 8 MV. Without a field-flattening filter in place, the 6 MV linac employed is capable of producing over 8 Gy/min at the axis of rotation, which is 85 cm from the source. There is very little rationale for multiple treatment energies for rotational IMRT.

The CT scanner is the most important type of imaging system for radiation therapy (Mackie 1995). CT-simulators are nearly ubiquitous in medium-sized and larger clinics. Having a CT scanner in the treatment room or on the treatment unit confirms that the treatment is set up according to the treatment plan. Helical tomotherapy was designed around the ring gantry of a helical CT scanner, because the slip-ring technology for passing power on board a continuously rotating gantry was already developed and the need for non-coplanar radiation fields is greatly diminished for IMRT delivery.

A CT scanner can accommodate the weight of the shielding required if the linac is compact and the field sizes are limited. Most importantly, a CT gantry is the ideal platform from which to obtain CT scans because the gantry is mechanically rigid enough to not require corrections for beam misalignment. Misalignment corrections must be made to the detector signal if the shifts are a significant fraction of the detector size (Jaffray et al. 1999). For example, when viewing a high contrast boundary, a 1% lateral shift in the detector position will masquerade as a 1% change in the contrast of the boundary. CT detector systems placed on linacs, which have isocentric stabilities on the order of 0.5 mm, will require significant corrections if their detectors have pixel dimensions of 5 mm and smaller. The corrections will not typically eliminate all the blurring and artifacts that misalignment motion will cause.

The CT capability on the UW Tomotherapy unit uses the linac as the source of radiation. The imaging quality is comparable with an older generation of CT scanners and, for example, enables such structures as the prostate and tumors in the lung to be visualized (see figures 18 and 21).

The software processes of helical tomotherapy are designed around its CT capability. Image fusion of the CT scan acquired before treatment with the planning CT is a way of determining the offset of the patient on a daily basis. It also enables postprocessing such as dose reconstruction, which determines the dose delivered with respect to the patient's CT scan acquired at the time of treatment. This, in turn, enables adaptive radiotherapy that alters the daily regimen to take account for delivery variation from day-to-day (Yan and Wong 1997; Wu 2002).

Figure 1 is a photograph of the helical tomotherapy unit now installed at M.D. Anderson Cancer Center-Orlando.

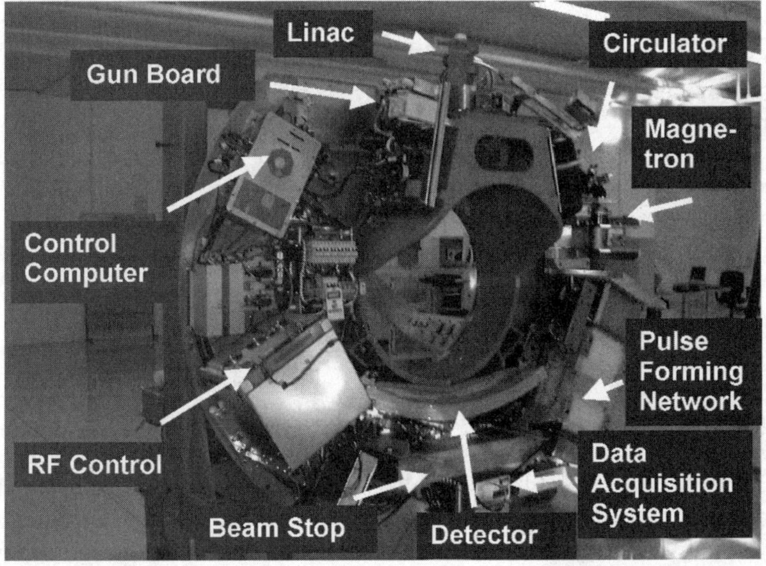


**Figure 1.** Photograph of a helical tomotherapy unit with components labeled. This unit is installed at the M.D. Anderson-Orlando clinic in Orlando, FL, and represents an improvement in the manufacturability and serviceability as compared to the UW prototype unit; however, the linac, jaw system, MLC, and detector system are nearly identical to the UW unit.

## Basic Principles Of Tomotherapy Beam Delivery

Tomotherapy is designed for IMRT delivery. Conventional irradiation techniques involving shaping the boundary of fixed fields cannot be delivered with tomotherapy.

There are a few ways in which the dose rate to the patient can be varied. The linac output can be varied, the jaw opening can be changed, the gantry speed can be altered, the couch speed can be modified, and the leaf states can be changed. It is impractical, due to its inertia, to change the gantry speed dynamically. The control software is built around a state file that specifies the linac output, couch speed, jaw positions, and on-off state of every leaf at few millisecond intervals. In the future any of these parameters could be changed during treatment, but today we have chosen to use the MLC as the only source of treatment modulation in real time.

## Intensity-Modulated Fan Beam Delivery

In a helical tomotherapy unit, an independent jaw pair integrated into the primary colli-mator of the machine forms the fan beam. This "clam-shell" design maximizes the shielding while maintaining compactness. The primary collimator and jaws are fabri-cated from an alloy containing 95% tungsten. In the forward direction, the thickness of the clamshell is about 22 cm, which reduces the leakage for IMRT with high numbers of monitor units to values typical for conventional delivery with conventional monitor units.

The jaws may be moved continuously between being completely closed or opened up to produce a 5 cm wide fan beam at the axis of the unit. Typical treatment fan beam opening widths are from 1 cm to 5 cm although field widths less than 1 cm could be used for very small target volumes. The CT scan jaw opening used up to now has been a width of 5 cm at the axis.

## Binary Multileaf Collimator (MLC) System

The tomotherapy system uses an MLC with 64 binary leaves. The motive power is compressed air. The interleaved design has the 32 even-numbered leaves powered from a piston block on one side of the assembly and the odd leaves powered by an identi-cal piston block from the other side. The valves are attached to the piston blocks with the air couplings utilizing carved channels in the piston block. This design minimizes the air volume between the valves and the pistons so that the latency to open or close the leaves is as short as possible. At 70 psi, the leaves cross over the field width in about 20 ms. The time it takes a relay to respond, a valve to open and for air to build up behind the piston takes about another 25 ms for a total leaf latency of about 50 ms. See figure 2. This is significantly faster than the NOMOS MIMiC binary collimator (see the chapter by Curran, *IMRT Delivery Using Serial Tomotherapy*). This latency is accounted for in the control system.

At the axis of rotation, the leaf thickness is 0.625 cm and the leaf height is 10 cm of 95% tungsten. The leaves have a tongue-and-groove design that results in an inter-leaf leakage less than 0.5% of its open intensity, which makes it the best-shielded radiotherapy unit used for IMRT.

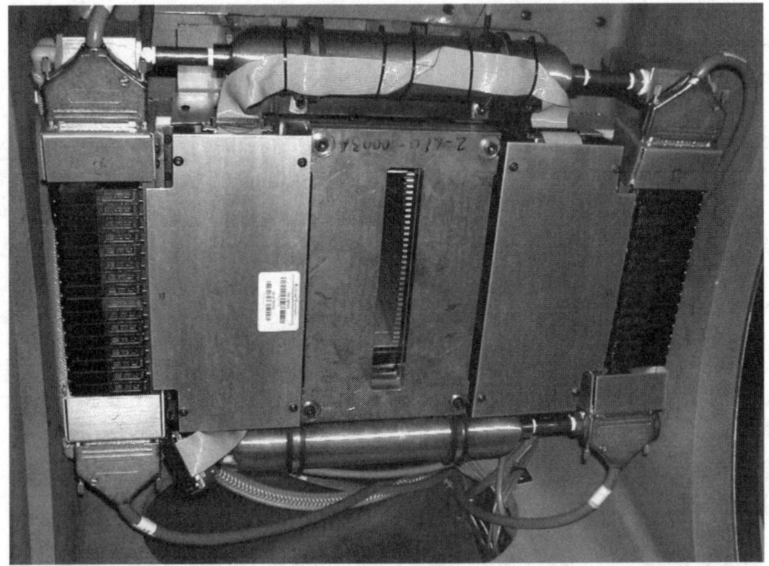

**Figure 2.** Photograph of the helical tomotherapy binary collimator mounted on the helical tomotherapy unit. One bank of leaves is visible. Sixteen of sixty-four valves are visible on both the left and right. Local high-pressure air reservoirs are visible above and below.

The modulation for a binary collimator is achieved by varying the leaf opening time. Each leaf is under independent control and currently we use the same method as serial tomotherapy (see the chapter herein by Curran). At the beginning and end of a projection all the leaves are closed. A full rotation is typically divided into 51 projections. A rotation period of 28 s, would mean that each projection lasts about 450 ms. If the intensity of a projection for a leaf is maximum, the leaf is commanded to open at the beginning of the projection and is commanded to close at a time equal to the total latency before the end so that it closes when the projection is over. For the minimum intensity the leaf is commanded to open at a time equal to the total latency before the half time of the interval and commanded to close at the half time. Assuming that half of the leaf movement time is considered open, if the latency is 50 ms and the projection lasts 450 ms, the minimum open time is about 10% and the maximum open time is about 90% of the projection time. Any continuous opening time between the minimum open and maximum open is valid. Of course not opening the leaf at all (i.e., a zero value) in the interval is also valid.

## Coplanar Delivery

The tomotherapy couch does not rotate; therefore, helical tomotherapy delivers beams in a coplanar fashion. In general, for treatments to the head and neck and below, coplanar delivery minimizes the integral dose because non-coplanar beams would typically have a longer pathlength through the body. In treatment of brain tumors, non-coplanar fields are sometimes useful, however the fields become difficult or even impossible to verify radiographically as the angle approaches the patient's zenith.

In general, there is so much more to be gained in adopting IMRT delivery than can be gained in using non-coplanar beam directions, that non-coplanar delivery is usually an unnecessary complication for extracranial sites. Another advantage of coplanar delivery is the simplicity of the trajectories used for treatment planning raytracing. It is possible to calculate and store the raytrace trajectories through the treatment geometry and greatly speed up raytracing. This is more difficult to do for non-coplanar trajectories.

The bore (opening through which the patient enters the unit) is 85 cm in diameter and so is large enough to accommodate a head support system to allow limited non-coplanar delivery for brain tumors for which non-coplanar delivery may truly be beneficial.

## Serial Vs. Helical Tomotherapy

Serial tomotherapy delivers the radiation with the couch stationary. Following each rotation the couch is carefully indexed so that the field junctions are precise. Imprecision results in hot spots when the couch is not moved far enough and cold spots if the couch is moved too much. In helical tomotherapy, the couch and gantry are moved continuously. The field boundary junction is continuously blurred together eliminating the possibility of severe hot and cold spots. Figure 3 illustrates film irradiated by serial and helical tomotherapy. There are reduced hot and cold spots in the field from helical delivery as compared to serial delivery. There is a small thread artifact in evidence that will be discussed in the section helical *Pitch And the Thread Artifact*.

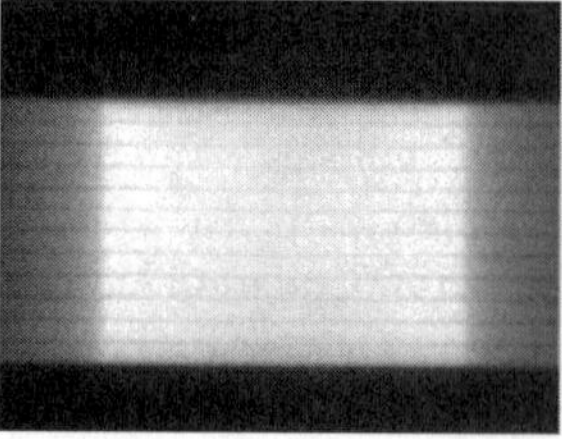

**Figure 3.** Film images of multiple serial fields and helical delivery. The left panel is a film image along the center of a cylindrical phantom following the delivery of 12 fan beams, each 1 cm wide junctioned together perfectly. The center is a film image from the same 12 fields junctioned together with a 0.2 mm gap. There is a sharp dose deficit between each of the fields. The right image is a film exposed to 26 helical rotations with a pitch of 0.5 (meaning that each field is 50% overlapping the prior and subsequent rotation).

One further problem with serial delivery is that the coverage in the longitudinal direction (the direction of couch motion) must be an integer multiple of the fan beam width. In helical delivery, the field coverage can be any length.

Unmodulated helical delivery produces a ramp function at the longitudinal edges of the field. This can be an advantage and a disadvantage. It is a disadvantage because the fall-off in the dose is slower than conventional radiotherapy along the longitudinal periphery of the field. This tends not to be a problem when there is sufficient beam overlap (i.e., small helical pitch) so that the ramp fall-off can be replaced by a steeper fall-off. A technique called a "running start and stop" can also eliminate the ramp function fall-off but this requires a careful synchronization of independent jaws during the delivery (Mackie et al. 1993). Modulated helical delivery can reduce somewhat the longitudinal penumbra. A ramp-like field junction can be an advantage if fields have to be junctioned. For example, the UW tomotherapy unit can irradiate up to a 160 cm long field. If a tall patient were to have his whole body irradiated, this could be done in two long helical fields that are junctioned by a nearly linear ramp up and ramp down so that positioning errors are reduced.

## Beam Characteristics Without A Field-Flattening Filter

There is no need for a field-flattening filter when the machine is designed for IMRT. The tomotherapy unit has instead a set of uniform thickness filters before and after the monitor chamber to provide buildup to the monitor chamber, to shield the monitor chamber from the jaws, and to remove extremely low-energy photons.

In the unlikely event that the optimizer selects a uniform energy fluence distribution to deliver, it is possible to modulate the distribution to be uniform. The absence of a field-flattening filter has many advantages. The energy fluence change is almost linearly decreasing as a function of distance from the center of the field. The rate of fall-off at a plane through the machine axis is about 2.5% to 3% per cm so that by the edge of the field (20 cm from the central axis) the output is 40% to 50% of its value at the center of the beam. The intensity variation leaf-to-leaf is about 2%, but this small discretization cannot be discerned dosimetrically.

The major advantage of a lack of a field-flattening filter is the beam quality. The thin set of filters produces far less head scatter than a conventional linac equipped with a field-flattening filter. This also improves the imaging characteristics of the beam. The energy spectrum at the center of the field is not significantly harder than the spectrum at the edge of the field. This means that the beam is easier to characterize with model-based dose calculation systems. See figure 4.

Of secondary importance is that the beam output is not wasted by the use of a field-flattening filter. Smaller fields can take advantage of the higher output offered by not having such a filter.

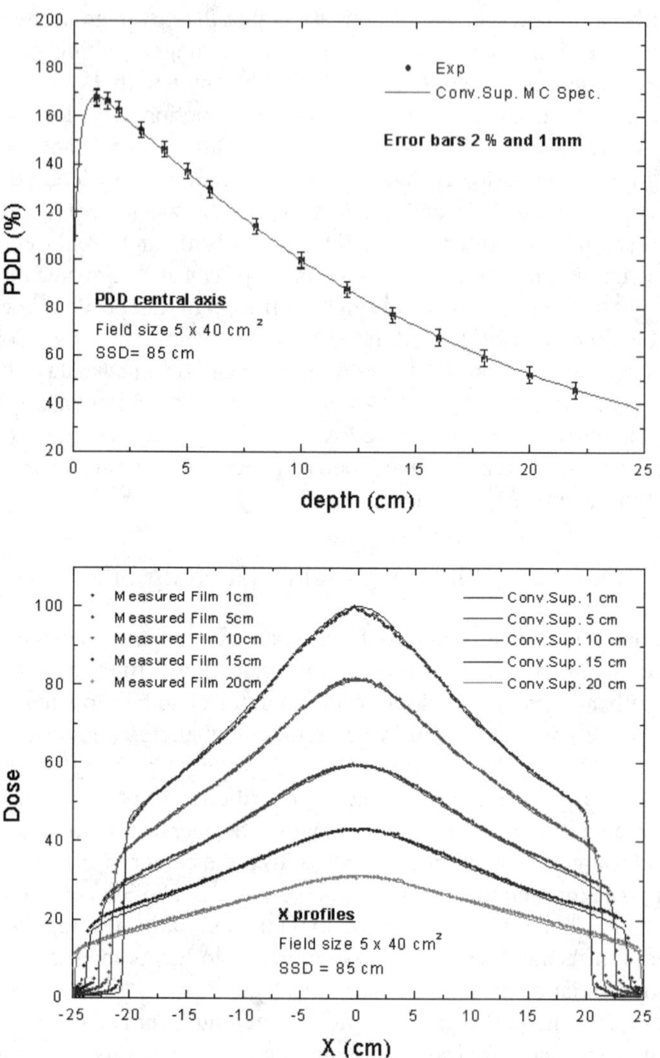



**Figure 4.** Measured and convolution/superposition computation depth-dose and lateral profiles for the UW Tomotherapy Unit. The triangular shape of the lateral dose profile is because there is no field-flattening filter used in the unit.

## Dependence Of Number of Beam Directions And Leaf Resolution

One notable characteristic of tomotherapy is that beams are issuing from many more directions than in conventional radiotherapy. Pirzkall found that rotational IMRT was slightly superior to fixed-field IMRT for complex-shaped targets (Pirzkall et al. 2000). If there are no considerations for normal tissues nearby the target volume, there is little need for multiple beam directions or even for modulation. Indeed, a uniform parallel-opposed pair of beams will often suffice as long as the normal tissue will not be harmed by the amount of radiation necessary to eradicate the tumor. Making these two fields intensity-modulated is a way to make the field flat at any depth. Adding more fields allows the entrance and exit doses to fall and the target volume to remain homogeneous. Having the fields non-opposed effectively increases the number of beams from having them opposed. For example, three fields or five fields are often better than two or three pairs of parallel-opposed fields, respectively. When there are enough fields, the choice of the field directions becomes inconsequential. Any reasonable odd number of directions equally distributed in angle will usually suffice. As the field boundaries overlap at the edge of the patient, there is negligible further reduction in the entrance or exit dose. For larger field sizes this overlap will happen with a smaller number of beam directions. For a cylindrical patient of diameter $d$ with a tumor volume of diameter $w$, overlap will approximately occur when the number of equally distributed fields $n$ is given by:

$$n = \pi d/w \, . \tag{1}$$

For a 30 cm diameter patient and a 10 cm diameter tumor, overlap will occur when the number of fields is greater than about 9. For a 5 cm tumor, the overlap will occur only when the number of fields is greater than 18.

The situation is more complicated when there are avoidance structures in or near the target volume. For example, first imagine a nine-field *non-IMRT* plan irradiating a target volume with an avoidance structure within it. If no beams were to pass through the sensitive structure, there would be a streak artifact produced from the deficit of energy fluence otherwise irradiating the avoidance structure. The deficit of dose would be greatest near the sensitive structure as several beams are occluded. Near the tumor boundary the deficit of dose would fall to 1/9 or about 10%. To reduce the deficit to 5% would require more than 18 fields or raising the energy fluence through the sensitive structure from zero to over 50%. For 51 beams the deficit in dose to the tumor would be under 3% with no increase in energy fluence through the sensitive structure.

It is possible to do something about the streak artifacts using IMRT other than allowing energy fluence through the sensitive structures. The optimizer views the streak artifacts as regions in which to increase the beam intensity using beams other than the occluded ones. However, close to the avoidance structure there is more than one beam being occluded. Indeed, next to the avoidance structure only beams traveling parallel to the boundary of the avoidance structure are not occluded. When there are only a few fields to modulate, a characteristic rosette pattern of inhomogeneous dose is formed around the avoidance structure. Using the nine-field example, within the target volume next to the avoidance structure, one beam has to supply nine times greater intensity. In turn, this will lead to an even more severe streak if there are not sufficient numbers of beams. Having more beams will repair the streak artifact until the projections of the avoidance occlusions at the tumor boundary overlap. In general, if the cylindrical avoidance structure has a diameter of $a$, at the center of a cylindrical tumor of diameter $w$, there is no further improvement in the dose homogeneity when the number of fields is larger than $n$, where $n$ is given by a formula similar in form to equation (1):

$$n = \pi w / a \ . \tag{2}$$

A 10 cm tumor diameter and a 2 cm avoidance structure will require 15 beams to produce dose homogeneity with maximum avoidance of sensitive structures. A 1 cm avoidance structure will require 30 beams. Having 51 beams will allow a 40 cm diameter target volume to be homogeneously treated with a 2.5 cm avoidance structure.

A fundamental radiobiological question arises when the number of beam directions increases. For the same amount of energy imparted (or integral dose deposited), is it really better to give a small dose to a large amount of normal tissue than a large amount to a small amount of normal tissue? Clearly, for serial structures this is true. For parallel structures the situation is unclear. The classical Lyman model (Lyman 1985) says that a little to a lot has the same consequence as a lot to a little so long as the integral dose is invariant. Radiobiological models with a threshold, such as that proposed by Niemierko (Niemierko and Goitein 1993), would favor high doses to a small volume for structures like lung and liver when the damage to a small part of the organ will not affect the performance of a whole. Obviously, surgeons employ this paradigm as well, but radiotherapy is often the only option when the patient cannot tolerate surgery. In any case, the use of a large number of directions is a different question than the opportunity to use a large number of directions if that is beneficial. In tomotherapy, it is entirely possible to have zero intensity for many of the beam directions.

As the collimator resolution gets finer, the amount of conformity of the target volume improves. Having a finer leaf resolution will allow finer structures to be avoided but as equation (2) shows, this will not be effective unless the finer resolution is accompanied by having more beam directions. It can be shown that halving the leaf size will achieve its increased ability to modulate only if the number of directions is doubled or if used with half the target volume size.

There are diminishing returns once the collimator resolution approaches the characteristic blurring size due to the finite source size and the lateral range of electrons set in motion, which increases in low-density tissue and for high-energy beams. There seems to be very little improvement in conformity for collimator sizes less than 4 mm. Figure 5 is a planning example with a variety of collimator sizes and beam directions, with an accompanying table.

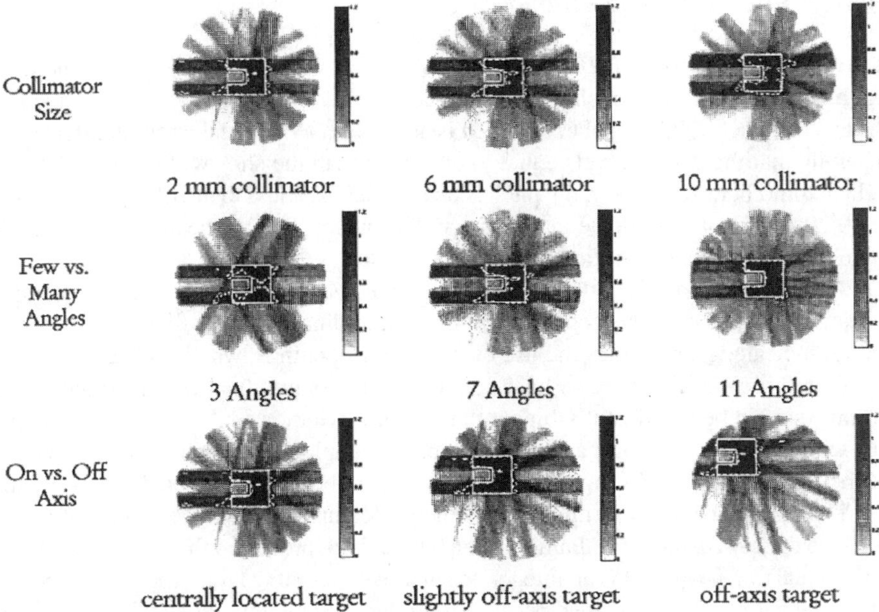



**Figure 5.** Planning example with a variety of collimator sizes and beam directions with accompanying table. A C-shaped target volume surrounds a square avoidance region on three sides. Unless otherwise noted, the plan uses seven beam directions, a collimator with a resolution of 6 mm, and is for a centrally located target volume. The resolution of a 6 mm collimator is not appreciably inferior to a 2 mm collimator; however, it is improved as compared to a 1 cm collimator. The dose homogeneity and normal tissue avoidance continues to improve with an increase in the number of beam directions. There is no need to locate the target at the center of the beam delivery axis. It is interesting to note that the integral dose (i.e., energy imparted) is nearly independent on the technique used to irradiate the tumor. [Reprinted from *Medical Physics,* vol 26, "A simple model for examining issues in radiotherapy optimization," D. M. Shepard, G. Olivera, L. Angelos, O. Sauer, P. Reckwerdt, and T. R. Mackie, pp. 1212–1221. © 1999 with permission from AAPM.]

| Number of Beam Directions | Objective Function Value | Standard Deviation In the Target Dose | Minimum Dose Covering 90% of the Target (1.0 = Max) | Mean Dose To the Region At Risk | Total Integral Dose |
|---|---|---|---|---|---|
| 3 | 0.665 | 0.124 | 0.747 | 0.488 | 2733 |
| 5 | 0.318 | 0.090 | 0.814 | 0.215 | 2564 |
| 7 | 0.242 | 0.064 | 0.867 | 0.206 | 2597 |
| 9 | 0.222 | 0.064 | 0.855 | 0.192 | 2599 |
| 11 | 0.202 | 0.058 | 0.879 | 0.186 | 2570 |
| 15 | 0.187 | 0.053 | 0.908 | 0.180 | 2542 |
| 21 | 0.176 | 0.049 | 0.912 | 0.171 | 2545 |
| 33 | 0.151 | 0.038 | 0.933 | 0.155 | 2544 |

## Helical Pitch And The Thread Artifact

The concept of pitch (actually the pitch ratio) is a key concept in helical tomotherapy. Pitch is the ratio of the couch travel distance per rotation to the field size defined at the axis. In a helical CT scanner the pitch is usually set to be equal or greater than one, meaning that the couch travels equal to or farther than the slice width. Contrarily, in helical tomotherapy delivery, the pitch is usually set to be less than 1/2. Typical values are 0.20 to 0.5 for a single helical delivery. This means that the beam irradiates each voxel throughout several rotations.

A pitch less than 1/2, with a voxel being irradiated during more than one rotation, effectively produces a finer resolution in the longitudinal direction than the jaw width would indicate. This enables the use of wider jaw openings, which makes the delivery more efficient although we have found that the longitudinal length of the target volume should be significantly bigger than the jaw width used. Note that axial delivery with tomotherapy using a single rotation is technically feasible when the length of the target volume is 5 cm or less, but this has not been implemented at this point.

The thread artifact is an unusual dosimetric feature of helical delivery that arises because of beam divergence. Parallel beams would not produce a thread artifact at any pitch equal to $1/n$ where $n$ is an integer because every point would sample every possible angle n times. It is so named because it produces a small modulation at the helical field boundary that resembles the thread on a bolt. It is most prominent outside the field, but it is in evidence even inside the field for larger irradiation diameters. The amplitude of the modulation increases with increased distance from the central axis, for larger field widths and for larger pitches. In a realistic diverging beam case, one might still expect the thread artifact magnitude to still be smallest when the pitch is close to $1/n$. However, with axial beam divergence, the function becomes complicated as the overlaps and gaps of beam edges at certain pitches can produce minima and maxima at unexpected pitches. The beam shape and degree of axial divergence are the most significant factors that determine the magnitude of this delivery artifact for pitches less than or close to 1. There is no thread artifact at the axis of rotation and it increases approximately linearly with radius from the central axis. The thread artifact is most prominent when the delivery is unmodulated. For a typical pitch of 0.2, 10 cm from the center of the field the amplitude of the thread modulation is on the order of $\pm 1\%$ when a 20 cm diameter cylindrical field is irradiated. When two helical deliveries are used, each starting 180 gantry degrees out of phase, the thread artifact nearly vanishes. Multiple helical deliveries each starting at a different gantry angle may employ higher pitches. Multiple loose helical pitches (with pitches as high as 3) with dephased started angles should be useful for lung irradiation (see the section herein *Lung Cancer*).

The pitch artifact is not always in evidence for intensity-modulated delivery in complicated irradiation volumes. With a modicum of care the pitch artifact is clinically inconsequential. Figure 6 demonstrates calculation of dose in a cylindrical phantom.

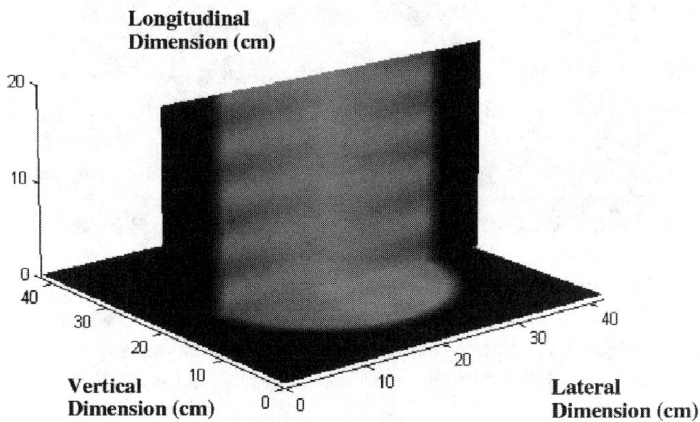


**Figure 6.** Calculation of the dose in a cylindrical phantom for a pitch of two. For single helical delivery, pitches less than 0.5 are recommended and pitches of 0.2 to 0.5 are typical. The calculated fan beam was uniform in intensity.

## Commissioning And Quality Assurance

The goals and principles of commissioning and quality assurance (QA) are the same for helical tomotherapy as for any other type of radiotherapy treatment unit in particular or medical device in general. The goal is to ensure that the unit is safe and is being operated so that it is as effective as possible. There are some aspects of tomotherapy that are quite novel and these will be emphasized. Many of the procedures derive from having an on-line sealed multiple channel ionization CT detector that is capable of independently detecting every linac pulse.

## Alignment Tests

The primary collimator has a narrower aperture than most linacs because it has been designed to produce a fan beam. The position of the linac in the longitudinal direction (couch movement direction) is therefore the most sensitive to misalignment.

If the linac is shifted longitudinally, the fully open aperture will be directed into or away from the rotation plane. If the shift is large it will also affect the output of the linac because part of the source will be occluded. Placing a film at a large distance from the source and shooting beams from opposed directions through the film can detect longitudinal misalignment. The nearer beam will have a smaller image on the film. The misalignment on the beams will be easily evident as a shift in the centers of the beam images. The results of one such test are shown in figure 7. A small misalignment that does not appreciably modify beam output can be compensated for by an offset in the position of the independent jaws. A twist in the face of the jaws can be detected with the same alignment procedure as used to detect the linac misalignment and shimmed to eliminate the twist.

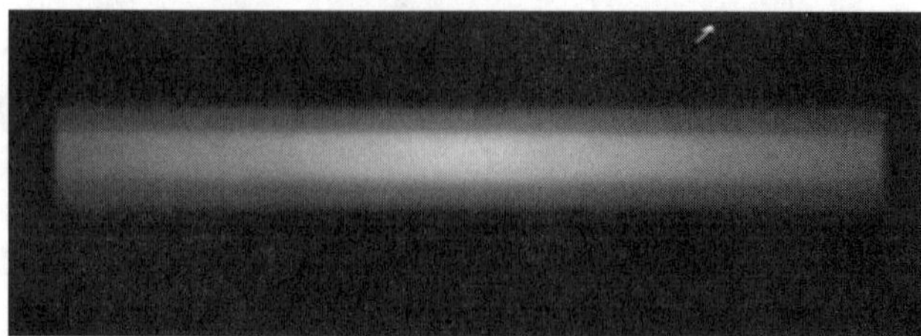

**Figure 7.** Film images of longitudinal alignment test. The narrower irradiation, which is nearer to the source, is bisecting the larger irradiation, which is farther from the source. This indicates that the source is aligned along the rotation plane defined by the fixed collimation system.

The MLC is pinned to the primary collimator and jaw assembly with no lateral adjustments. Therefore, the linac must be aligned to the MLC, not the other way around. A lateral misalignment of the linac can be detected with great precision using the binary MLC. A sequence of leaf motions is executed which maximizes the tongue-and-groove effect. First, all the odd leaves are open; they are then closed and all the even leaves are opened. Radiographic films or the CT detector signals acquired during the odd and then even deliveries are normalized to a delivery with all the leaves open. This reveals an image of the location of the tongue-and-groove positions projected onto the detector. When the linac is aligned the magnitude of the tongue and groove is approximately uniform. A small misalignment of the linac in the lateral direction can be accommodated in software by having an asymmetric beam penumbra and a leaf-dependent tongue-and-groove correction. An example of this measurement using film is shown in figure 8.

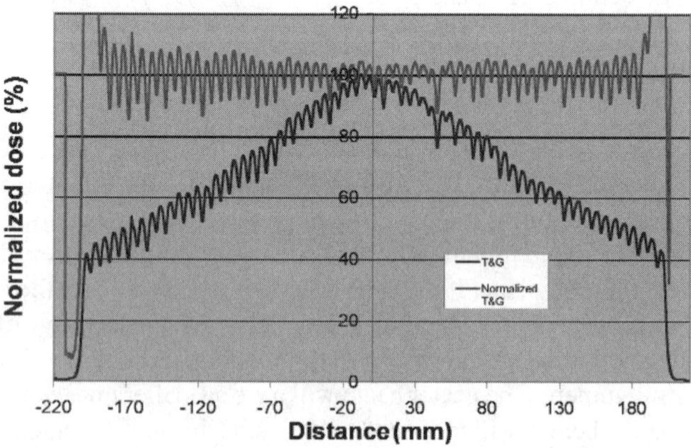


**Figure 8.** Use of the tongue-and-groove (T&G) effect to determine the lateral alignment. The result here indicates that the source is slightly on the positive side. This measurement was obtained using film, however, the on-board detector system can also be used to make this measurement. This degree of misalignment indicated by this test is small and can easily be accommodated in software.

## Beam Measurements

The dosimetry of helical tomotherapy has more similarities than dissimilarities to conventional radiotherapy. The beam can be delivered when the gantry and couch are static. This allows an unmodulated beam to be measured using a water or water-equivalent phantom. The largest field that can be delivered this way has a 5 cm width and a 40 cm length. Depth-dose curves for such fields are very comparable to a conventional linac beam. Lateral profiles reveal the triangle distribution of a beam that has not been flattened (see figure 4). As stated earlier, it is possible to modulate the beam so that it is uniform in intensity at a specific depth.

Cylindrical geometry is the most natural for a tomotherapy phantom. A 30 cm diameter × 18 cm long phantom has been developed for beam commissioning and for routine quality assurance (see figure 9). The phantom is split in half so that a radiographic film may be irradiated in the coronal or sagittal plane. Its shape is similar in size and shape to that of a cheddar cheese round so it has been dubbed the "cheese phantom." Small ion chambers may be placed along a line at several positions away from the axis of the phantom so that the film measurements can be supplemented with ionometry.

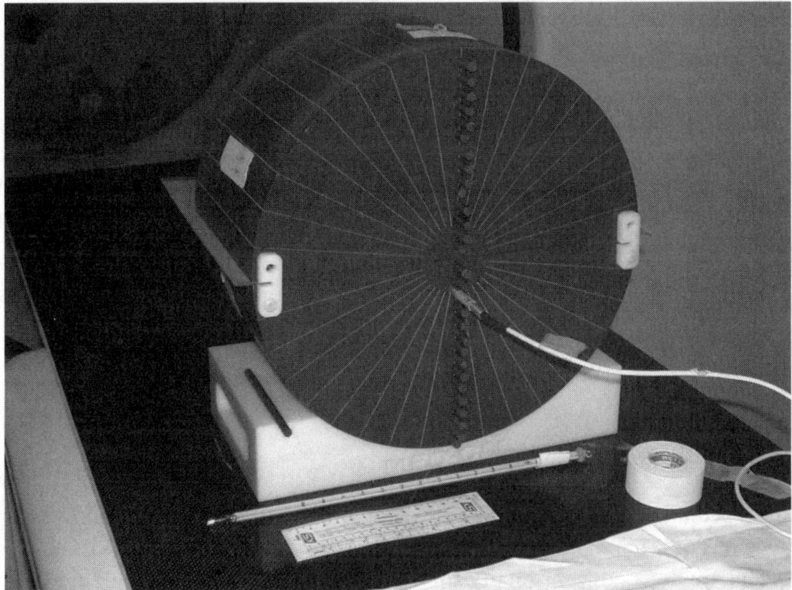

**Figure 9.** Photograph of the water-equivalent 30 cm diameter "cheese" phantom. A radiographic film is placed between two half cylinders. There are 29 holes spaced 1 to 1.5 cm apart drilled perpendicularly to the film plane. One or more ion chambers can be placed in the holes. Unused holes are plugged with water-equivalent rods.

Helical commissioning measurements are obtained using the "cheese" phantom. At the central axis of the phantom the dose distribution in the longitudinal direction for a single helical rotation is a convolution of a rectangle function describing the translation of the couch with a single static field to yield a characteristic triangular functional form. Two helical rotations join the distributions at the 50% point at the linear fall-off point to yield a nearly uniform field where they overlap.

Besides helical delivery of the beam, it is possible to deliver the beam with the couch fixed and the gantry rotating or with gantry fixed and the couch translating. The former is called "axial delivery" and the later is called "topotherapy." Axial delivery produces dose distributions identical to serial tomotherapy and is useful for QA confirmation of the treatment planning system. If the output of the accelerator is independent of angle, the axially delivered dose as measured at the center of a cylindrical phantom should also be invariant with gantry angle. Topotherapy delivery can be used to produce a field that is 40 cm wide by more than a meter long. An interesting feature of a topotherapy field is that, instead of inverse-square fall-off with depth, the fall-off is only inversely proportional to depth. When topotherapy is delivered to a cylindrical phantom, the dose distribution along the central axis is identical to a helically delivered plan. Topotherapy can be thought of as helical tomotherapy with an infinite pitch.

## Beam Calibration

The tomotherapy unit cannot produce a static 10 cm × 10 cm field at 100 cm from the source traditionally used to calibrate a conventional radiotherapy unit. The absorbed dose protocols were modified to calibrate the tomotherapy beam for a field size of 5 cm × 10 cm at 85 cm from the source. Monte Carlo simulation reveals that the stopping power ratio was unchanged from the values in AAPM Task Group 51. The TG-51 parameter $k_Q$ is approximately 0.995 to 0.998 depending on the ion chamber. The dose rate at the central axis with buildup for a 5 cm wide by 10 cm long field is currently set to a value of 8.5 Gy/min, which is slightly higher than the design specification of 8 Gy/min.

## Routine Quality Assurance

Running specialized imaging and treatment procedures performs routine quality assurance tests for a helical tomotherapy unit. Many of these procedures are similar to tests that are done conventionally such as directing static beams with normal incidence into a plastic phantom to determine beam output and to spot-check the change in dose with depth.

Some of the unconventional tests include using the intrinsic pulse-by-pulse detector system. One such test is running the unit without a phantom and letting the sealed detector system capture the beam as a function of angle. This can be normalized to the same procedure run previously. This reveals if the beam output is varying or whether there is significant change in the angular dependence of the output. For example, the UW tomotherapy system has the air compressor system on board and vibration from this system can affect the automatic frequency control as a function of angle if the vibration is not sufficiently damped (the next generation of tomotherapy units do not have an on-board air compressor). The mechanical axis of the unit is determined using the CT scan capability of the system. A high-contrast object such as a tungsten rod or an aluminum annulus is placed on the laser-indicated axis. A CT scan can determine the position of the circular-symmetric object with respect to the axis of rotation with an accuracy of about 0.5 mm. The leaf opening time is determined continuously by optical switches monitored by a computer on the rotating side of the gantry. This leaf verification can be checked using the detector signal to monitor the leaf opening dosimetrically.

## Patient-Specific Dosimetry Quality Assurance

The tomotherapy unit has been designed to accommodate the process of dose reconstruction (see the section herein *Dose Reconstruction*), which produces the dose actually delivered superimposed on the CT scan acquired at the time of delivery. Dose reconstruction is not yet released for clinical use so the dose verification has been performed for all the UW patients using the same "cheese" phantom shown in figure 9. A radiographic film can be placed in the film along a plane parallel to the axis of rotation. This orientation limits the number of rays that travel along the film plane, thereby limiting this type of artifact. Holes drilled into the phantom allow one or more small ion chambers to be placed in the phantom to get the absolute dose delivered to the phantom. Tissue-equivalent plastic rods are placed in all the holes when not penetrated by an ion chamber. The results from one such test are shown on figure 17.

When appropriate, several of our patients have also had thermoluminescent dosimeter (TLD) verification performed. On humans this has been with half-cylinder buildup caps over the TLDs. In sinus tumors in dogs (one of our research protocols is treating sinus tumors in client dogs from the UW Veterinary Radiotherapy program) we put TLDs encased in a tube in the dog's mouth. With a verification CT it is possible to visualize the exact position of the TLDs. The TLD results have been far less accurate than the phantom-based dosimetry because they are usually placed in high-dose gradients.

## Treatment Planning

The treatment planning system is specialized for the helical tomotherapy geometry and delivery methodology but the process of planning is nearly the same as other forms of IMRT. All patients must be CT planned and the CT image set transferred to the tomotherapy treatment planning station.

The target volumes and normal tissue regions of interest (ROIs) are contoured. They may be contoured on a CT-simulator or another treatment planning system and transferred to the tomotherapy planning system using the Digital Imaging and Communications in Medicine-Radiotherapy (DICOM-RT) protocol. The optimization system is capable of blocking or preventing beams going though any specified ROIs (e.g., the contralateral breast in breast radiotherapy). This feature can be used to set the beam intensity from beamlets traversing these ROIs to zero. ROIs can be overlapping so, for example, a voxel can be both contained within the tumor and a sensitive structure. A priority number (one being the highest priority) determines from which of the structures an overlapping voxel will subsume its optimization parameters.

Unlike a conventional or other IMRT treatment planning system, there is no selection of beam directions. Beams can be delivered from 51 equal-angularly spaced directions or projections. The treatment time is equal to the number of rotations times the rotation period, $R$. The number of rotations need not be an integer.

## Treatment Prescription And Dose Constraints

The dose prescription, dose and dose-volume constraints, optimization weighting factors, and avoidance penalties are specified to the system. These parameters have essentially a similar meaning as on other optimization systems for IMRT.

The dose prescription is usually set in terms of coverage to a target volume (ICRU Report 50 1993), typically the planning target volume (PTV). For example, a given dose to 95% of the volume is a typical specification. A minimum dose prescription specification would seek a given dose to 100% of the PTV. The optimizer guarantees that the prescription is met. In addition to the dose prescription, the minimum dose to the PTV, another dose-volume specification (set by default to be the same as the prescription), and the maximum dose to the PTV can be set along with a penalty factor if the criteria are not met. It is possible to have more than one target volume specified to treat with independent optimization goals. An overall importance is given for each of the target volumes. However, only one dose prescription specification is guaranteed to be met by the optimizer.

There can be multiple avoidance structures specified by the system, each of which is given an importance. Dose-volume constraints and a maximum dose can be specified with a penalty specified for each. Any of the optimization parameters can be reset without beginning the optimization again; however, at the beginning of the process it is often useful to start afresh so that the effect of changing a parameter can be better appreciated.

## Dose Rate, Rotation Speed, And Helical Pitch

For a given dose to deliver $D$, the calibrated dose rate $D_r$, rotation period $R$, and helical pitch $P$ are interrelated quantities given by:

$$D = c \, D_r \, R/(P \, M) \tag{3}$$

where $M$ is the modulation factor (discussed in the next section) and $c$ is a constant of proportionality that depends on the treatment plan and the dose prescription specified.

Having a longer rotation period increases the length of time that the beam travels over each point. Having a smaller pitch means that there are more rotations irradiating each point. Each dose rate produced by the unit requires a unique set of radiofrequency parameters.

The control system uses discrete rotation periods. We have typically used 20 or 28 sec rotation periods. We have most often used pitches of 0.2 to 0.33. A pitch of 0.5 produces a noticeable thread artifact unless the target volume is smaller than 10 cm in diameter. Smaller pitches also enable larger jaw widths to be used and this improves delivery efficiency.

## Modulation Factor

The modulation factor is the ratio of the maximum leaf opening time of any leaf to the average opening time of all of the non-zero leaf opening times. A modulation factor of one means that the leaves are not modulated. If not constrained by the optimizer the modulation factor could easily be 10 or even higher. In general, a higher modulation factor delivers higher dose gradients; however, the benefit of increasing the modulation factor quickly diminishes as the modulation factor increases above 3. We typically use modulation factors of 2 to 3, although modulation factors as low as 1.5 have been used. For comparison, in our observation of non-tomotherapy IMRT systems modulation factors higher than 2 are seldom used. If the modulation factor is high, the pitch is generally set low. The modulation factor is continuously variable and is tuned so that for a given dose rate, rotation period, and pitch, the dose can be delivered as efficiently as possible with the highest appropriate modulation.

## Convolution/Superposition Dose Calculation

The helical tomotherapy dose calculation engine uses the convolution/superposition method. It first models the incident energy fluence issuing from the MLC and interacting in the patient. Kernels, pre-calculated using the Monte Carlo method, model the charged particle transport and photon scatter.

Model-based methods like convolution/superposition and Monte Carlo are ideally suited to IMRT. The energy fluence issuing from each open leaf is a free parameter in these models. The amount of scatter issuing from the head does not have to be directly measured with a miniphantom or equilibrium buildup cap. Differences in the spectrum from the center of the beam to the periphery can be accounted for. For helical tomotherapy some of these advantages are reduced. There is very little head scatter because there is no field-flattening filter and its absence means that the spectrum is nearly invariant across the field.

Comparison of measured dose distributions and the results of the convolution/superposition dose calculation algorithm are shown in figure 4. The agreement is within 2% in low gradient regions and within 1 mm in high gradient regions.

The convolution/superposition method, while faster than Monte Carlo simulation, is still relatively time-consuming. Tomotherapy can employ tens of thousands of beamlets so the dose calculation burden is substantial. This problem was addressed using a parallel computer with 32 processors and gaining the ability to trade-off accuracy and speed by coarsening the calculation resolution at early phases in the optimization and becoming more accurate with finer resolution at later phases.

## Optimization

The system performs user-unattended pre-processing that, depending on the number of CT slices, takes 10 to 30 min to complete. Following this, the user-attended optimization is rapid with each iteration cycle typically taking about a second. The algorithm is a modification of the method described by Olivera (Olivera et al. 1999). Voxels for which the dose is too high request to the beamlets aimed at them to reduce their intensity. Whether any given beamlet is lowered in intensity depends on the requests of all of the voxels through which it traverses; similarly for the voxels for which the dose is too low.

    The dose-volume histogram (DVH) is updated in real-time to give the treatment planner rapid feedback. Any of the optimization constraints and weighting factors may be changed without requiring further pre-processing. This enables excellent user interaction to balance the degree of tumor dose homogeneity with the avoidance of critical structures. Figure 10 is an example of an optimization result for a conformal mantle field that spares the lungs and spinal cord.

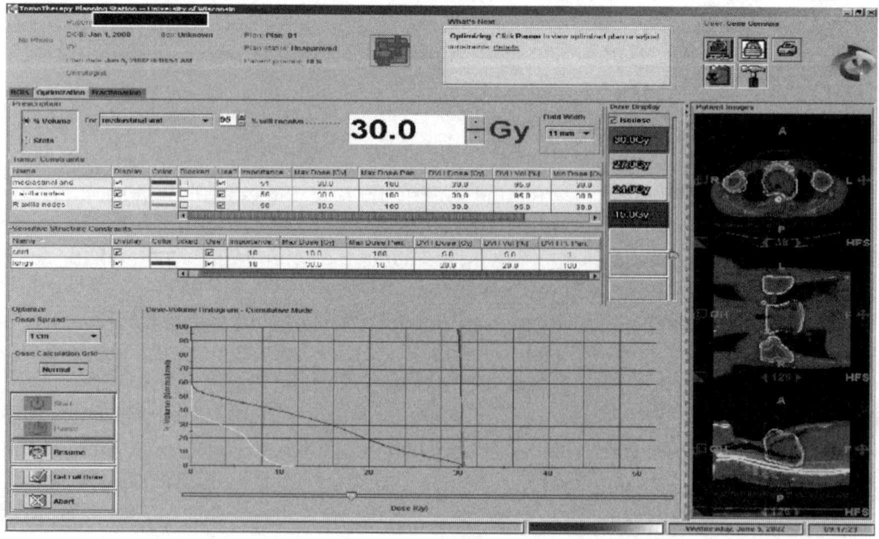

**Figure 10.** Optimization parameters, DVH, and dose distribution for a mantle field plan. The dose is very homogeneous to the nodal volumes irradiated yet the doses to the lung and the cord are low. In particular, the dose-volume constraint of the lung specified for less than 20% of the lung to a dose of 20 Gy or higher was met.

## Monitor Unit Calculations

Following approval of the optimization process the monitor unit calculation phase is initiated. The relative open time intervals are computed directly by the optimizer, taking into account the triangular-shaped energy fluence distribution that results from the absence of a field-flattening filter. The monitor unit calculation begins by computing the absolute opening and closing times. This determines the state of each leaf and its neighbors. The influence of the open neighbors is then taken into account with the opening and closing times adjusted. Specifically, if in any given leaf opening state one or both of a leaf's neighboring leaves are closed, the opening time for the leaf is increased because the neighbor will not contribute extra fluence. Any leaf, which is to be opened for a time shorter than the minimum in any given projection, is set to stay closed. This calculation takes only seconds. There is sufficient shielding on the helical tomotherapy unit to completely ignore the transmission through the leaves and jaws.

## Verification CT

The helical tomotherapy unit is not the first radiotherapy device to provide CT-guidance in a radiotherapy suite (Uematsu 1996) or to employ a megavoltage CT system (Swindell et al. 1983; Brahme, Lind, and Nafstadius 1987; Ruchala 1999; Ruchala et al. 2000a). The helical tomotherapy has a conventional xenon ion chamber CT detector system on board the system that acquires a transmission signal from the linac beam. The parameters of the linac radiofrequency system are adjusted for imaging from those for treatment so that the beam has a lower energy (about 3.5 MV), lower pulse repetition frequency, and smaller output. The typical dose rate to the patient is from 1.5 to 3 cGy. The data acquisition system (DAS) can read the ionization from each of the detector elements every 3 ms. As in some portal image detector systems, the pulsing of the linac is controlled by the DAS such that read-out synchrony of the detector elements is enforced.

The verification CT serves as the basis for most of the patient-specific QA processes. Having a CT scan at the time of treatment provides the capability for unprecedented knowledge of the patient during the course of therapy. Whether or not a CT scan is done every day depends on the reliability of setup. Likely, a CT scan will be done every day for a pelvic irradiation on an obese patient. However, a CT scan would likely be done only weekly on a cooperative head and neck patient. Between these extremes the frequency of acquisition will likely be highly patient- and practice-specific.

The linac and gantry systems of the tomotherapy system are highly favorable for CT. The gantry sag of the tomotherapy system is negligible so that no sag corrections are required. The size of the electron beam on the target is about 1 mm, as determined by physical and dosimetric measurements. These characteristics mean that the tomotherapy system approaches the resolution of a conventional CT scanner for high-contrast objects.

## Detector Characteristics For Verification CT

The tomotherapy unit's xenon gas detector, also used in an older generation of General Electric's CT scanners, has tungsten septa separating ionization cavities. The tungsten plates are the ion collection electrodes for the detector and were originally designed to block low-energy x-ray scatter and reduce channel-to-channel crosstalk. On the helical tomotherapy system the tungsten plates act as embedded converters to intercept the megavoltage photons and yet are thin enough to let an appreciable fraction of the electrons set in motion to deposit energy in the xenon gas. The interception of the beam by the tungsten means that the quantum efficiency of the system is about 25%, which is much more than the few percent collection efficiency of modern portal imaging systems.

## Contrast And Resolution Of Verification CT Images

In a CT scanner the contrast and resolution are related. Smaller objects are more visible when there is more image contrast. Smaller contrast differences can only be seen in larger objects. For high contrast objects, like an air cavity in a plastic phantom, the tomotherapy system has a resolution limit of about 1 to 1.2 mm (see figure 11), which will resolve the detailed shape of bone, sinuses, and lungs. When the object has a size of about 2.5 cm, it is possible to see density differences as small as 2% to 3% between it and its background for doses in the range from 1.5 to 3 cGy. Figure 11 shows an example of a 3% contrast object that is 2.9 cm in diameter. This means that the difference between fat and muscle, which has a density difference from 3% to 7%, can be easily resolved so that the prostate is identifiable and the difference between unit-density and fatty tissue in breast is resolved. The contrast between white and grey matter in brain is not visible.

## CT Number Calibration

Since the verification CT uses the megavoltage beam from the linac, the beam interacts almost exclusively by Compton interactions, which on a cross-section per electron basis, is material independent. The linear attenuation coefficient is linear with the electron density of the medium. This means that the conversion from CT number, which is a measure of the normalized difference in linear attenuation coefficient of the medium to water, to electron density should also be linear. Figure 12 indicates that the image density (as measured by a floating point relative CT#) is indeed linear with both the electron density and the gravimetric density.

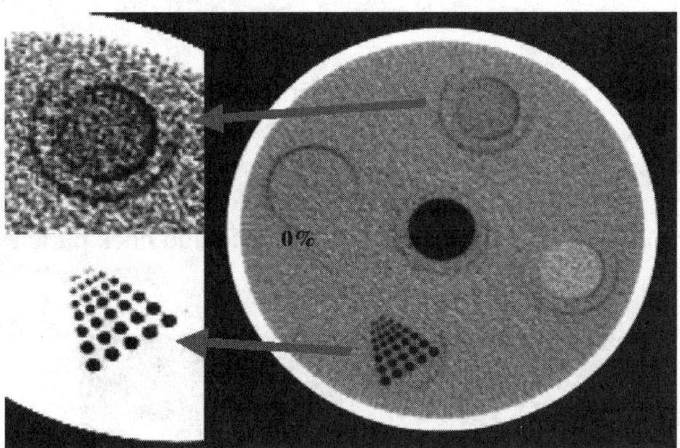



**Figure 11.** Verification CT of a Gammex-RMI contrast-resolution phantom. The percentage electron density contrast is 3% for the low contrast plug (that is also enlarged) and 6% for the brighter high contrast plug. The contrast plugs are about 2.9 cm in diameter. The 3% decrease in contrast is clearly seen. The smallest air cavities in unit density plastic, 0.8 mm in diameter, are not resolved. The 1.2 mm air cavities are fairly well resolved. The 1.6 mm air cavities are clearly resolved. In order of increasing size, the other cavity diameters are 2.0, 2.4, 2.8, and 3.2 mm. [Reprinted from *Medical Physics,* vol 29, "Methods for improving limited field-of-view radiotherapy reconstructions using imperfect *a priori* languages," K. J. Ruchala, G. H. Olivera, J. M. Kapatoes, P. K. Reckwerdt, and T. R. Mackie, pp. 2590–2605. © 2002 with permission from AAPM.]

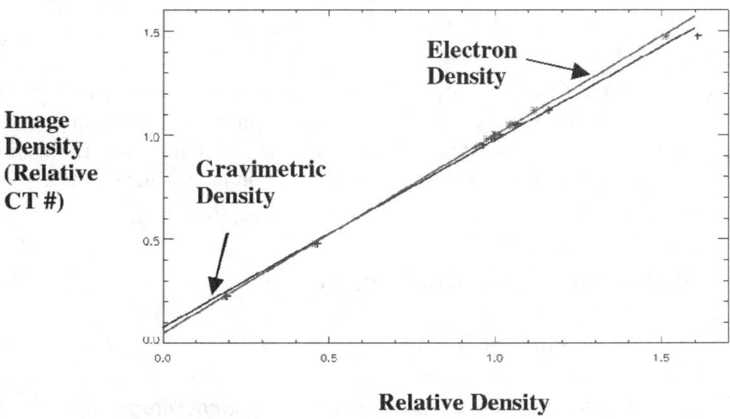



**Figure 12.** Graph of image density or relative CT number vs. relative density for the verification CT for various tissue-equivalent liquid and plastic mixtures. The image density, as well as gravimetric and electron densities, are normalized to water. The linear fit did not force the image density to be unity at a relative density of one. [Reprinted from *Physics in Medicine and Biology,* vol 45, "Calibration of a tomotherapeutic MVCT system," K. J. Ruchala, G. H. Olivera, E. A. Schloesser, R. Hinderer, and T. R. Mackie, pp. N27–36. © 2000, with permission from IOP Publishing.]

## Absence Of Metal Artifacts

Metal artifacts arise in conventional CT scanners because the attenuation of the metal is non-linear due to the photoelectric effect. In helical CT, the beam is penetrating enough to eliminate metal artifacts arising from hip prostheses and dental filings (see figure 13). This means that a verification CT could be a more reliable CT system for prostate patients with hip replacements and head and neck patients with cancer of the tongue.

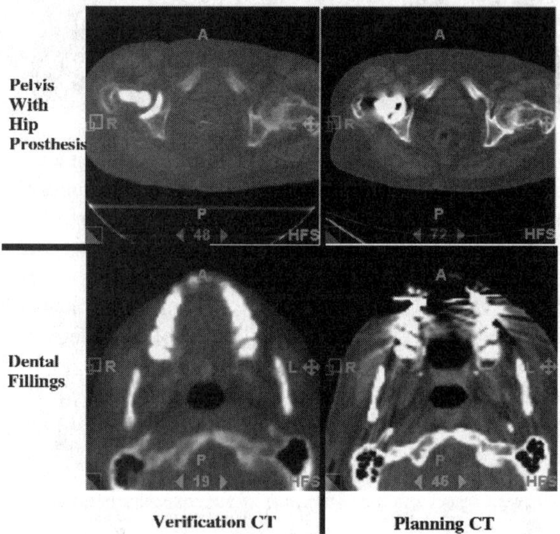


**Figure 13.** Verification CT and planning CT images of a pelvic site with a hip prosthesis and dental fillings. There are severe artifacts around the metal and bone in the planning CT of the pelvis. There are severe streak artifacts radiating from the metal fillings in teeth in the planning CT. These artifacts do not exist in the verification CT.

## Processes For Adaptive Radiotherapy

## Verification Of The Patient Setup

The verification CT is so named because it verifies the patient setup and, in that regard, has a role similar to a planar verification film. However, its capabilities far exceed a verification film. A digitally reconstructed radiograph (DRR), derived from the planning CT, can be useful to interpret a planar film. Even with DRRs, a verification film is extremely difficult to infer if the patient is rotated about an axis not perpendicular to the film. The soft-tissue contrast is usually insufficient to judge whether the target volume has the correct placement. Setup verification directly compares the planning CT with the verification CT using image fusion or registration.

At the time of treatment, if the patient is set up exactly as he was for the planning CT, the anatomy will be exactly registered between the verification and planning image sets. As in a diagnostic CT scanner, the patient is positioned using skin marks and lasers outside of the bore of the unit. A verification scan is taken that encompasses all or a representative sample of the treatment volume and the patient is returned to the same position outside of the gantry bore. The verification CT image set is then reconstructed. The verification image set is fused onto the planning image set and the translation and rotation offsets are reported. The image fusion can be done automatically using the mutual information algorithm (Ardekani et al. 1995; Maes et al. 1997; Ruchala et al. 2002b), manually, or a combination of both. Once the image registration is completed, the offsets also describe how the patient should be adjusted. Figure 14 shows an example of pre-registration and post-registration images of the planning and verification CT sets from a canine patient. The original set up was done without the aid of skin marks so the verification CT was the sole method to guide the treatment positioning.

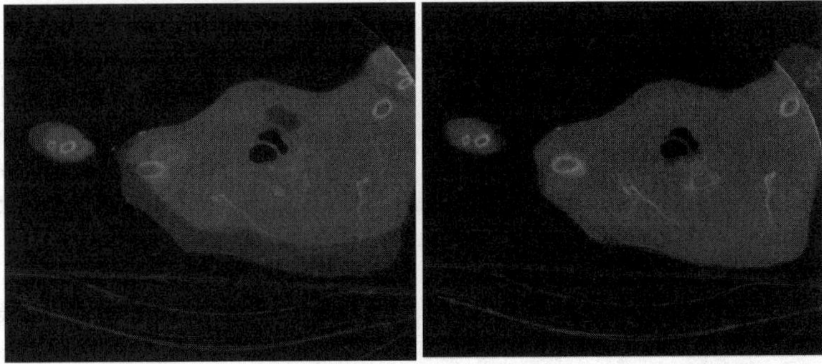

**Figure 14.** Pre-registration (left) and post-registration (right) of a canine patient. The darker gray image is the planning CT and the lighter image is the verification CT.

If the patient requires adjustment, the patient can be translated accordingly. A CT couch has vertical (elevation) and longitudinal movements. On the UW unit the couch top cannot be moved laterally. However, placing a slippery polyethylene sheet with handholds between the couch top and mattress can easily effect lateral movements. The next generation of couches on helical tomotherapy units has lateral adjustments.

Tomotherapy comes equipped with a set of moveable CT-simulator lasers so that the modified position of the patient can be confirmed.

## Dose Reconstruction

Dose reconstruction is a determination of the dose delivered superimposed on the CT at the time of treatment (McNutt, Mackie, and Paliwal 1997, Kapatoes et al. 2001). The CT detector runs at the time of treatment recording the treatment beam exiting through the patient and couch. Using the CT image set acquired just before treatment, the energy fluence incident on the patient can be computed. Using the incident fluence, the dose distribution is computed in the patient using the same convolution/superposition method used for helical tomotherapy treatment planning. The process is not accurate unless a CT of the patient at the time of treatment is used. Dose reconstruction has been tested using the UW tomotherapy benchtop unit but not yet implemented on the UW clinical unit.

## Deformable Registration And Autocontouring

The verification CT often reveals that the patient anatomy is not identical to the planning CT. When the anatomy is deformed, the dose distribution obtained from dose reconstruction cannot be directly compared to the planned dose distribution. Similarly, the regions of interest valid for the planning CT do not match the anatomy of the verification CT. Deformable registration matches, using a one-to-one mapping, the verification CT to the planning CT.

Deformable registration algorithms typically use common features such as contours or points that are identified automatically in both images (Blake and Isard 1998). The intervening space between identifiable features is deformed according to finite element methods using established elastic property parameters (Joshi and Miller 2000; Lu 2001). For example, high CT number voxels are likely bone and are therefore not elastic. If there are enough feature points, the methods are not sensitive to the accuracy of the elastic properties of the soft tissue. The method would have difficulty with the presence of contrast agents and severe distortion of the anatomy.

We have been exploring a multi-resolution method that uses a voxel-based objection function (Ruchala et al. 2002b) to produce a one-to-one transform of the new test image to make it appear like the prior reference image. Figure 15 illustrates deformable registration of a pelvic CT scan set. A test CT scan was deformed to appear like a reference CT scan. All the voxels of the deformed CT were obtained from the test CT scan but its appearance is much closer to the reference CT scan.

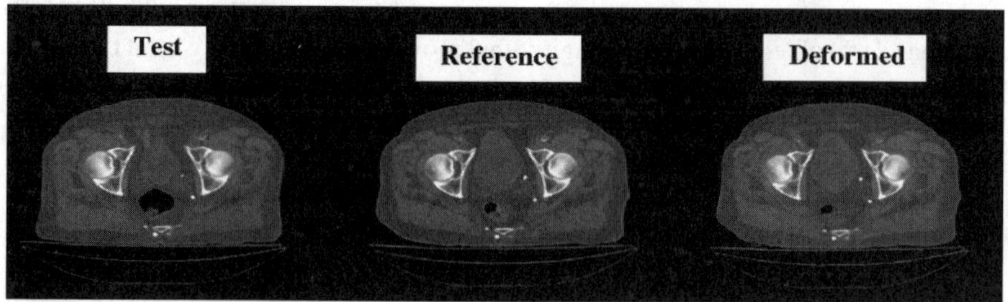


**Figure 15.** Example of deformable registration. The test and reference images are of the same patient CT scanned on different days. The rightmost image is the test image deformed to look like the reference image.

ROIs can be useful for deformable registration algorithms as *a priori* information. Perhaps in the future deformable registration will provide a method to autocontour the ROIs so that the reconstructed dose can be converted into a DVH with only operator approval. At the very least, the autocontoured ROIs provides a way to evaluate the accuracy of the deformable registration.

## Re-Optimization Of Subsequent Fractions

Re-optimization is the modification of subsequent treatment fractions on the basis of the dose reconstruction and deformable registration of the regions of interest and the dose distribution (Wu 2002). If the dose is too low to the target volume, the dose may be increased somewhat in the remaining fractions. While it is not possible to remove the excess dose delivered to a sensitive structure, it may be possible to take this into account in re-optimization so that the dose delivered in the whole course of therapy might be the same or only marginally higher. Re-optimization might also be done if it is decided that the target volume needs to change part way through the course of therapy. Re-optimization is a research topic and not yet being tested on the UW clinical unit.

Figure 16 is a simulation of re-optimization for a head and neck case following deformable registration for a two-fraction example. It is likely that the re-optimization would not be done on a daily basis as implied by figure 16 but the results for several fractions would be combined; for example, re-optimization could be done on a weekly basis.

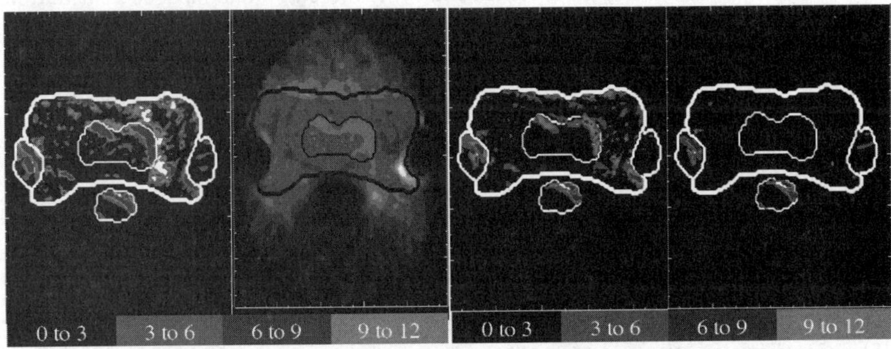


**Figure 16.** Reoptimization example following deformable registration. Panel A is an image of regions that are graded by a colorwash display into either % dose difference or mm of distance to agreement following a single fraction. Panel B is a dose image to deliver to make up for the dose errors shown in panel A. Panel C is the colorwash of the effect of the errors if nothing were done but the second fraction were delivered with no further errors. Panel D is the colorwash if the second fraction were to make up for errors in the first fraction as described by panel B and was delivered without further errors. Panel D shows that most of the errors after the first fraction in the target volume have been removed but there are still some errors in the avoidance structures but they are very similar to those of panel C.

## Clinical Examples

The UW helical tomotherapy prototype unit began human clinical use in August 2002. Despite the FDA (510k) approval we are committed to treating patients under research protocols or for compassionate use only. Our first prostate protocol has recently been approved and we expect to be treating prostate protocol patients soon. Even though some patients to be presented here have not been treated by tomotherapy, we have built up a large number of treatment plans on patients receiving conventional 3-D conformal, IMRT, and stereotactic radiosurgery.

## Palliative Treatments

The UW tomotherapy unit began clinical use with palliative patients, both veterinary and human, in order to carefully perfect the planning, delivery, and verification processes. The UW has an active radiotherapy program for pets and the first therapy use was canine oesteosarcoma treatments (begun in May 2002). The human palliative patients were bone metastases from breast, prostate and renal cell cancer.

Verification CT and setup adjustment were performed on each patient. In the canine cases this was done under general anesthesia with a vacuum bead-bag without the aid of skin marks. One of the human patients was morbidly obese and the target volume was as far as 2 to 4 cm from the position indicated by the skin marks.

Figure 17 is an example of tomotherapy applied to palliative treatment of a metastasis in the pubic bone. The isodose lines and DVH indicates that the dose distribution is both homogeneous and conformal to the target volume. The accompanying inset illustrates that the dose distribution was confirmed by irradiation of the cylindrical "cheese" phantom. The dose in the lateral direction approaches an inverse fall-off dependence with distance.

We think that our experience with palliative bone treatments provides valuable experience with extracranial spinal stereotactic radiosurgery (Hamilton et al. 1995).

## Prostate Cancer

Prostate cancer is one of the most common cancers treated with IMRT (Teh et al. 2001). Irradiation to the rectum and bladder has to be avoided despite their intimate proximity to the prostate. The central problem of prostate radiotherapy is the movement and deformation of the prostate due to differential filling of the rectum and bladder (Balter et al. 1993; Yan et al. 2001). Image guidance with verification CT to determine the location of the prostate on a daily basis is a particular strength of helical tomotherapy. Figure 18 illustrates a comparison between transverse views of a prostate patient acquired from a planning CT, a verification CT, and ultrasound echogram obtained through the anterior surface of the pelvis. The prostate can be clearly seen on the verification CT and the perspicuity of the prostate is superior to a pelvic ultrasound in this example.

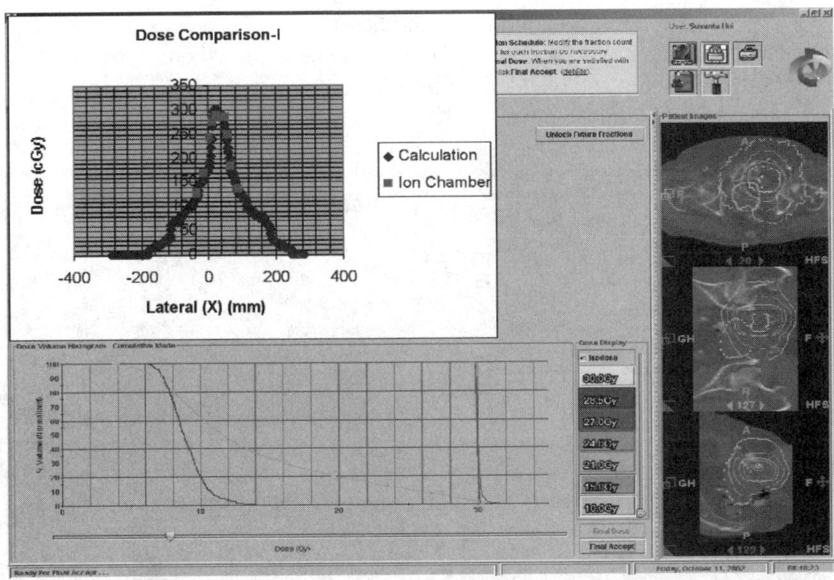

**Figure 17.** A screen shot of the treatment planning station illustrating the dose-volume histogram (DVH) and isodose lines on planning CT for a human case involving a bone metastasis in the pubic bone. The inset to the upper left is a dose comparison between calculation of the delivery to a cylindrical phantom and the ion chamber results.

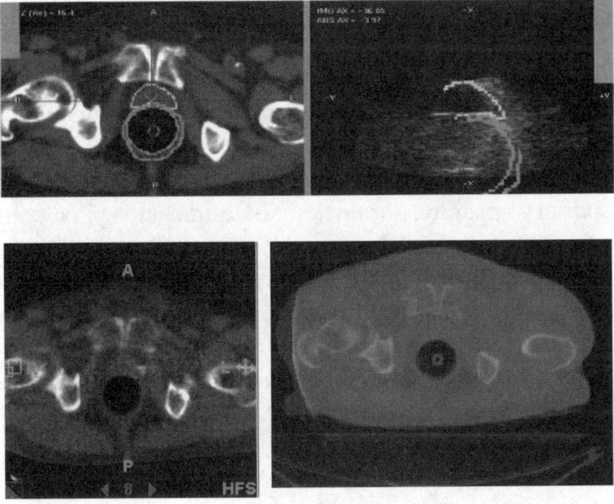

**Figure 18.** Transverse views of planning CT (upper left), ultrasound (upper right), verification CT (lower left) and fusion of planning CT (dark gray) and verification (light gray) images of the same prostate cancer patient.

The dose distribution for a helical tomotherapy plan for a prostate tomotherapy case is shown in figure 19. The dose is very homogeneous and there is excellent avoidance of both the rectum and bladder. Using a 2.5 cm jaw opening, the plan would take under 2 minutes of beam-on time.

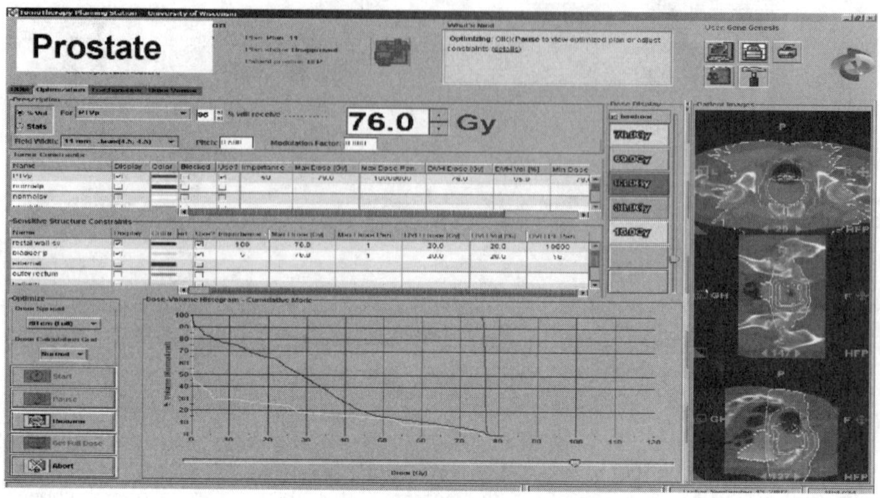

**Figure 19.** Prostate plan that would take under 2 minutes of beam-on delivery time. There is excellent dose homogeneity in the prostate and good avoidance of the rectum and bladder.

## Head And Neck Cancer

A complex target volume, with dual or even multiple prescription volumes as well as many surrounding avoidance structures, characterizes head and neck treatments. In head and neck radiotherapy the target volume may be extensive including both a large invading tumor and positive or suspected nodes. Avoidance structures include the optic chiasm, orbit, auditory apparatus, brainstem, parotids, and spinal cord. As compared to other forms of IMRT, for equal dose to avoidance structures, tomotherapy is capable of a more homogeneous dose to the target volumes, or for a given amount of dose homogeneity, tomotherapy can lower the dose to the avoidance structures.

Figure 20 is an example of the excellent sparing of the parotid and cord that can be achieved while maintaining dose homogeneity. Head and neck radiotherapy is a good example of a site where more beam directions is important.

## Lung Cancer

Lung is one of the most difficult sites to deliver IMRT (Balter et al. 1996). Lung motion, especially near the base, is substantial (Samson et al. 1999). Without arresting or accounting for the motion of the lung, IMRT delivered with a conventional MLC will result in hot and cold regions in the lung (Yu, Jaffray, and Wong 1998). Gating the delivery will reduce but not eliminate the artifacts. Breath-holding, either voluntary or assisted (Kubo and Hill 1996; Wong et al. 1999), is likely the best conventional solution at the moment to minimize the effect of breathing motion. Maximum inspiration breath-holding, while less reliable in lung displacement accuracy, has the advantage of expanding the lung to drive some normal lung out of the high-dose region (Mehta, Scrimger, and Mackie 2001). For tumors near the apex of the lung, motion is much less of a concern and so IMRT may be delivered with only shallow breathing in these cases.

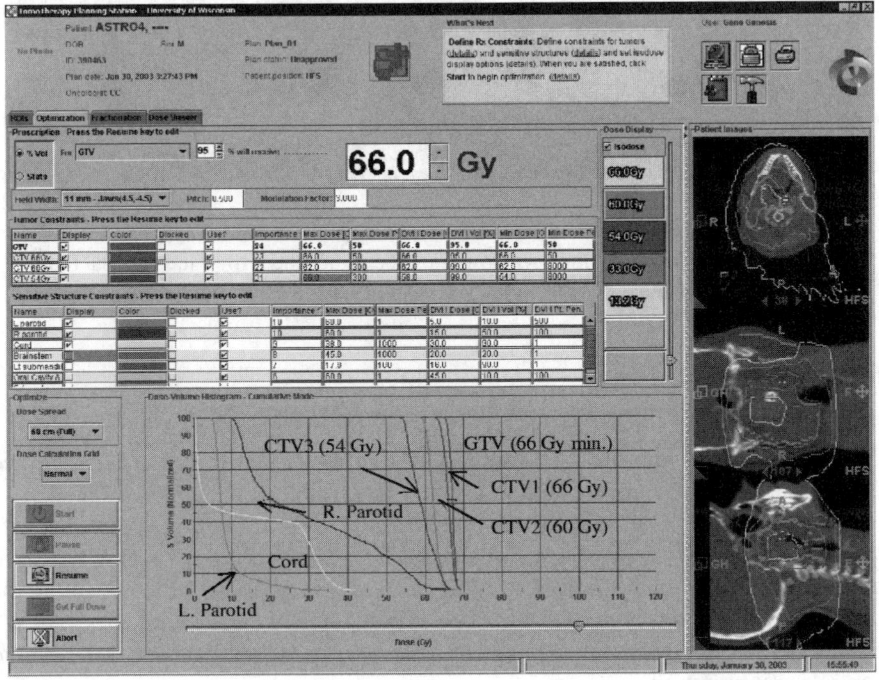

**Figure 20.** Head and neck helical tomotherapy treatment planning example of parotid, and cord sparing. There are multiple target volumes, each with own prescription as indicated on the figure. The helical tomotherapy planning system was able to reach each of the prescription values, which were specified as a minimum dose for the gross target volume (GTV) and 95% volume coverage level for the clinical target volumes (CTVs). The left parotid received less than 20% of its volume over 15 Gy. The spinal cord was less than 45 Gy. This example was distributed during a recent American Society for Therapeutic Radiology and Oncology (ASTRO)-sponsored intercomparison of IMRT planning systems.

There is a unique breath-holding strategy under development for helical tomotherapy. Rather than delivering the entire dose to a part of the target volume, it is possible to deliver a fairly uniform IMRT dose to the entire volume in one breath-hold. This is repeated for other breath-holds building up the dose until the total dose is reached. Each of the breath-hold deliveries has the same loose helical pitch but a different gantry start angle and end angle. Rather than a single helical source trajectory, the set of source trajectories resembles a loosely wound cable.

Figure 21 is a verification CT scan using a soft tissue window and a lung window. The lung tumor is clearly visible in the verification CT.

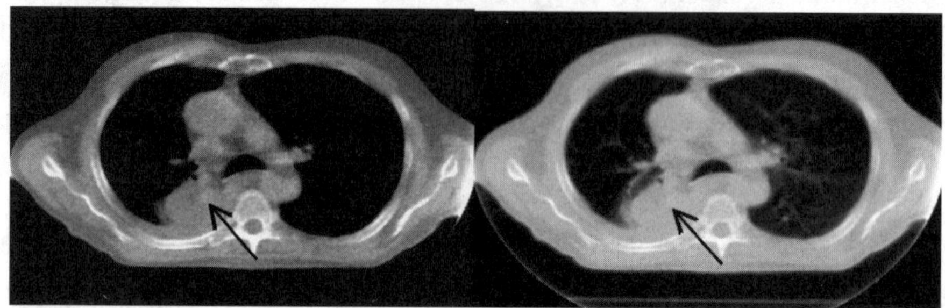

**Figure 21.** Transverse views of a slice from a verification CT of the lung. A soft tissue window is on the left and a lung window is on the right. The arrows indicate the tumor. The lung dose from the verification CT was only 3 cGy.

## Breast Cancer

From the standpoint of local tumor control there is little need for IMRT for breast radiotherapy. IMRT can improve the avoidance of normal tissue especially using limited field irradiation in the prone position. Limited-field irradiation has already been practiced successfully for some time using brachytherapy, and preliminary experience with IMRT has been reported by Baglan et al. (2003). We have been developing the capability to do limited-field irradiation in the prone position. In the prone position, the breast naturally assumes a position that is reproducible, is less mobile, reduces the possibility of dose-enhancing skin folds, and is more avoiding of the lungs, heart, and contralateral breast.

In conventional radiotherapy the prone breast is not easy to set up because of the difficulty in visualizing the medial skin marks on the sternum. The CT capability of helical tomotherapy should enable the prone breast setup to be imaged daily with a relatively low dose. A low dose is possible because of the high contrast between tissue and air. The woman would lie on a mattress raised 10 to 20 cm above the couch top of the unit with her involved breast falling through the mattress. Depending how pendulous her breast is, her back might not get imaged but that is inconsequential if beams do not enter through her back.

The lung, heart, and contralateral breast can be specified as blocking structures if necessary. Regions that are outside of the field of view are blocked as well so that beams cannot enter because of the indeterminacy of the depth the beam traverses. The skin may also be contoured as an avoidance structure. With the skin dose kept low, it may be possible to increase the dose per fraction but perhaps not as aggressively as is being done for breast brachytherapy (e.g., 34 Gy in 10 fractions given 2 fractions per day).

Figure 22 is an example of a limited-field right breast tomotherapy treatment planning in the prone position. An extra avoidance structure was contoured beneath the ipsilateral lung to aid in avoidance of that lung. Beams are allowed through only about one-third of the possible directions.

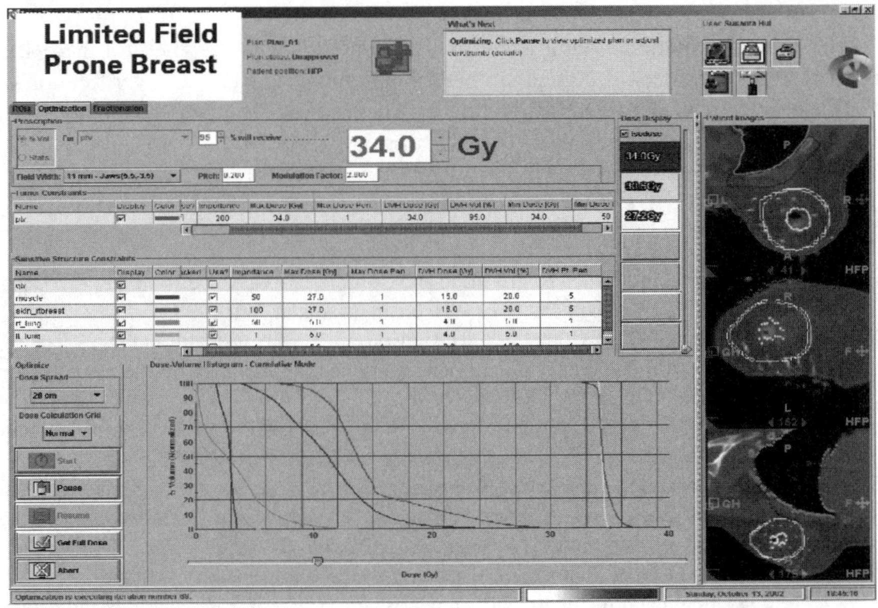

**Figure 22.** Planning example of limited-field prone breast that was treated with high-dose rate brachytherapy.

## Conclusions

Helical tomotherapy is the marriage of a linac to a CT scanner. A continuously rotating gantry delivers an intensity-modulated fan beam while the patient is translated through the bore of a CT-like ring gantry. The delivery geometry enables the acquisition of a CT scan using the treatment beam. Helical tomotherapy has entered clinical practice at the University of Wisconsin, with other institutions to follow shortly.

The dose distributions from tomotherapy are highly conformal with the target volume receiving a homogeneous dose and neighboring normal structures being well avoided. Just because the beam has the possibility of delivering radiation through 360 degrees does not mean that it must. The beam may be extinguished by the MLC nearly completely for large arc segments to avoid all but a negligible leakage component.

The CT capability enables several processes of adaptive radiotherapy. A verification CT acquired just before delivery is registered to the planning CT. The amount of setup variation reported provides guidance for improving the setup. The scan may be used as the basis for dose reconstruction whereby a calculation of the dose actually delivered is superimposed on the verification CT. The reconstructed dose is the basis for reoptimization of the delivery for subsequent fractions. However, organ deformation may have first to be taken into account. Deformable registration of the dose distribution enables the dose distribution to be accumulated on the planning CT reference frame.

The helical tomotherapy unit is the first integrated device designed for the delivery of IMRT. It has been designed so that the planning, delivery, and verification of IMRT can be done well, efficiently, and easily. The next few years will reveal how well the expectations for the design have been realized.

# References

Aldridge, J. S. Tomographic Patient Registration and Conformal Avoidance Tomotherapy. Deptment of Medical Physics. University of Wisconsin, Madison, WI, 1999.

Almond, P. R., P. J. Biggs, B. M. Coursey, W. H. Hanson, M. S. Huq, R. Nath, and D. W. Rogers. (1999). "AAPM's TG-51 protocol for clinical reference dosimetry of high-energy photon and electron beams." *Med. Phys.* 26:1847–1870.

Ardekani, B. A., M. Braun, B. F. Hutton, I. Kanno, and H, Iida. (1995). "A fully automatic multi-modality image registration algorithm." *J. Comput. Assist. Tomogr.* 19:615–623.

Baglan, K. L., M. B. Sharpe, D. Jaffray, R. C. Frazier, J. Fayad, L. L. Kestin, V. Remouchamps, A. A. Martinez, J. Wong, and F. A Vicini. (2003). "Accelerated partial breast irradiation using 3D conformal radiation therapy (3D-CRT)." *Int. J. Radiat. Oncol. Biol. Phys.* 55:302–311.

Balter, J. M., G. T. Chen, C. A. Pelizzari, S. Krishnasamy, S. Rubin, and S. Vijayakumar. (1993). "Online repositioning during treatment of the prostate: a study of potential limits and gains." *Int. J. Radiat. Oncol. Biol. Phys.* 27:137–143.

Balter, J. M., R. K. Ten Haken, T. S. Lawrence, K. L. Lam, and J. M. Robertson. (1996). "Uncertainties in CT-based radiation therapy treatment planning associated with patient breathing." *Int. J. Radiat. Oncol. Biol. Phys.* 36:167–174.

Blake, A., and M. Isard. *Active Contours.* Berlin: Springer-Verlag, 1998.

Brahme, A. (1988). "Optimisation of stationary and moving beam radiation therapy techniques." *Radiother. Oncol.* 12:129–140.

Brahme, A., B. Lind, and P. Nafstadius. (1987). "Radiotherapeutic computed tomography with scanned photon beams." *Int. J. Radiat. Oncol. Biol. Phys.* 13:95–101.

Carol, M. P., H. Targovnik, C. Campbell, A. Bleier, J. Streit, B. Rosen, P. Miller, D. Scherch, and R. Huber. "An Automatic 3D Treatment Planning and Implementation System for Optimised Conformal Therapy" in *Three-dimensional Treatment Planning.* P. Minet (ed.). European Association of Radiology Proceedings of the 5th Workshop by Commission Infomatique. Geneva, WHO Headquarters, pp. 173–187, 1993.

Hamilton, A. J., B. A. Lulu, H. Fosmire, B. Stea, and J. R. Cassady. (1995). "Preliminary clinical experience with linear accelerator-based spinal stereotactic radiosurgery." *Neurosurg.* 36:311–319.

ICRU Report 50. Prescribing, Recording and Reporting Photon Beam Therapy. Washington, DC: International Commission on Radiation Units and Measurements, 1993.

IMRTCWG (Intensity Modulated Radiation Therapy Collaborative Working Group). "Intensity-modulated radiotherapy: Current status and issues of interest." *Int. J. Radiat. Oncol. Biol. Phys.* 51:880–914.

Jaffray, D. A., D. G. Drake, M. Moreau, A. A. Martinez, and J. W. Wong. (1999). "A radiographic and tomographic imaging system integrated into a medical linear accelerator for localization of bone and soft-tissue targets." *Int. J. Radiat. Oncol. Biol. Phys.* 45:773–789.

Johns, H. E., and J. R. Cunningham. *The Physics of Radiology.* Springfield, IL: Charles C Thomas, 1983.

Joshi, S., and M. Miller. (2000). "Landmark matching via large deformation diffeomorphisms." *IEEE Trans. Image Processing* 9:1357–1370.

Kapatoes, J. M., G. H. Olivera, J. P. Balog, H. Keller, P. J. Reckwerdt, and T. R. Mackie. (2001). "On the accuracy and effectiveness of dose reconstruction for tomotherapy." *Phys. Med. Biol.* 46:943–966.

Kubo, H. D., and B. C. Hill. (1996). "Respiration gated radiotherapy treatment: A technical study." *Phys. Med. Biol.* 41:83–91.

Lu, W. Motion Detection and Correction for Image Guided Radiation Therapy. Ph.D. Dissertation. University of Wisconsin, Madison, 2001.

Lyman, J. T. (1985). "Complication probability as assessed from dose-volume histograms." *Radiat. Res.* 104:S13–S19.

Mackie, T. R., T. Holmes, S. Swerdloff, P. Reckwerdt, J. O. Deasy, J. Yang, B. Paliwal, and T. Kinsella. (1993). "Tomotherapy: A new concept for the delivery of dynamic conformal radiotherapy." *Med. Phys.* 20:1709–1719.

Mackie, T. R. "CT in Radiotherapy and Tomotherapy" in *Medical CT & Ultrasound: Current Technology and Applications.* L. W. Goldman and J. B. Fowlkes (eds.). Madison, WI: Advanced Medical Publishing, 1995.

Mackie, T. R., T. W. Holmes, P. J. Reckwerdt, and J. Yang. (1995). "Tomotherapy: Optimized planning and delivery or radiation therapy." *Int. J. Imaging Sys. Tech.* 6:43–55.

Mackie, T. R., J. Balog, K. Ruchala, D. Shepard, S. Aldridge, E. Fitchard, P. Reckwerdt, G. Olivera, T. McNutt, and M. Mehta. (1999). "Tomotherapy." *Semin. Radiat. Oncol.* 9(1):108–117.

Maes, F., A. Collignon, D. Vandermeulen, G. Marchal, and P. Seutens. (1997). "Multimodality image registration by maximization of mutual information." *IEEE Trans. Med. Imaging* 16(2):187–198.

McNutt, T. R., T. R. Mackie, and B. R. Paliwal. (1997). "Analysis and convergence of the iterative convolution/superposition dose reconstruction technique for multiple beams and tomotherapy." *Med. Phys.* 24:1465–1476.

Mehta, M., R. Scrimger, and R. Mackie. (2001). "A new approach to dose escalation in non-small-cell lung cancer." *Int. J. Radiat. Oncol. Biol. Phys.* 49:23–33.

Niemierko, A., and M. Goitein. (1993a). "Modeling of normal tissue response to radiation: The critical volume model." *Int. J. Radiat. Oncol. Biol. Phys.* 25:135–145.

Olivera, G. H., D. M. Shepard, K. Ruchala, J. S. Aldridge, J. Kapatoes, E. E. Fitchard, P. J. Reckwerdt, G. Fang, J. Balog, J. Zachman, and T. R. Mackie. "Tomotherapy" in *The Modern Technology of Radiation Oncology. A Compendium for Medical Physicists and Radiation Oncologists.* J. Van Dyk (ed.). Madison, WI: Medical Physics Publishing, pp. 521–587, 1999.

Pirzkall, A., M. Carol, F. Lohr, H. Hoss, M. Wannenmacher, and J. Debus. (2000) "Comparison of intensity-modulated radiotherapy with conventional conformal radiotherapy for complex-shaped tumors." *Int. J. Radiat. Oncol. Biol. Phys.* 48:1371–1380.

Ruchala, K. J. Megavoltage Computed Tomography for Tomotherapy Verification. Dept. of Medical Physics. Madison: University of Wisconsin, 1999.

Ruchala, K. J., G. H. Olivera, J. M. Kapatoes, E. A. Schloesser, P. J. Reckwerdt, and T. R. Mackie. (2000a) "Megavoltage CT image reconstruction during tomotherapy treatments." *Phys. Med. Biol.* 45:3545–3562.

Ruchala, K. J., G. H. Olivera, E. A. Schloesser, R. Hinderer, and T. R. Mackie. (2000b). "Calibration of a tomotherapeutic megavoltage CT system." *Phys. Med. Biol.* 45:27–36.

Ruchala, K. J., G. H. Olivera, J. M. Kapatoes, P. J. Reckwerdt, and T. R. Mackie. (2002a). "Methods for improving limited field-of-view radiotherapy reconstructions using imperfect a priori images." *Med. Phys.* 29:2590–2605.

Ruchala, K. J., G. H. Olivera, and J. M. Kapatoes. (2002b). "Limited-data image registration for radiotherapy positioning and verification." *Int. J. Radiat. Oncol. Biol. Phys.* 54:592–605.

Samson, M. J., J. R. van Sornsen de Koste, H. C. J. de Boer, H. Tankink, M. Verstraate, M. Essers, A. G. Visser, and S. Senan. (1999) "An analysis of anatomic landmark mobility and setup deviations in radiotherapy for lung cancer." *Int. J. Radiat. Oncol. Biol. Phys.* 43:827–832.

Shepard, D. M., G. Olivera, L. Angelos, O. Sauer, P. Reckwerdt, and T. R. Mackie. (1999). "A simple model for examining issues in radiotherapy optimization." *Med. Phys.* 26:1212–1221.

Swindell, W., R. G. Simpson, and J. R. Oleson. (1983) "Computed tomography with a linear accelerator with radiotherapy applications." *Med. Phys.* 10:416–420.

Teh, B. S., W.-Y. Mai, B. M. Uhl, M. E. Augspurger, W. H. Grant 3rd, H. H. Lu, S. Y. Woo, L. S. Carpenter, J. K Chiu, and E. B. Butler. (2001) "Intensity-modulated radiation therapy (IMRT) for prostate cancer with the use of a rectal balloon for prostate immobilization: Acute toxicity and dose-volume analysis." *Int. J. Radiat. Oncol. Biol. Phys.* 49:705–712.

Uematsu, M., T. Fukui, A. Shioda, H. Tokumitsu, K. Takai, T. Kojima, Y. Asai, and S. Kusano. (1996). "A dual computed tomography linear accelerator unit for stereotactic radiation therapy: A new approach without cranially fixated stereotactic frames." *Int. J. Radiat. Oncol. Biol. Phys.* 35:587–592.

Wong, J. W., M. B. Sharpe, D. A. Jaffray, V. R. Kini, J. M. Robertson, J. S. Stromberg, and A. A. Martinez. (1999. "The use of active breathing control (ABC) to reduce margin for breathing motion." *Int. J. Radiat. Oncol. Biol. Phys.* 44:911–919.

Wu, C. Treatment Planning in Adaptive Radiotherapy. University of Wisconsin Ph.D. Thesis. Madison, WI, 2002.

Yan, D., and J. Wong. (1997). "Adaptive modification of treatment planning to minimize the deleterious effects of treatment setup errors." *Int. J. Radiat. Oncol. Biol. Phys.* 38:197–206.

Yan, D., B. Xu, D. Lockman, K. Kota, D. S. Brabbins, J. Wong, and A. A. Martinez. (2001). "The influence of interpatient and intrapatient rectum variation on external beam treatment of prostate cancer." *Int. J. Radiat. Oncol. Biol. Phys.* 51:1111–1119.

Yang, J. N., T. R. Mackie, P. J. Reckwerdt, J. O. Deasy, and B. R. Thomadsen. (1997). "An investigation of tomotherapy beam delivery." *Med. Phys.* 24:425–436.

Yu, C. X., D. A. Jaffray, and J. W. Wong. (1998). "The effects of intra-fraction organ motion on the delivery of dynamic intensity modulation." *Phys. Med. Biol.* 43:91–104.

# Static MLC IMRT (Step And Shoot)

**Arthur L. Boyer, Ph.D.**
Department of Radiation Oncology
Stanford University
Stanford, California

## Intensity Modulation With Discrete Positions And Intensities

X-ray field modulation has been a commonly practiced radiotherapy technique for decades under the incarnation of wedges and missing tissue compensators. Wedges are almost universally constructed as one-dimensional piece-wise continuous modulators of x-ray fields. Compensating filters constructed from molds fabricated using ball end mills are also produced as continuous, two-dimensional x-ray beam modulators (Cunningham et al. 1976; Boyer 1983, Mageras et al. 1991). However, the Ellis-type compensating filter (Ellis, Hall, and Oliver 1959; Hendee and Garciga 1967) is a digital modulator in that both the levels of intensity attenuation and the spatial increments of those levels are made in a small number of discrete steps. The development of computer-driven multileaf collimators (MLCs) (Boyer et al. 1992; Galvin et al. 1992; Galvin, Smith, and Lally 1993; Jordan and Williams 1994; Klein et al. 1995; Frazier et al. 1995; Boyer 1996) has led logically to the modulation of x-ray fields with MLC leaves (Galvin, Chen, and Smith 1993; Chui, LoSasso, and Spirou 1994; Bortfeld et al. 1994). Control systems have been added to the mechanical MLCs that allow sequences of MLC positions to be generated as a function of monitor units delivered by the linear accelerator. The systems operate in two broad categories. On the one hand, there is a mode of operation that provides for continuous MLC motion synchronized with the continuous delivery of dose (Kijewski, Chin, and Bjarngard 1978; Tsai et al. 1998; Wang et al. 1996). On the other hand there are modes of operation that alternate rapidly between leaf motion without beam delivery and beam delivery with the leaves fixed at specified positions (Geis and Boyer 1996). The somewhat inappropriately-named "Static MLC IMRT" or "step-and-shoot IMRT" falls in the latter category, and delivers intensity modulation in both discrete levels of intensity and discrete spatial increments of those levels across the treatment field. Techniques falling in both categories have been used to compute delivery sequences for IMRT. In most cases these sequences have been computed using intensity patterns computed by inverse planning as a separate previous step. In this chapter we will consider details of the Static MLC (SMLC) method.

## Discrete Spatial Resolution Determined by Leaf Width

MLC configurations consist of small computer-controlled leaves that travel in opposed pairs along adjacent tracks. A number of entities, both accelerator vendors as well as independent companies, have developed MLC configurations that can be purchased along with exquisite computer control mechanisms. MLCs are offered by the accelerator vendors configured as built-in tertiary collimators, and configured as replacements for the upper or lower collimating jaws. MLCs are also available as add-on accessories that can collimate over a more restricted field size range. In any case, the fixed number of leaves necessarily implies a fixed number of discrete leaf tracks. The fact that the MLC is constructed from a fixed number of leaves determines a discrete step in the intensity modulation from leaf track to leaf track. The widths of the tracks projected to the plane at isocenter vary considerably. The widest tracks are the outer elements of the Siemens (Siemens Medical Systems, Inc., Concord, CA) system, projecting 6.5 cm in width at the isocenter (other leaves project 1.0 cm). The Elekta (Elekta Oncology Systems, Ltd., Crawley, England) and Varian systems (Varian Medical Systems, Palo Alto, CA) produce leaf tracks that are 1.0 cm and 0.5 cm wide. One variant of the Varian MLC consists of 1-cm leaf tracks produced by 40 pairs of leaves to cover the full range of the 40-cm extent of the treatment field with uniform tracks. Another variant of the Varian MLC contains 40 narrower 0.5-cm leaf tracks in the central 20 cm of the field, flanked on each side by 10 1.0-cm leaf tracks to cover the full 40cm wide field. This system contains a total of 120 leaves with their associated motors and position encoders. The MRC (MRC Systems, GmhH, Heidelberg, Germany) add-on system can produce 1.6mm tracks. The Brainlab m3® micro-MLC (BrainLAB Medical Computersysteme, GmbH, Heimstetten, Germany) can produce 3.0 mm tracks in the center of the field flanked by 4.5 mm tracks left and right of the 3mm leaves and 5.5 mm on the outside of the field. Radionics (Radionics, Inc., Burlington, MA) produces a micro-MLC with 31 pairs of leaves, each projecting a width of 4.0 mm.

To develop a mathematical description we will use an index $l$ to identify a specific leaf track in an MLC. For example, with an 80-leaf MLC consisting of 40 pairs of leaves, $l$ will run from $l = 1$ to $l = 40 = L$ where we have used $L$ to designate the total number of leaf pairs. Using this index, the spatial boundaries of the track of the $l^{th}$ leaf pair in a MLC will be designated as $y_l$ and $y_{l+1}$ in the plane at isocenter perpendicular to the axis of rotation of the collimator. These boundaries are diagramed in figure 1.

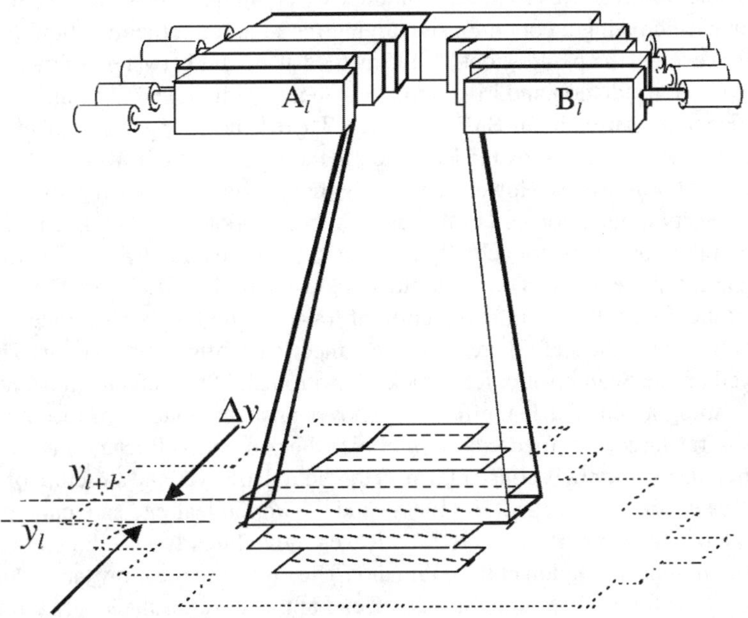


**Figure 1.** Schematic of motor-driven multileaf collimator leaves showing the lateral bounds of the discrete leaf track identified by the index $l$.

When one measures the dose variation across a leaf track, one finds that the dose does not vary as a step function. There are shoulders at the transitions from one dose level to another caused by the penumbra associated with the finite x-ray target size, the tongue-and groove cross section of the leaf, the scatter of radiation in the treatment head and in the patient, and the transport of radiation by the primary and secondary electrons as well as scattered photons generated by the x-ray fluence interacting in the patient. The resulting changes in intensity are not clean step functions but are more complex shapes that are affected by the leaf cross section, the depth in the patient, the size of the electron beam on the x-ray target, and the Source-to-Surface and Source-to-MLC distances (SSD and SCD). In addition, the incident fluence varies across the treatment field.

As the leaves decrease in size the width of the leaf tracks begin to approach the size of the shoulders in the beam intensity. Leaf tracks narrower than about $\Delta y = 1$ mm no longer produce a discrete step in intensity but rather produce a nearly monotonic gradient between intensity levels. Based on the use of sampling theory to relate leaf width to the width of the dose distribution produced by an elemental pencil beam, it has been argued that it makes no sense to use leaf tracks narrower than about 3 to 5mm in high-energy x-ray beams (Bortfeld, Oelfke, and Nill 2000; Otto, Clark, and Huntzinger 2002; Fiveash et al. 2002).

## Discrete Spatial Resolution Along Leaf Travel Direction

It is feasible for the leaves to move continuously along their tracks during an irradiation sequence creating a continuously varying modulation in the direction of the leaf track. However, the step-and-shoot SMLC method alternates between leaf motion increments without irradiation and irradiation increments without leaf motion. A sequence of leaf positions is used in the SMLC method. There is no strong logistical or strategic reason why the steps taken by the leaves along their direction of travel must be a fixed discrete size for all leaves. However, adopting this convention often makes calculation of the intensity modulation and of the leaf sequence simpler than the alternative.

Again the dose does not actually rise instantly at the end of a MLC leaf. As one would expect, there is also a dose shoulder at the end of the MLC leaf. The shape and width of the dose fall-off in the direction of travel of the leaf is also affected by the shape of the end of the leaf. There are two engineering configurations in use. The MLC employed on the Scanditronix Racetrack Microtron and the Siemens linear accelerator has a straight end. The leaf effectively moves on an arc that keeps the end aligned with the x-ray target, or "focused," to minimize the penumbra. Because the leaf moves on an arc, the penumbra is constant across the field. However, the structure of the leaf mechanics becomes complex. The Elekta and the Varian leaf ends are curved, taking the shape of segments from an arc. The leaves move linearly in a direction perpendicular to the axis of rotation of the collimator. The rays from the x-ray target that create the edge of the field roll around this curved end of the leaves as the leaves travel along the leaf tracks. This also produces a uniform penumbra across the entire range of leaf travel. The width of the penumbra observed for a particular MLC design depends on the design of the MLC. Even though one might expect the curved leaf end to produce a broader penumbra, when the leaves are positioned closer to the patient beneath the block collimators, the penumbra is about the same as a focused leaf positioned closer to the x-ray target (Huq et al. 2002).

## Discrete Intensity Levels

One can also require that the intensity modulation be composed of discrete intensity increments. The discrete intensity increments are frequently called "intensity levels" or "dose levels." Discrete intensity levels at discrete positions are produced by the SMLC method. They represent either absolute dose levels, or relative dose levels, or fraction of total monitor units delivered [e.g., fractional monitor units (fMUs)] depending on the context. There is no particular reason for all the level steps to be equal, but the equal step case is the easiest to handle mathematically.

The fluence is built up from the individual rectangular blocks delivered by the increment of monitor units delivered at each set of positions of the leaf pairs. The ideal fluence delivered across the field is then the two-dimensional sum of rectangular blocks of fluence down each leaf track stacked side-by-side.

The areal elements of the pixilated beam intensity patterns computed by inverse planning have been designated as "bixels." By setting the leaf ends to make small square elemental beams at each bixel and scanning the opening in a raster pattern across the area of the desired x-ray field, one could create an intensity pattern of any desired structure within the limitations imposed by the bixels. However, there are more efficient ways to produce the bixel intensity patterns required for intensity-modulated radiation therapy (IMRT). The x-ray intensity for the discrete position and discrete intensity level case is very much like the intensity produced by an ideal Ellis-type compensating filter.

## Combinations Of Delivery Sequences

## Possible Instances For One Maxima

It is fairly obvious that the shape of the one-dimensional profile is determined by the positions of the leaf ends set at each instance of the sequence. It is also easy to see that there is more than one way to achieve a given profile. This is illustrated in figure 2. Panel (a) depicts a simple one-dimensional ideal fluence pattern having a maximum of three levels at its center. Any completely described profile must by definition start at zero intensity and end at zero intensity. In order to reach a single maximum of $N$ levels, the profile must take $M = N$ steps up (going from left to right). Each step up is counted as a setting of the left-hand leaf (assume it is the A-leaf). Then the profile must take $N$ steps down at positions where the B-leaf has been positioned. The six panels (b) through (g) depict six different leaf sequences each consisting of three instance-pairs that all sum up to be the profile in panel (a). Yu et al. (1995) pointed out that any SMLC profile with a single maximum that requires $M$ leaf-end positions could be created by $M!$ unique sequences. For the first A-leaf position one may select $M$ B-leaf positions [for example (b) and (c), (d) and (e), and (f) and (g) in figure 2]. However this leaves only $M-1$ possible settings for the B-leaf for the next A-leaf position, and so forth until the last A-leaf position can be paired with only one B-leaf position. In the case illustrated in figure 2 there are $M! = 3! = 6$ unique sequences. The order in which the leaves are set in these sequences is not considered in this calculation. If you consider all permutations of the orders in which the positions are set there are $M!^2$ possible sequences.

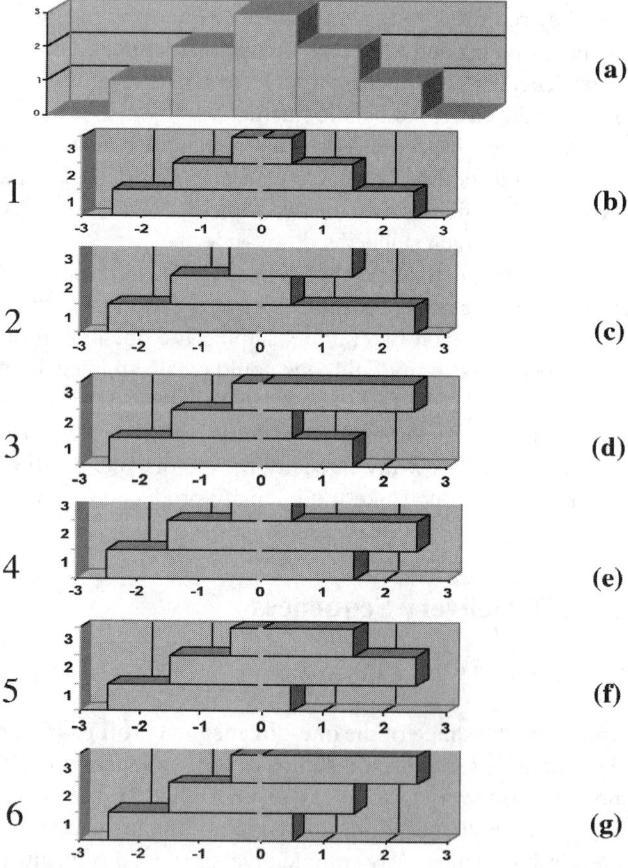

**Figure 2.** Six different sequences (b–g) that deliver the same one-dimensional single peak dose profile (a).

## Possible Instances For Multiple Maxima And Minima

Presumably as the profile becomes more structured, the number of possible sequences will increase. Webb (1998a,b) considered the more general case in which there are multiple maxima. The calculation is illustrated in figure 3. A one-dimensional profile is shown with peak intensities of levels $H_1$ and $H_2$. In general, there can be multiple maxima with levels $H_1$, $H_2$, $H_3$, ..., each peak characterized by a change in gradient of the profile from positive to negative. In general let *Max* be the total number of maxima. Between any two maxima is a minimum that drops to $P_1$, $P_2$, ...; each minimum is characterized by a change in slope of the profile from negative to positive. The two potential minima at the beginning and end of the profile are not counted. Thus there will be *Max*–1 such minima. Webb has shown that the number of physically achievable leaf sequences that produce the discrete profile is given by

$$A = \frac{H_1! \cdot H_2! \cdot H_3! \cdot \quad ... \quad H_{Max}!}{P_1! \cdot P_2! \cdot \quad ... \quad P_{Max-1}!}. \tag{1}$$

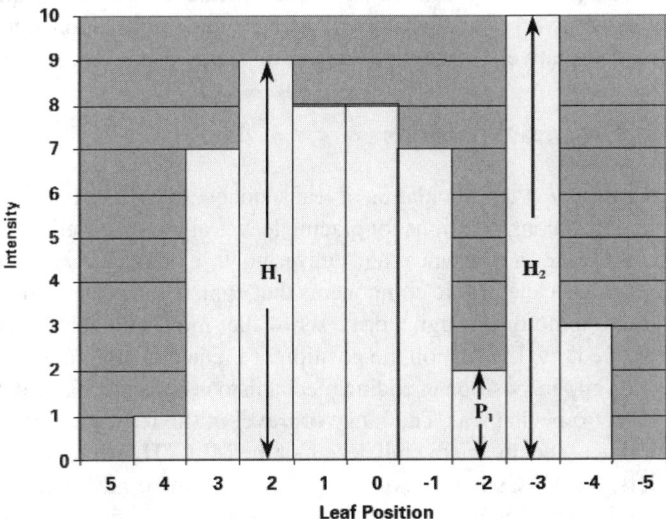


**Figure 3.** Illustration of number of levels in maxima and minima used to compute the number of possible sequences that create a step-and-shoot profile. The number of levels in the two peaks are $H_1$ and $H_2$. The number of levels in the enclosed minimum is $P_1$. The total number of different sequences that will produce the profile can be computed from these parameters.

This can be a very large number of possible step-and-shoot types of sequences that all create the same discrete profile. However, for the one-dimensional case, one can still carry out an exhaustive search for a solution that is, in some sense, optimal. For MLC systems that do not allow interdigitation and leaf end abutment, the number of physically achievable sequences is smaller. The reduction depends on the details of the MLC system. For the sake of formal expression, we will define a value $O_l \leq A$ that equals the number of physically achievable sequences once engineering constraints have been taken into consideration.

## Number Of Possible Combinations For Two Dimensions

When one considers all the leaf tracks together, the number of possible leaf sequences becomes even larger. Webb has shown that the number is

$$T = \prod_{l=1}^{L} O_l \cdot (M!)^L \tag{2}$$

Webb has calculated this value (Webb 1998a,b) for $O_l = 10^4$ typical for an Elekta MLC. In this case $T \approx 10^{94}$. In general, an exhaustive search of all possible two-dimensional leaf sequences for an optimum is impractical. Either the delivery sequences must be computed by some specific algorithm, or an efficient optimization algorithm must be used to search iteratively for an optimum in this large search space.

## Control Of Discrete Positions

Before looking further at the calculation of leaf sequences it will be helpful to consider some of the practical considerations for placing leaves at the specified positions under computer control in the *step* instances and delivering dose in the *shoot* instances. Figure 1 depicts the two basic electronic components that control the position of a leaf. Each leaf is attached to a motor through a drive screw that moves the leaf bi-directionally at a specified speed, ±v. In addition the position of the leaf at any time, x, is encoded. In the Elekta design, the position encoding mechanism is opto-mechanical. In the other systems it is electromechanical. The range of travel of the leaves and the constraints on the leaf motion are set by the overall design of the MLC. These characteristics differ among vendors. As MLCs have developed over time, there have been engineering design changes from one model to another, and this process continues up to the present moment. Therefore it is not possible to generalize about the most recent design specifics offered by any one vendor. One general type of design characteristic is the closest approach a leaf may make to its opposed leaf. This parameter ranges between 10 mm (in the isocenter plane projection) in earlier Elekta designs to 1mm in the Siemens system, to a user-selected value that may be as small as 0.0 mm with segmental delivery and 0.5 mm with dynamic delivery in the Varian designs. Obviously the value of this parameter impacts the delivery sequence. The Siemens and Elekta designs also disallow the interdigitization of a leaf with its opposing next nearest neighbors.

The elimination of interdigitization requires special considerations for leaf positioning in the delivery sequence. In the Varian system, the opposing sets of leaves, designated as "A-leaves" and "B-leaves," are mounted on two carriages that offset the starting points of the leaf extensions into the field. Although this design allows field boundaries to be set across the 40 cm field width with a physical leaf length smaller than the width of the field, it constrains the relative range of leaf extensions on each bank for any given carriage position. It may necessitate the repositioning of the carriages within a delivery sequence to cover the full field size. Currently, the Varian control system has no provision for repositioning a carriage within a field delivery sequence. The Varian sequence must be broken into two or more separate field sequences if the width of the intensity-modulated field exceeds about 15 cm in the direction of the leaf travel.

## Light Field Edge Position With Focused And Rounded Leaves

The projections of the position of leaves, A-leaf and B-leaf, must be accurately encoded for all positions of the leaves across their range of travel. This encoding must give a value of zero at the center of the field and must give an accurate, linear measure of the location of the effective radiation field edge at the end of each leaf. The engineering must be such that the encoding is linear with respect to the radiation field edge position. Once the encoding is linear, the encoded values must be calibrated with some offset and gain to produce a correspondence with the measured radiation field to within some specified accuracy and precision.

The positioning of straight-edged leaves would seem to be simpler than the determination of the effective edge of the field with curved ends. However, engineering details are even complex in this case, especially if the leaves are moving in an arc and the requirement is for the projected leaf position to be at a given location on a plane at the isocenter. The position encoding mechanisms still require calibration at multiple points. Computer look-up tables from which specific values are interpolated during operation are generally used. Although this level of sophisticated computer-control provides the required precision, it incurs an over-head in time needed to execute the command and control cycle for the *step* instances. This overhead contributes to the overall treatment time of the IMRT delivery. If the control systems are not critically damped, the computer controller will "hunt" for a setting that meets a preset accuracy, adding to the control over-head time.

The curved leaf has its own peculiar issues that must be addressed. To discuss this issue and its solution we will use figure 4, a schematic diagram of an MLC leaf with a rounded end placed at three positions. The distance from the x-ray source to the center of the leaf depth is designated as "SCD". The tip of the curve on the leaf end is shown at P at the centerline of the leaf depth. The distance to isocenter is designated as "SAD". The leaf end is shown with a radius of curvature R. In practice, the ends of the leaves are not strictly formed as a pure section of arc, but the approximation is adequate. The leaf is shown in three positions: collimating to the outside of the axis of rotation of the collimator such that $P$ projects to $a$; collimating to the axis of rotation of the collimator such that P projects to d; and collimating across the axis of rotation of the collimator such that $P$ projects to $e$. If $P$ is moved from the position projecting to $a$ to the position projecting to $d$, it moves a linear distance $W'/2$ perpendicular to the axis of collimator rotation at a distance SCD from the x-ray source, whereas its projection moves a distance $W/2$ in the isocenter plane at a distance, SAD. The projection of $W'$ to the isocenter plane is simply

$$W = W' \cdot \frac{SAD}{SCD}.$$

(3)

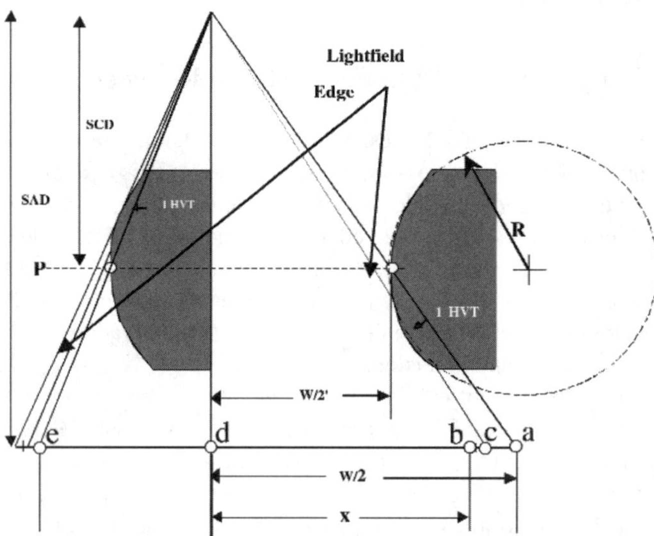


**Figure 4.** Schematic of leaf end showing relation of rays forming light field and radiation field boundaries relative to projection of leaf end. The distance from the field center to the light field is x, and the distance from the field center to the projection of the leaf tip is W/2.

This equation does not describe the position of the light field edge because it uses the tip of the curved leaf end, point $P$, as a reference. It has been shown (Galvin, Smith, and Lally 1993) that the light field width will be up to 5 mm smaller than this geometric dimension when curved leaves define the edge and equation (3) calculates the leaf position. This difference is illustrated by point b in figure 4 at the end of the ray line running from the center of the x-ray target tangent to the curved leaf face in figure 4. Point $b$ is a distance $x$ from the field center in the isocenter plane. There is a nonlinear difference between the light field projection x and the linear leaf displacement $W'/2$. This light field position $x$ is approximately (Boyer and Li 1997)

$$x = \frac{(W/2) \cdot SCD \pm R \cdot SAD \cdot \left( 1 - \dfrac{SAD}{\sqrt{SAD^2 + (W/2)^2}} \right)}{SCD \pm R \dfrac{W}{\sqrt{SAD^2 + (W/2)^2}}}. \tag{4}$$

The relationship is nonlinear with respect to the physical motion of the leaf. The plus sign corresponds to a leaf entering from the right as in figure 4 and the minus sign corresponds to a leaf entering from the left. Using this relationship reduces the size of the deviations between the selected leaf position and the light field projection of any leaf to a maximum of about 1 mm. This nonlinear relationship is currently accounted for by the leaf position encoding of the Varian MLC using a look-up table.

## Radiation Field Edge Offset

The edge of the light field does not correspond exactly to the effective edge of the radiation field. The x-ray fluence falls to 50% (relative to the value just inside the open portion of the field) along a ray line through a chord of the arc of the rounded leaf end that is equal to one half-value-layer (HVL). In figure 4, the ray ending at c is close to such a line. The attenuating chord of arc also rolls around the curved leaf end as the leaf is moved from one side of the field to the other. Thus the x-ray field is wider than the light field by a small value that is nearly constant for all leaves and for all positions of the leaves across the field. Calculation of the projection of the 1 HVT (half-value thickness) chord position puts it less than 1 mm outside the light field. More often than not, the MLC position specification is calibrated to correspond to the light field read out and the radiation field offset either ignored or included in the dose calculation algorithm.

One method for determining the offset between the light and radiation field is to measure the radiation beam profile relative to the light field using film or a diode detector. This measurement is difficult to make and may not result in a practical value. Occasionally within an SMLC delivery sequence one must abut two gap settings against each other in a leaf track. When this occurs, it is desirable to minimize the overdose or the under-dose that occurs at the junction. This requirement is a more practical criterion for determining the offset value. To determine the offset value one measures the radiation delivered along a line down the middle of a leaf track with film while abutting two gaps. One makes multiple measurements for minute differences between the specified positions of the leaves at the abutment point (see figure 5). To produce these curves multiple small fields were abutted along the track with offsets between the radiation field and the light field of 0.3 mm, 0.5 mm, 0.6 mm, and 0.7 mm as indicated in figure 5. In general one will observe both an over-dose and an under-dose at the juncture. The difference that produces the least over- and under-dose (figure 5c) is the most practical offset between the radiation field and the light field for IMRT.

This value should be used in the algorithm that computes the delivery sequence as an offset between the positions for the leaf ends entered into the control file and the positions one needs to place the effective radiation field boundaries at the leaf end. One must be careful with the sign convention used by the algorithm lest one add a double offset rather than removing the offset.

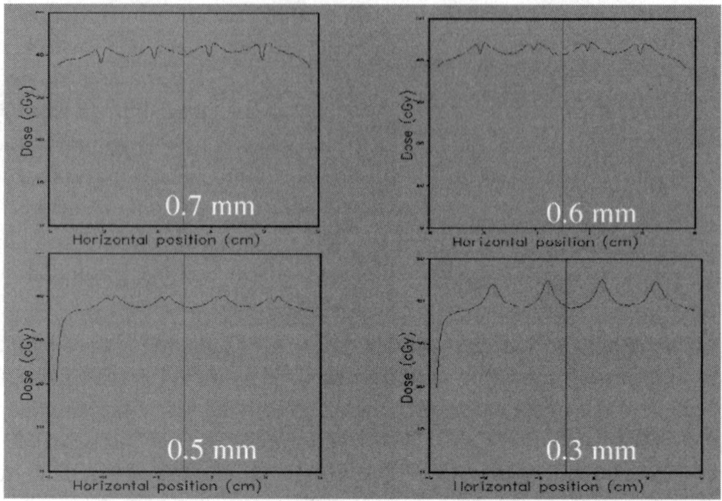


**Figure 5.** Film dosimetry profiles down center of a leaf track with small fields abutted with the indicated offsets between them.

## Control Of Discrete Monitor Units

The delivery of dose in a medical linear accelerator is controlled by a transmission parallel plate ionization chamber. The charge collected by the ionization chamber is measured by a solid-state electrometer. The electrometer and its associated digitization circuit must also be properly operating to provide monitor unit increments that are linear and a zero offset sufficiently small to be negligible with respect to the small increments of monitor units used to define a *shoot* instance in an SMLC IMRT delivery sequence. The precision of the Siemens and Elekta systems is one monitor unit (MU). Increments of monitor units less than 1.0 MU cannot be specified. The precision of the Varian system is one centi-monitor unit (cMU). The smallest monitor unit increment that can be specified is 0.01 MU.

### Electrometer Zero

An ionization current made up of pulses a few microseconds wide with amplitudes on the order of nano-Coulombs is produced by x-ray pulses passing through the transmission chamber in the linear accelerator. The circuitry that amplifies and digitizes the ionization current pulses from the transmission ionization chamber contains a series of solid-state electrometers. The electrometers are high-impedance, high-gain transistor circuits. Field service engineering support or the responsible physicist should verify that the electrometer zero is set as carefully as possible. This procedure is usually described by the vendor. The details depend on the design options selected for the particular medical linear accelerator. Usually the gain of an amplifying electrometer is set digitally or by an analog variable resistor to calibrate the dose per monitor unit. The pulse train amplified by this electrometer is integrated by a capacitor. The subsequent stage of the monitor unit electronics will be the digitization circuits. The voltage on the integrating capacitor is usually fed to a form of a Schmitt trigger circuit that fires when the voltage on the capacitor reaches a preset level. When the trigger circuit flip-flops, it produces a voltage that discharges the integrating capacitor to reset it to a zero value. The voltage used to discharge the integrating capacitor can be adjusted. If it is adjusted too high or too low, the dose as a function of monitor units will not pass exactly through zero. This effect can accumulate with the *step-and-shoot* method when many very small increments of dose are used in the delivery sequence.

## Electrometer End Effect

The classical term for the zero offset for a dose integration system is "End Effect." The standard method for measuring the end effect is a multiple exposure measurement. The method was established for calibrating $^{60}$Co teletherapy units whose source was driven into the "on" position by a pneumatic cylinder. The travel time of the source moving from the "off" position to the "on" position when a switch started the exposure, and then from the "on" position to the "off" position when an electrical timer ended the exposure, could be great enough to affect the dose delivered by short exposures. To measure the end effect, one selects a small number of monitor units $MU_1$ and a larger number of monitor units that is an integer multiple of the shorter exposure, $MU_2 = N \cdot MU_1$. One places an external ionization chamber in the x-ray field using standard calibration conditions and integrates charge with an external electrometer. One integrates over $N$ exposures using the smaller monitor unit setting. One collects charge as well as the small error multiple times when making the $N$ multiple exposures,

$$Q_1 = N \cdot MU_1 \frac{dQ}{dMU} + N \cdot \varepsilon. \tag{5}$$

One then sets an exposure $MU_2$ and collects charge over the single long exposure that contains only one end effect increment,

$$Q_2 = MU_2 \cdot \frac{dQ}{dMU} + \varepsilon = N \cdot MU_1 \cdot \frac{dQ}{dMU} + \varepsilon. \tag{6}$$

Subtracting equation (6) from equation (5) one finds the value of the end effect,

$$\varepsilon = \frac{Q_1 - Q_2}{N - 1}.$$  (7)

The charge digitization circuit should be adjusted to minimize the end effect. One will probably find slightly different optimal settings for each x-ray mode on multiple energy machines.

## Computer Control Of Delivery Of SMLCs

SMLC delivery sequences are simply extensions of the standard method of setting a field shape with the MLC (Du et al. 1994) and then delivering a set number of monitor units. However, the treatment sequence may contain a dozen or several score fields. In principle, the operator could draw each field into the MLC controller using computer operations available at the controller, set monitor units for each field, and initiate the treatment field manually. However, the time required to execute the large number of manual steps would lead to treatment times on the order of hours and would be prone to operator error. Consequently, computer-controlled systems have been provided to carry out the steps more efficiently and more accurately. These systems are under constant engineering revisions, so that generalizations specific to a given vendor are likely to become rapidly obsolete. However, the overall outline of the control system will appear similar to the generalized schematic in figure 6. The major components consist of the server that stores the patient-specific delivery sequence files in a database, a computer that interacts with the operator, a linear accelerator control computer, and a separate processor that is dedicated to controlling the MLC. The major components may in fact contain multiple processor chips at different levels of measurement and control.

## Anthropomorphic Design

One approach to automating the delivery sequence is to design a computer system to automate the functions of the operator. That is, delivery of an IMRT field sequence is viewed as automated operation of the linac control console that is used to deliver a static field. This will typically involve an external information management system (e.g., record and verify (R&V) system) that remotely controls the linac console. The console in turn communicates with an MLC controller subsystem. With this configuration the operator initiates the delivery of SMLC sequence, the R&V system sends the leaf settings and MU settings to the linac console one delivery instance at a time, replacing step-by-step human operations. Using the specifications of the MLC aperture for the step instance, the MLC controller moves each leaf into position. Comparators indicate the proximity of the leaves to their target positions. The MLC

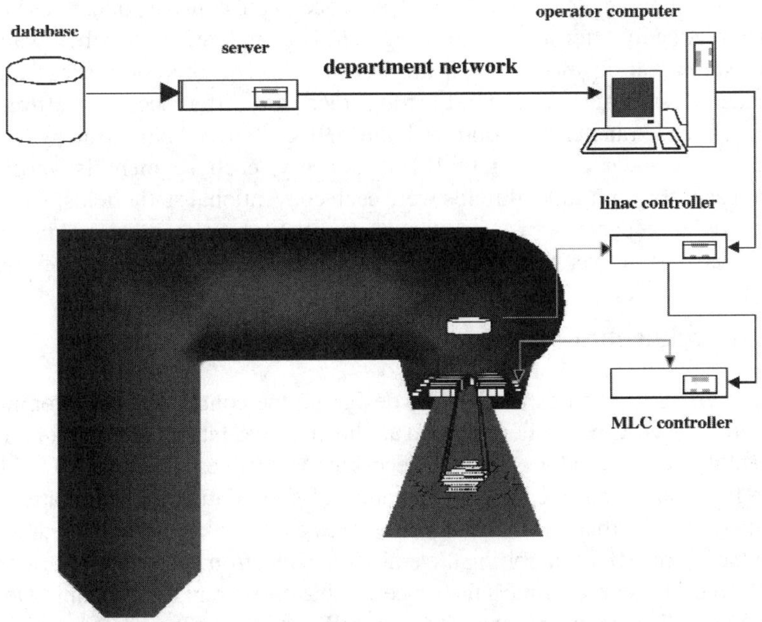



**Figure 6.** Schematic of MLC control system integrated with information management system and file server.

controller interrogates each comparator sequentially until all are within a preset tolerance. During this time, the other linac setup parameters are also set (if they are not already at the required setting) and verified. When the leaves and other linac settings are in position and verified, the linac controller automatically initiates the delivery of the increment of MUs associated with the shoot instance. The R&V system retrieves all machine parameters for the field just delivered and then initiates the next static field delivery. This process can be general, where automatic leaf/linac setup and beam initiation occurs even if parameters such as gantry, couch or collimator angle must be changed between fields. The process continues until all the apertures and their associated MUs have been delivered. The initial systems developed by Siemens and Elekta are generally designed along these lines. In the Siemens design, the automatic field sequence delivery mode suspends radiation during the step instances by de-phasing the RF in the wave guide with the gun pulses rather that turning off the gun and RF. This prevents acceptance of the electron pulses by the first accelerating cavity, but may allow some residual dark current within the wave-guide. An increase in IMRT delivery speed of the Siemens system has been achieved by customizing the control packets downloaded from the R&V system to the linac console. This modification takes advantage of the fact that, between segments within a field, only leaf positions will need to change. This reduces the amount of data to be sent and also the number of parameters to be verified after the beam is turned off. Also, since the order of segments is prede-

fined, segment parameters can be sent in advance to the console so that the MLC can
be set immediately after the previous segment is completed, rather than waiting for
the next set of leaf positions to be sent. So while this sort of system is essentially an
automated version of manual field setting, there are differences in the timing and
amount of data transfer that optimize the delivery speed. Note that with such a
segment-by-segment approach to IMRT delivery, each segment is verified and
recorded as if the multitude of fields were each conventional static fields. It should be
mentioned that, especially with a system such as this where segments are individually
downloaded, set and verified, efforts are made to minimize the number of segments.

## System Architecture

A gain in efficiency can be realized by designing the control system to optimize its
operation. The MLC controller can load all the instances into its memory upon initial-
ization of the sequence along with the necessary MU values. The total MU setting for
a given field can be checked by the operator before initiating the automatic delivery
of the sequence for that field. The *step* instances can be taken with the beam held off
by de-phasing the RF or inhibiting the emission of electron pulses with a gridded gun.
The MLC controller then directs the process using only a register containing the accumulated MUs. This register in the MLC controller is frequently updated (with a period
measured in milliseconds) by the linac controller. The master MLC control processor
assigns leaf positions to additional controllers that operate independently in parallel
while continuously polling the positions of each leaf to assess its status. These additional processors set the direction and speed of the motors so that the leaves move to
the desired position without overshooting the target, put the leaves in a braked condition when they arrive at the target position, and notify the master MLC control
processor that the leaf is in the target position. The MLC controller then allows the
linac controller to initiate the delivery of dose pulses. The arrival of these pulses at the
transmission ionization chamber results in the accumulation of values in the dose accumulation register. When the register reaches the value assigned to the current shoot
instance, the MLC controller inhibits the linac controller from delivering radiation and
reassigns the next set of leaf positions to the leaf positioning processors. The major
difference between the control system approach and the anthropomorphic approach
is that the MLC controller is the "conductor" of the control system approach process
once the sequence for the current field has been initiated. With the anthropomorphic
scenario, the MLC controller is essentially a slave to the linac controller, setting leaves
on command and verifying their positions to the linac console. Another important
distinction is that with the control system approach, a set number of MUs will be delivered within a field, where these total MUs are divided up between segments by the
MLC controller. The total number of MUs is guaranteed by the beam controller to be
correct, but there can be some uncertainty in the MU delivered per segment because
of the feedback mechanism (this is discussed further in the section *Effect Of Control
Loop Delay*). With the anthropomorphic design philosophy, the MU for each segment

is set independently and will be correct to the limit of the beam control system, but at the price of longer delivery time per segment.

## Effects Of Control System On Delivery Times

The details of the control system determine how quickly a leaf pattern can be set and then an MU increment delivered. This basic cycle time is determined by the means by which information is delivered to the MLC controller, how quickly the MLC leaves can be set and verified, how quickly a shoot instance can be initiated and terminated, and the time required to log the delivery of the instance. Either the speed of the leaf motion or the computer control over-head can be the rate limiting part of the cycle. The means by which the accelerator beam is activated also plays a major role. If the wave guide must be repowered for each MU increment, an additional over-head is added to the cycle time. Up to this point, the Siemens and Elekta systems cycle at a rate of about one step instance and one shoot instance every 7 seconds. With a rapid magnetron switching circuit, this time can be reduced by about 50%. The Varian system cycles at a rate of about one step-instance paired with one shoot-instance in about 1 second.

In addition, the MLC controller may control the secondary collimators. For most cases, the secondary collimators are kept fixed during the step-and-shoot IMRT deliveries. However, the secondary collimators plus additional backup diaphragms, such as those in the Elekta system, must be moved synchronously with the MLC leaves during each step of delivery. The control overhead for this control may also increase the time of delivery. For Siemens and Elekta systems, the time for driving the MLC leaves and other tertiary collimators is the rate limiting action of the step-and-shoot cycle time. This is in contrast to the Varian systems where the beam is turned off and on so rapidly that the mechanical motion is the rate-limiting portion of the cycle time. All vendors are continually upgrading their designs to reduce the cycle time.

## Effect Of Control Loop Delay

The control loop cycle time and the details of the data flow within that loop are important to the accuracy of the first and last instances in the delivery sequence. At the beginning of the delivery sequence, the leaves are set to the first aperture pattern. Radiation is initiated. If the number of MUs is very small in each instance, then slightly more than the specified discrete MU increment may be delivered in the first instance before the system can respond to interrupt radiation delivery. Thereafter, the beam is interrupted at regular intervals delivering a uniform small dose increment. However, at the last instance, the accelerator controller terminates the beam when the total number of set MUs have been delivered, not by the MLC controller. If a small over-dose occurred in the first instance, then the accelerator controller will terminate the sequence before the full final increment can be delivered in the last instance. This effect can be demonstrated by creating a test sequence consisting of a small number of subfields placed alongside one another (see figure 7). By delivering the fields at the maximum dose rate with a very small MU specified for each field, one can observe an over-dose in the first field (leaf-hand bar labeled 1 in figure 7) and an under-dose in the last field (right-hand bar labeled 5 in figure 7) using film to record the exposures. To better understand this effect, consider the details of delivery of figure 7. It was acquired with a *step-and-shoot* delivery file written to deliver 1.00 MU in each of the 1-cm wide strips by setting control points at 100 cMU, 200 cMU, 300 cMU, 400 cMU, and 500 cMU. The dose rate was set for 400 MU/min. During delivery, MLC controller received updates of the delivered dose every 50 milliseconds. A step-by-step description of the sequence of events is given in table 1. At this dose rate, the MLC was updated every 33 cMU. This is an ideal figure used in this example to illustrate the principle. Small variations in the electronics, calibrations, etc., will cause the update packets to vary by 1 or 2 cMU. Exactly 50 milliseconds after the beam is initiated, the dose accumulation register in the MLC controller was updated to 33 cMU (see first line in table 1). The MLC controller determined that the first 100-cMU control point had not been reached and allowed the irradiation to proceed for another 50 milliseconds. After the third update, the MLC controller accumulator was only 1 cMU short of the control point, but the MLC controller allowed the next packet to be delivered. When the next packet arrived, the controller determined that the goal of the first instance had been achieved (and indeed exceeded), and it inhibited the beam while the leaves were moved to the next strip (fifth line in table 1). By noting how cMU accumulated in the third column of table 1, one sees how the next three strips received approximately the correct dose. Then in the fifth strip, at the bottom of table 1, when the total dose of 500 cMU was reached, all exposure was terminated, leaving the dose in the last strip short by about 30%. In practice, using a lower dose rate can eliminate this effect. Then the packets will arrive in the MLC controller accumulator in approximately 8 cMU increments leading to a delivery error of about 4% in the first and last instance. Furthermore, the increments required within an instance in typical clinical cases are higher, leading to errors in only the first and last instance on the order of 1%, an insignificant effect. The dose rate at which the accelerator is set to run has a small effect on the time required to deliver *step-and-shoot* sequences that contain small MU increments since the majority of the time in the delivery cycle is occupied by the data management and process over-head.

## Computer Files For Delivery Of SMLCs

The files that control the SMLC process are often accessible in an ASCII format. However, there is no common file format for the computer files that create an SMLC IMRT among the different medical linear accelerator vendors. The concept of the SMLC sequence made of up instances is reflected in the format of the files available.

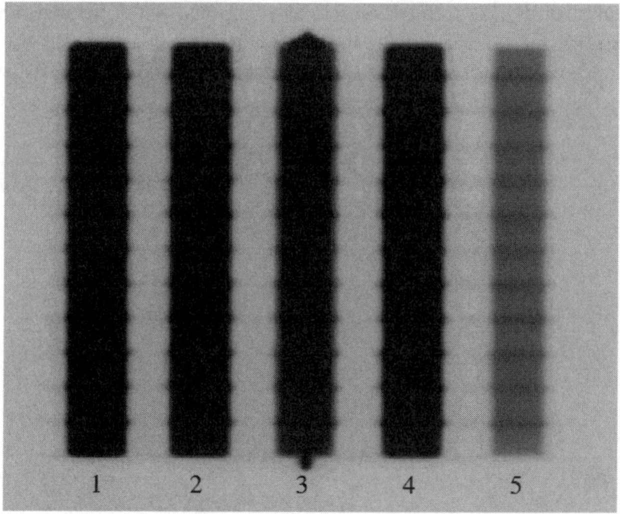



**Figure 7.** Film image of a 5-aperture step-and-shoot sequence irradiated at a high dose rate with 1 MU delivered through each aperture.

## Leaf Sequence File Structure

The data file that determines the treatment delivery sequence is depicted conceptually in table 2. At the $2m^{th}$ shoot-instance, the required pattern of leaves is given by the coordinates $x_{m,1}^A$, $x_{m,2}^A$, $x_{m,3}^A$,..., $x_{m,L}^A$ for the A-leaves and $x_{m,1}^B$, $x_{m,2}^B$, $x_{m,3}^B$,..., $x_{m,L}^B$ for the B-leaves. The leaf pattern represented by each row in table 2 is equivalent to a single static MLC aperture file. The aggregate of the leaf patterns constitutes the MLC treatment sequence. Note that every odd numbered row is a step in the step-and-shoot process. The fractional monitor unit, $fMU_i$, is zero in the first instance (first row of table 2) causing the first MLC aperture to be set with the x-ray beam inhibited. In the second instance (second row) the leaf positions are unchanged from the first row causing the aperture to remain unchanged whereas the fMU value changes to the first nonzero value, causing the beam to be uninhibited. Radiation is delivered until a number of MUs are accumulated equal to the product of MUs set for the field at the console with the value $fMU_1$. When this occurs, the beam is inhibited again marking the end of the second instance. The elapsed time since the initiation of the process will be 1 to 10 seconds depending on the details of the delivery system. At the beginning of the third instance a second aperture is specified in line 3 of table 2. The process continues with a repetition of the sequence of events that occurred in the first two instances until all the dose increments have been delivered through their specified apertures at the end of the last line of the table. A log is kept of the sequence that includes deviations between the target aperture and the set aperture and any interruptions caused by system errors or operator intervention.

**Table 1.** An Outline of an Extreme Example of a Step-and-Shoot Sequence Showing the Origin of Monitor Unit Delivery Errors in the First and last Instance. The second column contains the centi-monitor units (cMU) that appear in the MLC dose register every 50 milliseconds for a delivery sequence using an accelerator repetition frequency that produces 400 MU/min

| Control Point | cMU packet | Accumulated cMU | Total in Strip |
|---|---|---|---|
| | 33 | 033 | |
| | 33 | 066 | |
| | 33 | 099 | |
| 100 | 33 | 132 | 132 |
| Step to next strip | | | |
| | 33 | 165 | |
| | 33 | 198 | |
| 200 | 33 | 231 | 99 |
| Step to next strip | | | |
| | 33 | 264 | |
| | 33 | 297 | |
| 300 | 33 | 330 | 99 |
| Step to next strip | | | |
| | 33 | 363 | |
| | 33 | 396 | |
| 400 | 33 | 429 | 99 |
| Step to next strip | | | |
| | 33 | 462 | |
| | 33 | 495 | |
| Beam off at 500 | 05 | 500 | 71 |

**Table 2.** A representation of the Data in Leaf Sequence Specification File for a Step-and-Shoot Technique. The first column gives the instance number in the sequence, the second column gives the fractional monitor units to be delivered in that instance, the third and fourth columns give the positions of the leaves to be set before the monitor units are delivered, and the last column indicates whether the instance contains a *step* (positioning of the leaves) or *shoot* (delivery of the fractional monitor units)

| Instance | Fractional MU | Leaves of A Carriage | Leaves on B Carriage | |
|---|---|---|---|---|
| 1 | 0.00 | $X^A_{1,1}, X^A_{1,2}, X^A_{1,3}, \ldots, X^A_{1,L}$ | $X^B_{1,1}, X^B_{1,2}, X^B_{1,3}, \ldots, X^B_{1,L}$ | Step |
| 2 | $fMU_1$ | $X^A_{1,1}, X^A_{1,2}, X^A_{1,3}, \ldots, X^A_{1,L}$ | $X^B_{1,1}, X^B_{1,2}, X^B_{1,3}, \ldots, X^B_{1,L}$ | Shoot |
| 3 | 0.00 | $X^A_{2,1}, X^A_{2,2}, X^A_{2,3}, \ldots, X^A_{2,L}$ | $X^B_{2,1}, X^B_{2,2}, X^B_{2,3}, \ldots, X^B_{2,L}$ | Step |
| 4 | $fMU_2$ | $X^A_{2,1}, X^A_{2,2}, X^A_{2,3}, \ldots, X^A_{2,L}$ | $X^B_{2,1}, X^B_{2,2}, X^B_{2,3}, \ldots, X^B_{2,L}$ | Shoot |
| $\bullet$ | $\bullet$ | $\bullet$ | $\bullet$ | $\bullet$ |
| $\bullet$ | $\bullet$ | $\bullet$ | $\bullet$ | $\bullet$ |
| $\bullet$ | $\bullet$ | $\bullet$ | $\bullet$ | $\bullet$ |
| 2M-2 | $fMU_{M-1}$ | $X^A_{M-1,1}, X^A_{M-1,2}, X^A_{M-1,3}, \ldots, X^A_{M-1,L}$ | $X^B_{M-1,1}, X^B_{M-1,2}, X^B_{M-1,3}, \ldots, X^B_{M-1,L}$ | Shoot |
| 2M-1 | 0.00 | $X^A_{M,1}, X^A_{M,2}, X^A_{M,3}, \ldots, X^A_{M,L}$ | $X^B_{M,1}, X^B_{M,2}, X^B_{M,3}, \ldots, X^B_{M,L}$ | Step |
| 2M | $fMU_M$ | $X^A_{M,1}, X^A_{M,2}, X^A_{M,3}, \ldots, X^A_{M,L}$ | $X^B_{M,1}, X^B_{M,2}, X^B_{M,3}, \ldots, X^B_{M,L}$ | Shoot |

## Storage And Retrieval Of Leaf Sequence Files

The files associated with each treatment field must be placed on the server in a database such that the operator can retrieve them conveniently. Each vendor of medical linear accelerators has addressed this requirement with a specific software tool. The general problem of transferring information between different treatment planning systems and the database on the server of the different treatment delivery systems has been addressed by the development of a Digital Imaging and Communications in Medicine standard for radiotherapy (DICOM-RT). The standard makes it convenient to interface different systems, but it adds a layer of complexity to the software systems. To transfer files using DICOM-RT, the files must be translated by the vendor of the treatment planning system from its own internal proprietary format to a format compliant with the DICOM-RT standard. After transfer, within the treatment delivery file server software, the files must again be translated from the DICOM-RT format to the internal proprietary format of the treatment delivery system.

The DICOM-RT standard has a complex structure, but a brief description is in order here. The basic diagnostic DICOM records are based on a hierarchical structure appropriate for diagnostic imaging. The levels of the hierarchy are: (I) Patient, (II) Study, (III) Series, (IV) Image. The radiotherapy extension of DICOM (shown schematically in figure 8) applies a course of therapy as a Study and adds five objects to the DICOM structure that are not included in the diagnostic standard: (1) Radiotherapy Dose; (2) Radiotherapy Structure Set; (3) Radiotherapy Image; (4) Radiotherapy Plan; and (5) Radiotherapy Treatment Record. The Radiotherapy Plan specifications contain an External Beam module that provides for a description of dynamic and SMLC treatment sequences. The relevant portion of the structure of the External Beam module is given in table 3. The Beam module contains all the setup information such as beam energy, gantry angle, asymmetric jaw settings, collimator angle, and total monitor units to be delivered. In DICOM parlance, monitor units are called "Meter Set". Similarly, instances are designated as "Control Points". The structure of the Control Points within the DICOM-RT Beam Module is essentially the same as the SMLC delivery instance structure described in table 2. Each control point in table 3 corresponds to one line in table 2.

## Auto-Sequencing

The vendors have made provisions for delivering a super-sequence consisting of multiple beams. The data for each beam similar to the contents of table 1 are automatically transferred from the server to the linear accelerator controller. Some provision must be made to avoid collisions between the gantry and the patient or patient couch. One way of ensuring that collisions will not occur is for the movement of the gantry from one angle to the next to be inhibited until the operator activates a "dead-man" switch. The initiation of each beam is delayed until the operator activates a "beam-on" button. Alternatively, a "dry run" can be performed where the gantry and couch are set to the positions for each beam prior to a super-sequence being initiated. In practice, it is common for the gantry to be moved automatically but for the couch to be moved by the operator. In any case, all the beam delivery information is automatically transferred from the server to the linac controller, thereby reducing the chance of operator errors and improving the operational efficiency of the process. IMRT sequences can be embedded in the beam data as well. The auto-sequencing provision provides for rapid delivery of IMRT in the SMLC mode as well as in the dynamic delivery mode. It also provides for creating sequences of individual apertures and arcs. Thus, this level of automation enables a rich and flexible spectrum of opportunities for special treatment processes.

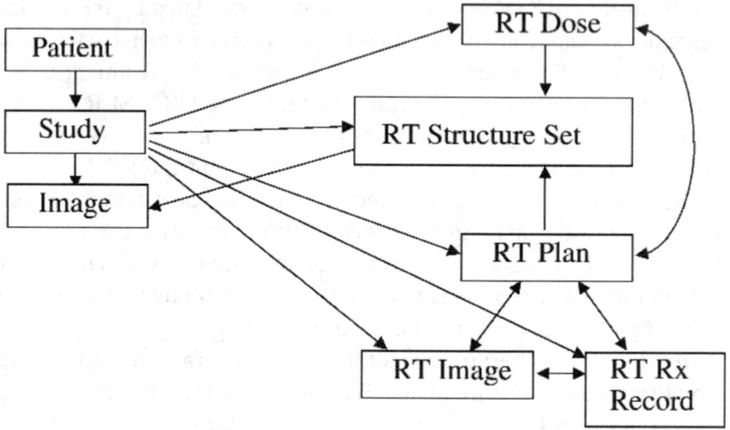


**Figure 8.** Schematic of DICOM-RT image object definition.

## Computation Of SMLC Sequence By Leaf Track

Given that one has at hand the technical means to create SMCL leaf sequences, and given that there are multiple sequences (in fact, thousands) possible for richly structured intensity-modulated beams, what is the best way to determine a leaf sequence to deliver a desired beam? Methods by which arbitrary x-ray beam intensity profiles may be produced through dynamic jaws or MLCs have been extensively investigated (Convery and Rosenbloom 1992; Galvin, Chen, and Smith 1993; Bortfeld et al. 1994; Chui, LoSasso, and Spirou 1994; Spirou and Chui 1994; Stein et al. 1994; Svensson, Källman, and Brahme 1994; Yu et al. 1995; van Santvoort and Heijmen 1996; Geis and Boyer 1996; Ma et al. 1998, 1999; Webb et al. 1997; Webb 1998a,b). The leaf setting methods have been investigated that use exhaustive searches, optimization iteration, linear programming, or direct best computation to minimize the total beam delivery time. As will be covered in this section, the determination of a leaf sequence is further complicated by physical constraints of the MLC and sometimes by strategies to correct for effects such as leaf leakage and the tongue-and-groove effect.

**Table 3.** Schematic Outline of the Data in a DICOM-RT File for a Leaf Sequence. The data begins with accelerator settings for all instances in the sequence. The instances following correspond to the lines in table 2

Beam

    Beam Name
    Radiation Type
    Beam Limiting Device
    (MLC, Collim.)
    Wedge
    Compensator
    Bolus
    Block
    Applicator
    Final Cumulative Meter Set
    # of Control Points
    Control Point

        Beam Energy
        Gantry Angle
        Rotation Direction
        Collimator Settings
        MLC Positions
        Cumulative Meter Set

    Control Point

        Beam Energy
        Gantry Angle
        Rotation Direction
        Collimator Settings
        MLC Positions
        Cumulative Meter Set .

## Determination Of Paired-Point Sequence

Consider first the strategy of determining the optimum leaf sequence for each leaf track independently, and then stepping through the sequences all at the same time. One should select a method that computes in some sense the optimal leaf sequence. Consider the simple case in figure 2. Figure 2b depicts what has been called the "close-in" technique. The first leaf-pair setting encompasses the entire width of the profile, and then succeeding settings close in on the maximum. When multiple maxima occur, the algorithm closes in on each one successively. Figure 2g depicts what has been called the "sweeping window" technique. The leaves form a gap that starts on the left side of the field and sweeps to the right side. The width of the gap is varied from step to step to produce the required maxima and minima.

To optimize a leaf sequence, methods have been investigated to minimize the delivery time, Siochi (1999) has considered two criteria for maximizing the efficiency of a sequence. One is based on the standard deviation of the gap sizes about the mean gap size of gaps for a given leaf pair. Another criterion is the minimization of the total travel of the leading leaf. Webb concluded that the sweeping window technique minimizes this standard deviation and also minimizes the travel of the leading leaf.

The algorithm that generates the sweeping window sequence is quite simple. Figure 9 depicts a simple example of an intensity pattern. This pattern was computed for the anterior field from a clinical case that treated a relatively small prostate. This example will be used to illustrate one of the step-and-shoot leaf sequencing methods. The intensity in a 9-cm × 5-cm field is expressed using eight nonzero discrete intensity levels, 10 through 80. Five 1-cm wide leaf tracks (numbered 18, 19, 20, 21, and 22 in figure 9) are to be used to generate the intensity pattern. The delivery sequence is first determined independently for each profile. We will use the profile required of leaf pair 19 in this example. The discrete intensity profile for leaf track 19 is shown separately in figure 10. One assumes that one will modulate the intensity along the profile by sweeping the leading leaf, 19B and the following leaf, 19A, from left to right along the X-axis. The first step in this procedure has already been taken; divide the total relative beam intensity into a number of equal intervals of width $\Delta\Phi$ as indicated in the illustration. In this case $\Delta\Phi = 10$. The second step in the procedure is to find the x-positions at which the profile passes through the centers of these increment bins as one traces the profile from left to right. These points are indicated by circles in figure 10a. The algorithm requires that an even number of such points be found. The third step is to divide the coordinate points into two groups. One group consists of those points lying on an ascending slope of the profile where there is a positive gradient (open circles in figure 10a), and the other group consists of those points lying on a descending slope of the profile where there is a negative gradient (filled circles in figure 10a). The fourth step is to rank order the points in each group as indicated with the black and white numbers in figure 10a. The numbers indicated are the $m$-index for the sequence for the $l = 19$ pair of leaves. Pairing together the coordinates of equal rank order and assigning the coordinates to the A- and B-leaves produces the desired leaf sequence, $\left\{ x_{l,m}^{A}, x_{l,m}^{B} \right\}$. The number of steps required to create the trajectories will not be the same for all leaf track profiles that make up a field. Steps must be added to the shorter sequences with the leaves abutting beneath a jaw at one end of the profile and/or the other so that all sequences for a field will have the same number of *step-and-shoot* instance pairs. A plot of the sequence derived from figure 10a is given in figure 10b. One can verify that the sequence will produce the desired profile by counting the total accumulated MU in each column of 10b.

When the sequences for each leaf track are combined, each step instance forms a treatment field consisting of one or more apertures. As the sequence evolves, these apertures form an irregularly shaped window that sweeps across the area to be irradiated. For this example, the 20 apertures required to deliver all five tracks are shown in figure 11 along with the fractional meter set used in each associated shoot instance. The $l = 19$ track is indicated by a dashed line in figure 11. This sequence of apertures is displayed for the operator during the delivery process. By examining the apertures

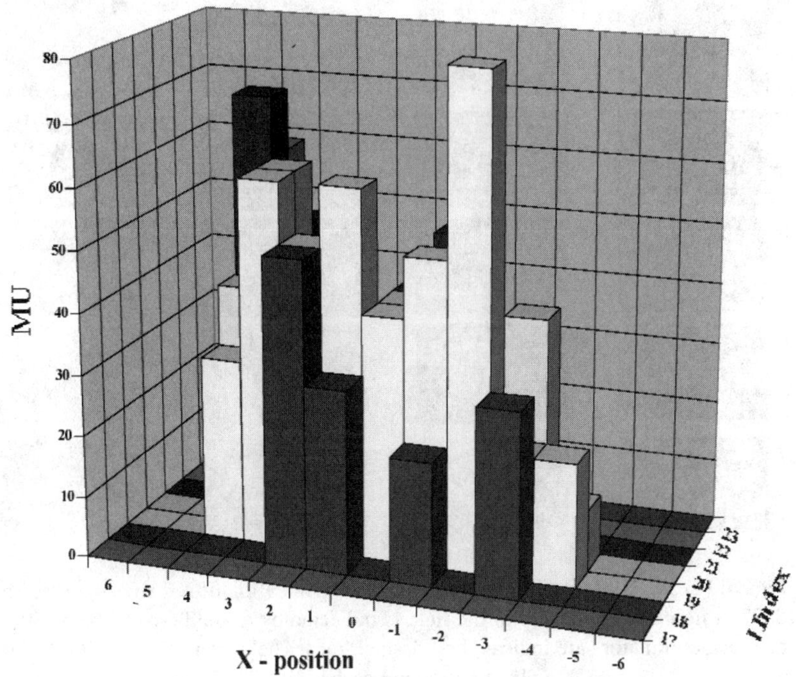



**Figure 9.** Depiction of an intensity pattern in MU units in a small x-ray field. The MLC leaf tracks are indicated by the indices 18–23.

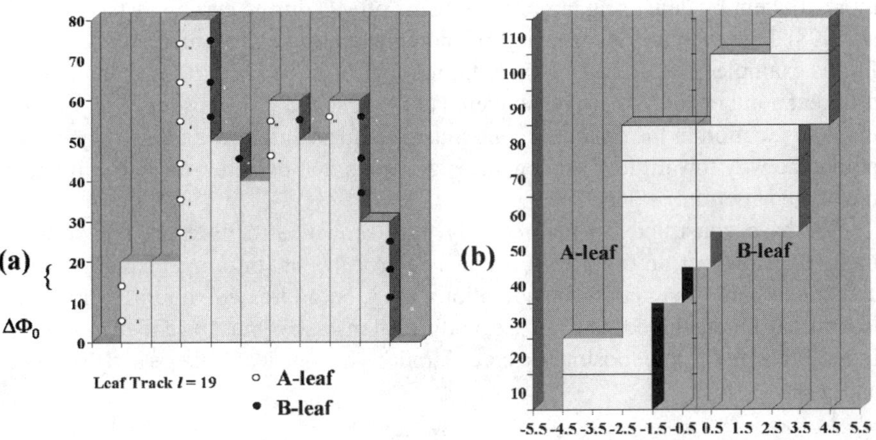



**Figure 10.** Method of leaf-sequence algorithm for the l = 19 track from figure 9. Panel (a) indicates the means by which the sequence of leaf ends is determined. Panel (b) indicates the resulting leaf sequence as a function of monitor units.

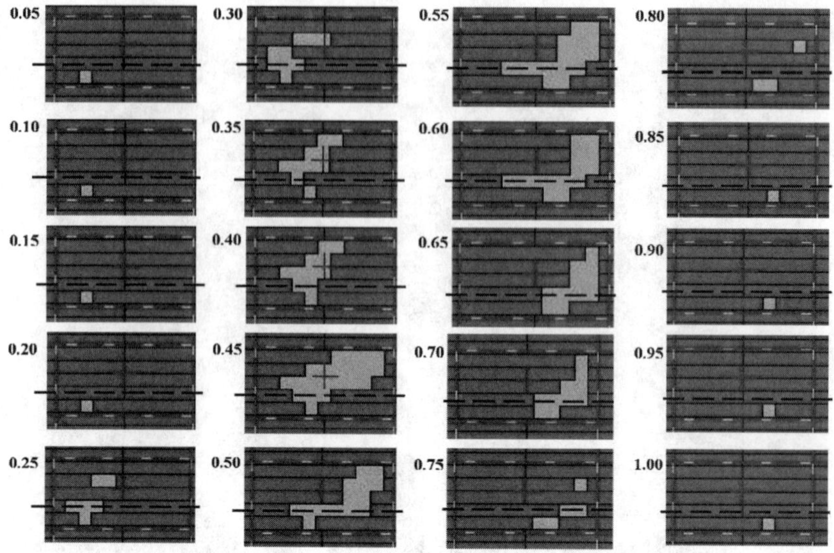

**Figure 11.** Sweeping window generated by the generation of sequences for leaves 18–22 in figure 9. The center of the field is indicated by a small cross. The positions of the block collimators are indicated by dashed lines. The center of track 19 is indicated by a horizontal dashed line.

in figure 11 one notices that the first four apertures are identical and the last four apertures are identical. These steps can be delivered as one step using four times the fractional meter set in each case. In general the step-and-shoot algorithm can be made more efficient by delivering larger increments of MU during certain instances (Ma et al. 1998). However, this increase in MU increment must be the same for all leaf tracks. In this example one can reduce the total number of steps from 20 to 14 by allowing different numbers of MUs to be delivered at the first and last steps. In order to implement a reduction in the instances, one must consider all the leaf tracks at once. This points the way toward leaf sequencing algorithms that consider the entire intensity-modulated aperture at once.

We have constructed a theoretically pure sequence to illustrate the principles involved. However, in order to form an effective irradiation sequence, a number of constraints and dosimetric considerations must be addressed. Inter-digitization of leaves may be precluded. In this case, additional instances must be added to avoid the inter-digitization. Other dosimetric considerations include leaf leakage and the tongue-and-groove effect.

## Corrections For Leaf Leakage

The idealized modulated fluence patterns do not take into consideration leakage through the leaves when they are used to attenuate the beam along their individual tracks. The material of choice for leaf construction is tungsten alloy because it has one of the highest densities of any metal as well as being hard, readily machinable, and reasonably inexpensive. Tungsten alloys also exhibit low coefficients of expansion, so that parts can be machined to exacting tolerances, an important consideration with regard to interleaf separations. Pure tungsten has a density of 19.3 $g/cm^3$, but alloys can be formulated having densities that range from 17.0 to 18.5 $g/cm^3$, with varying admixtures of nickel, iron, and copper. Pure tungsten is very brittle and the machinability of tungsten alloy improves with decreasing tungsten content. When the upper or lower jaws are replaced with leaves, the transmission requirements are the same as those of a set of collimating jaws. The requirements for the tertiary arrangement are somewhat different. When the adjustable photon jaws of the linac are used to set the overall size of the field, it is only necessary that the leaves of the tertiary MLC attenuate the primary beam to the same extent as customized blocks, i.e., <5% or between 4 HVL and 5 HVL. However, since there is transmission between the leaves, the transmission through the leaves should be lower than this to ensure that the overall transmission meets this criterion. This criterion is met by a minimum thickness of 5 cm of tungsten alloy. It is necessary to reduce the transmission by say, a further factor of 5 to 1% by increasing the thickness by approximately 2.5 to 3 cm. Thus for the tertiary MLC one has to trade off in-field attenuation against space between the collimator head and the couch.

The leakage through the leaves deposits a dose of about 1% to 2% of the total Meter Set at each shoot instance. However, in a given sequence there may be as many or more blocked instances as unblocked instances at any given point along the profile. The dose delivered by the leakage radiation cannot be neglected (Siebers et al. 2002). The leakage must be taken into consideration by the leaf-sequencing algorithm. A partial correction is possible. One may compute the sequence first ignoring the leakage. Once a preliminary sequence has been computed, the dose deposited by leakage can be computed. This will be a fairly uniform low dose across the field. The computed leakage fluence distribution can be subtracted from the desired profile to obtain a profile that must now be delivered assuming the leakage fluence distribution. This stratagem will produce a sequence that delivers a fairly accurate rendering of the desired fluence as long as the minima in the fluence distribution are not too close to zero. Given that a few percent dose will necessarily be delivered by the intra-leaf leakage, SMLC IMRT cannot deliver totally zero minima inside the field.

## Strategies To Remove The Tongue-And-Groove Effect

Other modifications of the leaf-setting sequence can correct for the tongue-and-groove effect. The origins of the tongue-and-groove effect will be explained in another discussion in the Summer School (***Dynamic MLC IMRT*** by Keall) and will not be repeated here. For dynamic MLC delivery, van Santvoort and Heijmen (1996) proposed an algorithm to remove this effect completely by synchronization of the motion of neighboring leaf pairs. Using their algorithm, the tongue-and-groove effect is limited in such a way that in each overlap region, the delivered beam intensity is always equal to the smaller of the two intensities determined by the two neighboring leaf pairs. In this definition, the tongue and groove effect is in fact not completely removed, but buried in the transition region of the two different intensities. This definition, on the other hand, is reasonable because the junction area between different intensities cannot be a sharp step function due to the physical nature of radiation. For SMLC delivery, since the speed of each leaf is not an adjustable parameter, the algorithm proposed for DMLC delivery cannot be used directly.

## Computation Of SMLC Sequence By Power-Of-Two Decomposition

Rather than sequence the one-dimensional leaf tracks one at a time, one may consider creating the sequence from the entire two-dimensional aperture areas. A number of methods have been investigated to carry out this strategy.

## Logarithmic Step Decomposition

An algorithm proposed by Xia (Xia and Verhey 1998) is an example of such an areal sequencing approach. A two-dimensional intensity distribution (or intensity matrix) is segmented into multiple subfields or apertures. We will use the same pattern of integers in the figure 9 to illustrate the basic ideas beneath this leaf-setting sequence. Figure 12a shows the monitor units to be delivered in the 9-cm $\times$ 5-cm field up to a maximum exposure of 80 MU and a minimum exposure within the field of 0 MU. The underlying principle of the algorithm for determining the sequence is that the most efficient way to subdivide a sequence is by halves. The sequence is to be delivered by MU increments that are powers of 2. In this case, the increments are $64=2^6$, $32=2^5$, $16=2^4$, $8=2^3$, $4=2^2$, $2=2^1$, and $1=2^0$. The first step is to set the leaves in a pattern that can deliver an exposure of 64 MU. There are two bixels in leaf tracks 19 and 21 of figure 12a with intensities of 64 or more. They are not contiguous, but leaves can be set to form two apertures around the two regions that each delivers an exposure of 64 MU. This constitutes a 64 MU shoot depicted in figure 12a. The residual exposure that needs to be delivered is shown in figure 12b. Leaf pattern can be found that expose bixels that require a residual exposure of 32 MU or more. However, two or three such regions exist on most of the leaf tracks so the delivery requires three separate sets of leaf settings. These are depicted in figures 12b, 12c, and 12d. The residual MU pattern then contains values up to 30 MU that can be reduced by exposures of 16 MU. Again, in order to expose all the bixels, multiple apertures are required, each delivering exposures of 16 MU. These are shown in figures 12e and 12f. A final setting to reach the bixel at −3 cm in track 18 finishes the 16 MU exposures. Then all the beamlet positions have either received their full exposure or have a residual of less than 16 MU. In all, 15 steps are required to deliver the intensity pattern (see figure 13). The single profile step-and-shoot leaf-setting algorithm requires 20 steps to deliver this pattern (14 if delivery of identical apertures is taken into consideration). In general the areal algorithm will take fewer steps than the pure single-track sequencing method to deliver the same pattern. The presence of the interleaf motion constraint increases the number of segments for both algorithms by approximately 25%. The advantage of such a constraint, however, is to synchronize the leaf motion, yielding a reduction of the tongue-and-groove effect.

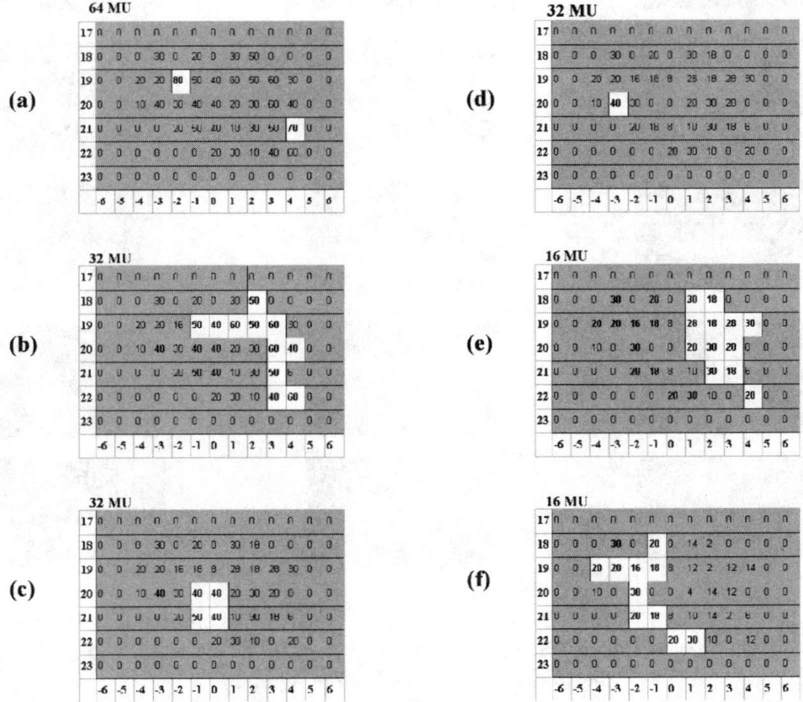

**Figure 12.** The first six steps taken to generate a logarithmic power-of-two decimation of the intensity pattern given in figure 9. The number of monitor units used in each step is shown at the top left of each field diagram.

## Optimization Of Sequence

The apertures in figure 13 do not form a window that sweeps systematically across the field. However, the aperture need not be delivered in any particular order. One may optimize the sequence to minimize the total leaf travel required to deliver the sequence. In addition, the sequence in figure 13 requires interdigitation and will produce tongue-and-groove effects. Extra steps can be added that eliminate these effects if needed. Optimization of the order of gantry, couch, and collimator angles can also be included in a total treatment optimization. This can be important, for example, if the gantry is to be moved automatically and the original plan, and hence DICOM control sequence, has unnecessarily large angle changes between beams.

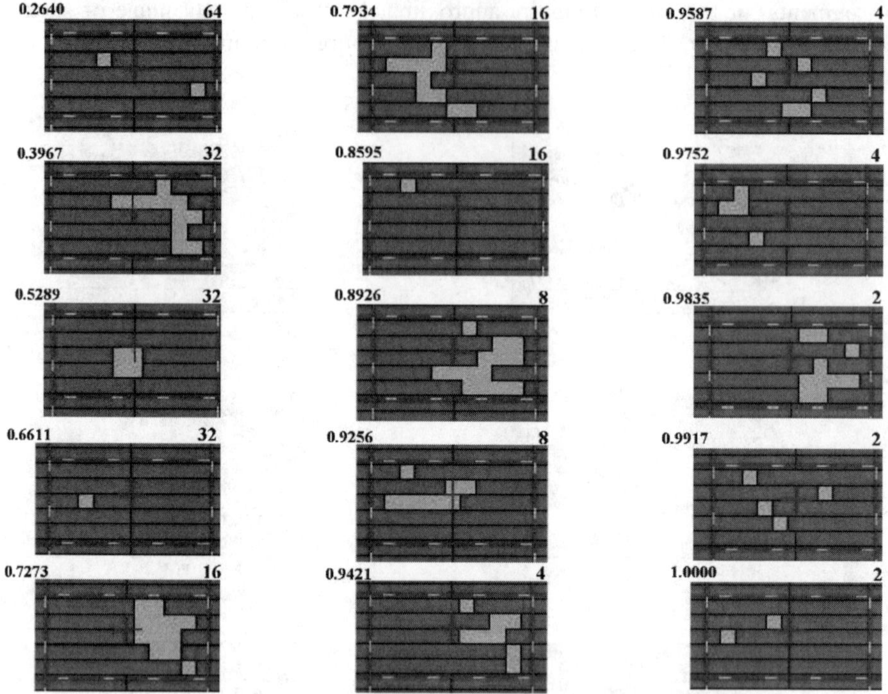

**Figure 13.** The 15 steps required to generate the intensity pattern in figure 9 by the logarithmic power-of-two decimation. These 15 steps generate the same pattern as the 20 (or 16) steps depicted in figure 11.

## Matrix Operator Method

The one-dimensional leaf track sequencing method and the two-dimensional decomposition leaf sequencing method are conceptually mathematical operations on a two-dimensional intensity matrix. The matrix operator method for leaf sequencing is along this line of thought (Ma et al. 1999; Ma 2002).

One noticeable feature of this matrix algorithm is that the aperture shape between sequential leaf segments typically changes gradually. This allows a user to combine some similar leaf apertures to reduce the number of leaf segments or further improve delivery efficiency without significantly impacting the dosimetry of a treatment plan. It can be shown that the total MU is minimized with the matrix operator algorithm but not necessarily the total number of segments. The matrix algorithm can be extended to accommodate certain delivery constraints and requirements (Ma 2002).

# Conclusion

The exploration of the implementation of IMRT with computer-controlled MLCs is a continuing process as the control systems and associated software applications evolve. New insights appear in nearly every new issue of the journals into the nature of inverse planning, the dosimetric characteristics of the delivery systems, and the architecture and optimization of the information management system. The medical physicist is presented with an opportunity to study and understand these systems in order to support their implementation and to illuminate obfuscations that arise over their operation.

# Acknowledgments

The author would like to acknowledge the contributions and critiques to this chapter contributed by Peter Hoban, Ph.D., Siemens Medical Systems; Calvin Huntzinger, M.S., Varian Medical Systems; and Lijun Ma, Ph.D., the University of Maryland.

# References

Bortfeld, T., U. Oelfke, and S. Nill. (2000). "What is the optimum leaf width of a multileaf collimator?" *Med. Phys.* 27:2494–2502.

Bortfeld, T. R., D. L. Kahler, T. J. Waldron, and A. L. Boyer. (1994). "X-ray field compensation with multileaf collimators." *Int. J. Radiat. Oncol. Biol. Phys.* 28:723–730.

Boyer, A. L. "Design and Use of Compensating Filters" in *Advances in Radiation Therapy Treatment Planning.* A. Wright and A. Boyer (eds.). New York: American Institute of Physics, pp. 185–200, 1983.

Boyer, A. L. "Basic Applications of a Multileaf Collimator" in *Teletherapy: Present and Future.* J. Palta and T. R. Mackie (eds.). AAPM 1996 Summer School Proceedings. Madison, WI: Advanced Medical Publishing, pp. 403–444, 1996.

Boyer, A. L., and S. Li. (1997). "Geometric analysis of light-field position of a multileaf collimator with curved ends." *Med. Phys.* 24:757–762.

Boyer, A. L., T. G. Ochran, C. E. Nyerick, T. J. Waldron, and C.J. Huntzinger. (1992). "Clinical dosimetry for implementation of a multileaf collimator." *Med. Phys.* 19:1255–1261.

Chui, C.-S., T. LoSasso, and S. Spirou. (1994). "Dose calculation for photon beam with intensity modulation generated by dynamic jaw or multileaf collimation." *Med. Phys.* 21:1237–1244.

Convery, D., and M. E. Rosenbloom. (1992). "The generation of intensity-modulated fields for conformal radiotherapy by dynamic collimation." *Phys. Med. Biol.* 37:1359–1374.

Cunningham J., D. J. Wright, H. P. Webb, J. A. Rawlinson, and P. M. K. Leung. (1976). "A semi-automatic cutter for compensating filters." *Int. J. Radiat. Oncol. Biol. Phys.* 1:355–360.

Du, M. N., C. X. Yu, M. Symons, C. Eng, D. Yan, R. Taylor, R. C. Matter, G. Gustafson, A. Martinez, and J. W. Wong. (1994). "Multileaf collimator prescription preparation system for conventional radiotherapy." *Int. J. Radiat. Oncol. Biol. Phys.* 30:707–714.

Ellis, F., E. J. Hall, and R. Oliver. (1959). "A compensator for variations in tissue thickness for high energy beams." *Br. J. Radiol.* 32:421–422.

Fiveash J. B., H. Murshed, J. Duan, M. Hyatt, J. Caranto, J. A. Bonner, R. A. Popple. (2002). "Effect of multileaf collimator leaf width on physical dose distributions in the treatment of CNS and head and neck neoplasms with intensity modulated radiation therapy." *Med. Phys.* 29:1116–1119.

Frazier, A., M. Du, J. Wong, F. Vicini, R.Taylor, C. Yu, A. Martinez, and D. Yan. (1995). "Dosimetric evaluation of the conformation of the multileaf collimator to irregular shaped fields." *Int. J. Radiat. Oncol. Biol. Phys.* 33:1229–1238.

Galvin, J. M., A. R. Smith, R. D. Moeller, R. L. Goodman, W. D. Powlis, J. Rubenstein, L. J. Solin, B. Michael, M. Needham, C. Huntzinger, and M. Kligerman. (1992). "Evaluation of multileaf collimator design for a photon beam." *Int. J. Radiat. Oncol. Biol. Phys.* 23:789–801.

Galvin, J. M., X.-G. Chen, and R. M. Smith. (1993). "Combining multileaf fields to modulate fluence distributions." *Int. J. Radiat. Oncol. Biol. Phys.* 27:697–705.

Galvin, J. M., A. Smith, and B. Lally. (1993). "Characterization of a multileaf collimator system." *Int. J. Radiat. Oncol. Biol. Phys.* 25:181–192.

Geis, P., and A. L. Boyer. (1996) "Use of a multileaf collimator as a dynamic missing-tissue compensator." *Med. Phys.* 23:1199–1205.

Hendee, W. R., and C. E. Garciga. (1967). "Tissue compensating filters for cobalt 60 teletherapy." *Am. J. Roentgen.* 99:939–943.

Huq, M., I. Das, T. Steinberg, and J. Galvin. (2002). "A dosimetric comparison of various multileaf collimators." *Phys. Med. Biol.* 47:N159–N170.

Jordan, T. F., and P.C. Williams. (1994). "The design and performance characteristics of a multileaf collimator." *Phys. Med. Biol.* 39:231–251.

Kijewski, P. K, L. E. Chin, and B. E. Bjärngard. (1978). "Wedge-shaped dose distributions by computer-controlled collimator motion." *Med. Phys.* 5:426–429.

Klein, E. E., W. B. Harms, D. A. Low, V. Willcut, and J. A. Purdy. (1995). "Clinical implementation of a commercial multileaf collimator: Dosimetry, networking, simulation, and quality assurance." *Int. J. Radiat. Oncol. Biol. Phys.* 33:1195–1208.

Ma, L. (2002). "Smoothing intensity-modulated treatment delivery under hardware constraints." *Med. Phys.* 29:2937–2945.

Ma, L., A. L. Boyer, L. Xing, and C.-M. Ma. (1998). "An optimized leaf-setting algorithm for beam intensity modulation using dynamic multileaf collimators." *Phys. Med. Biol.* 43:1629–1643.

Ma, L., A. Boyer, C.-M. Ma, and L. Xing. (1999). "Synchronizing dynamic multileaf collimators for producing two-dimensional intensity-modulated fields with minimum beam delivery time." *Int. J. Radiat. Oncol. Biol. Phys.* 44:1147–1154.

Mageras, G. S., R. Mohan, C. Burman, G. D. Barest, and G. J. Kutcher. (1991). "Compensators for three dimensional treatment planning." *Med. Phys.* 18:133–140.

Otto, K., B. Clark, and C. Huntzinger. (2002). "Exploring the limits of spatial resolution in radiation dose delivery." *Med. Phys.* 29: 1823–1831.

Siebers, J. V., P. J. Keall, J. O. Kim, and R. Mohan. (2002). "A method for photon beam Monte Carlo multileaf collimator particle transport." *Phys. Med. Biol.* 47:3225–3249.

Siochi, A. (1999). "Minimizing static intensity mmodulation delivery time using an intensity solid paradigm." *Int. J. Radiat. Oncol. Biol. Phys.* 43:671–680.

Spirou, S., and C. Chui. (1994). "Generation of arbitrary intensity profiles by dynamic jaws or multileaf collimators." *Med. Phys.* 21:1031–1041.

Stein J., T. Bortfeld, B. Dorschel, and W. Schlegel. (1994). "Dynamic x-ray compensation for conformal radiotherapy by means of multileaf collimation." *Radiother. Oncol.* 32:163–173.

Svensson, R., P. Källmann, and A. Brahme. (1994). "Analytical solution for the dynamic control of multileaf collimators." *Phys. Med. Biol.* 39:37–61.

Tsai, J. S., D. E. Wazer, M. N. Ling, J. K. Wu, M. Fagundes, T. DiPetrillo, B. Kramer, M. Koistinen, and M. J. Engler. (1998). "Dosimetric verification of the dynamic intensity-modulated radiation therapy of 92 patients." *Int. J. Radiat. Oncol. Biol. Phys.* 40:1213–1230.

van Santvoort, J., and B. Heijmen. (1996). "Dynamic multileaf collimation without 'tongue-and-groove' underdose effects." *Phys. Med. Biol.* 41:2091–2105.

Wang, X., S. Spirou, T. LoSasso, J. Stein, C. Chui, and R. Mohan. (1996). "Dosimetric verification of intensity-modulated fields." *Med. Phys.* 23(3):317–327.

Webb, S., T. Bortfeld, J. Stein, and D. Convery. (1997). "The effect of stair-step leaf transmission on the 'tongue-and-groove problem' in dynamic radiotherapy with multileaf collimator." *Phys. Med. Biol.* 42:595–602.

Webb, S. (1998a). "Configuration options for intensity-modulated radiation therapy using multiple static fields shaped by a multileaf collimator." *Phys. Med. Biol.* 43(2):241–260.

Webb, S. (1998b). "Configuration options for intensity-modulated radiation therapy using multiple static fields shaped by a multileaf collimator. II: Constraints and limitations on 2D modulation." *Phys. Med. Biol.* 43(6):1481–1495.

Xia, P., and L. J. Verhey. (1998). "Multileaf collimator leaf sequencing algorithm for intensity modulated beams with multiple static segments." *Med. Phys.* 25:1424–1434.

Yu, C. X., M. J. Symons, M. N. Du, A. A. Martinez, and J. W. Wong. (1995). "A method for implementing dynamic photon beam intensity modulation using independent jaws and a multileaf collimator." *Phys. Med. Biol.* 40:769–787.

# Dynamic MLC IMRT


**Paul Keall, Ph.D., Qiuwen Wu, Ph.D., Yan Wu, M.S.,
and Jong Oh Kim, Ph.D.**
Department of Radiation Oncology
Virginia Commonwealth University
Richmond, Virginia

# Scope

## Definition

**Dynamic multileaf collimator (DMLC)-intensity modulated radiation therapy (IMRT):** A method used to deliver intensity-modulated beams using an MLC, with the leaves in motion during radiation delivery. The *sliding window* technique is a form of DMLC-IMRT in which the window formed by each opposing pair of leaves traverses across the tumor volume while the beam is on (IMRTCWG 2001).

## What Is In This Chapter?

This chapter discusses the clinical application of the DMLC for IMRT. The designs and mechanics of DMLC are discussed, along with their dosimetric effects, including a comparison of dynamic vs. segmental multileaf collimation (DMLC vs. SMLC). This chapter also covers leaf sequencing and patient dose verification and presents DMLC-IMRT clinical implementation for the following tumor sites: head and neck, cervix, prostate, lung, and breast. Specific features of DMLC-IMRT and the application of DMLC for the management of respiratory motion are also included.

The contents of this chapter are biased towards the methods, materials, research findings, and clinical studies derived from our experiences in the Department of Radiation Oncology at Virginia Commonwealth University (VCU). In part, this is necessary as there are no nationally/internationally accepted guidelines for the application and use of DMLC-IMRT (Van Esch et al. 2002), and thus different groups are tackling problems in their own ways. Hopefully, when sufficient experience and clinical results are gained, such guidelines can be arrived at by consensus.

Due to space restrictions, not all aspects of DMLC are properly represented. The reference list will point those interested toward further reading. Throughout this chapter we have followed the suggested nomenclature of the IMRT Collaborative Working Group report (IMRTCWG 2001).

## What Is Not In This Chapter?

Helical and serial tomotherapy are examples of DMLC-IMRT; however, as these IMRT approaches are discussed in other chapters of this book, they will not be included in this chapter.

Quality assurance (QA) for IMRT is also covered in two dedicated chapters of this book, and except for patient-specific QA, will not be explicitly included in this chapter, though we wish to stress the importance of an effective QA program for the safe and accurate delivery of IMRT. Similarly, commissioning of the DMLC-IMRT system is an integral and necessary component of any IMRT program, but the in-depth discourse on commissioning and QA for IMRT planning is discussed in a separate chapter of this book.

## Introduction

### The "MLC" In DMLC-IMRT

Before further discussion of DMLC-IMRT it is important to briefly review the hardware, mechanics, and features of the MLCs used. Note that this section applies also to segmental MLC (SMLC) approaches. An ideal MLC for DMLC-IMRT would include the following features:

- Negligible leakage

- Small dosimetric penumbra

- Good patient clearance

- Fine leaf widths

- High maximum leaf speed and fast leaf acceleration

- Excellent mechanical accuracy, precision, and stability

For each MLC, two banks of independent tungsten alloy leaves face each other and travel either linearly perpendicular to the central axis (single focus) or in an arc about the x-ray target (double focus). Orthogonal to the direction of motion, the leaf edge is parallel to the ray line from the target. From the line of sight of the target, adjacent leaves overlap one other in order to reduce (1) the total amount of radiation leakage through the MLCs and (2) the variation in leakage dose across individual leaves. As shown in section *Tongue-and-Groove/Stepped-Edge Design* below, there are still variations in leakage dose beneath different parts of the MLC leaves.

Two MLC designs are shown schematically in figure 1, the Varian[1] Mark II 80-leaf MLC and Millennium™ 120-leaf MLC. Note that both of these are single-focused designs and thus have rounded leaf tips to ensure dosimetric penumbra similarity at different positions of the leaf. The 80-leaf MLC reduces radiation leakage using the tongue-and-groove design, whereas the 120-leaf MLC employs a stepped edge with alternating leaves having their thicker portion facing towards and away from the target to achieve the same end.

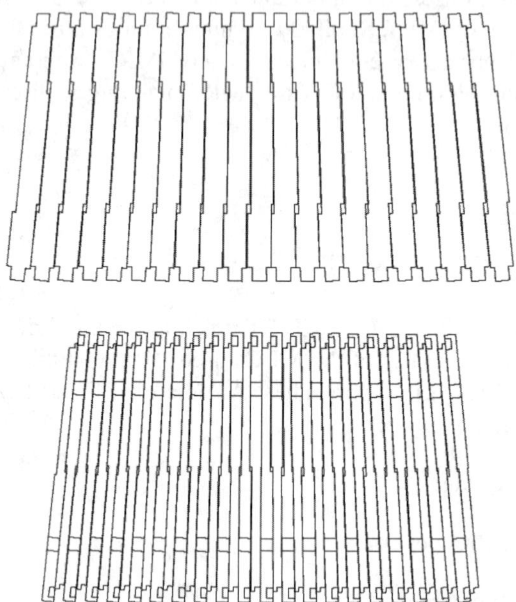

**Figure 1.** A cross-sectional view of the Varian Mark II 80-leaf MLC showing the end view (top) and the inner leaves of the Varian Millennium™ 120-leaf MLC (bottom). Orthogonal to the direction of motion the leaf thickness projected to isocenter is 1.0 cm for the 80 leaf and 0.5 cm for the inner leaves of the 120-leaf MLC. [Reprinted from *Medical Physics*, vol 28, "A Monte Carlo study of radiation transport through multileaf collimators," J. O. Kim, J. V. Siebers, P. J. Keall, M. R. Arnfield, and R. Mohan, pp. 2497–2506. © 2001, with permission from AAPM.]

## The "D" In DMLC-IMRT

The pioneering work in DMLC-IMRT has been attributed to several groups (Kallman et al. 1988; Convery and Rosenbloom 1992; Bortfeld et al. 1994; Spirou and Chui 1994; Stein et al. 1994; Yu et al. 1995). Since these important early works, DMLC

---

[1] Varian Medical Systems, Palo Alto, CA.

development at research, clinical and commercial centers has led to an ever-increasing clinical use of DMLC-IMRT. In some centers DMLC-IMRT is applied to virtually all tumor sites that are to be treated with curative intent (see the section *DMLC-IMRT Clinical Application*).

Though "dynamic" MLC motion implies that the leaf positions are changing with respect to time, in terms of the MLC controller it is the change in position with respect to monitor units (MUs) delivered that is important. The inputs required are the leaf positions at various control points, the fractional number of MUs to be delivered at each control point, and the total number of MUs to be delivered for that beam.

Each leaf is controlled by a separate motor. The leaf positions are indicated by encoders attached to the motors. An independent secondary feedback mechanism verifies correct leaf positioning. During DMLC delivery, the control software monitors the leaf positions and compares them to their prescribed positions. The beam is interrupted momentarily if any leaf position is outside tolerance [for Varian DMLCs this is a user-defined parameter selectable from 0.1 to 5.0 mm (LoSasso, Chui, and Ling 1998)].

An important factor for DMLC-IMRT leaf sequencing and delivery is the maximum leaf speed (position with respect to time). For the Varian MLCs this is approximately 3 cms$^{-1}$ at isocenter (LoSasso, Chui, and Ling 1998). If the requested leaf speed exceeds the dose rate used for the delivery of the DMLC field, then the dose rate will be reduced. If the dose rate is continually reduced, then the treatment time will increase.

For further information on MLC control, see other chapters of this book, Boyer (1996), or the manufacturer's documentation.[2] Subtleties of motion for single-focused MLCs are found in Boyer and Li (1997) and appendix A of Siebers et al. (2002a).

## Effects Of Leaf Design On Radiation Transport

*Tongue-And-Groove/Stepped-Edge Design*

The tongue-and-groove or stepped-edge design commonly used to design MLCs, and other additions to facilitate the use of MLCs as mechanical devices, result in different radiological path lengths across different parts of the leaves. The different radiological pathlengths manifest themselves as varying doses in a plane perpendicular to the leaf motion. An example of Monte Carlo N-Particle (MCNP) (Breismeister 1997) calculated leakage dose through the MLCs shown in figure 1 is given in figure 2. From this figure it is evident that (1) there are variations in leakage dose across a leaf on the order of 1% of the open field dose, (2) the amplitude of the undulations for the 120-leaf MLC is less than that of the 80-leaf MLC, and (3) the frequency of the undulations for the 120-leaf MLC is more than that of the 80-leaf MLC. The latter are due to the smaller interleaf separation distances and smaller leaf thickness, respectively.

---

[2] See for example "Integrated MLC (MLCi) for the Elekta Precise Treatment System (Elekta Oncology Systems) or "DMLC Implementation Guide" (Varian Oncology Systems).

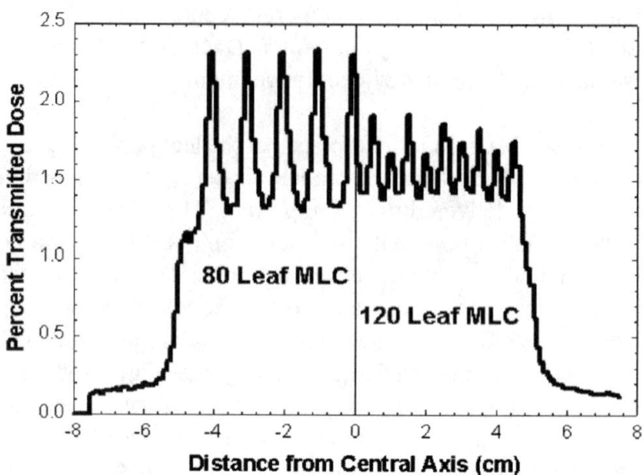



**Figure 2.** A profile curve perpendicular to the direction of leaf motion of the Monte Carlo computed radiation leakage from a MLC blocked 6 MV $10 \times 10$ cm$^2$ field at 5 cm depth in a water phantom for the 80-leaf (left side) and the 120-leaf (right side) MLCs. [Reprinted from *Medical Physics*, vol 28, "A Monte Carlo study of radiation transport through multileaf collimators," J. O. Kim, J. V. Siebers, P. J. Keall, M. R. Arnfield, and R. Mohan, pp. 2497–2506. © 2001, with permission from AAPM.]

As well as transmission of photons through the MLC, radiation interactions in the leaves act as a source of scatter. This scatter increases with field size, but is a small part of total leakage (up to 25% for a $20 \times 20$ cm$^2$ 6 MV field).

For the MLCs shown in figure 1, the average leakage dose through closed MLC leaves is between 1.5% and 2.2% of the open field dose that would be measured in the absence of the MLC. The leakage dose increases with field size (due to the increased contribution of MLC-scattered photons) and also increases with energy.

*Leaf Tips*

The rounded leaf edges employed on single-focused MLC designs will potentially act to broaden the penumbra. However, this potential source of broadening needs to be compared with other sources of penumbral broadening, namely the finite source size, and lateral electron transport. Studies have shown (e.g., Huq et al. 2002) that the MLC-patient distance, rather than the MLC design is the dominant factor in determining penumbral width. The rounded tip design of the MLC leaf ends yields dosimetric penumbras that are similar, independent of the position of the leaves with respect to central axis. A comparison of dose profiles through the leaf tips at different MLC positions is given in figure 3. This similarity in penumbra is useful for simplifying the complexity required to achieve accurate dose calculation in the patient (particularly when non-Monte Carlo methods are employed for dose calculation).

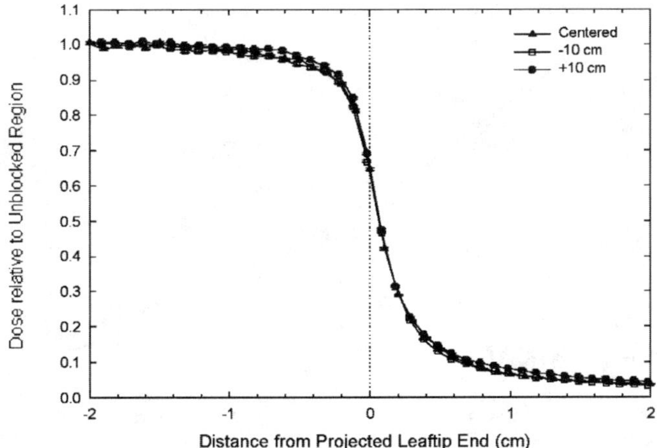


**Figure 3.** Monte Carlo calculated leaf tip dose profiles at a depth of 5 cm in a phantom at 95 cm SSD for the 120-leaf MLC leaf tips on the central axis, and at −10 and +10 cm from the central axis. [Reprinted from *Medical Physics*, vol 28, "A Monte Carlo study of radiation transport through multileaf collimators," J. O. Kim, J. V. Siebers, P. J. Keall, M. R. Arnfield, and R. Mohan, pp. 2497–2506. © 2001, with permission from AAPM.]

## Beam Hardening

As well as attenuating primary photons and acting as a source of scattered radiation, the combination of the polyenergetic beam, and the non-linear linear attenuation coefficient of the MLC material means that the lower energy (<~2 MeV) and to a lesser extent the higher energy photons (>~8 MeV) are preferentially attenuated, and thus beam hardening occurs.[3] The relative effect of the beam hardening on the MLC leakage depth dose curve compared to the open field depth dose curve for 6 MV and 18 MV beams is displayed in figure 4. This figure shows that though the beam hardening is dosimetrically significant for a 6 MV beam, the effect is much smaller for the 18 MV beam.

With the radiation effects of the MLC as described above, and the dynamic nature of delivery, accurate dose calculation requires knowledge of both the MLC geometry, as well as a thorough understanding of the leaf motion file to actual leaf motion conversion. Perhaps the most accurate way of calculating dose for DMLC-IMRT is to use Monte Carlo methods, as both the radiation interactions and complex time-varying geometry can be explicitly taken into account on a particle-by-particle basis (Chen, Boyer, and Ma 2000; Deng et al. 2001; Fix et al. 2001a,b; Keall et al. 2001b; Liu, Verhaegen, and Dong 2001; Siebers et al. 2002a).

---

[3] The mass attenuation coefficient as a function of energy for tungsten showing the minima between 2 and 8 MeV can be created using the XCOM program written by M. J. Berger, J. H. Hubbell, and S. M. Seltzer. See http://physics.nist.gov/PhysRefData/Xcom/Text/XCOM.html.

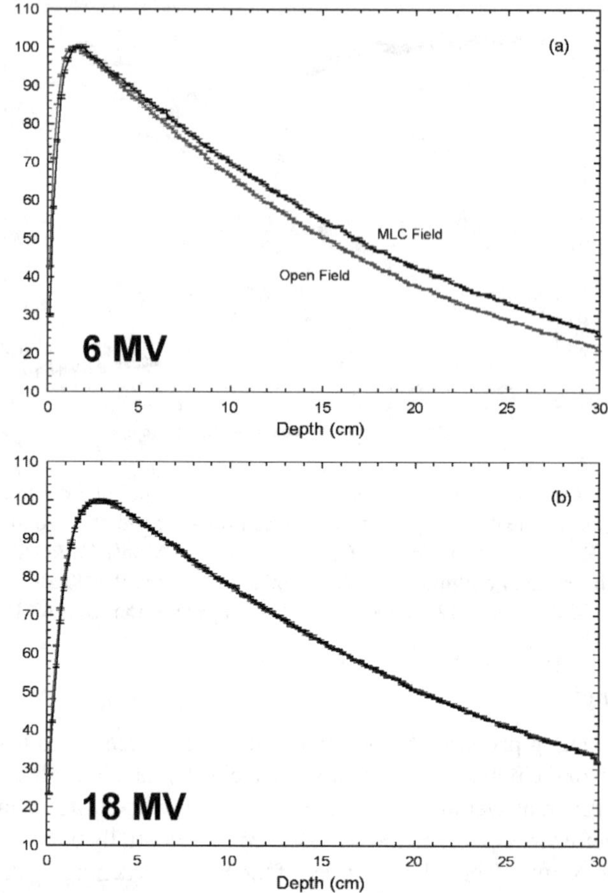

**Figure 4.** Monte Carlo calculated percent depth dose curves in a water phantom for $10 \times 10$ cm$^2$ field with and without MLC blocking for energies of 6 MV (top) and 18 MV (bottom). [Reprinted from *Medical Physics*, vol 28, "A Monte Carlo study of radiation transport through multileaf collimators," J. O. Kim, J. V. Siebers, P. J. Keall, M. R. Arnfield, and R. Mohan, pp. 2497–2506. © 2001, with permission from AAPM.]

If inaccurate dose calculation algorithms are used for DMLC-IMRT planning, there is a subtle penalty for using such algorithms during optimization, as well as the obvious limitation that the final dose calculation displayed on the treatment planning system does not represent the dose to the patient. This subtle limitation is that inaccurate dose calculation during IMRT optimization can lead to so-called "convergence errors," in which the "optimal" IMRT plan obtained with an inaccurate dose calculation algorithm converges to a different value than that obtained if a more accurate algorithm were used throughout the optimization (Jeraj, Keall, and Siebers 2002). A thorough discussion of these issues and other Monte Carlo dose calculation IMRT matters are the subject of an accompanying chapter in this book.

## DMLC Availability

Two vendors with DMLC-IMRT capability in current clinically released versions are BrainLab (Heimstetten, Germany) and Varian (Palo Alto, CA). Both clinically available DMLCs are examples of third level collimation (Boyer 1996) in that the MLC is added beneath both sets of jaws. The Elekta (Norcross, GA) MLC is capable of delivering DMLC-IMRT and is available for research purposes; however this technique is not yet available for clinical use. MRC (MRC Systems, Heidelberg, Germany) plans for a clinical release of DMLC-IMRT capability in early 2004.

3DLine Medical Systems (Owings Mills, MD) (to our knowledge) does not have DMLC-IMRT capability. Radionics (Tyco) (Burlington, MA) does not have DMLC plans at the current time. Siemens (Siemens Medical Solutions USA, Concord, CA) MLCs are technically capable of delivering DMLC-IMRT, however they are not available clinically. They envisage that future product releases will have DMLC capability though it is not in the immediate product plans.

Radionics (Tyco) gave the following explanations why they are not developing clinical DMLC-IMRT capability at the current time:

- The clinical advantage of dynamic vs. step and shoot has not been adequately demonstrated, particularly for miniature MLCs

- There are technical difficulties in interfacing an external MLC with the dose delivery control system of a linac

- Customers are interested in doing IMRT but are not demanding dynamic vs. static delivery.

Siemens gave these reasons for not pursuing clinical DMLC-IMRT capability at the current time:

- Communication and sampling rate limitations of DMLC (Xia, Chuang, and Verhey 2002)

- Delivery artifacts for high leaf velocity delivery (Low et al. 2001)

- Most Siemens users prefer the straightforward SMLC approach.

This discussion leads us into a further debate on the merits of DMLC vs. SMLC-IMRT.

## DMLC Vs. SMLC

Segmental MLC IMRT, also called "step-and-shoot IMRT," is the subject of a separate chapter in this book. However, it is worthwhile to take a minute to compare the two modalities, DMLC- and SMLC-IMRT. We need to be careful to separate the in-principle issues of DMLC vs. SMLC with the limitations of currently available hardware and software.

Xia and Verhey (2001) give the following arguments in the DMLC vs. SMLC debate.

Pro SMLC:

- Easy to understand [a simple extension of current three-dimensional conformal radiotherapy (3DCRT) practice]

- No requirement to control individual leaf speeds, thus simplifying the MLC control system

- An interrupted treatment is easy to resume

- It is easy to verify an intensity pattern for each field

- Fewer MUs are required in comparison with DMLC.

(The authors of this chapter would dispute the last three points, however they are included here for completeness.)

Pro DMLC:

- Shorter treatment time for complex intensity-modulated beam

- Reduction of dosimetric errors introduced by SMLC due to the discretization of a continuous intensity profile.

One perspective is that SMLC is a subset of DMLC (this is how SMLC is treated by the Varian MLC controller). In SMLC the leaf velocity (defined as change in position with dose) is either 0 or infinite velocity. For DMLC, the leaf velocity can be anywhere from 0 to infinite velocity inclusive. This adds a higher degree of freedom to any solution, and thus, in principle, the desired fluence can be more faithfully reproduced and/or the delivery time reduced. If a degree of freedom is added to the solution of any problem, then the best solution must be at least as good as that found in the more constrained space. This perspective is shown in figure 5. Using this argument it logically follows that the available solutions for 3DCRT, in which complex two-dimensional (2-D) varying fluences are not available to achieve desired dose distributions, is even more constrained. Of course, the limitation of this argument is that the solution space corresponds to a poorly defined problem, where the desired goals for the patient's treatment, which can vary due to the patient's disease, stage, site, anatomy, age, medical and genetic history, etc., are all coalesced into a few dose volume points or radiobiological parameters for various target and critical structures (Ebert 1997).

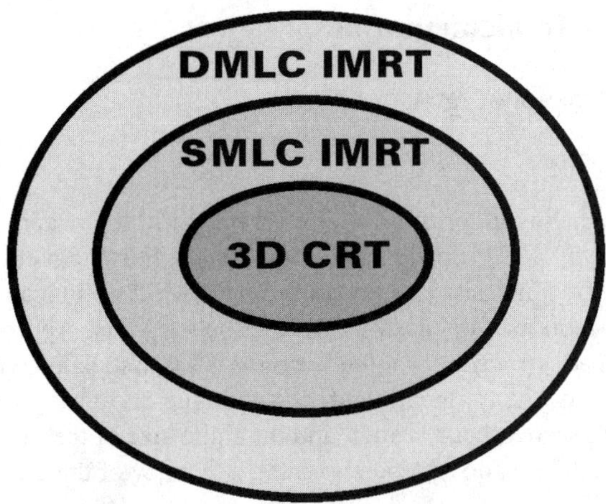


**Figure 5.** A schematic diagram showing the solution space of 3DCRT, SMLC-IMRT, and DMLC-IMRT. SMLC offers the advantage over 3DCRT in that the desired dose distribution can be achieved using a complex 2-D varying fluence that human planners and 3DCRT systems do not have the tools to deliver. DMLC has the advantage over SMLC in that the leaves can move while the beam is on. This increased degree of freedom, in principle, leads to improved resolution and/or faster beam delivery.

Though it is very hard to make an objective comparison between different treatment modalities, and the results are always dependent on the available equipment and implementation of the modalities, rather than a comparison of the modalities themselves, nevertheless a study was conducted by Chui et al. (2001) to compare DMLC- and SMLC-IMRT methods. They studied nine cases covering three treatment sites (prostate, nasopharynx, and breast). Though the SMLC results depended on the number of intensity levels and spatial resolution, in general a 5- to 10-level SMLC plan produced results comparable to that from a DMLC plan. The MUs were about 20% less for SMLC; however, the delivery time was about twice as long. Interestingly, in a respiratory gated study evaluating DMLC and SMLC-IMRT (Hugo, Agazaryan, and Solberg 2002), dynamic delivery was found to generate larger delivery errors than segmented delivery in most cases studied.

The argument between DMLC and SMLC becomes fairly meaningless when we consider other errors in radiotherapy. Studies have shown large inter- and intra-observer variations for target definition. Differences in target definition correspond to 100% differences between plans, whereas the difference between DMLC and SMLC is a few percent at most. Both DMLC and SMLC have been successfully clinically applied. Both techniques are evolving and improving. We believe that economics will be the winner. The technique of choice will be that which can treat the greatest number of patients in the smallest amount of time with the minimal overheads in terms of planning and QA time.

# DMLC-IMRT Implementation

## DMLC Leaf Sequencing Algorithms

*Introduction*

DMLC leaf sequencing algorithms (Kallman et al. 1988; Convery and Rosenbloom 1992; Bortfeld et al. 1994; Spirou and Chui 1994, 1996; Stein et al. 1994; Yu et al. 1995) convert desired intensity distribution from an IMRT optimization into leaf trajectories, i.e., leaf motion sequences as a function of MUs. Approximate empirical corrections are made to account for the various effects associated with the MLC characteristics, such as the rounded leaf tips, tongue-and-groove leaf design, leaf transmission, leaf scatter, head scatter, and the finite size of the radiation source. The accuracy of the delivered dose depends on the adequacy of these corrections.

*An Overview Of The Algorithms*

To simplify the discussions in this section on dynamic MLC, we will assume that all the leaves of the MLC are modeled using the transmission curve as shown in figure 6, i.e., all the leaves are double-focused and the tongue-and-groove effects are ignored unless specified otherwise. It is also assumed that all leaves will be sliding through the field uni-directionally.

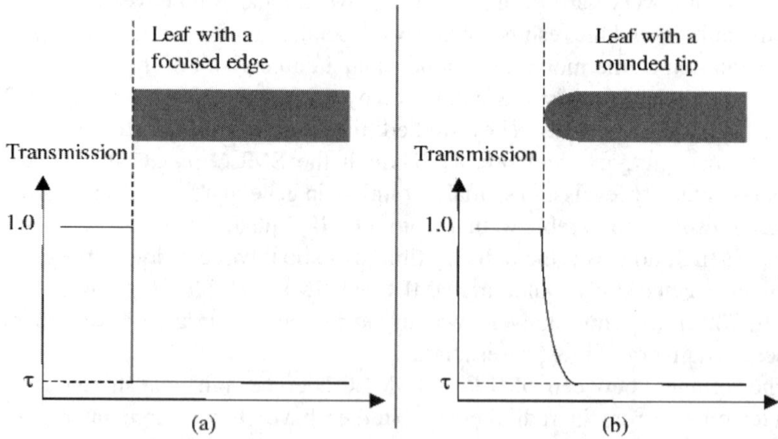


**Figure 6.** Transmissions of (a) a double-focused leaf (with a straight edge) and (b) a single-focused leaf (with a rounded tip).

Before introducing the formalism, let us first look at the simple situation of a pair of leaves starting at a closed position. If the following leaf keeps stationary while the leading leaf moves across the field at a constant speed, it will produce a downhill wedge intensity profile as shown in figure 7a, and the slope of the profile depends on the speed of the moving leaf. Another simple situation is a pair of leaves starting from an open position. If the leading leaf stays stationary while the following leaf moves across at a constant speed, an uphill wedge intensity profile will be created as shown in figure 7b, and again the slope of the profile is decided by the speed of the leaf. An arbitrary intensity profile across the field can therefore be generated using a combination of the leaf pair traveling at different speeds at different points in the field. It is worth noting that such a combination is not unique. A uniformed field with a given intensity could be generated with a pair of leaves moving across the field slowly with a narrow opening or quickly with a wide opening. It is intuitive that the maximum leaf speed should be used whenever possible to reduce the time (and MUs) needed.

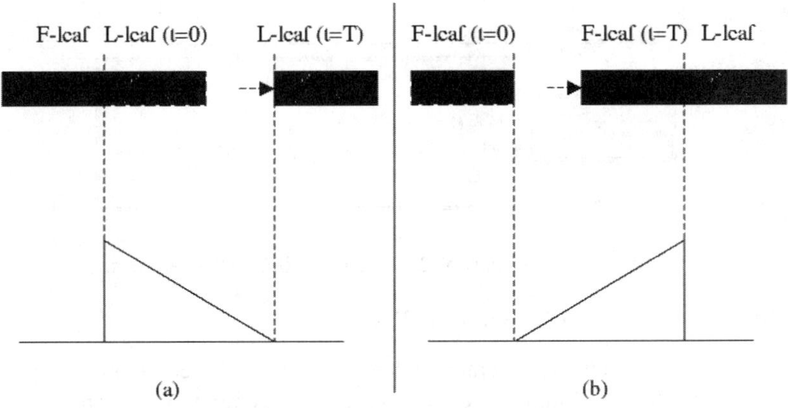


**Figure 7.** (a) A moving leading leaf creates a "downhill" intensity while (b) a moving following leaf generates an "uphill" intensity.

Due to the nonlinearity involved at the presence of the rounded leaf tip, leaf scatter, head scatter, and the finite source size, the DMLC leaf sequence generation is an iterative process consisting of two major functional blocks: intensity (or fluence) to leaf trajectories (F2T) and leaf trajectories to intensity (T2F) (figure 8). F2T generates leaf sequences $T(k)$ for the given intensity $\Phi(k)$ at the $k$th iteration ($\Phi(0) = \Phi_o$), assuming the leaves are of straight edges with constant leakage along the leaves as illustrated in figure 6a. The actual formulism for the generation of the leaf sequence will be given later in this section. The leaf sequences generated $T(k)$ are subsequently fed into T2F where the corrections for rounded leaf tips, head scatter, leaf scatter, and finite source size will be made for the reconstituted intensity (also called the deliverable intensity) $\Phi_d(k)$. The deliverable intensity is then compared with the desired intensity $\Phi_o$ from the IMRT optimization system. The iteration will terminate on one

                                **Paul Keall et al.**

of the three conditions: (1) the mean square error (MSE) between the desired and deliverable intensities is smaller than a user defined threshold $\varepsilon$; (2) the reduction of the MSE from last iteration to this iteration is considered too small; (3) MSE$(k)$ > MSE$(k-1)$, in which case, $T(k-1)$ and $\Phi(k-1)$ will be retained as the final results. The differences between the desired and deliverable intensities are fed back to adjust the intensity actually used to generate the leaf sequences in F2T.

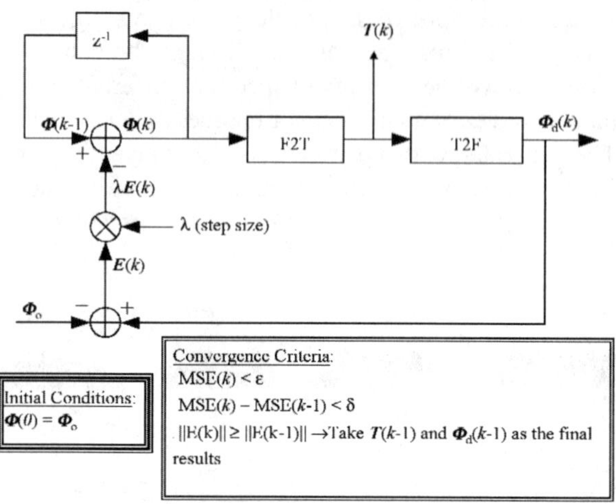


**Figure 8.** Flow chart of the dynamic MLC leaf sequencer.

*Intensity (Or Fluence) To Trajectories (F2T)*

The formalism used here to generate the leaf sequence is based on that of Spirou and Chui (1994, 1996). To facilitate an easy leaf sequence generation algorithm, the leaves are modeled with a straight edge shown in figure 6a. Only the primary contributions of the beam through both the opening and the leaves are considered, which also means each of the leaf pairs will generate the intensity profile underneath it independent of each other. We assume all the leaf pairs start with a closed position on one side of the field and finish with a closed position on the other side of the field. We also assume the starting and finishing points for both leaves of the pair under consideration are $x_0$ and $x_n$, and $x_i$ is an arbitrary point in $[x_0, x_n]$. We further let the MUs for the leading ($L$) leaf and following ($F$) leaf to reach a point $x_i$ for a leaf pair be $M_L(x_i)$ and $M_F(x_i)$. Then the intensity generated $\phi(x_i)$ by the leaf pair at $x_i$ will be

$$\phi(x_i) = [M_F(x_i) - M_L(x_i)] + \tau \times \{M - [M_F(x_i) - M_L(x_i)]\}, \tag{1}$$

where $\tau$ is the transmission through the leaf and $M$ is the total monitor units for the beam, which is not known *a priori*. It is obvious that the term $[M_F(x_i) - M_L(x_i)]$ is the direct contribution and the term $\tau \times \{M - [M_F(x_i) - M_L(x_i)]\}$ is the indirect contribution of the beam to the point. We can rewrite equation (1) as

$$\phi(x_i) = (1 - \tau) \times [M_F(x_i) - M_L(x_i)] + \tau \times M . \tag{2}$$

For a given leaf pair, as mentioned earlier, there is an infinite number of ways in which the required intensity can be generated. In order to deliver the treatment as rapidly as possible, we require that at any one point, one of the leaves of the pair travels at its maximum velocity permissible. Which of the leaves travels at its maximum speed depends on whether the required density is rising from point $i$ to $i+1$. If $\phi(x_{i+1})$ is greater than $\phi(x_i)$, then the L leaf must travel at its maximum velocity $v_{max}$ and vice versa. Thus for $\phi(x_{i+1}) > \phi(x_i)$

$$M_L(x_{i+1}) = M_L(x_i) + \frac{x_{i+1} - x_i}{v_{max}}, \tag{3}$$

and from equation (2) we get

$$M_F(x_{i+1}) = M_L(x_{i+1}) + \frac{\phi(x_{i+1}) - M \times \tau_i}{(1 - \tau)}. \tag{4}$$

Similarly, for $\phi(x_{i+1}) < \phi(x_i)$

$$M_F(x_{i+1}) = M_F(x_i) + \frac{x_{i+1} - x_i}{v_{max}}, \tag{5}$$

and from equation (3),

$$M_L(x_{i+1}) = M_F(x_{i+1}) + \frac{\phi(x_{i+1}) - M \times \tau_i}{(1 - \tau)}. \tag{6}$$

The total monitor units $M$ is determined as follows. We assume that, at the start of the beam, both the leading and following leaves of the pair are positioned at their starting closed position. The starting point is the grid point just before the first non-zero element of the corresponding row in the intensity matrix. The monitor units $M$ for the leaf pair is the MU value when the following leaf of the pair reaches its terminal position and the terminal position of the leaf pair is the grid point just after the last nonzero element.

We now attempt to develop an expression for computing the total beam-on time $M$. For those points for which $\phi(x_{i+1}) > \phi(x_i)$, substituting equation (3) in equation (4), we obtain

$$M_F(x_{i+1}) = M_L(x_i) + \frac{x_{i+1} - x_i}{v_{max}} + \frac{\phi(x_{i+1}) - M \times \tau}{1 - \tau}. \tag{7}$$

From equation (5) and equation (6)

$$M_L(x_i) = M_F(x_i) - \frac{\phi(x_i) - M \times \tau}{1 - \tau}. \tag{8}$$

Therefore

$$M_F(x_{i+1}) = M_F(x_i) - \frac{\phi(x_i) - M \times \tau}{1 - \tau} + \frac{x_{i+1} - x_i}{v_{max}} + \frac{\phi(x_{i+1}) - M \times \tau}{1 - \tau}, \tag{9}$$

or

$$M_F(x_{i+1}) = M_F(x_i) + \frac{x_{i+1} - x_i}{v_{max}} + \frac{\phi(x_{i+1}) - \phi(x_i)}{1 - \tau}. \tag{10}$$

Expressions equation (5) and equation (6) relate $M_F(x_{i+1})$ with $M_F(x_i)$ recursively for all values of the intensity under consideration. Using these, one can derive the MU reading for the terminal position $N$ of the leaf pair traveling, which can be shown to be

$$M_F(x_N) = (1 - \tau) \times \frac{x_{i+1} - x_i}{v_{max}} + \sum_{i=0}^{N-1} \{[\phi(x_{i+1}) - \phi(x_i)] \times H[\phi(x_{i+1}) - \phi(x_i)]\} \tag{11}$$

where $H(t)$ is the Heavyside function, i.e.,

$$H(t) = \begin{cases} 1 & \text{if } t > 0 \\ 0 & \text{otherwise}. \end{cases} \tag{12}$$

$M_F(x_N)$ is then the monitor units $M$ required to complete the trajectory of the leaf pair under consideration and the total beam-on time is just simply the maximum of all the leaf pairs involved.

    Figure 9 gives a more detailed description of the steps in F2T. Once the total beam MU is calculated using equation (11), the leaf sequences for all the leaf pairs can be generated independent of each other using equation (2) to equation (6). Leaf position synchronization (van Santvoort and Heijmen 1996; Webb et al. 1997; Ma et al. 1999) is then performed to reduce the tongue-and-groove effects. The most heavily pronounced algorithm is that of van Santvoort and Heijmen (1996), which eliminates the tongue-and-groove effects at the cost of total beam-on time. A more practical alternative to synchronize the leaf positions among the leaf pairs involved is the so-called "end-all-leaf-pairs-together" strategy, which basically just adjusts the speed of the leaf pairs accordingly to ensure all the leaf pairs will be at their terminating positions at the same time. The advantage of this simple strategy is that the total beam-on time will remain the same. The functionality of the procedure "Trim MU" is to ensure that the total number of control points needed does not exceed that of the maximum allowed by control software of the linear accelerator. The basic algorithms are just simply grouping points with close MU indices and then interpolate the leaf positions accordingly.

Fluence to leaf trajectories (F2T)

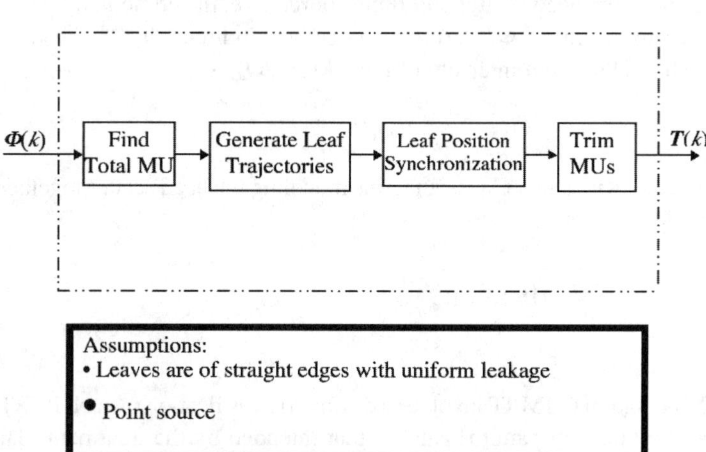


**Figure 9.** Procedures included in Fluence to Trajectories (F2T).

*Trajectories To Fluence (T2F)*

Figure 10 outlines the functions of T2F. This is basically the model of the delivery system of the linear accelerator. All the corrections for the nonlinearities are made in T2F. With leaf sequence generated from F2T, the transmitted intensity through the leaves $\Phi_t$ is calculated by integrating all the segments of the leaf trajectories with the leaves being modeled with rounded tips as shown in figure 6. The contribution of the leaf scatter $\ddot{O}_{Ls}$ is then added, i.e., the combined intensity, $\Phi_c$, is obtained as if the source of radiation is still a single point, i.e.,

$$\Phi_c = \ddot{O}_t + \Phi_{Ls} \tag{13}$$

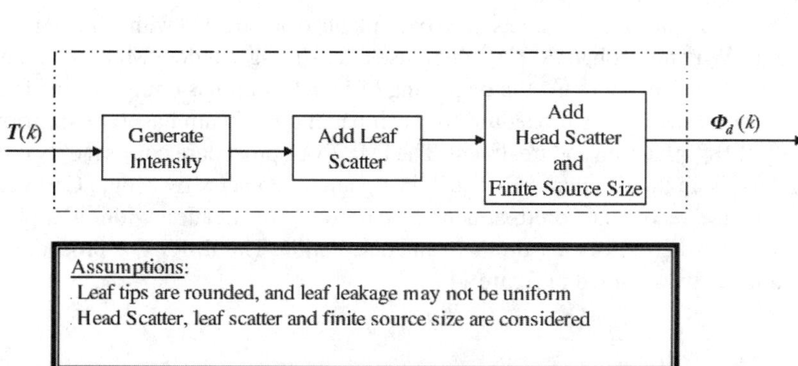


**Figure 10.** Procedures included in Trajectories to Fluence (T2F).

where $\Phi_{Ls}$ is proportional to the beam-on time and field size (Arnfield et al. 2000). To take into account of the head scatter and finite source size, the combined intensity $\Phi_c$ is then divided into the direct, $\Phi_c^{direct}$, (point source) and indirect, $\Phi_c^{indirect}$, (head scatter) components. The final output intensity of the DMLC, $\ddot{O}_d$, is

$$\ddot{O}_d = \ddot{O}_c^{direct} + \ddot{O}_c^{indirect} \otimes G_H , \tag{14}$$

where $G_H$ is a kernel with a few Gaussian terms modeling the head scatter together with the finite radiation source size.

## Pretreatment Dose Verification

### Introduction

Clinical implementation of IMRT involves a dosimetric verification of each IMRT field to ensure that the intensity pattern matches that intended by the treatment planning system and that the MUs specified by the treatment planning system will in fact deliver the intended dose. This QA step is typically completed using either film or ionization chamber dosimetry systems.

### IMRT QA With Film

Radiographic film is currently a practical dosimeter for IMRT delivered with DMLC because it provides excellent spatial resolution and integration of time-varying modulated dose. Although the film measurement is mostly selected as a state-of-the-art dosimetric verification method in clinic routine, it has some limitations in usage such as non-linearity of energy response due to over-response to low-energy photons and a relatively poorer reproducibility due to uncertainty in each dosimetric procedure including film positioning in the phantom, film development, scanning, and analysis. Also, a national/international standard film measurement protocol is not yet established for IMRT dose verification.

So far, a total of 150 patients have been planned and treated with our DMLC-IMRT system (Wu and Mohan 2000), which uses the sliding window MLC technique and optimization procedure. At the beginning of IMRT commissioning, we made a decision that an IMRT QA procedure for each patient and beam has to be performed to verify IMRT planning and treatment. The IMRT QA procedure consists of two phases. The first is an independent MU check in a patient geometry by Monte Carlo calculation and the second is a pretreatment dose delivery verification within flat phantoms by comparison of film measurement and calculation. The IMRT QA procedure at our institute is diagrammed in figure 11.

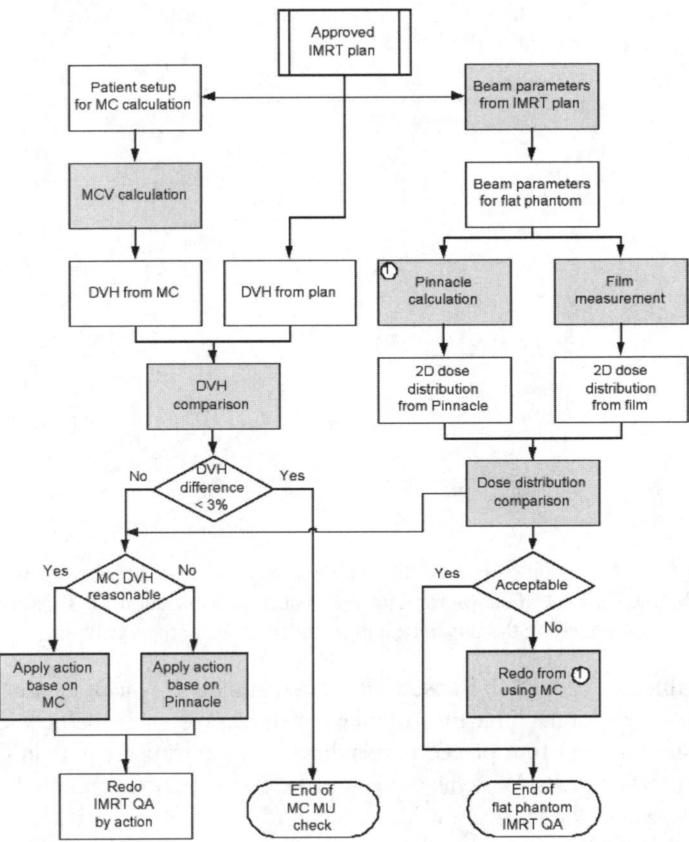

**Figure 11.** IMRT patient specific QA flow at VCU.

Phase I of the IMRT QA independently checks MUs in the patient. A Monte Carlo dose calculation is performed to obtain dose in the patient geometry with the DMLC code (Siebers et al. 2002a), using EGS4 (Nelson, Hirayama, and Rogers 1985; Nelson and Rogers (1988) user codes BEAM (Rogers et al. 1995) for the treatment head simulation upstream of the DMLC and DOSXYZ (Ma et al. 1995) for the patient dose calculation. Phase II of the IMRT QA measures absolute delivered dose in a flat phantom instead of the patient. The measured dose distribution is compared to the treatment planning system calculated dose distribution. As a result of the IMRT QA, a series of reports including dose-volume histogram (DVH) comparison, organ dose comparison, dose distribution, dose profiles, and dose difference histogram is filed in the patient's chart. We established action levels for when problems are found in DVH comparison or film measurement. A criterion on DVH difference between two dose calculation methods is limited to <3% at $D_{90}$ for the planning target volume(s) (PTV(s)). If the test fails to pass this criterion, an independent physicist reviews all procedures of the IMRT QA. Figure 12 shows an example DVH comparison for a head and neck tumor treatment.

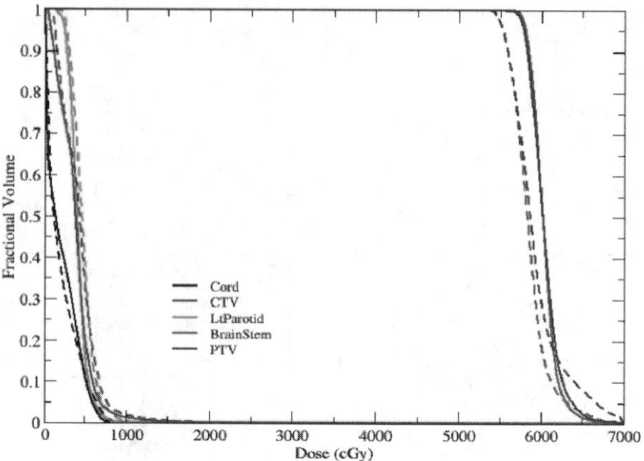

**Figure 12.** A DVH comparison of the treatment plan calculated using superposition and the Monte Carlo verification for a head and neck cancer treatment. This evaluation is signed by the physicist and included in the patient's chart.

Pretreatment DMLC-IMRT dose delivery verification in a phantom uses an extension of the conventional film measurement method. We use a perpendicular film configuration with the film placed perpendicular to the isoplane axis in flat water-equivalent plastic blocks. With the perpendicular configuration, film produces a 2-D dose distribution of the DMLC-IMRT irradiation.

The individual beams used in the patient plan are transferred from the patient to a flat phantom for dosimetric verification. All beams are rotated to a gantry angle of 0 degrees. At the treatment machine, films are be exposed for each field at a given depth and source-to-film distance (SFD). Typically, the SFD is 100 cm with a 5 cm depth in-phantom at both 6 MV and 18 MV energies.

One of the important procedures in film dosimetry is the film calibration so that optical density distribution of the film can be converted to a dose distribution to water. The configuration of film and plastic phantom for film calibration is the same as the configuration for dose verification. A $10 \times 10$ cm$^2$ field is exposed to the sandwich of film and phantoms. Because of non-linear optical density response to radiation dose, calibration points have to be carefully determined by film characteristics. X-OMAT V (XV) and EDR2 ready-packs from Kodak are currently used in our institute. The film calibration is performed from 0 to 80 MU at 10 MU intervals with the XV films because this film is near saturation at 80 MU. For the EDR2 film, higher MU spacing can be used because of the larger linear response, up to 300 MU. To establish the conversion table of optical density vs. dose, a $1 \times 1$ cm$^2$ area at the center of field is sampled and averaged. The calibration is performed on each day of IMRT QA and for each energy used.

Dose calculations are performed for the beams incident upon the flat phantom using the treatment planning system for the same geometry as the experimental film procedure outlined above. The dose grid at the measurement depth is extracted and compared with measurements using in-house film analysis software. This software automatically aligns two dose distributions by minimizing the root-mean-square dose difference.

Isodose contours, profiles, and dose-difference distributions are created by comparing the film measurement data with the calculated dose distribution. Isodose contours and profiles support visual inspection. Dose-difference distribution gives information regarding the center of the distribution, standard deviation of dose difference, and distribution itself. If these two distributions are identical, the dose-difference distribution must be a delta function at 0. From the center and width of the dose difference distribution the dose difference between measurement and calculation can be evaluated and quantified. Figure 13 shows an example of film measurement evaluation.

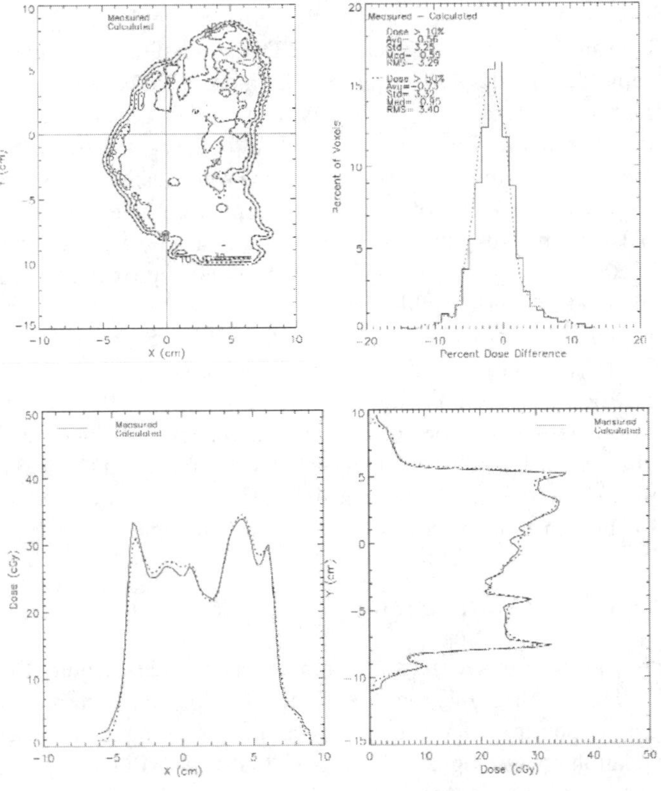

**Figure 13.** An example of film measurement vs. calculation evaluation for a VCU DMLC-IMRT patient. This evaluation is signed by the physicist and included in the patient's chart.

In addition, a distance-to-agreement test is performed with two modes of distance-to-agreement (DTA) which are 2% and 2 mm test criteria [see Low et al. (1988)] and 2% or 2 mm as our test criteria. In the 2% and 2 mm test, if a compared dose does not exceed an ellipse of 2% and 2 mm in dose difference and distance axis, it passes the criteria. In the 2% or 2 mm test, if the same dose is found on the other dose distribution within 2% or 2 mm in dose difference or distance coordinates, respectively, it passes the criteria.

The Monte Carlo dose verification is performed, analyzed, and approved before the patient treatment can start. The results of the film analysis are provided to the physicist responsible for the IMRT plan for approval and inclusion in the patient chart. The film dosimetry is completed and included in the patients chart (1) before 20% of the total patient dose is delivered and (2) before delivery of the sixth dose fraction.

### IMRT QA With An Electronic Portal Imaging Device (EPID)

Film measurements are currently the standard for IMRT dosimetric verification, however, film dosimetry is laborious and often error prone. Electronic portal image devices (EPIDs) are replacing films because EPIDs can acquire a real-time dose-image that allows rapid dosimetric verification. Furthermore, EPIDs can be used with the patient present for transmission dosimetry and the QA can (theoretically) be performed in few minutes. To verify IMRT dose delivery, the treatment planning system has to predict the absolute dose in the same setup as the EPID measurement. The energy dependent response of the EPID phosphor combined with the complex IMRT dose delivery, including the effects of treatment head scatter radiation, requires an accurate method to simulate the EPID with minimal approximations. The Monte Carlo (MC) method can perform this task.

We developed an MC module for a commercial EPID, aS500 from Varian and use it to compute IMRT pretreatment image for comparison with measurements for pretreatment IMRT dose verification. As an example of IMRT QA using EPID, pretreatment dose verification for a clinical head and neck IMRT patient plan, utilizing sliding window DMLC delivery, is presented in figure 14 (2-D images) and figure 15 (dose profiles). The MC simulation successfully reproduces measured pretreatment dose images with comparative accuracy to film measurement.

## Intratreatment Dose Verification

An exciting prospect for image-guided therapy is the ability to acquire EPID images during DMLC-IMRT delivery. This may aid in the development of tumor tracking/4-D radiotherapy and also for *ex vivo* IMRT verification. An example of the setup (figure 16) and verification results (figure 17) for breast DMLC-IMRT are given. An interesting note is that with breast IMRT, due to the slowly varying intensity modulation (contrast the head and neck example shown in figure 14) the anatomy of the chest wall and skin can be seen on both the calculated and measured images, allowing for the simultaneous dosimetric verification with the setup error assessment of the beam-target alignment.

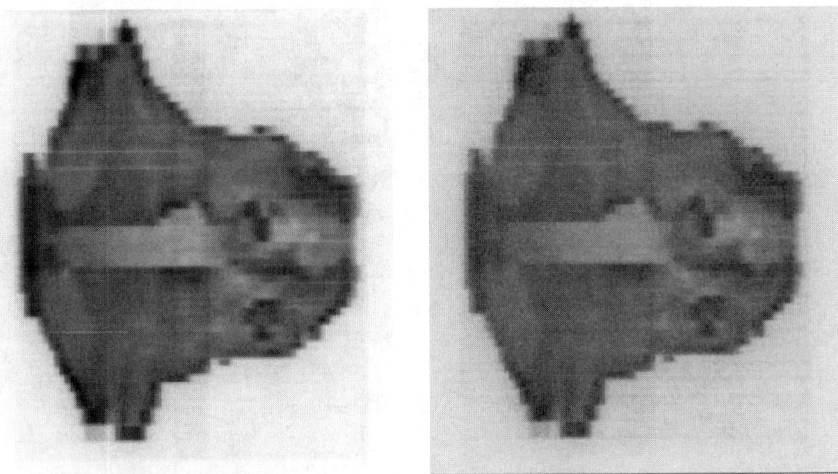

**Figure 14.** EPID measured (left) and Monte Carlo calculated (right) pretreatment DMLC-IMRT verification images.

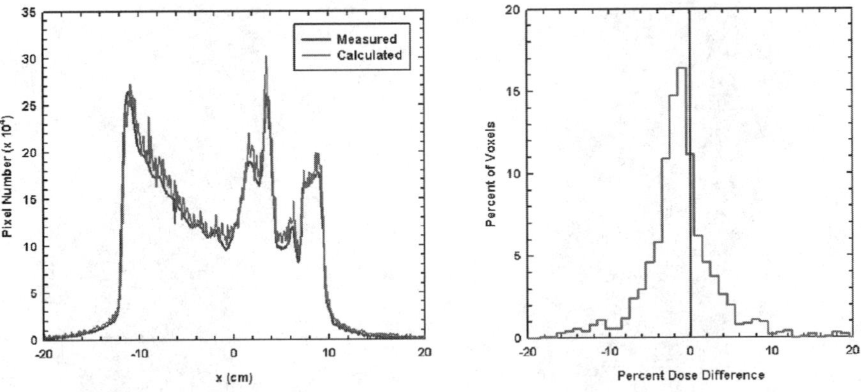

**Figure 15.** Measured and calculated profile curves taken from figure 14 (left), and percent pixel number difference histogram between EPID and Monte Carlo calculation (right). Note that absolute values are displayed (the Monte Carlo results are converted to EPID pixel values) and also the increased noise in the Monte Carlo calculation.

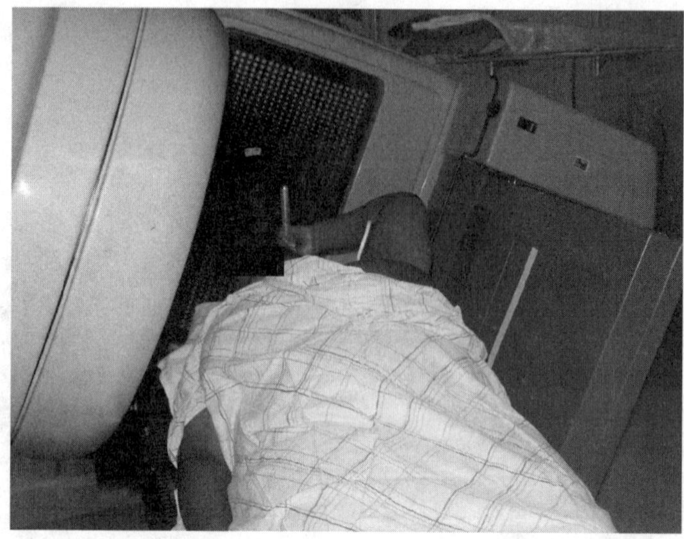

**Figure 16.** A DMLC-IMRT breast cancer patient setup for treatment.
Note the presence of the EPID during treatment to measure the transmitted dose.

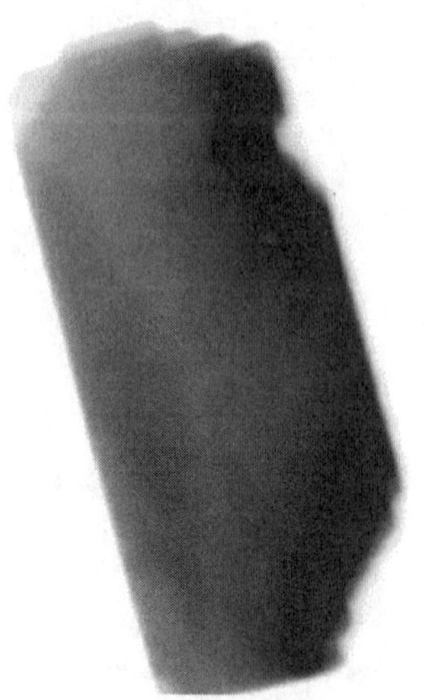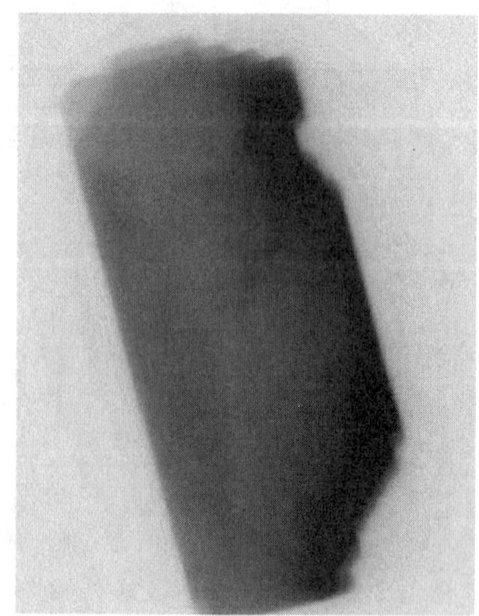

**Figure 17.** EPID measured (left) and Monte Carlo calculated (right) intra-treatment
DMLC-IMRT verification images.

# DMLC-IMRT Features

## Dynamic Feathering

In DMLC, each pair of opposing MLC leaves sweeps across the treatment field while the beam is on. The jaws and the MLC carriages do not move with the leaves. However, there is a limitation on the width of the fields that can be treated in one sweep. This limitation results from the fact that, for the Varian MLCs as used at VCU, the leaf length in the current model of the MLC is 14.5 cm (projected at the isocenter). Since each leaf pair must travel from the left boundary to the right boundary of the beam aperture and the back end of any leaf cannot travel past the edge of the jaw, the maximum width of the field aperture that can be accommodated in one sweep of leaves is also limited to 14.5 cm (in fact to a slightly smaller usable value). The MLC leaf width is 1 cm (0.5 cm for 120-leaf MLC) projected at the isocenter; therefore, the maximum IMRT field size that can be delivered in one sweep is 40 cm by 14.5 cm for an 80-leaf MLC (or a 120-leaf MLC) or 26 cm by 14.5 cm for a 52-leaf MLC.

IMRT can be used for the boost only or for the entire treatment course. It has been shown that, for certain treatment sites, IMRT produces more conformal dose distributions and is more efficient when used to plan and deliver the large and boost fields simultaneously (Mohan et al. 2000; Wu et al. 2000b), such as the cases presented in the next section. The required field sizes may be larger than 14.5 cm irrespective of the collimator rotation. To treat such large fields, they must be split into two or more smaller fields. A simple step "break" in the middle, as is usually done for static treatments with MLC, may be implemented. While this is certainly feasible, it would lead to field matching problems because uncertainties in setup and organ motion may cause undesirable hot or cold spots in the junction region. Since the intensity varies across the IMRT field, it is natural to consider splitting the beam into components with overlap between them and with variable intensity in the overlap region. We have developed a dynamic 'feathering' technique for splitting large fields (Wu et al. 2000a). In this method the intensity-modulated field is divided into two (or more) components. The components overlap each other, and the intensity gradually decreases in the overlap region for one component and increases for the other. The sum of intensities remains the same as for the original field. Each component is delivered using the sweeping window technique with the DMLC. This method provides a smooth transition from one field component to the next, thereby eliminating the field junction problems.

The intensity distributions in the overlap region can be split in an arbitrary manner as long as the total remains the same. We have chosen to split the beam intensity linearly and symmetrically. This may not be optimum for delivery but is very simple to implement and reasonably efficient for the DMLC delivery. The dynamic feathering technique may also be applied to split large static field treatments to minimize the junction problem, provided the machine is capable of dynamic delivery.

We illustrate the beam splitting using an example. It is one of the nine fields [anterior-posterior (AP)] used for the treatment of a head and neck cancer patient presented in a later section. The field is intended to be treated on a Varian Clinac 2100EX accelerator with a 120-leaf MLC. Figure 18 shows the intensity distributions for the large field and component fields. The large fields were used for the IMRT planning, and the split fields were used for the delivery, which was necessary for delivery by the DMLC. Note that the collimator is rotated through 90°, i.e., the leaves travel from the inferior to the superior direction ($x$ axis in the figures). The intensities for the component fields are generally smooth in the overlap region. Due to this characteristic, the sum of the MUs for the components is nearly the same as the MUs for the large original field, had it been deliverable. Thus, other than the time needed to remotely set up another field, there is virtually no increase in treatment time. The film dosimetry for the same beam on flat phantom at 5 cm depth is shown in figure 19, which compares the measured dose distribution for a composite of the two split fields with the corresponding calculated results; the agreement was found to be within 3%.

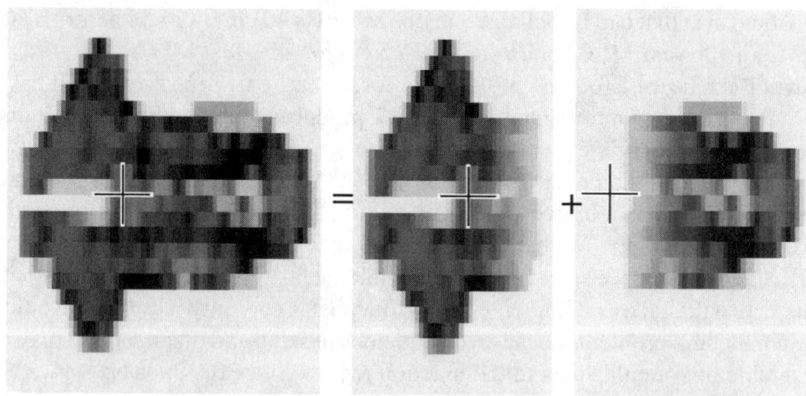

**Figure 18.** Intensity pattern for a typical anterior-posterior (AP) beam shown in gray scale. The beam was split into two subfields for delivery with DMLC. Notice the overlap regions in the middle. Cross hairs denote the isocenter. [Reprinted from *International Journal of Radiation Oncology Biology Physics*, vol 55, Q. Wu, R. Mohan, M. M. Morris, and R. Ullrich-Schmidt, "'Simultaneous boost IMRT' IMRT for advanced head and neck squamous cell carcinomas," In press, © 2003, with permission from Elsevier.]

In summary, DMLC delivery of IMRT allows the large field to be split with overlap regions. The smooth transition of intensities from one sub-field to another ensures that the overall intensity can be accurately delivered. The treatment time is increased slightly if a field is split, and the dosimetric verification takes longer. The film dosimetry performed demonstrated that this method works very well. We have applied the dynamic splitting technique to over one hundred DMLC-IMRT patients treated at our institution. A similar technique was also developed at Memorial Sloan-Kettering Cancer Center and is in clinical use (Hong et al. 2002).

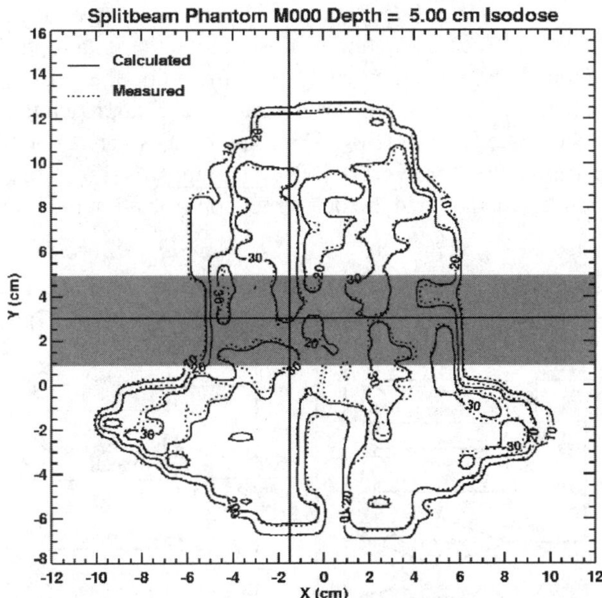


**Figure 19.** Comparison of calculated and measured dose distributions on a plane in phantom for the beam shown in figure 18. The measurement was performed with film. The shaded region indicates the overlap of the two split fields. Notice the collimator was reset to 0 degrees for the measurement. [Reprinted from *International Journal of Radiation Oncology Biology Physics*, vol 55, Q. Wu, R. Mohan, M. M. Morris, and R. Ullrich-Schmidt, "'Simultaneous boost IMRT' IMRT for advanced head and neck squamous cell carcinomas," In press, © 2003, with permission from Elsevier.]

## Deliverable-Based DMLC-IMRT Optimization

DMLC-IMRT (and other forms of IMRT in general) typically consider beam optimization and beam delivery as separate processes. Following optimization, the resultant intensities are transformed into leaf motion in order to achieve the desired dose distribution within the patient during treatment. However, due to the characteristics and limitations of the MLC, particularly related to leakage, the dose distribution that can actually be achieved in the patient is different to that desired. The resulting plan, though often still acceptable, may not be the best achievable.

Furthermore, separating optimization and leaf sequence conversion into two processes increases the amount of interaction time between the planner and the IMRT planning system, and can actually increase the number of "human" iterations, i.e., the number of times that objective function parameters, such as dose-volume constraints, have to be adjusted, and the plan re-optimized.

It seems somewhat intuitive (though non-trivial) to optimize what you actually can control, i.e., leaf positions as a function of dose rate, rather than optimize what you may not be able to deliver, i.e., an intensity grid. Including the delivery devices into the optimization leads to "deliverable" optimization. This approach to DMLC-IMRT was studied by Siebers et al. (2002b) and compared to so-called 'traditional' optimization (optimize-then-convert). Flow diagrams of the traditional optimize-then-convert method and the deliverable optimization method are shown in figure 20.

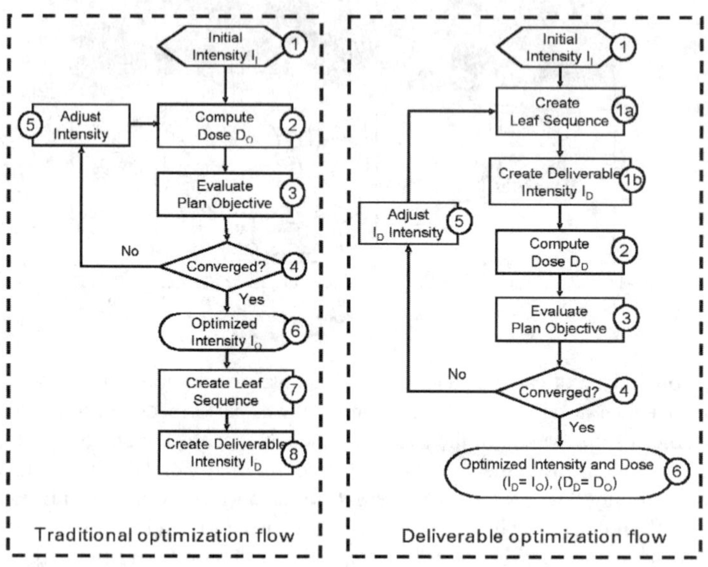


**Figure 20.** Flow diagram for traditional optimization (left) and deliverable optimization (right). Note that in deliverable optimization the intensity to MLC leaf sequence conversion is included inside the IMRT optimization loop. [Reprinted from *Medical Physics*, vol 29, J. V. Siebers, M. Lauterbach, P. J. Keall, and R. Mohan, "Incorporating multi-leaf collimator leaf sequencing into iterative IMRT optimization," pp. 952–959. © 2002, with permission from AAPM.]

Deliverable optimization was compared to traditional optimization for 17 patient IMRT plans spanning several tumor sites (e.g., head and neck, prostate, cervix, and lung). For all of these cases, where deliverable optimization followed traditional optimization [see table 1 of Siebers et al. (2002b)] an improved plan quality score was obtained. An example of DVHs from one of these patients is given in figure 21. This figure shows that even though the PTV dose for the two methods is equivalent, the deliverable optimization plan gives improved sparing of the critical organs.

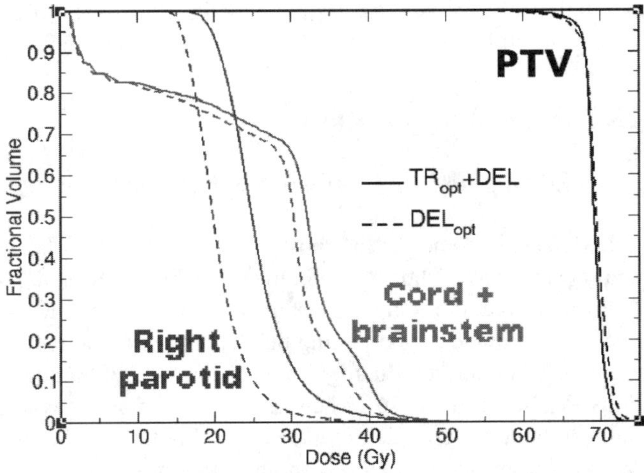


**Figure 21.** DVHs for the right parotid, cord+brainstem. and PTV for a nasopharyngeal cancer treatment plan. The solids lines correspond to the traditional optimization DVHs, and the dashed lines to the deliverable optimization DVHs. [Reprinted from *Medical Physics*, vol 29, J. V. Siebers, M. Lauterbach, P. J. Keall, and R. Mohan, "Incorporating multi-leaf collimator leaf sequencing into iterative IMRT optimization," pp. 952–959. © 2002, with permission from AAPM.]

## DMLC With Gantry And Collimator Rotation

As stated earlier, as the number of degrees of freedom used to solve a problem increases, then the solution found is at least as good as that obtained for the smaller space, provided local minima are not encountered. To this end, gantry rotation and collimator rotation have been proposed as techniques that can improve DMLC-IMRT.

Intensity-Modulated Arc Therapy, or IMAT, has been developed and clinically implemented by Yu and colleagues (Yu 1995; Li et al. 2001; Ma et al. 2001; Yu et al. 2002) and also studied by other researchers (Cotrutz, Kappas, and Webb 2000; Bratengeier 2001; Ramsey et al. 2001; MacKenzie and Robinson 2002; Wong et al. 2002). During IMRT, the gantry continuously rotates at a constant angular velocity and the DMLC leaf positions continually adjust to achieve the planned dose distribution. The gantry typically rotates several times during an entire treatment.

Incorporating collimator rotation during IMRT delivery was recently proposed by Otto and Clark (2002) to enhance IMRT through improved spatial resolution, reduced interleaf leakage size, and maximum deliverable field size over conventional techniques.

It should be noted that the number of degrees of freedom for IMRT can also be increased by several means other than gantry and collimator rotation. These include the addition of more beam angles (including non-coplanar beams with couch angle rotation), the reduction in the leaf thickness, the addition of multiple photon energies, the inclusion of intensity modulated electrons as well as photons, etc. The challenge for researchers and clinicians alike is to assess the benefits objectively of each possible option to improve plans with the hardware, software, planning, and delivery time costs.

## DMLC-IMRT Clinical Application

## Introduction To DMLC-IMRT Clinical Application

The use of the DMLC is in principle the most efficient method of delivering IMRT available currently (Spirou and Chui 1994; Stein et al. 1994; Svensson, Källman, and Brahme 1994). Furthermore, it has the highest resolution in the leaf motion direction, which may have the advantage of sharpening the beam penumbra, reducing margins assigned for the penumbra, and producing more conformal and homogeneous target dose distributions (Mohan et al. 1996). There are several advantages of DMLC that make it especially suitable for complex clinical cases. First, the radiation beam is on during the transitions from one segment to another; therefore there is no penalty on the treatment delivery time when many segments are used, i.e., there is no theoretical restriction on the number of segments one field can have. In practice, it is only limited by the MLC control software. Second, it is not required to discretize the intensity levels before it is converted to a leaf control sequence. Therefore, a high fidelity is maintained, i.e., the difference between the intensity from the optimization and the intensity from the converted leaf sequences is small, resulting in a deliverable dose distribution very close to the desired one. In summary, IMRT with DMLC allows highly modulated intensity patterns to be delivered; this makes it a desirable candidate for the demanding clinical cases where the clinical objectives are often complex and the resulting intensities are heavily modulated.

In this section, we present several typical clinical DMLC-IMRT cases that were implemented at our institution using in-house developed software (Wu and Mohan 2000) interfaced to the PINNACLE[3] treatment planning system.[4] The clinical rationale, IMRT planning techniques, and resulting dose distributions are shown to demonstrate DMLC-IMRT capability.

## Head And Neck Cancer

Because of the complex anatomy and numerous tissue types encountered, intensity-modulated treatment design for head and neck carcinomas is particularly challenging. Conventional treatments are often divided into two (or sometimes even more) phases: an initial large-field treatment followed by a boost to a reduced volume. In the large-field treatment, radiation is delivered not only to the gross disease but also to the regions of microscopic extensions and suspected disease. Towards the end of the treatment course, treatment volumes are reduced, partly with the assumption that microscopic disease requires a lower dose to control and partly to spare an overlap-

---

[4] Philips Radiation Oncology Systems, Milpitas, CA.

ping or adjacent normal structure. On the other hand, IMRT dose distributions are most conformal when designed to be delivered in the form of a "simultaneous integrated boost" or SIB (Wu et al. 2000b, 2003).

A VCU Radiation Oncology Phase I/II Head and Neck IMRT protocol utilizes this SIB strategy in which volumes of regional, suspected, and gross disease are all treated simultaneously. A dose of 68.1, 70.8, or 73.8 Gy is delivered to the gross tumor volume (GTV) in 30 fractions. Note the prescription dose varies as this is a dose escalation protocol. Over the same time course, the clinical target volume delineated by an approximate 1 cm margin around the GTV, the $CTV_{GTV}$, a region with a high risk of subclinical disease, receives 60 Gy. All uninvolved lymph node bearing tissues within the treated field, $CTV_{nodes}$, receive 54 Gy. The GTV includes the primary tumor and clinically involved lymph nodes. $CTV_{GTV}$ margins are edited as necessary to minimize critical normal tissue coverage, (e.g., mucosal surfaces in the oral cavity, oropharynx, and hypopharynx), to extend into areas at high risk for tumor infiltration (e.g., soft tissues of the tongue for tongue base carcinomas), or to exclude air. The $CTV_{nodes}$ include all lymph node groups electively irradiated, based on their risk of subclinical involvement. For reasons of consistency with the previous clinical experiences at our institution, target volume definitions are slightly different from those in International Commission on Radiation Units and Measurements (ICRU) reports 50 and 62 (ICRU 1993, 1999). In the ICRU reports, dose is prescribed to the PTV, not to the clinical target volume (CTV) or GTV. Our definitions of GTV and CTV also include a 2- to 3-mm margin for setup uncertainties and organ motion. Critical structures of relevance include the spinal cord, brainstem, parotid glands, portions of the larynx below the level of the hyoid bone, optic nerves/chiasm, and globes. Prescription dose levels and acceptable tolerance doses for organs-at-risk (OAR) are listed in table 1. To further ensure sparing of the spinal cord and brainstem due to setup uncertainties and patient motion, a 0.5 cm circumferential margin around each of these structures, except in the cranial-caudal direction, is added. A planning organ at risk volume (PRV) margin is only added to the cord and brainstem, and not other critical structures due to the serial nature of the cord and brainstem, and hence the chance for significant injury if a small volume receives a high dose. Such additions do not compromise the dose coverage of the target volumes. The typical IMRT planning parameters used during optimization are given in table 2 in Wu et al. (2003).

Nine 6-MV coplanar photon beams at equi-spaced gantry angles are used for the planning. While non-coplanar beams may provide some additional benefit, they are not considered for reasons of simplicity and delivery efficiency. The non-coplanar beam setup requires changing the couch angle, which, for our treatment machines, cannot be executed without entering the treatment room and prolonging the overall treatment time substantially.

**Table 1.** Prescription Doses and Tolerance Doses for Organs at Risk (OARs) for the VCU
Radiation Oncology Head And Neck IMRT Dose Escalation Protocol
(Note the Differences in GTV Dose Levels)

| Structures | Dose Volume Prescription |
|---|---|
| GTV | 68.1, 70.8, or 73.8 Gy to 98% of the volume |
| $CTV_{GTV}$ | 60 Gy to 95% of the volume |
| $CTV_{Nodes}$ | 54 Gy to 90% of the volume |
| Cord | Maximum dose <45 Gy, with 0.5 cm lateral margin |
| Brainstem | Maximum dose <55 Gy, with 0.5 cm lateral margin |
| Parotid gland | Volume (30 Gy) <50%, or as low as possible |

**Table 2.** Typical IMRT Planning Parameters for Various Targets
and Organs at Risk (OARs) for Lung IMRT at VCU

| Structures | Dose Volume Planning Parameters |
|---|---|
| $PTV_{GTV}$ | 100% >60 Gy, penalty = 20<br>100% <60.01 Gy, penalty = 5 |
| $PTV_{Nodes}$ | 100% >50.4 Gy, penalty = 20<br>100% <60.01 Gy, penalty = 5 |
| Lungs | 80% <20 Gy, penalty = 100 |
| Cord | 100% <45 Gy, penalty = 100 |
| Heart | 100% <60 Gy, penalty = 5 |

[Reprinted from *International Journal of Radiation Oncology Biology Physics*, vol 55, Q. Wu, R. Mohan, M. M. Morris, and R. Ullrich-Schmidt, "'Simultaneous boost IMRT' IMRT for advanced head and neck squamous cell carcinomas," In press. © 2003, with permission from Elsevier.]

The collimator angles are generally set to 90°; therefore, the MLC leaves move along the patient cranial-caudal direction. The reasons for this choice of collimator angle are two-fold: (1) this arrangement produces superior dose distributions since the computed tomography (CT) image slice thickness (3 mm) is usually less than the MLC leaf width (5 or 10 mm). If the collimator angle were set to the default (0°), each leaf pair would cover at least two CT slices. This would result in sub-optimal dose distributions in situations where the contours of volume(s) of interest changed substantially between adjacent slices. (2) In addition, at collimator angles set to 90°, the inter-leaf leakage and the tongue-and-groove effects through the MLC and parallel to the leaf motion direction, which could be significant in IMRT delivered by DMLC, are effectively smoothed by the presence of other beams, i.e., this unwanted leakage dose is averaged over different regions in the patient for each beam. On the other hand, if the collimators were set to 0° for all beams, then leakage from the same pair of MLC leaves would occur on the same CT slice.

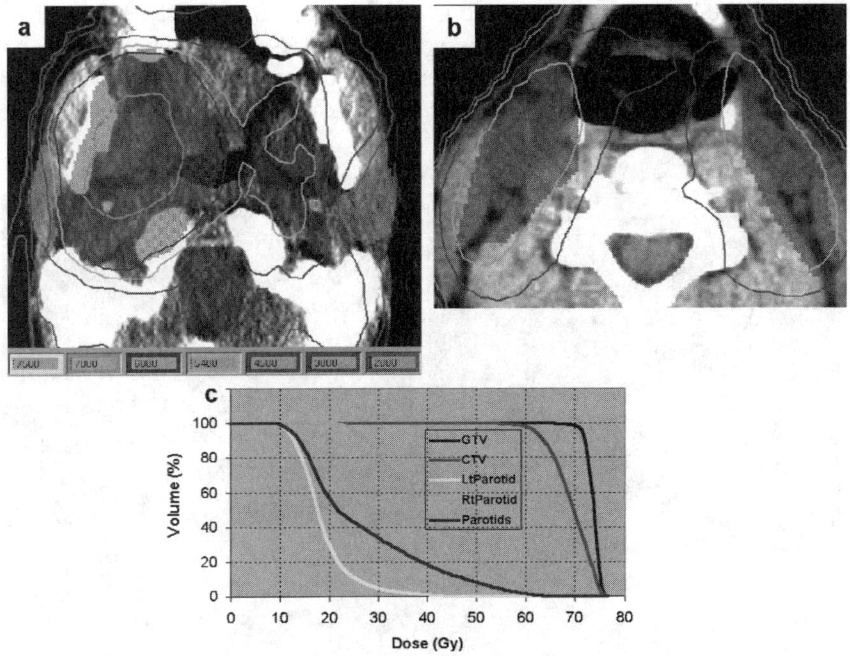



**Figure 22.** Dose distributions for one patient at the 70.8 Gy level. The gross tumor volume (GTV) is located on the right side; therefore, the left parotid gland is spared more than the right parotid gland. (a) Isodose distributions on one transverse CT slice at the GTV level with parotid glands. (b) Isodose lines on another slice that is 6 cm inferior; electively treated nodes and cord are shown. (c) Corresponding dose volume histograms (DVHs) for GTV, clinical target volume (CTV), and parotid glands. Structures shown include the GTV, brainstem, spinal cord, parotid glands, and uninvolved lymph nodes. [Reprinted from *International Journal of Radiation Oncology Biology Physics*, vol 55, Q. Wu, R. Mohan, M. M. Morris, and R. Ullrich-Schmidt, "'Simultaneous boost IMRT' IMRT for advanced head and neck squamous cell carcinomas," In press, © 2003, with permission from Elsevier.]

Figure 22 shows dose distributions for one patient who was treated at the 70.8 Gy level and for whom sparing of only the left parotid gland was considered feasible. The corresponding DVHs for the GTV, CTV, and parotid glands are also shown. Approximately 50% of the volume for the left parotid received 17 Gy, the right parotid received approximately 40 Gy, and both parotids combined received approximately 28 Gy. Doses to the GTV, $CTV_{GTV}$, and $CTV_{nodes}$ all met their prescriptions. Figure 23 shows similar data for another patient who was also treated at the 70.8 Gy level, and for which sparing of both parotid glands was attempted. In this case, 50% of the volume of each parotid gland received approximately 25 Gy.

In summary, SIB-IMRT of head and neck cancers yields highly conformal dose distributions. Significant sparing of at least one of the parotid glands can be achieved with this technique. Simultaneously, high target doses can be attained with satisfactory

352  Paul Keall et al.

coverage. Dose homogeneity achieved is also excellent. SIB-IMRT can be delivered efficiently using a DMLC. SIB-IMRT is more efficient, less error prone, and more accurate than traditional 3-D treatment planning and delivery. In addition, it may have biological advantages: the ability for dose/fraction escalation to tumor and conformal avoidance of normal tissues.

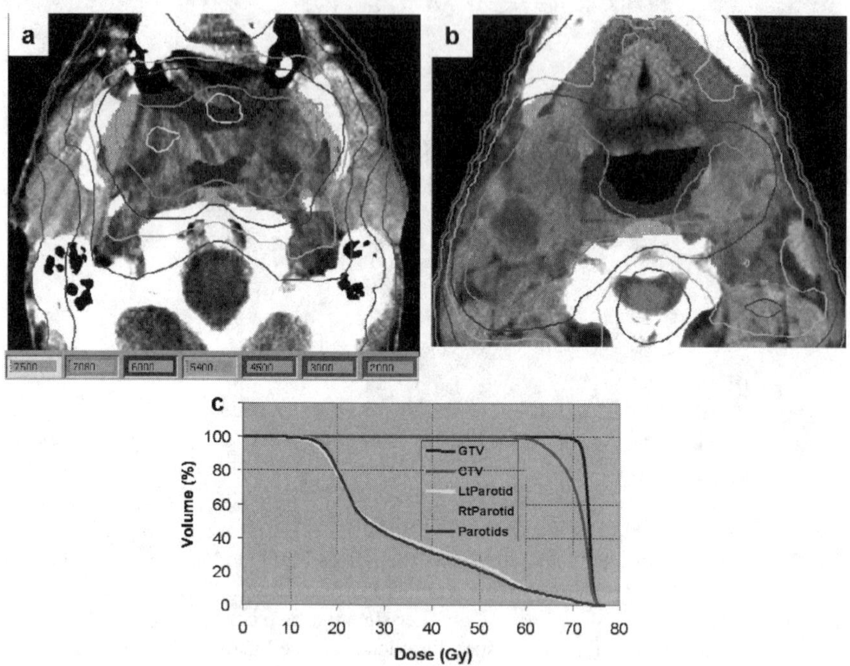

**Figure 23.** Dose distributions for another patient at the 70.8 Gy level. The tumor is located at the midline; therefore, doses to both parotid glands are minimized. (a) Isodose distributions on one transverse at CT slice with gross tumor. (b) Isodose distributions on another CT slice, which is 3.6 cm inferior, showing two involved nodes also prescribed at 70.8 Gy. (c) Corresponding dose volume histograms (DVHs) for gross tumor volume (GTV), clinical target volume (CTV), and parotid glands. The structures are shown in the same colors as in figure 22. [Reprinted from *International Journal of Radiation Oncology Biology Physics*, vol 55, Q. Wu, R. Mohan, M. M. Morris, and R. Ullrich-Schmidt, "'Simultaneous boost IMRT' IMRT for advanced head and neck squamous cell carcinomas," In press, © 2003, with permission from Elsevier.]

## Cervix Cancer

The current standard treatment strategy for patients with cervix carcinoma is 45 Gy of conformal external beam radiotherapy (CXRT) to the pelvis and weekly cisplatin (CDDP) chemotherapy prior to brachytherapy. Adding CDDP-based chemotherapy to

CXRT and brachytherapy improves survival when compared with radiotherapy alone, primarily because of improved local tumor control (Morris et al. 1999; Rose et al. 1999). It is hypothesized that IMRT can offer a means for improving local tumor control through enhancement of any CDDP-mediated radiosensitization and/or straightforward escalation of radiotherapy dose to the primary tumor. Furthermore, true radiosensitization more likely occurs during the fractionated external beam portion of radiotherapy rather than during any low dose rate brachytherapy, since *in vivo* studies have not revealed enhancement of continuous low dose rate irradiation by CDDP. Generally, radiosensitization is influenced by the dose per fraction, with greater effect at higher dose per fraction.

Improved pelvic disease control rates were achieved from results of a previous study in which concomitant boost accelerated radiotherapy was administrated using opposed lateral CXRT fields covering the primary tumor and parametria as a second fraction given 6 hours after treatment to the whole pelvis on selected days (Kavanagh et al. 1997, 2001). However, large volumes of normal tissue received high radiation dose, which presumably contributed to the very high rectal morbidity. It is expected that IMRT would allow improved conformal avoidance of adjacent critical normal structures so that when combined with CDDP, dose escalation to the primary might be achieved without excessive dose to sensitive regions along the rectal wall.

To account for inherent uncertainties, the gross target volume of the cervix cancer ($GTV_{cervix}$) is defined as all gross disease at the primary site, any contiguous lymph node involvement, and the remainder of the uterus, all of which is usually distinguishable from other structures in the pelvis by CT scan. Since the $GTV_{cervix}$ is a designated boost volume within a larger electively irradiated volume, it is considered equal to a clinical target volume of the cervix ($CTV_{cervix}$) without additional margin for microscopic adjacent extension. The $PTV_{cervix}$ includes the $CTV_{cervix}$ plus a 0.5 cm margin in all directions for positional uncertainty (Kavanagh et al. 2002; Schefter et al. 2002).

To account for occult microscopic spread of disease outside the uterus into adjacent soft tissue and regional lymph nodes, the whole pelvic clinical target volume for cervix, $CTV_{pelvis}$, includes the $PTV_{cervix}$ and the nodal regions in the internal and external iliac chains up to the lower common iliac nodes. The $PTV_{pelvis}$ includes the $CTV_{pelvis}$ plus a 0.5 cm margin for positional uncertainty.

Four 18-MV photon beams are used for the IMRT planning and delivery, the same number as for conventional 3D treatments; this is to facilitate the patient setup and treatment. The comparison of isodose distributions of conventional 3-D treatment and concomitant integrated boost IMRT plan for one axial CT slice is shown in figure 24. While the dose for $PTV_{pelvis}$ is almost identical at 1.8 Gy per fraction, the PTVcervix dose in the IMRT plan is raised to 2 Gy per fraction.

In summary, in the management of locally advanced cervix cancer, concomitant integrated boost IMRT offers the potential to improve the therapeutic ratio by enhancing chemotherapy-mediated radiosensitization and/or escalating radiotherapy doses preferentially to tumor tissue with minimal alteration of total dose to adjacent normal tissues.

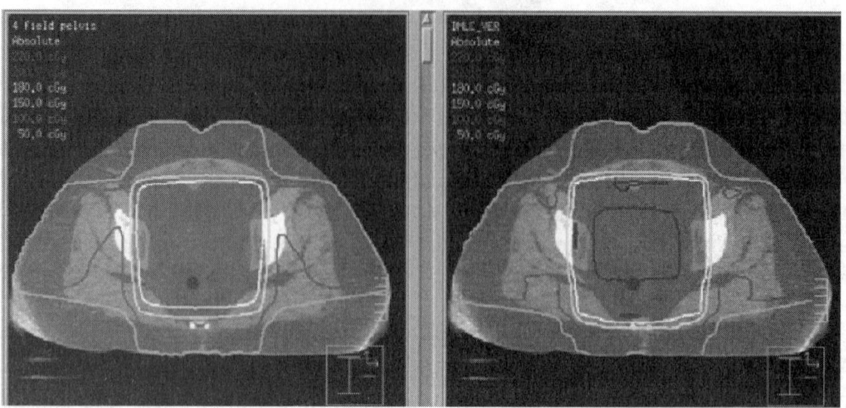

**Figure 24.** Isodose distributions from a standard four-field pelvis CXRT plan (left) compared with an IMRT plan using the same number and orientation of beams. The shaded pink volume is the PTV$_{\text{pelvis}}$, and the central red volume is the PTV$_{\text{cervix}}$. The gray isodose line on the right represents 2 Gy, and the white line represents 1.8 Gy. [Reprinted from *Seminars in Radiation Oncology*, vol 12, B. D. Kavanagh, T. E. Schefter, Q. Wu, S. Tong, F. Newman, M. Arnfield, S. H. Benedict, S. McCourt, and R. Mohan, "Clinical application of intensity-modulated radiotherapy for locally advanced cervical cancer," pp. 260–271. © 2002, with permission from Elsevier.]

## Prostate Cancer

A recent Radiation Therapy Oncology Group (RTOG) protocol (94-13) report (Roach et al. 2001) shows that for intermediate risk prostate patients, the inclusion of regional lymph nodes in the radiation treatment can improve the progression-free survival (PFS) by >15% comparing with prostate only (PO) treatment strategy.

However, in order to cover all possible regional lymph nodes, the radiation field size needs to be increased substantially. As a result, significant portions of critical structures are now inside the treatment volume. These structures include the small bowel, bladder, and rectum.

IMRT has been utilized for prostate radiotherapy at many cancer centers to (1) escalate the tumor dose and (2) spare critical structures (Zelefsky et al. 2000; Xia and Verhey 2001). Dose escalation for prostate patients has been shown to improve the disease-free survival (Pollack et al. 2000).

In this section, we describe the IMRT planning and delivery procedures implemented at our institution for prostate patients with simultaneous dose coverage to pelvic lymph nodes while increasing the sparing of small bowel and bladder beyond the capability of the standard 3-D conformal techniques.

For external beam radiotherapy, the GTV is limited to the prostate; the CTV includes the proximal 1.5 cm of seminal vesicles and 0.5 cm of peri-prostatic soft tissues expanded in all directions except toward the rectum. The PTV is the expansion of the CTV by 0.5 cm in all directions. For lymph nodes, it is extremely difficult to identify the GTVs on CT images. The CTV is constructed by contouring the vascular bundles and then expanding by 1.0 cm in all directions. A further expansion of 0.5 cm forms the PTV for nodal volumes. Treatments are to be delivered in 28 fractions. For $PTV_{Prostate}$, doses of 2.2 to 2.3 Gy per fraction are prescribed (nominal total dose of 61.6 to 64.4 Gy). To compute the biologically equivalent dose (BED) to 1.8 Gy per fraction, the LQ model is used. The BED becomes 69 Gy to 74 Gy if $\alpha/\beta = 1.5$ Gy; and 67 Gy to 71 Gy if $\alpha/\beta = 3.0$ Gy. In addition, a 6 Gy HDR (high dose rate) upfront boost is also delivered to patient (Wu et al. 2002).

Critical structures included the peri-prostatic rectum, bladder, small bowel, and 1 cm anterior skin fold. Seven coplanar 18 MV photon beams are used for the planning. Figure 25 shows the isodose distributions of one plan, and figure 26 shows the corresponding intensity maps for all seven beams. Each of the large fields is split into two smaller fields before the delivery, the splitting procedure is described in the section *Dynamic Feathering*.

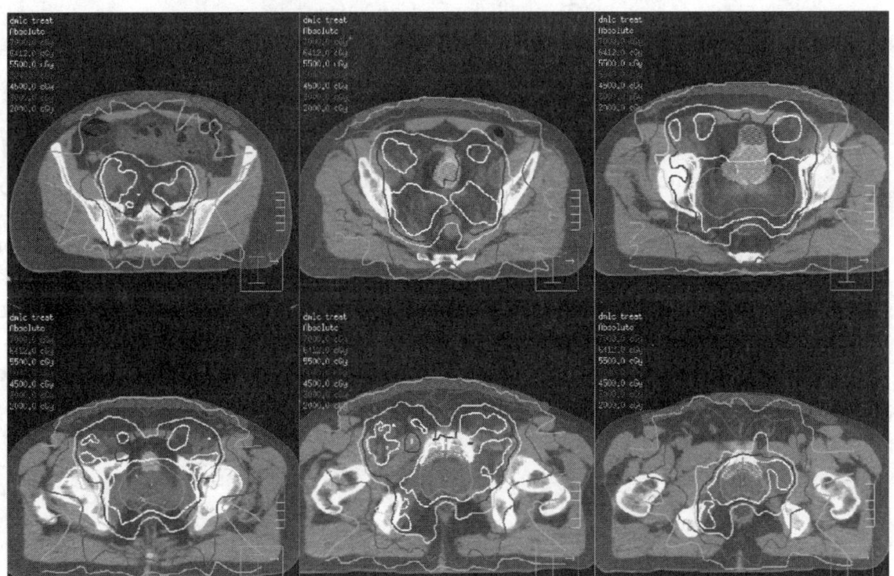

**Figure 25.** Isodose distributions on transverse CT slices for prostate case.

In summary, simultaneous coverage of regional lymph nodes and prostate is feasible with IMRT. Dynamic splitting, DMLC and auto-sequence can rapidly deliver the IMRT treatment accurately and efficiently.

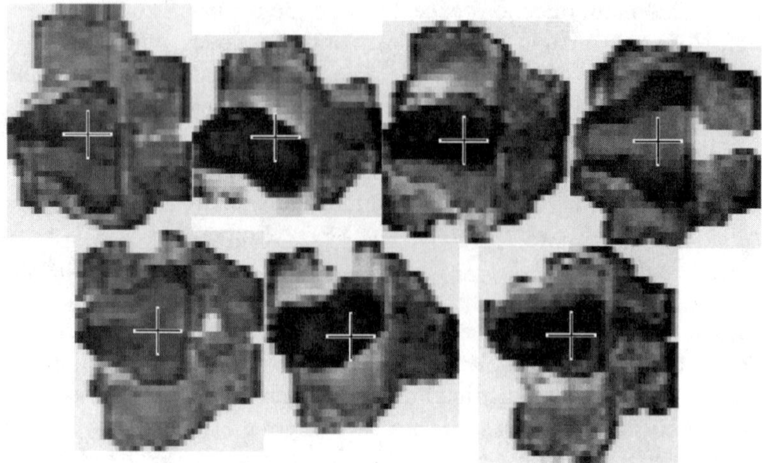

**Figure 26.** Intensity maps for beams gantry angles of 30°, 80°, 130°, 180°, 230°, 280°, and 330°, clockwise from upper left.

## Lung Cancer

The application of DMLC-IMRT for lung cancer treatments is described in this section. Two objections to the use of IMRT for lung cancer are (1) the effect of respiratory motion during dynamic IMRT delivery will cause unplanned significant high and low-dose regions (Yu, Jaffray, and Wong 1998; Keall et al. 2001a) and (2) the effect of inaccurate accounting for the MLC and the effect of heterogeneities during dose calculation will be magnified for lung IMRT causing significant dose calculation errors. The motion issue can be reduced through the use of breath-hold, respiratory gated, or 4-D/respiration synchronized methods (see *Respiratory Motion And DMLC-IMRT*). The dose calculation uncertainty can be reduced using Monte Carlo-based IMRT dose calculation methods (see the chapter herein ***Monte Carlo And IMRT*** by Siebers and Mohan).

*Conventional Radiotherapy Vs. IMRT For Lung Cancer*

Our procedures for DMLC-IMRT at VCU include for all patients a leaf-sequence-based Monte Carlo dose calculation (Siebers et al. 2002a), along with EGS4 (Nelson, Hirayama, and Rogers 1985; Nelson and Rogers 1988) user codes BEAM (Rogers et al. 1995) and DOSXYZ (Ma et al. 1995) to verify the planned dose distribution. For lung IMRT, a fluoroscopy study is performed to determine whether the magnitude of motion is sufficient to warrant gating (generally we use a 5 mm motion criterion above which we use respiratory gating).

Three-dimensional conformal radiotherapy (3DCRT) of the lung typically involves three different treatment plans: an AP-PA pair including the PTV$_{GTV}$ and mediastinum to cord tolerance, an oblique opposed field pair including the PTV$_{GTV}$ and the mediastinum, and a coned down oblique opposed field pair covering the PTV$_{GTV}$. The manual creation, checking and transfer of three plans is laborious. Using the SIB technique described previously it is possible to create a single DMLC-IMRT treatment plan that can treat the positive mediastinal nodes to at least 50.4 Gy in 1.8 Gy fractions, and the PTV to 60 Gy in 2.14 Gy fractions. It has been shown in a cohort of patients that treating only positive nodes (>1 cm) compared to elective nodal irradiation does not result in significant isolated nodal failure (Rosenzweig et al. 2001; Sensn et al. 2002). This approach allows a reduction in overall dose in order to limit toxicity, and was used here.

Though IMRT requires only one plan compared to the usual three for 3DCRT, it can be argued that IMRT requires more QA of both the chart and individual field measurements. Furthermore, for IMRT explicit contouring of the targets and critical structures is required, though the explicit contouring requirements are generally less for 3DCRT where the mediastinal anatomy to be treated can be implicitly defined using blocks. One may also argue that this implicit anatomical definition does not constitute a true 3-D approach where explicit anatomical definition is required.

*Lung Cancer DMLC-IMRT Example*

The example in this section is an 85-year-old male patient with stage $T_2N_2M0$ non-small cell lung cancer (NSCLC). The patient was treated with gated DMLC-IMRT, with the dose calculation verified by Monte Carlo calculation. The contoured geometry, as shown in figure 27, includes the $PTV_{GTV}$, $PTV_{Nodes}$, lungs, cord, esophagus, and heart. The field setup was a six-beam non-opposed coplanar arrangement as shown in figure 28. It is an important feature of any IMRT plan to use a "smart" beam arrangement. In this case, the beams were prominently from the anterior and posterior directions to limit the integral lung dose.

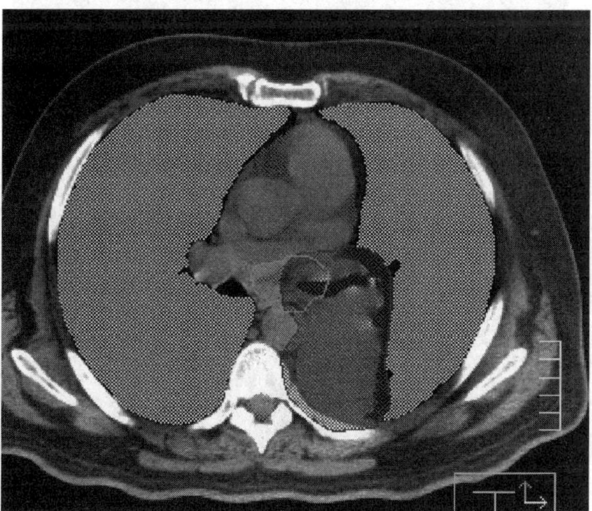

**Figure 27.** Geometry of the treatment. A CT slice at isocenter with the $PTV_{GTV}$, $PTV_{Nodes}$, lungs, cord, and heart outlined.

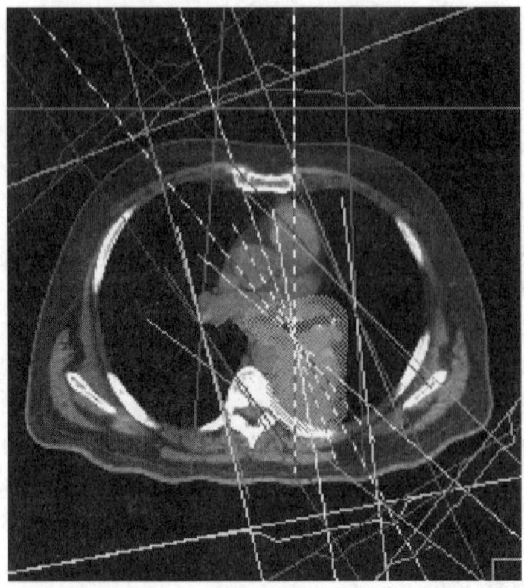

**Figure 28.** Six-field beam arrangement used for the DMLC-IMRT treatment. The combined PTV (based on the GTV and nodal expansions) is shown. The beam apertures are automatically generated to cover the combined PTV with a 0.5 cm margin.

The planning parameters used for the optimization are given in table 2. Note the use of the 100% criteria for the PTV specifications, and a uniform dose specification for the $PTV_{GTV}$, however a lower penalty for overdose than underdose. Isodose curves from the patient treatment plan and the Monte Carlo calculated dose verification plan are shown in figure 29. The superposition (solid lines) and Monte Carlo calculated (dashed lines) DVHs for the $PTV_{GTV}$, $PTV_{Nodes}$, lungs, cord, and heart are shown in figure 30. The similarity in isodose lines and DVHs between the Monte Carlo and superposition calculations, along with the film dosimetry results and the use of respiratory gating give us confidence that indeed the patient is receiving the planned dose.

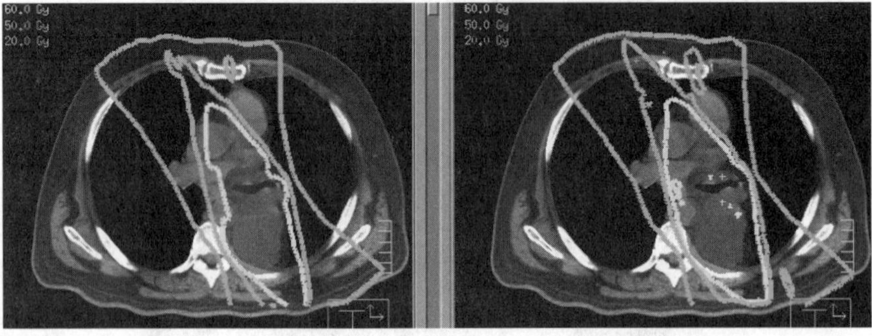

**Figure 29.** The dose distribution for the superposition-calculated plan (left) and the Monte Carlo calculated verification plan (right). The 20, 50, and 60 Gy lines are shown.

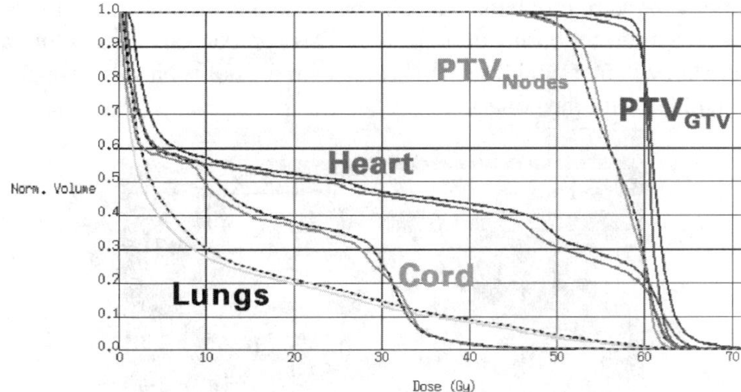


**Figure 30.** The dose-volume histograms for the superposition calculations (solid lines) and the Monte Carlo calculations (dashed lines). The structures from bottom left to upper right are, lungs, cord, heart, PTV$_{Nodes}$, and PTV$_{GTV}$.

## Breast Cancer

The use of parallel opposed tangential fields in the radiation treatment of early stage breast cancer is the current standard treatment approach. Although toxicity following tangential field irradiation is acceptable, with the increased use of Adriamycin, and longer follow-up times, it may be advantageous to further reduce dose to the heart and lungs during breast radiotherapy. Thus, the aim of this work was to develop a DMLC-IMRT technique with the following characteristics:

- Similar target dose homogeneity as compared to 3DCRT

- Lower heart, ipsilateral lung, and contralateral breast dose than 3DCRT

- Acceptable dose distributions in the presence of setup errors

- Efficient planning and delivery.

To achieve the desired criteria, an automated IMRT planning approach for DMLC delivery was developed. Parallel opposed beams are used. The desired PTV dose is 50 Gy, whilst the desired dose for the heart and ipsilateral lung is 0 Gy. For a given beam arrangement, the optimization algorithm finds the optimal compromise between the conflicting dose-volume constraints, with the PTV dose given a higher priority.

A problem with the literal application of the ICRU reports50/62 (ICRU 1993, 1999) formalism to breast planning is that the PTV extends outside the skin (see figure 31). Thus, most planning systems will assign the part of the PTV outside the skin to receive 0 dose. This complicates the IMRT optimization which will attempt to make up for this lack of dose by increasing beam intensities passing though this region for every iteration—a major problem. Our solution, as shown in figure 31, is to add virtual bolus to the breast surface during optimization. This approach also has its limitations—the optimal plan will be found for calculations with the bolus on, which differs to that when recalculated with the bolus off.

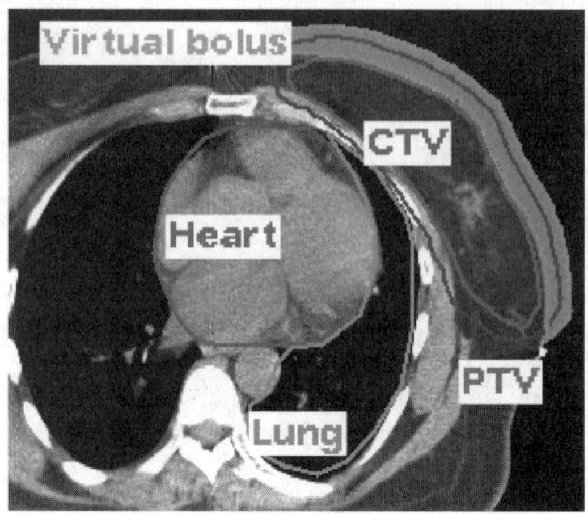


**Figure 31.** A contoured CT slice of the breast showing the PTV extending outside the skin and our planning solution of adding virtual bolus to extend outside the PTV for optimization purposes.

An illustration of the CTV-PTV and virtual bolus addition in beam view is given in figure 32. The results of this method (calculated with the bolus removed) are given in figure 33. The results of this DMLC-IMRT technique compared with 3DCRT are similar target coverage, however the DMLC-IMRT plan gives lower dose to the heart and lung. With auto-sequencing of the beam delivery, and obviating the need to change wedges and blocks between fields, DMLC-IMRT breast delivery can reduce treatment times compared to that of 3DCRT (Hong et al. 1999; chui et al. 2002).

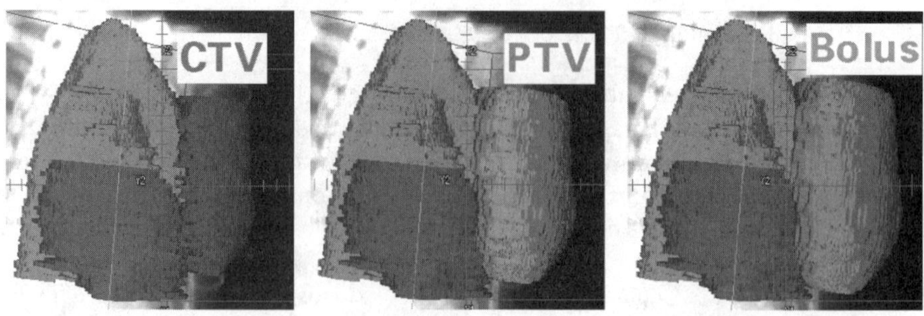


**Figure 32.** A beam view of the CTV-PTV expansion, and the added virtual bolus. The heart and ipsilateral lung are also shown.

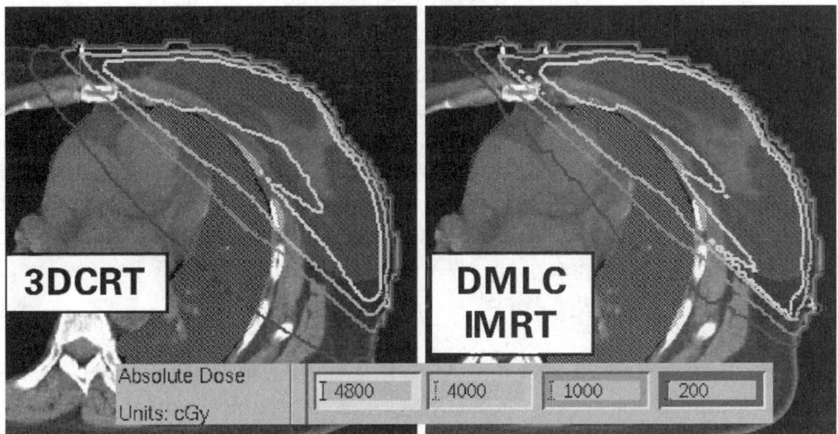


**Figure 33.** An isodose comparison of 3DCRT and DMLC-IMRT plans
for two-field whole breast radiotherapy.

The example in this chapter represents a 3-D delineation of anatomy. Due to the
laborious task of contouring, and the published intra- and inter-observer variability
(Hurkmans et al. 2001) in breast definition, there is a strong trend towards implicitly
defining the breast contour based on the tissue irradiated by the fields that physicians
are used to setting for both 2-D and 3-D breast radiotherapy.

## Respiratory Motion And DMLC-IMRT

### The Problems Of Respiratory Motion During Imaging, Planning, And Radiation Delivery

*Image Acquisition Limitations*

If respiratory motion is not accounted for during image acquisition, as is the case when
conventional radiotherapy techniques are applied in thoracic and abdominal sites, this
motion causes artifacts during image acquisition. These artifacts cause distortion of the
target volume and incorrect positional and volumetric information (Shepp, Hilal, and
Schulz 1979; Mayo, Müller, and Henkelman 1987; Tarver, Conces, and Godwin 1988;
Ritchie et al. 1994; Shimizu et al. 2001; Keall et al. 2002). These motion artifacts occur
because different parts of the object move in and out of the CT slice window during
image acquisition. Motion artifacts are commonly seen with thoracic CT images.

*Treatment Planning Limitations*

During treatment planning, margins need to be large enough to ensure coverage of the
target at the full extents of motion. Generally, for CT-planned lung cancer treatments,
the GTV (ICRU 1993, 1999) is outlined, from which a margin is added to include the

suspected microscopic spread (which added to the GTV creates the CTV). Thus, using ICRU 62 (ICRU 1999) nomenclature, obtaining the PTV from the CTV involves the addition of the internal margin and the setup uncertainty margin. Now, the internal margin by definition includes both intrafraction motion (due to respiration) and interfraction motion. Accounting for respiratory motion by adding treatment margins to cover the limits of motion of the tumor is clearly undesirable because this increases the volume of healthy tissues exposed to high doses. This increased treated volume increases the likelihood of treatment-related complications. However, if the margins are not sufficiently large, part of the CTV will not receive adequate dose coverage.

*IMRT Delivery Limitations*

During the IMRT of treatment sites affected by respiratory motion, the interplay between motion of the leaves of a DMLC[5] and the component of target motion perpendicular to the beam can lead to motion artifacts in dose distributions (Yu, Jaffray, and Wong 1998; Keall et al. 2001a). Yu, Jaffray, and Wong (1998) demonstrated this effect using a simple one-dimensional model. In this work, the integral photon fluence for a sinusoidally oscillating target irradiated by a moving pair of MLC leaves was numerically calculated. They found that in a "worst case" scenario the dose delivered can be up to 480% of that desired, and using clinically relevant parameters the difference can be over 100%. For several sites in the thorax and abdomen, the consequences of breathing motion may negate the potential benefits of IMRT. For maximum benefit, IMRT for such cases should be delivered using breathhold, respiratory gated, or 4-D techniques.

Note that illustrative movie clips showing the problems of respiration motion are listed in the appendix and can be found in the CD accompanying this book.

## Respiratory-Gated IMRT With DMLC

To alleviate the problems listed previously for DMLC-IMRT, a solution is to use respiratory gating. Mageras (2000) showed initial measurements that suggested respiratory gating had little effect on the intensity modulated beam profiles. A more thorough study was performed by Hugo et al. (2002), who quantified (1) the ability of the gating system to reproduce normal non-gated IMRT operation, and (2) errors of delivering a non-gated IMRT beam to a moving target. They found that delivery error was reduced with the use of gating, however due to residual motion within the gating window, that delivery errors did occur, and that these errors were related to the gating window size.

## 4-D Radiotherapy/IMRT With DMLC

Another proposed method to alleviate the respiratory motion problems is to use 4-D, or tumor tracking radiotherapy. 4-D radiotherapy is the explicit inclusion of the temporal

---

[5] Note that motion artifacts in dose distributions may be encountered with both DMLC- and SMLC-IMRT delivery.

changes in anatomy during the imaging, planning, and delivery of radiotherapy. 4-D radiotherapy/IMRT where the tumor is tracking intrafraction motion requires that the beam move with respect to the patient's skeletal anatomy. This relative motion can be performed by either moving the beam, or moving the patient (via couch motion). One advantage of moving the beam is that the deformation of the target during respiration can be explicitly included. Another advantage of moving the beam is that the patient is stationary, and thus less likely react to the applied forces if the couch is moving. On the other hand, the advantage of using the couch for 4-D radiotherapy is that, in principle, sub-millimeter motion accuracy can be achieved in 3-D, whereas with DMLC the resolution is limited by the leaf thickness. If the choice is to move the beam rather than move the couch, then DMLC is required.

The feasibility of using DMLC for 4D radiotherapy and 4D IMRT was studied by Keall et al. (2001a). In this work, a sinusoidally oscillating motion phantom was used to represent tumor motion, and leaf sequences were generated that tracked the tumor motion. Film measurements for a static target with 3-D IMRT (representing the control), moving target with 3-D IMRT (representing current practice), and moving target with 4-D IMRT delivery are given in figure 34 (isodose lines) and figure 35 (dose profile curves). These figures show that (1) 4-D IMRT is indeed feasible and (2) 4-D IMRT to a moving target is dosimetrically similar to delivering 3-D IMRT to a static target.

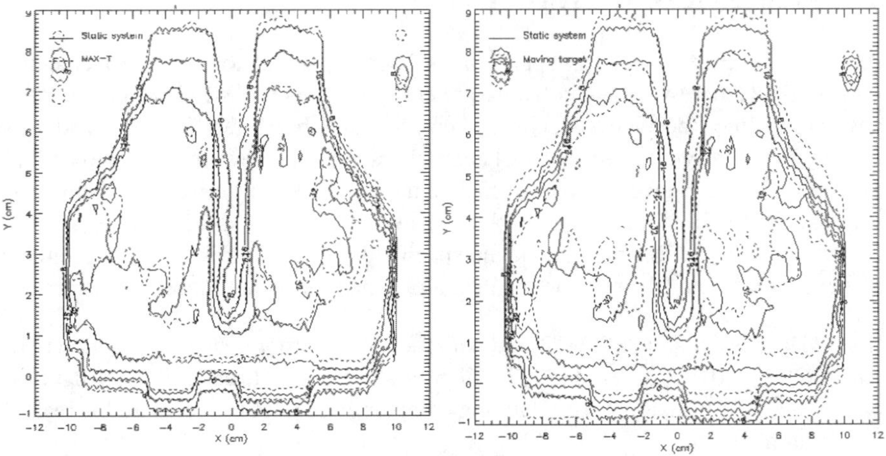


**Figure 34.** Isodose film measurements of an IMRT field with (a) 4-D IMRT (dashed line) and static target/3-D IMRT and (b) moving target/3-D IMRT (dashed line) and static target/3-D IMRT (solid line).

Note that illustrative movie clips showing the DMLC tracking tumors affected by respiration motion are listed in the appendix and can be found in the CD accompanying this book. There are also movie clips of a 4-D PTV on a 4-D CT scan.

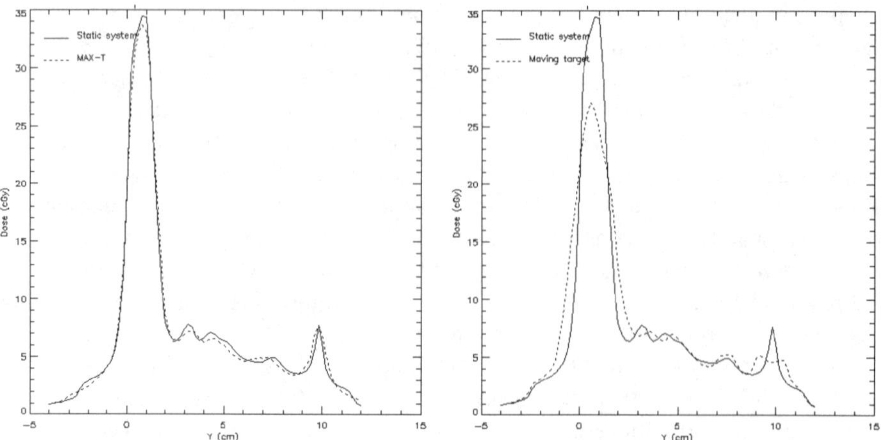



**Figure 35.** Dose profile film measurements taken from figure 34 at $x = 0$ with (a) 4-D IMRT (dashed line) and static target/3-D IMRT and (b) moving target/3-D IMRT (dashed line) and static target/3-D IMRT (solid line).

## The Future Of DMLC-IMRT

As you will learn in other chapters of this book, parallel to the improvements in DMLC-IMRT hardware and software are enhancements in SMLC-IMRT, tomotherapy, robotic linear accelerators, physical compensator-based IMRT, proton and heavy particle IMRT, as well as other novel approaches yet to be developed. It will be interesting to follow the developments of each of these modalities, both as a participant and a spectator. Which modality(ies) will ultimately be the most successful?

The future of IMRT in general, and specifically DMLC-IMRT, is very promising and exciting. Some advances on the near and distant horizon to look out for are:

- The combination of IMRT and both functional tumor image information (Chao et al. 2001; Xing et al. 2002; Alber et al. 2003) and functional normal tissue image information takes planning complexity beyond the comfortable realm of humans

- The combination of gene therapy (particularly radiation-inducible replication competent viruses) and IMRT will potentially substantially improve the therapeutic ratio

- Automated tissue segmentation will reduce the most laborious aspect of IMRT, contouring, and also serve to reduce the large inter- and intra-observer variations, acknowledged to be the greatest error in contemporary radiotherapy

- Class solutions will reduce the current trial-and-error approach to optimization

- Automated EPID-based IMRT QA will substantially reduce current QA time

- Optimization will include deliverable constraints (Siebers et al. 2002b) obviating the time and errors introduced by a separate leaf sequence conversion process

- Increased resolution and degrees of freedom during optimization (including couch, gantry, collimator, energy, modality, etc.) will result in significantly improved plans

- Delivery time will be reduced by more intelligent leaf sequencing

- Planning time will be close to real-time

- Real-time planning and delivery adaptation will be tied to image guidance

- 4-D radiotherapy will become the standard

- Monte Carlo dose calculation will become the standard.

We hope that these physics, dosimetric, technological, and molecular advances lead to improved patient outcomes.

## Acknowledgments

Grateful thanks to Devon Murphy for her careful editing of this manuscript under time pressure. Thank you to Dr. Art Boyer for discussions regarding the content of this chapter. We appreciate the contribution of Dr. Jeffrey Siebers for his ideas, data, and manuscript reviewing. We are grateful to Drs. Sastry Vedam and Vijay Kini for their help creating the movies enclosed in the accompanying CD. We acknowledge the publishers of the journals for their permission to reproduce some of the figures in this chapter. Some of the work presented here was funded by the NCI R01 grant #93626 *4D IMRT: Imaging, Planning and Delivery*.

Thanks also to Nader Salehi (3D Line), Carsten Raupach (BrainLab), Rajinder Dhada (Elekta), Jörg Stein (MRC), Zach Leber (Radionics/Tyco), Michelle Svatos (Siemens), and Cal Huntzinger (Varian) for their time and efforts responding to our questions regarding clinical DMLC-IMRT availability and future DMLC-IMRT plans for their products.

## Appendix: Movie Titles

A list of movies that are on the CD accompanying this book. Note that most of these video clips are best illustrated by using the continuous play mode of your movie software.

**2DmotionTracking.avi**   A 3DCRT field tracking a tumor moving with respiratory motion in two dimensions, as noted by Seppenwoolde et al. (2002).

**3D-CRTtracking.avi**   A 3DCRT field tracking a tumor moving with respiratory motion.

**4DaxialPTV.avi**   An axial view of a 4-D PTV on a 4-D CT scan.

**4DcoronalPTV.avi**   A coronal view of a 4-D PTV on a 4-D CT scan.

**4DsagittalPTV.avi**   A sagittal view of a 4-D PTV on a 4-D CT scan.

**4Dtracking.avi**   A beam view of the DMLC conforming to the 4-D PTV.

**IMRTstatic.avi**   A DMLC-IMRT field with no motion compensation.

**IMRTtracking.avi**   A DMLC-IMRT field tracking a tumor moving with respiratory motion.

**Lung.avi**   A fluoroscopy video showing a small tumor located above the dome of the diaphragm moving with normal respiratory motion.

**MlcCtv.avi**   A movie showing the CTV motion out of phase with the MLC motion. This causes dosimetric artifacts during IMRT delivery [see Yu, Jaffray, and Wong 1998; Keall et al. 2001a).

## References


Alber, M., F. Paulsen, S. M. Eschmann, and H. J. Machulla. (2003). "On biologically conformal boost dose optimization." *Phys. Med. Biol.* 48:N31–N35.

Arnfield, M. R., J. V. Siebers, J. O. Kim, Q. Wu, P. J. Keall, and R. Mohan. (2000). "A method for determining multileaf collimator transmission and scatter for dynamic intensity modulated radiotherapy." *Med. Phys.* 27:2231–2241.

Bortfeld, T., D. L. Kahler, T. J. Waldron, and A. L. Boyer. (1994). "X-ray field compensation with multileaf collimators." *Int. J. Radiat. Biol.* 28:723–730.

Boyer, A. L. "Basic Applications of a Multileaf Collimator" in *Teletherapy: Present and Future*, T. R. Mackie and J. R. Palta (eds.). Madison, WI: Advanced Medical Publishing, pp. 403–444, 1996.

Boyer, A. L., and S. Li. (1997). "Geometric analysis of light-field position of a multileaf collimator with curved ends." *Med. Phys.* 24:757–762.

Bratengeier, K. (2001). "Applications of two-step intensity modulated arc therapy." *Strahlenther. Onkol.* 177 394–403.

Briesmeister, J. F., (1997). MCNP- A General Monte Carlo N-Particle Transport Code, Version 4B, Report LA-13181 (Los Alamos, NM: Los Alamos National Laboratory).

Chao, K. S., W. R. Bosch, S. Mutic, J. S. Lewis, F. Dehdashti, M. A. Mintun, J. F. Dempsey, C. A. Perez, J. A. Purdy, and M. J. Welch. (2001d). "A novel approach to overcome hypoxic tumor resistance: Cu-ATSM-guided intensity-modulated radiation therapy." *Int. J. Radiat. Oncol. Biol. Phys.* 49:1171–1182.

Chen, Y., A. L. Boyer, and C.-M. Ma. (2000). "Calculation of x-ray transmission through a multi-leaf collimator." *Med. Phys.* 27:1717–1726.

Chui, C. S., M. F. Chan, E. Yorke, S. Spirou, and C. C. Ling. (2001). "Delivery of intensity-modulated radiation therapy with a conventional multileaf collimator: Comparison of dynamic and segmental methods." *Med. Phys.* 28:2441–2449.

Chui, C. S., L. Hong, M. Hunt, and B. McCormick. (2002). "A simplified intensity modulated radiation therapy technique for the breast." *Med. Phys.* 29:522–529.

Convery, D. J., and M. E. Rosenbloom. (1992). "The generation of intensity-modulated fields for conformal therapy by dynamic collimation." *Phys. Med. Biol.* 37:1359–1374.

Cotrutz, C., C. Kappas, and S. Webb. (2000). "Intensity modulated arc therapy (IMAT) with centrally blocked rotational fields." *Phys. Med. Biol.* 45:2185–206.

Deng, J., T. Pawlicki, Y. Chen, J. Li, S. B. Jiang, and C.-M. Ma. (2001). "The MLC tongue-and-groove effect on IMRT dose distributions." *Phys. Med. Biol.* 46:1039–1060.

Ebert, M. A. (1997). "Optimisation in radiotherapy I: Defining the problem." *Australas. Phys. Engr. Sci. Med.* 20:164–176.

Fix, M. K., P. Manser, E. J. Born, R. Mini, and P. Ruegsegger. (2001a). "Monte Carlo simulation of a dynamic MLC based on a multiple source model." *Phys. Med. Biol.* 46:3241–3257.

Fix, M. K., P. Manser, E. J. Born, D. Vetterli, R. Mini, and P. Ruegsegger. (2001b). "Monte Carlo simulation of a dynamic MLC: Implementation and applications." *Z Med. Phys.* 11:163–170.

Hong, L., K. Alektiar, C. Chui, T. LoSasso, M. Hunt, S. Spirou, J. Yang, H. I. Amols, C. C. Ling, Z. Fuks, and S. Leibel. (2002). "IMRT of large fields: Whole abdomen irradiation." *Int. J. Radiat. Oncol. Biol. Phys.* 54:278–289.

Hong, L., M. Hunt, C. Chui, S. Spirou, K. Forster, H. Lee, J. Yahalom, G. J. Kutcher, and B. McCormick. (1999). "Intensity-modulated tangential beam irradiation of the intact breast." *Int. J. Radiat. Oncol. Biol. Phys.* 44(5):1155–1164.

Hugo, G. D., N. Agazaryan, and T. D. Solberg. (2002). "An evaluation of gating window size, delivery method, and composite field dosimetry of respiratory-gated IMRT." *Med. Phys.* 29:2517–2525.

Huq, M. S., I. J. Das, T. Steinberg, and J. M. Galvin. (2002). "A dosimetric comparison of various multileaf collimators." *Phys. Med. Biol.* 47:N159–170.

Hurkmans, C. W., J. H. Borger, B. R. Pieters, N. S. Russell, E. P. Jansen, and B. J. Mijnheer. (2001). "Variability in target volume delineation on CT scans of the breast." *Int. J. Radiat. Oncol. Biol. Phys.* 50:1366–1372.

ICRU Report 50. Prescribing, Recording and Reporting Photon Beam Therapy. Washington, DC: International Commission on Radiation Units and Measurements, 1993.

ICRU Report 62. Prescribing, Recording and Reporting Photon Beam Therapy. Supplement to ICRU Report 50. Washington, DC: International Commission on Radiation Units and Measurements, 1999.

IMRTCWG (Intensity Modulated Radiation Therapy Collaborative Working Group). "Intensity-modulated radiotherapy: Current status and issues of interest." *Int. J. Radiat. Oncol. Biol. Phys.* 51:880–914.

Jeraj, R., P. J. Keall, and J. V. Siebers. (2002). "The effect of dose calculation accuracy on inverse treatment planning." *Phys. Med. Biol.* 47:391–407.

Källman, P., B. Lind, A. Eklöf, and A. Brahme. (1988). "Shaping of arbitrary dose distributions by dynamic multileaf collimation." *Phys. Med. Biol.* 33:1291–1300.

Kavanagh, B. D., H. L. Gieschen, R. K. Schmidt-Ullrich, D. Arthur, R. Zwicker, N. Kaufman, D. R. Goplerud, E. M. Segreti, and R. J. West. (1997). "A pilot study of concomitant boost accelerated superfractionated radiotherapy for stage III cancer of the uterine cervix." *Int. J. Radiat. Oncol. Biol. Phys.* 38:561–568.

Kavanagh, B. D., T. E. Schefter, Q. Wu, S. Tong, F. Newman, M. Arnfield, S. H. Benedict, S. McCourt, and R. Mohan. (2002). "Clinical application of intensity-modulated radiotherapy for locally advanced cervical cancer." *Semin. Radiat. Oncol.* 12:260–271.

Kavanagh, B. D., E. M. Segreti, D. Koo, A. Amir, D. Arthur, J. Wheelock, R. M. Cardinale, and R. K. Schmidt-Ullrich. (2001). "Long-term local control and survival after concomitant boost accelerated radiotherapy for locally advanced cervix cancer." *Am. J. Clin. Oncol.* 24:113–119.

Keall, P. J., V. R. Kini, S. S. Vedam, and R. Mohan. (2001). "Motion adaptive x-ray therapy: A feasibility study." *Phys. Med. Biol.* 46:1–10.

Keall, P. J., J. V. Siebers, M. Arnfield, J. O. Kim, and R. Mohan. (2001b). "Monte Carlo dose calculations for dynamic IMRT treatments." *Phys. Med. Biol.* 46:929–941.

Keall, P. J., V. R. Kini, S. S. Vedam, and R. Mohan. (2002). "Potential radiotherapy improvements with respiratory gating." *Australas. Phys. Engr. Sci. Med.* 25:1–6.

Kim, J. O., J. V. Siebers, P. J. Keall, M. R. Arnfield, and R. Mohan. (2001). "A Monte Carlo study of radiation transport through multileaf collimators." *Med. Phys.* 28:2497–2506.

Li, X. A., L. Ma, S. Naqvi, R. Shih, and C. Yu. (2001). "Monte Carlo dose verification for intensity modulated arc therapy." *Phys. Med. Biol.* 46(9):2269–2282.

Liu, H. H., F. Verhaegen, and L. Dong. (2001). "A method of simulating dynamic multileaf collimators using Monte Carlo techniques for intensity-modulated radiation therapy." *Phys. Med. Biol.* 46:2283–2298.

LoSasso T., C.-S. Chui, and C. C. Ling. (1998). "Physical and dosimetric aspects of a multileaf collimation system used in the dynamic mode for implementing intensity modulated radiotherapy." *Med. Phys.* 25:1919–1927.

Low, D. A., W. B. Harms, S. Mutic, and J. A. Purdy. (1998). "A technique for the quantitative evaluation of dose distributions." *Med. Phys.* 25:656–661.

Low, D. A., J. W. Sohn, E. E. Klein, J. Markman, S. Mutic, and J. F. Dempsey. (2001). "Characterization of a commercial multileaf collimator used for intensity modulated radiation therapy." *Med. Phys.* 28:752–756.

Ma, C.-M., P. Reckwerdt, M. Holmes, D. W. O. Rogers, B. Geiser, and B. Walters. (1995). DOSXYZ Users Manual. Report PIRS-0509b (National Research Council of Canada).

Ma, L., A. L. Boyer, C.-M. Ma, and L. Xing. (1999). "Synchronizing dynamic multileaf collimators for producing two-dimensional intensity-modulated fields with minimum beam delivery time." *Int. J. Radiat. Oncol. Biol. Phys.* 44:1147–1154.

Ma, L., C. X. Yu, M. Earl, T. Holmes, M. Sarfaraz, X. A. Li, D. Shepard, P. Amin, S. DiBiase, M. Suntharalingam, and C. Mansfield. (2001). "Optimized intensity-modulated arc therapy for prostate cancer treatment." *Int. J. Cancer* 96:379–384.

MacKenzie, M. A., and D. M. Robinson. (2002). "Intensity modulated arc deliveries approximated by a large number of fixed gantry position sliding window dynamic multileaf collimator fields." *Med. Phys.* 29:2359–2365.

Mageras, G. S. "Interventional Strategies for Reducing Respiratory-Induced Motion in External Beam Therapy" in *XIIIth International Conference on the Use of Computers in Radiation Therapy (XIII ICCR)*. Heidelberg, Germany. Heidelberg: Springer-Verlag, pp. 514–516, 2000.

Mayo, J. R., N. L. Müller, and R. M. Henkelman. (1987). "The double-fissure sign: A motion artifact on thin-section CT scans." *Radiol.* 165:580–581.

Mohan, R., Q. Wu, M. Manning, and R. Schmidt-Ullrich. (2000). "Radiobiological considerations in the design of fractionation strategies for intensity-modulated radiation therapy of head and neck cancers." *Int. J. Radiat. Oncol. Biol. Phys* 46(3):619–630.

Mohan, R., Q. Wu, X. Wang, and J. Stein. (1996). "Intensity modulation optimization, lateral transport of radiation, and margins." *Med. Phys.* 23:2011–2021.

Morris, M., P. J. Eifel, J. Lu, P. W. Grigsby, C. Levenback, R. E. Stevens, M. Rotman, D. M. Gershenson, and D. G. Mutch. (1999). "Pelvic radiation with concurrent chemotherapy compared with pelvic and para-aortic radiation for high-risk cervical cancer." *N. Engl. J. Med.* 340:1137–1143.

Nelson, W. R., H. Hirayama, and D. W. O. Rogers. (1985). The EGS4 Code System, Report SLAC-265 (Stanford, CA: Stanford Linear Accelerator Center).

Nelson, W. R., and D. W. O. Rogers. "Structure and Operation of the EGS4 Code System" in *Monte Carlo Transport of Electrons and Photons*. T. M. Jenkins, W. R. Nelson, and A. Rindi (eds.). New York: Plenum, pp. 287–305, 1988.

Otto, K., and B. G. Clark. (2002). "Enhancement of IMRT delivery through MLC rotation." *Phys. Med. Biol.* 47 3997–4017

Pollack, A., G. K. Zagars, L. G. Smith, J. J. Lee, A. C. von Aschenbach, J. A. Antolak, G. Starkschall, and I. Rosen. (2000). "Preliminary results of a randomized radiotherapy dose-escalation study comparing 70 Gy with 78 Gy for prostate cancer." *J. Clin. Oncol.* 18(23):3904–3911.

Ramsey, C. R., K. M. Spencer, R. Alhakeem, and A. L. Oliver. (2001). "Leaf position error during conformal dynamic arc and intensity modulated arc treatments." *Med. Phys.* 28:67–72.

Ritchie, C. J., J. Hseih, M. F. Gard, J. D. Godwin, Y. Kim, and C. R. Crawford. (1994). "Predictive respiratory gating: A new method to reduce motion artifacts on CT scans." *Radiol.* 190:847–852.

Roach, M., J. D. Lu, C. Lawton, I. C. Hsu, M. Machtay, M. J. Seider, M. Rotman, C. Jones, S. O. Asbell, R. K. Valicenti, S. Han Jr., and W. S. Shipley. (2001). "A phase III trial comparing whole-pelvic (wp) to prostate only (po) radiotherapy and neoadjuvant to adjuvant total androgen suppression (tas): Preliminary analysis of RTOG-9413 (abstract)." *Int. J. Radiat. Oncol. Biol. Phys.* 51:3.

Rogers, D. W. O., B. A. Faddegon, G. X. Ding, C.-M. Ma, J. We, and T. R. Mackie. (1995). "BEAM: A Monte Carlo code to simulate radiotherapy treatment unit." *Med. Phys.* 22:503–524.

Rose, P. G., B. N. Bundy, E. B. Watkins, J. T. Thigpen, G. Deppe, M. A. Maiman, D. L. Clarke-Pearson, and S. Insalaco. (1999). "Concurrent cisplatin-based radiotherapy and chemotherapy for locally advanced cervical cancer." *N. Engl. J. Med.* 340:1144–1153.

Rosenzweig, K. E., S. E. Sim, B. Mychalczak, L. E. Braban, R. Schindelheim, and S. A. Leibel. (2001). "Elective nodal irradiation in the treatment of non-small-cell lung cancer with three-dimensional conformal radiation therapy." *Int. J. Radiat. Oncol. Biol. Phys.* 50:681–685.

Schefter, T. E., B. D. Kavanagh, Q. Wu, S. Tong, F. Newman, S. McCourt, M. Arnfield, S. Benedict, and R. Mohan. (2002). "Technical considerations in the application of intensity-modulated radiotherapy as a concomitant integrated boost for locally-advanced cervix cancer." *Med. Dosim.* 27:177–184.

Senan, S., S. Burgers, M. J. Samson, R. J. van Klaveren, S. S. Oei, J. van Sornsen de Koste, P. W. Voet, F. J. Lagerwaard, J. Marten van Haarst, J. G. Aerts, J. P. van Meerbeeck. (2002). "Can elective nodal irradiation be omitted in stage III non-small-cell lung cancer? Analysis of recurrences in a phase II study of induction chemotherapy and involved-field radiotherapy." *Int. J. Radiat. Oncol. Biol. Phys.* 54:999–1006.

Seppenwoolde, Y., H. Shirato, K. Kitamura, S. Shimizu, M. van Herk, J. V. Lebesque, and K. Miyasaka. (2002). "Precise and real-time measurement of 3D tumor motion in lung due to breathing and heartbeat, measured during radiotherapy." *Int. J. Radiat. Oncol. Biol. Phys.* 53:822–834.

Shepp, L. A., S. K. Hilal, and R. A. Schulz. (1979). "The tuning fork artifact in computerized tomography." *Comput. Graph. Image Processing* 10:246–255.

Shimizu, S., H. Shirato, S. Ogura, H. Akita-Dosaka, K. Kitamura, T. Nishioka, K. Kagei, M. Nishimura, and K. Miyasaka. (2001). "Detection of lung tumor movement in real-time tumor-tracking radiotherapy." *Int. J. Radiat. Oncol. Biol. Phys.* 51:304–310.

Siebers, J. V., P. J. Keall, J. O. Kim, and R. Mohan. (2002a). "A method for photon beam Monte Carlo multileaf collimator particle transport." *Phys. Med. Biol.* 47:3225–3249.

Siebers, J. V., M. Lauterbach, P. J. Keall, and R. Mohan. (2002b). "Incorporating multi-leaf collimator leaf sequencing into iterative IMRT optimization." *Med. Phys.* 29:952–959.

Spirou, S. V., and C. S. Chui. (1994). "Generation of arbitrary intensity profiles by dynamic jaws or multileaf collimators." *Med. Phys.* 21:1031–1041.

Spirou, S. V., and C. S. Chui. (1996). "Generation of arbitrary intensity profiles by combining the scanning beam with dynamic multileaf collimation." *Med. Phys.*23:1–8.

Stein, J., T. Bortfeld, B. Dörschel and W. Schlegel. (1994). "Dynamic x-ray compensation for conformal radiotherapy by means of multileaf collimation." *Radiother. Oncol.* 32:163–173.

Svensson, R., P. Källmann, and A. Brahme. (1994). "Analytical solution for the dynamic control of multileaf collimators." *Phys. Med. Biol.* 39:37–61.

Tarver, R. D., D. J. Conces, and J. D. Godwin. (1988). "Motion artifacts on CT simulate bronchiectasis." *Am. J. Roentgenol.* 151:1117–1119.

Van Esch, A., J. Bohsung, P. Sorvari, M. Tenhunun, M. Fagundes, T. DiPetrillo, B. Kramer, M. Koistinen, and M. J. Engler. (2002). "Acceptance tests and quality control (QC) procedures for the clinical implementation of intensity modulated radiotherapy (IMRT) using inverse planning and the sliding window technique: experience from five radiotherapy departments." *Radiother. Oncol.* 65:53–70.

van Santvoort, J. and B. Heijmen. (1996). "Dynamic multileaf collimation without "tongue-and-groove" underdose effects." *Phys. Med. Biol.* 41:2091–2105.

Webb, S., T. Bortfeld, J. Stein, and D. Convery. (1997). "The effect of stair-step leaf transmission on the 'tongue-and-groove problem' in dynamic radiotherapy with multileaf collimator." *Phys. Med. Biol.* 42:595–602.

Wong, E., J. Z. Chen, and J. Greenland. (2002). "Intensity-modulated arc therapy simplified." *Int. J. Radiat. Oncol. Biol. Phys.* 53:222–235.

Wu, Q., and R. Mohan. (2000). "Algorithms and functionality of an intensity modulated radiotherapy optimization system." *Med. Phys.* 27:701–711.

Wu, Q., M. Arnfield, S. Tong, Y. Wu, and R. Mohan. (2000a). "Dynamic splitting of large intensity-modulated fields." *Phys. Med. Biol.* 45:1731–1740.

Wu, Q., M. Manning, R. Schmidt-Ullrich, and R. Mohan. (2000b). "The potential for sparing of parotids and escalation of biologically effective dose with intensity-modulated radiation treatments of head and neck cancers: A treatment design study." *Int. J. Radiat. Oncol. Biol. Phys.* 46:195–205.

Wu, Q., D. Arthur, S. Benedict, S. Tong, Y. Wu, and M. Hagan. (2002). "Intensity-modulated radiotherapy for prostate cancer treatment with nodal coverage (abstract)." *Int. J. Radiat. Oncol. Biol. Phys.* 54:321.

Wu, Q., A. Lauve, R. Mohan, M. M. Morris, and R. Schmidt-Ullrich. (2003). "'Simultaneous Boost IMRT' IMRT for advanced head and neck squamous cell carcinomas." *Int. J. Radiat. Oncol. Biol. Phys.* In Press.

Xia, P., and L. J. Verhey. (2001). "Delivery systems of intensity-modulated radiotherapy using conventional multileaf collimators." *Med. Dosim.* 26:169–177.

Xia, P., C. F. Chuang, and L. J. Verhey. (2002). "Communication and sampling rate limitations in IMRT delivery with a dynamic multileaf collimator system." *Med. Phys.* 29:412–423.

Xing, L., C. Cotrutz, S. Hunjan, A. L. Boyer, E. Adalsteinsson, and D. Spielman. (2002). "Inverse planning for functional image-guided intensity-modulated radiation therapy." *Phys. Med. Biol.* 47:3567–3578.

Yu, C. (1995). "Intensity modulated arc therapy with dynamic multileaf collimation: An alternative to tomotherapy." *Phys. Med. Biol.* 40:1435–1449.

Yu, C. X., D. A. Jaffray, and J. W. Wong. (1998). "The effects of intra-fraction organ motion on the delivery of dynamic intensity modulation." *Phys. Med. Biol.* 43:91–104.

Yu, C. X., X. A. Li, L. Ma, D. Chen, S. Naqvi, D. Shepard, M. Sarfaraz, T. W. Holmes, M. Suntharalingam, and C. M. Mansfield. (2002). "Clinical implementation of intensity-modulated arc therapy." *Int. J. Radiat. Oncol. Biol. Phys.* 53:453–463.

Yu, C. X., M. J. Symons, M. N. Du, A. A. Martinez, and J. W. Wong. (1995). "A method for implementing dynamic photon beam intensity modulation using independent jaws and a multileaf collimator." *Phys. Med. Biol.* 40:769–787.

Zelefsky, M. J., Z. Fuks, L. Happersett, H. J. Lee, C. C. Ling, C. M. Burman, M. Hunt, T. Wolfe, E. S. Venktraman, A. Jackson, M. Skwarchuk, and S. A. Leibel. (2000). "Clinical experience with intensity modulated radiation therapy (IMRT) in prostate cancer." *Radiother. Oncol.* 55(3):241–249.

# Functional Requirements For IMRT


**Timothy J. Waldron, M.S.**
Department of Radiation Physics
The University of Texas M. D. Anderson Cancer Center
Houston, Texas




## Introduction

Current implementations of first-generation intensity-modulated radiation therapy (IMRT) delivery systems have technological styles whose genesis result directly from the design of the machines on which they are based. Second-generation IMRT delivery systems are less constrained by existing design, while utilizing proven accelerator technology. Here is a brief review of the underlying principles of IMRT technology, together with descriptions of existing systems with emphasis on how these principles influence each implementation. By understanding some of the fundamental details underlying these systems, users might better manage the strengths and weakness of the IMRT implementation on their equipment.

## General Functional Considerations In IMRT Delivery Systems: Beam Production And Control

Production of a pulse of radiation in a linear accelerator (linac) involves the injection of electrons into the accelerator in the presence of a microwave accelerating potential. Turning the beam off and on again may be accomplished by manipulating the amplitude and/or timing of these two parameters. The particular techniques applied to this task in a particular linac design may significantly influence the potential and limitations for implementing IMRT on that platform.

The evolution of IMRT has placed more stringent requirements upon the control of the radiation beam used for delivery. For dynamic IMRT, the stability of dose rate in terms of both dose per pulse and dose per time play a critical role in synchronization of the beam modulator. Accurate dynamic IMRT delivery is based upon the presumption that the dose per pulse and dose per time are stable and/or well controlled.

In a stepwise IMRT delivery sequence, there is additionally a much greater number of beam on/off transitions than in conventional radiotherapy as the production of beam pulses is suppressed while the modulating device is re-positioned between segments. The characteristics of the beam on/off transition for a particular delivery system may influence the ways in which a stepwise delivery approach may be implemented. Some parameters of the beam on/off transition are run-up (or warm-up) time, dark current, and end effect.

The time period from beam initiation to the time when pulses of radiation begin exiting the machine is often referred to as "run-up" or "warm-up." During this time, typically the microwave accelerating potential is applied to the accelerator in the absence of coincident injection to allow tuning of the automatic frequency control. This tuning is necessary as the resistance of the copper accelerating structure creates heat, which changes the physical internal dimensions of the structure, necessitating some frequency adjustment to maintain resonance and/or correct propagation of the microwave energy. The length of this "run-up" period can vary from tens of milliseconds to seconds, depending upon design.

During the run-up period, or at other times when the microwave system is active but the beam is considered "off," it is not uncommon for stray charged particles to be dislodged from the walls of the accelerator or the injector. Depending upon their mass and charge, these might be captured in the accelerating potential and accelerated. This phenomenon is referred to as "dark current," and since these stray elements are not necessarily electrons, their direction and energy may be random. Those components of dark current that are not electron-like are generally absorbed in the shielding and materials surrounding the accelerator. For photon systems, most dark current that is transported through the accelerator will be absorbed or attenuated in the target or flattening filter. Photons produced through dark current phenomena that do exit the beam transport system perturb proper treatment and/or contribute to end effect. In general, dark current is not a major concern for photon IMRT, but may present future challenges for implementation of electron IMRT.

Characteristics of injection current control have a significant effect on beam control. As the stream of electrons is introduced into the accelerator, the accelerating potential expends work in accelerating them. If injection current is set sufficiently large, the work available at the microwave power level might be exceeded, resulting in a decrease in the average energy of electrons exiting the accelerator. This phenomenon is known as "beam loading," and it is one of the available means of controlling the beam energy spectrum. In machines equipped with bending magnets, excessive beam loading can result in low or unstable dose rate as the now lower-energy beam is blocked by the energy slits, and/or inplane asymmetry depending on the energy bandpass of the magnet. For non-bending magnet machines the flattening filter and target design are generally optimized for a specific electron spectrum; therefore, extremes in beam loading can produce unwanted effects in energy as well as cross-beam flatness, in the form of increased fluence at the outer edges of large fields (profile "horns").

Slew rate of injection or current is also a parameter that influences energy and stability of the beam. For this parameter it is desirable for the injection current to have the shortest possible slew rate, or on/off transition time. If correct beam loading is achieved at some peak value of injection current and the transition time is long, then the overall effect is a broadening of the electron beam energy spectrum (Karzmark 1984; Wangler 1998; Greene and Williams 1997).

## Dosimetry Monitoring Systems

Most current linacs employ a system of dual transmission ionization chambers and integrating electrometers to monitor radiation delivery. Many of these ionization chambers have multiple electrodes placed in such a way as to be able to monitor the differential beam intensity across one or more planes in addition to the gross quantity of radiation delivered. On some delivery system these differential signals are used to electromagnetically redirect or steer the electron beam in real-time to maintain maximum symmetry.

Dosimetric resolution of typical linacs in use today is from 1/64th to 1/100th of a monitor unit (MU), and most systems are calibrated such that 1 MU corresponds to an absorbed dose of 1 centiGray under specified conditions. As linac beams are pulsatile in nature, a more practical examination of this parameter might be made within the context of the available dose per pulse. For most delivery systems in use, the radiation per pulse might be from approximately 0.03 to 0.06 MU. Therefore, on a single beam pulse basis, the measured uncertainty in a single pulse is quite high, being as much as one part in three. Historically, treatment delivery typically involves the integration of hundreds of MUs in a measurement, but as segmentation of portals is increased and dose integration is performed over a smaller number of beam pulses, this uncertainty increases to significant levels. Using the values stated above and ignoring effects due to dark current and end effect, the minimum uncertainty available for a 3 MU segment is approximately 1%.

In the case of a delivery system with pulse-to-pulse beam control synchronized with the status of a beam-modulating device, the signal's timing and the timing nature of the dosimetry system may be a significant parameter. Recent work found that for a system of this type using a dynamic delivery, significant dose per segment errors were noted for cases of maximum dose rate and small numbers of MU per segment. One noteworthy conclusion of this work was that a significant contributor to the dose difference was the time delay in processing and communications between the linac control system and the modulating device. Another potential issue discussed is the effect of aliasing, or the inability of a digitizing system to resolve measurements as the signal frequency approaches one-half the sampling rate. Although aliasing in the dosimetry system studied was not found to be a perturbing factor in this instance, it remains as a limiting parameter for the increase of beam pulse rates and segmentation frequency (Xia, Chuang, and Verhey 2002).

In IMRT delivery systems, increased dose conformity can be achieved through increased segmentation of delivery sequence. Resultant increased delivery times might be maintained constant or decreased through increasing maximum dose rates. If this constitutes a trend in technological advancement of delivery systems, it follows that the current transmission ionization chamber-based dosimetry systems may become inadequate. Improved synchronization between the linac control system and beam modulation subsystems; as well as increased dosimetric sampling rates, increased MU resolution and decreased dose per pulse appear to be a prerequisite for technical evolution in this direction.

Strict use of ionometric beam monitoring as a means of determination of dose delivery has evolved from early linac technology in which dose rate controls were less effective. Elimination of ionometric dosimetry as the dependent variable for beam modulation is a possible avenue of development for second-generation IMRT delivery systems. Development in the overall technology of linacs and ancillary technologies may permit other means of monitoring as the primary determinant in segment delivery control.

Use of electronic portal imaging devices (EPIDs) to monitor and measure the exit portal can conceivably provide a segment-by-segment image of the distribution of exit fluence for comparison to on-line stored reference images. This approach has the potential to provide a two-dimensional confirmation of the distribution for each segment with the built-in transmission ionization chamber utilized as a back-up monitor. In this approach, additional beam pulses might be added or subtracted to the nominal amount for each segment to achieve the "correct" exit fluence map, with an "over" or "under" dose for the sequence falling within 1 or 2 MU of the planned number delivered. Currently, this technology is in use to verify IMRT delivery verification in the absence of the patient, but resolving the complexities of quantifying scatter and attenuation for individual patient's treatments remains to be achieved (Partridge et al. 1998).

Another ionometric-secondary approach is the use of time as the primary dependent variable for delivery. Most modern linac control systems maintain, or servo, dose rate using the dosimetry system as the primary feedback mechanism. The use of digital timing circuits implies that the resolution of a dose rate-based beam modulation scheme should be similar to that of the dosimetry system. For tomotherapy, delivery of the correct segment pattern as a function of beam angle may be more critical than the precise dose delivered to the pattern. In this case, segmentation control as a function of beam angle with strict limitation of dose rate and irradiation time may correctly displace ionometric monitoring as the primary IMRT synchronizing parameter.

## Beam Modulation Technologies

Currently available beam modulation technologies all utilize some form of multileaf collimator (MLC). Functionally, these devices can be divided into two broad groups. The grouping are Binary MLCs, in which each leaf is either in the retracted open state, or in an extended closed state. Binary MLCs have been successfully implemented as the modulation device for both first and second-generation tomotherapy IMRT delivery systems. Typical binary leaf widths are from 0.5 to 1.0 cm, and travel extents are on the order of 1 to 5 cm projected to the treatment plane. The second broad category of MLC is the cone beam type, in which each leaf can be extended and retracted over some range of travel within the beam. Typically leaves will have a projected width of 1.0 or 0.5 cm and have typical travel extents from 10 cm over the central axis to 20 cm retraction away as defined in the treatment plane.

Other means of categorizing MLCs are shape of the leaf ends, together with the trajectory of the leaf as it is extended or retracted. Ideally, the leaves of an MLC travel such that the leaf faces are always parallel to ray-lines emanating from the nominal source position of the machine. This type of motion results in a sharp or narrow penumbra cast by the leaf end. It can be achieved through the use of swiveling leaf faces; curved leaves traveling in an arc, or through the use of tangent or curved guides to tilt a rectangular leaf as it travels. This type of leaf design is referred to as a "double-focused approach." For binary MLC subsystems, this can be a trivial engineering problem due to the short travel distance involved. For cone beam collimation MLCs, there are unresolved engineering obstacles to implementing some of these techniques in a compact form. Another approach to resolving the penumbra problem is to use planar-travel leaves with curved ends. By selecting the proper curvature, the amount of partial-thickness leaf end that is intercepted by the beam is constant for all leaf positions, resulting in a wider, but nearly constant penumbra.

Both double-focused and curved-end MLC implementations are available as part of first-generation IMRT systems. In general, double-focus MLC subsystems are less compact along the beam axis than single-focus types. This has resulted in planar-travel MLC implementations both as tertiary collimators mounted below the rectangular photon jaws and jaw-replacement arrangements. The absolute static penumbra for a particular MLC may or may not fully represent the system's ability to conform dose delivery to a specific shape. The practical or effective penumbra for some particular field shape is a combination of the projected leaf end penumbra together with the uncertainty in leaf position. This is particularly important in fractionated treatment delivery, where positional uncertainty can have an unwanted cumulative influence. For a system with ±2 mm uncertainty in leaf position and a geometric penumbra of 4.0 mm, the total uncertainty or practical penumbra is dominated by the position uncertainty. Conversely, for a system with ±0.5 mm uncertainty in position and a geometric penumbra of 6 mm, effective penumbra is influenced mainly by the latter attribute. The magnitude of effective penumbra for these hypothetical systems does not significantly differ, despite the apparent differences in individual specifications (Boyer et al. 2001).

Geometric penumbra of the sides of the leaves also affects the delivery uncertainty. For most designs this phenomenon is minimized by utilizing a design that incorporates a tilt of the leaves and/or a proximal-to-distal increase in leaf width to align the sides as parallel as possible to imaginary radii emanating from the nominal source position. This side penumbra decreases the resolution of the fluence pattern formed by leaf sides. The magnitude of leaf side penumbra is a function of treatment head geometry together with the design technique used to reduce interleaf leakage. In IMRT delivery, tongue-and-groove features can produce strips of low-dose delivery resulting from the combined shielding of adjacent leaves sequentially occupying the same region (Balog et al. 1999).

Interleaf leakage, or radiation transport through the spaces between leaves, is reduced through the inclusion of "tongue-and-groove" features on the sides of the leaves and/or through the placement of bearing components between the leaves to act as attenuators. For the case of a leaf side forming a field or segment edge, these side features partially transmit radiation and widen the penumbra.

The presence of leaf side features affects the MLC subsystem in terms of leaf interdigitation, or the capacity for opposed-adjacent leaves to be extended next to one another. This ability is limited to planar-travel MLC subsystems, as damage would occur as the side features of curved-leaf subsystems intersect upon interdigitation. The consequence is that IMRT systems that interdigitate are able to produce isolated low-dose regions in a sequence delivery pattern more efficiently than non-interdigitating MLCs.

MLC leaf widths have evolved to provide higher spatial resolution in shaping beams. Earliest MLCs had leaves with projected widths of 1.0 to 4.5 cm at the treatment plane, whereas current systems offer projected leaf widths as narrow as 0.3 cm. Although a true limit is highly dependent upon clinical application and the treatment planning algorithm used, a recent linear systems analysis of the effects of decreased leaf width on dose conformity indicated that little practical benefit can be realized by decreasing projected widths below approximately 0.4 cm (Otto, Clark, and Huntzinger 2002; Bortfeld, Oelfke, and Nill 2000).

The significance of MLC leaf velocity is dependent upon both MLC design and IMRT implementation. For binary MLC subsystems, leaves travel short distances and occupy discrete positions. Leaf transit times are relatively instantaneous. For cone beam systems, leaf velocity may range from 1 to 3 cm/s. In IMRT implementations in which the leaves are motionless during beam on, leaf velocity affects overall throughput in treatment delivery only. For implementations involving leaf motion while the beam is on, the characterization and control of leaf velocity is a paramount aspect of the MLC subsystem.

Implementation of MLCs as beam modulators follows several general trends. For tomotherapy systems, leaves are generally used as binary devices, permitting a single narrow beam projection or beamlet to be either on or off. For cone-beam or first-generation systems, implementation is characterized by the manner in which leaf motion occurs together with the approach to beam synchronization applied. One technique characterized by leaf motion is the sliding window, in which a variable gap defined by each leaf pair begins at one end of leaf travel and sweeps across the field as the radiation is delivered. The other motion category is generally known as segmental MLC (SMLC), or step and shoot. Here the modulation occurs as a number of discrete field shapes, with no particular sweep, but instead segmental deposition of some cumulative fluence distribution.

In terms of beam synchronization, it is possible to deliver either type of motion pattern using discrete beam-on/beam-off steps. Implementation of one approach or the other depends strongly upon MLC leaf velocity, position certainty, and beam dose rate control. For binary MLC subsystems, intersegment time is fixed at the brief, relatively constant leaf transit time. Because this time may correspond to a small number of beam pulses, these systems allow practical implementation of dynamic beam delivery approach, and might be implemented with or without pulse-to-pulse dose rate synchronization. For cone-beam systems, the relationship between MLC leaf velocity and dose rate control is less straightforward. If pulse-by-pulse dose rate control is available, the sliding window approach lends itself to dynamic beam delivery. This is because for sliding window sequences, the MLC leaves make relatively small changes in position between segments, whereas for SMLC, there may be dramatic differences in leaf pattern in adjacent segments. These dramatic pattern adjustments require more variable intersegment time, and therefore less constant machine dose rate. By comparison the intersegment time for a sliding window sequence is more nearly constant, and machine dose rate can be approximately constant. Because much of the radiation field is closed during tomotherapy and sliding window delivery, these approaches generally require more MUs to deliver a particular fluence pattern than in SMLC mode. This can increase the head leakage contribution to whole-body radiation exposure in the course of treatment. For systems in which pulse-by-pulse dose rate control is unavailable the intersegment time may be dominated by the time required to turn the beam off and on, rather than the MLC velocity. For this type of system, the practical implementation of the sliding window approach is limited by the overall treatment delivery time. Efficiency in delivery can be realized by utilizing a small number of segments in each sequence, thereby limiting the number of beam-on and-off transitions. SMLC utilizing a small number of segments also lends itself to systems having smaller MLC leaf position uncertainty by limiting the number of times an uncertainty is contributed. Likewise the contribution of leaf position uncertainty as a per-segment fraction of field opening is decreased with a smaller number of generally larger openings (LoSasso, Chui, and Ling 1998; Chui et al. 2001).

## Delivery System Control

The evolution of IMRT delivery systems has been entirely dependent upon significant advances in embedded microprocessor and data communications technology. Medical linac technology is, for the most part, mature in terms of the linacs themselves. Therefore, any development that might occur will do so in the form of features and ancillary subsystems improving the efficiency and accuracy of delivery, as opposed to reliability and stability of beam parameters.

Since medical linear accelerators are treatment devices regulated by the Food and Drug Administration (FDA), significant changes to these systems can involve an expensive and time-consuming registration/approval process. This oversight has ensured the evolution of and continued availability of safe, stable, and reliable treatment platforms, and shaped the development of radiation delivery systems. While a stabilizing factor, the regulatory environment motivates delivery system original equipment manufacturers (OEMs) to avoid certain changes in design that affect how a machine controls, produces, and monitors radiation, and instead focuses on added features until market pressure dictates a complete redesign. Although this is not the only pressure upon linac OEMs, it figures prominently in the evolutionary process of delivery systems. Design of control system architecture for a delivery system platform must encompass foresight into years of ancillary technological developments, to maintain new technology compatibility without triggering the FDA re-certification process.

A medical linac control system involves both hardware and software. Functionally, it encompasses user interface, beam production, dosimetry, and safety. The control system also communicates with the other treatment subsystems, such as MLC or EPID, and Record and Verify (R&V) if present (hereafter referred to as delivery subsystems). Together the linac control system and delivery subsystems make up the delivery control system. The architecture of the linac control system ultimately determines the potential and limitations of any treatment mode for a particular treatment delivery system. This is particularly important in IMRT, where successful communication and synchronization with the delivery subsystems are as critical to proper operation as are the basic functions of user interface, beam production, dosimetry, and safety.

The functional aspects of linac control systems having the greatest impact on IMRT may be considered in two groups. The first grouping is dosimetry and beam control, which plays a significant role in the type of IMRT that may be implemented on a linac platform. A second grouping can be thought of as network and information systems (IS). This class of functional tasks impacts IMRT in terms of how efficiently and rapidly information such as treatment and machine parameters are communicated between the linac control system and the delivery subsystems. Beam control and dosimetry have already been referred to in terms of how they impact use of the MLC in IMRT. The time required for the beam to transit from the off to the on state, and the capacity of the control system to do so with accuracy and precision, can determine the available IMRT options for a particular delivery platform. The time required for the control system to monitor the dose delivered and pause the beam or turn it off can influence accuracy of sequenced delivery. As radiation therapy moves from conventional delivery to IMRT, the number of segments per portal might be increased 5 to 200 fold. This implies a minimum similar increase in opportunities for machine interlock as well as human error. Automated delivery through the use of computer R&V reduces the human error element, but shifts the burden of coordination and monitoring to the delivery control system. This places a number of additional functional requirements upon the linac control system. These are the IS aspects of functional requirements for IMRT.

To accommodate IMRT, the linac control system must incorporate fully functional interfaces to the delivery subsystems. This implies either built-in hardware communications ports with adequate speed, or the ability to add such technology. The linac control system must also monitor and interlock the function of these communications ports. Likewise, the linac control system must monitor and respond appropriately to hardware and software interlock conditions occurring within the delivery subsystems. The linac control system must also control and monitor segmented delivery, and interlock unwanted conditions specific to this process, and provide functional fault recovery for intra-sequence interruptions. All these additional functions must be incorporated into the linac control system in a fashion that does not compromise basic functionality and safety.

Furthermore, both the IS requirements and the more conventional requirements must function properly in concert. Timing among the elements of the delivery control system can become critical, particularly in the case of dynamic delivery systems. Here, if the time between beam pulses is less than the time required for the linac controller to process dosimetry status and signal the MLC controller, the result is an intrasegment dosimetry error. If undetected by the control system, this condition might manifest as spatial distortion in the delivered pattern. Errors in this particular timing relationship produce an effective decrease in resolution of the dosimetry system. Instead of resolving the dose due to a single beam pulse, the dosimetry system resolution is now equivalent to the dose resulting from the number of beam pulses produced during the controller-MLC processing and communication period. Increasing the number of devices that communicate in the control of IMRT delivery increases the opportunities for this type of degradation to occur. Another way to restate the above is to note that increasing the number of nodes on a given network without increasing bandwidth will degrade throughput. IMRT delivery systems are networks of specialized equipment. The ubiquitous challenges of bandwidth and standard means of communication are now a part of radiotherapy delivery technology. First-generation IMRT delivery systems incorporate a variety of communications protocols and network topology, sometimes involving incompatible protocols within the same system. This network fragmentation is a consequence of the OEM interest in avoiding both the cost of full re-design and the FDA certification process. Second-generation IMRT systems are designed as networks; therefore the challenges of bandwidth and communication protocol are currently less of an obstacle to development.

## Safety Considerations

Between 1985 and 1987, six patients were massively overdosed during radiotherapy treatment on AECL Therac 25 linear accelerators. The cause of these incidents is generally considered to be rooted in a lack of hardware-implemented safety functions as well as flaws in the software design and testing process used by Atomic Energy of Canada Limited (AECL). The Therac 25 was a departure from its predecessors, the Therac 6 and Therac 20. On the earlier units, the computer control acted as an overlay upon the already-functional linear accelerator in the form of an operator interface. In the case of the Therac 25, many functional controls and monitors were implemented in software rather than hardware. This absence of hardware-based safety interlocks set the stage for phase errors and race conditions occurring during program execution to allow beam-on while beam modifiers such as the target and scanning magnets were not properly placed in the beam path (Leveson 1995). One consequence of the Therac 25 catastrophe was that the remaining medical linear accelerator manufacturers responded by adopting a design philosophy that incorporates full implementation of controls and monitors or interlock functions in hardware are supplemented by, rather than supplanted by, the software. In this paradigm, the computer acts as a parallel or augmentative status monitor and operator interface, rather than as the immediate monitor/controller. Inclusion of this paradigm in first-generation IMRT delivery systems was inherent, as they are based on control systems that evolved immediately after the Therac 25 incident. Second-generation IMRT delivery systems also seem to be designed with hardware monitoring of critical processes augmented by software.

IMRT delivery itself presents few unique or additional safety challenges beyond those presented by physical differences from traditional radiotherapy. For first-generation systems, the treatment process differs in that the machine operator might make fewer trips into the treatment room to change physical beam modifiers or reposition the machine or patient. Intensity modulation replaces physical beam modifiers, and machine repositioning might be done from the control console after a trial run on the first treatment day. Therefore, in terms of physical safety, the introduction of IMRT may seems to reduce or eliminate the risk of patient or therapist injury through handling of heavy custom blocks and wedge compensators, and possibly increase the risk of gantry collision injury. Linear accelerators equipped with tertiary MLCs might be at particular risk in this regard due to the reduced clearance between isocenter and the external surfaces of the treatment head. Collision risk is greatly reduced for the current second-generation IMRT product, since nearly all moving parts of the machine are contained within the external housing. Here, physical safety risks may be limited to possible pinch points as the patient is translated into and out of the bore of the gantry.

# First-Generation IMRT Delivery Systems Implementation

The first generation of IMRT delivery systems are based on existing radiotherapy delivery systems. The following is a brief description of the salient features of the linear accelerator, linac control system, MLC and IMRT process as implemented on three major OEM platforms. The Elekta SL-25 (Elekta Oncology Systems, Ltd., Crawley, England), Siemens Primus (Siemens Medical Systems, Inc., Concord, CA), and Varian Clinac-21EX (Varian Medical Systems, Palo Alto, CA) products are covered. Some features common to all three systems are listed below:

Each of the machines is multimode; that is, capable or producing two or more photon beams and a number of electron beams. This implies sufficient complexity that accidents of the type experienced with the Therac 25 are possible.

For interlocks that may affect dosimetry or safety, all have some form of hardware implementation in addition to the software/computer control. Beam-on may be prevented through hardware interlocks regardless of the condition of the computer control system.

All three have some form of "watchdog" timing system that ensures computer events occur within certain time periods (i.e., if an event is "late," it may be due to some malfunction in communications or processing). This typically is implemented with more than one signal and monitoring scheme. Typically, this watchdog timer approach is used to trigger a hardware-implemented interlock

Each control system is designed such that the process of operation is divided into specific states, such as "On", "Setup", "Ready", "Beam On", "Normal Terminate", "Abnormal Terminate", etc.

The control system may only be in one state at a time, and it may only progress from the current state to the next state, or the last state (in some instances).

The transition from one state to anther is monitored by the control system, and deviations from proper transition result in "System" interlocks that may require additional diagnostic or service actions before resumption of use.

Each machine is based on a "C-arm" gantry configuration. That is, the rotating gantry is more or less in the shape of a letter "C", with the treatment head comprising the top of the "C" and a counterweight making up the bottom part.

## Elekta SL-25 IMRT Delivery System

The Elekta SL-25 is a dual-photon travelling-wave linear accelerator. Up to nine electron energies may be available. The microwave system is magnetron-based; the electron injector is a diode (non-gridded) type. The bending magnet is a 202.5° slalom arrangement made up of three alternating-direction sectors. Electron flattening is accomplished through dual foil scattering. A dual-channel, segmented ionization chamber is used for dosimetry monitoring.

*Elekta Control System Architecture*

The Elekta central control system comprises three Intel "X86" processors and peripherals at the console that reside on an "Intel Multibus 2" bus structure, that in turn communicate with distributed control elements in the linear accelerator via a dual serial communications link. This architecture is illustrated in figure 1. Machine Processor 1 controls the serial link between the console proper and the control areas of the linear accelerator. Control Processor 2 acts as the interface between the linac and operator console by communicating with Machine Processor 1. The Operator Processor 3 is the console interface between the user and the remainder of the control system.

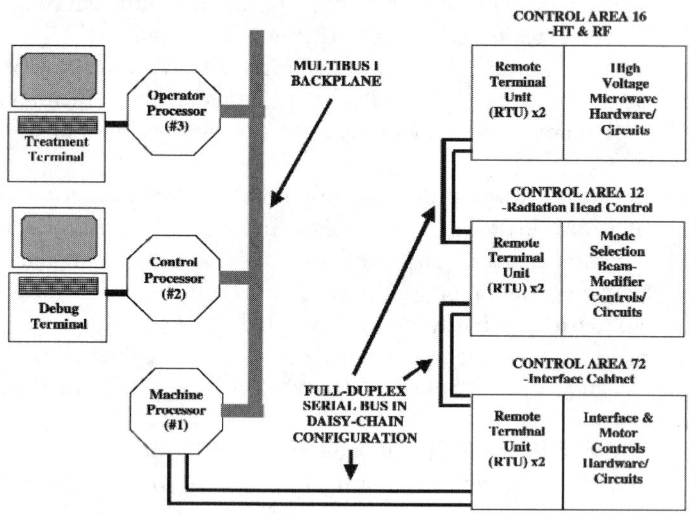


**Figure 1.** Elekta SL-25 Linac Control System Overall Diagram.

The distributed control elements are located in three functional areas of the linear accelerator, referred to as "Control Areas." These are connected to the Machine Processor by means of a full-duplex daisy chain serial communications link. The three Control Areas are the Interface Cabinet (ICCA), the Radiation Head (RHCA), and the High Tension and Radio Frequency (HTCA). Each Control Area has two processors called Remote Terminal Units (RTUs) whose function is to act as the interface between the various functional circuits in the Control Area and the Machine Processor 1. Each RTU contains a processor, or Multiplexer Terminal Unit (MTU), Analog to Digital (AD), Digital to Analog (DA), and signal conditioning circuitry as well as circuits specific to the function of the Control Area. Hardware logic for controls and interlocks is also implemented within each control area through the Field-Programmable Logic Arrays (FPLAs). Hardware interlocks are implemented locally within each Control Area, with status forwarded to the central control system through the serial link.

Logic implemented in the FPLAs controls the two high voltage interlock circuits that pass through each Control Area. The Control Area architecture is illustrated in figure 2.

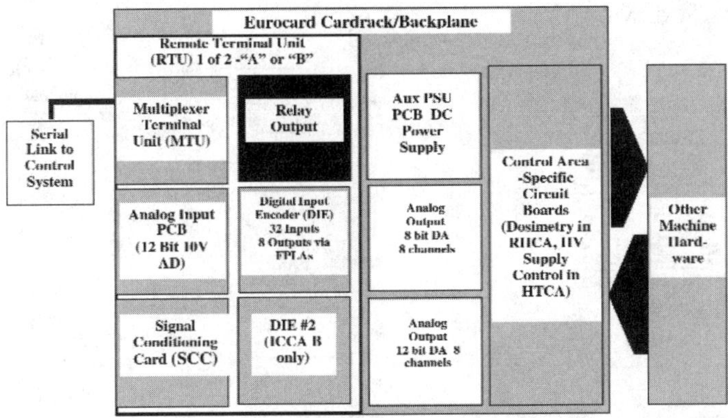


**Figure 2.** Elekta SL-25 Control Area Detail.

*Elekta Beam Modulation Subsystem*

An 80-leaf MLC forms the upper level of field collimation for the SL-25. The projection of each leaf is 1 cm wide in the isocentric plane. Leaf motion is planar; therefore, the leaf ends have a curved shape. Interleaf leakage is reduced through a single-step tongue-and-groove feature on the leaf sides. Interdigitation is not available for this subsystem. The range of leaf travel is +20.0 cm to −12.5 cm. Each leaf is screw driven by a DC motor; drive signals are multiplexed at the processor transmitted by serial communications and demultiplexed in the head of the machine. Leaf position is monitored through the use of a video feedback system. The reflective proximal surfaces of the leaves are viewed via a mirror and video camera arrangement in the head of the machine. A frame grabber digitizes the leaf pattern image 12.5 times per second. This digitized leaf pattern is processed by the MLC subsystem to drive the leaves to their planned positions. The MLC control subsystem comprises three processors connected through an Intel Multibus II bus. One of the processors is dedicated to the input-output processing of video leaf positions, and the remaining two are control processors. One of these provides in-room and console information about the MLC status, the other acts as the controller and interface to the linac control subsystem. The MLC control processor is connected to the linac control system Multibus through an Ethernet connection. The MLC control subsystem architecture is shown in figure 3.

*Elekta Beam Production And Control*

As Elekta uses a traveling-wave accelerating structure, the intrinsic beam energy (the beam energy proximal to the bending magnet) is chiefly a function of the microwave frequency. The microwave power level must be above the threshold necessary to accelerate the injected electron fluence, but otherwise power level does not primarily determine energy spectrum at the exit of the accelerator. The final energy spectrum is selected by a bending magnet system. This bending magnet consists of three alternating sections of 45° down, 45° up, and 112.5° down.

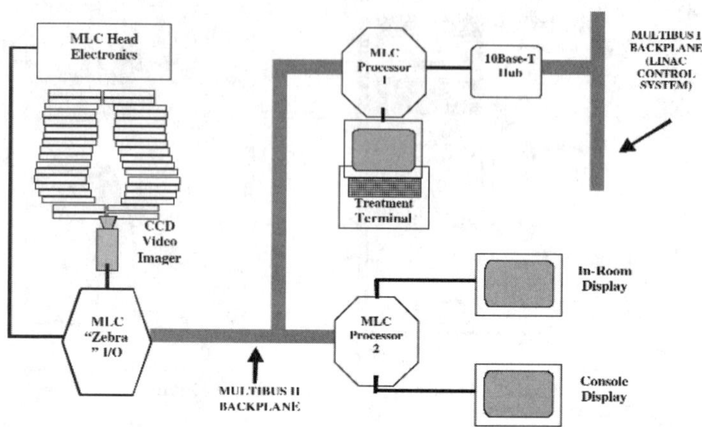


**Figure 3.** Elekta SL-25 Multileaf Collimator Subsystem Control Architecture.

In the SL-25, a gun/injector pulse is generated for every high voltage (HV)/microwave pulse. The pulse rate is 200 pulses per second (PPS) for a nominal dose rate of 400 MU/minute, or approximately 0.03 MU/pulse. Dose rate is selected by adjusting the HV and Injector pulse repetition frequency (PRF). The dose rate is not "servoed", or controlled for some specific value, but allowed to vary slightly. Dose rate may increase to the nominal value during the 4 second "run-up" period as the magnetron is tuned for the correct frequency and the injector and radio frequency (RF) system stabilize. In the case of machines used for IMRT, the magnetron may be equipped with electronic tuning, wherein the tuning plunger is moved by a linear actuation solenoid rather than by the more conventional chain/gear drive. This greatly reduces tuning time, resulting in more instantaneous nominal dose rate at beam on. Beam energy is monitored by comparing the signal on a pair of in-plane or radial electrodes in the ionization chamber. If the beam trajectory through the bending magnet system is correct, then so is the energy spectrum. When this occurs, the beam is centered on the ion chamber, and the signal difference between the electrodes is minimized. If the energy spectrum is not correct, the trajectory through the bending magnet will result in a deviation at the ion chamber, and a charge differential across the in-plane electrodes. This signal is used to adjust the injector current either up or down, resulting in the electron fluence increasing or decreasing. This adjustment of beam "loading" changes the energy spectrum, and so the trajectory through the bending magnet is altered, until the signal difference on the ion chamber sectors is minimized.

*Elekta IMRT Implementation And Delivery Process*

In IMRT mode, delivery is via a "step-and-shoot" technique. The MLC is positioned to the defined shape for the first segment and beam is initiated. Power is applied to the linac HV system and gun filaments and dose delivery commences after run up of 3 to 6 seconds. Once the segment MUs are delivered, the machine enters a PRF Pause state while the MLC is repositioned for the next segment. In the PRF Pause state, the gun filament voltage is kept at the nominal level while the HV system is not triggered. Holding the gun filament at the nominal value from the previous segment ensures that the injection current will be very nearly at the correct value to achieve specified dose rate when high voltage triggers resume. Upon resumption of high voltage triggers, the time required for the dose rate to stabilize is much less than the standard run-up time, in which the RF and energy control systems must tune to compensate for the heating of the accelerator structure, and achieve correct beam loading. High voltage triggers are resumed when the MLC reaches the target shape.

In this approach to IMRT, time in the intersegment Pause state is dependent upon the MLC leaf velocity, rather than the dosimetry system sampling time, machine dose rate, or beam pulse spacing. Overall treatment time limits the number of segments per sequence that can be delivered practically in the clinical setting. The MU end effect resulting from the Pause state may be significant and different from that in a non-Paused beam sequence. In a highly segmented sequence the cumulative end effect might be much more significant than for the case of fewer segments with the same total number of monitor units (Spitz, Personal communication).

## Siemens Primus IMRT Delivery System

The Siemens Primus series are dual photon standing-wave accelerators. Microwave excitation may be by either magnetron or klystron. Electron injection is by means of a triode (gridded) gun. The bending magnet system is a 270° loop with fixed slits. Dual scattering foils are used for electron field flattening of up to six electron beams. The mode motions are accomplished by several mode slides bars that translate to move the correct combination of target, filter, and foils into the beam path. Two slide-mounted dual-channel segmented ionization chambers provide dosimetry monitoring; one for photons and one for electrons.

*Siemens Control System Architecture*

The overall diagram of the Siemens digital control system is shown in figure 4. The console computer is an Intel X86-based PC. It is connected as the master Serial I/O Processor (SIP) to the machine via a serial communications link, and acts as the user interface to the machine. Control functions of the system are divided among eight 8051-based Function Controllers (FCs). These FCs are connected to the control console and each other via a full-duplex serial daisy chain topography. All the controllers are interrupted when polled by the master, but only the FC being addressed processes the data block and responds. The response is in the form of an "ack" (acknowledge) bit in the case of no data, or the appropriate data in response to the query. The serial link at each of the FCs is fed through to each of the others and will inhibit communications to all in the event any one of the controllers fails to respond.

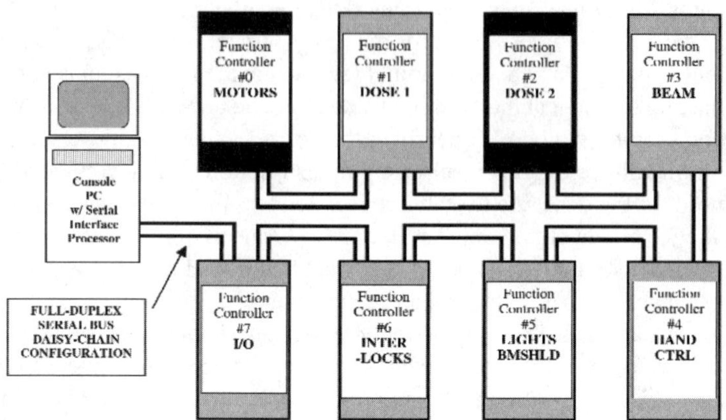


**Figure 4.** Siemens Primus Control System Architecture.

In addition to the serial connections, there are also four control signals lines of interest in terms of the Function Controller operation. The T1 "terminate" line and three "Supervisor" enable signals fed to function controllers numbers 0–4, 6, and 7. Their status enables or suppresses Rad On, HV On, or Gantry (motion). The condition of the three enable lines is a function of both the Logic Interface PCB and the function controllers themselves. Control and configuration information is sent to the input/output (I/O) function controller #7 from the console. These data are in turn sent to the Logic Control PCB (printed circuit board) where it is decoded with respect to current machine status. The result of this decoding determines the proper configuration of the three supervisor lines for the current machine state. In the event of an unexpected configuration of the three enable lines at one of the function controllers, that FC will "time out," and will not send its timing signal to the Watchdog PCB (see below). The operation of these "supervisor" signals enforces the machine state paradigm of proceeding from one state to another in the processing cycle.

The T1 or "terminate" line is controlled by the Watchdog PCB, which takes input of a timer signal from each of the function controllers at 20 ms intervals. In the event that one of the timing signals is late more than 100 ms, the Watchdog PCB will enable the T1 line to all function controllers, suppressing their transition to the HV On state and/or forcing transition out of the HV On state. The T1 line is also connected to the hardware interlock system via the Interlock PCBs, and so the T1 activates a hardware suppression of HV as well.

The Function Controllers are connected to the Machine Control circuits through Interface PC Boards, which encode and decode digital and analog values to and from frequency data. Differential and single-ended frequency encoding of voltages and digital data is used for noise immunity. The Machine Control Circuits consist of the analog and digital control circuitry needed to operate and monitor the linear accelerator, such as the dosimetry, mode selection, or motor control circuits.

Interlocks are implemented via Interlock PCBs, connected between the hardware and interface electronics. Safety and dosimetry functions are interlocked via hardware locally as well as through software, and interlocks may be asserted either via local hardware connected to the Interlock PCBs or by means of the function controller connected to the Interlock PCBs through interface electronics.

*Siemens Beam Modulation Subsystem*

A 58-leaf MLC forms the lower level of field collimation for the Primus. The projected width of each of the central 54 leaves is 1 cm in the isocentric plane, and the projected width of the 4 outer leaves is 6.5 cm. The MLC is a double-focused type; therefore, leaf motion is non-planar, and the leaves themselves are curved in shape. The ends of the leaves are flat, and oriented so as to be parallel to radiation beam ray-lines. Interleaf leakage is reduced through a double-step tongue-and-groove feature on the leaf sides. Interdigitation is not available for this subsystem. The range of leaf travel is +20.0 cm to −10.0 cm. Each leaf is driven by a DC motor and rotary gear arrangement that engages a tooth structure machined into the proximal or distal leaf surface. Position is monitored through a rotary potentiometer and absolute encoder in the gear train for each leaf. Leaf position resolution is ±2 mm per leaf in the isocentric plane. The MLC control subsystem hardware resides in a separate cabinet located in the treatment room. Here, the incoming motor control signals and outgoing position data are multiplexed onto a serial interface to the control console computer. Serial connection to the console control computer is through a "high speed" port, rather than through the function controller chain. Hardware connections also exist between the MLC controller and the linear accelerator motor control functions to ensure a hardware interlock path is maintained. The MLC control system layout is shown in figure 5.

A new version of this product is being marketed as the OptiFocus™ MLC. This version is to have 78 central leaves with 1 cm projected width and 4 outer leaves projecting 0.5 cm at the isocentric plane. Improved leaf position resolution and velocity are also specified for this version.

*Siemens Beam Production And Control*

The Primus is a standing-wave linac, therefore the energy spectrum exiting the accelerator structure is dependent primary upon the level of microwave power applied, and how that is "loaded" by the injection current. In terms of microwave frequency, the system operates at resonance, at which maximum power is transferred to the accelerator. Microwave power level is adjusted by means of setting the magnetron or klystron excitation current for the energy selected. Beam loading is a function of injection current. These are both fixed parameters for each beam. The final energy spectrum selection is made by the bending magnet, a 270° tri-sector with fixed slits at the point of maximum dispersion. These slits serve to block the unwanted highest and lowest energy spectra. Here, the current to the bending magnet coils determines the trajectory of a particular energy through the bending magnet, and so energy selection is adjusted by means of bending magnet current.

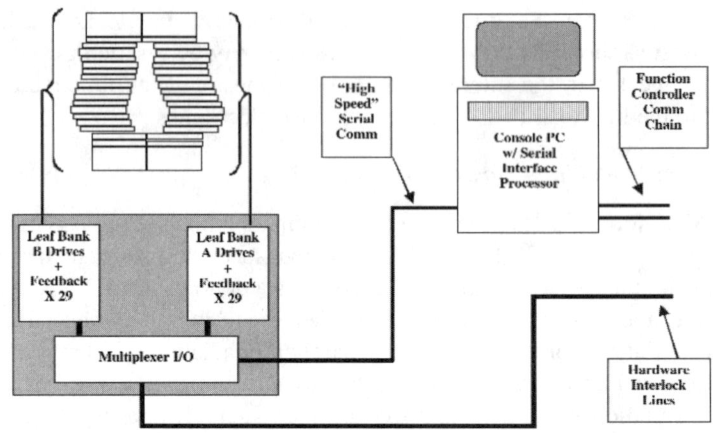


**Figure 5.** Siemens Primus MLC Subsystem Control Architecture.

In the Primus, a gun/injector pulse is generated for every HV/microwave pulse. Use of the grid in the triode gun allows rapid switching of the injector current. Immediately after high voltage is initiated, there is a run-up period of 2 to 6 seconds, during which the HV and RF are allowed to stabilize. During run-up, the trigger for the injector is occurring out of phase, or non-coincident in time with the RF pulse; this produces no accelerated beam pulse, but may produce some dark current. A defocusing lens coil around the proximal end of the accelerator is used to suppress dark current. At the end of run-up, the injector pulse is made coincident with the RF pulse, producing beam. Dose rate is controlled by adjusting the machine triggers PRF. It is servoed by adjusting PRF to maintain a constant dose rate as measured on dosimetry channel #2.

*Siemens IMRT Implementation And Delivery Process*

IMRT delivery is via a step-and-shoot/SMLC technique. The MLC is positioned to the defined shape for the first segment and beam is initiated. Power is applied to the linac HV system and dose delivery commences after run up of 2 to 6 seconds. Once the segment MUs are delivered, the machine enters a Pause state while the MLC is repositioned for the next segment.

During Pause, the injector pulse is made non-coincident in time with the RF pulse, HV remains on, and the HV amplitude is reduced to 80% of nominal to suppress dark current. Once the MLC or other devices reach their target positions, the HV amplitude is returned to 100% and the injection pulse timing is returned to a coincident state. This results in a return to nominal beam-on conditions within a fraction of a second.

In this approach to IMRT, time in the intersegment Pause state is dependent upon the MLC leaf velocity, and to a degree the speed of the linac control system. Communications in the daisy-chained function controller structure is accomplished in a strict polling sequence, effectively dividing the overall baud rate by the number of nodes. If leaf speed is sufficiently increased for the new MLC product, then it is possible that the speed of the linac control system may become the limiting factor in realizing any further decrease in intersegment time. The use of a timing shift rather than the removal of the RF excitation or electron injections reduces the time required to return to nominal beam-on from the Pause state. While less of an effect than for the Elekta traveling-wave accelerator presented here, the MU end effect resulting from the Pause state may be significant and different from that in a non-Paused beam sequence. In a highly segmented sequence the cumulative end effect might be much more significant than for the case of fewer segments with the same total number of MUs (Siemens Medical Systems 2000).

## Varian Clinac 21EX IMRT Delivery System

The Varian Clinac 21-EX is a dual-photon standing-wave linear accelerator. The microwave system is klystron based, and the electron injector is a triode (gridded) type. The bending magnet is a 270° tri-sector. Electron flattening is accomplished through dual foil scattering. A carrousel is used to position scattering foils for up to five electron beams and two flattening filters for mode selection. A dual-channel fixed segmented ionization chamber is used for dosimetry monitoring.

*Varian Control System Architecture*

The Varian control system utilizes two Intel X86-based processors and timing on a STD Bus as the core for the Clinac control system. Figure 6 shows an overall diagram of this control system. These processors are the Communications (Comm) Processor and the Control Processor. Both of these processors run programs stored in firmware. The Communications Processor handles communications between the control system and the machine hand and couch controls, the Console PC, and the gantry display unit. The Control Processor is the linac controller proper, and it sends commands to the circuits that make up the linear accelerator and processes information coming from them, via the programmable timers and general purpose I/O on the STD Bus. These two processors share a common block of random access memory (RAM) in which status of parameters and interlocks of system are posted. Each processor may fetch or modify data from the common RAM area in the course of normal operations, modifying a status byte associated with each location upon doing so. Commands from the console are posted in common RAM by the Comm Processor, then acted upon by the Control Processor. Results of the Control Processor actions are posted in common RAM for the Comm Processor to transmit to the console. The other critical circuit on the STD Bus is the Control Timer PCB. This is a 20-channel programmable timer through which the control system performs dosimetry monitoring and interlock generation, position readout timing, and machine triggers generation. Signals coming to and from the STD Bus units are processed through the Signal Conditioning Backplane, which, as the name implies, acts as a scaling and conditioning interface for I/O to the STD Bus. The Varian Cardrack contains circuits specific to the setup, operation, and interlock generation for the machine. Signal flow to the machine is both through the Signal Conditioning Backplane and the Varian Cardrack. Signal flow to the STD Bus circuits from the machine and the Varian Cardrack is through the Signal Conditioning Backplane. An Intel-based desktop PC serves as the operator interface for the machine. Configuration data and event logs are stored on the hard disk on this PC, as are the programs necessary for this unit to perform operator interface functions. Operator control of the machine is through a dedicated keyboard unit that communicates with the console PC through a serial port and is connected directly to the beam-on hardware through a keyswitch enable and hardware beam-off circuit (Varian Medical Systems 1998).

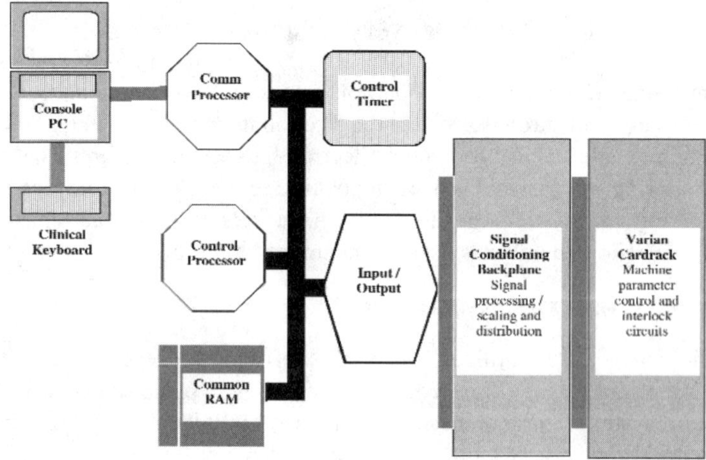


**Figure 6.** Varian 21-EX Control System Architecture.

*Varian Beam Modulation Subsystem*

The Varian MLC is a tertiary collimator, located distal to the upper and lower photon jaws of the treatment head. There are 120 leaves, of which the outer 40 project to 1 cm wide and the central 80 project 0.5 cm wide in the isocentric plane. The 0.5 cm wide leaves are tapered in width from one edge to central height, the full width portion of the leaf forming the 0.5-cm projection. The leaves are placed with the tapered edge alternating in the top or bottom orientation, allowing them to fit tightly in the head of the machine. A leaf can be extended 15 cm from the carriage on which each bank of 60 leaves is mounted. The range of carriage travel is from +20 cm to –20 cm. Leaf motion is planar, and the leaf ends are curved. Interleaf leakage is reduced through a double–step tongue-and-groove feature on the leaf sides, and the presence of the proximal photon jaws. Interdigitation of leaves is permitted. Each leaf is screw driven by a DC motor. Leaf position is monitored through a rotary pulse encoder mounted on each motor, and a pressure-sensitive linear potentiometer coupled to each leaf. Carriage position is monitored through a rotary pulse encoder mounted on each motor, and an optical position encoder. Leaf position accuracy is specified to be ±0.1 cm.

The MLC control subsystem consists of motor drives and position encoding and communications hardware located in the head of the machine and two processors located at the console. The MLC Control Processor is the MLC controller, and is linked to the hardware in the head of the machine by two full-duplex fiber optic communications links. All position, drive, and status information is passed over these links. The MLC Workstation functions as operator interface and information gateway. The Workstation has two communication connections to the MLC Controller. The first is an Ethernet connection to an FTP server running on the Controller for transfer of leaf pattern files. The second RS-422 connection transfers MLC and linac status information to and from the Millennium™ MLC application running on the Controller. The interface to the linac control system is through an RS-422 serial line and several hardware connections through the MLC Controller. A schematic this system is shown in figure 7. The hardware connection allows the MLC to assert a "beam holdoff" signal as well as the MLC interlock in the linac control system (Varian Oncology Systems 2001). As a tertiary collimator, the presence of this MLC decreases the distance from isocenter to the external surfaces of the treatment head by slightly less than 10 cm.

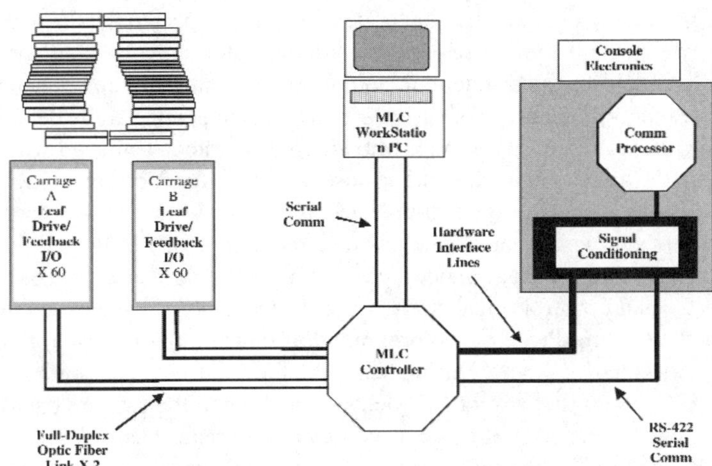


**Figure 7.** Varian MLC Subsystem Control Architecture.

*Varian Beam Production And Control*

The 21EX is a standing-wave accelerator linac; therefore, the energy spectrum exiting the accelerator structure is dependent primary upon the level of microwave power applied, and how that is "loaded" by the injection current. In terms of microwave frequency, the system operates at resonance, at which maximum power is transferred to the accelerator. Microwave power level is adjusted by means of setting the klystron to operate as a class A (linear) amplifier. In this mode the power output is a function of power input, and so adjusting the power level of the RF driver controls power out of the klystron. Another means of controlling energy in the 21EX is through the use of an "energy switch." The energy switch drives a plunger into one of the accelerator side cavities approximately one-third from the gun end. This effectively turns the remaining two-thirds of the accelerator into a drift tube, and little acceleration takes place.

Use of the energy switch allows a much higher power level to be applied to an effectively shorter accelerator. This permits acceleration of much higher beam currents needed to achieve the nominal dose rate of 600 MU/min. Final energy spectrum selection is made by the bending magnet, a 270° sector with fixed slits at the point of maximum dispersion. These slits serve to block the unwanted highest and lowest energy spectra. Here, the current to the bending magnet coils determines the trajectory of a particular energy through the bending magnet, and so energy selection is adjusted by means of bending magnet current.

In the 21EX the use of the grid in the triode gun allows rapid switching of the injector current. The injection system commences triggering of the gun upon mode selection for stable emission prior to beam-on. The microwave system and injector are operated at a constant PRF, 360 PPS for low-X and 180 PPS for high-X. At nominal max dose rate of 600 MU/min, this yields approximately 0.03 and 0.06 MU/pulse for low-X and high-X, respectively. Dose rate is controlled on a pulse-to-pulse basis by making the injected pulse timing either coincident or delayed with respect to the RF pulse timing. During the delayed injector pulse periods, dark current is suppressed by the focusing solenoid that encloses the accelerator, and an ionic vacuum pump connected to the space immediately distal to the injection area. Dose rate is selected by delaying some or all of the pulses in a 6-pulse train. Maximum dose rate is achieved when all 6 of the pulses in the train are coincident. The dose rate servo functions by delaying pulses based on dosimetry data during a 50-mSec control window. Once the proper dose has been recorded during a control window, the remainder of the injector pulses are delayed for that window. In all modes, cMU (centi-MU) dose counting occurs in the timer interface and control timer PCBs. The selected dose rate and dose information is used by the Control Processor to program the control timer to monitor dose, dose rate, dosimetry interlocks, etc. During beam-on, the Control Processor compares the desired MU count to the current MU delivery, and when the two are equal, sends a complete signal to the control timer, which then terminates beam via hardware and software paths through the timer interface PCB. The control timer also performs the dose rate servo and dose rate counting functions.

*Varian IMRT Implementation And Delivery Process*

In IMRT or dynamic beam delivery mode, the time aspect of the dose rate control window is simply augmented with some other segmented input, such as MLC position, gantry angle for arc therapy, photon jaw position for dynamic wedge, or gating input for gated therapy. In SMLC mode, the number of MUs are delivered for each segment field shape and the beam holdoff line is asserted by the MLC as leaves are moved to the next segment field shape. This delays the injection pulses to suppress beam until the field shape is achieved. Upon release of the beam holdoff by the MLC, control of this input returns to the Dose Rate Servo. In dynamic beam delivery mode, the beam is on continuously as the MLC leaves are moved. Each leaf trajectory as a function of MU delivered is subdivided into control points. During delivery, leaf velocity and dose rate are modulated on a pulse-by-pulse basis to achieve delivery as a linear function between control points within a user-prescribed leaf position tolerance.

Note that this approach to dynamic beam delivery can be described as a step-and-shoot technique approaching the limit in the number of segments per sequence. Here, the intersegment time can be as short as 50 ms, which is MLC position sampling time (Varian Medical Systems 2001).

## Second-Generation IMRT Delivery Systems Implementation

The second generation of IMRT delivery systems are radiotherapy delivery systems designed specifically for IMRT. Currently, the TomoTherapy Hi-Art system is the only second-generation product available with FDA approval. The following is a brief description of the salient features of the delivery system in terms of control, beam delivery, and IMRT implementation as was presented for the first-generation systems.

## TomoTherapy Hi-Art IMRT Delivery System

The Hi-Art delivery system is based on tomotherapy, in which narrow axial regions are serially treated by rotating the beam delivery system around the patient and moving the patient for the next treatment "slice" between rotations. This system delivers treatment in a helical pattern by continuously rotating the delivery system while the patient is translated longitudinally on the treatment couch. A megavoltage computed tomography (MVCT) imaging system is incorporated into the delivery system for anatomic delivery verification. The linac and imaging subsystems are mounted on a supporting ring much like an imaging CT unit. A system of slip rings supplies power and control signals to the rotating components. The Hi-Art linac subsystem uses a single-photon linear accelerator. The microwave system is magnetron based, and the electron injector is a triode (gridded) type. A dual-channel fixed segmented ionization chamber is used for dosimetry monitoring. A 500-detector array permits $512 \times 512$-pixel megavoltage imagery with a 40-centimeter field of view (Mackie et al. 1993).

*TomoTherapy Control System Architecture*

The Hi-Art delivery control system comprises three control computers connected by local Ethernet: The On Board Computer (OBC) mounted on the rotating portion of the gantry, the Stationary Computer (STC), and the Data Receiver Server (DRS). The OBC controls the collimator jaws, MLC, and the linac subsystem. A diagram of the control system is shown in figure 8. The STC controls the couch subsystem and supports control and data transfer from the rotating components to the stationary components. The DRS processes image data from the CT detector subsystem and acts as an interface between the delivery system, the operator workstation, and a central database server. The three computers that compose the delivery control system run the VxWorks real-time operating system, and are synchronized in a distributed state machine pattern. When a procedure is selected by the operator, the appropriate machine parameters are retrieved by the DRS and parsed out to functional elements of the delivery subsystems through a specialized object-oriented interface developed for distributed control systems. After all the subsystems are initialized, they signal the master state controller that allows the transition to the next machine state. A number of such setup states may occur prior to the radiation delivery state. Once in the radiation delivery state, hardware synchronization is used to trigger the couch motion, gantry rotation, linac triggers, MLC leaf motion, and image detector acquisition. The synchronization signal is shown in figure 8 as a heavy dashed line. Communications with external devices is suppressed during irradiation. An interlock subsystem with hardware and software paths monitors system performance and interrupts the high voltage circuit in the case of interlock condition. Completion of the high voltage interlock chain requires the closing of relay contacts by the room door switch, console treatment enable switch, the STC, and the OBC. Software interlocks are additionally implemented through the OBC and STC run-time environment, and a local area network watchdog timer is implemented in software to monitor and interlock any loss of communication. The interlock subsystem is shown in figure 9. Hardware interlocks paths are shown as heavy dashed lines, and software interlocks are shown as solid lines. Upon termination of irradiation, a postprocessing machine state is entered, in which delivery data is written back to the central database. This allows the correct data for an interrupted irradiation to be re-entered upon resumption of treatment.

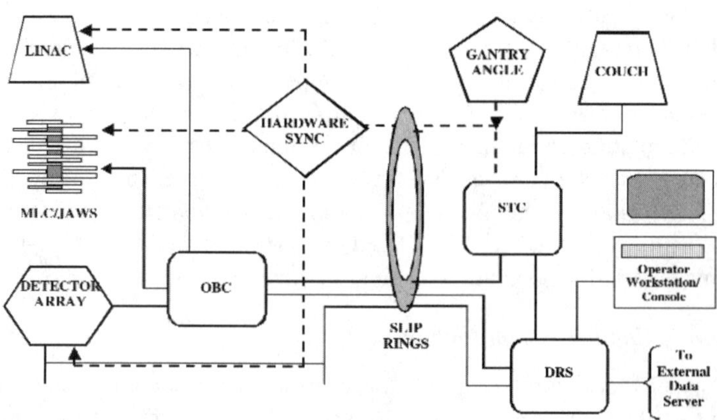



**Figure 8.** TomoTherapy Hi-Art Control System Architecture.

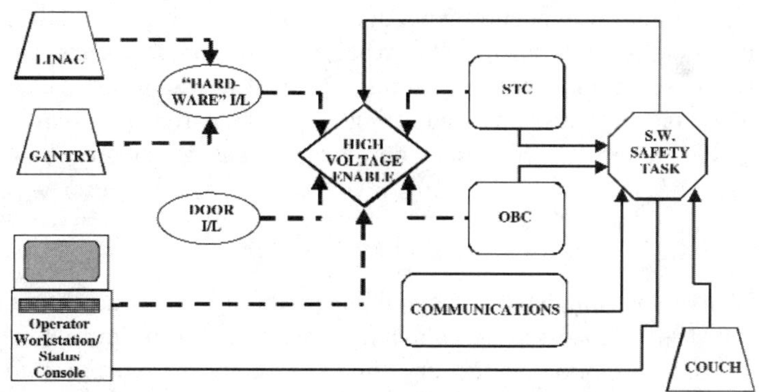


**Figure 9.** TomoTherapy Hi-Art Interlock Subsystem.

## TomoTherapy Beam Modulation Subsystem

A compressed-air-driven binary MLC is used to modulate the Hi-Art x-ray beam. The MLC has two opposed banks of 32 interlaced leaves, each projecting to a width of approximately 0.625 cm in the isocentric plane. The leaves include a double-step tongue-and-groove feature to reduce interleaf leakage. The ends of the leaves need not be curved, since they are always either in the "open" or "closed" state. Leaf position is monitored optically, and the status of each leaf is "open", "closed", or "in transit." Transit time is specified to be 50 ms. In addition to the MLC, a pair of double-focused collimators can be positioned to adjust the slit, or slice width from 0.5 to 4.0 cm at the isocentric plane.

## Tomotherapy Beam Production And Control

The Hi-Art uses a standing-wave linac; therefore, the energy spectrum exiting the accelerator structure is dependent primary upon the level of microwave power applied, and how that is loaded by the injection current. In terms of microwave frequency, the system operates at resonance, at which maximum power is transferred to the accelerator. Microwave power level is adjusted by means of setting the magnetron excitation current. No bending magnet is used, resulting in a broader intrinsic electron spectrum than machines equipped with bending magnets. A desirable photon spectrum is achieved through careful target and filter design. The target consists of a rotating water-cooled tungsten disk. A rotating target theoretically allows higher electron beam current and therefore higher dose rate with a fixed target. A beam filter is present to adjust photon spectrum rather than intensity distribution. Beam intensity distribution is controlled instead as part of IMRT delivery (Balog et al. 1999).

In the Hi-Art linac subsystem, a gun/injector pulse is generated for every HV/microwave pulse. Use of the grid in the triode gun allows rapid switching of the injector current. Immediately after high voltage is initiated, there is a run-up period of 2 to 6 seconds, during which the HV and RF are allowed to stabilize. During run-up, the trigger for the injector is occurring out of phase, or non-coincident in time with the RF pulse; this produces no accelerated beam pulse, but may produce some dark current. At the end of run-up, the injector pulse is made coincident with the RF pulse, producing beam. Dose rate is controlled by adjusting the machine triggers PRF. It is servoed by adjusting PRF to maintain a constant dose rate as measured on one of the dosimetry channels.

*TomoTherapy IMRT Implementation And Delivery Process*

Treatment delivery is completed as a spiral pattern through the couch being continuously translated as the linac is rotated about the patient with the beam on. Leaf motion, linac triggers, couch motion, and gantry angular velocity are synchronized in time, rather than measured delivered dose. The delivery sequence downloaded to the DRS from the central database is arranged in terms of leaf pattern as a function of timing, which is, in turn, related to gantry angle through the hardware triggers system. The ionometric dosimetry subsystem acts as a backup means of dose monitoring and is used to maintain a constant dose rate (Murray, Personal communication 2003).

As a designed-for-purpose system, the second-generation approach to IMRT delivery is unburdened by compromise inherent in adaptation of existing technology. The choice of a compact single-energy linac minimizes the hardware support and space required by larger multi-mode systems, at loss of other treatment modes such as electron beams.

Mounting the system in a ring gantry structure may eliminate the gantry sag that occurs with C-arm gantry systems. This approach to the mechanical configuration also offers some advantage from the perspective of radiation shielding design, in that the fixed geometry can allow the use of narrower primary barriers. Likewise, geometry and small field sizes reduce the thickness of secondary barriers needed. Increased workload, on the other hand, necessitates thicker primary barriers for this type of system, some portion of which may be incorporated in the machine counter weight (Robinson et al. 2000). A second geometric disadvantage may be the lack of available couch rotation. While adjustment of couch angle about isocenter is used to match field edges and avoid critical structure irradiation on conventional and first-generation IMRT delivery systems, it is not available on the second-generation system. It may be that these functions might eventually be successfully implemented instead with IMRT, but under current practice this remains an open question. A tomotherapy configuration lends itself to the use of a binary rather than a cone-beam style MLC. Since the leaves are either "open" or "closed," the leaf ends are not involved in field shaping, effectively eliminating issues surrounding penumbra and focus. The binary MLC further culls the technological problem set by simplifying leaf position tracking, calibration, and leaf velocity. In the case of the Hi-Art system reviewed, the control system functionality is structured as an information system network of specific functions operating according to a planned topology. This network has an overlay of hardware interlocks and timing signals to ensure fail-safe operation. This seems to fulfill the paradigm requiring hardware implementation of critical interlocks, yet emphasizes the information systems approach rather than hardware. In terms of clinical flexibility, first-generation systems retain some superiority in the ability to offer electron beams and conventional styles of treatment not available with second-generation systems. Whether this represents a greater liability to the first generation or second generation OEMs remains to be seen.

# References


Balog, J. P., T. R. Mackie, P. Reckwerdt, M. Glass, and L. Angelos. (1999). "Characterization of the output for helical delivery of intensity modulated slit beams." *Med. Phys.* 26:55–64.

Bortfeld, T., U. Oelfke, and S. Nill. (2000). "What is the optimum leaf width of a multileaf collimator?" *Med. Phys.* 27:2494–2502.

Boyer, A., P. Biggs, J. Galvin, E. Klein, T. LoSasso, D. Low, K. Mah, and C. Yu. (2001). Basic Applications of Multileaf Collimators. Report of AAPM Task Group No. 50 Radiation Therapy Committee. AAPM Report 72. Madison, WI: Medical Physics Publishing.

Chui, C.-S., M. F. Chan, E. Yorke, S. Spirou, and C. C. Ling. (2001). "Delivery of intensity-modulated radiation therapy with a conventional multileaf collimator: Comparison of dynamic an segmental methods." *Med. Phys.* 28:2441–2449.

Greene, D., and P. C. Williams. *Linear Accelerators for Radiation Therapy.* Bristol, UK: Institute of Physics Publishing, 1997.

Karzmark, C. J. (1984). "Advances in linear accelerator design for radiotherapy." *Med. Phys.* 11:105–128.

Levenson, N. *Safeware: System Safety and Computer.* Boston, MA: Addison-Wesley, Appendix A, 1–49, 1995.

LoSasso, T., C.-S. Chui, and C. C. Ling. (1998). "Physical and dosimetric aspects of a multileaf collimation system used in the dynamic mode for implementing intensity modulated radiotherapy." *Med. Phys.* 25:1919–1927.

Mackie, T. R., T. Holmes, S. Swerdloff, P. Reckwerdt, J. O. Deasy, J. Yang, B. Paliwal, and T. Kinsella. (1993). "Tomotherapy: A new concept for the delivery of dynamic conformal radiotherapy." *Med. Phys.* 20:1709–1719.

Murray, D. C. (2003). Personal communication. TomoTherapy Inc., Madison, WI.

Otto, K., B. G. Clark, and C. Huntzinger. (2002). "Exploring the limits of spatial resolution in radiation dose delivery." *Med. Phys.* 29:1823–1831.

Partridge, M., P. M. Evans, A. Mosleh-Shirzi, and D. Convery. (1998). "Independent verification using portal imaging of intensity-modulated beam delivery by the dynamic MLC technique." *Med. Phys.* 25:1872–1878.

Robinson, D., J. W. Scrimger, G. C. Field, and B. G. Fallone. (2000). "Shielding considerations for tomotherapy." *Med. Phys.* 27:2380–2384.

Siemens Medical Systems. *Linear Accelerator System Manual.* Concorde, CA: Siemens Medical Systems Inc., 2000.

_______. *Multileaf Collimator System Manual.* Concorde, CA: Siemens Medical Systems Inc., 1998.

Spitz, F. Personal communication. (2002). Department of Radiation Oncology, Thomas Jefferson University Hospital, Philadelphia, PA.

TomoTherapy Inc. *TomoTherapy Hi-Art System Product Data Shee*t. Madison, WI, 2002.

 **Timothy J. Waldron**


Varian Medical Systems. *CLINAC 2100C/D, 2300C/D, 21EX, 23EX Systems Manual*. Palo Alto, CA: Varian Medical Systems, 1998.

———. *DMLC Implementation Guide*. Palo Alto, CA: Varian Medical Systems, 1999.

———. *Millenium MLC User Guide*. Palo Alto, CA: Varian Medical Systems, 2001.

Wangler, T. *RF Linear Accelerators*. New York: Wiley & Sons, 1998.

Xia, P., C. Chuang, and L. Verhey. (2002). "Communication and sampling rate limitations in IMRT delivery with a dynamic multileaf collimator system." *Med. Phys.* 29:412–423.

# Radiation Shielding For IMRT


**Daniel A. Low, Ph.D.**
Associate Professor of Radiation Oncology
Washington University School of Medicine
St. Louis, Missouri




## Conventional Shielding Protocols

Linear accelerators used for radiation therapy are designed to deliver tumorcidal doses to the patient using well-controlled apertures. Unfortunately, the process of producing and delivering the radiation causes unwanted stray radiation. If unshielded, this radiation would present an unnecessary hazard to radiation personnel and the general public, so linear accelerator vaults are heavily shielded to attenuate the radiation to a point at which it is considered safe. The radiation therapy or medical health physicist is generally responsible for designing the vault that complies with the regulatory limits of radiation levels in an area.

The stray radiation is typically broken down into three categories: (1) Transmission through the patient or direct beam that misses the patient (flash). This radiation is termed "primary" radiation because it consists mostly of unscattered photons from the radiation source. (2) Radiation that has been scattered within the patient or other object and is subsequently emitted. This component is termed "scattered radiation." (3) Radiation that has escaped through the linear accelerator shielding, termed "leakage radiation." The three types of radiation have different spectral and angular distribution signatures that significantly affect the shielding calculations.

The basic purpose of radiation shielding calculations is to assure that the shielding material and thickness is adequate to reduce the intensity by virtue of attenuation and scatter. The protocol for determining the dose rate outside a barrier depends on whether the barrier attenuation concerns primary, scatter, or leakage radiation. Primary barriers are those that shield from the direct beam. For conservative estimates, the beam is assumed not to be attenuated by the patient on its way to the primary barrier. Secondary barriers are those that are intended to block scattered and leakage radiation. They typically consist of all room walls, floors, and ceiling that do not intercept the primary beam.

**Daniel A. Low**

The equation for determining barrier thickness of a primary barrier is

$$B_p = \frac{Pd_{pri}^{\;2}}{WUT} \tag{1}$$

where $B$ is the transmission fraction through the barrier, $P$ is the exposure rate limit, $d$ is the distance from the radiation source to the evaluation point (McGinley 2002), $W$ is the workload to scatter within the treatment room [Sv wk$^{-1}$], $U$ is the user factor, and $T$ is the occupancy factor found in the National Council on Radiation Protection and Measurements (NCRP) report 49 (NCRP 1976). The units of these values are selected to be convenient: $P$ [Sv wk$^{-1}$], $d$ [m], $W$ [Sv wk$^{-1}$], $U$ [unitless], and $T$ [unitless].

The barrier thicknesses are based on two time scales, hourly and weekly. The hourly limit is used to restrict dose to transient personnel or the general public. For example, a waiting area on the other side of a barrier wall will typically have different people sitting over the course of a week. If most of the dose is given in a short time scale (for example, if the linear accelerator is placed in an operating room), a large portion of the weekly limit could be delivered within 1 hour. Regulatory agencies account for this by restricting the exposure averaged over a 1-hour period. For the case when personnel are stationed at a location more permanently (such as an office), the weekly limit is more appropriate.

The workload is defined as the dose equivalent per week at isocenter. For photon beams, the quality factor (ratio between dose equivalent and dose) is typically assumed to be 1. For linear accelerators up to 10 MV, NCRP report 49 (NCRP 1976) suggested a value of 1000 Gy per week. For higher energy linear accelerators, NCRP report 51 (NCRP 1977) suggested 500 Gy per week. These values were based on techniques used in the 1970's and the values were intended for use by departments that could not determine their actual workloads. Kleck and Elsalim (1994) surveyed four departments with 10 dual- and 3 single-energy linear accelerators. They found that the single (typically 6 MV) and multimodality linear accelerators had workloads of less than 350 Gy per week, and less than 250 Gy per week, respectively, indicating that the NCRP workloads are conservative. Note that the shielding requirements for clinical electron beams are significantly less than for photon beams, so the workloads should include only photon beam treatments. In our clinic, patients are typically scheduled for 10-minute time slots with 2 Gy per treatment. Therefore, in a 40-hour week, we would deliver 480 Gy. Allowing for some special treatments, this value would be conservative. Of course, the designed vault will typically be used well beyond the current technical and clinical standards of practice, and the incremental cost of shielding is relatively small compared against the cost of retrofitting a room, so a conservative estimate of workload is warranted.

The use factor is intended to subdivide the workload as a function of beam orientation. Because the primary barrier attenuates direct radiation, the barrier is designed for the times when the linear accelerator points at it. Applying a use factor allows the shield to be thinner than it would be if the beam were permanently pointing in its direction. Typically, use factors of 0.25 are used for walls and the ceiling, but the floor (beam straight down) is assigned a conservative value of 1.0 (NCRP 1976). Special circumstances (for example, a fixed beam direction or a unit that primarily treats whole-body irradiation) would require a modification of this practice. When the 1-hour dose rate is being considered, a conservative practice is to set the use factor to 1.0.

Many locations, such as hallways, beyond the shielding barrier will be occupied infrequently. For these areas, a modifying factor, termed the "occupancy factor," allows for a reduction in the barrier thickness. In the absence of other data, table 1 shows typical occupancy factors (NCRP 1976; Horton 1987). The occupancy factor is set to 1 when the 1-hour dose rate is being considered.

**Table 1.** Occupancy Factors Recommended by NCRP Report 49 for Planning in the Absence of Other Data [Reprinted from *Handbook of Radiation Therapy Physics*, J. L. Horton, © 1987 Prentice-Hall, with permission from Prentice-Hall.]

| Occupancy | Area |
|---|---|
| Full (T = 1) | Work areas such as offices, laboratories, shops, wards, nurses' stations, living quarters, children's play areas and occupied space in nearby buildings |
| Partial (T = 1/4) | Corridors, rest rooms, elevators with operators, unattended parking lots |
| Occasional (T = 1/16) | Waiting rooms, toilets, stairways, unattended elevators, janitor's closets, outside areas used only for pedestrians or vehicular traffic |

The distance that appears in equation (1) refers to the distance from the point that the workload is specified (isocenter) to the point that the exposure rate is being determined. However, primary barriers are quite thick and the internal scatter within the barrier acts as its own source, effectively reducing the distance from which the radiation appears to emanate (McGinley 2002). Because the inverse-square fall-off is taking place at a location that is effectively closer than isocenter, the dose fall-off is faster than that predicted by equation (1), so the equation remains somewhat conservative.

Calculation of barrier thickness due to patient-scattered radiation requires a different equation (McGinley 2002):

$$B_p = \frac{P}{aWT}\left(d_{\text{sec}}^{\,2}\right)\left(d_{sca}^{\,2}\right)\frac{400}{F} \tag{2}$$

where the subscript $p$ indicates patient scatter, $a$ refers to the scattered fraction by the object, $F$ is the field size (in cm$^2$) at the patient, $d_{sca}$ refers to the distance from the target to the scatterer, and $d_{\text{sec}}$ refers to the distance from the scatterer to the point being evaluated. Note that equation (2) has no use factor.

A similar equation is defined for scatter from a barrier.

$$B_s = \frac{P}{\alpha A W U T}\left(d_{sec}^{2}\right)\left(d_{sca}^{2}\right)$$

(3)

where $\alpha$ is the reflection coefficient (fraction per square meter) of the shielding material, and $A$ is the radiation beam's cross-sectional area at the barrier.

Finally, the equation used to calculate barrier thickness due to linear accelerator leakage is:

$$B_l = \frac{1000\,P}{W T}\left(d_{pri}^{2}\right)$$

(4)

where the factor of 1000 is based on the specification that linear accelerator leakage is 0.1% of the dose rate at isocenter. While leakage emanates from the radiation source, the average position of the source is at isocenter, so the primary distance is used.

Each equation has a dose limit $P$ that must be adhered to. The dose limits $P$ where the public can be exposed is 1.0 mSv per year (1.0 mSv = 100 mrem and is equivalent for calculation purposes to 0.02 mSv per week) (McGinley 2002). These areas are termed "uncontrolled." In addition to the annual limit, the maximum permissible in any one hour is 0.02 mSv, or 2 mrem, with no allowance for reduced occupancy ($T = 1$).

The allowable exposure for areas where radiation workers operate is significantly greater. These areas are assumed to be populated by workers that are trained in the handling of radioactive materials or in the processes of avoiding radiation exposure. They are also typically monitored for radiation exposure to assure they remain within the allowable limits. For these controlled areas (controlled by signage and/or physical barriers), the value is 0.05 Sv per year (corresponding to 1 mSv per week, or 50 times the value for the general public). While this value is legally allowed, a concept called ALARA (As Low As Reasonably Achievable) was developed based on the concept that the radiation levels should be kept at a reasonable minimum. The ALARA value is typically one-tenth the regulatory limit, so in this case the radiation levels are limited to 0.10 mSv per week. The occupancy factor is typically taken as 1.0 for controlled areas. These limits are recommendations and individual states can further restrict the radiation levels for uncontrolled and controlled areas.

Equations (1) through (4) provide the attenuation required by the barrier to reduce the primary or scattered radiation to the acceptable level. The source of that attenuation is the shielding wall, typically constructed of a relatively high-density material. Because of its low cost, and the ability to design relatively thick walls, new facilities make liberal use of concrete. The transmission characteristics of these materials have been published for use in shielding calculations. For primary beams, the tables are arranged as a function if incident electron energy on the linear accelerator target (NCRP 1977; Williams and Thwaites). Because of spectral changes in the relatively thick barriers, the first tenth-value layer (TVL) is independently calculated relative to the remaining layers. If $N$ tenth-barrier thicknesses are required to attenuate the beam, the total barrier thickness $S$ required is

$$S = T_1 + (N-1)T_e \qquad (5)$$

where $T_1$ and $T_e$ are the first and subsequent TVLs, respectively. Figures 1 through 3 show graphs of $T_1$ and $T_e$ for concrete, steel, and lead.

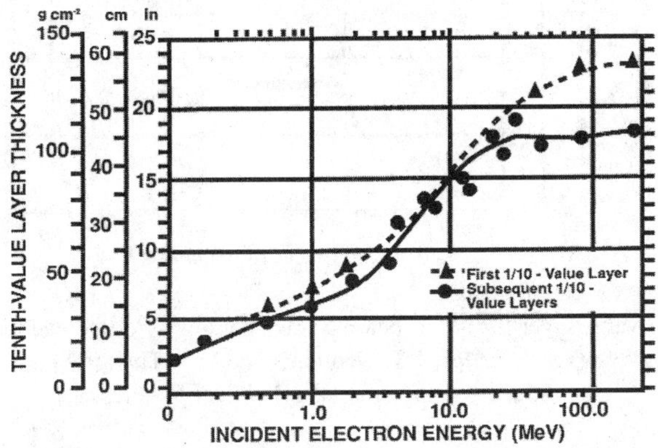

**Figure 1.** Tenth-value layer for broad-beam X rays passing through concrete. [Reprinted from *Radiotherapy Physics in Practice*, J. R. Williams and D. I. Thwaites (editors). © 2000, with permission from Oxford University Press.]

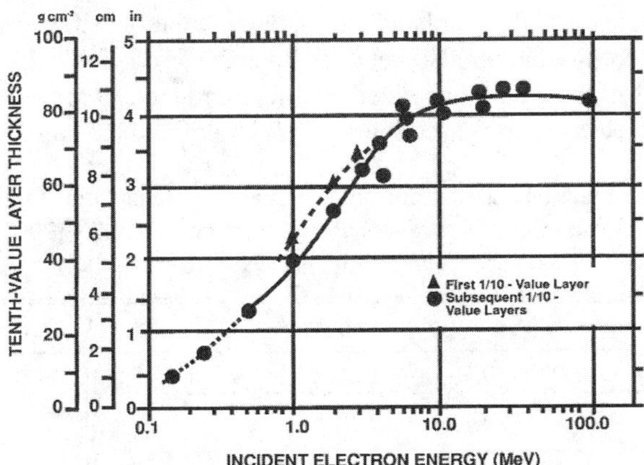

**Figure 2.** Tenth-value layer for broad-beam X-rays passing through steel [Reprinted from *Radiotherapy Physics in Practice*, J. R. Williams and D. I. Thwaites (editors). © 2000, with permission from Oxford University Press.]

Daniel A. Low

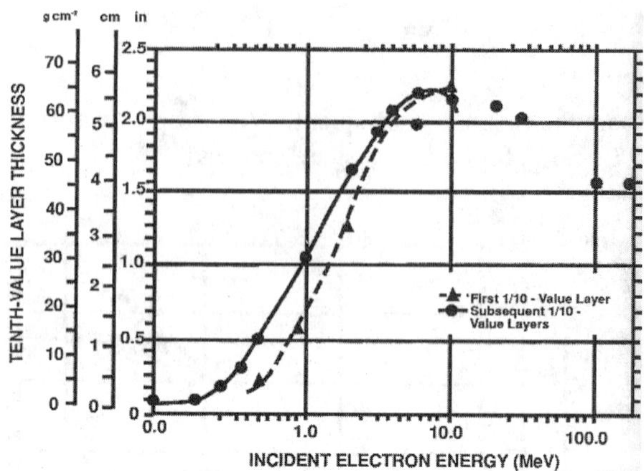



**Figure 3.** Tenth-value layer for broad-beam X-rays passing through lead [Reprinted from *Radiotherapy Physics in Practice*, J. R. Williams and D. I. Thwaites (editors). © 2000, with permission from Oxford University Press.]

The energy of the leakage beam is assumed to be the same as the primary beam, so the data from figures 1 through 3 can be used to compute shielding for leakage radiation. For patient tissues, megavoltage radiation scatters primarily via Compton scattering. The maximum energy of Compton scattered X rays is 0.511 MeV and 0.255 MeV for 90° and backscattering directions, respectively. This is significantly less than the primary and leakage radiation energies and it is generally assumed that leakage shielding can more than adequately block scattered radiation. However, for some short mazes, the scattered radiation also needs to be considered. Table 2 shows the scatter fractions (a) at 1 m from a human-sized phantom and table 3 shows the mean energy of patient-scattered radiation (McGinley 2002; Taylor and Rodgers 1999).

**Table 2.** Scatter Fractions (a) at 1 m from a Human-Sized Phantom, Target-to-Phantom Distance of 1 m and Field Size of 400 cm² [Data from McGinley (2002) and Taylor and Rodgers (1999)]

| Angle (deg) | 6 MV | 10 MV | 18 MV | 24 MV |
|---|---|---|---|---|
| 10 | $1.04 \times 10^{-2}$ | $1.66 \times 10^{-2}$ | $1.42 \times 10^{-2}$ | $1.78 \times 10^{-2}$ |
| 20 | $6.73 \times 10^{-3}$ | $5.79 \times 10^{-3}$ | $5.39 \times 10^{-3}$ | $6.32 \times 10^{-3}$ |
| 30 | $2.77 \times 10^{-3}$ | $3.18 \times 10^{-3}$ | $2.53 \times 10^{-3}$ | $2.74 \times 10^{-3}$ |
| 45 | $1.39 \times 10^{-3}$ | $1.35 \times 10^{-3}$ | $8.64 \times 10^{-4}$ | $8.30 \times 10^{-4}$ |
| 60 | $8.24 \times 10^{-4}$ | $7.46 \times 10^{-4}$ | $4.24 \times 10^{-4}$ | $3.86 \times 10^{-4}$ |
| 90 | $4.26 \times 10^{-4}$ | $3.81 \times 10^{-4}$ | $1.89 \times 10^{-4}$ | $1.74 \times 10^{-4}$ |
| 135 | $3.00 \times 10^{-4}$ | $3.02 \times 10^{-4}$ | $1.24 \times 10^{-4}$ | $1.20 \times 10^{-4}$ |
| 150 | $2.87 \times 10^{-4}$ | $2.74 \times 10^{-4}$ | $1.20 \times 10^{-4}$ | $1.13 \times 10^{-4}$ |

Table 3. Mean Energy of Patient-Scattered Radiation as a
Function of Scattering Angle and Megavoltage Beam Energy
[Data from McGinley (2002) and Taylor and Rodgers (1999)]

| Beam Energy (MV) | Scatter Angle (deg) | | | | | | | |
|---|---|---|---|---|---|---|---|---|
| | **0** | **10** | **20** | **30** | **40** | **50** | **70** | **90** |
| 6 | 1.6 | 1.4 | 1.2 | 0.9 | 0.7 | 0.5 | 0.4 | 0.2 |
| 10 | 2.7 | 2.0 | 1.3 | 1.0 | 0.7 | 0.5 | 0.4 | 0.2 |
| 18 | 5.0 | 3.2 | 2.1 | 1.3 | 0.9 | 0.6 | 0.4 | 0.3 |
| 24 | 5.6 | 3.9 | 2.7 | 1.7 | 1.1 | 0.8 | 0.5 | 0.3 |

Megavoltage linear accelerators operating at energies greater than 10 MV have the potential for producing high-energy neutrons. In general, the shielding required for photons is sufficient for the neutron flux. NCRP report 79 (NCRP 1984) concludes:

> Since practical therapy rooms need concrete walls at least two X-ray tenth-value layers thick, adequate concrete shielding for the photons will always be adequate for the neutrons as well.

Of course, this is not appropriate for other materials, such as lead or steel. As pointed out by Williams and Thwaites (2000), attenuation of neutrons is poorer than photons and $(\gamma,n)$ and $(n,\gamma)$ interactions in iron and lead can create problems.

The previously outlined formalism was developed for conventional therapy and has also been used after the development of conformal therapy, which in principle, provided a greater distribution of gantry angles and often a larger number of beams. With the introduction of intensity-modulated radiation therapy (IMRT), the concepts behind the shielding protocols were reexamined.

## IMRT Shielding Protocols

Very little has been published concerning room shielding formalisms for IMRT (Rodgers 2001; Mutic et al. 2001). Our group (Mutic et al 2001) published a manuscript that provided an initial formalism for IMRT conducted using conventional linear accelerators and linear-accelerator based tomotherapy. Difference in treatment delivery between dynamic multileaf (DMLC) and static multileaf (SMLC) were not considered. Helical tomotherapy and the Accuray CyberKnife® (Sunnyvale, CA) were also not considered. As in the conventional shielding formalism, the analysis was broken into primary and secondary shielding barriers, with the secondary barriers further broken down into patient scatter and head leakage.

Rodgers (2001) subdivided the linear accelerator workloads into conventional and special, high monitor unit (MU) procedures (IMRT and total-body irradiation) and determined the total workload as a sum of the individual workloads. This technique provided a convenient formalism for evaluating mixed-use facilities.

One important consideration for IMRT was the decoupling of the workload from the dose at isocenter. It is assumed that the total energy delivered to the patient is roughly the same with IMRT than with conventional therapy, although the greater conformality of high dose may lead to reduced integral energy. The dose is delivered either through a sequence of complex overlapping portals [multileaf collimator (MLC)], sequential slices (tomotherapy), physical filtering, or by narrow pencil beams (CyberKnife). The amount of photon fluence created at the electron-stopping target will not be the same with IMRT as conventional therapy. Because of the inefficient delivery with IMRT, the more photons are created at the target per unit dose to the patient. This relationship is often presented as a ratio of tumor dose $TD$ (representing the prescription isodose surface) to the number of monitor units $MU$ required to deliver that dose.

$$TD = E\ MU \tag{6}$$

where $E$ is the treatment efficiency and is a number that is typically less than 1. For conventional therapy the value of $E$ is nearly 1, so the concept of workload could use either the tumor dose or the MUs when computing primary, secondary or leakage radiation shielding requirements. Table 4 shows estimates of the value of $1/E$ (termed "$C$" in Rodgers' manuscript (Rodgers 2001) for different treatment situations (Followill, Geis, and Boyer 1997).

**Table 4.** Ratio of MUs to Tumor Dose ($1/E$) for Typical Conventional and IMRT Deliveries [Data from Followill, Geis, and Boyer 1997]

| Beam Energy (MV) | Conventional | | Beam Intensity Modulated | |
|---|---|---|---|---|
| | Unwedged (MU/cGy) | Wedged (MU/cGy) | MLC (MU/cGy) | Serial Tomotherapy (MU/cGy) |
| 6 | 1.2 | 2.4 | 3.4 | 9.7 |
| 18 | 1.0 | 1.5 | 2.8 | 8.1 |
| 25 | 1.0 | 1.5 | 2.8 | 8.1 |

The decoupling of MUs and TDs requires separate analysis of the workloads for primary, scattered, and leakage radiation.

## Primary Barriers

As mentioned above, the integral energy delivered to a patient is assumed to be roughly the same with IMRT and conventional conformal therapy. The difference between the two is that with IMRT, the dose is delivered in a different temporal sequence from conventional conformal therapy. With conformal therapy, the dose is subdivided among a few portals with relatively homogeneous fluences. A primary barrier blocks the radiation delivered from one of these portals during its delivery, and when the gantry is rotated, other primary barriers attenuate the other beams. The use factor (U) accounts for this distribution of primary fluence. The gantry angle distribution is not expected to change significantly with the use of IMRT. Therefore, for MLC-based IMRT, no modifications are required to the primary shielding protocols. However, the selection of energies for a multimodality linear accelerator may be affected by the use of IMRT. Because of the increased neutron dose, many facilities select 10 MV or lower energy beams rather than the more conventional higher energy beams to avoid whole-body neutron irradiation of the patient. The change of energy selections may influence the dose rates outside the shielding walls.

Experimental validation of this was provided by Mutic et al. (2001), who modeled a sliding window technique with static portals and determined that the integral dose-to-MU relationship was the same outside a primary barrier as it was at isocenter.

Tomotherapy is available as serial tomotherapy from the NOMOS Corporation (Cranberry Township. PA) and helical tomotherapy from TomoTherapy, Inc. (Madison, WI). The helical tomotherapy device has a built-in beamstopper, so no primary radiation is released from the unit (Kapatoes et al. 1999). Serial tomotherapy (Low et al. 1998a,b) uses a tertiary collimator attached to a conventional linear accelerator. Therefore, unless the linear accelerator has a beamstopper, the primary shielding protocol needs to be addressed.

Serial tomotherapy delivers fluence while the linear accelerator is operating in arc mode. Assuming that the fluence is delivered uniformly throughout rotation, the primary beam points at a specific barrier for only a fraction of the total gantry rotation. The field size is limited to 20 cm width, corresponding to an angle of 11.4°. Total gantry rotation angles range from 180° to 340°, corresponding to a fractional collimator opening angle of 0.063 to 0.034, respectively. This quantity was termed "$\kappa$" in Mutic et al. (2001). These values have similar meanings as the use factor, which is 0.25 for beam angles excluding straight down. Mutic et al. (2001) defined the changes in workload calculation protocols as modifications to the use factor calculation. The smaller effective use factors are compensated by the fact that serial tomotherapy dose is delivered in a slice-by slice sequence. The patient is moved between slices (indexing), but the primary beam hits the same location on the shielding wall. If the number of indexes is $I$, then the primary barrier will be struck $I$ times for each patient treatment. The serial tomotherapy use factor $U_t$ definition was suggested to be modified to

$$U_t = \eta\, I\, \kappa\, \lambda \tag{7}$$

where $\eta$ is the ratio of output (dose per MU) from the open tomotherapy field to that of the field size used in the conventional primary shielding calculations as measured outside the barrier, and $\lambda$ is a factor that corrects the geometric projection approximation for scatter within the shielding barrier [1.1 to 1.6 in Mutic et al. (2001)]. This modification to the use factor was valid only for primary shielding calculations where the time-averaged dose rate was desired. For cases where the use factor would not normally be applied (e.g., for determinations of dose in any 1 hour), the use factor needs to be modified to

$$U_t = \eta\, I \tag{8}$$

Mutic et al. (2001), determined that, while $\kappa$ was very small, and $I$ could be as large as 12 (although in our clinic the average value is 7), the combination led to a use factor based on equation (7) of 0.15 or less, which is smaller than the value of 0.25 used for conventional calculations. However, if the use factor in equation (8) is used, the value is 1.68 for 7 indexes and 2.88 for 12 indexes, considerably greater than 0.25. This assumes that the 1-hour calculation should include the number of indexes but not the angular distribution of beams. Because tomotherapy uses only rotating beams, use of equation (7) would be appropriate for both weekly and hourly dose estimates.

The cross-sectional length of the tomotherapy beam is significantly smaller than what is available with a conventional field size (3.4 cm vs. 40 cm), so a facility designed exclusively for tomotherapy could have narrower primary shields. However portal images and other uses of the linear accelerator may necessitate use of standard primary shielding dimensions.

## Secondary Barriers—Patient Scatter

The patient scatter is assumed to be proportional to the integral energy delivered to the patient. IMRT is assumed to deliver approximately the same integral energy as conformal therapy, so the amount of scattered radiation is unchanged. The distribution of that radiation into the room may change slightly if the distribution of gantry angles is different than conformal therapy, but this is unlikely to be significant for MLC-based IMRT.

For serial or helical tomotherapy, as in MLC-based IMRT, the gantry rotates in a single plane, so the gantry angle distribution may not be significantly different than for MLC-based IMRT. The fact that the treatment is delivered for multiple slices will distribute the radiation in time more evenly than for MLC-based IMRT, but this will probably significantly affect the assumptions used in shielding calculations. Unless the integral energy is shown to change dramatically with the use of IMRT, or the selection of beam energy changes dramatically, it is unlikely that a change in patient-scattered radiation calculation protocols are required.

## Secondary Barriers—Leakage

The influence of IMRT on head leakage is profound (Rodgers 2001; Mutic et al. 2001). With dynamic IMRT systems, the linear accelerator is producing leakage radiation even when very small amounts of primary beam are exiting the head. The use of MUs to determine the workload for leakage radiation is appropriate for these calculations. The energy distribution or angular distributions will not be affected by IMRT. As shown in table 4, the increase in MUs when using IMRT is significant. The weekly MUs would be used in conjunction with the expected head leakage fraction to determine the barrier thickness [equation (4)]. Compared against a conventional installation, between 2 and 3 additional half-value layers (HVLs) would be required if the installation was expected to treat 100% of their patients with IMRT. These conclusions are appropriate for any IMRT system, but may require some modification based on the final definition of a monitor unit for helical tomotherapy.

## Neutron Contamination

Neutron contamination needs to be considered for facilities greater than 10 MV (NCRP 1984). Vault mazes are designed to attenuate both photon and neutron radiation, but the vault door is typically designed with neutron shielding in mind. Typically, the source of neutrons are ($\gamma$,n) reactions in linear accelerator head components. These reactions have minimum energy thresholds, which is why lower energy linear accelerators are not affected. Photoneutrons are produced roughly isotropically and penetrate shielding in all directions (McGinley 2002). For purposes determining the influence of IMRT on neutron shielding, it is treated the same as leakage radiation, so the dose rate due to neutrons will increase substantially when high-energy IMRT is used. Boyer and collaborators (Boyer, personal communication) surveyed an 18 MV linear accelerator for neutron levels just beyond the vault door. They used portable neutron rem counters and a moderated $BF_3$ counter. Two IMRT treatment plans were irradiated, one treating an abdominal sarcoma, and one treating breast cancer. Both used 1.8 Gy per fraction and had an average value of $1/E = 8.5$ and 7.6 for the abdomen and breast case, respectively. The abdomen case was irradiated twice, once with the correct gantry angles and once with the gantry pointing down. The breast cancer case was irradiated with the gantry pointing down. As a control, a closed field, $20 \times 20$ cm$^2$ and $40 \times 40$ cm$^2$ fields were irradiated using various gantry angles. Table 5 shows the resulting neutron equivalent doses in nSv/MU.

As table 5 shows, the abdomen IMRT with seven angles yielded similar neutron levels to the open fields. The same treatment, when using only a vertical gantry angle, yielded a greater neutron flux, indicating that there is some direction sensitivity to the flux. This can also be seen comparing the $40 \times 40$ cm$^2$ fields at their three gantry angles. The 270° beam delivered the greatest flux, followed by 0° and 90°. Even with this variation, the results were remarkably consistent, with the IMRT delivering an average of only 25% more than the large fields and slightly less than the closed-jaw irradiation. While these results indicate that neutron fluxes are relatively constant as a function of MUs and that the IMRT and conventional therapy fluxes are not too dissimilar (when normalized by the MUs), they clearly indicate that the total number of delivered MUs needs to be considered when designing the neutron shielding (primarily the maze and door).

**Table 5.** Neutron Equivalent Dose and Photon Dose Outside the Treatment Room Door for Some Tested Beam Configurations [Data courtesy of A. L. Boyer (private communication)]

| Field Size (cm × cm) | Gantry angle (deg) | Neutron Rem (nSv/MU) | Photon Dose (nGy/MU) |
|---|---|---|---|
| 0×0 | 0 | 1.12 | 0.77 |
| 20×20 | 0 | 0.98 | 0.70 |
| 40×40 | 0 | 0.78 | 0.73 |
| 40×40 | 90 | 0.60 | 0.80 |
| 40×40 | 270 | 0.83 | 0.80 |
| Abdomen IMRT | (7 angles) | 0.85 | 0.54 |
| Abdomen IMRT | 0 | 1.14 | 0.48 |
| Breast IMRT | 0 | 1.02 | 0.58 |

## Conclusions

The influence of IMRT on shielding calculation protocols is primarily in the calculation of barriers that attenuate head leakage. For these cases, an additional 2 to 3 HVLs may be required. Rodgers (2001) presented a table (a modified version is shown in table 6) that shows the added leakage shielding required as a function of the fraction of clinical IMRT treatments and MU efficiency of the IMRT protocol. They showed that for 100% IMRT cases, with an MU efficiency of 10% ($E = 0.1$), a TVL may need to be added to all secondary shielding walls. This thickness can be considerable (approx. 40 cm) and would be expensive to retrofit in the case of an existing vault. Careful review of the shielding capacity of existing clinics is warranted as they transition to IMRT. The results for neutrons are similar, although more studies are warranted before definitive recommendations can be made.

**Table 6.** Additional TVLs Required to Shield a Conventionally
Designed Vault when IMRT Is Introduced
[Data from Rodgers (2001)]

| r (%) | 1/E Additional | TVLs |
|-------|----------------|------|
| 0 | — | 0 |
| 50 | 4 | 0.40 |
| 50 | 10 | 0.74 |
| 100 | 4 | 0.60 |
| 100 | 10 | 1.0 |

$r$ refers to the fraction of treatments using IMRT. $E$ is the
monitor unit efficiency, expressed as the ratio of tumor dose
to delivered monitor units.

# References

Boyer, A. L. Personal communication.

Followill, D., P. Geis, and A. Boyer. (1997). "Estimates of the whole-body dose equivalent
produced by beam intensity modulated conformal therapy." *Int. J. Radiat. Oncol. Biol. Phys.*
38:667–672.

Horton, J. L. *Handbook of Radiation Therapy Physics.* Englewood Cliffs, NJ: Prentice-Hall,
1987.

Kapatoes, J. M., G. H. Olivera, P. J. Reckwerdt, E. E. Fitchard, E. A. Schloesser, and T. R.
Mackie. (1999). "Delivery verificaiton in sequential and helical tomotherapy." *Phys. Med.
Biol.* 44:1815–1841.

Kleck, J. H., and M. Elsalim. (1994). "Clinical workloads and use factors for medical linear
accelerators." Abstract. *Med. Phys.* 21:952–953.

Low, D. A., K. S. Chao, S. Mutic, R. L. Gerber, C. A. Perez, and J. A. Purdy. (1998a). "Quality assurance of serial tomotherapy for head and neck patient treatments." *Int. J. Radiat.
Oncol. Biol. Phys.* 42:681–692.

Low, D. A., S. Mutic, J. F. Dempsey, R. L. Gerber, W. R. Bosch, C. A. Perez, and J. A. Purdy.
(1998b). "Quantitative dosimetric verification of an IMRT planning and delivery system."
*Radiother. Oncol.* 49:305–316.

McGinley, P. H. *Shielding Techniques for Radiation Oncology Facilities*, 2nd edition. Madison,
WI: Medical Physics Publishing, 2002.

Mutic, S., D. A. Low, E. E. Klein, J. F. Dempsey, and J. A. Purdy. (2001). "Room shielding for
intensity-modulated radiation therapy treatment facilities." *Int. J. Radiat. Oncol. Biol. Phys.*
50:239–246.

National Council on Radiation Protection and Measurements (NCRP) Report 49. Structural
Shielding Design and Evaluation for Medical Use of X Rays and Gamma Rays of Energies up to 10 MeV. Bethesda, MD: NCRP, 1976.

National Council on Radiation Protection and Measurements (NCRP) Report 51. Radiation
Protection Design Guidelines for 0.1–100 MeV Particle Accelerator Facilities. Bethesda,
MD: NCRP, 1977.

National Council on Radiation Protection and Measurements (NCRP) Report 79. Neutron Contamination from Medical Linear Accelerators. Bethesda, MD: NCRP, 1984.

Rodgers, J. E. (2001). "Radiation therapy vault shielding calculational methods when IMRT and TBI procedures contribute." *J. Appl. Clin. Med. Phys.* 2:157–164.

Taylor, L., and J. E. Rodgers. (1999). "Scatter fractions from linear accelerators with x-ray energies from 6 to 24 MV." *Med. Phys.* 26:1442–1446.

Williams, J. R., and D. I. Thwaites (editors). *Radiotherapy Physics in Practice.* 2nd edition. Oxford, England: Oxford University Press, 2000.

# Dosimetry Metrology For IMRT

**Jean M. Moran, Ph.D.**
Department of Radiation Oncology
University of Michigan, Ann Arbor. Michigan



## Introduction

This chapter focuses on the measurements and dosimeters necessary to commission intensity-modulated radiation therapy (IMRT). Acceptance and commissioning techniques are described primarily for multileaf collimator (MLC)-based IMRT delivery systems. The advantages and disadvantages of dosimetric devices for commissioning IMRT are discussed. Then, a number of specific tests are described, ranging from simple geometry tests to anthropomorphic verification of IMRT delivery. Finally, some potential pitfalls that may arise during commissioning are presented.

Conventional commissioning has focused on verifying safe and accurate accelerator operation and on acquiring beam data for treatment planning (Fraass et al. 1998). As new technology is implemented clinically, the commissioning requirements should be adjusted accordingly. For example, when MLCs were added for beam shaping, commissioning tests were updated to verify the accuracy and reproducibility of leaf positioning, and characteristics such as the penumbra were compared to measurements with blocks (Boyer et al. 1992; Galvin et al. 1998; Galvin, Han, and Cohen 1992; Klein, Harms, and Low 1995; LoSasso and Kutcher 1995; Palta, Yeung, and Frouhar 1996). Dose calculation algorithms were adapted to calculate dose for MLC-shaped fields, and tested fields included clinical examples and geometric shapes (Fraass et al. 1998).

With IMRT, the situation is more complicated for both treatment planning and treatment delivery. Because computerized optimization is used to obtain intensity maps, a wider range of intensity maps is possible. To test the true limitations of a calculation algorithm and delivery system would require substantial (exhaustive) testing. In addition, several commercial systems have developed new algorithms for their optimization software and calculations that may not have been thoroughly tested for conventional treatment planning. In addition, a leaf sequencing algorithm converts intensity maps into a deliverable MLC file with leaf positions and fractional monitor units. Tools are needed to accurately compare calculations and measurements. Finally, record-and-verify systems are another critical part of delivery that also required testing.

Whereas the majority of dosimetric commissioning measurements for conventional therapy can be made with a scanning water phantom system with an ionization chamber, such measurements are insufficient for fields where the intensity varies across the field. To obtain profile information, an ionization or linear diode array is required. It is no longer a straightforward task to acquire the necessary information for machine commissioning, and modeling and verification of beams in the treatment planning system. Because the delivery involves leaf motion, multiple field deliveries are required to measure a depth dose curve or profile with an ionization chamber. Because of intensity variation across the field, film has re-emerged as a major component of routine dosimetry, and electronic portal imaging devices (EPIDs) are being investigated to make some of the time-consuming quality assurance (QA) tasks more efficient. For MLC-based IMRT delivery, the system performance must be thoroughly evaluated. Factors include leaf speed, beam linearity, symmetry, and flatness for low doses, dose rate, leaf position reproducibility and accuracy, and small field output. Dosimetric measurements must be assessed with respect to the dose calculation algorithm, leaf sequencing, IMRT delivery method, and accelerator hardware.

## Acceptance Testing

When a linear accelerator is installed, acceptance tests are performed to verify that the machine is functioning as specified by the manufacturer. Prior to installation of the accelerator, the manufacturer's acceptance tests should be reviewed. If the tolerances and tests provided by the manufacturer are determined to be inadequate, an agreement should be worked out in writing in advance with the manufacturer to allow for additional testing or stricter limits at the acceptance testing stage.

For IMRT delivery with MLC systems, it is important to know the basic design of the system. MLC designs depend on the manufacturer and the MLC model. Some of the basic design information and dosimetric characteristics have been compared between manufacturers (Arnfield et al. 2001; Galvin et al. 1992; Huq et al. 2002; Xia and Verhey 2001). The main differences include whether or not the leaves are single- or double-focused and whether or not the leaves have a straight or rounded leaf end. In addition, the MLC location in the treatment head varies and has an impact on the physical size of the leaves (and therefore the projected leaf width at isocenter) and the necessary leaf position accuracy. Some systems allow interdigitation of leaves whereas others do not. This information is relevant to how IMRT fields are sequenced for delivery. For add-on IMRT delivery systems, such as the MIMiC®, the integration of the device with the accelerator must be verified (Low et al. 1998; Saw et al. 2001).

Acceptance testing of MLC-based delivery systems should begin with the static collimation system. Using IMRT capabilities prior to verifying the static MLC carriage and leaf positions could result in mechanical damage to the collimation system. Static MLC tests include:

1. Carriage skew: orientation of MLC carriages in the accelerator head.

2. Physical gap between carriages.

3. Leaf position offset/radiation vs. light field.

4. Leaf position reproducibility and accuracy.

5. Transmission beneath and between leaves.

The carriage skew and leaf position offset (with respect to central axis) should be adjusted with the engineer using feeler gauges for a very small field (LoSasso, Chui, and Ling 1998). Once set, the carriage positions and leaf positions with respect to the central axis should be verified with film. The carriage skew and the leaf position offset are typically stored in files on the MLC controller. For systems with rounded leaf ends and linear leaf motion, the radiation leaf position offset corrects the leaf position across the field because of the dependence of the field width on the leaf position (Boyer and Li 1997).

The accuracy and reproducibility of leaf positions should first be evaluated in static mode. Leaf positioning should be within 0.025 cm (LoSasso, Chui, and Ling 1998). The transmission should be measured beneath and between the leaves for all energies. These characteristics are typically measured with high monitor units (MUs) delivered to ready-pack film at depth in solid water where the dose through closed leaves is compared to an open field. Typical values for static fields vary by the leaf design and can range from 1.5% to 2% (Arnfield et al. 2000; Clark et al. 2002; Galvin, Chen, and Smith 1993; LoSasso, Chui, and Ling 1998). Profiles should be extracted both off-axis and near the central axis across the field and evaluated. Interleaf leakage has been measured to be approximately 2.7% for one system ( LoSasso, Chui, and Ling 1998).

Most treatment planning systems require an average transmission value because the physical characteristics of the MLC are usually not modeled. Typically, the tongue-and-groove effect is also not modeled. The tongue-and-groove design of adjacent leaves can result in small regions of a field being blocked and therefore having reduced dose. Some leaf sequencing algorithms synchronize leaves to minimize the effect. To account for these effects, more sophisticated Monte Carlo methods are being developed that model both the physical design of the collimator head and leaves.

For IMRT delivery, additional acceptance tests include assessment of the following characteristics in dynamic and/or segmented MLC (DMLC and/or SMLC) mode:

1. Leaf speed.

2. Dose rate evaluation.

3.  Leaf position tolerance and reproducibility.

4.  Leaf acceleration/deceleration.

5.  Leaf switch rate for MIMiC system.

6.  Rounded leaf tip transmission.

7.  Beam stability (output, symmetry, flatness) and linearity for low MUs.

8.  Treatment interrupts.

MLC test files should be provided by the manufacturer to evaluate mechanical functions such as the leaf speed. Along with the files, the range of MUs and dose rates for proper and safe MLC function should be included. In addition, the manufacturer should provide an MLC implementation guide. The user may need to add additional tests at this stage or make dosimetric measurements of the actual tests. The user should evaluate the accelerator in both step-and-shoot and dynamic sliding window modes if both methods may be used in patient care.

The leaf speed is measured by determining the time it takes for leaves to travel a specific distance. Systems with different leaf thicknesses within the same MLC may measure different maximum speeds. For some of the acceptance tests, it is appropriate to use the optimization system and leaf sequencer to arrive at a set of files for testing at different dose rates and to deliver different doses. Because the leaf sequencing is dependent on the specific hardware constraints, it is important that the correct monitor units and dose rate are used for delivery of dynamic sliding window files (Litzenberg, Moran, and Fraass 2002).

The relationship between dose rate and leaf position tolerance is dependent on the communications timing between the accelerator and MLC controller. For example, in the current Varian system it takes up to 50 ms for the excursion of a beam hold-off if a leaf position is out of tolerance. The dosimetric error may be greater for higher dose rates since more dose can be delivered prior to a beam hold-off. To minimize the effect of the communications delay, the leaf position tolerance must actually be set larger (0.2 to 0.25 cm) for more accurate delivery for dynamic sliding window delivery (Litzenberg, Moran, and Fraass 2002a; LoSasso, Chui, and Ling 1998). Setting a smaller leaf position tolerance value results in numerous beam hold-offs since the leaves are unable to stay within tolerance for the full delivery of the field. The effect of tolerance setting on delivery should be assessed for each delivery mode that will be used clinically. The reproducibility of leaf positioning in dynamic mode should also be evaluated. Analysis of the machine's record of MLC delivery (dynamic log files in the Varian system) is another method of evaluating the MLC performance. The information in the log file can be useful in identifying the cause of dosimetric errors and in understanding leaf motion effects such as acceleration and deceleration.

Rounded leaf end MLC-based IMRT delivery systems also require measurement of the leaf end transmission. This can be determined from the average measured transmission or from a regression analysis of small field width data (LoSasso, Chui, and Ling 1998). Measurements at several centers have found values ranging from a leaf offset of 0.7 to 1 mm to approximate the effect. (Arnfield et al. 2000; Cadman et al. 2002; Graves et al. 2001; Kung and Chen 2000; LoSasso, Chui, and Ling 1998; Zygmanski and Kung 2001).

After calibration of the accelerator, beam linearity should be investigated for small monitor unit settings with static fields (Hansen et al. 1998). A chamber can be placed with full buildup in air. Measurements should be normalized to a $10 \times 10$ cm$^2$ field. For example, measurements can be made for monitor unit settings from 1 MU to 100 MUs (e.g., 1, 2, 3, 4, 5, 6, 7, 8, 9, 10, 20, 30, 50, and 100) (Hansen et al. 1998). The values should then be plotted to assess the linearity of the beam. The user should also evaluate the beam flatness for low monitor unit settings to determine if the beam behavior at the beginning of a delivery is stable enough for dynamic delivery. This can be done with an ion chamber placed off-axis, a chamber array, or film. Flatness and symmetry for low dose segments may vary by as much as 9% (Hansen et al. 1998). A service engineer should be contacted if the behavior is unacceptable. Also, limits can be put on the number of monitor units allowed per segment (Wong et al. 2001).

Additional tests include measuring the delivery for fields where the beam is interrupted and restarted during delivery and comparing to the measurements from the uninterrupted treatment (Dirkx and Heijmen 2000; Essers et al. 2001). The record of the partial delivery should be checked in the record-and-verify system and the monitor unit settings on the mechanical counters should be checked for accuracy.

If clinical treatments will occur with a record-and-verify system, delivery should be tested using that system to verify that the results of the tests defined above are still accurate. For example, it is important to verify that the user-defined leaf position tolerance setting is used by the record-and-verify system during delivery rather than a default setting at the treatment unit. If the system does not work as expected, the acceptance stage is a good time to alert the manufacturer so that problems can be corrected prior to commissioning and patient treatments. Finally, tests in dynamic mode should include situations in which delivery should fail. For example, if an MLC file is modified in a text editor (not the regular software), the system should not be able to run the field.

## Commissioning Measurements

This section describes the specific equipment and software as well as tests for IMRT commissioning. Simple commissioning tests are described for measurements in air or a simple geometry to assess the components of correct IMRT delivery. More complicated tests are also described in similar geometry. Finally, the use of anthropomorphic tests as part of the commissioning process is discussed.

## Equipment And Software

After acceptance of the accelerator, beam data are required for both beam fitting and testing of beam models. IMRT commissioning requires the use of multiple detectors because it is difficult and time-consuming to accurately acquire two- and three-dimensional (2-D and 3-D) data in a water phantom system. Measurements of profiles and depth dose curves require stepping an ion chamber or array across the field or up the field. This information is still insufficient for commissioning the system. If such systems are used, the detector response should be thoroughly tested and verified for static fields. An ideal system would have excellent spatial resolution, accuracy, tissue equivalent response, ability to provide 3-D information, portability to multiple phantoms, and ease of use. No single detector meets all the needs of IMRT commissioning. Therefore, the advantages and disadvantages of 1-D, 2-D, and 3-D dosimetric methods are described.

### Detectors

When a new detector is purchased for IMRT, it is critical that the detector response is characterized for both static and dynamic fields for linearity, energy dependence, and angular response. If the chamber will be used for absolute measurements, then the chamber and electrometer should be calibrated by a calibration laboratory (Almond et al. 1999).

There are a number of ion chambers available for IMRT measurements. The necessary resolution of the detector depends on the resolution of the beamlet grid that is using for planning and sequencing fields for delivery. Chambers with smaller volumes are more sensitive to position and will have a higher response when positioned at an opposing leaf pair junction and between adjacent leaves. Ionization chambers should typically be placed in low gradient regions (IMRTCWG 2001; Low et al. 1998). To minimize the effect of volume averaging, the detector should be smaller than the homogeneous region of dose to be measured.

**Small-Field Detectors**. A number of smaller chambers have been developed specifically for radiosurgery measurements and are applicable to small field IMRT measurements (Bank 2002; Gotoh et al. 1996; Lee et al. 2002; Martens, De Wagter, and De Neve 2000). Ionization chambers are required for absolute point dose measurements. Basic information about detector specifications is shown in table 1 for several detectors that have been evaluated for small fields.

Silicon diodes and pinpoint chambers over-respond to low-energy photons due to the interactions in silicon and the steel central electrode, respectively. This effect can be minimized for the pinpoint chamber by normalizing output measurements to a $5 \times 5$ cm field at 5 cm$^2$ depth (Martens, De Wagter, and De Neve 2000). The diamond detector has been shown to have excellent characteristics with respect to angular dependence, energy response ($Z = 6$), and penumbra (Rustgi 1995). However, the resolution of the diamond detector is slightly worse than that of a silicon diode detector, and the response must be corrected for dose rate dependence (Fidanzio et al. 2000; Haryanto et al. 2002; Laub et al. 2000; Laub, Kaulich, Nüsslin 1999; Rustgi 1995). The detector cost should be considered against the gain in accuracy.

**Table 1.** Summary of Small-Field Detector Specifications

| Detector | Measurement Volume (cm³) | Sensitive Area (cm²) | Diameter (cm) | Thickness (cm) | Effective Point of Measurement (cm) |
|---|---|---|---|---|---|
| Micro-chamber | 0.009 | 0.24 | 0.6 | NA | 0.2 |
| p-type Si diode | 0.3 | 0.49 | 0.4 | 0.06 | 0.6 |
| Stereotactic diode | NA | 0.011 | 0.45 | 0.006 | 0.07 |
| Pinpoint chamber | 0.015 | 0.010 | 0.2 | NA | 0.06 |
| MOSFET | NA | 0.04 | NA | 0.1 | NA |
| Diamond | 0.0019 | 0.056/0.073 | 0.73 | 0.026 | 0.1 |

Metal oxide silicon field effect transistors (MOSFETs) have also been applied to IMRT measurements, and phantoms are now available commercially to accommodate the small detectors. The primary advantages of MOSFETs are their excellent spatial resolution (due to their small size), automatic and immediate readout, and ability to be reused immediately when compared with thermoluminescent dosimeters (TLDs) and film (Chuang, Verhey, and Xia 2002; Francescon et al. 1998; Kron et al. 2002). An earlier design showed an over-response for the phantom scatter factor for small fields (Francescon et al. 1998). A later commercial version of a low-sensitivity MOSFET was recently characterized with a high-voltage power supply (Chuang, Verhey, and Xia 2002). The MOSFET response was found to have ±3% reproducibility, ±2.5% angular dependence, linear response for doses greater than 30 cGy, and agreed with ion chamber depth dose measurements to within ±3%. A drawback for this configuration was decreased linearity for doses less than 30 cGy limiting the MOSFET to high dose applications. The specific application and measurement conditions should be carefully assessed and the device should be used in the appropriate dose range.

Another detector that has been used for IMRT commissioning measurements are TLDs. TLDs are versatile and easy to use in multiple phantoms. The advantages include the small size, versatility in placement, and readily available readout equipment. However, TLDs must be characterized, which is time-consuming, and accuracy is limited to 2% to 3%. Use of an automatic TLD reader is recommended when using TLDs for IMRT field verification due to the large number of TLDs required for verification in a measurement plane (60 or more) (Low et al. 1998; Van Esch et al. 2002). It is important that the additional equipment be routinely monitored, such as TLD reader response and oven temperature, to maintain consistent TLD response.

Ion chamber arrays and linear diode arrays have been applied to measurements for scanned beams and commissioning of dynamic wedge. For IMRT, 1-D detector arrays have limited utility since they still only provide a profile of information. The arrays can be used to benchmark some 2-D systems for specific parts of a distribution and to determine the flatness and symmetry of static and uniform dynamic fields. However, 2-D data are needed for commissioning and can be obtained by acquiring a profile at one position during delivery, stepping across the field to the next position, and then repeating the delivery as necessary. The dosimetric characteristics have been found to be acceptable for both ion chamber and silicon diode arrays (Martens, De Wagter, and De Neve 2001; Martens et al. 2001; Sidhu 1999).

Electrometers that are used with measurement equipment should be periodically tested and calibrated regularly (Blad, Wendel, and Nilsson 1998). In addition, cables should be in good working order and have low noise properties.

**Two-Dimensional Detectors**. Due to availability and advantages in obtaining 2-D information, film plays a critical part in IMRT commissioning at many centers. Radiographic film has excellent spatial resolution and can be used for relative dosimetry measurements. Disadvantages of radiographic film include over-response to low energies because of its composition, dependence on processor and laser digitizer QA, sensitivity to storage conditions, and need for a measured dose response curve for accurate measurements. Because radiographic film responds to light, it must be sealed from light with opaque tape when cut to fit in phantoms. Whenever possible, ready-pack film should be used, a corner of the film packet should be punctured, and the packet should be compressed to remove the air.

Due to variability in processor performance and other characteristics, the dosimetric response of film should be measured each time under the calibration conditions to obtain accurate dosimetric information over the dose range of interest for data analysis. Methods have been developed to measure multiple dose levels per film (Childress, Dong, and Rosen 2002). When done accurately, this method saves both time and film. All measurements for an experiment should be made with the same batch of film. To identify problems within a film batch, a sensitometer can be used to expose the film to multiple optical densities in the dark room prior to processing (LoSasso, Chui, and Ling 1998). When using film for relative dosimetry, the equipment must be maintained correctly to minimize errors in the analysis process. The film processor should be warmed up prior to use for data analysis films. Processor maintenance is a concern as centers begin to use electronic portal imagers instead of film on a daily basis. Several films should be run through the system in advance, an appropriate amount of chemicals should be in the processor so additional chemicals do not need to be added in the middle of processing films for data analysis, and the temperature should be stable. Rate of films fed into the processor should be consistent. Routine processor quality assurance must be performed.

In the United States the primary types of radiographic film used are Kodak XV and EDR (enhanced dynamic range). The response of EDR film has recently been characterized for photon beams (Chetty and Charland 2002; Dogan, Leybovich, and

Sethi 2002; Esthappan et al. 2002; Olch 2002; Zhu et al. 2002). When compared to XV film, EDR film has less dependence on the processor, field size, and less response to low energy photons. EDR film also has been found to have better reproducibility and agreement with ion chamber measurements than XV film. Because of the decreased sensitivity of EDR film, it can be used to measure a complete fraction of an IMRT delivery.

Radiochromic film has also been used for dosimetric measurements. The recommendations of AAPM Task Group 55 should be followed in using radiochromic film (Niroomand-Rad et al. 1998). The advantages of radiochromic film include decreased sensitivity to low-energy photons compared to radiographic film because of composition, no processing (the film changes color with irradiation), insensitivity to visible light, and high spatial resolution. However, there are a number of disadvantages that have limited its use when compared with radiographic film. The response of the film to radiation is non-uniform (a double exposure technique minimizes some of the effect) and is dependent on factors such as time and temperature. Radiochromic film is far more expensive than radiographic film.

When using either radiographic or radiochromic film, accurate positioning of the film in the phantom is important for registration in the treatment planning system. Some errors can be decreased by using a solid-water slab designed for film. Other phantoms have pins between slabs that puncture the film where the pinholes are used as registration marks. These methods align the film with respect to the phantom but not with respect to the beam. Another system uses the leakage between leaves to align the film. It is important that delivery problems are not masked by using the alignment process to remove actual differences between the delivery and the calculation. For example, a skew in the MLC might not be identified if automated alignment tools are used.

Another part of performing accurate film dosimetry is quality assurance of the digitizer or scanner system. The spatial intensity, characteristic response, and noise due to large changes in optical density need to be verified (Dempsey et al. 1999; Halpern 1995; Meeder, Jaffray, and Munro 1995; Teslow 1997). For radiochromic film analysis, the response of a digitizer is dependent on the light source of the digitizer as well as other design characteristics (Gluckman and Reinstein 2002). These factors should be considered in choosing and maintaining a laser digitizer for accurate film dosimetry.

Other detectors have been used for relative 2-D IMRT measurements. Ma et al. described a beam imaging system located in the block tray of the accelerator to measure the fluence distribution for comparison to calculation (Ma, Geis, and Boyer 1997). A similar system was developed in water using a charge-coupled device (CCD) camera system and a scintillator (Li, Boyer, and Ma 2001). The screen has a 30 cm diameter, resolution of 0.586 cm (512 × 512 pixels), and linear dose response after correction for background and blurring. EPID systems using CCDs, liquid ion chambers, and amorphous silicon flat panel detectors have also been used to measure 2-D distributions. These devices have been primarily applied to patient-specific pre-treatment field verification and MLC QA (Partridge et al. 1998; Partridge,

Symonds-Tayler, and Evans 2002; Partridge, Ebert, and Hesse 2002). For measurements at different depths in a solid water phantom, an amorphous silicon flat panel detector (AMFPD) has been adapted for dosimetric measurements, including IMRT applications (El-Mohri et al. 1999; Moran et al. 2002; Nurushev et al. 2001). The detector area is $26 \times 26$ cm$^2$ and has a resolution of 0.508 mm.

**Gel Dosimetry.** As treatment planning and delivery have become more complex, obtaining additional dosimetric information than can be obtained from point and 2-D dosimeters has become more important. Gel dosimetry has been further developed from initial Fricke dosimeters to polymer gels. McJury et al. (2000) recently reviewed methods and applications of polymer gel dosimetry. Gels can be made in a lab facility or purchased as a ready-to-mix package (MGS, Guildford, New Haven, CT). Great care and specialized equipment are required to do accurate gel dosimetry. The response of polymer gels is dependent on exposure to light and oxygen, the composition, and the temperature of the gel during readout. The optimum readout time is also a factor and was found to be 3 to 4 days after irradiation for a particular system (McJury et al. 1999). Readout equipment includes either a magnetic resonance imaging (MRI) scanner (expensive to use and readout time might be limited) or an optical scanner. Similar to film, a dose response curve must be measured for each experiment. For 0-10 Gy irradiations of BANG® polymer gels (MGS, Guildford, New Haven, CT), the dosimetric accuracy is approximately within 3% to 5% and the spatial resolution is approximately 2 to 5 mm when an MR scanner is used with a T2-weighted imaging sequence (McJury et al. 2000). Optical CT scanning may make use of polymer gels more widespread since the cost is substantially less than that of an MR scanner. Several investigators have been developing CT scanning systems based on either CCD detectors or laser scanning (Doran et al. 2001; Gore et al. 1996; Kelly, Jordan, and Battista 1998; Oldham et al. 2001). There are technical challenges to overcome with both methods.

Gel dosimetry measurements have been made for stereotactic and/or IMRT treatment plans by a number of investigators and compared to calculations and other dosimeters (De Deene 2002; Gum et al. 2002; Low et al. 1999; Oldham et al. 1998). The accuracy of the readout was found to be increased for higher doses (Oldham et al. 1998). Perhaps the greatest potential for gel dosimetry is for use in inhomogeneous phantoms where the sensitivity and density of the gel can be varied. The gel can be shaped to fit in the phantom. For example, an anthropomorphic phantom of the thorax was developed and different densities of Fricke gel were used for the lung and spinal cord, and other parts of the phantom (Gum et al. 2002). Due to the large size of the phantom, the dosimetric accuracy was limited to approximately 5%, which was obtained after a 10-hour MR scan time.

Prior to general use throughout the community, further development of more robust polymer gels requiring less sensitive conditions is required along with readily available and accurate readouts. Because of the multiple steps involved and the time dependence of the readout, gel dosimetry requires additional time from the preparation of gels to data analysis.

*Phantoms For IMRT Measurements*

Commissioning of IMRT requires a more flexible geometry than a simple water-filled phantom since multiple dosimeters are required and irradiation from different gantry angles must be thoroughly verified. Many manufacturers allow phantoms to be customized by the user for different detectors. For example, special holders have been made out of square slabs for holding TLDs or MOSFET detectors (Chuang, Verhey, and Xia 2002; Low et al. 1998). Cylindrical phantoms offer a straightforward geometry for absolute ion chamber measurements of a full-field IMRT delivery. Appropriate factors should be applied to convert to dose in water if necessary (Tello, Tailor, and Hanson 1995).

A few phantoms have been developed specifically for IMRT commissioning and patient dosimetric verification. A water-filled cylindrical phantom that can be rotated was developed which allows for different positions of an ion chamber in the phantom (Xing et al. 1999). Another example is a water-equivalent square phantom that was developed for TLD and ion chamber measurements (Low et al. 1998). The phantom allows the position of the ion chamber in the slab to be varied through the use of different spacers of the water-equivalent material. Special consideration should be given to the use of fiducials for film alignment and scribe lines on the phantom for a reproducible setup. A cylindrical phantom was designed to use film and an ion chamber simultaneously (Paliwal et al. 2000). An ion chamber is placed at the center of the phantom for an absolute dose measurement and a piece of film winds in a spiral from the center to the outside of the phantom. An entire treatment plan can be delivered and then evaluated by comparing the irradiated film to the measurements. Special software is required (or can be developed by the user) to do the data analysis.

Anthropomorphic phantoms still play an appropriate role for testing the process from CT-simulation to optimization and full-field IMRT delivery. They can be used for limited measurements to evaluate the process of patient treatment planning and delivery and to identify problems that are not evident in simple homogeneous geometric phantoms. There are disadvantages to using such phantoms since they still do not accurately represent the phantom geometry and often have thick slices.

*Dosimetry Analysis Software*

The final piece of a comprehensive dosimetry system is software for 2-D dosimetric data analysis. Optimized fluence maps must be easily transferred from a patient plan to the phantom geometry for field and plan verification at specific planes. Dosimetric data must be imported into the planning system, or the dose calculation at the specified plane must be exported to another software program for comparison to the measurements. As mentioned above, the registration of the data to the calculation is important. Tools that have been developed for dosimetric analysis of measurements and calculations include:

1. Isodose overlay.

2. 2-D dose difference displays with colorwash.

3. Dose difference histograms.

4. Distance-to-agreement.

5. Combination of dose difference display and distance-to-agreement.

6. Highlight of specific regions of disagreement or agreement on a dose difference display.

7. Gamma evaluation.

A number of these tools have been routinely used in the past for commissioning and evaluation of new dose calculation algorithms (Fraass, Martel, and McShan 1994; Harms et al. 1998; Low et al. 1998). When appropriate, relative detector measurements should be normalized to ionization chamber measurements and then compared with calculations rather than normalizing the measurements to a point on the calculation plane.

The gamma evaluation tool has most recently been applied to IMRT as an easy-to-use tool for interpreting the complicated difference displays of IMRT fields (Depuydt, Van Esch, and Huyskens 2002; Low et al. 1998). The user sets the criteria for dose difference and distance-to-agreement values. Using this information, a composite distribution is calculated which shows regions that did not meet either criteria. Several tools are automated to quickly identify discrepancies between measurements and film (Kapulsky, Mullokandov, and Gejerman 2002). Another tool is a filter that has been developed to compare intensity maps for new patient plans against repetitive patterns for prostate IMRT fields (De Brabandere et al. 2002).

At this time, more versatile phantoms and detectors are still required. Additional software analysis and computational tools are needed to identify the cause of discrepancies between delivery and measurements and to determine the impact on patient treatment.

## Simple Geometry

For commissioning tests in a simple geometry, the tests developed by Chui et al. and LoSasso et al. can be used for both commissioning and developing a routine quality assurance program for MLC-based IMRT delivery systems (Chui, Spirou, and LoSasso 1996; LoSasso, Chui, and Ling 1998, 2001). Others have used the same or similar tests as required for their own applications (Dirkx and Heijmen 2000; Essers et al. 2001; Van Esch et al. 2002). These tests focus on verifying that the leaf motions are dosimetrically accurate and reproducible for a range of geometric situations. The following simple tests can be used to assess correct MLC function:

1.  Leaf position reproducibility in dynamic mode.

2.  Effect of gravity on leaf position accuracy and reproducibility.

3.  Sweeping gap test.

4.  Fence test.

5.  Leaf speed stability.

6.  Leaf acceleration/deceleration.

7.  Output checks from small to large fields.

8.  MLC limits, e.g., field size restrictions.

9.  Depth-dose curve measurements.

Leaf position and gap width reproducibility should be tested in both static and dynamic modes. In static mode, the light field can be projected on graph paper at isocenter. Leaf positions should be within 0.25 mm (LoSasso, Chui, and Ling 1998). In dynamic mode, all leaves can be tested at multiple positions using a narrow band test (Chui, Spirou, and LoSasso 1996). The leaves are programmed to stop at specific positions for the same pattern for right and left leaves with a time lag between the opposing leaves. For rounded leaf end systems, the result is additional transmission through the leaves where they are stopped. Incorrect leaf positions are easily seen as hot or cold spots on film (or EPID).

The influence of gravity on MLC function should be assessed with measurements with a cylindrical ion chamber in air. For example, a $10 \times 10$ cm$^2$ field can be delivered with a 0.5 cm wide scanning slit (or SMLC field) at multiple gantry and collimator angles and normalized to an open $10 \times 10$ cm$^2$ field at the same gantry angles. Errors in gap width of approximately 0.001 cm can be detected by a 2.5% deviation in dose (LoSasso, Chui, and Ling 1998). Measurements have been reported to be within $\pm 2\%$ for multiple centers (LoSasso, Chui, and Ling 1998; Van Esch et al. 2002). The sweeping gap test only evaluates the center leaves and the region close to the ion chamber. To test the positioning of all leaves, a fence test can be used to show errors of 0.02 cm on film, an EPID, or 2-D ion chamber array (Van Esch et al. 2002). All leaf pairs are moved at constant speed across the field and then stopped at regular intervals. Increased dose regions should appear like a fence. Position inaccuracies can be identified as misalignment on the film or other measurement device.

The speed of leaf pairs can be evaluated using a ramp or stepwise dose delivery test for different dose levels such as 10, 20, 30, 40, 50, 60, 70, 50, and 20 MUs (Chui, Spirou, and LoSasso 1996). The intensity map should be made in the optimization system and then sequenced with the correct dose rate to determine the appropriate monitor units for delivery. Film (or other 2-D device) can be used for dosimetric evaluation. Dose profiles should be extracted across each single leaf pair and should show a constant dose. Fluctuations in the profiles indicate instability in the leaf speed. The ramp or stepwise test can also be used to assess acceleration and deceleration effects by rotating the field 90 degrees and re-sequencing and interrupting the treatment during delivery (Chui, Spirou, and LoSasso 1996; Van Esch et al. 2002).

As mentioned earlier, measurements should also be made for interrupted treatments since such an event may occur in the midst of a patient treatment. Interruptions can range from simple interruption of the field to a loss of power. Measurements should be made with both film and an ionization chamber at depth to verify that the accelerator resumes the treatment accurately (Dirkx and Heijmen 2000; Essers et al. 2001).

Because small fields are a part of IMRT delivery, output factors should be measured for fields ranging from $1 \times 1$ cm$^2$ to larger fields (e.g., $15 \times 15$ cm$^2$) for all energies (Hansen et al. 1998; LoSasso, Chui, and Ling 1998; Sharpe et al. 2000). An appropriate detector and technique should be used. Measurement of extra-focal radiation is particularly difficult to measure with a mini phantom. It may be necessary to make these measurements at extended distances. These measurements are useful for thoroughly testing how the dose calculation algorithms handle head scatter and to set appropriate limits for IMRT segment sizes if appropriate.

The effect of physical limits of the MLC such as carriage motion or over-travel of individual leaves should also be investigated and the correction method evaluated (Wu et al. 2000; Xia, Wang, and Verhey 2002). For example, if optimized fields are split at the leaf sequencing stage due to leaf positioning limits, 2-D measurements should be made at depth in a phantom to verify that the abutment region is not over- or underdosed.

Finally, measurements should be made at multiple depths for a few sample fields. For example, it is straightforward (although time-consuming) to measure with an ion chamber at multiple depths for a $10 \times 10$ cm$^2$ uniform field and then to compare to the static field measurement. Film can be placed at multiple depths in a phantom and then interpolated using the ion chamber curve to evaluate a 3-D distribution (Stern et al. 1992). This is an important check at the commissioning stage since once the system is routinely used, pre-treatment QA measurements are usually limited to one depth.

## Complex Cases: Simple Phantom Geometry

As part of commissioning, complicated intensity patterns should be developed in the optimization system and transferred to the delivery system to irradiate a simple phantom geometry such as a cylindrical phantom or stack of solid water. Both a point chamber and film should be used to compare measurements and calculations. The phantom should be CT scanned and used for treatment planning. As mentioned earlier, the treatment planning system must be able to import the measured data for evaluation or export dosimetric data at the appropriate plane for analysis. All tests should be performed at the dose rate and monitor units that will be used clinically. In addition, a range of clinically relevant fractionation values should be tested.

Film and ion chamber measurements should be made at multiple depths for tests ranging from different geometry tests to those developed using the optimization system for patient-type cases. Both individual field measurements and full-field delivery should be assessed. A range of tests has been developed at a number of centers. Tests with a simple geometry include: uniform, single step, steps in $x$ and $y$ directions (as described in a previous section), roof shape, intensity well, checkerboard, and fields with low-intensity regions in the midst of a square (Papatheodorou et al. 2000; Van Esch et al. 2002; Xing et al. 1999). Another example is the chair test which has leaf pairs that move at constant and maximum speeds and tests the leaf function under different conditions (Van Esch et al. 2002). Dosimetric profiles should be extracted and compared to measurements to evaluate the effect of approximations in dose modeling and delivery effects. Tests should be adapted as necessary depending on the optimization and delivery method to define the limitations of the optimization and delivery systems.

Another test of the system focuses specifically on how the output varies upon the degree of modulation in the field. For example, a test field with multiple intensities can be used. The central axis region can be held constant. The modulation in a different portion of the field can be set to a low intensity, equal intensity, and higher intensity than the central axis intensity. The dosimetric results may show some variation depending on how the fields are sequenced and delivered.

Evaluation of the tests for both individual fields and full-field delivery at this stage is important to help the physicist identify the significance of some errors. It is possible that the effect of individual beam errors may be washed out during the full-field delivery. However, it is difficult to then extrapolate this information to the patient situation with heterogeneities and irregular geometry. Therefore, commissioning should include both individual field and full-field delivery measurements.

## Complex Geometry

A final commissioning check for IMRT includes complex geometries such as anthropomorphic phantoms. Although anthropomorphic phantoms do not accurately represent the geometry of individual patients, such tests can be used to check the overall accuracy of the patient planning process (IMRTCWG 2001). It is critical that calculation and measurements have been evaluated and understood for the situations described above in cylindrical and cubic homogeneous phantoms. The expected agreement between calculations and measurements will depend on the phantom geometry and whether or not the dose calculation algorithm accounts for heterogeneities. When conducting such tests, it is also important to perform the pre-treatment quality assurance tests with film (or other 2-D dosimeter) and an ion chamber prior to delivery on the complex phantom.

Anthropomorphic phantoms with heterogeneities have been used by several centers effectively to commission IMRT and to verify the process from CT scan and treatment planning to immobilization and delivery (Lee et al. 2002; MacKenzie et al. 2002; Tsai et al. 1998; Van Esch et al. 2002; Verellen et al. 1997). In addition to standard dosimetric checks, the accuracy of immobilization has been evaluated as well as technique changes (Lee et al. 2002; Verellen et al. 1997). Other centers have used the tests to identify the source of discrepancies by using heterogeneous and homogeneous phantoms of the same shape (Tsai et al. 1998). Detectors have included TLDs, film, gel dosimetry, and alanine crystals. Testing in anthropomorphic phantoms for IMRT has been shown to be useful in identifying clinical issues that may not have been identified otherwise. It is an appropriate final check prior to the start of patient treatments with IMRT.

## Potential Pitfalls

Finally, there are a number of potential pitfalls when commissioning an accelerator and optimization system for IMRT. As mentioned earlier, it is critical that all equipment used for commissioning is checked on a routine basis for correct functioning. Detectors, electrometers, processors, digitizers, TLD readers, and other equipment need to be maintained properly to minimize errors. Pre-treatment QA tests do not replace routine quality assurance of the accelerator and IMRT delivery equipment. Checks should also be performed and documented after any changes to software such as for optimization, leaf sequencing, or record-and-verify systems.

For absolute measurements, small ion chambers are very sensitive to position. For routine measurements, the ionization chamber should not be used to measure the tongue-and-groove of adjacent leavesbecause the magnitude of this effect will depend on the detector size. Extra care is needed because ion chamber measurements are often used to normalize film measurements and systematic errors could be introduced into the dosimetric evaluation. For phantom plans, digitally reconstructed radiographs (DRRs) can be generated in the planning system and compared against film or portal images for phantom positioning. For relative measurements, care should be taken in film registration to the phantom and the beam.

Several authors have found systematic errors with different delivery systems that may affect many users. While the patient-by-patient significance of such discrepancies varies, such discrepancies are part of why pre-treatment quality assurance is regularly performed at many centers. Delivery issues, several of which are related, include timing issues for MLC leaf positioning (Budgell 1999; Budgell et al. 2000; Litzenberg et al. 2002; LoSasso, Chui, and Ling 2001), high leaf velocity effects (Low et al. 2001), effect of the leaf switch rate (Hossain, Houser, and Galvin 2002; Tsai, Rivard, and Engler 2000), end-effect due to small discrepancies for small monitor units (Verhey 2001), dose overshoot phenomenon for SMLC (Ezzell and Chungbin 2001), and abutment regions for serial tomotherapy (Dogan et al. 2000; Leybovich et al. 2000; Low et al. 1999). The dosimetric effects due to tongue-and-groove (up to 29% in an extreme case) (Essers et al. 2001; Sykes and Williams 1998) and leaf abutment regions (Low and Mutic 1997; Low et al. 1999, 2001) are also of concern in treatment planning. Several of these problems can be minimized by adding constraints to the leaf sequencing algorithm or by more accurate models of the effects such as the leaf-switch rate.

Finally, the IMRT Collaborative Working Group has recently published a document that can be used to guide decisions related to IMRT (IMRTCWG 2001). When setting agreement criteria between measurements and calculations, the limitations of detector accuracy to approximately 2% to 3% need to be considered. The limitations of an optimization system, dose calculation algorithms, and delivery methods should be determined at the commissioning stage so that appropriate values for the agreement criteria can be set for pre-treatment QA. Anthropomorphic tests help quantify the potential error to a patient from dosimetric errors found from flat phantom measurements at one depth. Development of more accurate algorithms, phantoms, software tools, and delivery systems is expected to continue as the number of IMRT users also increases.

# References


Almond, P. R., P. J. Biggs, B. M. Coursey, W. H. Hanson, M. S. Huq, R. Nath, and D. W. Rogers. (1999). "AAPM's TG-51 protocol for clinical reference dosimetry of high-energy photon and electron beams." *Med. Phys.* 26:1847–1870.

Arnfield, M. R., J. V. Siebers, J. O. Kim, Q. Wu, P. J. Keall, and R. Mohan. (2000). "A method for determining multileaf collimator transmission and scatter for dynamic intensity modulated radiotherapy." *Med. Phys.* 27:2231–2241.

Arnfield, M. R., Q. Wu, S. Tong, and R. Mohan. (2001). "Dosimetric validation for multileaf collimator-based intensity- modulated radiotherapy: A review." *Med. Dosim.* 26:179–188.

Bank, M. I. (2002). "Ion chamber measurements of transverse gamma knife beam profiles." *J. Appl. Clin. Med. Phys.* 3:12–18.

Blad, B., P. Wendel, and P. Nilsson. (1998). "A simple test device for electrometers." *Phys. Med. Biol.* 43:2385–2391.

Boyer, A. L., and S. Li. (1997). "Geometric analysis of light-field position of a multileaf collimator with curved ends." *Med. Phys.* 24:757–762.

Boyer, A. L., T. G. Ochran, C. E. Nyerick, T. J. Waldron, and C. J. Huntzinger. (1992). "Clinical dosimetry for implementation of a multileaf collimator." *Med. Phys.* 19:1255–1261.

Budgell, G. J. (1999). "Temporal resolution requirements for intensity modulated radiation therapy delivered by multileaf collimators." *Phys. Med. Biol.* 44:1581–1596.

Budgell, G. J., J. H. L. Mott, P. C. Williams, and K. J. Brown. (2000). "Requirements for leaf position accuracy for dynamic multileaf collimation." *Phys. Med. Biol.* 45:1211–1227.

Cadman, P., R. Bassalow, N. P. Sidhu, G. Ibbott, and A. Nelson. (2002). "Dosimetric considerations for validation of a sequential IMRT process with a commercial treatment planning system." *Phys. Med. Biol.* 47:3001–3010.

Chetty, I. J., and P. M. Charland. (2002). "Investigation of Kodak extended dose range (EDR) film for megavoltage photon beam dosimetry." *Phys. Med. Biol.* 47:3629–3641.

Childress, N. L., L. Dong, and II. Rosen. (2002). "Rapid radiographic film calibration for IMRT verification using automated MLC fields." *Med. Phys.* 29:2384–2390.

Chuang, C. F., L. J. Verhey, and P. Xia. (2002). "Investigation of the use of MOSFET for clinical IMRT dosimetric verification." *Med. Phys.* 29:1109–1115.

Chui, C. S., S. Spirou, and T. LoSasso. (1996). "Testing of dynamic multileaf collimation." *Med. Phys.* 23:635–641.

Clark, C. H., C. D. Mubata, C. A. Meehan, A. M. Bidmead, J. Staffurth, M. E. Hunphreys, and D. P. Dearnaley. (2002). "IMRT clinical implementation: prostate and pelvic node irradiation using Helios and a 120-leaf multileaf collimator." *J. Appl. Clin. Med. Phys.* 3:273–284.

De Brabandere, M., A. Van Esch, G. J. Kutcher, and D. Huyskens. (2002). "Quality assurance in intensity modulated radiotherapy by identifying standards and patterns in treatment preparation: a feasibility study on prostate treatments." *Radiother. Oncol.* 62:283–291.

De Deene, Y. (2002). "Gel dosimetry for the dose verification of intensity modulated radiotherapy treatments." *Z Med. Phys.* 12:77–88.

Dempsey, J. F., D. A. Low, A. Kirov, and J. F. Williamson. (1999). "Quantitative optical densitometry with scanning-laser film digitizers." *Med. Phys.* 26:1721–1731.

Depuydt, T., A. Van Esch, and D. P. Huyskens. (2002). "A quantitative evaluation of IMRT dose distributions: refinement and clinical assessment of the gamma evaluation." *Radiother. Oncol.* 62:309–319.

Dirkx, M. L., and B. J. Heijmen. (2000). "Testing of the stability of intensity modulated beams generated with dynamic multileaf collimation, applied to the MM50 racetrack microtron." *Med. Phys.* 27:2701–2707.

Dogan, N., L. B. Leybovich, and A. Sethi. (2002). "Comparative evaluation of Kodak EDR2 and XV2 films for verification of intensity modulated radiation therapy." *Phys. Med. Biol.* 47:4121–4130.

Dogan, N., L. B. Leybovich, A. Sethi, M. Krasin, and B. Emami. (2000). "A modified method of planning and delivery for dynamic multileaf collimator intensity-modulated radiation therapy." *Int. J. Radiat. Oncol. Biol. Phys.* 47:241–245.

Doran, S. J., K. K. Koerkamp, M. A. Bero, P. Jenneson, E. J. Morten, and W. B. Gilboy. (2001). "A CCD-based optical CT scanner for high-resolution 3D imaging of radiation dose distributions: equipment specifications, optical simulations and preliminary results." *Phys. Med. Biol.* 46:3191–3213.

El-Mohri, Y., L. E. Antonuk, J. Yorkston, K. W. Jee, M. Maolinbay, K. L. Lam, and J. H. Siewerdsen. (1999). "Relative dosimetry using active matrix flat-panel imager (AMFPI) technology." *Med. Phys.* 26:1530–1541.

Essers, M., M. de Langen, M. L. Dirkx, and B. J. Heijmen. (2001). "Commissioning of a commercially available system for intensity-modulated radiotherapy dose delivery with dynamic multileaf collimation." *Radiother. Oncol.* 60:215–224.

Esthappan, J., S. Mutic, W. B. Harms, J. F. Dempsey, and D. A Low. (2002). "Dosimetry of therapeutic photon beams using an extended dose range film." *Med. Phys.* 29:2438–2445.

Ezzell, G. A., and S. Chungbin. (2001). "The overshoot phenomenon in step-and-shoot IMRT delivery." *J. Appl. Clin. Med. Phys.* 2:138–148.

Fidanzio, A., L. Azario, R. Miceli, A. Russo, A. Piermattei. (2000). "PTW-diamond detector: Dose rate and particle type dependence." *Med. Phys.* 27:2589–2593.

Fraass, B., K. Doppke, M. Hunt, G. Kutcher, G. Starkschall, R. Stern, and J. Van Dyk. (1998). "American Association of Physicists in Medicine Radiation Therapy Committee Task Group 53: Quality assurance for clinical radiotherapy treatment planning." *Med. Phys.* 25:1773–1829.

Fraass, B. A., M. K. Martel, and D. L. McShan. "Tools for Dose Calculation Verification and QA for Conformal Therapy Treatment Techniques" in *XIth International Conference on the Use of Computers in Radiation Therapy.* A. R. Hounsell, J. M. Wilkinson, and P. C. Williams (eds.). Mar 20-24, 1994. Manchester, UK. Manchester: Christie Hospital NHS Trust, pp. 256–257, 1994.

Francescon, P., S. Cora, C. Cavedon, P. Scalchi, S. Reccanello, and F. Colombo. (1998). "Use of a new type of radiochromic film, a new parallel-plate micro-chamber, MOSFETs, and TLD 800 microcubes in the dosimetry of small beams." *Med. Phys.* 25:503–511.

Galvin, J. M., X. G. Chen, and R. M. Smith. (1993). "Combining multileaf fields to modulate fluence distributions." *Int. J. Radiat. Oncol. Biol. Phys.* 27:697–705.

Galvin, J. M., K. Han, and R. Cohen. (1998). "A comparison of multileaf-collimator and alloy-block field shaping." *Int. J. Radiat. Oncol. Biol. Phys.* 40:721–731.

Galvin, J. M., A. R. Smith, R. D. Moeller, R. L. Goodman, W. D. Powlis, J. Rubenstein, I, J, Solin, B. Michael, M. Needham, C. J. Huntzinger and M. Kligerman. (1992). "Evaluation of multileaf collimator design for a photon beam." *Int. J. Radiat. Oncol. Biol. Phys.* 23:789–801.

Gluckman, G. R., and L. E. Reinstein. (2002). "Comparison of three high-resolution digitizers for radiochromic film dosimetry." *Med. Phys.* 29:1839–1846.

Gore, J. C., M. Ranade, M. J. Maryanski, and R. J. Schulz. (1996). "Radiation dose distributions in three dimensions from tomographic optical density scanning of polymer gels: I. Development of an optical scanner." *Phys. Med. Biol.* 41:2695–2704.

Gotoh, S., M. Ochi, N. Hayashi, S. Matsushima, T. Uchida, S. Obata, K. Minami, K. Hayashi, T. Matsuo, M. Iwanaga, A. Yasunaga, and S. shibata. (1996). "Narrow photon beam dosimetry for linear accelerator radiosurgery." *Radiother. Oncol.* 41:221–224.

Graves, M. N., A. V. Thompson, M. K. Martel, D. L. McShan, and B. A. Fraass. (2001). "Calibration and quality assurance for rounded leaf-end MLC systems." *Med. Phys.* 28:2227–2233.

Gum, F., J. Scherer, L. Bogner, M. Solleder, B. Rhein, and M. Bock. (2002). "Preliminary study on the use of an inhomogeneous anthropomorphic Fricke gel phantom and 3D magnetic resonance dosimetry for verification of IMRT treatment plans." *Phys. Med. Biol.* 47:N67–77.

Halpern, E. J. (1995). "A test pattern for quality control of laser scanner and charge-coupled device film digitizers." *J. Digit. Imaging* 8:3–9.

Hansen, V. N., P. M. Evans, G. J. Budgell, J. H. Mott, P. C. Williams, M. J. Brugmans, F. W. Wittkamper, B. J. Mijnheer, and K. Brown. (1998). "Quality assurance of the dose delivered by small radiation segments." *Phys. Med. Biol.* 43:2665–2675.

Harms, W. B., Sr., D. A. Low, J. W. Wong, and J. A. Purdy. (1998). "A software tool for the quantitative evaluation of 3D dose calculation algorithms." *Med. Phys.* 25:1830–1836.

Haryanto, F., M. Fippel, W. Laub, O. Dohm, and F. Nüsslin. (2002). "Investigation of photon beam output factors for conformal radiation therapy—Monte Carlo simulations and measurements." *Phys. Med. Biol.* 47:N133–143.

Hossain, M., C. J. Houser, and J. M. Galvin. (2002). "Output variation from an intensity modulating dynamic collimator." *Med. Phys.* 29:1693–1697.

Huq, M. S., I. J. Das, T. Steinberg, and J. M. Galvin. (2002). "A dosimetric comparison of various multileaf collimators." *Phys. Med. Biol.* 47:N159–170.

IMRTCWG (Intensity Modulated Radiation Therapy Collaborative Working Group). "Intensity-modulated radiotherapy: Current status and issues of interest." *Int. J. Radiat. Oncol. Biol. Phys.* 51:880–914.

Kapulsky, A., E. Mullokandov, and G. Gejerman. (2002). "An automated phantom-film QA procedure for intensity-modulated radiation therapy." *Med. Dosim.* 27:201–207.

Kelly, B. G., K. J. Jordan, and J. J. Battista. (1998). "Optical CT reconstruction of 3D dose distributions using the ferrous-benzoic-xylenol (FBX) gel dosimeter." *Med. Phys.* 25:1741–1750.

Klein, E. E., W. B. Harms, D. A. Low, V. Willcut, and J. A. Purdy. (1995). "Clinical implementation of a commercial multileaf collimator: Dosimetry, networking, simulation, and quality assurance." *Int. J. Radiat. Oncol. Biol. Phys.* 33:1195–1208.

Kron, T., A. Rosenfeld, M. Lerch, and S. Bazley. (2002). "Measurements in radiotherapy beams using on-line MOSFET detectors." *Radiat. Prot. Dosim.* 101:445–448.

Kung, J. H., and G. T. Chen. (2000). "Intensity modulated radiotherapy dose delivery error from radiation field offset inaccuracy." *Med. Phys.* 27:1617–1622.

Laub, W. U., T. W. Kaulich, and F. Nüsslin. (1999). "A diamond detector in the dosimetry of high-energy electron and photon beams." *Phys. Med. Biol.* 44:2183–2192.

Laub, W., M. Alber, M. Birkner, and F. Nüsslin. (2000). "Monte Carlo dose computation for IMRT optimization." *Phys. Med. Biol.* 45:1741–1754.

Lee, H. R., M. Pankuch, J. C. Chu, and. J. J. Spokas. (2002). "Evaluation and characterization of parallel plate microchamber's functionalities in small beam dosimetry." *Med. Phys.* 29:2489–2496.

Lee, N., C. Chuang, J. M. Quivey, T. L. Phillips, P. Akazawa, L. J. Verhey, and P. Xia. (2002). "Skin toxicity due to intensity-modulated radiotherapy for head-and-neck carcinoma." *Int. J. Radiat. Oncol. Biol. Phys.* 53:630–637.

Leybovich, L. B., N. Dogan, A. Sethi, M. J. Krasin, and B. Emami. (2000). "Improvement of tomographic intensity modulated radiotherapy dose distributions using periodic shifting of arc abutment regions." *Med. Phys.* 27:1610–1616.

Li, J. S., A. L. Boyer, and C.-M. Ma. (2001). "Verification of IMRT dose distributions using a water beam imaging system." *Med. Phys.* 28:2466–2474.

Litzenberg, D. W., J. M. Moran, and B. A. Fraass. (2002). "Incorporation of realistic delivery limitations into dynamic MLC treatment delivery." *Med. Phys.* 29:810–820.

Litzenberg, D. W., J. M. Moran, and B. A. Fraass. (2002). "Verification of dynamic and segmental IMRT delivery by dynamic log file analysis." *J. Appl. Clin. Med. Phys.* 3:63–72.

LoSasso, T., and G. J. Kutcher. (1995). "Multileaf collimation versus alloy blocks: analysis of geometric accuracy." *Int. J. Radiat. Oncol. Biol. Phys.* 32:499–506.

LoSasso T., C.-S. Chui, and C. C. Ling. (1998). "Physical and dosimetric aspects of a multileaf collimation system used in the dynamic mode for implementing intensity modulated radiotherapy." *Med. Phys.* 25:1919–1927.

LoSasso, T., C.-S. Chui, and C. C. Ling. (2001). "Comprehensive quality assurance for the delivery of intensity modulated radiotherapy with a multileaf collimator used in the dynamic mode." *Med. Phys.* 28(11):2209–2219.

Low, D. A., and S. Mutic. (1997). "Abutment region dosimetry for sequential arc IMRT delivery." *Phys. Med. Biol.* 42:1465–1470.

Low, D. A., R. L. Gerber, S. Mutic, and J. A. Purdy. (1998). "Phantoms for IMRT dose distribution measurement and treatment verification." *Int. J. Radiat. Oncol. Biol. Phys.* 40:1231–1235.

Low, D. A., W. B. Harms, S. Mutic, and J. A. Purdy. (1998). "A technique for the quantitative evaluation of dose distributions." *Med. Phys.* 25:656–661.

Low, D.A., S. Mutic, J. F. Dempsey, R. L. Gerber, W. R. Bosch, C. A. Perez, and J. A. Purdy. (1998). "Quantitative dosimetric verification of an IMRT planning and delivery system." *Radiother. Oncol.* 49:305–316.

Low, D. A., J. F. Dempsey, R. Venkatesan, S. Mutic, J. Markman, E. Mark Haacke, and J. A. Purdy. (1999). "Evaluation of polymer gels and MRI as a 3-D dosimeter for intensity-modulated radiation therapy." *Med. Phys.* 26:1542–1551.

Low, D. A., S. Mutic, J. F. Dempsey, J. Markman, S. M. Goddu, and J. A. Purdy. (1999). "Abutment region dosimetry for serial tomotherapy." *Int. J. Radiat. Oncol. Biol. Phys.* 45:193–203.

Low, D. A., J. W. Sohn, E. E. Klein, J. Markman, S. Mutic, and J. F. Dempsey. (2001). "Characterization of a commercial multileaf collimator used for intensity modulated radiation therapy." *Med. Phys.* 28:752–756.

Ma, L., P. B. Geis, and A. L. Boyer. (1997). "Quality assurance for dynamic multileaf collimator modulated fields using a fast beam imaging system." *Med. Phys.* 24:1213–1220.

MacKenzie, M. A., M. Lachaine, B. Murray, B. G. Fallone, D. Robinson, and G. C. Field. (2002). "Dosimetric verification of inverse planned step and shoot multileaf collimator fields from a commercial treatment planning system." *J. Appl. Clin. Med. Phys.* 3:97–109.

Martens, C., C. De Wagter, and W. De Neve. (2000). "The value of the PinPoint ion chamber for characterization of small field segments used in intensity-modulated radiotherapy." *Phys. Med. Biol.* 45:2519–2530.

Martens, C., C. De Wagter, and W. De Neve. (2001). "The value of the LA48 linear ion chamber array for characterization of intensity-modulated beams." *Phys. Med. Biol.* 46:1131–1148.

Martens, C., W. De Gersem, W. De Neve, and C. De Wagter. (2001). "Combining the advantages of step-and-shoot and dynamic delivery of intensity-modulated radiotherapy by interrupted dynamic sequences." *Int. J. Radiat. Oncol. Biol. Phys.* 50:541–550.

McJury, M., M. Oldham, M. O. Leach, and S. Webb. (1999). "Dynamics of polymerization in polyacrylamide gel (PAG) dosimeters: (I) Aging and long-term stability." *Phys. Med. Biol.* 44:1863–1873.

McJury, M., M. Oldham, V. P. Cosgrove, P. S. Murphy, S. Doran, M. O. Leach, and S. Webb. (2000). "Radiation dosimetry using polymer gels: Methods and applications." *Br. J. Radiol.* 73:919–929.

Meeder, R. J., D. A. Jaffray, and P. Munro. (1995). "Tests for evaluating laser film digitizers." *Med. Phys.* 22:635–642.

Moran, J. M., T. S. Nurushev, D. L. Litzenberg, L. Antonuk, Y. El-Moghri, and B. Fraass. (2002). "Commissioning of an A:Si active matrix flat panel dosimeter for IMRT quality assurance." *Med. Phys.* 29:1367.

Niroomand-Rad, A., C. R. Blackwell, B. M. Coursey, K. P. Gall, J. M. Galvin, W. L. McLaughlin, A. S. Meigooni, R. Nath, J. E. Rodgers, and C. G. Soares. (1998). "Radiochromic film dosimetry: Recommendations of AAPM Radiation Therapy Committee Task Group 55. American Association of Physicists in Medicine." *Med. Phys.* 25:2093–2115.

Nurushev, T. S., J. M. Moran, I. Chetty, L. Antonuk, Y. El-Moghri, and B. Fraass. (2001). "Relative dosimetry for DMLC Treatment delivery with An A-Si AMFPI-based dosimetry system." *Med. Phys.* 28:1267.

Olch, A. J. (2002). "Dosimetric performance of an enhanced dose range radiographic film for intensity-modulated radiation therapy quality assurance." *Med. Phys.* 29:2159–2168.

Oldham, M., I. Baustert, C. Lord, T. A. Smith, M. McJury, A. P. Warrington, M. O. Leach, and S. Webb. (1998). "An investigation into the dosimetry of a nine-field tomotherapy irradiation using BANG-gel dosimetry." *Phys. Med. Biol.* 43:1113–1132.

Oldham, M., J. H. Siewerdsen, A. Shetty, and D. A. Jaffray. (2001). "High resolution gel-dosimetry by optical-CT and MR scanning." *Med. Phys.* 28:1436–1445.

Paliwal, B., W. Tomé, S. Richardson, and T. R. Mackie. (2000). "A spiral phantom for IMRT and tomotherapy treatment delivery verification." *Med. Phys.* 27:2503–2507.

     **Jean M. Moran**

Palta, J. R., D. K. Yeung, and V. Frouhar. (1996). "Dosimetric considerations for a multileaf collimator system." *Med. Phys.* 23:1219–1224.

Papatheodorou, S., J. C. Rosenwald, S. Zefkili, M. C. Murillo, J. Drouard, and G. Gaboriaud. (2000). "Dose calculation and verification of intensity modulation generated by dynamic multileaf collimators." *Med. Phys.* 27:960–971.

Partridge, M., M. Ebert, and B. M. Hesse. (2002). "IMRT verification by three-dimensional dose reconstruction from portal beam measurements." *Med. Phys.* 29:1847–1858.

Partridge, M., P. M. Evans, A. Mosleh-Shirazi, and D. Convery. (1998). "Independent verification using portal imaging of intensity-modulated beam delivery by the dynamic MLC technique." *Med. Phys.* 25:1872–1879.

Partridge, M., J. R. Symonds-Tayler, and P. M. Evans. (2000). "IMRT verification with a camera-based electronic portal imaging system." *Phys. Med. Biol.* 45:N183–196.

Rustgi, S. N. (1995). "Evaluation of the dosimetric characteristics of a diamond detector for photon beam measurements." *Med. Phys.* 22:567–570.

Saw, C. B., K. M. Ayyangar, R. B. Thompson, W. Zhen, and C. A. Enke. (2001). "Commissioning of Peacock System for intensity-modulated radiation therapy." *Med. Dosim.* 26:55–64.

Sharpe, M. B., B. M. Miller, D. Yan, and J. W. Wong. (2000). "Monitor unit settings for intensity modulated beams delivered using a step-and-shoot approach." *Med. Phys.* 27:2719–2725.

Sidhu, N. P. (1999). "Interfacing a linear diode array to a conventional water scanner for the measurement of dynamic dose distributions and comparison with a linear ion chamber array." *Med. Dosim.* 24:57–60.

Stern, R. L., B. A. Fraass, A. Gerhardsson, D. L. McShan, and K. L. Lam. (1992). "Generation and use of measurement-based 3-D dose distributions for 3-D dose calculation verification." *Med. Phys.* 19:165–173.

Sykes, J. R., and P. C. Williams. (1998). "An experimental investigation of the tongue and groove effect for the Philips multileaf collimator." *Phys. Med. Biol.* 43(10):3157–3165.

Tello, V. M., R. C. Tailor, and W. F. Hanson. (1995). "How water equivalent are water-equivalent solid materials for output calibration of photon and electron beams?" *Med. Phys.* 22:1177–1189.

Teslow, T. N. (1997). "The laser film digitizer: density, contrast, and resolution." *J. Digit. Imaging* 10:128–132.

Tsai, J. S., M. J. Rivard, and M. J. Engler. (2000). "Dependence of linac output on the switch rate of an intensity-modulated tomotherapy collimator." *Med. Phys.* 27:2215–2225.

Tsai, J. S., D. E. Wazer, M. N. Ling, J. K. Wu, M. Fagundes, T. DiPetrillo, B. Kramer, M. Koistinen, and M. J. Engler. (1998). "Dosimetric verification of the dynamic intensity-modulated radiation therapy of 92 patients." *Int. J. Radiat. Oncol. Biol. Phys.* 40:1213–1230.

Van Esch, A., J. Bohsung, P. Sorvari, M. Tenhunun, M. Fagundes, T. DiPetrillo, B. Kramer, M. Koistinen, and M. J. Engler. (2002). "Acceptance tests and quality control (QC) procedures for the clinical implementation of intensity modulated radiotherapy (IMRT) using inverse planning and the sliding window technique: experience from five radiotherapy departments." *Radiother. Oncol.* 65:53–70.

Verellen, D., N. Linthout, D. van den Berge, A. Bel, and G. Storme. (1997). "Initial experience with intensity-modulated conformal radiation therapy for treatment of the head and neck region." *Int. J. Radiat. Oncol. Biol. Phys.* 39:99–114.

Verhey, L. J. "Commissioning and Quality Assurance of Siemens IMRT System" in *3-D Conformal and Intensity Modulated Radiation Therapy: Physics & Clinical Applications*. J. A. Purdy, W. H. Grant, J. R. Palta et al. (eds.). Madison, WI: Advanced Medical Publishing, pp. 305–310, 2001.

Wong, J. W., M. Sharpe, D. Yan. "Commissioning and Quality Assurance of Elekta IMRT System" in *3-D Conformal and Intensity Modulated Radiation Therapy: Physics & Clinical Applications*. J. A. Purdy, W. H. Grant, J. R. Palta et al. (eds.). Madison, WI: Advanced Medical Publishing, pp. 325–331, 2001.

Wu, Q., M. Arnfield, S. Tong, Y. Wu, and R. Mohan. (2000). "Dynamic splitting of large intensity-modulated fields." *Phys. Med. Biol.* 45:1731–1740.

Xia, P., and L. J. Verhey. (2001). "Delivery systems of intensity-modulated radiotherapy using conventional multileaf collimators." *Med. Dosim.* 26:169–177.

Xia, P., A. B. Hwang, and L. J. Verhey. (2002). "A leaf sequencing algorithm to enlarge treatment field length in IMRT." *Med. Phys.* 29:991–998.

Xing, L., B. Curran, R. Hill, T. Holmes, L. Ma, K. M. Forster, and A. L. Boyer. (1999). "Dosimetric verification of a commercial inverse treatment planning system." *Phys. Med. Biol.* 44:463–478.

Zhu, X. R., P. A. Jursinic, D. F. Grimm, F. Lopez, J. J. Rownd, and M. T. Gillin. (2002). "Evaluation of Kodak EDR2 film for dose verification of intensity modulated radiation therapy delivered by a static multileaf collimator." *Med. Phys.* 29:1687–1692.

Zygmanski, P., and J. H. Kung. (2001). "Method of identifying dynamic multileaf collimator irradiation that is highly sensitive to a systematic MLC calibration error." *Med. Phys.* 28:2220–2226.

# Intensity-Modulated Radiation Therapy: The Good, The Bad, And The Misconceptions

**James M. Galvin, D.Sc.**
Thomas Jefferson University Hospital
Jefferson Medical College
Philadelphia, PA



## Background

*IMRT has existed in various forms for decades.* This statement is not meant to include the common use of wedges to modify intensity to obtain homogeneous dose distributions when beam orientations are not geometrically balanced, or when wedges are used to compensate for missing tissue. The use of wedges to modulate beams is not usually categorized as intensity-modulated treatment. A less frequently encountered treatment technique, that is a more appropriate precursor of IMRT, has been used by some centers for many years. This is the insertion of partial transmission blocks into otherwise open fields for the purpose of shaping dose distributions. A typical example is the use of blocking over the spinal cord to bend isodose lines around this important critical structure and reduce the dose it receives relative to target tissues. Another example is the technique of treating *ethmoid* sinus tumors that push between the eyes by either partially or fully blocking these critical structures for both lateral fields and a single anterior field. This partial irradiation of the target for different field directions is a fairly common planning approach that bends the isodose lines around the eyes while treating a target that surrounds and pushes against them.

It is interesting that the early evolution of our current form of inverse planning for IMRT did not start with such simple intuitive approaches. Instead, beamlet-based inverse planning (Censor, Powlis, and Altschuler 1987) (see also the chapter by Yair Censor in this book, ***Mathematical Optimization For The Inverse Problem Of Intensity-Modulated Radiation Therapy***) generalized the problem and did not attempt to work with each gantry angle individually. That is, beamlet-based inverse planning separates the problem into many hundreds or even thousands of small beamlets during the optimization, and works with the entire set as the process proceeds. In taking this approach, the intuitive nature of the solution can be lost as the optimization shifts beamlet weights from one gantry angle to the next as it drives toward a solution. A limitation of beamlet-based inverse planning is that it introduces many unnecessary complications that can be avoided if a more intuitive inverse planning approach is taken.

It is possible to build an inverse treatment planning technique on the idea of placing partial transmission blocks, or by using a multileaf collimator (MLC) equivalent for these blocks, over structures that are to receive a reduced dose relative to target structures. This inverse planning approach is interesting because it shows that current IMRT efficiency in terms of patient total body dose, multileaf wear and tear, and overall quality assurance (QA) burden can easily be improved. This issue is discussed in the chapter in this book that describes aperture-based or contour-based inverse planning (see ***Aperture-Based Inverse Planning*** by Shepard and Yu et al.).

## Indications For IMRT

IMRT is labor intensive relative to three-dimensional conformal radiation therapy (3DCRT). There are a number of contributing factors that make this the case, but one major reason is the increased workload involved with verifying IMRT treatments. Port filming for 3DCRT gives the clinician a fairly easily interpreted visual representation of what is being treated with the different radiation beams that make up the treatment plan. It is possible to verify the isocenter position for IMRT, but techniques that are much more complex than simple port filming must be used to guarantee that correct beam apertures are applied or that the dynamic sweep of an MLC is correct. For this reason, at least at this stage in the evolution of this new technology, it is not wise to use IMRT when it is not needed. Doing so can lead to errors that are easily avoided by employing simpler treatment methods. This section outlines the indications for using intensity-modulated treatment so that decisions to shift from 3DCRT to IMRT can be based on clear dosimetric advantages.

There are four major advantages or indications for IMRT relative to 3DCRT. First, as illustrated with the two simple examples above, modulated beams can be used to produce invaginations in otherwise convex dose clouds. This feature can be used to protect critical structures that push against and cause concavities in the surface of a clinical target volume (CTV) and that overlap with the corresponding planning target volume (PTV). This ability to protect invaginating critical structures is the major feature of IMRT that cannot be duplicated with 3DCRT techniques. Second, in situations where the location of a target or combination of targets relative to nearby critical structures requires a complex arrangement of non-coplanar beams, inverse planning techniques coupled with intensity-modulated dose delivery can be used to obtain an acceptably homogeneous dose distribution. This second application can prove helpful when the beam geometry is so complex that it is not easy to select, orient, and weight standard fields that may or may not use conventional wedges. The third indication for IMRT is somewhat related to the second advantage. In situations where the geometry of missing tissue makes it difficult to apply standard wedges to compensate for thickness deficits, inverse planning and intensity-modulated dose delivery can solve an otherwise difficult planning problem with significantly reduced effort on the part of the dosimetrist.

The fourth indication for IMRT is easily misunderstood. It is often stated that IMRT can produce more compact isodose lines than 3DCRT. It is better to say that IMRT can be used to control the positioning of sharp dose gradients within a dose distribution. For example, if a target touches a critical structure, IMRT can place a sharp dose gradient just at the point of contact of these two regions.

Figure 1 illustrates this point. This figure shows a gray target abutting a black critical structure. As shown in the figure, it is possible to use a simple parallel-opposed beam arrangement to obtain a rapid dose fall-off at the position of the shared boundary where the critical structure touches the target. This simple field arrangement will best accomplish the task of protecting the critical structure as long as dose to the regions falling within the path of the opposed beams can receive a dose that is the same as or somewhat higher than the dose delivered to the target. If this is not the case, more field directions must be added. The end result is that the parallel opposed beam dose gradient in the region where the target and critical structure touch will decrease to some degree. Adding more and more field directions will decrease the sharpness of the dose gradient still further while increasing the overall dose conformality around the target. The task of finding the weights of the fields that give the best possible conformality consistent with the sharpest possible dose gradient at the position where the critical structure pushes against the target quickly becomes unmanageable as more beam directions are added, and the process of developing an acceptable dose distribution requires the use of inverse planning to move the dose gradient into position while sparing the critical structure shown in the figure as well as any other dose limiting structures in the region. Thus, inverse planning and IMRT are useful in moving tight dose gradients to the exact position where they are needed.

Only the first feature of IMRT discussed above is truly unique relative to 3DCRT. However, the ability of inverse planning and intensity-modulated dose delivery to handle complex treatment planning problems (e.g., non-coplanar field arrangements, highly irregular contour changes at beam entry surfaces, or manipulation of sharp dose gradients) represents an important advancement and enhances the well-documented advantages of traditional 3DCRT (Smith and Purdy 1991).

The improved treatment automation that has accompanied the introduction of IMRT also represents a significant change in the way radiation is delivered and has generally led to more conformal dose distributions. However, this change has also resulted in considerable confusion when comparing modulated beam treatment to 3DCRT, and is not listed here as one of the advantages or indications for IMRT. It is now standard practice to carry out IMRT treatments with a single button push that avoids any reentry of the treatment room until the process is complete. The automation includes not only MLC leaf movement, but also gantry and collimator rotation, couch longitudinal position changes, and couch rotation. This complete automation of the process means that it is easy to increase the number of beam orientations used to create a treatment plan. This change alone accounts for much of the improvement in dose conformality seen for IMRT, but it is important to point out that similar improvements are possible as more field directions are added for standard 3DCRT. Thus, this feature is an indication for IMRT only when this level of automation is restricted to that treatment modality. This could be the case when a tertiary binary collimator is added to a standard linear accelerator and automated field shaping coupled with gantry rotation is only available for the IMRT treatment mode.

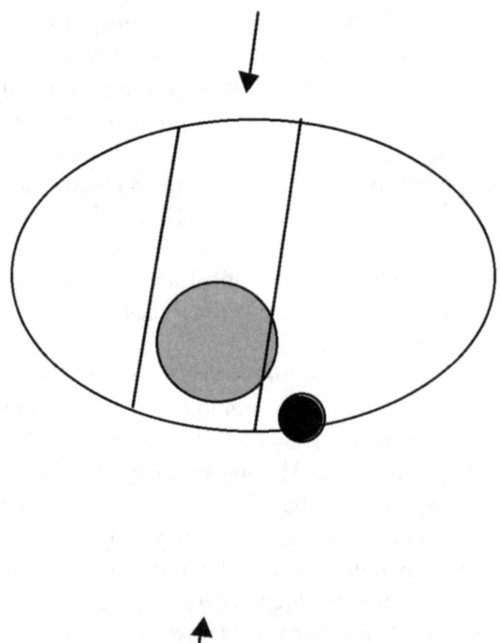

**Figure 1.** Depiction of using IMRT to control positioning of sharp dose gradients within a dose distribution.

In summary, although the introduction of inverse planning techniques and intensity modulated dose delivery has dramatically changed the character of the dose distributions now obtainable for radiation treatment, the major indication for using this technology instead of 3DCRT should be situations where a target pushes into or invaginates a target.

## Potential Problems With IMRT

### Is It Ever Possible To Obtain An Optimum Treatment Plan?

There is a common misconception that inverse treatment planning will automatically generate an optimum dose distribution, and that IMRT plans must be better than standard 3DCRT plans. For a number of reasons, optimum dose distributions can never be achieved. Also, plans that are grossly inferior to traditional plans are often returned by inverse planning systems.

It must be remembered that any inverse planning solution is dependent on the dose constraints and objective functions specified by the user. Thus, although a mathematically optimum solution might be obtained, the quality of the result depends on the physician's specification of dose constraints and the treatment planner's understanding of how these parameters might be used to obtain the desired result. Inverse planning in its current form requires a clear definition of the problem and does not include a mechanism for dynamically ensuring that the best plan has been obtained.

### What Steps Can Be Taken To Find An Acceptable Inverse Treatment Plan?

At least in the early stages of starting a new IMRT program and as each new disease site is approached, the user should gain experience through a laborious process of iteratively generating and comparing alternative plans. This simple approach is a major safeguard against unknowingly accepting poor results. In addition, there are currently available many excellent training courses like the one documented in this book that provide important information on the implementation of an IMRT program. The best of these include strong physics and clinical components, and provide a mechanism for hands-on treatment planning activities. The clinical component should be conducted by clinicians who have extensive experience using IMRT for the specific disease sites being considered for treatment with a new IMRT program. It is also recommended that training for IMRT be undertaken as a team approach where dosimetrists, physicists, and physicians from the same institution attend as a group.

Another important method for guarding against accepting inferior IMRT treatment plans uses past experience, as determined through examination of the plans previously generated at a particular institution, to develop the dose constraints used for the inverse planning. This approach assures that the IMRT plans are at least as good as traditional plans. An extension of this approach is to use the information available in cooperative group IMRT protocols whenever possible to guarantee that a final plan is near optimal relative to the experience of the individuals who wrote the study protocol.

Examples are the oropharynx and nasopharynx protocols developed by the Radiation Therapy Oncology Group (RTOG) (see www.rtog.org). It should be remembered that such protocols can usually be downloaded from cooperative group websites used as a template without being a part of the protocol group. However, working within a multi-institution cooperative group is highly recommended.

There is now a great deal of information available describing the use of IMRT to treat both the prostate and head and neck tumors. Careful study of such publications allows the extraction of data that can be used for dose constraints and the gaining of an appreciation for the dose-volume histograms (DVHs) that might be obtained. A literature review should be considered as a minimum requirement for starting an IMRT program.

Inferior IMRT treatment plans can often be detected by carefully examining the entire dose distribution instead of relying on DVHs and dose statistics to judge an inverse plan. For 3DCRT, the treatment plans for a particular disease site do not show a lot of variation because the treatment planner usually solves the problem in the exact same way for each patient. In many ways, these plans are well behaved and examining DVHs and dose statistics is a fast way for determining that a dose distribution is acceptable. Inverse plans can be dramatically different from 3DCRT plans or more standard plans. Even for the same treatment site, the exact target geometry can vary and dose distributions for an IMRT plan can differ widely as a result. It is essential for new users of inverse planning systems to develop a full appreciation for the character of inverse plans for a particular disease site or target geometry. This is best accomplished through careful examination of the treatment plans without relying on shortcut methods. As experience is gained, the clinician might decide to modify this approach, but it is strongly recommended that this not be done in the early stages of a new IMRT program.

## The Tendency Toward Target Underdose When Using IMRT

IMRT offers the possibility of moving and bending isodose lines to achieve improved critical structure sparing relative to 3DCRT. It can be argued that this new feature makes it very tempting to decrease target margins without modifying any other aspects (e.g., immobilization) of the patient's previous treatment, or to thread isodose lines between a target and critical structure when there is no space between them. Without introducing improvements in either patient positioning and target localization, this temptation should be resisted.

The technology surrounding IMRT is changing rapidly. Image-guided techniques are now in common use for defining the target position for IMRT, and PTV margins for some target locations are decreasing. However, unless one is able to duplicate the techniques used for image-guided target localization as described in the peer reviewed literature, it is unwise to decrease margins to the extend reported in these studies.

Another problem is the increased dose inhomogeneity encountered with IMRT (see discussion below). This difference for inverse plans compared to 3DCRT plans has led to the practice of allowing a small underdose for IMRT. It is now typical to prescribe IMRT plans to achieve coverage of 95% of the planning target volume.

## Approximations Introduced In The IMRT Process

Another reason why inverse treatment plans are never optimum is that many approximations must be made to move from a calculated intensity map to the step of dose delivery. For example, beamlet-based inverse planning involves such a large number of individual fields (beamlets) that it is hard, given current available technology, to carry out the inverse planning with dose calculation algorithms that fully and accurately account for scattered radiation. A common method for handling this problem is to use a fast but crude algorithm to initially derive an intensity map. This intensity distribution is then translated to a more manageable number of field apertures (Galvin et al. 1993). As a follow-up step to improve the quality of the final result, these apertures can be combined with a more precise calculation algorithm and the dose distribution recalculated. This step can also use an additional "weight" optimization to help meet desired dose constraints. However, the complicated nature of this process can make the desired result hard to reach without numerous attempts at re-optimization that might not prove to be successful.

## The Inevitable Trade-Offs Of IMRT

## Character Of Intensity Maps

It is possible to control the smoothness of intensity maps in various ways, and some investigators have built this process into the optimization itself (Spirou et al. 2001). The motivation for doing this is that busy intensity patterns with many internal low intensity regions abutting high intensity regions can require excessive monitor units (MUs), force an unnecessarily high number of field segments for a step-and-shoot approach, or produce gross approximations when dynamic MLC delivery is used.

Intuitive intensity patterns are also desirable in that they can decrease the QA burden otherwise required. As mentioned previously, there is a long tradition in radiation oncology for visual verification of the fields used to treat the patient. The use of "portal imaging" accomplishes two things. First, these images check the position of the isocenter for the different fields. Second, they are used to verify the shape and orientation of the field aperture at each gantry angle. Although various techniques have been devised to verify IMRT treatment, none currently duplicate the simplicity or relatively unambiguousness of standard portal imaging.

The problem with treatment verification of IMRT is that the intensity patterns can sometimes appear random and may not be easily recognizable as conforming to known patient anatomy. That is, even when fields appear to conform to a target or combination of targets, there is no protection against having the beamlets along the aperture edge turned off so that the beam is not truly conformal. This difficulty leads to a requirement that additional labor-intensive QA steps must be taken to guarantee correct dose delivery.

Smoothing intensity patterns can compromise the quality of the final treatment plan. For this reason, the relationship between behavior in terms of the overall number of extrema for the intensity patterns and the quality of the treatment plan should be determined for different disease sites when an IMRT treatment planning system is being commissioned for first use. Also, when considering purchase of an inverse planning system, the tendency for a particular IMRT system to produce busy intensity patterns should be considered as a negative when dose delivery and monitor unit efficiency are compromised as a result.

## Monitor Unit Efficiency Of IMRT

One of the earliest reports on IMRT (Galvin et al. 1993) recognized the inherent problem of low monitor unit efficiency for inverse planning and intensity modulated dose delivery. Increases on the order of a factor of 3 were projected in this early paper. This increase in MUs is related to both the inefficiency of modeling busy intensity patterns containing numerous extrema, and to the splitting of fields to create concavities in otherwise convex dose clouds. As mentioned above, it is possible to improve monitor unit efficiency by using inverse algorithms that create a smoother intensity distribution. Aperture-based or contour-based inverse planning accomplishes this by restricting the number of apertures considered in the optimization process. However, it is important to point out that there is a limit to how smooth an intensity map can be in that creating concavities in a dose distribution requires the use of split segments that tend to increase monitor units. This increase in monitor units is often unavoidable when the desired result is the bending of an isodose line around a critical structure and a standard MLC must be used to accomplish beam modulation. Unlike the insertion of a physical compensator or a partial transmission block, using an MLC can require the splitting of fields when creating a concavity in a dose cloud.

The increase in MUs for IMRT is a direct result of partial treatment of the target volume. That is, compared to conformal treatment where the entire target is encompassed in each field, IMRT often splits fields to protect critical structures. This also happens when the collimator has limited reach and cannot cover the entire target. The best example here is tomotherapy. The binary collimator used for this dose delivery method is restricted to two banks of moving leaves. Typically, each leaf-bank covers a 1.0 cm cross section of anatomy as the gantry rotates. This means that the target plus margin must be treated with abutting modulated fields of 2.0 cm width. Thus, in general, for a target that extends 10 cm including a margin, five gantry rotations are required. This results in an increase in MUs that is higher by a factor of approximately 5 compared to a step-and-shoot method. Of course, if the standard MLC used for step-and-shoot delivery is not able to reach all parts of a large target, the difference in MUs will not be this great because some delivery efficiency will be wasted in splitting fields to extend the reach of the MLC.

This loss in monitor unit efficiency for tomotherapy is handled by increasing the thickness of the MLC to compensate for the extra MUs and/or by removing the flattening filter to decrease any wasting of photons. However, especially for add-on binary collimator systems, it is the responsibility of the user to guarantee that placing extra shielding effectively subtends the beam for all parts of the patient's body. This is particularly important when monitor units that are as much as a factor of 10 higher than traditional values are used for IMRT. When a new IMRT program is started, it is helpful to compare the IMRT monitor units to the monitor units that would have been used traditionally as an easy but crude estimate of the potential increase in the patient's total body dose.

## Increase In The Number Of Field Segments

The modern design of the multileaf collimator as it appeared on both Varian and Elekta (previously Philips) equipment in the early 1990's did not consider IMRT, but was instead aimed at simple block replacement. Relative to 3DCRT, IMRT techniques can significantly increase the number of different field shapes used for each patient. It is not uncommon to have on the order of 50 to 150 field changes per patient treated. If an accelerator treats just 20 patients per day, this translates to about 2,000 field changes per day. This number far exceeds the design limits for any MLC, and can lead to excess MLC wear and tear. Additionally, treatment times can be excessive when using step-and-shoot delivery techniques for complex target arrangements with invaginating critical structures. Adopting a dynamic MLC dose delivery technique can minimize the treatment time problem, but this change is made at the expense of an increased QA burden.

## Dose Heterogeneity

The point was made in a previous section that a major advantage associated with IMRT is the ability to bend isodose lines around critical structures that are near or push into a target or combination of targets. Bending isodose lines in a 2-D projection or creating an indent in a 3-D dose cloud is accomplished by casting a shadow over the regions needing protection and then spreading the effect of this shadow by employing numerous beam directions. A trade-off for this approach is that the different shadows spread through the surrounding regions to produce dose heterogeneity that exceeds that seen for standard 3DCRT techniques.

The typical increased dose variation for IMRT that occurs across the target has lead to changes in the way dose is prescribed for this treatment modality. It is common practice when using IMRT (see the RTOG IMRT protocols for oropharynx and nasopharynx at www.rtog.org) to write a prescription so that the intended dose covers 95% of the volume of the target instead of the 100% coverage used previously. That is, underdose to 5% of the volume of the target is allowed. For the RTOG protocols, additional dose limits are used to control the amount of underdose. This limit is established by not allowing more than 1% of the volume to receive a dose that is less than 93% of the prescribed dose value. Dose limits are also placed on any overdose within the target.

## Conclusions

There is little doubt that the introduction of inverse treatment planning and intensity-modulated dose delivery has dramatically changed our ability to control dose distributions for radiation therapy. However, like any other technological advancement, there are the unavoidable trade-offs, compromises, and even hazards that must be understood to guard against a negative impact instead of the widely anticipated and already partially proven positive advantages. New users should not approach IMRT casually. This technology turns a great deal of the decision-making for radiation therapy treatment planning over to a computer. This is both good and bad. It is good in that much more difficult problems that might have gone untreated or been treated with less than desirable plans in the past can now be dealt with more effectively. The drawback is that IMRT systems are not yet completely automated, and poorly defining a particular treatment planning problem will produce inferior and potentially hazardous results. The problem is made more difficult by the fact that particular IMRT treatment planning systems might not be completely optimized to minimize factors like leakage radiation reaching the patient. The most effective way out of this quandary is study of the peer-reviewed literature, attending training courses that included a strong clinical component, and hands-on investigation of the characteristics of the particular treatment planning system available.

## References

Censor, Y., W. D. Powlis, and M. D. Altschuler. "On the Fully Discretized Model for the Inverse Problem of Radiation Therapy Treatment Planning" in *Proceedings of the 13th Annual Northeast Bioengineering Conference.* Vol 1. K.R. Foster (Ed.). New York: IEEE Press, pp. 211–214, 1987.

Galvin, J. M., X.-G.Chen, and R. M. Smith. (1993). "Combining multileaf fields to modulate fluence distributions. *J. Radiat. Oncol. Biol. Phys.* 27:697–705.

Radiation Therapy Oncology Group (RTOG). www.rtog.org.

Smith, A. R., and J. A. Purdy (Eds.). No authors listed. (1991). "Three-dimensional photon treatment planning." Report of the Collaborative Working Group on the Evaluation of Treatment Planning for External Photon Beam Radiotherapy. *Int. J. Radiat. Oncol. Biol. Phys.* 21(1):1–265.

Spirou, S. V., N. Fournier-Bidoz, Y. Jie, C.-S. Chui, and C. C. Ling. (2001). "Smoothing intensity-modulated beam profiles to improve the efficiency of delivery." *Med. Phys.* 28:2105–2112.

# Commissioning And Quality Assurance For IMRT Treatment Planning


**Michael B. Sharpe, Ph.D., DABMP**
Department of Radiation Oncology,
Princess Margaret Hospital and University of Toronto
Toronto, Ontario, Canada




## Introduction

Modern radiotherapy is driven by the need to target diseased tissue accurately while controlling normal tissue complications. Intensity-modulated radiation therapy (IMRT) tailors radiation delivery by deriving non-uniform beam intensity patterns with numerical optimization methods and delivering these patterns with a limited number of fixed beams, arc-based tomotherapy techniques, or other novel approaches (Bortfeld et al. 1994; Brahme 1999; Brahme, Roos, and Lax 1982; Carol et al. 1996; Convery and Rosenbloom 1992; Galvin, Chen, and Smith 1993; Mackie et al. 1999; Oelfke and Bortfeld 2001; Powlis et al. 1989; Siochi 1999; Spirou and Chui 1994; Stein et al. 1994; Webb 1999, 2001; Wu et al. 2001; Yu 1995; Yu et al. 1995). In tandem with advances in medical imaging, this promising but complex treatment modality is positioned to reduce normal tissue toxicity substantially, and in turn, to generate new clinical opportunities that broadly challenge the classical concepts of radiotherapy practice (Leibel et al. 2002; Ling et al. 2000; Macklis, Weinhous, and Harnisch 2000).

Systematic commissioning and quality assurance (QA) are integral to the implementation of the technologies used in radiation oncology (Kutcher et al. 1994; Thwaites et al. 1995). Vigilant QA procedures have had a measurable impact on the magnitude and frequency of serious errors, and their importance is reinforced by the consequences of a small number of major incidents occurring over the last decade (Cosset 2002; Macklis, Meier, and Weinhous 1998). In addition to minimizing error rates, several publications have also emphasized the need to optimize the accuracy and precision of dosimetry and geometry to maximize the effectiveness of therapy (Brahme 1984; Cunningham 1982; Dutreix 1987; ICRU 1976; Mijnheer, Batterman, and Wambersie 1987). Van Dyk and Purdy have published an excellent review of the need for accuracy and precision in radiotherapy, the principles of internationally recognized quality systems, as well as a broad perspective on the cycles of technology development and integration in medicine (Van Dyk 1999; Van Dyk and Purdy 1999).

## Unique Aspects Of An IMRT Treatment Planning System

Computer-based treatment planning systems with IMRT capability are the central element for supporting medical decisions, and for the optimization and technical implementation of the radiotherapy prescription. From a clinical perspective, IMRT represents a radical change in practice because it provides a unique power to manipulate dose gradients, and because it requires adherence to detailed quantitative treatment objectives. Furthermore, the high-dose gradients and associated collimator movement during treatment delivery emphasize the need to control and determine treatment margins through objective measurement of setup uncertainties' internal organ motion (Keall et al. 2001a; Ten Haken et al. 1997; van Herk, Remeijer, and Lebesque 2002; Yan et al. 2001; Yan and Lockman 2001). The increased leakage radiation from higher number of treatment monitor units also gives cause to revisit the risks of secondary cancers and occupational exposure (Followill, Geis, and Boyer 1997; Mutic et al. 2001; Mutic and Low 1998). To maximize the anticipated benefit of IMRT, all aspects of the radiotherapy process should be re-examined under more stringent requirements for accuracy and precision (IMRTCWG 2001). From a technology perspective, however, IMRT can be viewed as a natural evolution of three-dimensional conformal radiation therapy (3DCRT) because it stands incrementally on the foundations of volumetric imaging technologies [e.g., computed tomography (CT), magnetic resonance (MR), positron emission therapy (PET)], advanced dose calculation algorithms, utilizing tools that aid in visualization and segmentation of tissue volumes, and the evaluation of treatment plans (IMRTCWG 2001; Verhey 2002).

## Quality Assurance In IMRT Treatment Planning

IMRT is a nascent technology and no specific consensus has emerged regarding the most effective commissioning and QA practices. General practice guidelines have been or will soon be issued by the National Cancer Institute (NCI), American Association of Physicists in Medicine (AAPM), and American Society for Therapeutic Radiology and Oncology (ASTRO). Due to the inherent complexities, diversity of implementation, and interdependence of IMRT planning and delivery technologies, it will still be some time before definitive procedures are recommended. For these reasons, these interim guidance documents have recommended a *patient-specific* approach to verification and QA.

Patient-specific QA captures the integrated results of image acquisition, image segmentation, planning, agreement with the dose prescription, as well as the geometric and dosimetric calibration of the treatment planning and delivery systems. This approach validates the performance of the combined systems by performing a series of measurements at the final stages of the planning process and is aimed at identifying problems in the overall procedure. Patient-specific QA procedures are currently labor intensive, but do not preclude the need for more extensive testing of the individual key technologies that make IMRT possible. Detailed commissioning and QA of the individual components and algorithms lead to a deeper understanding and a greater capacity to respond to the problems detected with procedures that verify the cumulative results of the combined system.

## Scope And Goals Of Chapter

This chapter summarizes the current state of procedures for commissioning and QA of treatment planning systems in general, and reviews the current thinking on potential extensions for IMRT treatment planning systems. The goal is to highlight how IMRT changes the process of commissioning and validating the performance of a treatment planning system.

## Acceptance And Commissioning Guidelines

To a large extent, the tasks and concerns surrounding the clinical implementation of a system capable of generating IMRT treatment plans are the same as those encountered when implementing 3DCRT. All treatment planning systems, for example, have the same basic requirements for the collection and proper association of patient demographics with images, contours, modeling of treatment geometry, dose distributions, and other data imported or generated by the system. Preparing an IMRT treatment planning system for clinical use involves:

1. Initial acceptance of hardware and software.

2. Measurement and entry of basic dosimetric data.

3. Collection and entry of machine geometry data and other operational parameters (e.g., wedge angle and orientation, leaf travel constraints, etc.).

4.  Tuning of algorithm parameters to achieve the best performance over the range of anticipated clinical situations.

5.  Verification of the dose algorithms and associated configuration parameters.

6.  Configuration of import interfaces to external imaging systems.

7.  Verification of image quality and geometric fidelity following data transfer from all sources of image data.

8.  Configuration of export interfaces to treatment machines.

9.  Learning how to interact with the system and apply it to clinical cases.

Following the receipt and basic installation, it is important to verify that the hardware and software meet or exceed the tendered specifications. Once the features of the system are confirmed, the task of preparing the system for clinical use can proceed. Dose calculations are a central component of a much broader treatment planning process, and a significant amount of effort is required to configure and validate the dosimetric components of a planning system. The planning computer has also evolved into the central system in an extended network of devices for image acquisition, visualization, and for accumulating the technical aspects required to implement the medical prescription. There are also a host of geometric and other non-dosimetric parameters to configure and validate, including network connectivity with external sources of imaging and contouring data. The function of network interfaces for exporting electronic plans, dose distributions, and derived images such as digitally reconstructed radiographs (DRRs) must also be configured and verified prior to clinical use (Born et al. 1999; Craig, Brochu, and Van Dyk 1999; Fraass et al. 1998; Shaw 1996; Van Dyk et al. 1993). At the same time, it is important to verify that the purchased dose algorithms perform in a manner consistent with the stated specifications and the published literature.

The inverse planning system is a complex configuration of hardware components, algorithms, and procedures involving personnel with diverse training. The quality achieved during clinical use will depend on the quality of the data used to configure the system, and on the user's ability to discover dose or biological constraints, treatment geometry, and other parameters that adequately guide the optimization process. Training and experience are an essential element of the commissioning process. The experience of learning to interact with an IMRT treatment planning system to achieve quality treatment plans is discussed in detail in other chapters.


## Establishing Acceptance And Commissioning Criteria

Commissioning of a treatment planning system requires measurement and entry of institution-specific dosimetric data, geometric parameters describing the treatment machines, and other non-dosimetric information. Published experience suggests that IMRT imposes more stringent requirements on the accuracy of data collected for beam modelling, including beam penumbra measurements and small-field output factors (Cadman et al. 2002; Van Esch et al. 2002). It is important to review techniques and detectors for making accurate measurements of the beam penumbra. Once the basic data requirements have been fulfilled, the model and data entered by the user must be verified against independent measurements and tests. Task Group 53 of the AAPM has produced a widely cited report to guide the commissioning and QA of 3DCRT planning systems (Fraass et al. 1998). Reports from other agencies have recommended similar procedures for the commissioning and QA of 3DCRT treatment planning systems (Born et al. 1999; Mayles et al. 1998; Shaw 1996). Much of what is contained in these reports can be applied directly to IMRT systems.

The definition of acceptance criteria is an important aspect of determining the scope, time, and resources required to complete the acceptance and commissioning process, and the subsequent tolerances established for QA activities. Configuration of geometric and other non-dosimetric parameters are typically evaluated by a functional pass-fail criteria. For example, by comparing to true machine movements and motion limits, the geometric accuracy of the machine model can be verified.

Validation of dosimetry models typically involves comparing samples of calculated dose distributions with measurements under a variety of conditions. For a 3DCRT system, this process typically begins with verification of single fields over a range of field sizes and depths, as well as simple blocking arrangements in simple geometric phantoms. The verification process progresses systematically to test beam modifiers, corrections for variations for patient surface contour, tissue heterogeneity corrections, and more complex multifield geometries in anthropomorphic phantoms. Based on the work of Van Dyk et al. (1993) Task Group 53 has recommended a combination of dose difference and distance to agreement criteria for the comparison of measured and calculated dose in the high-dose region, buildup regions near the phantom surface, low-dose region outside of the fields, and the high-gradient transition regions (Fraass et al. 1998). Recognizing the increasing complexity of IMRT dose distributions, and the need for more objective methods to compare dose distributions, several groups have developed and refined automated techniques for comparing measured and calculated dosimetric data (Depuydt, Van Esch, and Huyskens 2002; Harms et al. 1998; Low et al. 1998a). Such objective formalisms expedite the validation of the dosimetry parameters of the planning system and are gradually being incorporated into commercial planning systems.

## Imaging And Treatment Geometry

IMRT treatment planning is guided by prescriptions that are expressed in terms of physical dose objectives in volumes. Dose and volume criteria can be incorporated directly, or implicitly through biological effect models. The anatomical structures are *patient specific*, and as a consequence, volumetric imaging modalities are a central component of the planning process. Access to a CT scanner is considered a minimum imaging requirement for implementing an IMRT program. A scanner dedicated to the radiation oncology practice is highly desirable because it fosters better integration into the radiotherapy process and greater latitude with scheduling, accessories, and procedures when circumstances require it. CT scans are the principal method of mapping patient anatomy, and also provide the electron density maps of tissues, which are required for accurate dose calculations. Increasingly, MR images and PET are available to provide complimentary visualization of the patient's anatomy and physiology. In a multimodality imaging environment, tools for the quantitative registration of images are necessary. For information regarding the commissioning and QA of medical imaging equipment and image registration tools, the reader is once again directed to AAPM Task Group reports for additional information and references (Frass et al. 1998; Kutcher et al. 1994).

From a systems perspective, network communication must be established with each source of imaging information. Bid specification should insist on DICOM-RT (Digital Imaging and Communications in Medicine-Radiotherapy) compliance with the existing equipment. Tests must be performed to verify the functional aspects of image transfers, image quality, the registration of image and planning coordinate systems, and geometric orientation, image scale, and slice thickness. The transfer of images and contour data between computer systems involves a sequence of electronic query, transmission, and storage events that could result in corruption of the data. A planning system may, for example, reduce the image resolution in order to conserve memory. This process may be acceptable when the IMRT planning system is not the primary tool for the segmenting the images into volumes of interest, but it generates a risk of degrading image resolution, and possible data corruption as data moves between different network nodes, especially when software and hardware updates of the various systems fall out of synchrony. Prior to clinical use, each interface must be thoroughly tested for the anticipated imaging parameters and patient orientations.

From a process perspective, it is important to assure that the imaging parameters adopted for patients with a particular disease are used in a consistent manner, and that deviations from these parameters are vetted under controlled circumstances. In addition to image quality, image orientation and the fidelity of the image geometry must be validated regularly to assure image quality and robust conservation of the image orientation and image geometry. Deviations in slice thickness from patient to patient, for example, could lead to changes in partial volume averaging, and a misinterpretation of structure volumes. This could lead to an incorrect optimization result and a misinterpretation of dose-volume histogram (DVH) data when evaluating the compliance of a plan to the dose-volume criteria documented in a clinical protocol. For each imaging modality, therefore, effort is required to establish and maintain a set of acquisition parameters that remain consistent within a group of patients treated based on the same clinical experience.

As radiotherapy increasingly relies on delineated tissue volumes to describe patient anatomy, the segmentation of images into anatomical structures becomes more involved and more crucial to the planning process. Segmented structures are used to aid beam placement, guide plan optimization, compute DVHs, and in some systems to delineate the external surface of the patient. Most treatment planning systems offer tools to automatically segment structures on the basis of variations in the image intensity. In many cases, it is possible to apply these tools to MR or PET scans to aid in the delineation of target volumes. Caution must be exercised, however, to understand how the specific nature of the intensity variations, and how variations in image acquisition parameters or interpretation, can influence the accuracy of computer-assisted segmentation (Erdi et al. 1997; Nehmeh et al. 2002). With respect to IMRT, it should be emphasized that there is a greater need to assure diligent care and accuracy of the segmented structures. Presuming that the segmentation guidelines outlined by AAPM Task Group 53 have been addressed (Fraass et al. 1998), the interaction of segmentation with the processes of IMRT becomes one of staff awareness, adequate time, and resources to facilitate diligent adherence to the segmentation requirements of clinical protocols.

The geometry of the treatment unit represents another major area requiring configuration and validation of geometric parameters. IMRT imposes an expanded reliance on electronic transfer of treatment parameters, and consequently, the representation of machine movements and physical limits must accurately follow the geometric conventions and constraints adopted by the manufacturer of the treatment unit. These conventions must remain consistent within the record and verify (R&V) database as well. Craig, Brochu, and Van Dyk (1999) have published novel phantom designs for comprehensively testing the geometric aspects of the treatment planning process, beginning with the acquisition of CT data, transfer to the planning system, examination of image geometry, slice thickness, digital reconstruction of radiographs, export to an R&V system, and following through treatment machine, and electronic portal imaging system. Similar functionality can be found in a variety of commercially available phantoms.

## Dose Calculations

Accuracy of dose calculated for high-energy photon beams has been a central preoccupation in the evolution toward conformal radiotherapy and remains a critical consideration for the implementation of IMRT. Several authors have reviewed how photon beam dose calculation algorithms have evolved over the past 20 years, and Monte Carlo algorithms still represent the benchmark for accuracy and general applicability (Ahnesjo and Aspradakis 1999; Battista et al. 1997; Mackie et al. 1996; Wong and Purdy 1990). Several groups have demonstrated a role for Monte Carlo methods in the optimization and verification of IMRT plans, but widespread clinical use has remained elusive because of the prohibitive amount of computation time required (Aaronson et al. 2002; Keall et al. 2001b; Laub et al. 2000; Pawlicki and Ma 2001).

*Heterogeneity Corrections*

The use of tissue heterogeneity corrections has been a matter of active discussion for a number of years (Klein et al. 1993; Orton et al. 1998; Papanikolaou and Klein 2000). There is concern that past clinical experience has been accumulated without accounting for variations in tissue density and it is unclear how dose prescriptions should be modified when corrections are applied. Until recently, it may also have been difficult to get routine access to CT scanners for treatment planning. As algorithms continue to evolve, there is concern that the inadequacies and variability of calculation methods prevent the adoption of uniform standards for estimating tissue heterogeneity corrections. However, there is a growing consensus that tissue heterogeneity corrections should be included in IMRT optimization (IMRTCWG 2001). The growing support for heterogeneity corrections is based on the observations that the necessary electron density information is becoming widely accessible with the use of dedicated CT scanners, that the shortcomings of dose calculations have largely been addressed by a shift from measurement-based to model-based algorithms (Mackie et al. 1996). There is also speculation that the accumulated experience from the past will not translate robustly into the era of IMRT, and applying prescriptive corrections from state-of-the-art algorithms will reduce the uncertainty in dose reporting for patients enrolled in clinical studies (Papanikolaou and Klein 2000).

Institutions that do not currently use tissue heterogeneity corrections will need to acquire phantoms to calibrate the conversion of CT numbers to electron density, and use simple slab and phantoms with cavities filled with air and bone-equivalent materials to verify that the algorithms integrated into the planning system perform in a manner consistent with vendor claims. Retrospective planning studies and measurements in anthropomorphic phantoms should be performed for each relevant treatment technique to understand how to interpret treatment plans that include heterogeneity corrections, and how to support any required adjustments of the physician's prescription or clinical procedures.

Occasionally, it is useful to use contrast agents to aid in image segmentation, and from time to time metal prostheses and dental amalgams are encountered in some clinical situations. The electron density of these materials generally falls beyond the dynamic range of calibration for CT number to electron density conversion. More importantly, the resulting attenuation can generate streaking artifacts and signal dropout. These artifacts have a negative effect on image quality, visibility of structures, and can potentially render CT data unsuitable for dose computation. As part of the commissioning process, the physicist should evaluate planning tools to override the density determined from CT data, in order deal with any contrast agents used during imaging, or imaging artifacts introduced by metallic prostheses.

*Dose Calculations And Optimization Algorithms*

As outlined previously, IMRT differs from 3DCRT in two major respects: the use of numerical optimization methods to achieve prescription goals; and the leaf motion calculators used to determine a sequence of radiation fields, which vary in shape and in the number of monitor units (MUs) applied. It is important to recognize how these components interact with the more familiar components of the planning system, including heterogeneity corrections as discussed above. The IMRT Collaborative Working Group (IMRTCWG) of the NCI has discussed the influence of optimization and leaf sequencing on the treatment planning process (IMRTCWG 2001). Briefly, dose distributions calculated for each set of candidate plan parameters are fed into the cost function and evaluated against the prescribed objectives. The cost function is a mathematical formalism that permits an objective evaluation of the plan parameters and their influence over the dose distribution. A review of the details regarding the design of cost functions, and the mathematics of optimization can be found elsewhere (Oelfke et al. 2001; Webb 2001).

Optimization of the plan parameters can require iterative computation and evaluation of thousands of dose distributions. During the iterative phase, considerable approximations are needed to streamline the dose calculation in order to achieve results in a reasonable amount of time. For example, few treatment planning systems optimize the treatment machine or multileaf collimator (MLC) settings directly. Rather, pencil beams represented by a matrix of elemental *beamlet* intensities and the matrix elements are optimized instead. The beamlet intensity matrix is a surrogate for the machine parameters, and to take the physical aspects of the treatment machine into account, a secondary computation is required to optimize a sequence of field shapes and associated MUs after the beamlet optimization has completed.

Dose calculations and plan evaluation may also be accelerated by simplifying tissue heterogeneity corrections, by ignoring scattered radiation, and by adopting random sampling techniques for evaluating DVHs. It is important to understand the approximations adopted to accelerate the optimization software. The method used for DVH sampling, for example, can be extremely important for critical structures with a small volume. The resolution and extent of the dose calculation grid can also have an enormous influence on the speed and accuracy of dose calculations and DVH reconstructions. Decreasing the dose grid resolution significantly reduces the dose calculation time required for each iteration and reduces the number of points that must be sampled to reconstruct the DVH. The influence of the dose grid on the accuracy of dose distributions, DVH reconstructions, and the stability of the optimization should be evaluated during the commissioning phase. If it is possible to interrupt the iterative optimization and restart it, it is also important to assess how this feature influences the quality of the plan if the interruptions are combined with changes in the plan objectives.

Following the optimization phase, the need for rapid calculations can be relaxed and it is possible to assess the dose distribution that will be delivered to the patient by feeding the results of the leaf motion calculator into a more sophisticated dose calculation algorithm. Dose calculations in the final stages of plan evaluation can more accurately model the effects of tissue heterogeneity, scattered radiation, and, with the leaf motion calculation, the physical characteristics and limitations of the treatment machine. It is important to understand the approximations employed in the optimization process. Physicists should develop a high degree of "algorithm aware-ness," and attention must be given to the interplay and compromises imposed on dose algorithms integrated into the IMRT planning system. Some commercial planning systems offer recalculation with more accurate algorithms, or apply corrections during the leaf motion calculation. More research is needed to find the best overall compro-mise between accuracy and speed. Currently, dosimetric approximations are a necessary component of the optimization phase, and can be expected to compromise the mathematically optimized plan solutions. Recovery from these approximations will inevitably change the optimized solution, and it is important to assure that the final machine delivery sequence still meets the required plan objectives in final stages of plan evaluation.

Figure 1 demonstrates a sequence of phantoms for probing the algorithms of the inverse planning system. A small volume is placed at a depth of 20 cm in isocentric geometry. This target exposed to a $20 \times 20$ cm$^2$ field in a water phantom (a), a medi-astinum phantom with large air or cork-filled cavities (b), a surface modified to generate a $5 \times 5$ cm$^2$ tower, or spike (c), and a narrow $1 \times 1$ cm$^2$ spike (d). Simple calcu-lations and optimization of the dose to the small volume will probe algorithms for dealing with tissue heterogeneities and surface contour variations. Comparison of results from (a) and (b) will demonstrate how the algorithms deal with off-axis density variations and the loss of scattered radiation. Differences between (a) and (c) will probe surface contour corrections and the loss of scatter integration, while differences between (c) and (d) will determine if the system is capable of estimating dose in the absence of electronic equilibrium. These tests should be applied to single open fields, and to modulated fields that are optimized to achieve an equal dose to the small volume in the four geometries. If the system offers the opportunity to recompute the dose following a leaf motion calculation, this aspect of the system should be tested as well. The results of these tests will give an appreciation for the approximations made at the various phases of the treatment planning process. These tests represent extreme geome-tries, and the differences noted may not bear out in clinical situations, but the information is valuable for probing the behavior of the underlying algorithms.

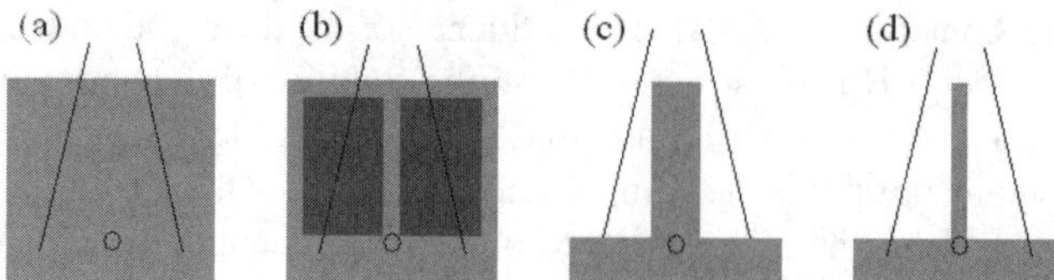


**Figure 1.** A sequence of phantoms for probing the optimization and dose algorithms of a planning system. (a) A small volume is positioned isocentrically at a 20 cm depth in a uniform water phantom, 25 cm on a side; (b) a mediastinum phantom with large air or cork cavities; (c) a surface modified to generate a $5 \times 5$ cm$^2$ spike; and (d) a narrow $1 \times 1$ cm$^2$ spike.

Figure 2 is a schematic example of four phantom geometries used in the treatment planning tests and modeled after Van Esch et al. (2002). The white regions in each figure represent a rectangular slab that should receive a uniform dose when adjacent (a), staggered (b), in the presence of a surface contour variation (c), and with overlying cavities filled with cork or air.

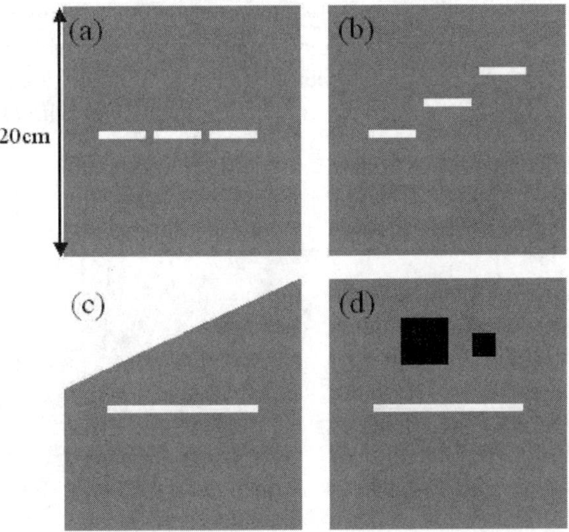

**Figure 2.** Schematic of test phantoms used to assess the capabilities of an inverse planning system and leaf motion calculator (Van Esch et al, 2002). The white boxes represent rectangular target regions that should receive a uniform dose when (a) adjacent, (b), staggered, (c) below an oblique surface, and (d) below air or cork heterogeneities. [Modeled after Van Esch et al. (2002). "Acceptance tests and quality control (QC) procedures for the clinical implementation of intensity modulated radiotherapy (IMRT) using inverse planning and the sliding window technique: Experience from five radiotherapy departments." *Radiother. Oncol.* 65:53–70. © 2002 Elsevier Science.]

Simple geometric phantoms are also helpful for evaluating how the planning system deals with targets that encroach on the skin, and when the planning target volume (PTV) extends beyond the surface of the patient. Care must be taken when the target encroaches on the skin because doses calculated in the build-up region near the surface are commonly inaccurate, and typically err on the side of underestimation. If the build-up region is subject to a high-dose objective, the optimization software will drive up the intensity of beamlets in this region.

Multiple field arrangements in symmetrical cube and cylindrical geometries are also useful for probing the algorithms of the treatment planning system. Consider the examples in figure 3. For a symmetrical cube target located at the center of a cube of water and treated with a four-field box (figure 3a), all four beams have an equivalent source-to-surface distance (SSD) and field size, and it seems intuitive that prescribing a uniform dose to the cube target should result in symmetrical beam intensity distributions and equal beam weights. Similar symmetries should be obtained for the cylindrical phantom and unopposed field arrangement shown in figure 3b. Variations of this test can include a larger number of fields or even arc-based delivery techniques. Various dose constraints and penalties can be applied to the surrounding normal tissue, and the problem can be made progressively more complex by moving the target to an asymmetric position, or by introducing a symmetric adjacent structure to be spared preferentially. Such tests will lead to clinically meaningful strategies for driving the optimization, and are satisfying when the outcome is consistent with clinical experience and intuition.

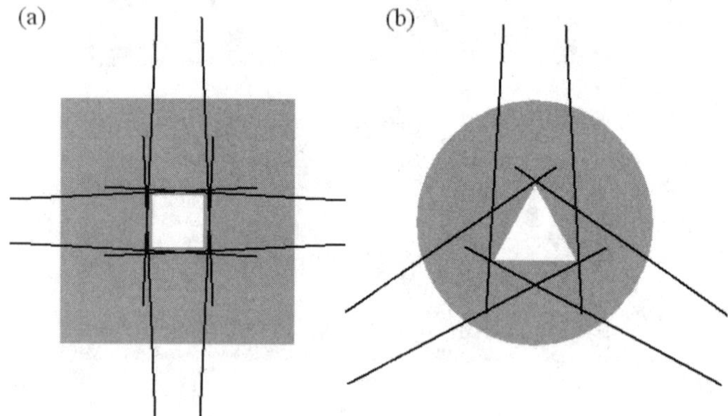

**Figure 3.** Examples of simple geometric phantoms and beam arrangements for testing optimization algorithms.

Hunt et al. (2002) of the Memorial Sloan-Kettering Cancer Center have used ideal concave target geometries to explore the interaction of the number of fields, beam energy, proximity to a cylindrical normal tissue structure interact, and selection of dose constraints, and how these factors influence the conformity and uniformity of the dose distribution in the target. The observations from this work were used to develop a strategy for guiding the optimization of clinical plans with similar characteristics.

## Dose Calculations And Leaf Sequencing Algorithms

Leaf motion calculators generate a sequence of physically realizable radiation field shapes and associated beam intensities, which are to be delivered using a field-based "step and shoot" delivery approach (Galvin, Chen, and Smith 1993; Siochi 1999; Wu et al. 2001), or a leaf trajectory based "dynamic" approach (Convery and Rosenbloom 1992; Spirou and Chui 1994; Yu et al. 1995). When such sequences of smaller radiation fields are superimposed during delivery, the accuracy of the calculated beam penumbra and leaf transmission can have a significant influence on the overall plan accuracy. Dose calculations have required a number of refinements to accurately account for the effects of head scatter, penumbra of the leaf ends, tongue-and-groove effects, transmission, leakage, the interplay of leaf speed with dose rate, and other physical constraints on MLC and jaw motion. When generating field shapes from the beamlet intensity matrix, there is the potential for fields that are much smaller than those normally used in radiation therapy, and there is a need to determine the dose delivered per MU for these small fields (Boyer et al. 1999; Sharpe et al. 2000). Dynamic MLC techniques require special attention to the interplay between the accuracy of the leaf penumbra, transmission, and tongue-and-groove effects. The accuracy of the dose calculation algorithm with regard to these factors is crucial to the quality of the calculated dose distribution, and the degree of confidence placed in final plan results following the optimization and leaf sequencing. There is a growing body of experience with the commissioning of step-and-shoot and dynamic leaf motion IMRT delivery systems (Cadman et al. 2002; LoSasso, Chui, and Ling 1998; MacKenzie et al. 2002; Mohan et al. 2000; Potter et al. 2002; Van Esch et al. 2002). There is also a large body of literature dealing with the dosimetry of small fields, and valuable experience can be translated from the radiosurgery field (Beddar, Mason, and O'Brien 1994; Heydarian, Hoban, and Beddoe 1996; Kubsad et al. 1990; Letourneau, Pouliot, and Roy 1999; Ramani et al. 1994).

Cadman et al. (2002) have reported their experience in using film measurements to refine a beam model for a segmented, or step-and-shoot IMRT approach. These authors found that the planning system under study did not account for the curved ends of the MLC leaves, but adjusting the leaf positions to account for the effective widening of the leaf openings can significantly improve the agreement between calculations and measured doses. Van Esch et al. (2002) have published a multi-institutional experience in the implementation of dynamic IMRT planning and delivery systems. This paper describes the approach taken by five institutions that purchased the same equipment and adopted a similar approach to the implementation of IMRT. In refining the beam modeling parameters, the authors advise that basic dosimetry measurements should be performed using small-volume ion chambers or solid-state dosimeters.

Extensive experience with the clinical implementation of an IMRT treatment planning system for *serial* tomotherapy has been published by Low et al. (Low et al. 1998b, 2001; Low and Mutic 1998). This system employs a measurement-based dose calculation model, and by and large, the commissioning process follows the steps outlined at the beginning of this section. Unique issues include precise characterization of the beam penumbra for matching abutting delivery slices, and consideration of the amount of leakage dose received by the patient. *Helical* tomotherapy is an emerging system of IMRT technologies under development at the University of Wisconsin (Mackie et al. 1993, 1999). A limited number of tomotherapy systems have only recently become available, but from a verification and QA perspective, the TomoTherapy (Madison, WI) approach is innovative in that it includes a number of algorithms and measurement systems for real-time patient imaging, active delivery verification, and dose reconstruction (Kapatoes et al. 2001).

From this discussion it should be apparent that the measurement and entry of basic dosimetry data for IMRT treatment planning is similar to a 3DCRT system. In general however, it is reasonable to anticipate expanded requirements for the dosimetry of small radiation fields and for characterization of the dose outside the field, in and beyond the penumbra region. The specific aspects of system acceptance and commissioning will depend on the treatment planning system purchased. The accuracy of the planning results will depend on the beam model implemented in the system, and on how much effort is put into the measurement of the MLC beam penumbra and small field output factors. In this regard, model-based systems handle these effects explicitly. Additional geometric information may also be required for the leaf motion calculator, in order to assure it will derive treatment delivery sequences. To avoid confusion, it is important to understand the specific data requirements of the particular planning system under consideration. In a recent review article, Low (2002) cites the example of MLC leaf leakage. Interleaf leakage can be measured to a high resolution with film or a small-volume ionization chamber, but if the planning system does not account for interleaf leakage explicitly, the *average* transmission may be a more appropriate value to enter into the system, rather than the transmission through the leaf body *per se*.

## Plan Evaluation

Normalization of the isodose distribution is central to the interpretation of an IMRT plan, and for establishing the parameters for MU calculations. IMRT dose distributions are characterized by sharp gradients near critical structures, and aggressive conformation to the surface of irregularly shaped target volumes. Often, these capabilities come with the cost of "noisy" high-dose regions, greater dose variation within the target volume, and a tendency to spread low-dose regions over large volumes of normal tissue. The marked advantages of the IMRT plan can alter the focus of plan evaluation, and a temptation to overlook the inferior aspects of the dose distribution. For example, the dose at the plan normalization point can vary over the course of the optimization, and from patient to patient treated with the same optimization parameters. The variations in the dose at the normalization point can be large enough to distort isodose distribution and interpretation of normalized DVHs. These variations can be avoided by evaluating and ranking plans according to absolute dose, rather than relative to a normalization point.

When considering 3DCRT plans, it is possible to separate the interpretation of the dose distribution from the MU calculation, but the complexity of IMRT makes this difficult. Determination of the MUs and absolute dose delivered depends on the leaf sequencing, relative beam weights, method of plan normalization, and the method of dose prescription. A thorough understanding of the principles underlying the dose calculation is required to assure the prescription and plans are interpreted, as they will be delivered. The commissioning and acceptance of an IMRT treatment planning system must include tests of relationship between the absolute dose prescribed and the number of MUs estimated by the planning system. These tests should follow the standard practice of working progressively from single fields in simple phantoms, and follow a progression to more complex geometries and realistic clinical cases. This relationship should be tested under reasonable clinical conditions, and with more extreme geometric phantoms, and with the normalization point placed in high-gradient regions, under blocks, and within non-target structures. If the planning system offers different options for plan normalization, each method must be tested, and different hand calculation techniques and independent computations should be used to check the MUs determined by the planning system.

Once the accuracy of the beam model has been confirmed for single beams, and for multiple field arrangements in symmetrical phantom geometries, the system must be validated with realistic patient data over the anticipated range of clinical application. These tests are best performed for situations that closely emulate specific clinical techniques. These tests should span the entire treatment process and check the system components that are most important to the design and implementation of realistic treatment plans. This includes optimization of imaging parameters for the anatomical site, verification of contouring tools, prescription entry, and plan normalization. This aspect of commissioning highlights another unique aspect of IMRT compared to 3DCRT, in that physician involvement is necessary to establish plan optimization goals for realistic clinical testing. Determination of plan objectives can be an iterative and time-consuming process of running plans and evaluating the resulting dose distributions and DVH data, but this is a vital part of the learning process and training required to use the system in an effective and efficient manner. Once a set of viable plan objectives has been established, it is possible to validate the accuracy of dose calculations and MU settings in appropriate anthropomorphic phantoms.

## Export And Documentation

When a treatment plan has been completed and approved, implementation of the plan requires thorough documentation and transfer of the parameters determined by the planning system to the actual settings of the treatment unit. The complexity of IMRT treatment plans generates a vast amount of information, and imposes a greater reliance on the electronic exchange of machine parameters.

Proprietary interfaces between equipment have gradually been replaced by the open DICOM standard, with extensions to support the exchange of radiotherapy information between different planning systems, treatment management systems, clinical trial databases, and treatment machines (i.e., DICOM-RT). Conformance to standards for information exchange give confidence that information moving between systems will be preserved and remain consistent, but it does not necessarily guarantee the integrity of the information. Without adequate training or support, the technical challenges of establishing a functional and reliable communication network can be daunting, especially in a multi-vendor environment. A basic understanding of the underlying communication protocols and nomenclature can aid in assuring that the conventions used in the radiotherapy treatment planning (RTP) system match the coordinate and scale conventions of the treatment unit. Review of the protocols will also give an appreciation for the conventions used to represent parameters such as beam names, geometric units, scaling, and resolution.

The electronic transfer of machine settings improves efficiency and reduces the frequency of manual transcription errors, but reduced user interaction does not prevent other errors, such as failure to select the delivery sequence corresponding to the medically approved plan or failure to clearly communicate a plan modification. Reduced human interaction can even delay the detection of systematic planning errors, deficiencies in the system configuration, or errors introduced by software or equipment changes in the planning system or "upstream" image sources. In addition to accurate patient demographics, all storage media, networking, and paper documentation for treatment plans should include detailed information to identify all staff participating in the planning process, as well as a unique revision code or time stamp that can be used to assure that the machine settings downloaded from the planning system originated from the approved treatment plan. It is vital to recognize the interdependence of the various systems required for imaging, planning, delivery, and administration of radiotherapy procedures. Because of the critical reliance on electronic data exchange, it may also be prudent to monitor and manage the supporting communication infrastructure as an extension of the medical devices used in treatment planning.

## Staff Training And Experience

The treatment planning system operates in an environment requiring staff with a diverse set of training and experience to perform a complex array of tasks. All staff members require adequate initial training, periodic refresher courses, and technical support to assure effective interaction with the planning system. As already outlined, involvement of physicians and treatment planning staff in the commissioning of IMRT treatment techniques serves the dual role of validating a process for treatment planning, and providing a mechanism for staff training. A high degree of confidence can be gained from well-documented clinical procedures developed during the commissioning of specific treatment techniques.

When situations require deviations from the commissioned clinical process, this confidence should be accompanied by attentive system operation and diligent awareness of the system's limitations. Unexpected software deficiencies and incorrect interpretation of features are inevitable. Staff must be vigilant about unexpected software behavior, and maintain communication with the system manufacturer and user groups so that these situations can be addressed as they are discovered, and appropriate workarounds can be employed.

## Quality Assurance Guidelines

The goals of treatment planning system QA is to assure proper use of the system, consistent software behavior, integrity of beam modeling and patient data, and to detect possible corruption of electronic data imported or exported between external systems. QA procedures should be designed with consideration of the tests recommended by the manufacturer of treatment planning system, assessment of the relevant sections of AAPM Task Group reports (Fraass et al. 1998; Kutcher et al. 1994), the level of control or cooperation over external sources of imaging data, and by identification of other unique aspects of the local clinical environment. The aim is to assure the integrity of the systems and data spanning the entire chain of treatment planning and delivery.

### Establishing Baseline Performance

To develop an effective QA program, the physicist should make an assessment of the planning system, external source of imaging data, and the treatment units supported by the planning system. It is useful to keep a system QA log to document the results of QA tasks and to verify current software versions on all imaging, planning, and delivery systems. Service engineers should be encouraged to record their activities in the log in order to track hardware maintenance and software changes that may influence image quality or data integrity. It is valuable to examine computer system log files periodically to understand the manner in which the systems interact, and the status and error codes documented in the system log file.

QA activities should include participation by the clinical staff using the equipment on a daily basis who are most familiar with the systems. At a minimum, it is valuable to send a simple geometric phantom through the planning process on a weekly or monthly basis. A known phantom geometry should be aligned to lasers, scanned, and the images transferred to the planning system. If a separate CT-Simulation package is used for contouring and beam placement, it should be included in the test. Simple measurement tools in the planning system and CT-Sim can serve as a quick check for geometric distortions, image scale, and orientation.

The phantoms shown in figure 4 are examples from a QA system designed to monitor the non-dosimetric aspects of the treatment planning process, as described by Craig, Brochu, and Van Dyk (1999). A number of commercially available phantoms are capable of performing similar tests. The phantoms can be used to perform a basic CT to electron density conversion check, and to verify the geometric accuracy of volume segmentation and DVH calculations. It is also possible to validate and monitor the registration of image, planning, and treatment coordinate systems. Rotating components can be used to verify machine geometry parameters, beam display, and accuracy of DRR and multi-planar reconstructions. DRRs of the rotating components can be generated for any combination of gantry and couch rotation. The DRRs can be exported to electronic portal imaging software to check the correspondence of the planning coordinates, treatment geometry, and portal image verification devices.

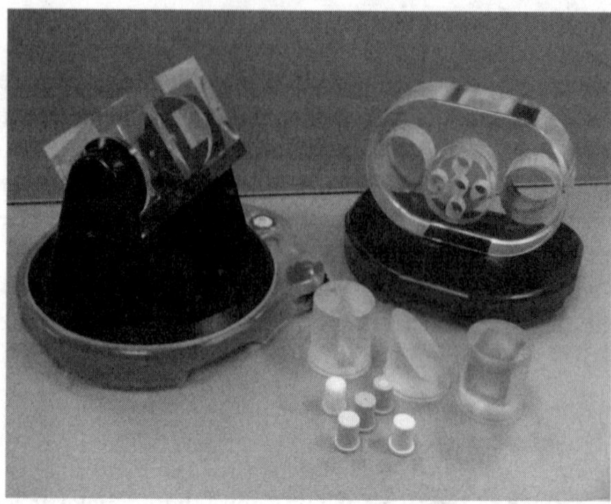

**Figure 4.** A pair of phantoms designed for QA of the non-dosimetric aspects of
the treatment planning process, as described by Craig, Brochu, and Van Dyk (1999).
The phantom on the right supports QA of CT to electron density conversion, geometric
accuracy of volume segmentation, and DVH calculations. The phantom on the left is used
to validate and monitor the registration of image, planning, and treatment coordinate
systems. Rotating components can be used to verify machine geometry parameters
and accuracy of DRR and multi-planar reconstructions.

Because of the distributed nature of the systems that supply information or rely
on information derived from the planning system, there is a need to monitor the
computing infrastructure supporting the treatment planning application, and to verify
the integrity of beam modeling data and patient records. With support from an information systems specialist, it is important to monitor network security, network
performance, system hardware performance, memory usage, and disk space. The
integrity of backup systems and patient record archiving should also be monitored.
Federal initiatives dealing with patient privacy are also raising the standards for security of patient records and the configuration and maintenance of user accounts.
Physicists may find it necessary to seek the assistance of computer security and support
specialists in order to meet these standards, and to assure the integrity of system security, machine modeling data, active patient records, and data archives.

Routine dosimetric QA of the planning system can be achieved by maintaining a
database of representative clinical cases completed during system commissioning.
These cases are re-planned, documented, and delivered periodically to confirm the
system produces the same results and that plan export tools are functioning properly.
Such tests are valuable for confirming consistent system performance, but may be too
coarse to detect subtle changes in algorithms following software patches or major
version upgrades. Following software updates, some of the detailed tests performed
during commissioning should be repeated, and compared with the original commissioning results.

## Frequency And Scope Of Periodic QA

AAPM Task Groups 40 and 53 provide detailed discussions regarding the frequency and scope of periodic treatment planning system QA (Fraass et al. 1998; Kutcher et al. 1994). The main aims are to confirm the integrity and security of the machine modeling data and to verify the import and export of data with peripheral devices, imaging modalities, and treatment delivery devices. Both reports recommend QA tests at regular intervals, primarily to detect changes caused by external factors, but Task Group 53 has concluded that after the planning system has been configured and validated for clinical use, the most important aspect of a QA program is inclusion of QA practices into the day-to-day aspects of planning and delivery, for every patient and every plan (Fraass et al. 1998). Based on the multi-institutional experience from Europe, the clinical implementation of IMRT only heightens the need for integrated approaches, and patient-specific QA (Van Esch et al. 2002).

Treatment planning QA should continue in the context of the development of treatment techniques. With each new technique, it is possible to adopt new sources of patient imaging data, and to adopt procedures or system features that have not been assured by prior testing. When this approach is adopted, treatment procedures are refined and documented in a manner that generates a clear understanding of treatment goals and procedures. This greatly facilitates the maintenance of planning skills and training of new staff.

## Dealing With Exceptions

Because of the complexity of planning software, unexpected behaviors can be discovered from time to time. All staff interacting with the system should be vigilant and conscientious about reporting unexpected software behavior. Detailed information describing the exact nature of the activities that generated the concern should be documented and reported to the manufacturer. Vendors maintain a database of user reports to assess the frequency and any risks associated with the observed problem. If warranted, the vendor will communicate the nature of the problem and any workaround that should be adopted until the issue can be addressed in a software revision. Clinical staff should be encouraged to document and track problems in the QA log book.

## Summary

The acceptance tests and the procedures for commissioning any 3-D planning system are complex and time consuming. To successfully implement IMRT in a timely fashion, adequate resources and training must be put in place, and realistic targets for system accuracy must be identified. This discussion is intended to highlight issues that should be evaluated by the individuals responsible for the technical aspects and assurance of the appropriate use of IMRT treatment planning. It must be emphasized that currently there are no prescribed tests to evaluate and control risks for IMRT treatment planning systems. While specific tests for the optimization and leaf sequencing components of the system evolve, the AAPM Task Group 53 Report remains the benchmark for the commissioning and quality assurance of modern radiotherapy treatment planning systems.

Because of the complexity and magnitude of the testing required, it is almost infeasible for a single institution to test all aspects of a modern treatment planning system. Therefore, it is important to concentrate local efforts on establishing an accurate configuration of the geometric and dosimetric parameters required to support the local clinical environment. It is also important to understand the underlying algorithms and operational aspects of the planning system. Efforts to validate and characterize the systems algorithms should be coordinated with the QA practices and diligence of the system vendor, and it is important to exchange information with institutions using the same system.

## Acknowledgments

The author wishes to thank Gary Ezzell, Dan Low, Ramani Ramaseshan, John Jezioranski, Paul Keall, and Yan Wu for helpful discussions.

## References

Aaronson, R. F., J. J. DeMarco, I. J. Chetty, and T. D. Solberg. (2002). "A Monte Carlo based phase space model for quality assurance of intensity modulated radiotherapy incorporating leaf specific characteristics." *Med. Phys.* 29:2952–2958.

Ahnesjo, A., and M. M. Aspradakis. (1999). "Dose calculations for external photon beams in radiotherapy." *Phys. Med. Biol.* 44:R99–155.

Battista, J. J., M. B. Sharpe, E. Wong, and J. Van Dyk. (1997). "A New Classification Scheme for Photon Beam Dose Algorithms" in *XIIth International Conference on the Use of Computers in Radiation Therapy*. (XII ICCR). D. D. Leavitt and G. Starkschall (eds.). Salt Lake City, May 27–30, 1997. Madison, WI: Medical Physics Publishing, pp. 103–107, 1997.

Beddar, A. S., D. J. Mason, and P. F. O'Brien. (1994). "Absorbed dose perturbation caused by diodes for small field photon dosimetry." *Med. Phys.* 21:1075–1079.

Born, E., A. Fogliata-Cozzi, F. Ionescu, V. Ionescu, and P. A. Tercier. *Recommendations #7: Quality Control of Treatment Planning Systems For Teletherapy*. Swiss Society of Radiobiology and Medical Physics, 1999).

Bortfeld. T., A. L. Boyer, W. Schlegel, D. L. Kahler, and T. J. Waldron. (1994b). "Realisation and verification of three-dimensional conformal radiotherapy with modulated fields." *Int. J. Radiat. Oncol. Biol. Med. Phys.* 30:899–908.

Boyer, A., L. Xing, C.-M. Ma, B. Curran, R. Hill, A. Kania, A. Bleier. (1999). "Theoretical considerations of monitor unit calculations for intensity modulated beam treatment planning." *Med. Phys.* 26:187–195.

Brahme, A. (1984). "Dosimetric precision requirements in radiation therapy." *Acta Radiol. Oncol.* 23:379–391.

Brahme, A. (1999). "Optimized radiation therapy based on radiobiological objectives." *Semin. Radiat. Oncol.* 9:35–47.

Brahme, A., J. E. Roos, and I. Lax. (1982). "Solution of an integral equation encountered in rotation therapy." *Phys. Med. Biol.* 27:1221–1229.

Cadman, P., R. Bassalow, N. P. Sidhu, G. Ibbott, and A. Nelson. (2002). "Dosimetric considerations for validation of a sequential IMRT process with a commercial treatment planning system." *Phys. Med. Biol.* 47:3001–3010.

Carol, M., W. H. Grant 3rd, D. Pavord, P. Eddy, H. S. Targovnik, B. Butler, S. Woo, J. Figura , V. Onufrey, R. Grossman, and R. Selkar. (1996). "Initial clinical experience with the Peacock intensity modulation of a 3-D conformal radiation therapy system." *Stereotact. Funct. Neurosurg.* 66:30–34.

Convery, D. J., and M. E. Rosenbloom. (1992). "The generation of intensity-modulated fields for conformal therapy by dynamic collimation." *Phys. Med. Biol.* 37:1359–1374.

Cosset, J. M. (2002). "ESTRO Breur Gold Medal Award Lecture 2001: Irradiation accidents — lessons for oncology? *Radiother. Oncol.* 63:1–10.

Craig, T., D. Brochu, and J. Van Dyk. (1999). "A quality assurance phantom for three-dimensional radiation treatment planning." *Int. J. Radiat. Oncol. Biol. Phys.* 44:955–966.

Cunningham, J. R. "Tissue Inhomogeneity Corrections in Photon-Beam Treatment planning" in *Progress in Medical Radiation Physics* C. G. Orton (ed.). New York: Plenum Press, pp. 103–131, 1982.

Depuydt, T., A. Van Esch, and D. P. Huyskens. (2002). "A quantitative evaluation of IMRT dose distributions: Refinement and clinical assessment of the gamma evaluation." *Radiother. Oncol.* 62:309–319.

Dutreix, A. (1987). "Prescription, precision, and decision in treatment planning." *Int. J. Radiat. Oncol. Biol. Phys.* 13:1291–1296.

Erdi, Y. E., O. Mawlawi, S. M. Larson, M. Imbriaco, H. Yeung, R. Finn, and J. L. Humm. (1997). "Segmentation of lung lesion volume by adaptive positron emission tomography image thresholding." *Cancer* 80:2505–2509.

Followill, D., P. Geis, and A. Boyer. (1997). "Estimates of whole-body dose equivalent produced by beam intensity modulated conformal therapy." *Int. J. Radiat. Oncol. Biol. Phys.* 38:667–672. [Published erratum appears in *Int. J. Radiat. Oncol. Biol. Phys.* 39(3):783].

Fraass, B., K. Doppke, M. Hunt, G. Kutcher, G. Starkschall, R. Stern, and J. Van Dyk. (1998). "American Association of Physicists in Medicine Radiation Therapy Committee Task Group 53: Quality assurance for clinical radiotherapy treatment planning." *Med. Phys.* 25:1773–1829.

Galvin, J. M., X. G. Chen, and R. M. Smith. (1993). "Combining multileaf fields to modulate fluence distributions." *Int. J. Radiat. Oncol. Biol. Phys.* 27:697–705.

Harms, W. B., Sr., D. A. Low, J. W. Wong, and J. A. Purdy. (1998). "A software tool for the quantitative evaluation of 3D dose calculation algorithms." *Med. Phys.* 25:1830–1836.

Heydarian, M., P. W. Hoban, and A. H. Beddoe. (1996). "A comparison of dosimetry techniques in stereotactic radiosurgery." *Phys. Med. Biol.* 41:93–110.

Hunt, M. A., C. Y. Hsiung, S. V. Spirou, C. S. Chui, H. I. Amols, and C. C. Ling. (2002). "Evaluation of concave dose distributions created using an inverse planning system." *Int. J. Radiat. Oncol. Biol. Phys.* 54:953–962.

ICRU Report 24. Determination of Absorbed Dose in a Patient Irradiated by Beams of X or Gamma Rays in Radiotherapy Procedures. Washington, DC: International Commission on Radiation Units and Measurements, 1976.

Kapatoes, J. M., G. H. Olivera, K. J. Ruchala, J. B. Smilowitz, P. J. Reckwerdt, and T. R. Mackie. (2001). "A feasible method for clinical delivery verification and dose reconstruction in tomotherapy." *Med. Phys.* 28:528–542.

Keall, P. J., V. R. Kini, S. S. Vedam, and R. Mohan. (2001a). "Motion adaptive x-ray therapy: A feasibility study." *Phys. Med. Biol.* 46:1–10.

Keall, P. J., J. V. Siebers, M. Arnfield, J. O. Kim, and R. Mohan. (2001b). "Monte Carlo dose calculations for dynamic IMRT treatments." *Phys. Med. Biol.* 46:929–941.

Klein, E. E., L. M. Chin, R. K. Rice, and B. J. Mijnheer. (1993). "The influence of air cavities on interface doses for photon beams." *Int. J. Radiat. Oncol. Biol. Phys.* 27:419–427.

Kubsad, S. S., T. R. Mackie, M. A. Gehring, D. J. Misisco, B. R. Paliwal, M. P. Mehta, and T. J. Kinsella. (1990). "Monte Carlo and convolution dosimetry for stereotactic radiosurgery." *Int. J. Radiat. Oncol. Biol. Phys.* 19:1027–1035.

Kutcher, G. J., L. Coia, M. Gillin, W. F. Hanson, S. Leibel, R. J. Morton, J. R. Palta, J. A. Purdy, L. E. Reinstein, G. K. Svensson, M. Weller, and L. Wingfield. (1994). "Comprehensive QA for radiation oncology: Report of AAPM Radiation Therapy Committee Task Group 40." *Med. Phys.* 21:581–618.

Laub, W., M. Alber, M. Birkner, and F. Nüsslin. (2000). "Monte Carlo dose computation for IMRT optimization." *Phys. Med. Biol.* 45:1741–1754.

Leibel, S. A., Z. Fuks, M. J. Zelefsky, S. L. Wolden, K. E. Rosenzweig, K. M. Alektiar, M. A. Hunt, E. D. Yorke, L. X. Hong, H. I. Amols, C. M. Burman, A. Jackson, G. S. Mageras, T. LoSasso, L. Happersett, S. V. Spirou, C. S. Chui, and C. C. Ling. (2002). "Intensity modulated radiotherapy." *Cancer J.* 8:164–176.

Letourneau, D., J. Pouliot, and R. Roy. (1999). "Miniature scintillating detector for small field radiation therapy." *Med. Phys.* 26, 2555–2561.

Ling, C. C., J. Humm, S. Larson, H. Amols, Z. Fuks, S. Leibel, and J. A. Koutcher. (2000). "Towards multidimensional radiotherapy (MD-CRT): Biological imaging and biological conformality." *Int. J. Radiat. Oncol. Biol. Phys.* 47:551–560.

LoSasso T., C.-S. Chui, and C. C. Ling. (1998). "Physical and dosimetric aspects of a multileaf collimation system used in the dynamic mode for implementing intensity modulated radiotherapy." *Med. Phys.* 25:1919–1927.

Low, D. A. (2002). "Quality assurance of intensity-modulated radiotherapy." *Semin. Radiat. Oncol.* 12:219–228.

Low, D. A., and S. Mutic. (1998). "A commercial IMRT treatment-planning dose-calculation algorithm." *Int. J. Radiat. Oncol. Biol. Phys.* 41:933–937.

Low, D. A., W. B. Harms, S. Mutic, and J. A. Purdy. (1998a). "A technique for the quantitative evaluation of dose distributions." *Med. Phys.* 25:656–661.

Low, D.A., S. Mutic, J. F. Dempsey, R. L. Gerber, W. R. Bosch, C. A. Perez, and J. A. Purdy. (1998b). "Quantitative dosimetric verification of an IMRT planning and delivery system." *Radiother. Oncol.* 49:305–316.

Low, D. A., S. Mutic, J. F. Dempsey, J. Markman, K. S. Chao, and J. A. Purdy. (2001). "Abutment dosimetry for serial tomotherapy." *Med. Dosim.* 26:79–82.

MacKenzie, M. A., M. Lachaine, B. Murray, B. G. Fallone, D. Robinson, and G. C. Field. (2002). "Dosimetric verification of inverse planned step and shoot multileaf collimator fields from a commercial treatment planning system." *J. Appl. Clin. Med. Phys.* 3:97–109.

Mackie, T. R., J. Balog, K. Ruchala, D. Shepard, S. Aldridge, E. Fitchard, P. Reckwerdt, G. Olivera, T. McNutt, and M. Mehta. (1999). "Tomotherapy." *Semin. Radiat. Oncol.* 9(1):108–117.

Mackie, T. R., T. Holmes, S. Swerdloff, P. Reckwerdt, J. O. Deasy, J. Yang, B. Paliwal, and T. Kinsella. (1993). "Tomotherapy: A new concept for the delivery of dynamic conformal radiotherapy." *Med. Phys.* 20:1709–1719.

Mackie, T. R., P. J. Reckwerdt, T. R. McNutt, M. Gehring, and C. Sanders. "Photon Beam Dose Computations" in *Teletherapy: Present and Future*. J. R. Palta and T. R. Mackie (eds.). Proceedings of the AAPM 1996 Summer School. Madison, WI: Advanced Medical Publishing, pp. 103–135, 1996.

Macklis, R. M., T. Meier, and M. S.Weinhous. (1998). "Error rates in clinical radiotherapy." *J. Clin. Oncol.* 16:551–556.

Macklis, R., M. Weinhous, and G. Harnisch. (2000). "Intensity-modulated radiotherapy: Rethinking basic treatment planning paradigms." *Int. J. Radiat. Oncol. Biol. Phys.* 48:317–318.

Mayles, W. P. M., R. A. Lake, A. L. Mackenzie, E. M. Macaulay, H. M., Morgan, and S. K. Powley. Report 81 Physics Aspects of Quality Control in Radiotherapy. York, UK: Institute of Physics and Engineering in Medicine, 1998.

Mijnheer, B. J., J. J. Battermann, and A. Wambersie. (1987). What degree of accuracy is required and can be achieved in photon and neutron therapy?" *Radiother. Oncol.* 8:237–252.

Mohan, R., M. Arnfield, S. Tong, Q. Wu, and J. Siebers. (2000). "The impact of fluctuations in intensity patterns on the number of monitor units and the quality and accuracy of intensity modulated radiotherapy." *Med. Phys.* 27:1226–1237.

Mutic, S., and D. A. Low. (1998). "Whole-body dose from tomotherapy delivery." *Int. J. Radiat. Oncol. Biol. Phys.* 42:229–232.

Mutic, S., D. A. Low, E. E. Klein, J. F. Dempsey, and J. A. Purdy. (2001). "Room shielding for intensity-modulated radiation therapy treatment facilities." *Int. J. Radiat. Oncol. Biol. Phys.* 50:239–246.

IMRTCWG (Intensity Modulated Radiation Therapy Collaborative Working Group). "Intensity-modulated radiotherapy: Current status and issues of interest." *Int. J. Radiat. Oncol. Biol. Phys.* 51:880–914.

Nehmeh, S. A., Y. E. Erdi, C. C. Ling, K. E. Rosenzweig, O. D. Squire, L. E. Braban, E. Ford, K. Sidhu, G. S. Mageras, S. M. Larson, and J. L. Humm. (2002). "Effect of respiratory gating on reducing lung motion artifacts in PET imaging of lung cancer." *Med. Phys.* 29:366–371.

Oelfke, U., and T. Bortfeld. (2001). "Inverse planning for photon and proton beams." *Med. Dosim.* 26:113–124.

Orton, C. G., S. Chungbin, E. E. Klein, M. T. Gillin, T. E. Schultheiss, and W. T. Sause. (1998). "Study of lung density corrections in a clinical trial (RTOG 88-08). Radiation Therapy Oncology Group." *Int. J. Radiat. Oncol. Biol. Phys.* 41:787–794.

Papanikolaou, N., and E. E. Klein. (2000). "Heterogeneity corrections should be used in treatment planning for lung cancer." *Med. Phys.* 27:1702–1704.

Pawlicki, T., and C.-M. Ma. (2001). "Monte Carlo simulation for MLC-based intensity-modulated radiotherapy." *Med. Dosim.* 26:157–168.

Potter, L. D., S. X. Chang, T. J. Cullip, and A. C. Siochi. (2002). "A quality and efficiency analysis of the IMFAST segmentation algorithm in head and neck "step & shoot" IMRT treatments." *Med. Phys.* 29:275–283.

Powlis, W. D., M. D. Altschuler, Y. Censor, and E. L. Buhle Jr. (1989). "Semi-automated radiotherapy treatment planning with a mathematical model to satisfy treatment goals." *Int. J. Radiat. Oncol. Biol. Phys.* 16:271–276.

Ramani, R., A. W. Lightstone, D. L. Mason, and P. F. O'Brien. (1994). "The use of radiochromic film in treatment verification of dynamic stereotactic radiosurgery." *Med. Phys.* 21: 389–392.

Sharpe, M. B., B. M. Miller, D. Yan, and J. W. Wong. (2000). "Monitor unit settings for intensity modulated beams delivered using a step-and-shoot approach." *Med. Phys.* 27:2719–2725.

Shaw, J. Report 68: A Guide to Commissioning & Quality Control of Treatment Planning Systems. York, UK: Institute of Physics and Engineering in Medicine, 1996.

Siochi, R. A. (1999). "Minimizing static intensity modulation delivery time using an intensity solid paradigm." *Int. J. Radiat. Oncol. Biol. Phys.* 43:671–680.

Spirou, S. V., and C. S. Chui. (1994). "Generation of arbitrary intensity profiles by dynamic jaws or multileaf collimators." *Med. Phys.* 21:1031–1041.

Stein, J., T. Bortfeld, B. Dorschel, and W. Schlegel. (1994). "Dynamic x-ray compensation for conformal radiotherapy by means of multi-leaf collimation." *Radiother. Oncol.* 32:163–173.

Ten Haken, R. K., J. M. Balter, L. H. Marsh, J. M. Robertson, and T. S. Lawrence.(1997). "Potential benefits of eliminating planning target volume expansions for patient breathing in the treatment of liver tumors." *Int. J. Radiat. Oncol. Biol. Phys.* 38:613–617.

Thwaites, D., P. Scalliet, J. W. Leer, and J. Overgaard. (1995). "Quality assurance in radiotherapy. European Society for Therapeutic Radiology and Oncology Advisory Report to the Commission of the European Union for the 'Europe Against Cancer Programme'." *Radiother. Oncol.*, 35:61–73.

Van Dyk, J. "Radiation Oncology Overview" in *The Modern Technology of Radiation Oncology. A Compendium for Medical Physicists and Radiation Oncologists.* J. Van Dyk (ed.). Madison, WI: Medical Physics Publishing, pp. 1–17, 1999.

Van Dyk, J., J. A. Purdy. (1999). "Clinical Implementation of Technology and the Quality Assurance Process" in *The Modern Technology of Radiation Oncology. A Compendium for Medical Physicists and Radiation Oncologists.* J. Van Dyk (ed.). Madison, WI: Medical Physics Publishing, pp. 19–51, 1999.

Van Dyk, J., R. B. Barnett, J. E. Cygler, and P. C. Shragge. (1993). "Commissioning and quality assurance of treatment planning computers [see comments]." *Int. J. Radiat. Oncol. Biol. Phys.* 26:261–273.

Van Esch, A., J. Bohsung, P. Sorvari, M. Tenhunun, M. Fagundes, T. DiPetrillo, B. Kramer, M. Koistinen, and M. J. Engler. (2002). "Acceptance tests and quality control (QC) procedures for the clinical implementation of intensity modulated radiotherapy (IMRT) using inverse planning and the sliding window technique: experience from five radiotherapy departments." *Radiother. Oncol.* 65:53–70.

van Herk, M., P. Remeijer, and J. V. Lebesque. (2002). "Inclusion of geometric uncertainties in treatment plan evaluation." *Int. J. Radiat. Oncol. Biol. Phys.* 52(5):1407–1422.

Verhey, L. J. (2002). "Issues in optimization for planning of intensity-modulated radiation therapy." *Semin. Radiat. Oncol.* 12:210–218.

Webb, S. (1999). "Conformal intensity-modulated radiotherapy (IMRT) delivered by robotic linac—testing IMRT to the limit?" *Phys. Med. Biol.* 44:1639–1654.

Webb, S. *Intensity-Modulated Radiation Therapy.* (1st ed.) Bristol, UK: IOP Publishing, 2001.

Wong, J. W., and J. A. Purdy. (1990). "On methods of inhomogeneity corrections for photon transport. [Review]." *Med. Phys.* 17:807–814.

Wu, Y., D. Yan, M. B. Sharpe, B. Miller, and J. W. Wong. (2001). "Implementing multiple static field delivery for intensity modulated beams." *Med. Phys.* 28:2188–2197.

Yan, D., and D. Lockman. (2001). "Organ/patient geometric variation in external beam radiotherapy and its effects." *Med. Phys.* 28:593–602.

Yan, D., B. Xu, D. Lockman, K. Kota, D. S. Brabbins, J. Wong, and A. A. Martinez. (2001). "The influence of interpatient and intrapatient rectum variation on external beam treatment of prostate cancer." *Int. J. Radiat. Oncol. Biol. Phys.* 51:1111–1119.

Yu, C. X. (1995). "Intensity-modulated arc therapy with dynamic multileaf collimation: An alternative to tomotherapy." *Phys. Med. Biol.* 40:1435–1449.

Yu, C. X., M. J. Symons, M. N. Du, A. A. Martinez, and J, W. Wong. (1995). "A method for implementing dynamic photon beam intensity modulation using independent jaws and a multileaf collimator." *Phys. Med. Biol.* 40:769–787.

# Clinical Implementation Of IMRT Treatment Planning


**Gary A. Ezzell, Ph.D.**
Mayo Clinic Scottsdale
Scottsdale, Arizona




## Introduction

Once the IMRT system has been commissioned for accuracy, the problem remains of learning how to use it well. This is a nontrivial exercise, and one that challenges experienced treatment planners to develop a new set of skills. Indeed, a common lament of IMRT planners is a frustrated "How do I steer this thing?". The goals of this chapter are to illustrate some of the characteristics of inverse planning, point out some potential pitfalls, and suggest a process for developing expertise with this new way of thinking.

Inverse planning differs from conventional forward planning in its basic approach. When planning conventionally, the planner directly tries different solutions (i.e., beam combinations) and compares the resulting dose distribution to the desired outcome. When planning with an inverse system the planner tries different problem statements that the optimizer then turns into solutions. The planner influences the result indirectly. If the resulting dose distribution does not satisfy the clinical goal, the planner needs to change the way the problem is described so that the optimizer returns a better solution. Knowing what to change can be difficult, and sometimes the correct choice is counter-intuitive. For example, sometimes asking for less tissue sparing can result in more. There are reasons for this behavior, to be sure, and it is possible to develop an effective process and eventually an intuitive feel for inverse planning.

When discussing inverse planning, it is useful to differentiate between three concepts, all of which are sometimes called "prescription." The first is the statement of the clinical problem and the physician's goals. The second is the set of planning parameters entered into the radiotherapy treatment planning (RTP) system. The third is the final planned distribution that is accepted for treatment.

A naïve IMRT user might assume that he can enter the physician's goals into the inverse planning system and that the optimizer software will automatically return the best possible result that then can be used without further investigation. This assumption is likely to be wrong for three reasons. First, the clinical goals may not be achievable. Second, the overall problem may have been incompletely described to the planning system, so that the answer makes mathematical but not clinical sense. Or, the optimizer may return results that differ from the stated goals, requiring that the planning parameters be adjusted accordingly. In practice, all these problems frequently occur, so the inverse planning process is necessarily iterative.

This chapter will first describe some of the difficulties in adequately converting the clinical problem into planning parameters required by the inverse planning system. Then the discussion will turn to suggestions for learning how the system performs as planning parameters are changed. Finally, some aspects of overall clinical implementation of the IMRT plans are discussed.


## Modeling The Clinical Problem

All treatment planning is numerical modeling. We start with a numerical model of the patient, of the treatment unit and its radiation beams, and of the interactions of the radiation with the patient. In conventional planning, we choose the details of the beams to be applied and calculate the resulting dose distribution. We then compare the numerical model of the dose to our mental understanding of the clinical problem, and alter our choice of beams accordingly.

Inverse planning inserts another layer of numerical modeling into this process, and that is a model of "what we want to achieve." This model then chooses the details of the beams. This model is complicated. It includes descriptions of the target tissues, normal tissues, and uncertainties in their positions; dose and volume goals for these tissues; and the value judgments to be made in balancing competing goals. As complicated as the model is, it is not clairvoyant. Much that is implicit in conventional planning needs to be made explicit in this new model for the results to be clinically useful.

## Defining Targets

All targets need to be explicitly defined. To use the terminology of ICRU reports 50 and 62 (ICRU 1993, 1999), this includes the gross target volume (GTV) and the clinical target volume (CTV). The major difficulty comes in defining CTV regions, because the tumor there, by definition, is not imaged. The CTV includes areas of potential direct extension and lymph node spread. To define these areas to an inverse planner, physicians often need to convert their experience in drawing portal shapes on simulator films to drawing target volumes on computed tomography (CT) images. There are recent publications (Gregoire et al. 2000; Chao et al. 2002) that aid the clinician to recognize and contour lymph node levels in the head and neck region and to decide how much of the seminal vesicles to include for prostate irradiation (Kestin et al. 2002). Routine use of intravenous contrast agents may be needed in order to reliably distinguish nodes from vessels, and this may present a challenge for departments that manage their own CT simulators but have not implemented contrast injection. Contouring targets post-operatively is always challenging and may require image fusion with pre-operative images.

There is a real challenge in balancing the dangers of contouring too little and having a geographic miss and contouring so much that there are few normal tissues that can be spared. Contrast in the bladder may also be needed for accurate prostate definition. Distinguishing the base of the prostate from the bladder wall is difficult on CT without the use of contrast. In conventional planning, over-contouring the prostate base may not lead to excessive bladder complications, but if doses are escalated with IMRT, such may not be the case. In addition, if ultrasound is used to locate the prostate daily, then the accurate determination of the prostate base on CT becomes crucial. It is the interface between bladder and prostate that most clearly shows on ultrasound, and an overly generous CT contour could cause a systematic misalignment in the daily targeting.

Creating CTV expansions of the GTV to account for potential direct extension can also be problematic if automatic expansion tools are used. In some cases, internal barriers, such bony compartments, may limit the actual expansion. A human planner who is directly controlling beam shapes can trim the beams accordingly. When inverse planning, the CTV contours need to be trimmed to avoid targeting tissues unnecessarily. Note that the planning target volume (PTV) could cross such barriers, since that accounts for positioning uncertainty.

## Defining Normal Tissues

All tissues to be spared need to be explicitly defined. In conventional planning, physicians design ports to exclude tissues that need not be treated. For example, in many head and neck treatments, parallel-opposed lateral fields usually exclude the oral mucosa. If a parotid-sparing protocol is implemented using IMRT, then many other beam directions will be used, and significant dose may be given to the oral mucosa unless that area is explicitly contoured and assigned dose limits. Planners often need to define new avoidance regions in addition to well-established structures such a spinal cord or lenses.

Structures such as rectum, bladder, and lungs need to be defined consistently if dose-volume limits are to be used in planning. Requiring, for example, that no more than 30% of the rectum can receive more than 65 Gy implies that the entire rectum has been segmented. If the dose-volume limits are taken from the literature, then the structure needs to be segmented in a fashion that is consistent with the reference. This is less true for structures such as the spinal cord in which the dose is limited by localized hot spots, but very important for structures with large volume effects, such as the lung.

## Defining Margins

IMRT, like any other form of conformal radiotherapy, must take into account uncertainties in the location of targets and structures. ICRU reports 50 and 62 use the terms planning target volume (PTV) and planning organ at risk volume (PRV) to express this concept. Choosing the margins to use when expanding a CTV into a PTV requires decisions to be made about the uncertainties occasioned by internal organ motions and by daily setup variations. IMRT does not inherently demand or permit tight margins; in fact, the margins are determined by the patient, imaging technique, and immobilization technique and are independent of the type of beam delivery. However, since IMRT can be used to wrap dose around critical structures, the temptation may be strong to use tight margins in planning. The treatment team needs to make sure that the use of such tight margins is, in fact, justified. This may require changes in imaging to better define the anatomy, changes in immobilization, and changes in treatment verification, such as more frequent portal imaging.

The PTV concept is frequently not used in conventional planning. Instead, clinicians may be accustomed to designing fields with a particular block margin around the target. This is not the margin that should be used when inverse planning, however, since it includes the beam penumbra. The margins allocated to the PTV must not include the penumbra, because the optimizer will account for the penumbra when planning. Confusion about this point would cause the treated volumes to be unnecessarily large. Clinics that use margins to block edge can determine their effective PTV margins by inspecting conventional plans and measuring the distance from target to a specified isodose line, such as 99% or 95% of the isocenter dose. That distance corresponds to the PTV expansion, and the isodose value chosen would then represent the minimum dose to the PTV for IMRT planning of the same case.

## Targets In The Buildup Region

A special problem arises in inverse planning if targets are drawn or expand into the buildup region. In such a case, the inverse planner will see lower doses in that region and will increase localized beam intensities in order to increase them. This will likely have two deleterious effects. One is that the overall plan quality will likely diminish since those higher intensities will cause higher doses elsewhere in the patient. A second is that the patient's skin dose will be increased, probably more than represented by the plan since the effects of tangential beams and immobilization devices may not be well modeled in the dose calculations. This problem can be mitigated if the skin region, say 5 to 6 mm deep, is contoured as a separate structure and given dose limits (Lee et al. 2002). If the target really does extend close to the skin surface, then bolus should be used in that area so that the dose is well controlled. Whenever possible, it is best to image the patient with the bolus in place so that it is accurately represented.

## Different Targets Receiving Different Doses

It is common in radiotherapy for primary targets to receive larger total doses than secondary targets, and for this to be accomplished by shrinking fields so that each receives a standard daily dose. IMRT invites, and sometimes requires, that such targets be treated simultaneously over the same number of fractions. Hence, they receive different daily doses. The radiobiological consequences of that nonstandard fractionation need to be appreciated by the clinician, and the prescribed total doses perhaps changed accordingly (Mohan et al. 2000; Brahme 1999; Wu et al. 2002).

## Target Dose Inhomogeneity

With IMRT, doses to the primary target may be much less homogeneous than has been the norm in radiation oncology. The degree of inhomogeneity will depend on the concavity of the dose distribution and the slope of dose gradients required. Physicians will often be in unfamiliar territory in deciding how to balance competing risks. Acute reactions may increase with IMRT, especially in the head and neck region where the PTV often includes sensitive mucosa (Balter et al. 1999), although acute reactions may decrease with the use of IMRT for prostate treatments (Shu et al. 2001; Zelefsky et al. 2000). The risk of late complications because of higher maxima or of recurrences because of lower minima is unknown for many treatment sites. For that reason, it is important that dose distribution data be summarized so that any effect on outcome can be established.

## Defining Realistic Planning Goals

Inverse planning systems need a numerical model of "what is desired." Inverse planning is more likely to be successful if that model is realistic. Of course, the user does not know *a priori* what is achievable and may be tempted to ask for something that is overly optimistic. The problem with this approach is that the optimizer may not be steered toward useful plans if no plan looks good to it. For example, asking for no dose to the spinal cord may cause the system to regard a plan that gives 60 Gy to the cord to be better than one that gives 40 Gy, if some other constraint is better met by the 60 Gy plan.

One strategy for dealing with a new planning situation is to first develop a reasonable 3-D conformal plan and use it to establish the baseline for IMRT planning. Another is to refer to goals used by a relevant multi-institutional protocol, if one exists.

In any case, it is imperative that the clinician expresses to the planner what dose-volume criteria must be met for a plan to be acceptable and what criteria are to be optimized. (Of course, the physician's goals may change during the planning process once the possibilities and compromises become clearer.) For example, for a tumor near the spine, the clinician may define the problem thusly: keeping the cord dose to a maximum of 45 Gy, and the target dose uniformity to 15%, maximize the mean dose to the target. Or perhaps the cord and target doses will be specified, and the target dose uniformity is to be maximized. Compromises are nearly always needed for difficult planning problems, so the planner needs to understand the clinician's thinking so he can build the model of "what is desired" as well as possible. This need is not limited to IMRT, to be sure, but is inescapable with inverse planning.

Adding to the difficulty is the need to make decisions about dose-volume relationships at a level of detail that may be unfamiliar. Questions that may arise include:

How large a hotspot is clinically significant: a single voxel, 1 $cm^3$?

How much of the PTV can be allowed to receive less than the desired dose?

How much variation in target dose is acceptable?

For a particular normal structure (e.g., rectum), what dose-volume histogram (DVH) points most influence the outcome?

Only after such questions are answered can the planner begin to work on the clinical problem using the parameters offered by the inverse planning system.

## Dealing With A Plethora Of Planning Parameters

Once the clinical problem has been defined (volumes drawn, margins chosen, goals specified), the planner can then begin to select the various parameters used by the inverse planning system. Depending on the system employed, these may include:

1.  Dose-volume constraints for targets

2.  Dose-volume constraints for normal tissues

3.  Importance or weighting factors for these targets and tissues

4.  Beamlet size

5.  Beam energy

6.  Number of beams or arcs

7.  Beam directions or arc limits

8.  Number of intensity levels

9.  Delivery limitations, e.g., minimum monitor units (MUs) per segment or minimum segment dimensions

10. Delivery mechanism, e.g., static or dynamic MLC motion

11. Optimization method, e.g., gradient descent or simulated annealing

Clearly, choosing the best combination of these parameters is a non-trivial meta-optimization problem. A later section in the chapter suggests some exercises that can help a new user develop some experience with altering the parameters and observing the effects on plan quality and efficiency of delivery. However, many of these parameters interact non-linearly, and each new type of planning problem (prostate, head and neck, peri-spinal, brain, etc.) may have its own preferred subset of parameters. IMRT planning can be very efficient once the huge set of possibilities has been winnowed down, but getting to that point may require a significant investment in time.

## Choice Of Beam Directions

Choice of beam directions still matters for IMRT, especially if the number of fields is to be limited to fewer than seven. This has been demonstrated in a number of studies (Kulik et al. 2002; Price et al. 2002), and is actually intuitively reasonable. Choosing beam directions that separate the targets and critical structures means that less modulation will be required of the fields, resulting in more efficient plans, and almost certainly will improve factors such as target dose uniformity. Similarly, choosing collimator angles that reduce stair-step effects will improve planning.

## Plan Evaluation

Since the inverse planning system designs the beams and intensity patterns, there is the possibility of hotspots and cold spots occurring in unexpected areas. Inspection of DVHs will not necessarily identify troublesome areas, since all geometric information is removed. A cold spot in the center of the target will have the same effect on the DVH as the same cold spot on the periphery of the PTV, but the clinical impact could be quite different. Similarly, hot spots may occur in normal structures distant from the target. The isodose distribution on each imaging plane needs to be reviewed individually to look for such anomalies. If hot spots do occur in normal tissue outside of previously defined structures, then additional avoidance areas can be created to prevent them. It is useful, although not sufficient, to inspect the DVH for "all tissue not otherwise assigned to a structure," if the planning system permits such a calculation.

Another point with respect to plan evaluation relates to the question of whether IMRT should be used at all. IMRT is preferred if normal structures invaginate the target, but if the target is convex then forward-planned conformal beams may provide a better plan (Hsiung et al. 2002; Vineberg et al. 2002). In principle, inverse planning should always return a result at least as good as any forward-planned alternative (Chui and Spirou 2001), but this is certainly not true in these early days of inverse planning and IMRT. It is important to compare the IMRT and forward-planned alternatives on an equal basis: same targets, same margins, same acceptability criteria. It is not always easy if there are two planning systems involved that differ in their details of creating volumes and handling margins. Nevertheless, since IMRT delivery usually requires many more MU than conventional delivery, the IMRT plan should be sufficiently better to justify the decreased departmental efficiency, increased whole-body dose, and increased wear on the treatment unit.

## Dose Reporting

The reporting and documentation of the dose distribution should parallel the statement of the treatment goals. If the physician has determined acceptability criteria for specific organs (e.g., dose to 30% of the rectum to be less than 65 Gy and less than 2 cm$^3$ more than 80 Gy), then the plan report should tabulate those parameters. Target dose distributions also need to be summarized. Dose to a point, such as the isocenter, are less relevant than a statement of mean dose along with some indication of dose uniformity. For example, one might decide to report the minimum dose to the PTV, dose that covers 95% of the PTV, dose that covers 5% of the PTV, and maximum dose to the PTV. As mentioned above, the consequences of inhomogeneous target doses are not well known and should be a focus of clinical study.

## Building Experience With Inverse Planning Using Artificial Problems

This section suggests a series of exercises that can aid the user in building experience with inverse planning. The objective is to explore the capabilities and limitations of the system and observe how the various planning parameters impact plan quality and delivery efficiency. The exercises use a progression of geometries beginning from simple, idealized shapes. These exercises are, of course, only suggestions and would need to be customized to the characteristics of the specific planning system.

When embarking on these tests, it is useful to standardize some measures of plan quality. For example, target dose uniformity may be expressed in terms of ratio between the maximum and minimum points, or perhaps the ratio of the highest dose covering 5% of the target to that covering 95%.

### Simple Cylindrical Geometry

The first idealized shape is shown in figure 1. It is a cylindrical phantom with a single, cylindrical CTV at its center and four cylindrical critical structures. It can be used to perform baseline tests for situations in which the good results can be obtained with forward planning.

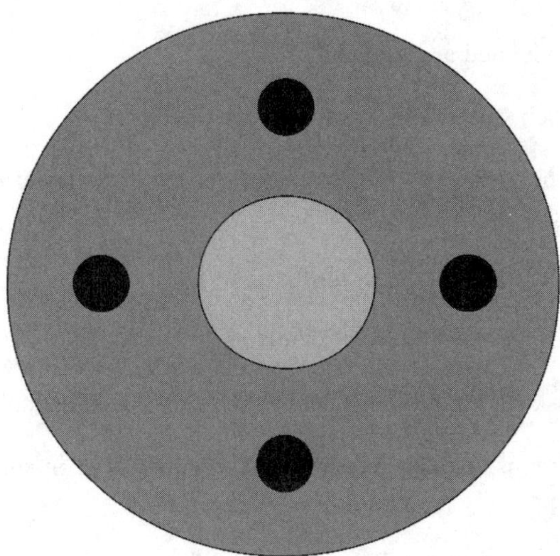

**Figure 1.** Cross section through a 20 cm diameter cylindrical phantom with a 6 cm central target and four 2 cm peripheral normal structures.

*With no constraints on the structures, can the IMRT system create dose uniformity for a single target and simple beam arrangements?*

Create a 10 mm PTV margin around the CTV. Initially, with no dose constraints set for the regions of interest, how does the system perform if it is asked to irradiate the target to a uniform dose? As a preliminary step, calculate a dose distribution with a forward plan so the limits on achievable uniformity are known.

    a.   Start with relaxed goals for target uniformity, e.g., –5% to +5% and three symmetrically arranged fields.

       How well do the DVHs for the CTV and PTV meet the stated DVH goals?

       Is the result more uniform than requested, the same, or less?

       What is the mean dose to the target?

       Where do hot and cold spots appear in the CTV and PTV?

       Where do hot spots appear in the surrounding tissue?

       If there are hot spots in tissue, can they be mitigated by imposing additional constraints?

       How modulated are the beams?

       How much variation is there between the beams?

       If there are delivery efficiency controls, how do they affect the plan quality and degree of modulation?

    b.   Increase the goals for target uniformity.

       If you ask for the achievable limits, are they found?

       If you ask for better than achievable results, what happens?

       If you impose absurd requirements, e.g., no dose in surrounding tissues, what happens?

    c.   Repeat the test with parallel-opposed fields.

       Can the inverse planning system impose symmetry on opposing beamlets?

    d.   Repeat the test with two fields at 90° from each other.

       Can the inverse planning system meet or beat the results for a wedged pair?

*How does the IMRT system behave with easily achievable constraints on the critical structures?*

a.  Impose equal dose constraints on the critical structures at 50% of the target dose. Use four fields at 45° intervals so that two irradiate the critical structures and two do not (e.g., 0°, 45°, 90°, and 135°).

   Does the inverse planning system return a result that mimics the obvious wedged pair solution?

   How large are the doses outside the targets? How does the result compare to a wedged pair?

   If the dose constraints are raised to 75% of the target dose, does the optimizer redistribute intensities to the beams that go through the structures or still heavily favor the fields that do not?

b.  Impose equal dose constraints on the critical structures at 20% of the target dose and moderate target dose uniformity. Use at least 9 equally spaced fields, preferably 15.

   How well do the DVHs for the structures match the constraints? Are the structures spared more than requested, less, or neither?

   Are the intensities distributed in an intuitive fashion?

   Do hot spots occur in the normal tissue between the structures? Can they be suppressed by changing tissue parameters or defining additional structures?

   How is the dose uniformity to the target affected? Can it be improved if tighter uniformity criteria are imposed?

   If you impose more restrictive constraints on one of the structures, how are the DVHs affected?

   How low can you drive the dose to one of the structures?

## C-shaped target

The next series of tests uses the geometry of figure 2. It has a cylindrical phantom, a central cylindrical critical structure, and a C-shaped target partially surrounding it with a 10 mm gap between them.

   Starting with 15 equally spaced fields, 10 intensity levels, a 5 mm expansion for the PTV and no expansion for the structure, test how the target uniformity and structure dose varies with increasing constraints on the structure.

**Gary A. Ezzell**

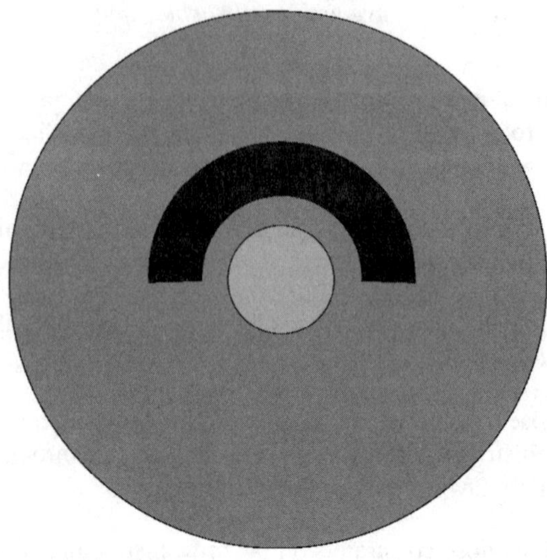

**Figure 2.** Cross section through a 20 cm diameter cylindrical phantom with a 4 cm central target and C-shaped normal structure, 2 cm in thickness, spaced 1 cm from the target.

   a.  For a structure goal of 50% of the target dose, how do the target and structure DVH change with parameters such as importance factors or the shape of the structure DVH constraint?

       Physics requires a dose gradient across the structure. How does the plan quality vary as the structure DVH constraint becomes unrealistic?

   b.  Starting with a structure dose limit of 50% of the target, how do the target and structure DVH change as the structure dose limit is decreased?

       Does relaxing the target dose uniformity constraints influence the result?

   c.  Keeping the other factors constant, how do the target and structure DVHs change as the number of fields is reduced.

       How does the required number of fields needed to achieve a certain degree of target dose uniformity change as the difference between target and structure doses increases?

   d.  Keeping the other factors constant, how do the target and structure DVHs change as the number of intensity levels is increased or decreased? What is the effect on the number of segments and MUs?

   e.  Keeping the other factors constant, how do the target and structure DVHs change as the beamlet size is changed? What is the effect on the number of segments and MUs?

For 10 mm beamlets, does shifting the isocenter by 2.5 or 5 mm affect the plan quality?

f.  If you change the geometry so that the PTV overlaps the structure, which is given priority by the optimizer? Can that be changed?

How is the overlap region handled when reporting the DVH? Is it associated with one or the other structure or both?

Can an uncertainty margin be associated with a critical structure, creating a PRV?

g.  If you change the geometry to demand more concavity or tighter margins, how is plan quality affected?

Are more beams required to achieve acceptable target dose uniformity?

What target dose uniformity can be achieved?

## Target In Buildup Region

Figure 3 shows a cylindrical phantom with an off-center target that is 10 mm from the nearest surface. Develop five-field plans using the beam direction on the phantom-target axis and ±30° and ±60° from it.

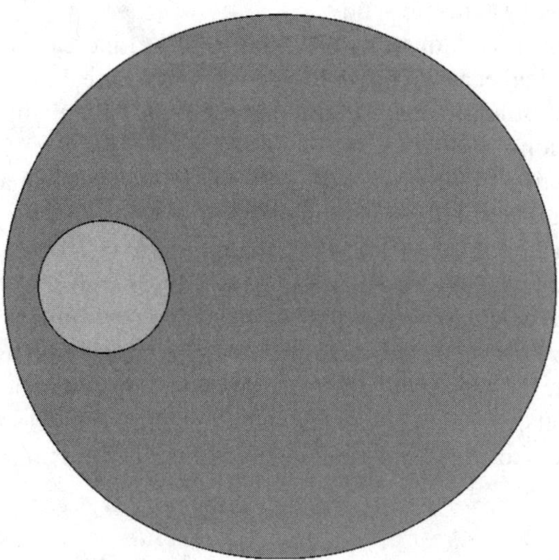

**Figure 3.** Cross section through a 20 cm diameter cylindrical phantom with a 6 cm target placed 1 cm from the surface.

a. How does the plan quality change as you increase the PTV expansion from 0 to 10 mm?

b. Can you improve the plan quality by defining a skin region and assigning it dose limits?

How thick does that skin region need to be to be effective?

## Comments On These Idealized Tests

Experienced planners will likely begin these exercises with some expectations about how the inverse planning system will behave. One might expect that given a simple problem, the inverse planner would find the obvious simple solution. If it does not, the reason may well be that the "simple" problem has implicit characteristics that have not been adequately represented in the numerical model of "what we want to achieve." For example, if the user specifies target goals only, the optimizer may throw significant hot spots in distant normal tissue because it has not been told that this is a bad thing to do. Working on these simple problems can be instructive because it can help the new user understand how to model the complete clinical situation.

On the other hand, it may also be the case that the optimizer will never settle on a solution as simple as intuition suggests. This might be caused by details of the cost function or search algorithm that are hidden from the user. It would certainly be useful and interesting to know how the optimizer would evaluate the forward planned alternative in terms of the elements of its cost function. That is a feature not often available on inverse planning systems presently.

One would also expect that the plan quality would increase with the number of fields applied (Pirzkall et al. 2002). This may not be the case, however, if adding more fields increases the solution space to the point that the optimizing algorithm fails to find the best solutions.

Careful inspection of where low doses in the PTV occur can also be instructive. One would expect them to occur near the critical structures. If they also occur along edges distant from the structures, then that would seem to be an unnecessary deficiency that would need to be handled by increasing the PTV margins.

In general, one would expect that the difficulty of the problem would increase as the required concavity increases and/or the slope of the required dose gradient increases (Hunt et al. 2002). More difficult problems should benefit from more beams, more intensity levels, or smaller beamlets (although that would need to be confirmed) at the cost of increased complexity and decreased target dose uniformity.

## An Approach To Developing An Inverse Planning Protocol For A Particular Disease Site

The previous exercises will give a new user some basic experience with inverse planning. With that in hand, efforts can then be focused on developing an inverse planning protocol for the particular disease site(s) of interest to the department.

Most of these topics were discussed earlier in this chapter, so here is simply a sequential list of the tasks to be performed. Note that these tasks relate specifically to planning; other elements of clinical implementation are discussed in the section on clinical implementation.

a.  Determine conventions for defining targets and structures.

b.  Determine margins.

c.  Decide on the criteria for determining an acceptable plan.

   Dose-volume criteria for target.

   Dose-volume criteria for structures.

d.  Decide on the element(s) of the dose distribution to be optimized (e.g., dose to 50% of parotids).

e.  Develop a 3-D conformal forward plan that would be the alternative treatment were IMRT not used. This helps to set baseline expectations and gives a starting point for DVH constraints.

f.  Systematically work through different combinations of planning parameters, documenting the combinations tried and the results. Start with relaxed constraints and gradually tighten them.

g.  Repeat the process on enough patients to establish a robust methodology.

The outcome of this process should be:

a.  A type of class solution in which many of the possible planning parameters have been specified and will be rarely changed, and

b.  A sense of which planning parameters can be used to efficiently drive the solution in a desired direction for individual patients.

The results of such a process have been published for prostate irradiation (Ezzell, Schild, and Wong 2001).

# Clinical Implementation Of IMRT

Implementing IMRT impacts all members of the radiation oncology staff: physicians, physicists, dosimetrists, therapists, schedulers, etc. From the outset, an implementation team should be established to plan, execute, and review IMRT procedures. The many aspects to consider have been discussed at length in the IMRT subcommittee report *Guidance Document on Delivery, Treatment Planning, and Clinical Implementation of IMRT* (Ezzell et al. 2003):

a. Equipment and space requirements

b. Time and personnel requirements

c. Changes in treatment planning practice

d. Changes in treatment delivery practice

e. Quality assurance of equipment and individual patient treatments

f. Staff training and patient education

g. Changes in scheduling, billing, and charting practice

h. Overall integration

This section highlights some of the most important elements.

## Immobilization And Localization

The team will need to consider how the patients are to be immobilized for treatment. If the implementation of IMRT is part of a new emphasis on high-precision radiotherapy, then there may be new immobilization devices and techniques to be mastered. Part of this process should be a quantitative assessment of the positioning uncertainty associated with the technique. Such an assessment may be needed for well-established techniques as well as to justify any proposed reduction in treatment margins.

If the patient is to be imaged daily for target localization (e.g., with ultrasound, CT, or electronic portal imaging) then that process will need to be validated and the operators trained.

## Imaging For Planning

Imaging for IMRT planning may be more demanding because of the need to use contrast agents in CT and/or images from other modalities. In addition, CT images may need to be taken at finer increments to better define anatomy and to produce good quality digitally reconstructed radiographs (DRRs). More slices may be needed to cover the entire range of potential beam entry if non-axial beams are considered.

Patient preparation for the imaging procedure may change as well, especially if margins are to be reduced. For example, a long-standing practice of putting contrast in the rectum may systematically displace the prostate enough to be a concern if doses are increased and margins decreased.

## Portal Imaging During Treatment And Isocenter Verification

The department will need to decide how intensity-modulated fields are to be filmed. Many treatment systems permit the filming of the outer bounding shape of the MLC field, and this can be compared to DRRs from the planning system. Note that if each field's intensity patterns are separately verified, there is still the need to ensure that the field is properly oriented with respect to the patient.

An element of the process should be isocenter verification with orthogonal fields, even if those fields are not used for treatment. It is critical that those images be checked against DRRs of similar fields generated by the inverse planning system for the treatment geometry used in the plan. There is always the possibility that the isocenter was shifted during the planning, either deliberately or inadvertently, from its original location. If that shift is not implemented, then serious treatment errors could occur. Such a shift would not be recognized if the portal image is compared to the original simulator image.

## Transfer Of Information From The Planning
## To The Delivery System

The safe delivery of complex IMRT treatments requires that the field parameters and multileaf collimator (MLC) sequences be accurately transferred from the planning system to the delivery system. This is best accomplished using electronic methods that minimize the need for human transcription of data. The implementation team should validate and mandate the use all available methods to reduce this source of error.

## Quality Assurance

A comprehensive discussion of IMRT QA is beyond the scope of this chapter, but there are some points to be made here relevant to the overall issue of clinical implementation. The first point is that implementing IMRT does require additional tests of the delivery system (i.e., accelerator and MLC) to be incorporated into routine practice — daily, weekly, monthly, and annually. Time and resources need to be allocated to these tasks. Furthermore, the quality assurance for each patient is significantly more time-consuming for IMRT than for conventional treatments. Time and resources also need to be allocated to these tasks. Finally, periodic review of IMRT procedures is an important element of quality assurance. Of course, this is true for radiation oncology and medicine in general, but it is especially necessary for processes that are new and rapidly changing. New software versions of planning systems and delivery systems may make new tools available, eliminate some sources of error, and create others. The implementation team should not stop meeting after the first patient is treated.

## Maintenance And Downtime

IMRT puts more demands on the linear accelerator and MLC components, and this may impact the frequency of maintenance, both planned and unplanned. Clinics may want to invest in more staff training and spare parts in order to cope with unexpected problems. A backup plan should be established to handle the situation of an IMRT-capable machine being unavailable for an extended time.

## Training

This chapter explained a number of ways in which IMRT planning differs from conventional planning. Other chapters have concentrated on how IMRT delivery differs from conventional delivery. These differences can accrue to the patient's advantage or detriment, depending on how well they are understood, mastered, and controlled. Initial education of physicians, physicists, and other allied health staff is needed to implement IMRT successfully, and continued education will be necessary as IMRT evolves.

## References


Brahme, A. (1999). "Optimized radiation therapy based on radiobiological objectives." *Semin. Radiat. Oncol.* 9(1):35–47.

Butler, E. B., B. A. Teh, W. H. Grant III, B. M. Uhl, R. B. Kuppersmith, J. K. Chiu, D. T. Donovan, and S. Y. Woo. (1999). "Smart (simultaneous modulated accelerated radiation therapy) boost: A new accelerated fractionation schedule for the treatment of head and neck cancer with intensity modulated radiotherapy." *Int. J. Radiat. Oncol. Biol. Phys.* 45:21–32.

Chao, K. S., F. J. Wippold, G. Ozyigit, B. N. Tran, and J. F. Dempsey. (2002). "Determination and delineation of nodal target volumes for head-and-neck cancer based on patterns of failure in patients receiving definitive and postoperative IMRT." *Int. J. Radiat. Oncol. Biol. Phys.* 53(5):1174–1184.

Chui, C. S., and S. V. Spirou. (2001). "Inverse planning algorithms for external beam radiotherapy." *Med. Dosim.* 26:189–197.

Ezzell, G. A., S. E. Schild, and W.W. Wong. (2001). "Development of a treatment planning protocol for prostate treatments using intensity modulated radiotherapy." *J. Appl. Clin. Med. Phys.* 2:59–68.

Ezzell, G. A., D. Low, J. R. Palta, I. Rosen, M. B. Sharpe, P. Xia, Y. Xiao, L. Xing, C. X. Yu, and J. M. Galvin. (2003). "Guidance document on delivery, treatment planning, and clinical implementation of IMRT: Report of the IMRT Subcommittee of the AAPM Radiation Therapy Committee." *Medical Physics.* In press.

Gregoire, V., E. Coche, G. Cosnard, M. Hamoir, and H. Reychler. (2000). "Selection and delineation of lymph node target volumes in head and neck conformal radiotherapy. Proposal for standardizing terminology and procedure based on the surgical experience." *Radiother. Oncol.* 56:135–150.

Hsiung, C. Y., E. D. Yorke, C. S. Chui, J. Hu, J. P. Xiong, M. A. Hunt, C. C. Ling, E. Y. Huang, C. C. Sung, Y. J. Huang, C. J. Wang, H. C. Chen, S. A. Yeh, H. C. Hsu, and H. I. Amols. (2002). "Intensity modulated radiation therapy versus conventional three-dimensional conformal radiotherapy for the boost or salvage treatment of nasopharyngeal carcinoma." *Int. J. Radiat. Oncol. Biol. Phys.* 53(3):638–647.

Hunt, M. A., C. Hsiung, S. V. Spirou, C. Chui, H. I. Amols, and C. C. Ling. (2002). "Evaluation of concave dose distributions created using an inverse planning system." *Int. J. Radiat. Oncol. Biol. Phys.* 54:953–962.

ICRU Report 50. Prescribing, Recording and Reporting Photon Beam Therapy. Washington, DC: International Commission on Radiation Units and Measurements, 1993.

ICRU Report 62. Prescribing, Recording and Reporting Photon Beam Therapy. Supplement to ICRU Report 50. Washington, DC: International Commission on Radiation Units and Measurements, 1999.

Kestin, L. L., N. S. Goldstein, F. A. Vicini, D. Yan, H. J. Korman, and A. A. Martinez. (2002). "Treatment of prostate cancer with radiotherapy: Should the entire seminal vesicles be included in the clinical target volume?" *Int. J. Radiat. Oncol. Biol. Phys.* 54:686–697.

Kulik, C., J.-M. Caudrelier, M. Vermandel, B. Castelain, S. Mauoche, and J. Rosseau. (2002). "Conformal radiotherapy optimization with micromultileaf collimators: Comparison with radiosurgery techniques." *Int. J. Radiat. Oncol. Biol. Phys.* 53:1038–1050.

Lee, N., C. Chuang, J. Quivey, T. Philips, P. Akazawa, L. Verhey, and P. Xia. (2002). "Skin toxicity due to intensity-modulated radiotherapy for head-and-neck carcinoma." *Int. J. Radiat. Oncol. Biol. Phys.* 53:630–637.

Mohan, R., Q. Wu, M. Manning, and R. Schmidt-Ullrich. (2000). "Radiobiological considerations in the design of fractionation strategies for intensity-modulated radiation therapy of head and neck cancers." *Int. J. Radiat. Oncol. Biol. Phys* 46(3):619–630.

Pirzkall, A., M. P. Carol, B. Pickett, P. Xia, M. Roach III, and L. J. Verhey. (2002). "The effect of beam energy and number of fields on photon-based IMRT for deep-seated targets." *Int. J. Radiat. Oncol. Biol. Phys.* 53:434–442.

Price Jr. R. A., G. E. Hanks, S. W. McNeeley, E. M. Horwitz, and W. H. Pinover. (2002). "Advantages of using noncoplanar vs. axial beam arrangements when treating prostate cancer with intensity-modulated radiation therapy and the step-and-shoot delivery method." *Int. J. Radiat. Oncol. Biol. Phys.* 53:236–243.

Shu, H. K., T. T. Lee, E. Vigneauly, P. Xia, B. Pickett, T. L. Phillips, and M. Roach. (2001). "Toxicity following high-dose three-dimensional conformal and intensity-modulated radiation therapy for clinically localized prostate cancer." *Urol.* 57:102–107.

Vineberg, K. A., A. Eisbruch, M. M. Coselmon, D. L. McShan, M. L. Kessler, and B. A. Fraass. (2002). "Is uniform target dose possible in IMRT plans in the head and neck?" *Int. J. Radiat. Oncol. Biol. Phys.* 52:1159–1172.

Wu, Q., R. Mohan, A. Niemierko, and R. Schmidt-Ullrich. (2002). "Optimization of intensity-modulated radiotherapy plans based on the equivalent uniform dose." *Int. J. Radiat. Oncol. Biol. Phys.* 52:224–235.

Zelefsky, M. J., Z. Fuks, L. Happersett, H. J. Lee, C. C. Ling, C. M. Burman, M. Hunt, T. Wolfe, E. S. Venktraman, A. Jackson, M. Skwarchuk, and S. A. Leibel. (2000). "Clinical experience with intensity modulated radiation therapy (IMRT) in prostate cancer." *Radiother. Oncol.* 55(3):241–249.

# Patient-Specific Quality Assurance In IMRT

**Ping Xia, Ph.D., and Cynthia Chuang, Ph.D.**
Department of Radiation Oncology
University of California at San Francisco
San Francisco, California



## Introduction

Intensity-modulated radiation therapy (IMRT) is an advanced form of three-dimensional conformal therapy (3DCRT). Unlike conventional conformal therapy, the beam intensity of each IMRT field is modulated in a rather complex way. Delivery of intensity-modulated fields relies on the use of computer controlled multileaf collimators (MLCs) equipped on modern linear accelerators. Because of the complex beam intensity modulation, each IMRT field often includes many small, irregular, off-axis fields resulting in isodose distributions for each IMRT plan that are more conformal to the tumor target volume than those from conventional treatment plans. These features impose new requirements for quality assurance (QA) in IMRT delivery, including machine-specific and patient-specific issues. This chapter is focused on issues of patient-specific QA.

## Procedure Of IMRT Treatment

Figure 1 is a flow chart for an IMRT procedure. Similar to conventional conformal therapy, processes of IMRT treatment include treatment setup, patient immobilization, computed tomography (CT) image acquisition, treatment planning, treatment verification, and the actual treatment. In the following sections, we will discuss each process, emphasizing special considerations for patient-specific QA in IMRT treatment.

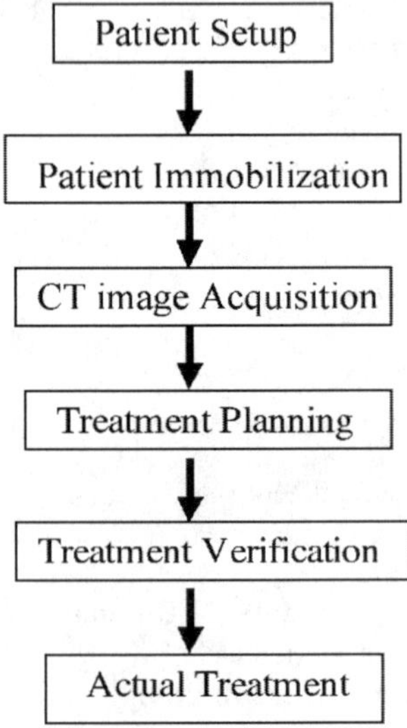


**Figure 1.** An IMRT procedure flow chart.

## Treatment Setup And Patient Positioning

During treatment setup, patients should be in a comfortable position since IMRT treatment may take longer than conventional treatment. The location of the isocenter is usually placed at the center of the tumor volume if IMRT is delivered with conventional MLCs. If IMRT is delivered with an add-on collimator, placement of the isocenter should also consider clearance between the patient and the add-on collimator. For example, if IMRT is delivered with the MIMiC® collimator (NOMOS Corporation, Cranberry Township, PA) utilizing arcs of more than 200 degrees; the distance from the treatment couch to the isocenter should be less than 14 cm when treated with a Siemens linear accelerator to prevent a gantry-couch collision.

## Patient Immobilization

Stringent patient immobilization is required for IMRT treatments because IMRT plans are highly conformal and often include high-dose gradient regions at the boundaries between the tumor and sensitive structures. Dosimetric effect of patient movement and setup uncertainties in IMRT treatment are greater than those in conventional treatment (will be discussed in the next section).

At our institution, we have introduced an index patient positioning method for IMRT treatment, particularly for head and neck IMRT. Figure 2 shows a base plate (S-type board, Med-Tec Inc., Orange City, IA) for a head-neck-shoulder mask that can be directly connected to the treatment couch, as well as to the CT couch top. The location of the S-type board on the couch is indexed. Figure 3 shows a head and neck cancer patient immobilized with the head-neck-shoulder mask, with part of the neck mask removed. Indexing patient positioning simplifies the treatment setup procedure, thus reducing the probability of setup error. Moreover, it prevents large patient movement during treatment. Using this S-type board made of carbon fiber, we are able to set up a patient's head-neck-shoulder region suspended at one end of the treatment couch, as shown in figure 2, allowing us to have access to all coplanar beam angles. This beam angle accessibility is particularly important for head and neck IMRT treatment since seven to nine coplanar beam angles are often used at our institution. The attenuation through the board is approximately 2% to 3% with a 6 MV photon beam.

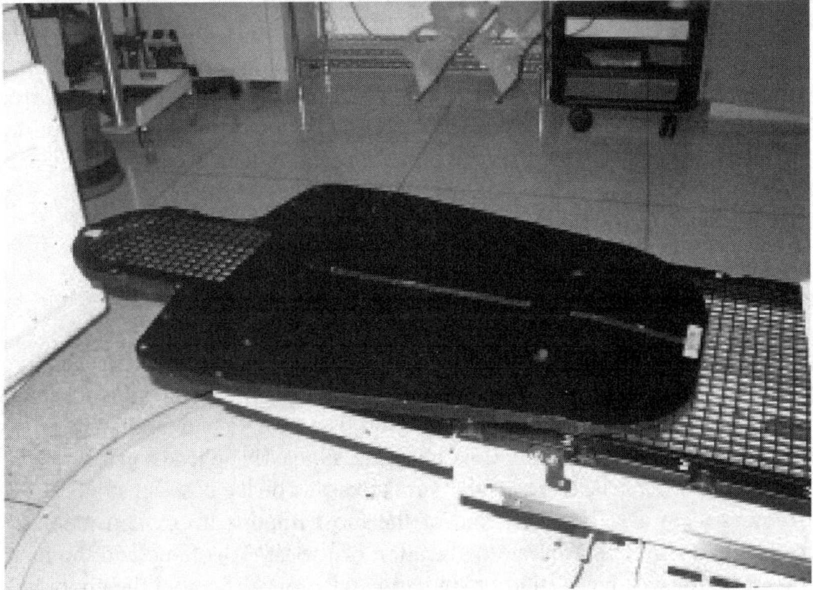

**Figure 2.** The base plate (S-type board, Med-Tec) used for a head-neck-shoulder mask.

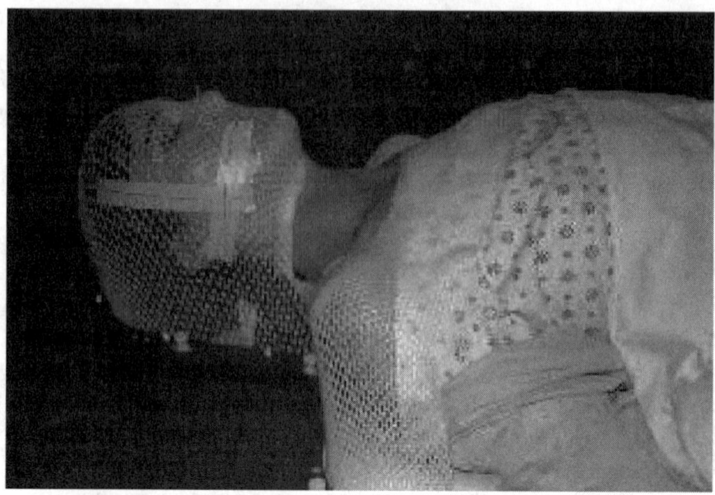

**Figure 3.** A head and neck cancer patient immobilized using the head-neck-shoulder mask, with part of the neck mask removed.

## CT Acquisition

In IMRT, especially in inverse planned IMRT, delineation of the target volume and its nearby sensitive structures becomes very important because the computer optimization process in inverse planning critically depends on the accuracy of this information. In treatment planning CT acquisition, thinner image slice (i.e., 3 mm) is preferred for IMRT treatment so that radiation oncologists and treatment planners can outline the tumor volume and sensitive structures more accurately. Furthermore, thinner image slice is also preferred for the creation of better quality digitally reconstructed radiographs (DRRs).

## Treatment Planning

Treatment planning of IMRT can be done via forward or inverse planning. The forward planning method is the same as conventional 3DCRT planning, except that each beam direction may consist of two or more subfields. The inverse planning concept is very different from the conventional 3DCRT planning. It heavily depends on the delineation of target volume and the nearby sensitive structures, and on the dose constraints imposed upon these structures. Therefore, one of the most important QA considerations in inverse planned IMRT is accurate delineation of the target volume and the involved sensitive structures. At our institution, radiation oncologists contour the tumor volume directly on the treatment planning station. The treatment planners contour the involved sensitive structures, which are verified by the attending radiation oncologist.

Although facilitated by computer optimization, inverse-planned IMRT plans are not always optimal. The choice of objective functions and the specification of dose constraints are two key components in obtaining an optimal plan in inverse planning. In addition, during plan evaluation, examination of dose-volume histograms (DVHs) alone is not sufficient. It is necessary to carefully exam isodose distributions on each axial slice, and pay particular attention to hot and cold spots.

## Treatment Verification

### Treatment Information Transfer

Prior to patient treatment, it is essential that all treatment data, including beam configuration and patient information, be directly sent through a local network from a treatment planning system to a record and verify (R&V) system. Initially, it is necessary to verify that there is no treatment information lost or modified during this data transferring process. Due to incorrect default settings in some R&V systems, it is possible that the transferred data could be lost or altered.

### Patient Setup Verification

With the use of CT simulation during the initial patient setup, a second patient setup verification may be omitted in some situations, provided the treatment isocenter is the same as the CT isocenter. If the treatment isocenter is different from the initial CT isocenter, a patient setup verification procedure is necessary to shift the marked isocenter from the CT isocenter to the treatment isocenter. A second set of orthogonal simulation films is taken using the treatment isocenter. This set of simulation films is compared with the orthogonal DRRs of the treatment isocenter created from the treatment planning system or from the CT simulator, to assure that this newly shifted isocenter agrees with the treatment isocenter. At our institution, this patient setup verification procedure is performed for most of our patients, regardless of whether the treatment isocenter is the same as the CT isocenter or not. If there is no isocenter shift, we use this procedure to verify patient setup reproducibility.

### First-Day Treatment Verification

On the first day of treatment, the treatment isocenter is re-verified on the treatment couch. For conventional treatment, the block shapes would also be verified at the same time. For IMRT treatment, whether or not to verify and record the intensity patterns on film is debatable. The physician may like to view and record the treatment regions, similar to the conventional treatment. However, using any commercially available films, it is difficult to obtain a good quality image with an intensity pattern superimposed on the patient anatomy information. For example, if IMRT is delivered with static MLC, an intensity pattern is composed of a series of segments, each assigned with a different monitor unit (MU). Directly delivering the treatment intensity pattern to any type of commercially available films cannot obtain an image with good contrast for both the intensity pattern and patient anatomy, even with an added open field using up to 5 MUs at the end of each beam direction. Alternatively, using the regular portal film, one can record the outer boundary of the intensity pattern as a substitute for the block shape in conventional treatment, although the intensity variation across the field is not recorded. Unfortunately, most commercial treatment planning systems do not provide tools for obtaining a special field (let us say portal film field) with the outside boundary of each intensity pattern. Some institutions have developed in-house software to create such a special portal film field for each beam direction. At our institution, we tape a ready-pack EDR2 film on the reticle for each beam direction, obtain a fluence intensity pattern without patient anatomy, and compare it to the printed map, as shown in figure 4. Simple visual inspection of the fluence map can easily reveal gross errors in treatment delivery or field identification. The advantages of this method are that there is no need to create special portal fields and it can be done during the treatment. The drawback of this method is that physicians cannot view the intensity pattern in relationship with the patient anatomy.

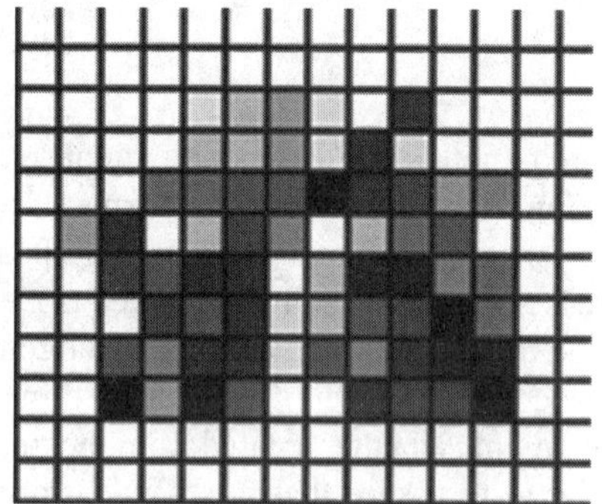 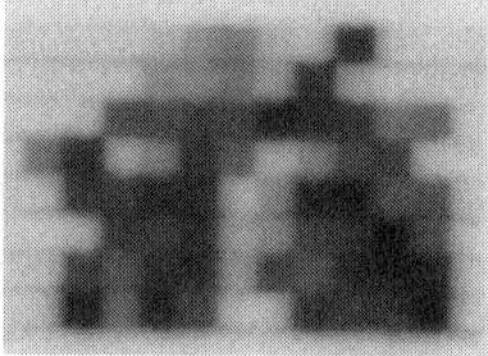

**Figure 4.** A comparison of a printed and a measurement fluence map.
(a) A printed fluence map produced by the planning system;
(b) a fluence intensity pattern from an EDR2 film taped to the reticle.

## Isocenter Verification Frequency

Early in the course of treatment, patients are often nervous and unaccustomed to their treatment positions. At our institution, the treatment isocenter is verified every day for the first 3 days of the treatment, and every week thereafter.

## Patient-Specific Dosimetric Verification

Patient-specific dosimetric verification includes phantom plan verification and an independent MU check. For each IMRT plan, a dosimetric check at multiple specific points in a phantom is currently required to ensure that each treatment portal of each treatment plan is correct. A patient-specific phantom plan is created within the treatment planning system using the beam configurations of the patient plan but recalculated with the phantom geometry, a feature now present in most IMRT treatment planning systems. The phantom plan can be measured using a single or multiple ionization chambers, in conjunction with diodes, thermoluminescent dosimeters (TLDs), and/or film. Such measurements are best made in regions with relatively uniform dose intensity to prevent errors caused by small displacements in dosimeter positions. Similarly, smaller volume dosimeters are preferred. At our institution, we have chosen to use a 0.147 cc (IC-10, Wellhöffer Dosimetries, Schwarzenbruck, Germany) ionization chamber to measure the high dose region. For other dose regions, we usually use metal oxide semiconductor field effect transistor (MOSFET) detectors for dosimetric verifications, except for special cases in which film measurement might be required.

## MOSFET Dosimeter

The MOSFET dosimeter offers several advantages over conventional dosimeters, including its small detector size (approximately 0.04 mm$^2$), and a simple and fast readout process as compared to either TLDs or film. In addition, with the commercial MOSFET system, multiple detectors can be used simultaneously. Figure 5 shows the photograph of a patient dose verification system TNRD50 (Thomson & Nielson, Ottawa, Canada). It includes the reader, the bias box, and five MOSFETs. To evaluate the feasibility of MOSFET for routine IMRT dosimetry, a comprehensive set of experiments has been reported (Chuang, Verhey, and Xia 2002), to investigate the stability, linearity, energy, and angular dependence of the MOSFETs. It showed that the MOSFETs presented a linear response from dose range of 0.3 Gy to 4.2 Gy. The measured dose variation from 0° to 180° is about 2.5%.

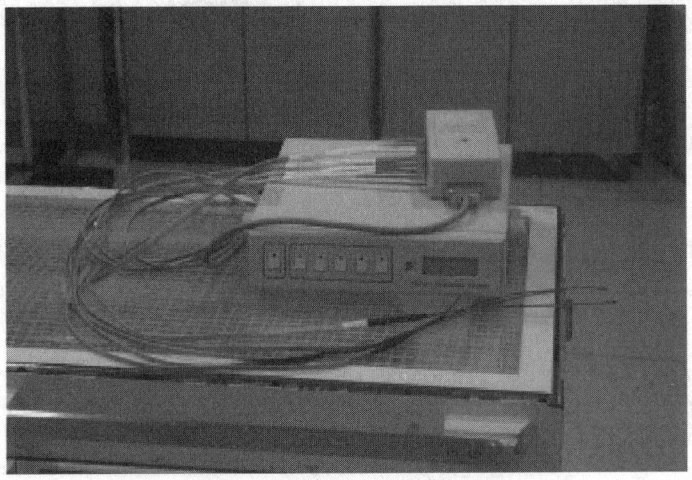

**Figure 5.** A photograph of a patient dose verification system TNRD50 (Thomson & Nielson, Ottawa, Canada).

   **Ping Xia and Cynthia Chuang**

## EDR2 Film

A new ready-pack film with enhanced dynamic range from Eastman Kodak (Eastman Kodak Co., Rochester, NY) is the EDR2 film, different from the XV2 film from the same company. The EDR2 film has an AgBr grain size of 1/10 and is more uniform in shape than those used for XV2 film. In addition, the silver content of the EDR2 is about one-half that of the XV2 film, significantly lowering the sensitivity of the film, thus increasing the dynamic range of the film. It has been reported that this new film has a larger dynamic range, from 0 up to 700 cGy (Olch 2002). Furthermore, due to the reduced sliver content and smaller grain size, the problem of energy dependence in EDR film is reported to be reduced. Because of its large dynamic range, EDR2 film can be used to measure the same daily fraction dose as delivered to the patient, without saturation (Esthappan et al. 2002; Olch 2002; Zhu et al. 2002). It is also reported that the EDR2 film is more resistant to film processor condition changes than the XV2 film.

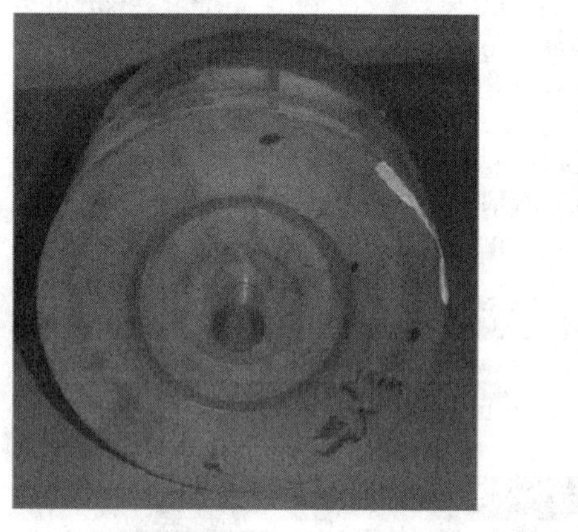
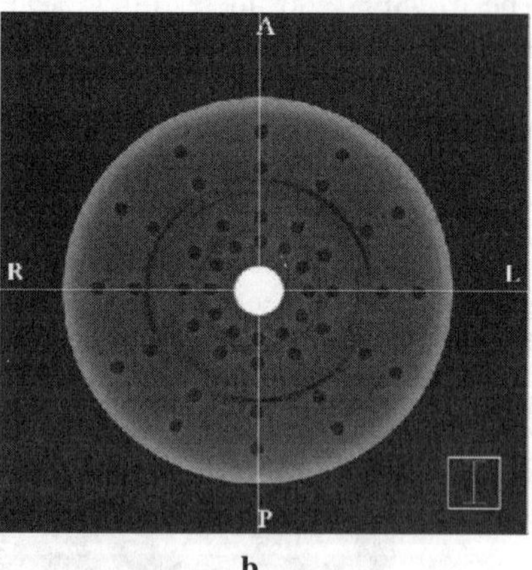


a.    b.

**Figure 6.** (a) A photograph of a concentric cylindrical acrylic phantom.
(b) An axial image of the phantom with ion chamber insertion in the middle
and 48 possible MOSFET placement locations.

## Phantoms

Figure 6 shows a concentric cylindrical phantom made of acrylic. At the center is the insertion location for an ionization chamber (IC-10, Wellhöffer Dosimetries, Schwarzenbruck, Germany). Forty-eight smaller circles (3 mm diameter) represent the possible locations for MOSFETs. The center cylinder is an ionization chamber holder, which can be moved in and out along the axis. The longitudal locations of MOSFETs are fixed.

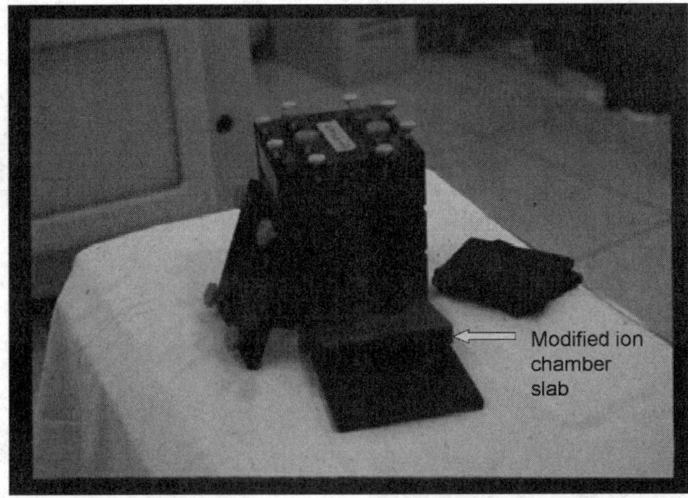


**Figure 7.** A box phantom made of solid water that is lightproof
(NOMOS Corporation) with a modified plate for ion chamber measurement.

Figure 7 shows a box phantom made of solid water that has previously been used
for IMRT dosimetric verification studies (Low et al. 1998b). The phantom manufactured by NOMOS (NOMOS Corporation, Cranberry Township, PA) is designed as a
light proof film phantom. Films can be loaded in axial, coronal, or sagittal orientation
in a dark room. With one side-wall of the box phantom removed and a home-made
solid-water slab with an ion chamber hole in it, this modified box phantom can also
be used for ion chamber measurement. At our institution, this box phantom is primarily used for phantom measurements for small tumors in the brain or head and neck
regions. For small tumors, it is often difficult to find multiple measurement points that
are located in relatively uniform dose regions, thus one point dose measurement with
an ion chamber in conjunction with film measurement is used.

Figure 8a shows a large phantom made by stacking together 30 cm of solid-water
slabs, each with a $30 \times 30$ cm$^2$ cross sectional area. A special 1.0 cm thick slab was
drilled with a slit at the center that is 1 cm in width and 15 cm in length from the edge
of the slab (shown in figure 8b), for an ion chamber placement. This slot allows the
ionization chamber with a buildup cap to slide in and out in the superior to inferior
direction. Additional small blocks of 1, 2, 3, 4, 5 cm in length can be used to fill the
space between the tip of the ion chamber to the to edge of the slot. Another special
1.0 cm slab was drilled with 81 holes (3 mm width $\times$ 7 mm length $\times$ 3 mm height)
arranged at an equal spacing of 3 cm for MOSFET dosimeter, as shown in figure 8c.
To identify these possible MOSFET locations in the treatment planning system, small
staples were placed in the slits during CT image acquisition. This large solid-water
phantom is used for dose measurement of large tumors in the thorax and the abdominal regions. The measurement can be conducted using a combination of an ion
chamber with five or more MOSFETs, or an ion chamber with films.

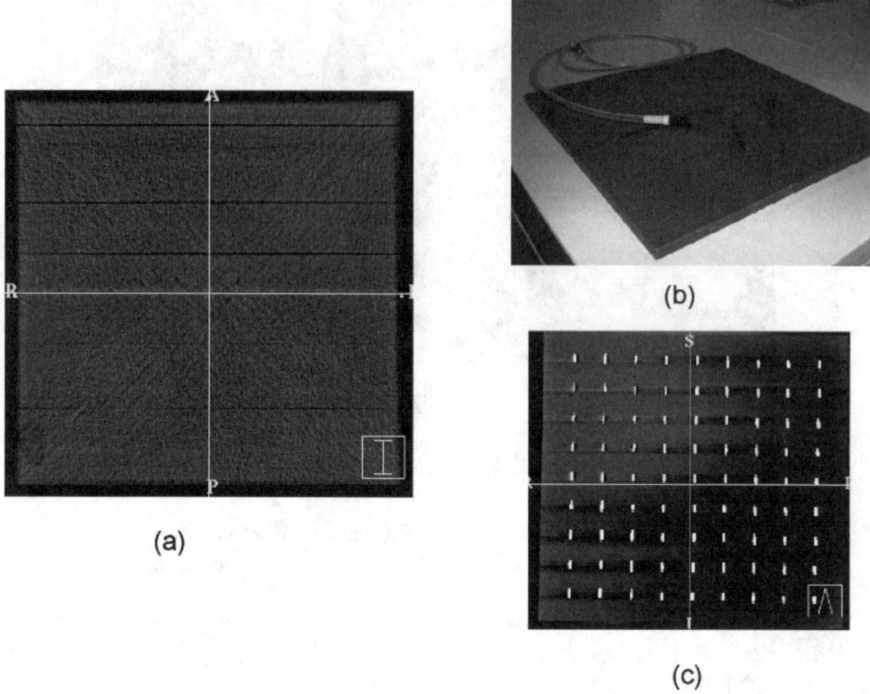

**Figure 8.** (a) A CT reconstructed axial image of large solid water phantom.
(b) A photograph of a special 1.0 cm-thick slab drilled with a slit that is 1 cm in width
and 15 cm in length from the edge of the slab, for an ion chamber placement.
(c) A coronal image of a special 1.0 cm slab that has 81 holes
(3 mm width × 7 mm length × 3 mm height) drilled into the slab,
with the holes arranged at an equal spacing of 3 cm for MOSFET
dosimeter placements.

## Ion Chamber Measurement

At our institution, an ion chamber is always used in IMRT phantom verifications. Due
to the size of the ion chamber used (IC-10, Wellhöffer Dosimetries, Schwarzenbruck,
Germany), the ion chamber is generally placed at a high dose, relatively homogeneous
region. For these regions, the results of ion chamber measurements are usually within
4% deviation from the calculations, as shown in figure 9. Using the ion chamber, we
also have tried to measure the low-dose region for critical structures such as the spinal
cord. Partly due to the fact that the planning system's calculation algorithm often
cannot model transmission, leakage, and scattering dose accurately in low-dose regions
and partly due to the difficulty in finding a relatively uniform dose area for these
regions, the ion chamber measurements in low-dose regions often showed higher dose
than predicted by the planning system. Table 1 shows the measurement results of

low-dose regions at 30% to 50% of the planned maximum dose for nine phantom plans. It is noted that the absolute dose deviations shown in table 1 depended on the measured dose. Deviations greater than 10% were noted on some plans. The lower the measured dose, the more sensitive the absolute dose deviation. Therefore, in table 1 we also listed relative deviations normalized to the planned maximum dose. Deviations normalized to the maximum dose were sometimes greater than 4%. Ion chambers are ideally used in the low gradient of both high- and low-dose regions and are more reliable compared to the film measurements.

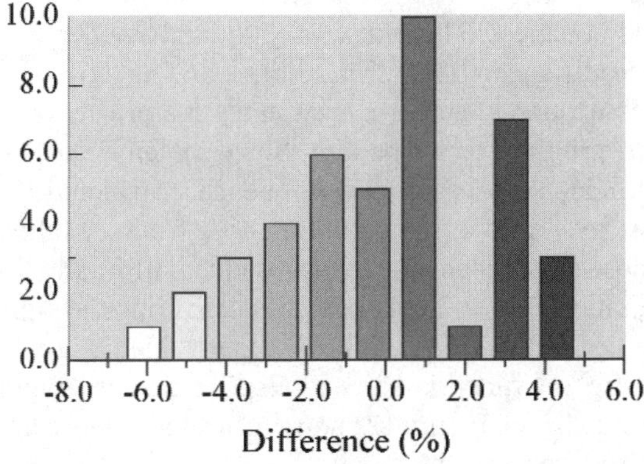



**Figure 9.** Histogram of ion chamber measurement results in the high-dose regions.

**Table 1.** Ion Chamber Measurements in Low-Dose Region

|  | Plan 1 | Plan 2 | Plan 3 | Plan 4 | Plan 5 | Plan 6 | Plan 7 | Plan 8 | Plan 9 |
|---|---|---|---|---|---|---|---|---|---|
| Plan Maximum Dose (Gy) | 2.40 | 2.40 | 2.40 | 1.00 | 1.00 | 1.00 | 2.40 | 2.40 | 2.40 |
| Measured Dose (Gy) | 1.14 | 1.12 | 1.16 | 0.39 | 0.39 | 0.29 | 0.79 | 1.02 | 0.85 |
| Planned Dose (Gy) | 1.09 | 1.09 | 1.14 | 0.40 | 0.43 | 0.33 | 0.79 | 0.91 | 0.79 |
| Deviation (%) | 4.40 | 2.40 | 1.60 | 3.00 | 10.00 | 14.00 | 0.00 | 11.70 | 7.90 |
| Deviation Relative to Max Dose (%) | 2.00 | 1.10 | 0.10 | 1.00 | 4.40 | 4.40 | 0.00 | 4.50 | 2.60 |

## Film Measurements

Films are ideal for measurements in the high-dose gradient, where the quality metric can be easily quantified as distance to agreement of a given dose value. For film measurements of IMRT fields, one should be particularly cognizant of possible film calibration errors due to the large amounts of low-energy scatter radiation that are present in the highly modulated IMRT fields (radiographic film over-responds to low-energy X-rays because of its high silver content). Because of variation in film processor conditions and the film batch itself, it is recommended that a film calibration should be conducted every time. To speed up the calibration process, we have created an eight-strip pattern, as shown in figure 10. Each strip is 2 cm wide, with 1 cm gap in between the strips. The MU assigned to each strip as well as the measured doses associated with these strips are listed in table 2. The film was calibrated at a depth of 3 cm with 100 cm source-to-surface distance (SSD). The corresponding dose for each strip was measured using an ionization chamber placed under the projection of each strip at 3 cm depth while delivering the entire pattern. Since the entire pattern was delivered during each measurement, the measured dose for each strip included the primary dose from the measured strip as well as the scattering dose from the other strips. Once we have measured the dose under each strip, the subsequent film calibration is performed by setting up a calibration film at 3 cm depth and delivering the eight-strip pattern to the film. The Hurter & Driffield (H&D) curve was obtained by finding average optical density of each strip as a function of its corresponding dose. Figure 11 is an H&D curve for a 6 MV photon beam. Figure 12 shows measured isodose lines superimposed with the calculated isodose lines.

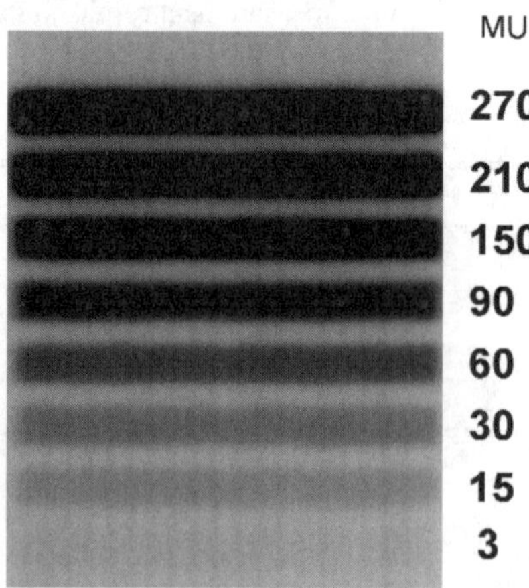



**Figure 10.** Calibration film pattern consisting of eight strips.

**Table 2.** MU and Dose for the Eight-Strip Pattern Calibration Film

| Strip Number | MU | Dose (Gy) |
|:---:|:---:|:---:|
| 1 | 1 | 10.8 |
| 2 | 5 | 21.9 |
| 3 | 10 | 36.9 |
| 4 | 20 | 63.8 |
| 5 | 30 | 91.3 |
| 6 | 50 | 150.0 |
| 7 | 70 | 208.6 |
| 8 | 90 | 264.0 |

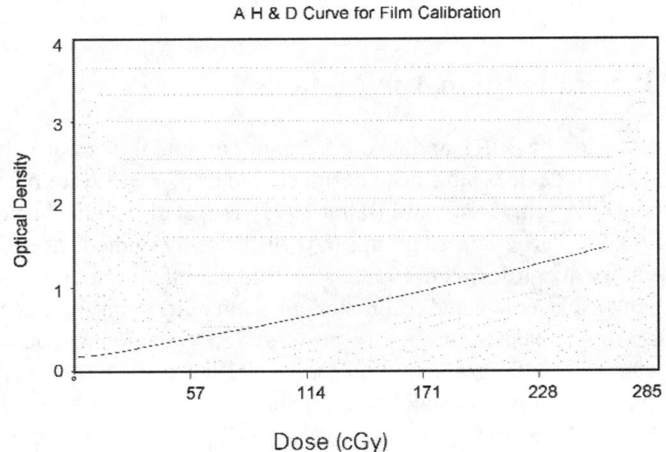


**Figure 11.** An H&D curve for a 6 MV photon beam.

## MLC Plan  Isodose Verification

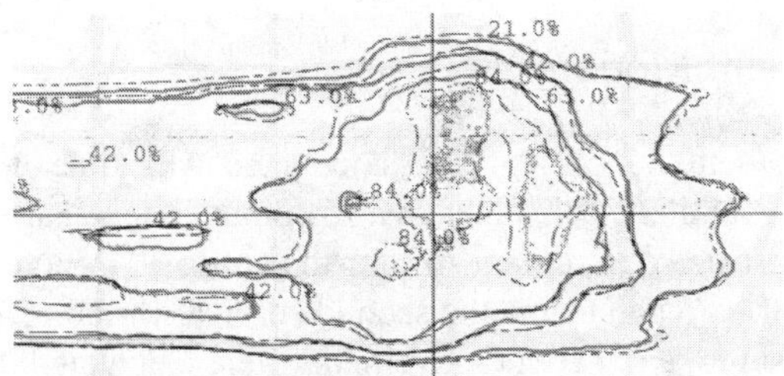


**0.40 Gy, 0.30 Gy, 0.20 Gy, 0.10 Gy**

**Figure 12.** A comparison of isodose distributions of measured isodose lines superimposed onto the calculated isodose lines.

## Independent MU Check

The phantom plan dosimetric measurement verifies the beam configuration of a patient plan, but does not verify the relationship between the beam configuration and patient geometry. If there is an error in this relationship, measurement of a phantom plan could not reveal the error. A quick check of this relationship is to verify the SSD of each beam. A comprehensive check of this relationship is to verify the MU of each beam independently. Because of the inclusion of the many subfields in one IMRT field, a conventional MU check using manual calculation becomes infeasible. Some institutions have developed their in-house software to do this MU check. Commercial software is also available now to do independent MU checks. Another chapter will discuss this in more detail (***Monitor Unit Calculation And Plan Validation For IMRT*** by Xing et al.).

## Effect Of Patient Position And Motions

With the introduction of IMRT and its conformality around the tumor volume, more rigid immobilization devices have been designed and implemented for head and neck IMRT treatment (Marsch, Evans, and Balter 1997; Tsai et al. 1999; Chao et al. 2000; Saw et al. 2001). Similarly, various groups have also closely studied patient setup variation and the subsequent dosimetric effects. A study simulating possible dosimetric effects of patient displacement and collimator and gantry angle misalignment on IMRT showed that a 3 mm movement in anterior-posterior (AP) positioning could contribute up to a 38% decrease in the minimum target dose (Xing et al. 2000). Another study determined that with 5 mm translational shifts in all six directions [superior-inferior (SI), AP, and right lateral (RL)], the incorporation of planning organ at risk volume (PRV) could indeed decrease the average volume of contralateral parotid receiving greater than 30 Gy from 22% to 4% (Manning et al. 2001).

At our institution, we have conducted one study to investigate the uncertainties in patient immobilization and patient positioning, in patients with nasopharyngeal carcinoma, and the subsequent dosimetric effects in the delivery of an IMRT plan.

## Intrafraction Patient Motion

The intrafractional patient motion study was conducted at the time of verification setup. Three sets of orthogonal films were taken in a 15-minute interval after the initial setup. The patients were instructed to remain still for the entire 30 minutes, if possible. The distance and angle of hard palate and the second cervical vertebra, axis (C2) from the isocenter were measured, and patient movements were calculated. For most patients, movements seem to be random and the average movement is approximately 1 to 2 mm, although patients tend to be able to stay still for the first 15 minutes, but not as well into the second 15 minutes. The teatment plan of each patient was then recalculated to simulate such intrafractional patient movement by shifting the original isocenter according to the movement obtained from the motion study. It was concluded that for both gross target volume (GTV) and clinical target volume (CTV), the planned DVH, and the recalculated DVHs according to patient movement do not differ significantly; however, for small sensitive structures such as the chiasm, the difference could be significant, as can be seen on figure 13.

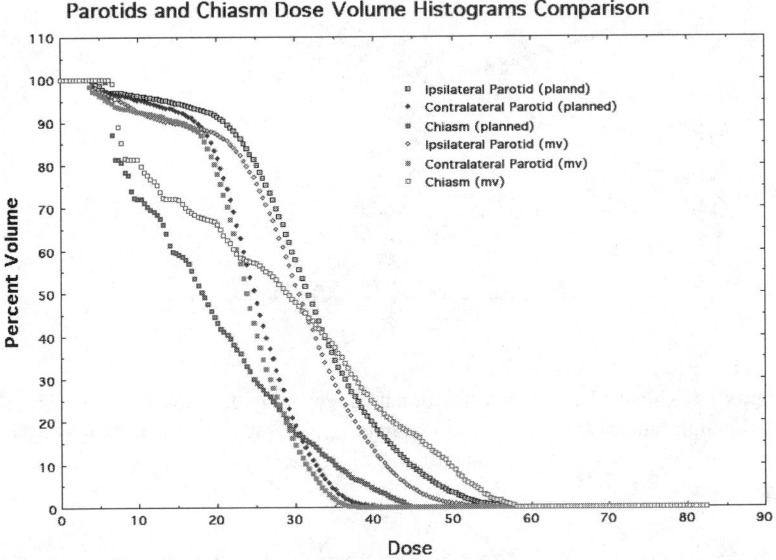


**Figure 13.** The results from intrafractional patient movement study showing that for small sensitive structures such as the chiasm, the dose received and planned could differ significantly.

## Interfraction Patient Position

Weekly port films from IMRT patients were analyzed to study the intertreatment patient positioning uncertainties. The distance and angle of hard palate and or C2 from the isocenter were measured, and interfractional patient setup uncertainties were calculated. For most patients, the interfractional positioning is accurate to within 1.5 mm, but there were patients who showed larger positioning discrepancies, up to 3 mm. Thus, we have since employed the patient positioning indexing system to improve the ease of repetitive patient setup. The treatment plan of each patient was then recalculated to simulate such interfractional patient setup uncertainties by shifting the original isocenter according to the movement obtained from the port film study. Although tumor coverage did not change significantly, the brainstem dose could have quantifiable changes, as shown in figure 14.

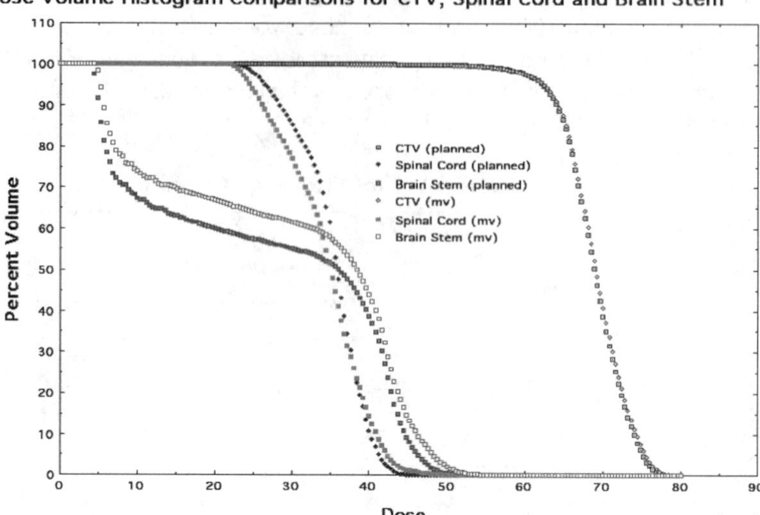


**Figure 14.** The results from interfractional patient setup discrepancy study showing that although tumor coverage does not change significantly, the brainstem dose shows quantifiable changes.

## Dosimetric Effects Of Patient-Positioning Uncertainties

We have determined that 3 mm positioning error is the worst situation observed in our patients' port film study, and that with the patient's head and neck immobilized in the head mask, it is estimated that the most likely head motion is rotation with the chin up or down. IMRT plans of five head and neck patients were recalculated by simultaneously shifting the original isocenter 3 mm posterior and 3 mm superior to simulate patient chin up movement, and to shift the isocenter 3 mm anterior and 3 mm inferior simultaneously to approximate chin down rotation (Xia et al. 2000). Figure 15 shows the changes in the GTV coverages between a normal plan, plans with chin-up (superior-posterior isoshift) and chin-down (inferior-anterior isoshift) motions, and the average effects over these three plans. Similarly, figure 16 shows the changes in the maximum dose encompassing 1% of the brain stem volume. From the results of this study, it was shown that changes in dose coverage to both the GTV and the CTV were not very sensitive to random patient motion and setup errors of up to 3 mm. In this circumstance, the average changes in dose to sensitive structures were also not significant. However, systematic setup errors such as chin-up motion could introduce significant changes in dose to sensitive structures such as the brain stem and the chiasm.

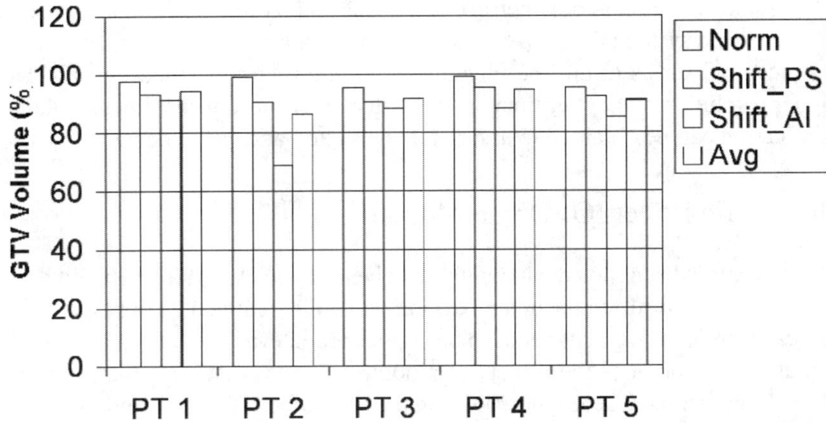


**Figure 15.** Bar graph of the percentage of the GTV volume receiving ≥70 Gy for five head and neck patients' plans. Norm represents the original plan without isocenter shift; Shift_PS plan represents a simulated plan with isocenter shifted in posterior and superior directions; Shift_AI represents a simulated plan with isocenter shifted in anterior and inferior directions. Avg represents the average effect of the three plans with and without isocenter shifts.

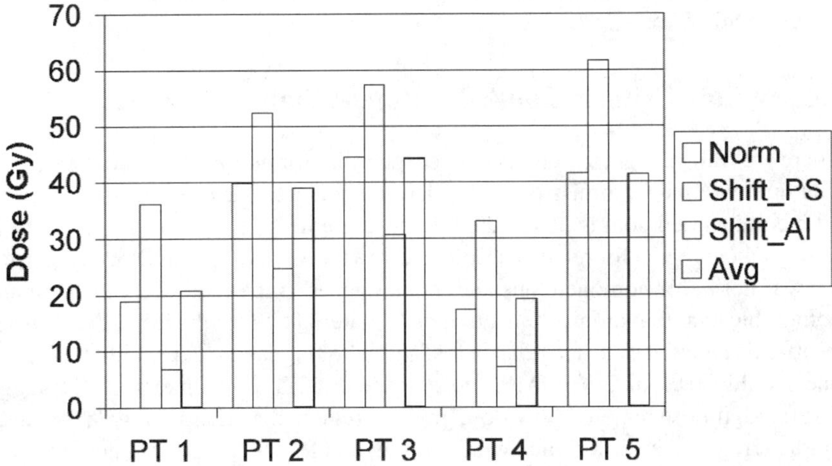


**Figure 16.** Bar graph of the Maximum dose received by 1% of the brain stem for five head and neck patients' plans. Norm represents the original plan without isocenter shift; Shift_PS plan represents a simulated plan with isocenter shifted in posterior and superior directions; Shift_AI represents a simulated plan with isocenter shifted in anterior and inferior directions. Avg represents the average effect of the three plans with and without isocenter shifts.

With these possible dosimetric consequences, it is important that care should be taken to avoid systematic setup errors and large intrafractional patient movement. With the recent advances in on-line imaging using amorphorous silicon panels that have higher resolution and better image quality than previous on-line imagers, daily setup verification can be obtained to assure that no systematic errors occur.

## Dosimetric Effects Of Organ Motion

The preceding discussion dealt mainly with head and neck IMRT treatment. However, more and more institutions are embarking on IMRT treatment for prostate cancer. In this case, organ movement needs to be considered in evaluation of treatment plans. A recent study examines the effects of random and systematic geometric errors (van Herk, Remeijer, and Lebesque 2002). In the study, the CTV was randomly displaced and rotated with respect to the planned position to simulate systematic geometric errors, i.e., the difference in CTV position from initial CT for planning and the actual treatment position. It was concluded that a margin of 10 mm between the CTV and the planning target volume (PTV) is needed for maintaining the same level of tumor coverage [tumor control probability (TCP)]. Margin reduction will lead to loss of coverage, and more dose is needed to achieve the same TCP, and will only reduce the dose received by normal tissue at the high-dose gradient regions. The study also simulated random errors and found that random errors do not contribute as much impact as systematic errors.

## Acceptance Criteria For A Treatment Plan

There are well-recognized criteria of acceptability for photon beam dose calculations. The International Commission on Radiation Units and Measurements (ICRU) report 42 recommended goal is 2% in the low-dose gradient region and 2 mm in the high-dose gradient region for relative absorbed doses (ICRU 1987). Van Dyk suggested quite a few criteria, for homogeneous and inhomogeneous materials, as well as in anthropomorphic phantom or uncertain composite materials. Since the last criteria also apply to off-axis calculations, irregular fields, and inhomogeneities, it should be the criteria one should first look at for IMRT acceptance criteria. In his paper, it was suggested that for high-dose region or low-dose gradient region, the criterion is 4%; for high dose gradient region, the criterion is within 4 mm; and for small dose gradient in low-dose region, the criterion is 3%. For inhomogeneity corrections, central axis calculations should be 3% (Van Dyk et al. 1993).

However, such criteria were designed for single field photon calculations, so they might not all be applicable for IMRT. As mentioned earlier, each IMRT field consists of many small segments; many of them are off-axis and irregular shaped. It is difficult to find a uniform dose region for each IMRT field so that it cannot be accurately measured individually by an ionization chamber. Uniform dose regions in IMRT plans are the collective effect of all IMRT fields, in which a single IMRT field may not enclose a uniform region applicable for measurement. Another method of verifying the dose calculation is by measuring planar dose distributions and superimposing the measurements onto the corresponding planned isodose distribution. In low-dose gradient regions, the comparison is straightforward, and the doses can be compared directly. However, in high-dose gradient regions, small spatial displacement can result in a large dose difference between the calculation and the measurement. Therefore, in these regions, the concept of a distance-to-agreement (DTA) distribution is often used to determine the acceptability of the dose calculation. Low et al. (1998a) have suggested a numerical quality index, gamma, that incorporates both dose difference and DTA, and measures the disagreement in the regions that fail the acceptance criteria, thus quantifying the quality of the agreement between the desired calculated and measured isodoses.

# References


Chao, K. S., D. A. Low, C. A. Perez, and J. A. Purdy. (2000). "Intensity-modulated radiation therapy in head and neck cancers: The Mallinckrodt experience." *Int. J. Cancer* 90(2):92–103.

Chuang, C., L. J. Verhey, and P. Xia. (2002). "Investigation of the use of MOSFET for clinical IMRT dosimetric verification." *Med. Phys.* 29(6):1109–1115.

Esthappan, E., S. Mutic, W. B. Harms, J. F. Dempsey, and D. A. Low. (2002). "Dosimetry of therapeutic photon beams using an extended dose range film." *Med. Phys.* 29(10):2438–2445.

ICRU Report 42. Use of Computers in External Beam Radiotherapy Procedures with High-Energy Photons and Electrons. Washington, DC: International Commission on Radiation Units and Measurements, 1987.

Low, D. A., W. B. Harms, S. Mutic, and J. A. Purdy. (1998a). "A technique for the quantitative evaluation of dose distribution." *Med. Phys.* 25(5):656–661.

Low, D. A., S. Mutic, J. F. Dempsey, R. L. Gerber, W. R. Bosch, C. A. Perez, and J. A. Purdy. (1998b). "Quantitative dosimetric verification of an IMRT planning and delivery system." *Radiother. Oncol.* 49:305–316.

Manning, M. A., Q. Wu, R. M. Cardinale, R. Mohan, A. D. Lauve, B. D. Kavanagh, M. M. Morris, and R. K. Schmidt-Ullrich. (2001). "The effect of setup uncertainty on normal tissue sparing with IMRT for head-and-neck cancer." *Int. J. Radiat. Oncol. Biol. Phys.* 51(5):1400–1409.

Marsch, R., J. Balter, and V. L. Evans. (1997). "Design and analysis of an immobilization and repositioning system for treatment of neck malignancies." *Med. Dosim.* 22(4):293–297.

Olch, A. J. (2002). "Dosimetric performance of an enhanced dose range radiographic film for intensity-modulated radiation therapy quality assurance." *Med. Phys.* 29(9):2159–2168.

Saw, C. B., R. Yakoob, C. A. Enke, T. P. Lau, and K. M. Ayyangar. (2001). "Immobilization devices for intensity-modulated radiation therapy (IMRT)." *Med. Dosim.* 26(1):71–77.

Tsai, J. S., M. J. Engler, M. N. Ling, J. K. Wu, B. Kramer, T. Dipetrillo, and D. E. Wazer. (1999). "A non-invasive immobilization system and related quality assurance for dynamic intensity modulated radiation therapy of intracranial and head and neck disease." *Int. J. Radiat. Oncol. Biol. Phys.* 43(2):455–467.

Van Dyk, J., R. B. Barnett, J. E. Cygler, and P. C. Shragge, (1993). "Commissioning and quality assurance of treatment planning computers." *Int. J. Radiat. Oncol. Biol. Phys.* 26(2):261–273.

van Herk, M., P. Remeijer, and J. V. Lebesque. (2002). "Inclusion of geometric uncertainties in treatment plan evaluation." *Int. J. Radiat. Oncol. Biol. Phys.* 52(5):1407–1422.

Xia, P., C. Chuang, F. Hguyen-Tan, K. K. Fu, and L. J. Verhey. "Computer Simulated Patient Motion and Setup Uncertainties in Intensity Modulated Radiotherapy" in *XIII International Conference on the Use of Computers in Radiation Therapy*. (XIII ICCR). W. Schlegel and T. Bortfeld (eds.). May 2000, Heidelberg, Germany. Berlin: Springer, 2000.

Xing, L., Z. Lin, S. S. Donaldson, Q. T. Le, D. Tate, D. R. Goffinet, S. Wolden, L. Ma, and A. L. Boyer. (2000). "Dosimetric effects of patient displacement and collimator and gantry angle misalignment on intensity modulated radiation therapy." Radiother. Oncol. 56(1):97–108.

Zhu, X. R., P. A. Jursinic, D. F. Grimm, F. Lopez, J. J. Rownd, and M. T. Gillin. (2002). "Evaluation of Kodak EDR2 film for dose verification of intensity modulated radiation therapy delivered by a static multileaf collimator." *Med. Phys.* 29(8):1687–1692.

# Monitor Unit Calculation And Plan Validation For Intensity-Modulated Radiation Therapy

Lei Xing, Ph.D.[1], Yong Yang, Ph.D.[1], Jonathan G. Li, Ph.D.[2], Yan Chen, Ph.D.[3], Gary Luxton, Ph.D.[1], Zhe Chen, Ph.D.[4], Y. Song[1], and Arthur L. Boyer, Ph.D.[1]

[1]Department of Radiation Oncology, Stanford University School of Medicine, Stanford, California

[2]Department of Radiation Oncology, University of Florida, Gainesville, Florida

[3]Department of Radiation Oncology, Thomas Jefferson University Hospital, Philadelphia, Pennsylvania

[4]Department of Radiation Oncology, Yale University School of Medicine, New Haven, Connecticut



## Introduction

Intensity-modulated radiation therapy (IMRT) is being developed into an important radiation therapy modality (Ling et al. 1996; Wang et al. 1996; Tsai et al. 1998; Xing et al. 2000b; Webb 2001; IMRTCWG 2001; Cheng and Das 2002; Xia et al. 2000) and methods for the plan optimization and delivery have evolved to a high level of sophistication (Xing et al. 1999; Lian, Cotrutz, and Xing 2002; Wu et al. 2002; Pugachev and Xing 2002; Shepard et al. 1995; Hou et al. 2003). However, the development of means for quality assurance (QA) has lagged behind. At present, the verification of IMRT treatment plans remains a labor-intensive and institution-dependent process. Considerable confusion exists regarding what dosimetric tests are needed to validate an IMRT plan and how to efficiently execute these tests in a routine

clinical environment. Generally, the methods of IMRT plan validation can be classified into two categories: experimental measurement and independent calculation.
While the former method is, in principle, more reliable, the latter approach has a
number of advantages and may be more suitable for routine application. Instead of
using ionization chamber and/or radiographic films to actually perform the dosimetric
measurements, it attempts to simulate the treatment on a computer and independently
calculates the dosimetric quantities, such as the spatial doses or fluence maps. The
philosophy here is similar to that used in plan validation in three-dimensional (3-D)
conformal radiation therapy (3DCRT), where a manual or simple computer calculation is employed to double check the monitor units (MUs) of a treatment. In this
chapter, we review different techniques used for computer-based IMRT plan validation and summarize our experience in implementing the technique.

## Review Of IMRT Dose Validation Algorithms

## Dose Calculation In IMRT

It is useful to first summarize the dose calculation algorithms that are widely used in
IMRT treatment planning systems. There are two major types of dose calculation algorithms: correction-based and model-based (IMRTCWG 2001). Correction-based
models compute the dose distributions in patients by correcting the dose distributions
of similar geometries in a homogeneous water phantom for the beam modifiers, patient
contours, tissue heterogeneities, and volume scattering effect. The type of heterogeneity corrections includes the 1-D method, in which only densities along the primary
photon path are considered, and the equivalent tissue-air ratio method. The volume
scattering effects (scatter dose as a function of field size and shape) are often computed
by using the equivalent square field method and/or Clarkson integration. Some pencil
beam methods, like the finite-size pencil beam algorithm (Bourland and Chaney 1992),
are also classified as the correction-based models.

Model-based models can directly calculate the dose distributions in a patient for
a given beam energy, geometry, beam modifiers, patient contour, and tissue heterogeneities. The kernel-based convolution/superposition (Mackie, Scrimger, and Battista
1985; Mackie et al. 1988; Boyer and Mok 1985; Boyer et al. 1989) and Monte Carlo
method (Ma et al. 2000; Jeraj and Keall 1999; Solberg et al. 1998) are representatives
of the kind. In the convolution/superposition techniques, the dose deposition is viewed
as a superposition of appropriately weighted kernels to point irradiations and the superposition can be efficiently evaluated by means of convolution if the kernels are
considered as spatially invariant. The kernels, representing the energy transport and
dose deposition of secondary particles stemming from a point irradiation, can be calculated by Monte Carlo simulation. Monte Carlo method computes the dose distributions
by simulating particle transport in a patient. Model-based models are capable of
accounting for the electronic disequilibrium effects and therefore are more accurate
in dealing with the tissue inhomogeneity and calculating the dose in the electron disequilibrium regions.

Despite the fact that kernel-based models are superior to the correction-based models in calculation accuracy, the correction-based models are still useful, especially as a means for independent check of the treatment planning calculations because of their simplicity and efficiency. Pencil beam algorithms, which are the hybrid of the two approaches, are also useful for IMRT dose optimization and for independent IMRT dosimetric check because of their flexibility to model lateral fluence variations and their computational efficiency.

## A General Formalism For MU Or Point Dose Check

A few simplified algorithms have been proposed for the independent dose (or MU) calculation (Xing et al. 2000a; Kung and Chen 2000; Watanabe 2001; Chen, Xing, and Nath 2002). Here we briefly review a general algorithm developed by our group (Xing et al. 2000a; Yang et al. 2003). This method provides a clear physical picture and allows implementation of the MU calculation at a different level of sophistication to meet the specific requirements of different systems. For a single incident beam, the dose at a given point, $(x, y, z)$, can be expressed as a sum of the contributions from all beamlets (Xing et al. 2000a),

$$D(x, y, z) = MU \sum_{m}^{M} C_m D_m^0 , \tag{1}$$

where $MU$ is the total monitor unit of the field, is the dose per unit MU from the $m$th beamlet when it is open, $C_m$ is called the dynamic modulation factor (DMF), which represents the fractional MU of the $m$th beamlet when the beam is assigned with a unit MU, and $M$ is the total number of beamlets. The DMF, $C_m$, can be calculated by

$$C_m = \sum_{k}^{K} [S_{c,m,k} + \alpha S_c'(1 - \delta_{m,A_k})] f_k , \tag{2}$$

with

$$\delta_{m,A_k} = \begin{cases} 1 & \text{if} \quad m \in A_k \\ 0 & \text{if} \quad m \notin A_k \end{cases}, \tag{3}$$

where $K$ is the number of segments of the field, $f_k$ is the fractional MU of the $k$-th segment, $A_k$ is the field boundary defined by the $k$-the segment, $S_{c,m,k}$ is the head scatter factor of the beamlet $m$ in the $k$th segment, $S_c'$ is the head scatter factor for the rectangular field defined by the jaws, and $\delta$ is the average transmission factor (Arnfield et al. 2000). Here we have ignored the tongue-and-groove and MLC leaf end effects. When the head scatter is negligible, equation (2) becomes (Xing et al. 2000a)

$$C_m = \sum_k^K [\delta_{m,A_k} + \alpha(1 - \delta_{m,A_k})] f_k \tag{4}$$

To accurately compute the dose, it is also required to know the beamlet kernel, $D_m^0$. The formalism described above is general enough and allows using beamlet kernels derived from any method. We have implemented a Clarkson summation method, in which equation (1) is re-written as the sum of the contributions of the primary radiation and the scatter radiation:

$$D(x,y,z) = MU[C_{m_0} D_{p,m_0}^0 (x,y,z) + \sum_{m \neq m_0}^M C_m D_{s,m}^0 (x,y,z)], \tag{5}$$

where the first term is the primary dose and the second one is the scatter contribution. We treat the primary dose by a weighted average of the intensities in the surrounding 16 beamlets (a $2 \times 2$ cm$^2$ square). The $D_{p,m0}^0(x,y,z)$ can be calculated using

$$D_{p,m_0}^0 (x,y,z) = (\frac{100}{100 - z})^2 C_f S_p(0) TMR(d_{eff},0) POAR(d_{eff},x,y), \tag{6}$$

where $C_f$ is the calibration factor of the linac, $d_{eff}$ is the water equivalent depth of the calculation point, $S_p(0)$ and $TMR(d_{eff},0)$ are the phantom scatter factor and tissue-maximum ratio (TMR) for zero field size, respectively. $POAR(d_{eff}, x, y)$ is the primary off-axis ratio at the calculation point (Gibbons and Khan 1995). As was described earlier (Xing et al. 2000a), the scatter dose contribution is computed by summing over the contributions from all the scatter sources. We use $0.5 \times 0.5$ cm$^2$ sub-beamlets as the elementary calculation units. The $D_{s,m}^0(x,y,z)$ can be obtained by

$$D_{s,m}^0(x,y,z) = (\frac{100}{100 - z})^2 C_f [S_p(r + \Delta r) TMR(d_{eff}, r + \Delta r) - S_p(r) TMR(d,r)] POAR(d_{eff}, m), \tag{7}$$

where $r$ is the distance between the center of the $m$th sub-beamlet and the projection of the calculation point on the isocenter plane, $\Delta r = 0.5^2/2\pi r$, $POAR(d_{eff}, m)$ is the primary off-axis ratio at the center of the $m$th sub-beamlet in water equivalent depth $d_{eff}$.

Figure 1 shows the intensity map of a clinical IMRT treatment field (figure 1a) and the absolute dose profiles along the four lines marked in figure 1a were computed using the above algorithm in isocenter plane at 3.0 cm depth in the cubic water equivalent phantom. The results are shown in figures 1b, 1c, 1d, and 1e as solid dots. The film measurements and CORVUS® calculations were also performed in the phantom using a Varian Clinic 2300C/D with 80-leaf MLC and 15 MV photon beam. The results are shown in figure 1. While the overall agreement between our calculations, the CORVUS plans and the ion chamber measurements is excellent, there are regions (region A, B, C in figure 1) where the dosimetric discrepancies between the three are more than 5%.

In these regions, it seems that our program yielded closer doses to the measured values in comparison with that of the CORVUS calculation. Furthermore, as can be seen from figure 1, the penumbra regions are modeled adequately by our calculation.

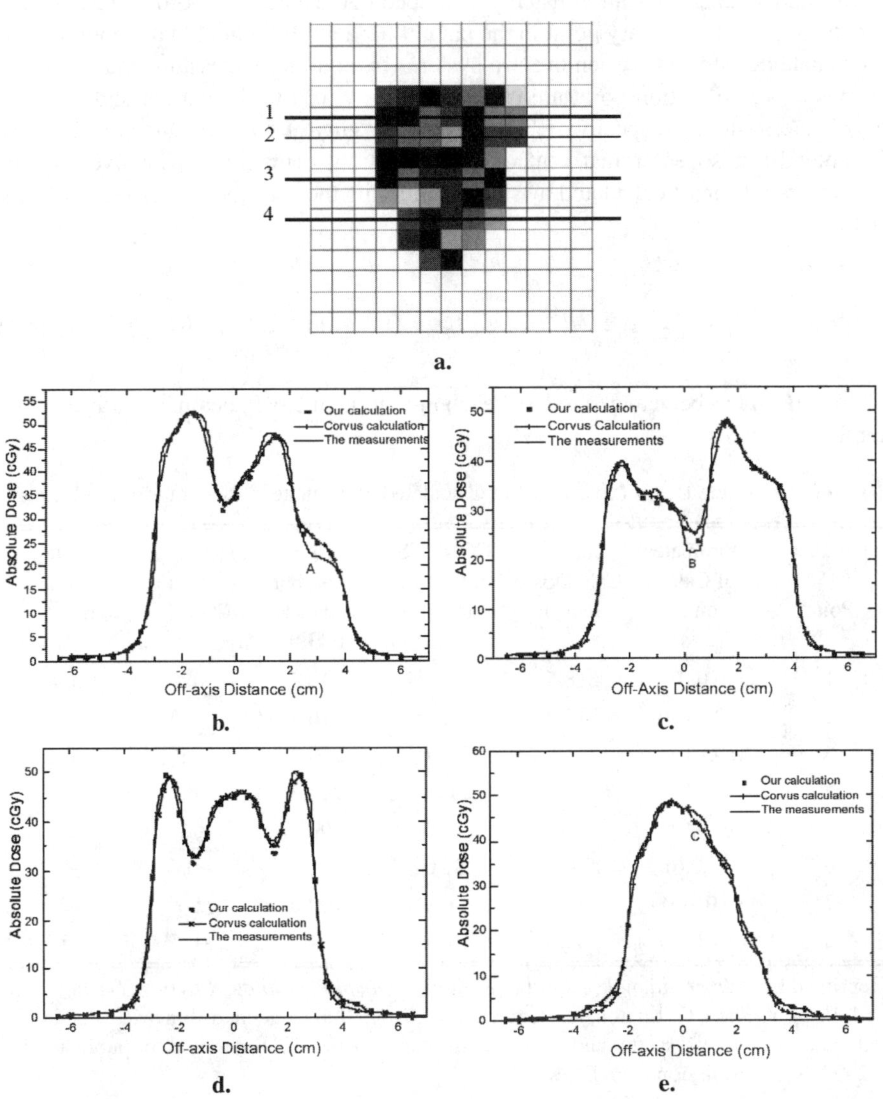


**Figure 1.** Comparison of our calculations with ion chamber measurements and CORVUS® plan for a clinical intensity-modulated field. The intensity map of the field and the four lines along which the doses were compared are shown in (a). The absolute dose profile for line–1, –2, –3, and –4 are shown in panels b, c, d, and e, respectively. [Reprinted from *International Journal of Radiation Oncology Biology Physics*, Y. Yang, J. G. Li, J. Palta, Y. Chen, G. Luxton, A. Boyer, and L. Xing, "Independent dosimetric calculation with inclusion of head scatter and MLC transmission for IMRT," Submitted for publication. © 2003, with permission from Elsevier.]

## Point Dose Calculation For Multifield IMRT

A point of interest (POI) is conveniently specified using a patient-fixed coordinate system and a radiation beam is usually described in the machine coordinate. To calculate the dose at an arbitrary point in the patient for a multiple field IMRT treatment, a coordinate transform between the two systems is required. We assume that the coordinates of a verification point are $(x,y,z)$ and $(x', y', z')$ in the patient and machine coordinate systems, respectively, and that the origins of two systems are set at the isocenter. In an isocenter treatment, only rotation transformations are involved and the dose at a point can be calculated by simply summing the contributions from all beams, that is

$$D(x,y,z) = \sum_{j=1}^{J} D_j(x',y',z') = \sum_{j=1}^{J} MU_j \left( C'_{m_0,j} D^0_{p,m_0 j}(x',y',z') + \sum_{m \neq m_0}^{M} C'_{m,j} D^0_{s,m,j}(x',y',z') \right), \quad (8)$$

where index $j$ has been added to label each individual incident beam, and $J$ is the total number of beams.

**Table 1.** Absolute Doses Measured and Calculated in a Lucite™ Phantom for the Case 1

| Number of Calc Point | Coordinates of Calc Points (cm) | Current Calc Dose (cGy) | CORVUS Calc Dose (cGy) | Ion Chamber Measurement (cGy) | Deviation with CORVUS | Deviation with Measurement (%) |
|---|---|---|---|---|---|---|
| 1 | (0,0,0) | 218.5 | 217.0 | 216.7 | 0.7 | 0.8 |
| 2 | (2,0,0) | 212.2 | 215.0 | 216.7 | −1.3 | −2.1 |
| 3 | (0,2,0) | 211.4 | 209.0 | 210.9 | 0.9 | 0.2 |
| 4 | (0,0,2) | 210.6 | 211.0 | 207.2 | −0.2 | 1.6 |
| 5 | (0,0,6) | 78.6 | 74.0 | 78.1 | 6.2 | 0.6 |
| 6 | (−6,0,6) | 78.5 | 80.0 | 79.2 | −0.6 | −0.9 |
| 7 | (6,0, −5) | 97.8 | 96.0 | 100.6 | 1.9 | −2.8 |
| 8 | (−6,2,−5) | 102.5 | 103.0 | 104.3 | −0.5 | −1.7 |

[Reprinted from *International Journal of Radiation Oncology Biology Physics*, Y. Yang, J. G. Li, J. Palta, Y. Chen, G. Luxton, A. Boyer, and L. Xing, "Independent dosimetric calculation with inclusion of head scatter and MLC transmission for IMRT," Submitted for publication. © 2003, with permission from Elsevier.]

The dosimetric validation of the above algorithm for a six-field IMRT prostate treatment plans was performed on the cylindrical Lucite™ phantom. The gantry angles of the six beams are 0°, 55°, 145°, 180°, 215°, and 305°, respectively, and the corresponding intensity maps are shown in figure 2. We independently computed the doses at eight pre-selected spatial points inside the phantom. The coordinates of the points of interest relative to the isocenter are listed in table 1, along with the results from the CORVUS calculation and the ion chamber measurements. Our calculations agree with the measurements to within 3.0% for all eight verification points. The agreement between our calculations and the CORVUS plans are also within 3.0% for all the points except point 5. At point 5, the deviation of the CORVUS dose from the measurement was found to be 5.6%, whereas our calculated dose for the point is only 0.6% different from the measured value. We attribute the superior performance of our system to the better modeling of head scatter contributions.

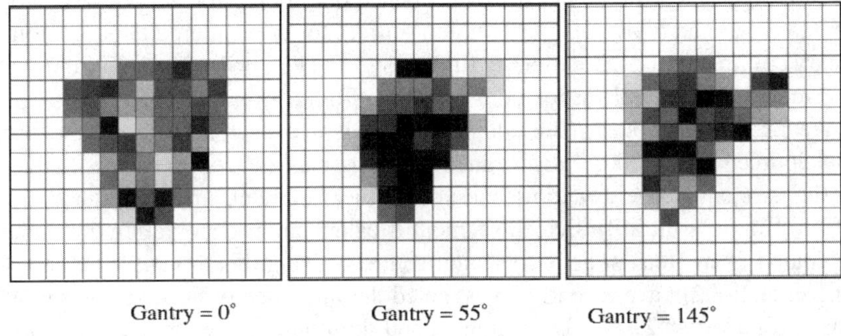


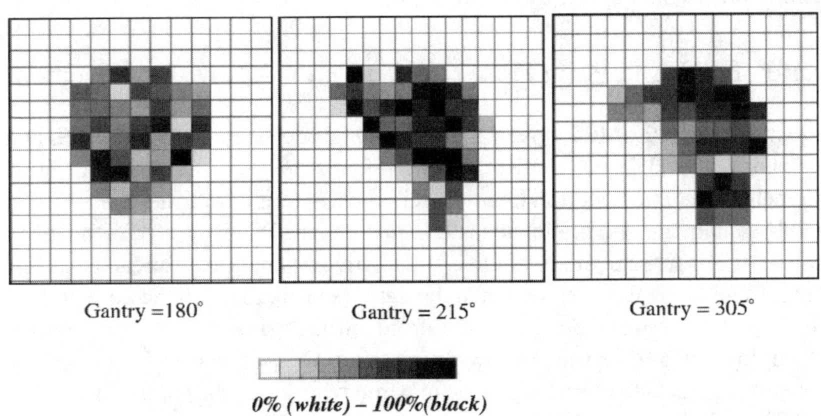


**Figure 2.** The intensity maps for a six-field IMRT prostate treatment. Intensity level of a beamlet is characterized by its gray level, ranging from 0 (white) to 100 (black). [Reprinted from *International Journal of Radiation Oncology Biology Physics*, Y. Yang, J. G. Li, J. Palta, Y. Chen, G. Luxton, A. Boyer, and L. Xing, "Independent dosimetric calculation with inclusion of head scatter and MLC transmission for IMRT," Submitted for publication. © 2003, with permission from Elsevier.]

## Role Of Scatter From MLC Segments

To compute the spatial doses of an IMRT field, it is critical to model the MLC transmission and scatter accurately. The calculation of head scatter for irregularly shaped MLC segments is challenging and, up to this point, its effect has not been accounted for adequately in many commercial systems. Recently, Yang et al. (2002) have reported an effective three-source model for the calculation and it is claimed that less than 0.3% of accuracy can be achieved for the measured and calculated head scatter factors for a variety of testing fields. In this model, the photon radiation to the point of calculation is treated as if from three effective sources: one source for the primary photons from the target and two extra-focal photon sources for the scattered photons from the primary collimator and the flattening filter, respectively. The intensity distributions of the scatter sources and their positions and the off-axis difference of the scatter radiation are taken into account in the calculation model on a machine- and energy-specific basis. Source parameters are determined by fitting the head scatter factors to the data of a series of square fields and no backscatter measurements are needed. Head scatter factor for an arbitrarily shaped segment is calculated by integrating the radiation contributed from areas in the two scatter sources. Using this model, Yang and Xing (Yang et al. 2002) have recently investigated the influence of head scatter on IMRT delivery for a Varian 2100 C/D accelerator and showed that an error of 3% to 5% error can result if the head scatter from a MLC shaped segment is ignored. It is anticipated that the inclusion of head scatter will be even more crucial for Siemens and Elekta machines due to their specific MLC designs.

## Inverted Field And Point Dose Calculation In A Low-Dose Region

Our experience with IMRT dose validation in high-dose regions indicated that dose agreement within 3%~5% is adequate and reflects the current standard of practice. Implementation of the criterion for all IMRT cases is complicated, however, by the fact that the beam intensity is modulated and frequently, the POI is located in the low-dose region of one or more treatment fields. The relative dosimetric error can be as high as 5% to 30% in a low-dose region when the data are normalized to the dose at the POI. In reality, a large relative error may rise from a true dosimetric error or simply from the "amplification" effect in the low-dose region. One method to better portray the dosimetric impact is to normalize to the maximum dose (see the chapter herein by Xia and Chuang, *Patient-Specific Quality Assurance in IMRT*). Another way is to be able to draw a more decisive conclusion based on the independent dose calculation; it is desirable to have a unified QA criterion for both high- and low-dose regions.

We introduce a useful concept of the inverted field for IMRT. For each intensity-modulated field (primal field), there exists a unique inverted field whose beamlet weights are defined as

$$W_i(n) = W_{max} - W_p(n) , \tag{9}$$

where $W_i(n)$ and $W_p(n)$ are the weights of the $n$th beamlet in the inverted and primal fluence maps, respectively, and $W_{max}$ is the maximum beamlet weight of the primal beam. By convention, we set the maximum beamlet weight of the primal field to be 100. The inverted field plus the primal field constitutes a uniform open field defined by setting the weights of all beamlets under the collimator jaws to be 100. As a result of the inversion relation defined by equation (9), the low-dose region of the primal field corresponds to the high-dose region of its inverted field, and vice versa. This complementary relation bridges what appears to be two independent schemes and allows us to validate the MU setting of the primal field by using the dosimetric data of the inverted field. That is, instead of directly evaluating the primal field, we may proceed by assessing the dose of the inverted field when the POI is located in a low-dose region of the primal field. Because the POI is in the high-dose region of the inverted field, the commonly used QA criterion can be readily employed for QA decision-making. Without the criterion based on the inverted field, it would be difficult to judge whether a QA action should be taken if we were to rely only on a relative dose error of the primal field dose.

Three intensity maps, consisting of a wedged field and two well-shaped fields, are shown in figure 3 to illustrate the inverted field approach. The dose distributions of the three intensity-modulated beams in a circular Lucite phantom were computed using the CORVUS planning system. The gray scale intensity maps of the inverted fields are plotted in figures 3d through 3f. The total MUs of each beamlet from the two fields were set to 100 MU. In table 2 we list the isocenter dose for the three primal and inverted fields. In these three cases, the sum of the primal and inverted fields constituted a $10 \times 10$ cm square field. In table 2, we also list the results of ion chamber measurement. For comparison, we have also computed directly the dose distributions of the three inverted fields using the CORVUS system. The CORVUS isocenter doses for the three sets are listed in the table.

The wedged field represents an intuitive example and it is easy to conceive that, when the positive and negative wedges shown in figures 3a and 3d are combined, a uniform open field is the result. Indeed, as shown in table 2, the summation of the isocenter doses of the primal and inverted wedged fields is equal to that of the uniform $10 \times 10$ cm field to within 2.0% for both ion chamber measurements and theoretical calculations The two well-shaped fields are similar except that the central four beamlets are zero for the field shown in figure 3c. The isocenter is located in a low-dose region in both cases. Once again, the sum of the primal and inverted field doses for the two cases was found to be equal to that of the open field dose to within 2.5% for both energies. For the third case shown in figure 3c, the isocenter dose is completely from scatter and transmission. The disagreement between the ion chamber measurements and the direct calculations was found to be large, ~5.1% for 6 MV photon beam and 13.2% for 15 MV photon beam when normalized to the measurement data. The relative discrepancy between the independent calculation and the CORVUS calculation was also found to be excessive (~18%) for the 15 MV photon beam. Similarly, for the 6 MV photon beam shown in figure 3b, the relative discrepancy between the independent calculation and the CORVUS calculation was found to be ~11%. As we have mentioned earlier, in reality, a large relative error may rise from a true dosimetric error or simply because the point is in a low-dose region which "enhances" the relative error. The concept of the inverted field provides an effective method to properly evaluate the error. For these two particular cases, we found that the relative discrepancies were all within 4.0% when normalized to the inverted field dose. It is thus concluded that the CORVUS calculation for these fields meets the QA criterion

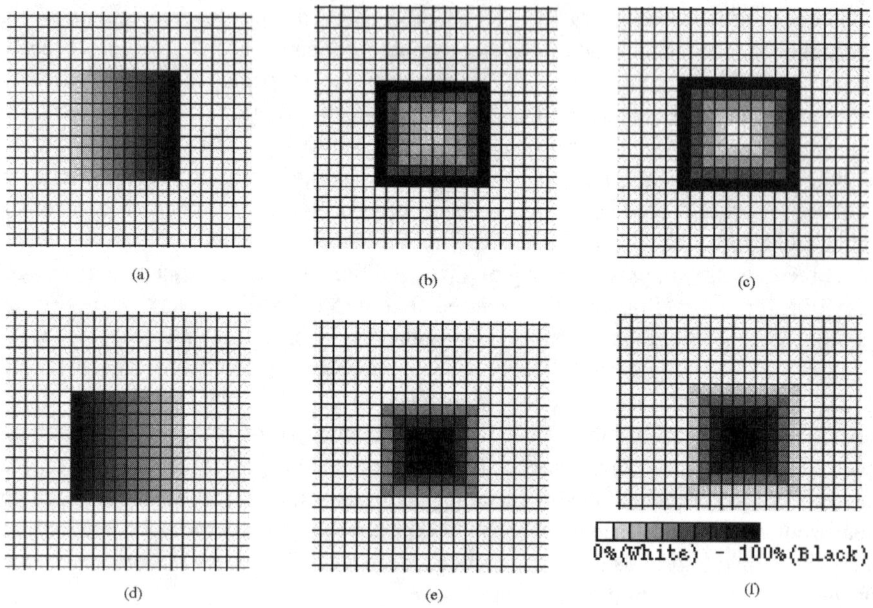



**Figure 3.** Fluence maps of a wedged field (a) and two well-shaped fields [(b) and (c)]. The intensity levels for the wedged field are 10, 20, 30, 40, 50, 60, 70, 80, 90, and 100 from right to left. The intensity levels for figure 1b are 0, 10, 30, 60, and 100 from inside to outside. For figure 3c, the intensity levels are 10, 20, 30, 60, and 100 from inside to outside. The inverted fields for the primal fields are shown in 3d, 3e, and 3f.

**Table 2.** Measured and Calculated Doses at the Center of a Cylindrical Lucite™ Phantom for the Intensity-Modulated Beams Shown in Figure 3

The top of each row shows the 6 MV data and the bottom row shows the data for 15 MV photons. The data shown in the third column is obtained using the complementary relation of the primary and inverted fields. The dose of the $10 \times 10$ cm open field at the center of the phantom is 0.627 Gy for 6 MV photon beam and 0.781 Gy for 15 MV photon beam, which is consistent with an ion chamber measurement and a simple hand calculation

| Field Name | Direct Calculation (Gy) | Calculation Using Inverted Field (Gy) | Ion Chamber Measurement (Gy) | CORVUS Calculation (Gy) |
|---|---|---|---|---|
| **6 MV Photon** | | | | |
| Wedged field (fig. 3a) | 0.315 | 0.311 | 0.314 | 0.318 |
| Inverted wedged field (fig. 3d) | 0.316 | 0.312 | 0.318 | 0.321 |
| Well-shaped field (fig. 3b) | 0.100 | 0.091 | 0.106 | 0.111 |
| Inverted well-shaped field (fig. 1e) | 0.536 | 0.527 | 0.522 | 0.528 |
| Well-shaped field (fig. 3c) | 0.074 | 0.066 | 0.078 | 0.071 |
| Inverted well-shaped field | 0.561 | 0.553 | 0.548 | 0.565 |
| **15 MV Photon** | | | | |
| Wedged field (fig. 3a) | 0.399 | 0.383 | 0.391 | 0.399 |
| Inverted wedged field (fig. 3d) | 0.398 | 0.381 | 0.394 | 0.398 |
| Well-shaped field (fig. 3b) | 0.111 | 0.092 | 0.116 | 0.115 |
| Inverted well-shaped field (fig. 3e) | 0.689 | 0.670 | 0.665 | 0.672 |
| Well-shaped field (fig. 3c) | 0.072 | 0.056 | 0.083 | 0.059 |
| Inverted well-shaped field (fig. 3f) | 0.725 | 0.709 | 0.712 | 0.731 |

## Is A Point Dose Enough For Validating
## An IMRT Treatment Plan?

### Necessity Of Multiple Points Validation For IMRT

Let us start by discussing the independent dosimetric verification procedure in conventional 3-D conformal radiation therapy (3DCRT). In 3DCRT, the verification is mainly concerned with the MU calculation for each incident field. An independent calculation of the dose or MU at a point based on primitive machine data is recommended by AAPM Task Group 40 (Kutcher et al. 1994). Because the fluence of a uniform/wedged field is spatially correlated, information of the dose at a spatial point can in principle be used to estimate the dose in other spatial points provided that the off-axis information is known. This is, however, not the case for an intensity-modulated field since the weights of the beamlets across the field are independent. The correctness of the dose at a spatial point only warrants, at most, the correctness of the beamlets passing through or nearby that point. Because of the independence of the beamlets, the doses at multiple points must be verified to ensure the correctness of the whole field. An independent fluence map check is also highly recommended to ensure the integrity of the field. This is addressed in the following.

### Independent Fluence Map Calculation And Its Utility
### For IMRT Plan Validation

The fluence map check can yield valuable information about the spatial correlation of the beamlets and thus complements the point dose check. In the past, the verification of a fluence map has been done using radiographic film, an electronic portal imaging device (EPID) (Pasma et al. 1999; Curtin-Savard and Podgorsak 1999; Partridge et al. 1998) or a beam imaging system (BIS) (Ma, Geis, and Boyer 1997) by actually delivering the leaf sequence file. While the measurement provides a reliable test on whether the leaf sequence file is deliverable and whether the execution of the file reproduces the intended fluence map, it is a labor-intensive and time-consuming process. Furthermore, the electronic devices are suitable only for a step-and-shoot delivery. They may have difficulty in verifying dynamic delivery because of finite dead-time of the electronics. Xing and Li (2000) have pointed out that it is more practical to use a computer simulation for the independent verification of the leaf sequences or fluence map. It is proposed to separate the IMRT treatment plan verification and the QA of the dynamic MLC. In the independent fluence map calculation, the program reads in the leaf sequence file generated by the planning system and recalculates the fluence map. The calculation is then compared quantitatively with the intended fluence map from the treatment planning system. The goal of the simulation is to warrant that, assuming that a rigorous independent QA of the MLC system has been performed so that the dynamic MLC can accurately execute the instruction of a leaf sequence file, the execution of the leaf sequence will generate the desired fluence map should it pass the simulation test. This eliminates the experimental verification for each treatment field and each patient and significantly simplifies the QA procedure. The philosophy here is similar to that of using an independent dose calculation to replace the ion chamber or film measurements.

We consider the QA of dynamic MLC delivery a separate important issue. In practice, the point doses and fluence maps should be verified for every patient treatment. The frequency and the extent of the MLC QA are, on the other hand, independent issues and should be determined by the need to maintain the normal operation of dynamic delivery. This does not require an actual delivery check for every IMRT patient treatment field, similar to that we do not usually check dynamic jaw movement for every treatment involved with a dynamic wedge in conventional radiation therapy.

The fluence map calculation for both step-and-shoot and dynamic deliveries has been discussed by Xing and Li (2000). Computationally, the fluence map of a field can simply be obtained by normalizing the DMF distribution with respect to its maximum value. To quantitatively compare the independently computed fluence map and the intended fluence map from the treatment planning system, we have introduced two indices. The first one is the maximum difference between the two maps. The pixel value difference is reported. In addition, a global quantity that has proved useful in IMRT is the correlation coefficient defined as (Ma, Geis, and Boyer 1997; Xing and Li 2000)

$$r = \frac{\sum_n (F_n - \overline{F})(R_n - \overline{R})}{\sqrt{\sum_n (F_n - \overline{F})^2}\sqrt{\sum_n (R_n - \overline{R})^2}}, \tag{10}$$

where $F_n$ and $R_n$ are the pixel values of the computed and the reference images, respectively, $\overline{F}$ is the average of $F_n$ and $\overline{R}$ is the average of $R_n$. The correlation coefficient measures the strength of the association between the two images and tests the linear predictability of the calculation from its reference image, and vice versa. The correlation coefficient is not very sensitive to the variation of the individual pixel value, but may provide valuable information on the global behavior of the fluence map.

Depending on the MLC manufacturer, different MLCs may have different specifications and constraints. These physical restrictions also need to be checked by the software to ensure that the leaf sequences not only reproduce the intended fluence map in a computer simulation, but also meet the machine constraints. A warning should be issued if these limitations are exceeded in an MLC file. This will prevent scheduling an undeliverable treatment from taking place since the MLC application cannot load a faulty file.

## Conclusions

In this chapter we have discussed the rationale and methods for independent point dose and fluence map check. From the IMRT dosimetry point of view, we believe that it is necessary to perform these two tests to validate an IMRT treatment plan. The validation of fluence map is unique to IMRT and ensures the integrity of the IMRT field (or the correctness of the relative planar distribution of the beamlets). Furthermore, we have argued that both types of tests can be more efficiently done using a computer and summarized our previous work on how to carry out these calculations. We emphasize that the proposed computer verification of the MU and fluence map is not intended to replace the QA of the MLC delivery system. A rigorous QA procedure for MLC must be established independent of the proposed software development to achieve the desired fluence/dose distribution through the actual delivery. The QA items for a dynamic MLC delivery system should include various mechanical and dosimetric properties as well as the proprietary software that controls the movement of the MLC leaves during radiation delivery.

## Acknowledgments

This work was partly supported by a Research Scholar Award from the American Cancer Society (RSG-01-022-01-CCE) and Department of Defense (DAMD17-01-0635). Table 1 and figures 1 and 2 are from a submitted manuscript to the *International Journal of Radiation Oncology, Biology, Physics*. We would like to thank Elsevier Science for permission to use the figures and the table.

## References

Arnfield, M. R., J. V. Siebers, J. O. Kim, Q. Wu, P. J. Keall, and R. Mohan. (2000). "A method for determining multileaf collimator transmission and scatter for dynamic intensity modulated radiotherapy." *Med. Phys.* 27:2231–2241.

Bourland, J. D., and E. L. Chaney. (1992). "A finite-size pencil beam model for photon dose calculations in three dimensions." *Med. Phys.* 19:1401–1412.

Boyer, A., and E. Mok. (1985). "A photon dose distribution model employing convolution calculations." *Med. Phys.* 12:169–177.

Boyer, A. L., Y. P. Zhu, L. Wang, and P. Francois. (1989). "Fast Fourier transform convolution calculations of x-ray isodose distributions in homogeneous media." *Med. Phys.* 16:248–253.

Chen, Z., L. Xing, and R. Nath. (2002). "Independent monitor unit calculation for IMRT using MIMiC multileaf collimator." *Med. Phys.* 29:2041–2051.

Cheng, C. W., and I. J. Das. (2002). "Comparison of beam characteristics in intensity modulated radiation therapy (IMRT) and those under normal treatment condition." *Med Phys.* 29:226–230.

Curtin-Savard, A.J., and E. B. Podgorsak. (1999). "Verification of segmented beam delivery using a commercial electronic portal imaging device." *Med. Phys.* 26:737–742.

Gibbons, J. P., and F. M. Khan. (1995). "Calculation of dose in asymmetric photon fields." *Med. Phys.* 1995; 22:1451–1457.

Hou, Q., J. Wang, Y. Chen, and J. Galvin. (2003). "An optimization algorithm for intensity modulated radiotherapy—The simulated dynamics with dose–volume constraints." Med. Phys. 30: 61–68.

IMRTCWG (Intensity Modulated Radiation Therapy Collaborative Working Group). "Intensity-modulated radiotherapy: Current status and issues of interest." Int. J. Radiat. Oncol. Biol. Phys. 51:880–914.

Jeraj, R., and P. Keall. (1999). "Monte Carlo-based inverse treatment planning." Phys. Med. Biol. 44:1885–1896.

Kung, J., and G. Chen. (2000). "A monitor unit verification calculation in intensity modulated radiotherapy as a dosimetric quality assurance." Med. Phys. 27:2226–2230.

Kutcher, G. J., L. Coia, M. Gillin, W. F. Hanson, S. Leibel, R. J. Morton, J. R. Palta, J. A. Purdy, L. E. Reinstein, G. K. Svensson, M. Weller, and L. Wingfield. (1994). "Comprehensive QA for radiation oncology: Report of AAPM Radiation Therapy Committee Task Group 40." Med. Phys. 21:581–618.

Lian, J., C. Cotrutz, and L. Xing. (2002). "Therapeutic treatment plan optimization with probalistic dose prescription." Med. Phys. 27: In press.

Ling, C. C., C. Burman, C. S. Chui, G. J. Kutcher, S. A. Leibel, T. LoSasso, R. Mohan, T. Bortfield, L. Reinstein, S. Spirou, X. H. Wang, Q. Wu, M. Zelefsky, and Z. Fuks. (1996). "Conformal radiation treatment of prostate cancer using inversely-planned intensity-modulated photon beams produced with dynamic multileaf collimation." Int. J. Radiat. Oncol. Biol. Phys. 35:721–730.

Ma, L., P. B. Geis, and A. L. Boyer. (2000). "Quality assurance for dynamic multileaf collimator modulated fields using a fast beam imaging system." Med. Phys. 24:1213–1220.

Ma, C.-M., T. Pawlicki, S. B. Jiang, J. S. Li, J. Deng, E. Mok, A. Kapur, L. Xing, L. Ma, and A. L. Boyer. (2000). "Monte Carlo verification of IMRT dose distributions from a commercial treatment planning optimization system." Phys. Med. Biol. 45:2483–2495.

Mackie, T. R., J. W. Scrimger, and J. J. Battista. (1985). "A convolution method of calculating dose for 15-MV x rays." Med. Phys. 12:188–196.

Mackie, T. R., A. F. Bielajew, D. W. Rogers, and J. J. Battista. (1988). "Generation of photon energy deposition kernels using the EGS Monte Carlo code." Phys. Med. Biol. 33:1–20.

Partridge, M., P. M. Evans, A. Mosleh-Shirazi, and D. Convery. (1998). "Independent verification using portal imaging of intensity-modulated beam delivery by the dynamic MLC technique." Med. Phys. 25:1872–1879.

Pasma, K. L., M. L. Dirkx, M. Kroonwijk, A. G. Visser, and B. J. Heijmen. (1999). "Dosimetric verification of intensity modulated beams produced with dynamic multileaf collimation using an electronic portal imaging device." Med. Phys. 26:2373–2378.

Pugachev, A., and L. Xing. (2002). "Incorporating prior knowledge into beam orientation optimization." Int. J. Radiat. Oncol. Biol. Phys. 54:1565–1574.

Shepard, D. D., M. A. Earl, X. A. Li, S. Naqvi, and C. X. Yu. (1995). "Direct aperture optimization: A turnkey solution for step-and-shoot IMRT." Med. Phys. 29:1007–1018.

Solberg, T. D., J. J. DeMarco, F. E. Holly, J. B. Smathers, and A. A. DeSalles. (1998). "Monte Carlo treatment planning for stereotactic radiosurgery." Radiother. Oncol. 49:73–84.

Tsai, J. S., D. E. Wazer, M. N. Ling, J. K. Wu, M. Fagundes, T. DiPetrillo, B. Kramer, M. Koistinen, and M. J. Engler. (1998). "Dosimetric verification of the dynamic intensity-modulated radiation therapy of 92 patients." Int. J. Radiat. Oncol. Biol. Phys. 40:1213–1230.

Wang, X., S. Spirou, T. LoSasso, J. Stein, C. Chui, and R. Mohan. (1996). "Dosimetric verification of intensity-modulated fields." Med. Phys. 23(3):317–327.

Watanabe, Y. (2001). "Point dose calculations using an analytical pencil beam kernel for IMRT plan checking." *Phys. Med. Biol.* 46:1031–1038.

Webb, S. *Intensity-Modulated Radiation Therapy.* Bristol, UK: Institute of Physics Publishing (IOP), 2001.

Wu, Q., R. Mohan, A. Niemierko, and R. Schmidt-Ullrich. (2002). "Optimization of intensity-modulated radiotherapy plans based on the equivalent uniform dose." *Int. J. Radiat. Oncol. Biol. Phys.* 52:224–235.

Xia, P., K. K. Fu, G. W. Wong, C. Akazawa, and L. J. Verhey. (2000). "Comparison of treatment plans involving intensity-modulated radiotherapy for nasopharyngeal carcinoma." *Int. J. Radiat. Oncol. Biol. Phys.* 48:329–337.

Xing, L., and J. G. Li. (2000). "Computer verification of fluence maps in intensity modulated radiation therapy." *Med. Phys.* 27:2084–2092.

Xing, L., J. G. Li, A. Pugachev, Q. T. Le, and A. L. Boyer. (1999). "Estimation theory and model parameter selection for therapeutic treatment plan optimization." *Med. Phys.* 26: 2348–2358.

Xing, L., Y. Chen, G. Luxton, J. G. Li, and A. L. Boyer. (2000a). "Monitor unit calculation for an intensity modulated photon field by a simple scatter-summation algorithm." *Phys. Med. Biol.* 45:N1–7.

Xing, L., Z. Lin, S. S. Donaldson, Q. T. Le, D. Tate, D. R. Goffinet, S. Wolden, L. Ma, and A. L. Boyer. (2000b). "Dosimetric effects of patient displacement and collimator and gantry angle misalignment on intensity modulated radiation therapy." *Radiother. Oncol.* 56(1):97–108.

Yang, Y., L. Xing, A. Boyer, Y. Song, and Y. Hu. (2002). "A three-source model for the calculation of head scatter factors." *Med. Phys.* 29:2024–2033.

Yang, Y., J. L. Li, J. Palta et al. (2003). "Independent dosimetric calculation with inclusion of head scatter and MLC transmission for IMRT." *Int. J. Radiat. Oncol. Biol. Phys.* Submitted.

# Monte Carlo And IMRT

**Jeffrey V. Siebers, Ph.D.[1] and Radhe Mohan, Ph.D.[2]**
[1]Medical College of Virginia
Virginia Commonwealth University
Richmond, Virginia
[2]Department of Radiation Physics
UT M.D. Anderson Cancer Center
Houston, Texas




## Introduction

Monte Carlo (MC) methods solve complex, analytically intractable problems, such as radiation transport and dose deposition, by using statistical sampling techniques to simulate processes according to known laws of nature. Therefore, MC methods are often termed as the "first principles" methods. Given some known inputs and a set of probability distributions describing the events that occur, MC methods utilize multiple random samples of the probability distributions to determine a probable outcome of some event. As applied to radiation therapy photon dose calculation, for instance, typical inputs would be electrons incident upon the radiation therapy accelerator bremsstrahlung target, the geometry and materials of the radiation therapy accelerator (including patient-specific beam modifiers) and the geometry and materials of the radiation therapy patient. The probability distributions are the cross sections for various photon and electron interactions for the materials in the accelerator and the patient. The event that is being simulated is the radiation therapy treatment process, and the outcome that is scored is the radiation dose deposited in the patient. To get a good estimate of the radiation dose, a very large number ($10^8$ or more) of initial events may need to be sampled.

The assumptions inherent in MC simulations are that the geometry, materials and their associated cross sections, and characteristics of initial particles are known to a high degree of accuracy. Accelerator geometry and material information should be obtainable from the linear accelerator manufacturers. For patients, methods have been developed to translate computed tomography (CT) Hounsfield numbers into materials and cross-sectional data (Kawrakow, Fippel, and Friedrich 1996; Schneider, Bortfeld, and Schlegel 2000). Material cross-section data are available in the form of libraries compiled over the last half a century and are based on measurements and calculations of well-established nuclear models. The accuracy of data in competing libraries is sometimes debated. However, for the most part, these data are more than adequately accurate for radiotherapy dose computation needs. For the initial particle states, although the energy, angular, and spatial distributions of initial particles (electrons) exiting the accelerator might differ from the nominal values quoted by the accelerator manufacturers, procedures have been developed to empirically solve for these parameters by adjusting them so that MC calculations match measured dose distributions in water phantoms under controlled conditions (Sheikh-Bagheri and Rogers 2002). Alternatively, source models describing the photon energy fluence impinging on the patient have been developed and tuned to match MC calculations with measurements (Schach von Wittenau et al. 1999).

For the most part, the consequences of the assumptions made in MC dose calculations are small. For this reason, it is commonly acknowledged that MC techniques provide the most accurate means of predicting dose distributions used for designing and optimizing radiation treatment plans. Were it not for limitations of computer speed, MC methods would likely be in routine clinical practice for all three-dimensional (3-D) treatment planning. With the spectacular increase in computer speed and the development of clever algorithms and variance reduction techniques, MC methods are now becoming practical for routine use for 3D and intensity-modulated radiation therapy (IMRT) treatment planning.

This chapter focuses on the use of MC techniques for IMRT. MC may play an important role in IMRT since it is generally accepted that a higher level of accuracy for IMRT is desirable since reduced margins are often used and dose gradients may be large near critical structures. The importance of accurate prediction and delivery of optimal dose distributions will increase as biological/molecular imaging is used to better delineate targets, subtargets, and normal structures. It is through MC's superior dose-calculation accuracy that the full benefits of IMRT's superior dose distributions will be realized. At the simplest level, MC methods may be used for re-computing dose distributions for IMRT plans optimized previously using conventional dose computation methods. This will provide a more accurate estimate of deliverable dose distribution, which may be used to prescribe the treatment monitor units (MUs) or to simply verify the treatment in place of laborious measurements. Ultimately, however, using MC in the optimization process is expected to maximally exploit the potential of IMRT. MC will enable us to locate areas of dose deficiencies and dose excesses in targeted tissues and adjacent normal critical structures accurately, and the IMRT optimization process, using the MC dose algorithms, will tailor the dose to best achieve the treatment goals.

## Monte Carlo For IMRT Dose Calculations

Led by advances in imaging during the last 20 years, our understanding of how heterogeneities influence patient dose distributions and recognition of the limitations of various dose-calculation algorithms have greatly increased. Three-dimensional dose-calculation algorithms have advanced from simple correction-based methods, such as tissue-air ratio (TAR) or pencil-beam (PB), to advanced model-based algorithms including superposition/convolution (SC) and MC (Mackie et al. 1996). For IMRT, the choice of dose-calculation algorithm poses a dilemma. Since optimization is an iterative process, which may require repeated dose calculations for each of a very large number (ranging from a few tens to few thousands) of iterations, there is a strong need for the dose algorithms to be very fast. On the other hand, since IMRT relies on accurate accounting of the dose to both targets and critical structures (either of which may have rather small margins surrounding them), the need for high dose accuracy also exists. As is usually the case, the requirements of speed and accuracy are contradictory goals.

Most IMRT implementations use fast PB algorithms to compute dose. PB methods use the effective radiological path-length correction to account for heterogeneities. For non-IMRT cases, they can have dose errors of 10% or more (Mackie et al. 1985; Woo and Cunningham 1990). However, PB methods are very fast, requiring less than 1 second to compute dose distribution for a beam. More sophisticated SC algorithms are slower (~30 seconds/beam) and account for heterogeneities using the local density variations to scale an energy deposition kernel. SC is more accurate than PB; however, inaccuracies persist under certain circumstances (Yu, Mackie, and Wong 1995). MC algorithms are slower still (minutes to hours per beam), but account for heterogeneities more accurately by transporting incident and scattered photons and electrons directly through a realistic representation of the patient geometry.

The potential impact of MC techniques for IMRT is perhaps greatest when one considers that IMRT is typically delivered through a sequence of small, possibly dynamically shaped multileaf collimator (MLC) apertures with high-intensity gradients. For such fields, assumptions used in conventional algorithms regarding scatter equilibrium and output factor variation with field size typically break down. Also, for IMRT, a significant fraction of the dose within anatomic structures is due to MLC scattered or leakage radiation (Mohan et al. 2000). It is precisely under these circumstances that calculated dose distributions have the greatest uncertainties due to approximations inherent in conventional methods of transforming intensities into MLC leaf sequences.

The following two sections will cover the effect of the MLC on dose distributions and methods used to integrate MLCs into MC dose-calculation algorithms.

## Effect Of IMRT On Dose Distributions

In addition to modulating the intensity distributions, the MLC also changes the spectral characteristics of the radiation emerging from the accelerator and incident upon the patient. Consider, for example, the photon energy spectrum for a uniform intensity field generated using an open field and generated using a dynamic MLC (DMLC) field with 1.0 cm and 0.25 cm sliding window gaps (figure 1). As the MLC window width decreases, the energy spectrum of photons from the target is hardened (panel a) mainly due to an increase in the amount of attenuating material in the beam. In addition, as the window width decreases, the scatter contributions from both the Primary Collimator (panel b) and Flattening Filter (panel c) become harder and decrease in terms of their total contribution. The MLC scatter contribution (panel c), however, increases with decreasing window width.

The spatial distribution of radiation leaking through the MLC is shown in figure 2, which shows the dose profile due to total radiation leakage through an MLC configured to completely block a $10 \times 10$ cm$^2$ radiation field. It also shows the components of the radiation transmitted through and scattered from the MLC. Within the field defining jaws, the majority of the dose is due to MLC transmitted radiation; however, outside the field edge, the dose is almost entirely due to MLC scatter. The fractional component of MLC scatter is broad, diffuse, and increases as the area of the MLC exposed increases. The MLC leakage as a function of field size (as defined by jaws) is given in table 1 for the Varian 120 leaf MLC. The increase in MLC scatter radiation is responsible for the MLC leakage increasing from 1.557% of the open field dose for a $5 \times 5$ cm$^2$ MLC blocked field to 1.898% of the open field dose for a $20 \times 20$ cm$^2$ MLC blocked field at 6 MV. MLC scatter radiation accounts for ~25% of the MLC leakage radiation for a $20 \times 20$ cm$^2$ 6 MV beam.

It should also be noted that electrons generated and escaping from the MLC contribute substantially to the surface dose. For instance, for a $10 \times 10$ cm$^2$ MLC blocked field, at 6 MV, 18% of the surface dose is due to electrons generated in the MLC, while at 18 MV, 35% of the surface dose is due to MLC electrons. Assuming that, for a typical IMRT case, two-thirds of the beam is blocked but that the number of MUs is about three times the number for conventional treatments, the electron contribution to surface dose might be non-negligible and may require MC to be estimated accurately.

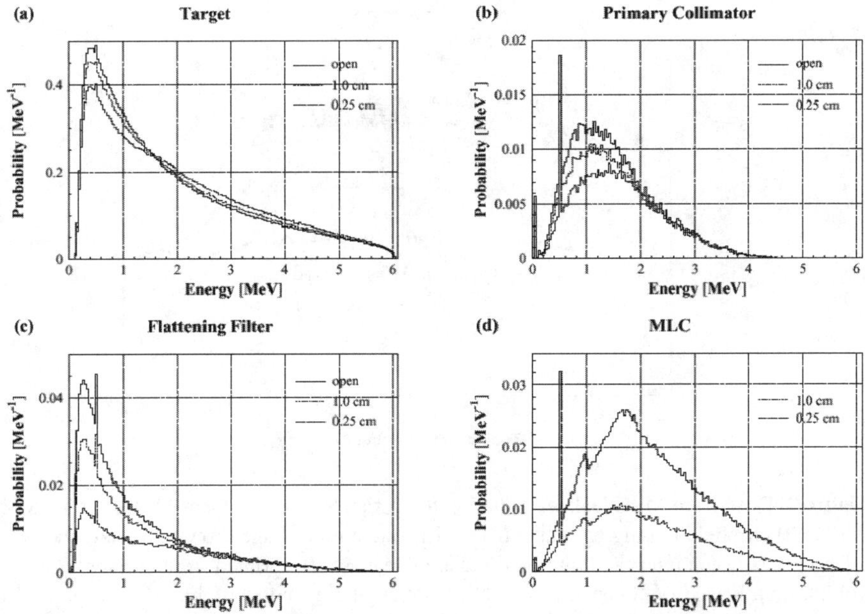



**Figure 1.** Contributions of main treatment head scatter components to the total energy spectrum of a 6 MV open beam and beams created by dynamically sweeping a 1.0 and 0.25 cm MLC window (a) target, (b) primary collimator, (c) flattening filter, and (d) MLC. Scatter components from the target, primary collimator, and flattening filter decrease and become harder as the MLC slit width decreases. The MLC scatter contribution, on the other hand, increases with decreasing slit width. [Reprinted from *Physics in Medicine and Biology*, vol 46, M. K. Fix, P. Manser, E. J. Born, R. Mini, and P. Ruegsegger, "Monte Carlo simulation of a dynamic MLC based on a multiple source model," pp. 3241–3257. © 2001, with permission from IOP Publishing.]

For clinical IMRT beams, the amount of MLC beam hardening and leakage radiation will depend upon field size and efficiency (defined as ratio of the number of MUs required to deliver the field to the number of MUs required to deliver the same maximum dose with an open field, also sometimes referred to as the "modulation factor") of the IMRT field. As the efficiency decreases, the primary energy spectrum becomes harder and the contribution due to MLC scatter and contaminant electrons increases. Conventional methods of including intensity modulation into dose calculations ignore such spectral changes and, therefore, are less accurate than MC methods, for which such changes can be properly accounted. Methods that have been used to incorporate MLCs into MC dose calculation are covered in the next section.

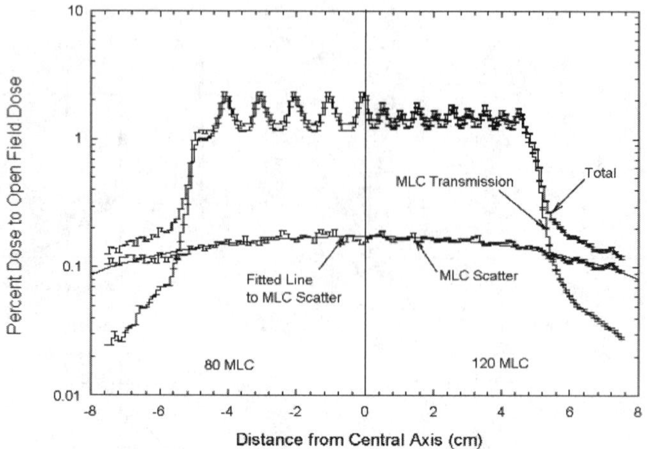


**Figure 2.** Dose from MLC leakage radiation for Varian 80- and 120-leaf MLCs for a 6 MV $10 \times 10$ cm² field impinging on the MLC. The radiation leakage shows structure due to differences between inter- and intra-leaf radiation leakage. [Reprinted from *Medical Physics*, vol 28, J. O. Kim, J. V. Siebers, P. J. Keall, M. R. Arnfield, and R. Mohan, "A Monte Carlo study of radiation transport through multileaf collimators," pp. 2497–2506. © 2001, with permission from AAPM.]

**Table 1.** MC Computed Radiation Leakage Components as a Function of Field Size for 6 MV and 18 MV Fields Blocked by the MLC One-standard-deviation statistical uncertainties are given in parenthesis. [Adapted from Kim et al. 2001.]

| 120 MLC – 6 MV | $5 \times 5$ | $10 \times 10$ | $15 \times 15$ | $20 \times 20$ |
|---|---|---|---|---|
| Total | 1.557(0.011) | 1.620(0.013) | 1.737(0.012) | 1.898(0.019) |
| MLC Transmission | 1.486(0.011) | 1.444(0.011) | 1.427(0.011) | 1.427(0.011) |
| MLC Scatter | 0.071(0.002) | 0.176(0.006) | 0.310(0.006) | 0.471(0.014) |

| 120 MLC – 18 MV | $5 \times 5$ | $10 \times 10$ | $15 \times 15$ | $20 \times 20$ |
|---|---|---|---|---|
| Total | 1.730(0.012) | 1.825(0.013) | 1.975(0.014) | 2.142(0.015) |
| MLC Transmission | 1.670(0.012) | 1.657(0.012) | 1.657(0.012) | 1.672(0.012) |
| MLC Scatter | 0.060(0.002) | 0.168(0.004) | 0.318(0.006) | 0.470(0.008) |

## Methods For Incorporating Intensity Modulation Into Monte Carlo

As mentioned above, the impact of MC, relative to SC algorithms, on the accuracy of predicted deliverable dose distributions is likely to be greatest when the effect of scattering from and transmission through the intricate MLC geometry is to be accounted for. As will be shown, exact modeling of the MLC and exact tracking of each and every particle through the MLC may be prohibitively time-consuming even with the largest and the fastest cluster of affordable computers available today. Therefore, it is necessary to resort to approximations and variance reduction techniques. Different investigators have adopted different strategies in this regard. It is important that the approximations and variance reduction techniques be appropriately validated, else they may lead to uncertainties in calculated dose distributions. The following sections discuss some of the published strategies.

## Intensity Matrix Method

One frequently used approach for IMRT MC is to directly use the treatment planning system's intensity matrix (IM) $I$ (or a similarly produced IM) to account for intensity modulation during the MC simulation, i.e., use the same intensity matrix to modulate the incident particle stream as the one used for the non-MC IMRT dose calculations (Ma et al. 2000; Aaronson et al. 2002; Wang, Yorke, and Chui 2002). In this strategy, during the MC simulation, as a particle encounters the MLC, instead of explicitly transporting the particle through the MLC, the statistical weight of the incident particle $w_i$ is modified by the intensity value $I(x,y)$ at the corresponding $x,y$ location to compute the final weight $w_f$, using

$$w_f(x, y) = w_i(x, y) \times I(x, y).$$
(1)

While the IM method is extremely fast for MC, it also is overly simplistic. When the treatment planning system's IM is used for MC dose calculation, any errors inherent in the leaf segmentation/trajectory-to-fluence conversion process are promulgated through to the patient calculation. In this mode, the MC only effectively accounts for the patient heterogeneities and not the incident fluence prediction, and thus may have only a modest accuracy advantage over SC algorithms.

Alternatively, the IM can be developed independent of the treatment-planning system (Ma et al. 2000; Aaronson et al. 2002). The MLC-leaf sequence file is read in and the MLC transmission is integrated into a two-dimensional (2-D) matrix, typically defined at the isocenter plane. The method to do this can be demonstrated for a segmented MLC (SMLC) IMRT plan. For a given sMLC segment, the IM is a map of the relative transmission values corresponding with the leaf positions for the MLC field shape $s$. Transmission values are determined using the leaf thickness for the corresponding leaf shape, either including leaf-edge tongue-and-groove effects (Aaronson et al. 2002) or ignoring them (Ma et al. 2000). The transmission at point $x,y$ is equal to

$$T(x, y)_s = \exp(-\overline{\mu}_W(x, y) \times l(x, y)_s),$$
(2)

where $\bar{\mu}_W(x, y)$ is the effective linear attenuation coefficient for the MLC material ($W$) and $l(x,y)$ is the path length though the MLC. $\bar{\mu}_W(x, y)$ varies as a function of the distance from the beam central axis to account for the off-axis energy dependence of the incident beam. Note, beam hardening caused by the MLC is ignored when the effective attenuation coefficient is used, since individual components of the incident energy spectrum are not individually attenuated.

In practice, the intensity matrix method for MC is not applied to individual segments, but instead is applied for the combination of segments at a given beam angle. In this case, the composite intensity grid is the weighted sum over the $s$ individual segments

$$I(x, y) = \sum_s T(x, y)_s \times f_s, \tag{3}$$

where $f_s$ is the fraction of the monitor units (MUs) delivered through segment $s$.

The resultant intensity matrix is similar to the one produced for dose computations by conventional treatment-planning systems. The uniform-field photon particles incident on the patient are then assigned weights proportional to intensities using equation (1). Although this method of incorporating intensity modulation in MC is independent of the treatment planning system, it is not likely to be an improvement over the use of treatment planning system's IM.

The weakness of the IM approach is that it does not account for scattered photons and electrons produced in the MLC. To account for MLC leaf leakage, an empirical correction term can be introduced (Ma et al. 2000), however, this neglects the energy and angular dependence of the scattered radiation.

## Full Simulation Method

The most rigorous method for the use of MC for calculating dose distributions for intensity-modulated fields is the direct use of the leaf-sequence file and leaf positions during the radiation transport simulation. There are numerous published examples of modeling MLCs for MC calculations. The BEAM system (Rogers et al. 1995) includes the MLCQ module, which uses simplified, focused leaf edges and the VARMLC module (Kapur, Ma, and Boyer 2000), which includes the details of the leaf edges for the 80-leaf Varian MLC. Monte Carlo N-Particle (MCNP) (Briesmeister 1997) has a full combinatorial geometry package, which has been used by Kim et al. (2001) for MLC modeling. However, as mentioned above, detailed transport through the full MLC geometry is computer-time prohibitive. For MCNP, for instance, an estimated 100 GHz×hours would be required to transport enough particles for sufficient statistical precision (2%) through the full MLC geometry. To increase the dose-calculation speed, simplifying geometric assumptions are typically made. For example, DMLC-IMRT fields may be simulated as a sequence of many (hundreds of) static fields (Fix et al. 2001). Other geometric simplifications include ignoring details of the leaf sides (tongue-and-groove) (Liu, Verhaegen, and Dong 2001) or including the leaf edges but approximating the rounded MLC leaf tip with a focused leaf tip with an effective offset Fix et al. 2001).

## Monte Carlo MLC Models Designed Specifically For IMRT

Two MLC models designed specifically for IMRT have been described in the literature. These models make varying simplifying assumptions regarding geometry of the MLC and physics of the radiation transport to ensure that they are efficient and accurate. They are described in the following sections.

### Probability-Based DMLC Model

One model designed specifically for IMRT is Keall's probability based DMLC model (Keall et al. 2001). The model uses the MLC-leaf sequence file and the phase space of particles incident upon the MLC as inputs. [The phase space consists of the particle type, energy, positional coordinates $(x,y,z)$, directional coordinates $(u,v,w)$, and the statistical importance or weight $(W)$ of each particle.] For each incoming particle, the MLC leaf with which the particle intersects at the mid-plane of the MLC is selected; thus, in effect, the MLC is collapsed to a plane. If the particle is a photon, its statistical weight is reduced by the probability that the MLC leaf attenuates it. The photon attenuation probability at a given $x,y$ location is determined by integrating the leaf positions (open, closed, leaf tips) at that $x,y$ position over time. The proper energy-dependent photon attenuation coefficient is used, hence, accounting for the effects of the MLC on the energy spectrum.

For an electron, the statistical weight is reduced by its probability of intersecting the MLC. Electron transport in the MLC is altogether neglected.

The output of the model is the phase space of particles exiting the MLC, which can then be used for patient or phantom dose calculations. This model properly accounts for leaf transmission, leaf-tip profiles, and beam hardening. Because the model collapses the MLC to a single plane, it does not include cross-leaf transport. It neglects tongue-and-groove–type leaf-edge effects that occur when the leaves are not synchronized. Scatter from the MLC leaves is approximated by first Compton scatter, and other scatter mechanisms and secondary electron production are ignored.

### Transport-Based DMLC Model

Another approach to incorporating dynamic MLC in MC dose calculations is the use of simplified particle transport. Such a model has been proposed by Siebers et al. (2002a). The model uses plausible physical and geometric approximations to achieve fast, yet accurate, results and is applicable for both DMLC and SMLC IMRT delivery.

The general flow for incorporating the MLC model into MC dose calculation is shown in figure 3. The positions of the MLC leaves are read from the MLC leaf-sequence file that is normally sent from the treatment planning system to the linear accelerator for treatment delivery. The sequence of subfields in the file can result in static beam delivery, SMLC-IMRT beam delivery, or DMLC-IMRT beam delivery. The positions specified in the leaf-sequence file are translated into physical leaf coordinates using the same scheme as the linear accelerator's control system. This results in a table of physical leaf positions as a function of monitor units. Incoming particles are read from the phase space of particles exiting the treatment jaws and are transported though the MLC using some geometry and physics approximations. Surviving exiting particles are written to an exiting phase space file that is used as input for Monte Carlo patient dose calculations. The transport of particles through the MLC continues until a specified number of particles, derived from the incident phase space, has been transported.

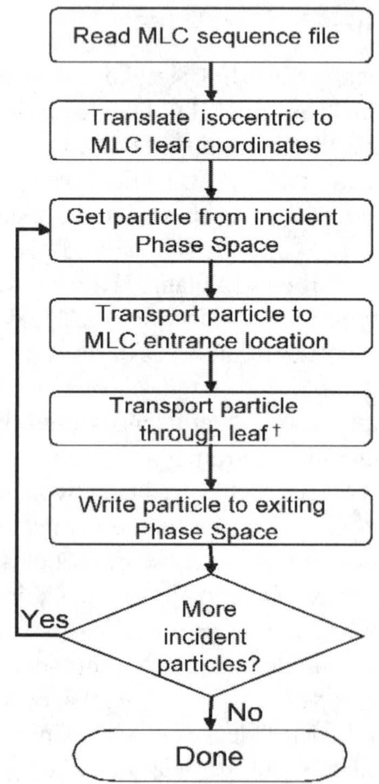


**Figure 3.** Flow diagram for including the MLC into MC dose calculation.

The model separates the complex MLC geometry into simple non-reentrant geometric regions, each of which readily lends itself to simplified radiation transport. For Varian MLCs, two non-reentrant regions are required. At each of $n$ of $N$ different randomly selected number of fractional monitor units, the new position of the MLC leaves is determined. The total path length of attenuating material encountered by an individual particle while traversing the entire MLC is the sum of the individual thicknesses traversed in each of the geometric regions. The thickness traversed in an individual region is correctly evaluated for particles emanating from the target, but, in some MLC configurations, can be incorrect for highly divergent particles since cross-leaf transport in a given MLC region is ignored in this model.

The statistical weight of an incident MC photon ($w_i$) is modified to account for the attenuation through the total path length ($t_n$) traversed for sample $n$. Using the $N$ different fractional MU settings (different times and leaf positions), the average attenuation and statistical weight ($w_f$) of the exiting photon is

$$w_f = \frac{w_i}{N} \sum_{n=1}^{N} e^{-\mu(E)t_n / \cos\theta_z} \tag{4}$$

where $\mu(E)$ is the attenuation coefficient of the MLC material at energy $E$, and $\cos\theta_z$ is the $z$-direction cosine of the photon.

For photons, only attenuation and first Compton scatter interactions are considered. Photoelectric effect and pair production in the MLC are ignored. Compton scatter is sampled based upon the total MLC thickness traversed and is sampled from EGS4-derived functions. Transport of Compton-scattered photons from the MLC presumes a slab-beam type geometry.

All electron transport in the MLC is ignored. The weight of incoming electrons is reduced by the probability that they intersect any portion of the MLC.

The MC-MLC model was tested for 6-MV and 18-MV photon beams by comparing it with measurements and MC simulations that incorporate the full physics and geometry for fields blocked by the MLC, for fields with the maximum possible tongue-and-groove and tongue-or-groove effect, for static test cases and for sliding windows of various widths. The MLC model predicts the field size dependence of the MLC leakage radiation within 0.1% of the open-field dose. The entrance dose and beam hardening behind a closed MLC are predicted to within ±1% or 1 mm. Dose undulations due to differences in inter- and intraleaf leakage are also predicted to within ±1% or 1 mm. For the worst-case scenario test of the tongue-and-groove effect, the MC MLC model predicts the tongue-and-groove effect within ±1% or 1 mm for 95% of the points at 6 MV and 88% of the points at 18 MV. The dose through a static leaf tip is also predicted to within ±1% or 1 mm. Tests with dynamic delivery verified that the model reproduced measurements to within 0.5%.

## Monte Carlo For Plan Verification

Monte Carlo can be used as an independent dose calculation for verification of IMRT plans. The reliability of this method of plan confirmation depends upon the depth of detail of the MC simulation. Application of MC on the patient geometry inherently accounts for the patient heterogeneities, provided that the patient CT image set is converted into a sufficient number of tissue-like materials. The ability to accurately account for the modulated fluence distribution incident on the patient depends upon the rigor of the MC source model and of the transport of particles through the beam modifiers, including the MLC.

This section will review verification of IMRT plans designed with conventional dose-calculation algorithms with MC simulations. The effect of rigorousness of the MLC transport on the results will also be discussed.

## Intensity Matrix Approximation

When an intensity matrix approximation is used to account for the intensity modulation, the effect of patient heterogeneities is accounted for in the MC simulation, but the effects of MLC scatter and transmission are only approximated. Both Ma et al. (2000) and Wang et al. (Wang, Yorke, and Chui 2002) used variations of the IM approach to re-compute dose distributions with MC for IMRT plans, designed originally with PB algorithms. Wang et al. directly re-used the intensity matrix produced by the treatment-planning system for 10 IMRT cases (9 patients). Figure 4 shows differences in the dose to 95% of the planning target volume (PTV) ($D_{95}$), the fraction of the PTV receiving 95% of the dose ($V_{95}$) and the mean dose ($D_{mean}$). For the five lung patients (patients 1–5), a systematic decrease in each dose parameter was observed for each patient. The extreme case was lung patient 5, who showed a nearly 10% decrease in $D_{95}$ and a 20% decrease in $V_{95}$. The five head and neck plans did better, on average, with the extreme being a 9% increase in $D_{95}$ for patient 6. Similar differences were observed by Ma et al. (2000).

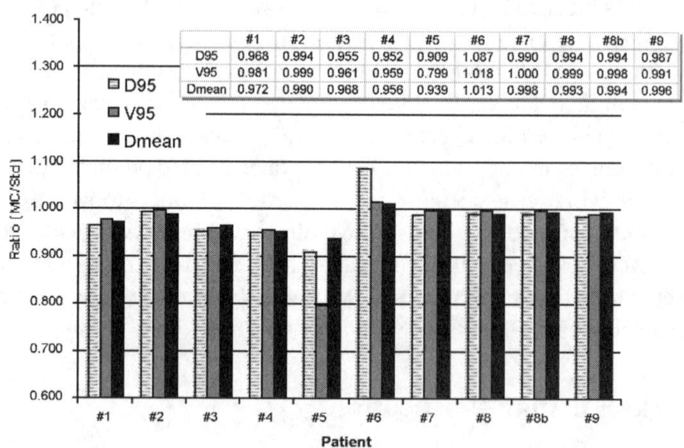


**Figure 4.** Ratio of MC to pencil beam doses for 10 IMRT plans (patients 1–5, lung cases; patients 6–9 head and neck cases). [Reprinted from *Medical Physics*, vol 29, L. Wang, E. Yorke, and C.-S. Chui, "Monte Carlo evaluation of 6 MV intensity modulated radiotherapy plans for head and neck and lung treatments," pp. 2705–2717. © 2002, with permission from AAPM.]

The ability of MC to correctly account for heterogeneities is highlighted in figure 5, which shows an upper thoracic spine case computed with the IMRT planning system's PB algorithm and with MC (Pawlicki and Ma 2001). The combination of the electron transport through the low-density lung tissue and the titanium rods in the vertebral bodies significantly affected the dose-volume histogram (DVH), resulting in a 9% lower mean dose to the target.

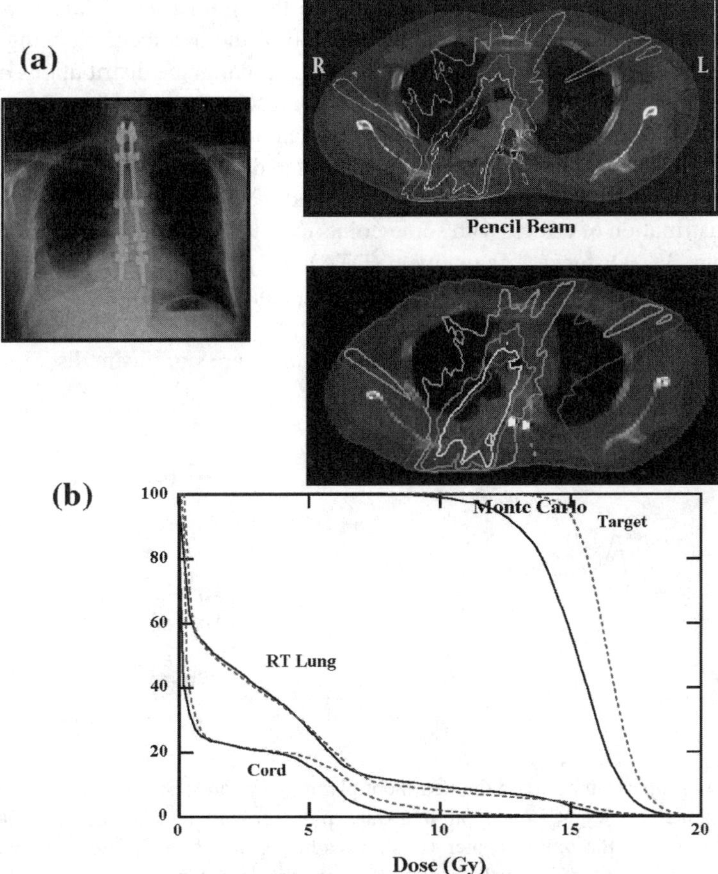


**Figure 5.** MC and PB dose distributions for a patient treated with 8 coplanar 4-MV IMRT fields. The patient has titanium rods inserted in the vertebral column. Dose values in (a) are 16.2, 14.4, 12.6, 9.0, 5.4, and 1.8 Gy. The DVHs in (b) show a large difference between the target coverage computed using the PB algorithm (dashed line) and MC (solid line). [Reprinted from *Medical Dosimetry*, vol 26, T. Pawlicki and C.-M. Ma, "Monte Carlo simulation for MLC-based intensity-modulated radiotherapy," pp. 157–168. © 2001, with permission from Elsevier Science.]

## Verification Including IMRT MLC Models

MC can be used not only for verifying the patient dose distributions, but also for confirmation of in-phantom quality assurance measurements. An example of this is shown in figures 6 through 9. To assess the accuracy of the predicted "deliverable" fluence and the actual fluence realized at the treatment machine, computed IMRT dose distributions are compared with measurements of individual beam dose distributions at 5 cm depth in a flat phantom oriented normal to the beam axis. Figure 6 compares measurements with the results of the SC method of the treatment-planning system. Figure 6a compares a profile through the isocenter point in the distributions of one of the beams. Qualitatively, this graph suggests reasonable agreement between the measured and the SC dose results. However, quantitative analysis of a histogram of the difference between the measured and computed dose distributions for all (not just those along the profile of figure 6a) calculated and measured points (figure 6b) shows a broad distribution of errors, with some points exceeding ±10% and the mean difference being –3%. Distance-to-agreement (DTA) analysis and percent dose difference analysis (figure 6c) find that only 54% of the calculated values are within ±2% or 2 mm of the measurements and that some points with 5% to 10% dose differences have DTAs that exceed 2 cm. This clearly shows that there are significant discrepancies in the SC-computed phantom dose distributions.

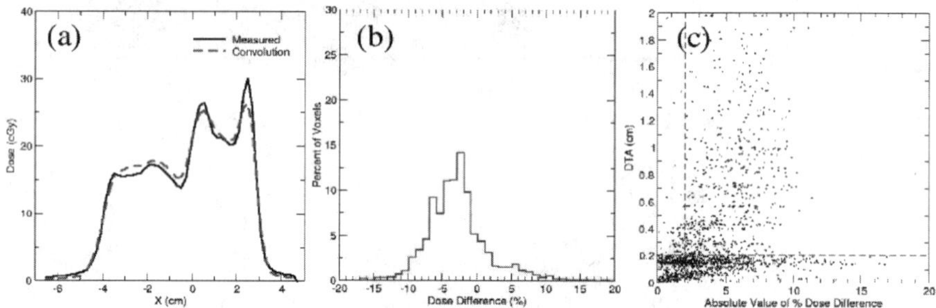


**Figure 6.** Comparison between the treatment planning system's SC dose distribution for a single beam computed at 5 cm depth in a water phantom with measurements. (a) shows a single dose profile through isocenter, (b) shows a histogram of the difference between the measured and computed dose values, and (c) shows the dose difference and the distance to agreement (DTA) for each point. The dashed lines indicate that DTA=2 mm and a dose difference of 2%. For this case, only 54% of points fall within ±2% or 2 mm.

Figure 7 shows that changing to MC for just the transport of radiation in the phantom, while still using the intensity matrix (IM) produced using conventional methods, does not materially change the result. Discrepancies remain for the IM approach regardless of whether MC or SC (or PB) is used in the phantom. This is not surprising since a properly commissioned SC or PB algorithm should be nearly as accurate as MC in a homogeneous water phantom.

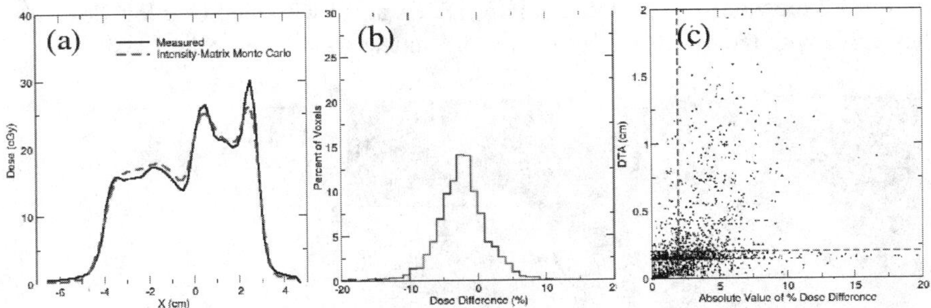

**Figure 7.** Comparison between MC using IM approximation and measurement. Note MC with the IM approximation does not improve agreement with the measured dose profile.

When MC is also used to transport incident particles through the moving MLC (MC-MLC), dose differences with respect to measurement are greatly reduced (figure 8). The mean dose difference (figure 8b) is zero, and the width is dominated by the 2% statistical precision in the MC dose computation. Ninety-seven percent of the points agree within ±2% or 2 mm. The MC, including transport through the moving MLC on the homogeneous phantom, has uncovered a fluence prediction error. This error is not detected when the treatment-planning system's intensity matrix is used for MC intensity modulation.

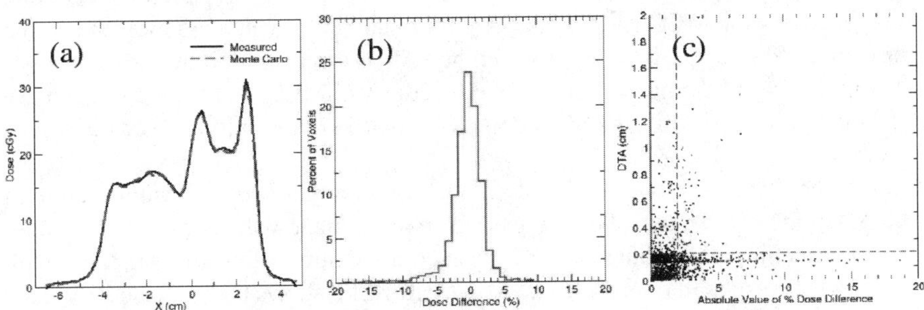

**Figure 8.** Comparison between MC that includes MLC transport and measurements. The MC reproduces the measurements, and 97% of the points fall within ±2% or 2 mm.

Dose distributions for the patient for whom the dosimetry data are shown in figures 6, 7, and 8 are shown in figure 9. These deliverable IMRT plans were computed using SC and MC. The MC plans were computed with both the intensity matrix approximation (MC-IM) and using the more accurate MLC transport model (MC-MLC) discussed above. The MC-MLC result exhibits a 66 Gy hot spot and poor coverage of the PTV by the 57 Gy line, features that are missing from SC. The PTV DVHs show that with the SC plan, compared with the "true" patient dose (assuming that MC-MLC represents the truth), there is a 4.5% dose deficit at the $V_{95}$ and a ~5% increase in dose for 15% of the volume. The MC-IM PTV DVHs agree with the SC at low doses, but they agree with the MC-MLC results for the hottest 15% of the volume.

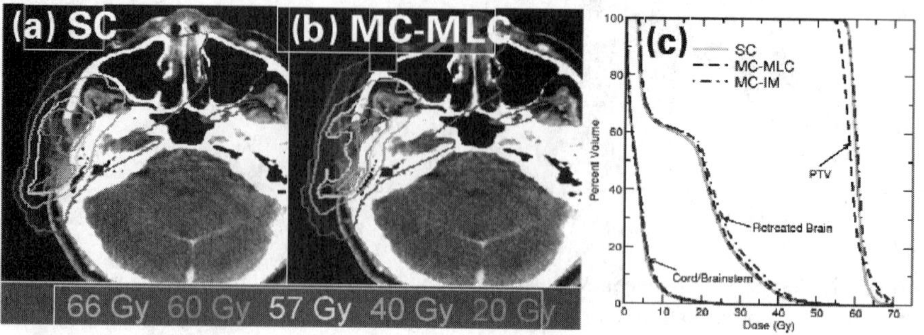


**Figure 9.** Comparison of isodose profiles for (a) SC, (b) MC-MLC dose computations, and (c) DVHs for these computations and intensity matrix-based MC (MC-IM). The MC-IM isodose (not shown) is similar to that for SC.

In another head and neck example (figure 10), DVHs for the PTV are compared for SC computations, MC using the IM approximation, and IM using the moving MLC (i.e., delivery based on sliding window technique). The MC-IM calculation agrees with the treatment planning system's SC dose-calculation algorithm. From these results, one might incorrectly presume that the SC method is accurate for this patient's treatment. However, when the MLC and its effects on the incident fluence are included in the simulation, a 9% dose deficiency at $V_{90}$ in the PTV is discovered. Film measurements in a homogeneous flat phantom confirmed that the MC-MLC result agreed within 2% of the measurements, while the SC and intensity matrix MC results showed up to 10% differences.

Another such comparison involving a commercial IMRT planning system ($P^3$IMRT) and SMLC mode of delivery is a case of a patient with a recurrent, left sphenoid wing meningioma. Pinnacle's SC dose computation results are compared with the MC-MLC results in figure 11. The MC-MLC result shows that the true PTV dose is more inhomogeneous than that indicated by SC and that doses to the PTV and left eye are elevated. The physician responded to this discrepancy by reducing the monitor units to reduce the risk of optic nerve damage.

These cases demonstrate that one source of discrepancy between the measured and deliverable IMRT dose distributions is the incorrect prediction of the radiation fluence on the patient. MC can only account for this if explicit transport through the MLC occurs during particle simulations. When the MLC is included in the MC verification calculation, the MC can be useful for determining dose discrepancies due to both patient heterogeneities and fluence perturbations caused by the MLC.

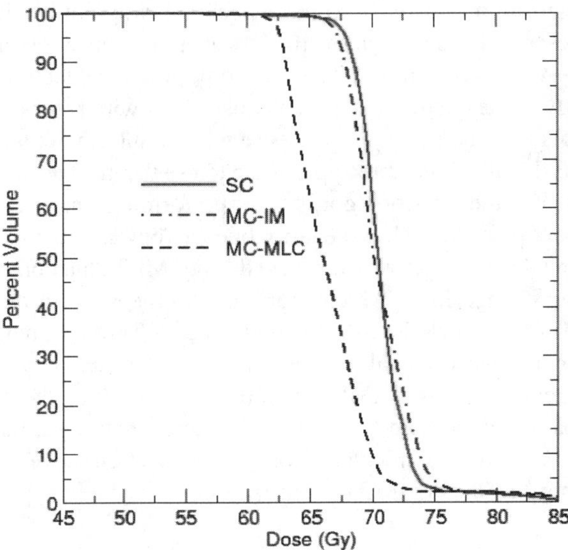


**Figure 10.** PTV DVHs for a head and neck case computed with the SC algorithm, with MC with the IM approximation (MC-IM) and with MC with direct transport through the MLC (MC-MLC). For this patient, dose errors are almost entirely due to incorrect fluence prediction by the SC and MC-IM methods.

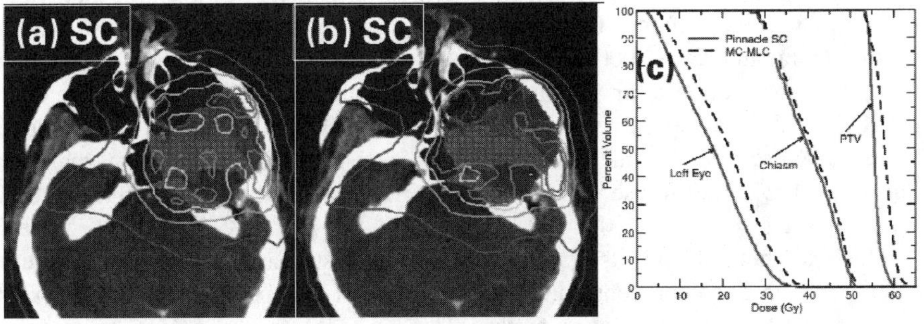


**Figure 11.** Comparison of (a) SC and (b) MC dose computations for a patient planned with P³IMRT. The MC computation shows poorer dose homogeneity in the PTV and a higher dose to the left eye.

## Use Of Monte Carlo During IMRT Optimization

While using MC to verify final IMRT treatment plans is useful, it is akin to planning a patient using hand calculations and then verifying the final plan using a 3-D dose-calculation algorithm. Since MC is more accurate, why not use it as the basis for defining the prescribed dose and allow the less accurate conventional methods to serve as secondary verification tools? There is some initial reluctance to take this approach, due partly to the desire to maintain consistency with prior experience and ongoing IMRT trials and due partly to the desire to wait until there is greater confidence in MC results. Ideally, it is more appropriate to use the most accurate algorithm for patient planning and the inferior algorithm for performing a cursory check of the final IMRT treatment plan. In such a scenario, one can envision using MC (including transport through the beam delivery devices) during IMRT plan optimization, then using either a PB or SC algorithm (which approximates the effect of radiation transport through the MLC) to check the MC dose calculation. Thus, although use of MC for plan verification is a worthy goal to avoid improper dose delivery, MC can help exploit one of the real strengths of IMRT plan optimization, i.e., IMRT's ability to use multiple beams to compensate for dose deficiencies that might be revealed by more accurate dose distribution calculations. This section covers the various approaches for using MC during IMRT optimization.

## Bixel Method

One method to incorporate MC into IMRT optimization is to use MC to pre-compute individual pencil beams in the patient geometry (bixels). The IMRT optimization process then adjusts the weights of the individual beamlets to minimize the objective function and hence determine the optimal plan. The advantage of the bixel approach is that the MC calculations need to be performed only once; however, the statistical uncertainty in each computed bixel must be small to avoid artifacts due to insufficient statistics (Jeraj and Keall 2000).

To avoid truncation error, ideally the bixels should be saved over the entire dose grid. This leads to a very large memory requirement ($N_{bixels} \times N_{DoseGridElements}$). To reduce this memory requirement, methods have been proposed to save sparse bixel matrices (Thieke et al. 2002) or to use wavelets to store the bixels (Deasy, Wickerhauser, and Picard 2002).

The bixel method lends itself to segmented MLC (step-and-shoot) beam delivery or delivery with fixed compensators. One limitation of the bixel method is that bixels are computed on a fixed resolution pattern. This limits the ability of IMRT to produce dose distributions with sharp gradients. Another limitation of the bixel method concerns beam delivery. Bixels are typically computed using the energy spectrum of the open beam; however, the device used to modulate the beam (MLC or compensators) both hardens the beam energy spectrum and introduces scattered radiation. Without *a priori* knowledge of the beam modulation, the consequences of this beam hardening and scattered radiation are difficult to assess. Thus, the bixel method with MC-computed bixels can properly account for patient heterogeneities in the dose calculation, but it cannot include effects from radiation transport through the beam delivery device. Given its limitations, it has seen only limited applicability.

Using the bixel approach, Jeraj et al. (Jeraj, Keall, and Siebers 2002) studied the effect of dose-calculation accuracy on IMRT plans. A 2-D lung case was studied using PB, SC, and MC algorithms. Optimization was performed using each algorithm separately, resulting in different optimal fluence patterns for each dose algorithm. It was observed that the optimization with the various dose-calculation algorithms each converged to equivalent DVHs. Following optimization, each final dose distribution was re-computed using Monte Carlo. The resultant DVHs differed (figure 12). From the study, two types of dose-calculation errors were defined: Systematic errors are the differences in dose distributions computed using two different algorithms (e.g., PB and MC) with the same incident fluence distributions. Systematic errors are observed when dose verification calculations are performed. The second error is termed the "convergence error," which is when IMRT optimization converges to a different solution than that found when optimization is performed with an algorithm that has systematic errors. True convergence errors can only be determined by optimizing with a dose-calculation algorithm that has no systematic errors. In place of that utopian algorithm, MC can be used as a surrogate to estimate the convergence error of non-MC algorithms. Panel (b) of figure 12 shows the impact of convergence errors on a treatment plan.

It is important to note that when MC-computed bixels are used for optimization, they can only avoid convergence errors caused by patient heterogeneities. Pre-computed MC bixels do not include the effect of the MLC on the dose distribution; thus, convergence errors due to the MLC persist for this approach.

## Pre-Computed Leaf Segments

Another method for MC-based IMRT optimization is to pre-compute MC dose distributions for given leaf segments and then optimize the weights of these pre-selected leaf segments to minimize the plan objective function. The leaf segments used for the MC dose computation are determined by a pre-optimization with some other faster, more approximate dose-calculation algorithm. This method is implemented in the Hyperion family of MC IMRT optimization codes (Fippel et al. 2000). The memory storage requirements for this approach are modest in comparison with the bixel approach, requiring only $N_{Segments} \times N_{DoseGridElements}$.

The pre-computed segment method with MC can properly account for both the patient heterogeneities and the effects from radiation transport through the beam delivery device in the dose calculation during the optimization process. This is a key advantage of the pre-computed segment approach. The MC dose calculation for each segment can fully include the MLC leaf configuration for that segment. Thus, full transport through the MLC can occur, and MLC-induced beam hardening, scatter, and inter- and intraleaf leakage can be explicitly included in the dose calculation. The major disadvantage of this approach is that the solution space during MC optimization is limited by the segments selected during initial pre-optimization. Another disadvantage of this method is that it is limited to SMLC delivery.

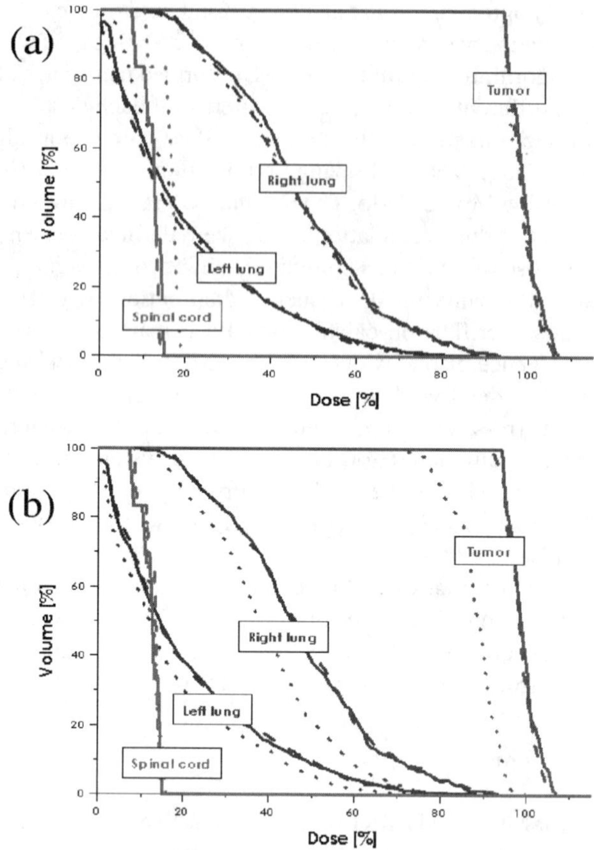


**Figure 12.** DVHs for 2-D IMRT lung case. (a) compares DVHs for the plan optimized using the stated dose algorithm [MC (Solid), SC (Dotted), and PB (Dashed)]. In (b), the doses for each plan were re-computed with MC showing the convergence error. [Reprinted from *Physics in Medicine and Biology*, vol 47, R. Jeraj, P. J. Keall, and J. V. Siebers, "The effect of dose calculation accuracy on inverse treatment planning," pp. 391–407. © 2002, with permission from IOP Publishing.]

## IMCO Method

The inverse Monte Carlo optimization method (IMCO) has been proposed and tested as a method for performing IMRT optimization with MC (Bogner, Scherer, and Herbst 1999). This method completes IMRT optimization in the time required for two MC calculations. The first MC simulation is performed for an open beam from each pre-selected beam angle. During this computation, the correlation between the point at which the particle passes through the beam modulator plane and the energy deposited in a given voxel is determined. This is termed the "inverse kernel" ($\Phi_{i,k}$) and contains elements $\varphi_{i,k}(x,y)$ that are the relative total energy deposited in voxel $i$ relative to the total energy deposited in the target volume (TV) or organ at risk (OAR) by the fluence element at $(x,y)$ for a beam with gantry angle $k$. Using the computed dose along with the plan objective function, an initial estimate for the beam modulation intensity matrix $M_k^0$ for each $k$ beam is determined.

A new MC simulation is then started in a stepwise fashion using $M_k^0$ for its initial intensity modulation. This simulation only requires storage of dose values in the TVs and OARs (and not their point of origin). The calculation is performed in $S$ steps. For each substep $s$ of the calculation, $N_{total}/S$ particles are simulated, where $N_{total}$ is the anticipated total number of particles required for sufficient statistics in the final result. After each substep, the objective function is reevaluated and the inverse kernels are used to update the intensity matrix for the next substep $M_k^{s+1}$. Substeps are further simulated and evaluated (without zeroing the intensity matrix) until $N_{total}$ particles are simulated. Typically, 10 substeps are used in the optimization. The total beam modulation is the sum of the individual beam modulations used for each substep.

Use of the inverse kernels in the IMCO method results in accurate determination of the gradient of the dose with respect to the incident fluence; hence, rapid convergence of the IMCO method is observed. IMCO will properly account for patient heterogeneities during MC dose calculation and optimization, but, since the optimization is based upon delivery fluence maps, it does not include radiation leakage and scatter effects from the MLC in the optimization dose calculation. Such effects can be included in a post-optimization, post-segmentation forward MC calculation of all segments (requiring a third MC simulation).

### Iteration-Specific Monte Carlo

The brute force approach of performing a full MC dose calculation for each iteration of the optimization can also be used. The brute force approach can properly account for patient heterogeneities and the effects from radiation transport through the beam delivery device in the dose calculation during the optimization process. One must be careful to ensure that sufficient particles are simulated so as to ensure that the derivatives used to compute intensity updates are not adversely affected by the statistical noise inherent in the MC dose calculation (this is true for all methods). Several methods have been developed for iteration-specific MC dose calculations, and each of these methods is described in greater detail in the following subsections.

### Intensity Matrix Approximation Approach

The simplest method to use MC for IMRT optimization is to use the intensity matrix produced by the treatment planning system during optimization to adjust the statistical weights of particles incident upon the patient. At each iteration, a new IM is used during the MC simulation.

*Optimization Including MLC Transport*

When IMRT optimization includes explicit transport through the MLC during the dose calculation, the general flow of the optimization changes as indicated in figure 13. Figure 13a shows the typical optimization process where beam optimization (shaded region) and beam delivery technique (cross-hatched region) are considered as separate steps. To correctly include the MLC in an MC dose calculation used during optimization, the beam delivery technique and conversion to leaf sequences must occur as indicated in figure 13b. This scheme is necessary since MC calculations use leaf positions at different points in time to accurately compute dose distributions. This technique has been termed deliverable-based optimization (Siebers et al. 2002b). An advantage to deliverable optimization is that at the completion of the optimization sequence, the optimized beams are ready for delivery to the patient. Changes in the intensity or dose distribution due to post-optimization leaf sequence generation are avoided.

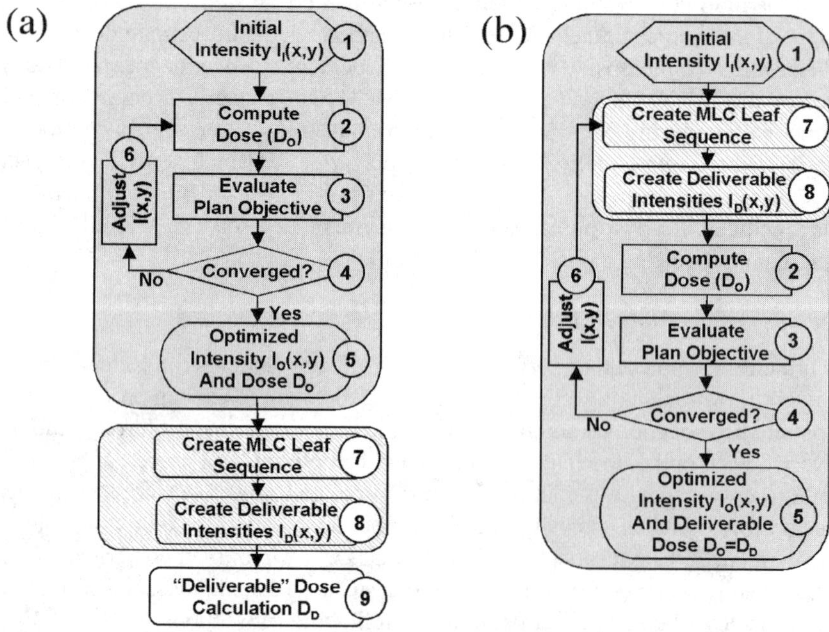


**Figure 13.** Flow diagrams for IMRT optimization processes. The typical optimization process is shown in (a), where optimization occurs independent of beam delivery. When MC is used, including explicit transport through the MLC leaves, a deliverable optimization sequence such as that listed in (b) is required. Box labels are similar in the two diagrams to aid interpretation. [Adapted from Siebers et al. (2002b).]

An example of MC deliverable-based optimization is given in figure 14. This is the same patient case as described in figures 6 through 9. Note that the deliverable optimization restores the dose coverage of the PTV and essentially eliminates the hot spot.

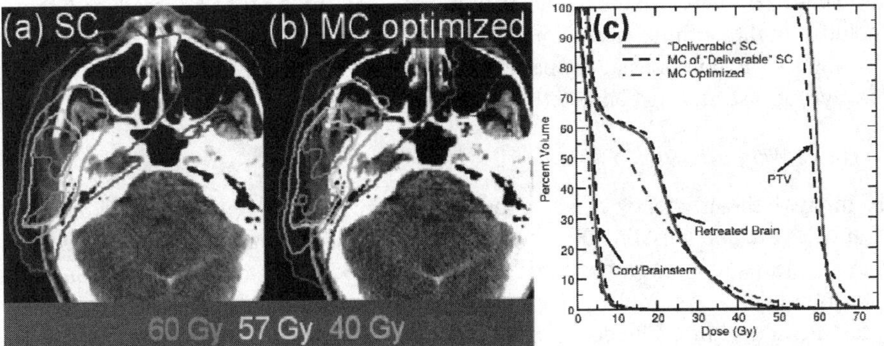



**Figure 14.** MC deliverable-based optimization. (a) Isodose curves for non-deliverable optimization with the SC algorithm. This dose is an error as indicated in figure 9. (b) Isodose profile for the MC deliverable-based optimized plan. Panel (c) shows selected DVHs. The MC optimized DVH restores the PTV coverage or the original SC optimized plan.

A second example showing MC deliverable-based optimization is shown in figure 15. The plan was initially optimized using an SC algorithm ($ND_{opt}$, i.e., "non-deliverable" optimization). Conversion to an SC deliverable plan ($ND_{opt}+DEL$) resulted in apparent poorer dose homogeneity to the PTV, with the majority of the PTV receiving a higher overall dose. MC simulations of this SC deliverable plan showed that the SC, in fact, had a lower dose to the PTV. Optimization with MC, however, results in a DVH that is nearly identical to the original optimized plan.

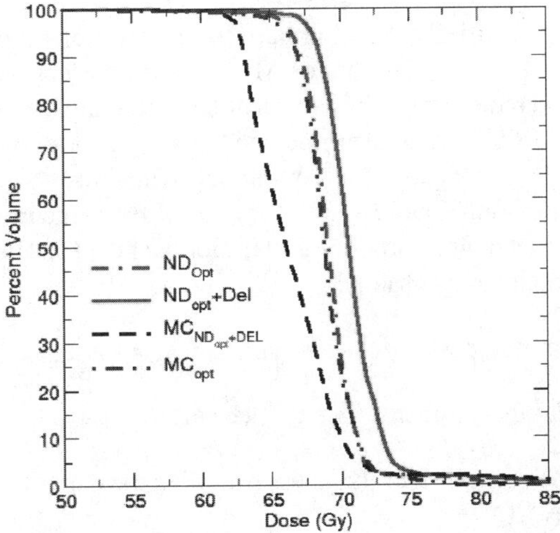



**Figure 15.** PTV DVHs for non-deliverable optimization ($ND_{opt}$), incorporating beam delivery ($ND_{opt}+DEL$), MC simulation of $ND_{opt}+DEL$, and MC optimization of the plan ($MC_{opt}$).

These test cases demonstrate that if both MC and MLC leaf sequencing are included in the optimization loop, the optimization process can adjust IMRT fluence distributions to compensate for patient heterogeneities, beam delivery limitations and leakage, and scattering characteristics of the MLC.

### Negative Weight Particle Method

To improve the efficiency of MC simulations during IMRT optimization, Laub et al. (Laub, Bakai, and Nüsslin 2001) and Fippel et al. (2000) have proposed methods that may be termed the "negative particle weight methods." Prior to using MC, an initial pre-optimization is completed with some faster, less-accurate algorithm, for example, a fast PB algorithm. Fluences from this pre-optimization are used in an initial MC calculation of the deliverable plan. Following MC, the plan objective function is evaluated and the desired change in fluence for the next MC calculation is determined. This fluence update can be either positive or negative, with the negative fluence bounded by the minimum fluence that can be produced (e.g., the leakage corresponding to MLC being closed for the entire irradiation). In the MC dose calculation for the next iteration, particle weights are assigned based on the differential fluence such that at the completion of that iteration the desired total beamlet weights are achieved. Positive weight particles result in dose increases, while negative weight particles reduce the dose. This method corrects the dose distribution from the previous iteration step to that required for the present step. The MC optimization is iteratively repeated until the objective function converges.

Applying the negative weight particle method without considering beam delivery is relatively straightforward and has the potential to substantially improve MC dose computation efficiency. However, in this mode, the effects of MLC leakage and scatter are ignored.

As an example, we briefly describe here the method of Fippel et al. (2000) to include the effects of a compensator (or MLC) using the negative particle weight method. This method requires: (a) the same source producing the exact same particles incident upon the IMRT beam delivery device (compensator or MLC) for iteration $k$ and iteration $k+1$; (b) storage of the compensator thicknesses or MLC leaf positions/sequences at iteration $k$ and $k+1$; and (c) use of the same random numbers and random number sequence for particle $i$ in iteration $k$ and $k+1$. The method proceeds as follows (assuming a compensator):

Using initial random number $R^i$, get source photon $i$ ($i=1, N_{SourceParticles}$) and

- Transport it to the compensator entrance surface

- Determine the compensator thickness $t^i$ for both the current ($t^i_{k+1}$) and the previous iterations ($t^i_k$)

- If $t^i_{k+1}$ is not equal to $t^i_k$ then

  - Store the current state of the random number generator $R^i_{step}$

  - Set the particle weight negative and transport particle $i$ through compensator thickness $t^i_k$ and the patient geometry (following all secondary products)

  - Reset random number generator to $R^i_{step}$

  - Set the particle weight positive and transport particle $i$ through compensator thickness $t^i_{k+1}$ and the patient geometry

- Return to top of loop and select the next source photon

The efficiency of this method depends on the intensity modulation change between iteration $k$ and $k+1$. For a compensator with $B$ elements, the efficiency $\varepsilon$ can be written as

$$\varepsilon \propto \frac{B}{2\Delta B} + S$$

where $\Delta B$ is the number of elements that change and $S$ is a small quantity required to account for the source sampling time. When $\Delta B$ is small (few compensator elements change), the method is extremely efficient, however, as $\Delta B\Delta B$, the efficiency drops and the calculation takes twice as long as a stand-alone calculation.

*Hybrid Approaches*

Hybrid dose-calculation techniques involve combining results from two or more different dose-calculation algorithms to effectively accelerate dose calculation. As developed, these techniques involve using fast dose-calculation algorithms (e.g., PB algorithms) for the majority of the dose calculations and periodically correcting the dose with more accurate but slower methods (e.g., SC and MC) (Siebers et al. 2002c).

The simplest method is the multi-stage sequential dose-calculation method. It uses a fast PB calculation for initial optimization iterations followed by more accurate SC or MC dose calculations for final optimization iterations (Siebers et al. 2001, 2002c). The sequence method results in a ~60% reduction in the optimization time. The sequence method is not a true hybrid method since the PB algorithm is used just to obtain a better initial guess for the SC or MC dose optimization.

The true hybrid methods are the ratio-matrix method and the dose-correction method (Siebers et al. 2002c). These methods use both slow and accurate and fast and less accurate algorithms throughout the optimization process.

The basic flow of the ratio-matrix hybrid method is given in figure 16. A correction matrix $R$ is applied to fast dose-calculation results (presumed to be PB in the figure) to approximate the results that would be obtained using the MC algorithm. Initially, the voxel-by-voxel dose-correction matrix ($R$) for each beam is set to unity for each voxel (box 1). The optimization proceeds (box 2) using the PB (or SC) algorithm in the deliverable-based optimization scheme with $D_R = D_{PB}\_R$ for the dose. Following convergence of the optimization, the dose is computed using the MC dose-calculation algorithm (box 4). This step can include the MLC-leaf motion. Results of the MC and corrected PB (or SC) dose computations are compared (box 5). If the results differ (plan scores differ by more than the convergence criteria), the ratio matrix is updated to be the ratio of the two dose computations ($D_{MC}/D_{PB}$), and the optimization continues. Otherwise, the ratio matrix has converged, and optimization is completed.

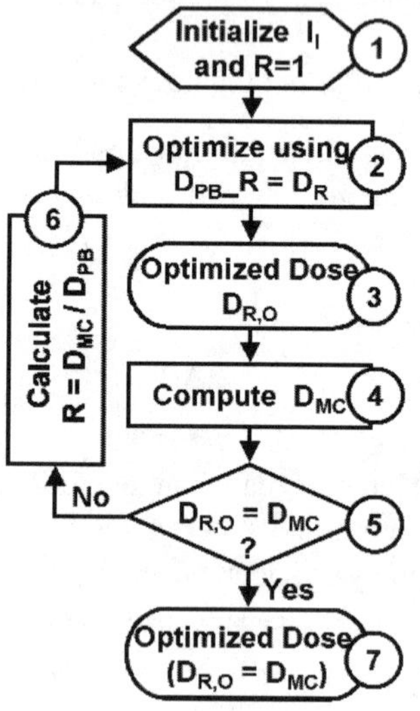


**Figure 16.** Flow of the ratio-matrix method used to speed up MC IMRT optimization.

It is important to note that once the ratio matrix is set to $R = D_{MC}/D_{PB}$, the next new iteration in box 2 is executed with the MC algorithm, $D_{PB} \times R = D_R = D_{MC}$. The terma (Ahnesjo, Andreo, and Brahme 1987), $T$, used in the PB calculation algorithm (Mohan, Chui, and Lidofsky 1986) is directly proportional to the intensity, $I$; therefore, $D_R = (T_I \otimes K) \times R$, where $K$ is the 2-D point spread function. With $I_{R_{MC}}$ being the intensity when $R$ is defined, for further optimization iterations, $I_n = I_{R_{MC}} + \Delta I_n$. Using the distributive of property convolution, it can be shown that

$$D_R = (T_{I_n} \otimes K) \times R = (T_{I_{R_{MC}}} \otimes K) \times R + (T_{\Delta I_n} \otimes K) \times R = D_{MC} + (T_{\Delta I_n} \otimes K) \times R. \quad (5)$$

Only the change in intensity and associated PB dose modify the MC dose distribution. As convergence approaches, the optimization is effectively completed using MC (as $\Delta I_n \to 0$, $D_R \to D_{MC}$). The accuracy of the MC calculation is preserved, and convergence error should be eliminated.

The dose-correction method is similar to the ratio method except that during the optimization $D_C = D_{PB} + C$ is used in box 2 with $C = D_{MC} - D_{PB}$ defined in box 6. When used with PB and SC algorithms, the ratio and dose-correction methods were found to maintain both the accuracy and the optimality of full iterative SC optimization, while requiring only 2 to 3 SC computations. This results in a 2- to 10-fold total optimization speed increase. Use of the hybrid methods with MC is still under development.

## Other Methods To Reduce Monte Carlo Dose Computation Time

Another set of dose-computation acceleration techniques, specific to MC methods, involves smoothing or de-noising results of the MC dose computation (Deasy 2000; Kawrakow 2002). Smoothing/de-noising reduces statistical noise inherent in MC dose calculations, trading it off for possible systematic bias of the results. The overall result is a reduction of the dose-computation time for a given total (systematic plus random) dose uncertainty. Due to the large variations intrinsic in the intensity within a single treatment field, these techniques must be used with caution. An example of a smoothed IMRT intensity profile is shown in figure 17. In this example, the smoothing method of Kawrakow was applied to in-phantom single-beam IMRT profiles. The advantage of Kawrakow's method is that the smoothed data are compared with respect to the original data with its known statistical uncertainties to determine the acceptability of the smoothed data set. Local smoothing parameters can change based upon this comparison, and, in some cases, smoothing can be entirely rejected. After smoothing is applied to the MC results with 5% statistical noise, little difference between it and the 2% statistical noise results remain.

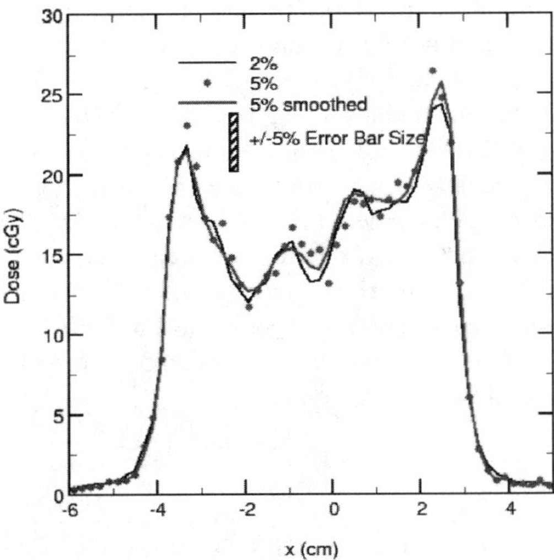


**Figure 17.** In-phantom IMRT profile computed to 2%, 5%, and 5% smoothing using Kawrakow's method (Kawrakow 2002). Note: Statistics are with respect to maximum dose.

## Summary And Future Directions

It is commonly acknowledged that MC techniques provide the most accurate means of predicting dose distributions used for designing and optimizing radiation treatment plans. Furthermore, it is generally accepted that a higher level of accuracy for IMRT is desirable. Therefore, the application of MC for IMRT is of a greater importance than for conventional treatments. Dose accuracy may be more important for IMRT since reduced margins are often used and dose gradients may be large near critical structures. With small margins, dose errors could diminish the potential advantages of IMRT. The value of MC techniques is further accentuated considering that IMRT is typically delivered through a sequence of small, possibly moving apertures in which high intensity gradients are achieved. A significant fraction of the dose within anatomic structures is due to MLC scattered or leakage radiation. As is clear from the examples shown, it is under these circumstances that calculated dose distributions have the greatest uncertainties and where MC would have the greatest impact. If MC is used to accurately transport radiation through the MLC, and if the leaf sequence generation is incorporated into the optimization process, the optimized and deliverable dose distributions are not only the most accurate but also truly optimum. Ultimately, using MC in the optimization process is expected to maximally exploit the potential of IMRT. MC will identify areas of dose deficiencies and dose excesses in targeted tissues and adjacent normal critical structures, and the IMRT optimization process, using the MC dose algorithms, will tailor the dose to best achieve the treatment goals.

While there is a strong case for the use of MC in IMRT, there are also major challenges as compared with its use for conventional radiotherapy. This is because the optimization process needs to repeatedly (perhaps hundreds to thousands of times, depending upon the optimization algorithm and the nature of the optimization problem being solved) to obtain dose distributions for new sets of intensity distributions and for different beam configurations for beam configuration optimization. Thus, even though the speed of MC calculations for a given treatment plan is now within acceptable times, the use of MC for IMRT optimization may require some special variance reduction techniques and dose computation acceleration strategies. There is a continued need for the further development of these methodologies. Nevertheless, limited implementations of MC methods for IMRT are already taking place in some academic institutions. As commercial vendors incorporate MC dose calculations into their IMRT planning systems, the use of this important technique is likely to become widespread. The use of MC is essential not only for improved patient care but also to produce higher quality dose-response data.

## References

Aaronson, R. F., J. J. DeMarco, I. J. Chetty, and T. D. Solberg. (2002). "A Monte Carlo based phase space model for quality assurance of intensity modulated radiotherapy incorporating leaf specific characteristics." *Med. Phys.* 29:2952–2958.

Ahnesjo, A., P. Andreo, and A. Brahme. (1987). "Calculation and application of point spread functions for treatment planning with high energy photon beams." *Acta Oncol.* 26:49–56.

Bogner, L., J. Scherer, and M. Herbst. (1999). "An inverse Monte Carlo optimization algorithm for conformal radiotherapy." *Physica Medica* XV:111–119.

Briesmeister, J. F. MCNP-A General Monte Carlo N-Particle Transport Code. Version 4B. Report LA-13181. Los Alamos, NM: Los Alamos National Laboratory, 1997.

Deasy, J. O. (2000). "Denoising of electron beam Monte Carlo dose distributions using digital filtering techniques." *Phys. Med. Biol.* 45:1765–1779.

Deasy, J. O., M. V. Wickerhauser, and M. Picard. (2002). "Accelerating Monte Carlo simulations of radiation therapy dose distributions using wavelet threshold de-noising." *Med. Phys.* 29:2366–2373.

Fippel, M., M. Alber, M. Birkner, W. Laub, F. Nüsslin, and I. Kawrakow. (2000). "Inverse Treatment Planning for Radiation Therapy Based on Fast Monte Carlo Dose Calculation." Monte Carlo 2000 Conference, (Lisbon).

Fix, M. K., P. Manser, E. J. Born, R. Mini, and P. Ruegsegger. (2001). "Monte Carlo simulation of a dynamic MLC based on a multiple source model." *Phys. Med. Biol.* 46:3241–3257.

Jeraj, R., and P. Keall. (2000). "The effect of statistical uncertainty on inverse treatment planning based on Monte Carlo dose calculation." *Phys. Med. Biol.* 45:3601–3613.

Jeraj, R., P. J. Keall, and J. V. Siebers. (2002). "The effect of dose calculation accuracy on inverse treatment planning." *Phys. Med. Biol.* 47:391–407.

Kapur, A., C. M. Ma, and A. L. Boyer. (2000). "Monte Carlo simulations for multileaf-collimator leaves: Design and dosimetry." *Med. Phys.* 27:1410.

Kawrakow, I. (2002). "On the de-noising of Monte Carlo calculated dose distributions." *Phys. Med. Biol.* 47:3087–3103.

Kawrakow, I., M. Fippel, and K. Friedrich. (1996). "3D electron dose calculation using a voxel based Monte Carlo algorithm (VMC)." *Med. Phys.* 23:445–457.

Keall, P. J., J. V. Siebers, M. Arnfield, J. O. Kim, and R. Mohan. (2001). "Monte Carlo dose calculations for dynamic IMRT treatments." *Phys. Med. Biol.* 46:929–941.

Kim, J. O., J. V. Siebers, P. J. Keall, M. R. Arnfield, and R. Mohan. (2001). "A Monte Carlo study of radiation transport through multileaf collimators." *Med. Phys.* 28:2497–2506.

Laub, W. U., A. Bakai, and F. Nüsslin. (2001). "Intensity modulated irradiation of a thorax phantom: comparisons between measurements, Monte Carlo calculations and pencil beam calculations." *Phys. Med. Biol.* 46:1695–1706.

Liu, H. H., F. Verhaegen, and L. Dong. (2001). "A method of simulating dynamic multileaf collimators using monte carlo techniques for intensity-modulated radiation therapy." *Phys. Med. Biol.* 46:2283–2298.

Ma, C. M., T. Pawlicki, S. B. Jiang, J. S. Li, J. Deng, E. Mok, A. Kapur, L. Xing, L. Ma, and A. L. Boyer. (2000). "Monte Carlo verification of IMRT dose distributions from a commercial treatment planning optimization system." *Phys. Med. Biol.* 45:2483–2495.

Mackie, T. R., E. El-Khatib, J. Battista, J. Scrimger, J. Van Dyk, and J. R. Cunningham. (1985). "Lung dose corrections for 6- and 15-MV x rays." *Med. Phys.* 12:327–332.

Mackie, T. R., P. Reckwerdt, T. McNutt, M. Gehring, and C. Sanders. "Photon Beam Dose Computations" in *Teletherapy: Present and Future.* T. R. Mackie and J. R. Palta (eds.). Madison, WI: Advanced Medical Publishing, 1996.

Mohan, R., C. Chui, and L. Lidofsky. (1986). "Differential pencil beam dose computation model for photons." *Med. Phys.* 13:64–73.

Mohan, R., M. Arnfield, S. Tong, Q. Wu, and J. Siebers. (2000). "The impact of fluctuations in intensity patterns on the number of monitor units and the quality and accuracy of intensity modulated radiotherapy." *Med. Phys.* 27:1226–1237.

Pawlicki, T. and C.-M. Ma. (2001). "Monte Carlo simulation for MLC-based intensity-modulated radiotherapy." *Med. Dosim.* 26:157–168.

Rogers, D. W. O., B. A. Faddegon, G. X. Ding, C.-M. Ma, J. We, and T. R. Mackie. (1995). "BEAM: A Monte Carlo code to simulate radiotherapy units." *Med. Phys.* 22:503–524.

Schach von Wittenau, A. E., L. J. Cox, P. M. Bergstrom Jr., W. P. Chandler, C. L. Hartmann Siantar, and R. Mohan. (1999). "Correlated histogram representation of Monte Carlo derived medical accelerator photon-output phase space." *Med. Phys.* 26:1196–1211.

Schneider, W., T. Bortfeld, and W. Schlegel. (2000). "Correlation between CT numbers and tissue parameters needed for Monte Carlo simulations of clinical dose distributions." *Phys. Med. Biol.* 45:459–478.

Sheikh-Bagheri, D., and D. W. Rogers. (2002). "Sensitivity of megavoltage photon beam Monte Carlo simulations to electron beam and other parameters." *Med. Phys.* 29:379–390.

Siebers, J. V., S. Tong, M. Lauterbach, Q. Wu, and R. Mohan. (2001). "Acceleration of dose calculations for intensity-modulated radiotherapy." *Med. Phys.* 28:903–910.

Siebers, J. V., P. J. Keall, J. O. Kim, and R. Mohan. (2002a). "A method for photon beam Monte Carlo multileaf collimator particle transport." *Phys. Med. Biol.* 47:3225–3249.

Siebers, J. V., M. Lauterbach, P. J. Keall, and R. Mohan. (2002b). "Incorporating multi-leaf collimator leaf sequencing into iterative IMRT optimization." *Med. Phys.* 29:952–959.

Siebers, J. V., M. Lauterbach, S. Tong, Q. Wu, and R. Mohan. (2002c). "Reducing dose calculation time for accurate iterative IMRT planning." *Med. Phys.* 29:231–237.

Thieke, C., S. Nill, U. Oelfke, and T. Bortfeld. (2002). "Acceleration of intensity-modulated radiotherapy dose calculation by importance sampling of the calculation matrices." *Med. Phys.* 29:676–681.

Wang, L., E. Yorke, and C.-S. Chui. (2002). "Monte Carlo evaluation of 6 MV intensity modulated radiotherapy plans for head and neck and lung treatments." *Med. Phys.* 29:2705–2717.

Woo, M. K., and J. R. Cunningham. (1990). "The validity of the density scaling method in primary electron transport for electron and photon beams." *Med. Phys.* 17:187–194.

Yu, C. X., T. R. Mackie, and J. W. Wong. (1995). "Photon dose calculation incorporating explicit electron transport." *Med. Phys.* 22:1157–1165.

# IMRT Delivery System QA

**Thomas J. LoSasso, Ph.D.**
Memorial Sloan-Kettering Cancer Center
New York, New York



## Introduction

Multileaf collimator (MLC) use is increasingly common in radiation therapy clinics throughout the world. These devices are well established as a replacement for conventional blocks in the majority of treatment sites where static field techniques are used for conventional 3-D conformal radiation therapy (3DCRT). At the present time only a small percentage of MLC-equipped centers are using the MLC for intensity-modulated radiation therapy (IMRT), even though the technology has been commercially available for almost 10 years. The hesitance is in large part due to the complexity of the technical aspects of planning and delivery. Before this new technology can be safely implemented, each component of the process must be understood by the users, and a comprehensive quality assurance (QA) program should be in place. A QA program will need to address treatment-planning systems, delivery issues involving

MLC mechanics, electronics, and software, and patient treatment verification. Only delivery issues will be presented here.

In the broad sense, QA for IMRT delivery encompasses acceptance testing, commissioning, routine MLC QA, and patient-specific QA. It begins at the time of installation of new equipment or at the time an existing MLC is upgraded for use with IMRT in order to affirm the capability for accurate IMRT with the specific MLC. Commissioning implies the accurate acquisition of the treatment planning parameters specific to IMRT, rigorous testing of the dose calculation algorithm under the increased demands of intensity modulation, and ancillary techniques such as respiration gating and the splitting of large fields. Periodic MLC-specific QA checks of the stability of the mechanical aspects of the MLC, i.e., leaf positioning, and the dosimetric aspects of the linac for small numbers of monitor units (MU), i.e., linearity and symmetry, ensure that when the treatment parameters are correctly set, the correct dose is delivered. Verification of the integrity of the treatment plan from the planning through the delivery stages (patient-specific QA) is the last component. These procedures complement each other, and together they ensure accurate dose delivery.

The QA for MLC used in static mode, conventional 3DCRT, is relatively simple. Similar to the procedures required for jaws and blocks, the QA checks involve mechanical alignment of the MLC to the accelerator and leaf position reproducibility (Mubata, Childs, and Bidmead 1997; Hounsell and Jordan 1997). The QA procedures specific to the use of IMRT present special issues for dose delivery compared to 3DCRT. Hardware and software for MLC are still relatively new to the end users in the clinic, and the potential for dosimetric errors is still not well understood, while the consequences of such errors may be clinically significant. Individual treatment centers should expect a learning curve for understanding novel treatment planning and QA issues. The urge to implement IMRT at individual therapy centers should be tempered while these issues come into focus and are addressed at each center.

In general, when MLCs are used to perform intensity-modulated treatments, they require more stringent tolerances and, in turn, a more involved QA program. Tests used for static QA of the MLC need to be redesigned to achieve the required accuracy. This emphasis is justified if one considers that for static treatments these parameters only define the dose near the borders of the field; depending upon the proximity of abutting critical tissues, 1 to 2 mm uncertainty of the leaf positions is acceptable. Periodic checks of the projected leaf positions with graph paper at isocenter are sufficient for this purpose. However, for IMRT, the leaves modulate the dose delivered throughout the target volume; more specifically, the dose delivered with IMRT is sensitive to the width of the gap defined by each leaf pair. Then, it is only a matter of assuring that the leaves are in the correct position at each moment during treatment. Regardless of MLC designs, or whether the delivery mode is segmental (SMLC) or dynamic (DMLC), these tests should stress the precise execution of the gap width defined by opposing leaf positions; and for DMLC, the ability of the leaves to maintain their specified leaf speed is also important.

It is necessary to identify sources of leaf positioning error for the specific MLC design, and to develop QA tests and frequencies to detect these mechanical problems before dose errors become significant. Analysis of QA data to track the long-term stability of MLC performance can reveal patterns of MLC failure. These areas then need to be monitored closely to ensure that the planned dose is delivered accurately and reproducibly. Manufacturer's modifications to MLC hardware and software often follow from an analysis of the frequency and severity of malfunctions during clinical use.

This chapter will focus on dose delivery related QA procedures applicable to acceptance testing and routine MLC QA specific to IMRT. Some of these methods use static fields; they are applicable to all three MLC designs, Siemens, Elekta, and Varian. However, many of the tests rely on dosimetric measurements using the dynamic mode, and so are only applicable to the Varian MLC.

## MLC Alignment

As for the movable jaws and conventional metal-alloy blocks, the alignment of the MLC leaves affects the spatial uncertainty between the peripheral extent of the radiation beams and the perimeter of the target volume. For IMRT, MLC alignment in the direction of leaf travel affects the registration of the intensity-modulation (IM) patterns between fields altering the composite dose distribution for the plan and also shifts the IM dose distribution for each individual field relative to the patient's anatomy. In some regions, such as when the spinal cord is to receive a low dose, dose gradients may be very large within an IMRT field, as much as 10% per millimeter, similar to using a metal conventional block to shield the cord. Fortunately, the effect from one field is, in general, diluted by the dose from the other IM beams; on the other hand, IMRT fields have more frequent gradients than conventional fields. Misalignment of the MLC in the direction perpendicular to leaf motion typically shifts the dose distributions for all the fields in the same direction with respect to the patient anatomy, comparable to a systematic patient setup error.

Alignment in the direction of leaf motion, including leaf bank skewness and center-line offset can be readjusted via leaf calibration using the alignment of the jaws as a guide. Alignment in the direction perpendicular to leaf motion is fixed at the factory. Even optimal alignment of the MLC does not ensure perfect registration between fields. Gantry sag, the displacement of the field in the radial direction, is maximal at gantry angles of 0° and 180°, while gantry roll is maximal at 90° and 270° and shifts these fields vertically downward. Similar problems exist for IM fields delivered with fixed compensators.

Misalignment of the MLC relative to the isocenter can be evaluated with the following procedure. A film is irradiated with two complementary leaf patterns, which nominally suggest a uniform field. For MLC with an interleaf space coincident with the central axis (Varian and Elekta), the patterns are similar to those illustrated in figure 1. For this leaf configuration, the fields match at the central axes. When the center leaf overlies the central axis (Siemens), the match line perpendicular to leaf motion is shifted off the axis by 0.5 cm. Ideally, the image would appear as in figure 2a, a uniform field with a low-density strip from Top to Bottom, corresponding to tongue-and-groove underdosage. MLC leaves with rounded edges (Varian and Elekta) will yield a high-density strip from Left to Right if their digital readouts are calibrated to the light field edge, corresponding to added leakage through the rounded edges of the opposed leaves. If the leaves are calibrated using the radiation field edge, then the high-density region will appear relatively uniform. Doubly focussed MLC leaves (Siemens), in theory, should also be uniform from Left to Right. A second image is produced with the same leaf patterns (center leaf reversed for the Siemens MLC), but with the collimator rotated exactly 180° between fields. The density change of the strips in this image is proportional to the misalignment of the MLC and can be calibrated with a third image, figure 2b, using the same two fields as for figure 1, but introducing a 1 mm shift in each directions, simulating an 0.5 mm misalignment (0.5 mm is a reasonable tolerance limit), in both the radial and transverse directions. These images may be visually evaluated or scanned. These images may be obtained at other gantry angles as well.

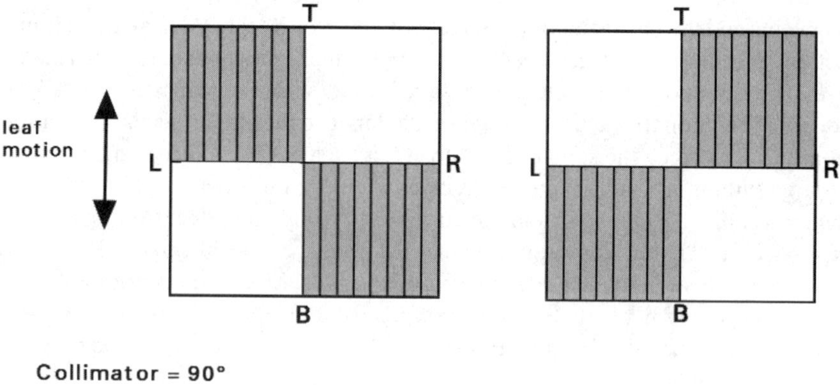


**Figure 1.** Complimentary leaf patterns to test the MLC alignment.

## Leaf Positioning

For conventional 3DCRT, the accuracy of static field edges, whether defined by the MLC, blocks, or the jaws, only affects the high gradient regions near the borders of the target volume or critical structures. In these static treatments, 1 mm errors are usually tolerated. In contrast, the dose delivered with IMRT, whether SMLC or DMLC, can be very sensitive to errors in the calibration of leaf position (Budgell et al. 2000). Therefore, leaf movements must be executed much more precisely.

For DMLC, the impact of leaf calibration is illustrated in figure 3. Dose errors for fixed width gaps moving at constant speed are proportional to gap errors and inversely proportional to the gap width (ignoring leaf transmission). For example, if the nominal gap width is 2 cm, then a gap error of 1 mm, introduced by one or both leaves of a pair, will produce a 5% dose error. In clinical DMLC fields, neither the gap width

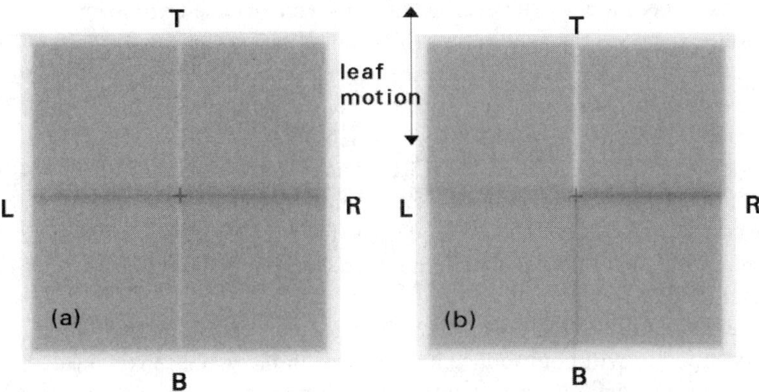



**Figure 2.** Composite images testing the alignment of the MLC using the leaf patterns from figure 1 for a Varian MLC. (a) Uniform field is interrupted by a tongue-and-groove underdose (vertical band) and leakage between leaf faces (horizontal band) when the leaves are calibrated using a feeler gauge or the light field. If the calibration is to the radiation field edge, the dark band should disappear. In either case, symmetry indicates perfect alignment. (b) The asymmetry shown here corresponds to 0.5 mm misalignments both perpendicular and parallel to leaf motion.

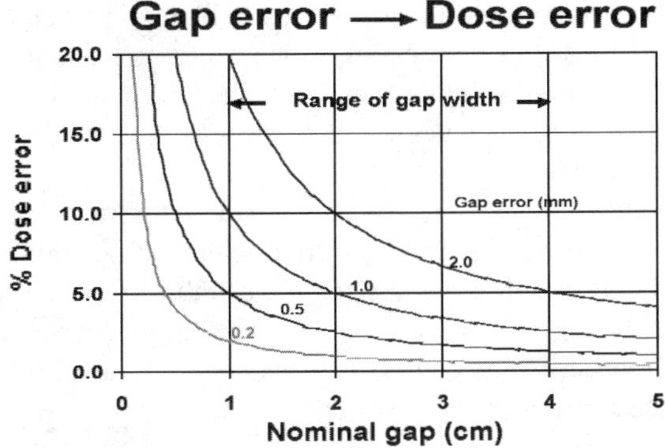



**Figure 3.** Relationship between dose error and gap error for DMLC fields. For the range of gap widths typical of DMLC fields, dose errors as a percent of dose delivered are shown as a function of the gap width error. Gap calibration error of ~0.2 mm translates to dose error of ~1% for typical DMLC fields. These numbers apply to SMLC as well, although the gap and dose errors are distributed differently. These curves do not account for transmission through the leaves, which will reduce the percent dose errors somewhat. [Reprinted from *A Practical Guide to Intensity-Modulated Radiation Therapy*, MSKCC staff. © 2003, with permission from Medical Physics Publishing.]

nor the leaf speeds are fixed; nevertheless, the average dose error is inversely proportional to the average gap width, for which 1 to 4 cm is typical (LoSasso, Chui, and Ling 1998). For SMLC, overlapping or underlapping of abutting field segments lead to hot or cold spots in the abutment regions of approximately 13% $mm^{-1}$ and 17% $mm^{-1}$ of the average dose for the abutting segments, for 6 and 18 MV photon beams, respectively (Low et al. 2001). SMLC fields, which approach the resolution of DMLC fields, will experience the same average dose error throughout the field, although the errors will be concentrated in the abutment regions. For both SMLC and DMLC, if average gap calibration error is less than 0.2 mm, then the average dose error from this source in typical fields will be less than 1%.

A leaf calibration error, which shifts both leaves of a pair in the same direction by the same amount, will not produce a dose error in the usual sense; instead, the dose distribution for the individual leaf pair will be shifted. Potential problems may become apparent when the modulated fields are combined depending upon the magnitude of the shift, although such errors will be reduced more or less by the other fields. This scenario demonstrates the subtle, but important distinction between leaf position errors, which may be offsetting, and gap width errors. Precision QA test methods should focus on the stability of the gap width, rather than the leaf position, since gap width is a better indicator of dose delivery, and because it is easier to measure on a periodic schedule using mechanical and dosimetric procedures.

Calibration of MLC leaf positions should be performed with methods suggested by the manufacturer (Boyer et al. 2001). However, the manufacturer's specifications for leaf positioning accuracy, while adequate as a block replacement in static fields, may not be suitable for IMRT applications. Fine calibration and periodic checking of the leaf position and gap width calibration should be performed over the clinically used range of travel. There are many ways to carry out these checks; a few categorical examples will be described here.

Many of the following tests may be performed at different gantry and collimator angles to observe the effect of gravity and friction on leaf positioning and speed. It is important to establish baseline values for undesirable backlash as all mechanical systems have inherent tolerances, which allow their components to move without binding. It is wise for physicists and engineers to acknowledge and understand the effects that these tolerances introduce into treatments.

## Light Field Projection

Prior to implementation of IMRT, periodic QA procedures for leaf position may have consisted of simply checking the field sizes using the field light projections of the leaf ends onto graph paper at the isocenter, similar to the calibration of the jaws. Unlike the jaws however, the light field and radiation field may not agree. The rounded leaves of the Varian and Elekta MLC allow significant transmission in the first millimeter; consequently, the radiation field edge defined by the 50% dose is shifted under the leaf by a fraction of a millimeter. The correct position of the leaves as measured by the light field will obviously depend upon whether the calibration of the digital readout is based upon the light field or the radiation field. This procedure is consistent with the sole function of the MLC for static fields, that is, to shape the field edges. While this test is coarse by IMRT standards, it does provide a quick visual assessment of the MLC to a precision of about 0.5 mm, both on and off the axis and is useful when troubleshooting problems and machine down time is critical.

## Mechanical Measurement Of The Gap (Feeler Gauge)

Since the delivered dose in IMRT fields is critically dependent upon the gap width, a direct independent measurement of the gap is worthwhile. The absolute calibration of the gap width defined by an opposed pair of leaves is obtained by setting a small gap, perhaps 1 mm (at isocenter distance). A feeler gauge having good precision (0.001 in. or 0.025 mm) is then inserted between the ends of opposing pairs of leaves. For rounded leaves (Varian and Elekta), the gap is measured at the center of the leaf; for focused leaves (Siemens), the measurement point is at the leaf edge closest to isocenter. The gauge should indicate the value of the gap demagnified to the aperture defining point at the MLC (e.g., 0.51 mm for a 1 mm gap for the Varian MLC, which is centered at 51 cm from the source). Each of the pairs of leaves can be measured in the same way (although by other methods), but observing the projections of the light field or the radiation field is more practical for determining the relative calibration of the remaining leaf pairs. The exception is the Varian MLC, where the leading edges of the leaves always form a straight line. Then by equalizing the gap between two pairs of leaves, the banks of leaves will be parallel to each other; the skewness and centerline offset can then be adjusted using the light field.

Alternatively, the Millennium™ MLC series features a "Field Alignment Tool"[1], which when attached to the head of the machine between the banks of leaves, can be used with the feeler gauge to adjust the skewness and offset of the leaves as well as the gap. Using the feeler gauge at other gantry and collimator angles will assess the effects of gravity on the gap. Mechanical backlash due to gravity affects opposing leaves in the same direction and, therefore, the effect of backlash on the gap width should be less than its effect on the positions of the corresponding leaves individually.

The above procedure can also be used to verify the gaps at off-axis positions. Once again, this is quick to do for a single leaf pair. Narrow gaps at isocenter for the range of leaf travel can be defined as individual fields and consecutively set and measured at the MLC with the feeler gauge. The measured gaps should correspond to the set gaps demagnified to the MLC (with an additional off-axis correction provided for the Varian MLC from the MLCtable.txt file). Such a series of measurements is shown in figure 4 for a Varian Millennium 120 MLC. Upper and lower bounds correspond to the widths of the gauge, which are slightly larger and smaller than the gap, respectively.

---

[1] "MLC User Guide", (1999). Varian Associates, Inc., Oncology Systems, Palo Alto, CA

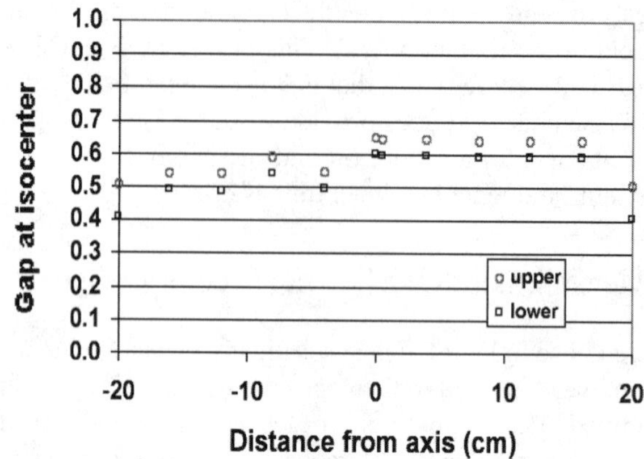


**Figure 4.** Verification of 0.5 mm (at isocenter) gap widths at off-axis positions using a feeler gauge. Measurements at the Varian MLC are magnified to the isocenter with an additional correction provided from the MLCtable.txt file. Values are plotted for widths of the gauge that are slightly larger (upper) and smaller (lower) than the gap.

## Film Techniques

Radiographic film is a useful tool for verifying relative leaf position and gap width accuracy with the so-called "picket fence." There are many variations of this technique, but they all provide an assessment of the positioning of each MLC leaf individually relative to the alignment of the other leaves. Some methods irradiate abutting fields to generate uniform patterns at the junctions (Boyer et al. 2001; Low et al. 2001). Others irradiate narrow bands at specified intervals (Chui, Spirou, and LoSasso 1996). In either case, the technique is to irradiate a film-loaded cassette or Kodak Ready Pack film without additional buildup at isocenter using the lowest energy available, probably 6 MV X-rays, to obtain the sharpest image. After a brief series of irradiations using abutting fields or narrow bands using static, segmented fields or dynamic fields, the film can be processed and evaluated. The dose uniformity along the match lines and bands is sensitive to even small deviations of individual leaves. Discontinuities between adjacent leaves are easily detected with the naked eye as in figure 5 for a Varian Mark 2 MLC, where relative errors, ±0.5 and ±0.2 mm, in leaf positions are intentionally introduced for demonstration purposes in the image on the right. The reference image on the left does not contain errors. Figure 6 shows bands extending to ±14 cm laterally for a Varian Millennium MLC. An accurate scale can be superimposed upon the film image to observe the absolute accuracy of the leaves; a 4 × 4 cm grid is superimposed on the bands in this image. These films may be obtained at other gantry angles to observe the variations in leaf positions as when influenced by gravity. Commercial scanning and digital analysis routines[2] are available for those who prefer a more objective evaluation.

---

[2] Radiological Imaging Technology, Denver, CO.

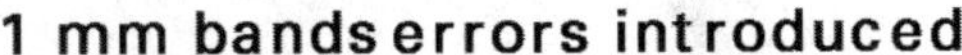


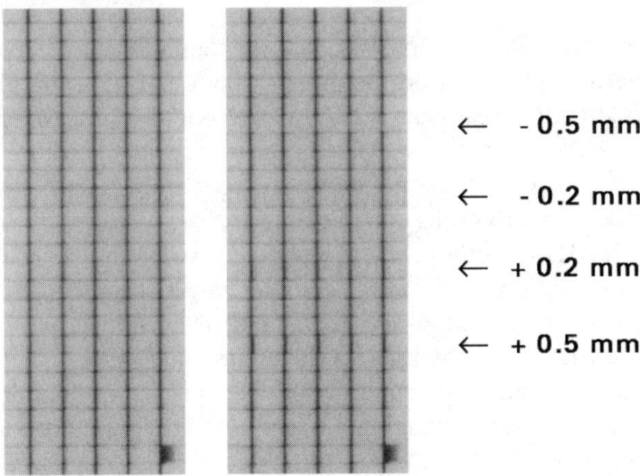


**Figure 5.** Film test to determine relative leaf positioning. The film image on the right has leaves intentionally shifted by –0.5 to +0.5 mm to demonstrate the method. The image on the left does not have errors. [Reprinted from *A Practical Guide to Intensity-Modulated Radiation Therapy*, MSKCC staff. © 2003, with permission from Medical Physics Publishing.]

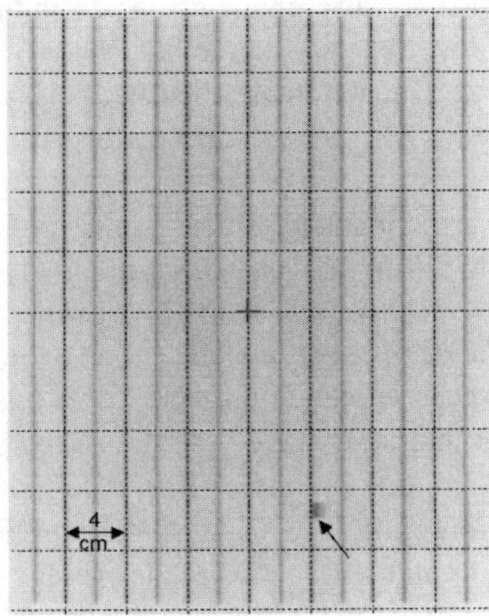


**Figure 6.** Film test to determine absolute leaf positioning accuracy. The bands extend to ±14 cm laterally for a Varian Millennium™ MLC. An accurate scale can be superimposed upon the film image to observe the absolute accuracy of the leaves; a 4 × 4 cm grid is superimposed on the bands in this image.

## Clinically Oriented Test Fields

Identifying the source of a problem is not always straightforward, especially if more than one component of the IMRT process may be the source of the problem. A prerequisite for accurate IMRT treatment is careful and ongoing assessment of the dose delivery as compared with the dose calculations for standard treatment conditions. However, dose calculations are based upon assumptions and approximations, which may not hold under more rigorous conditions.

Hypothetical IMRT test cases and clinical dose distributions selected from actual patient's fields for a variety of simple to complex targets can be planned, delivered, and measured to evaluate the overall accuracy of the system (Xing et al. 1999; LoSasso, Chui, and Ling 2001; Van Esch et al. 2002). Verification of these fields using two-dimensional high-resolution techniques, such as film in flat, cylindrical, or cubic phantoms or electronic portal imaging devices (EPIDs), should be appended to a routine QA program. Methods are described in detail in the chapter *Patient-Specific QA* by Xia. Such dose distribution comparisons evaluate the overall performance of the MLC at the level of dose and dose variation actually received by the patient, and they provide a direct link to the treatment planning system dose calculations. Another advantage is that the use of dose distributions overlays and differences are more familiar than standard QA data to many physicians, therapists, and physicists alike. Repeated use of the same fields demonstrates the stability of the delivery system over time. For departments equipped with multiple MLC, they can also be the basis for an IMRT intercomparison of MLC. Discrepancies can be indicative of irregularities in the delivery system or the dosimetry measurement system, as well as the dose calculation algorithm or the leaf sequencer. Such tests should be performed periodically as well as for new MLC, new MLC software, and modifications of the treatment planning algorithms.

As is common in most new clinical treatment strategies, IMRT at Memorial Sloan-Kettering Cancer Center (MSKCC) began with a relatively undemanding treatment site, the prostate (Ling et al. 1996). Before IMRT treatments began at MSKCC, we acknowledged three specific parameters, which needed to be re-commissioned for the IMRT dose calculations. These were: (1) the MLC transmission (primary plus scatter) through the leaves and interleaf spaces; (2) the added transmission through the rounded leaf edges; and (3) output factor for small MLC-shaped fields simulated by an analytical source function (LoSasso, Chui, and Ling 1998). These factors have minor influences for conventional static fields as the average MLC transmission, 1.5% to 2.0%, is less than that for metal alloy blocks, ~3.5%, the round edge only slightly broadens the penumbra in these cases, and MLC output factor for a tertiary collimator can be ignored in most cases. In contrast for IMRT, transmissions through the leaves and the rounded leaf edges contribute 4% and 10%, respectively, to the delivered dose to the target volume in typical IMRT fields, and small variable gaps between leaves produce local output variations.

Concurrently, as IMRT fields increased in size, modulation, and irregularity, periodic QA for clinical fields showed increasing discrepancies in certain cases. QA was gradually intensified to look at different components of the MLC and to try to identify the problem. After some time we concluded that commissioning parameters needed to be reevaluated. The average value for MLC scatter, based upon prostate and head and neck field sizes, was included in the MLC transmission that is applied to all fields; however, it is not accurate for larger IMRT fields. We have refined the source function, to more accurately calculate MLC output for very small gaps. Additionally, we modeled the interleaf spaces giving the planner the option to evaluate tongue-and-groove effects in individual plans.

Clinical dose measurements indicate potential problems in highly modulated and irregularly shaped fields. Recently, a multi-institution comparison of calculated and measured clinical dose distributions indicated that the center-specific dose kernels derived from deconvolution of ion chamber profiles were inadequate (Van Esch et al. 2002). One of the more extreme cases at MSKCC, an IMRT lung field, calculated and measured in a flat homogeneous phantom, is illustrated in figure 7. The overlay of calculations and measurements shows large variations in dose, 15 to 60 cGy within the field, with an average dose of about 30 cGy. The dose difference in figure 7a shows that discrepancies can be 25% of the average dose (15% of the local dose) in such fields. Most differences are found near the high dose gradients and can be attributed to inaccuracies in the extra-focal source distribution. Calculations comparing the source distribution used for figure 7 with a new source distribution are shown in figure 8. The modification appears to have resolved most of the discrepancy. It should be noted that these discrepancies would be less in the composite dose distribution due to the smoothing influence of other fields.

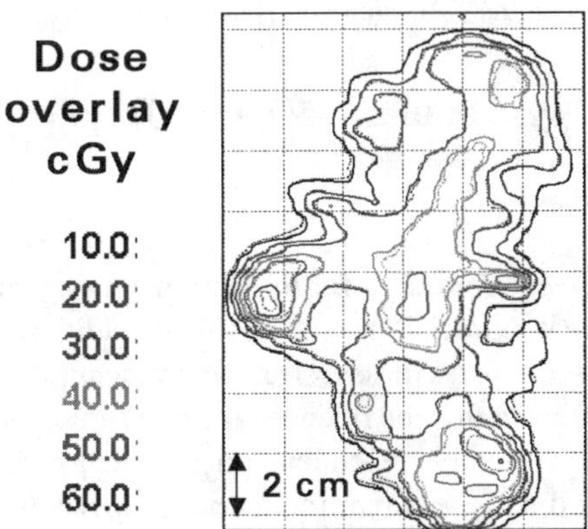


**Figure 7.** Overlay comparison of calculation (solid lines) and film measurement (dotted lines) for a posterior-anterior (PA) lung field used in an IMRT treatment. The intensity-modulated dose varies from 10 to 60 cGy.

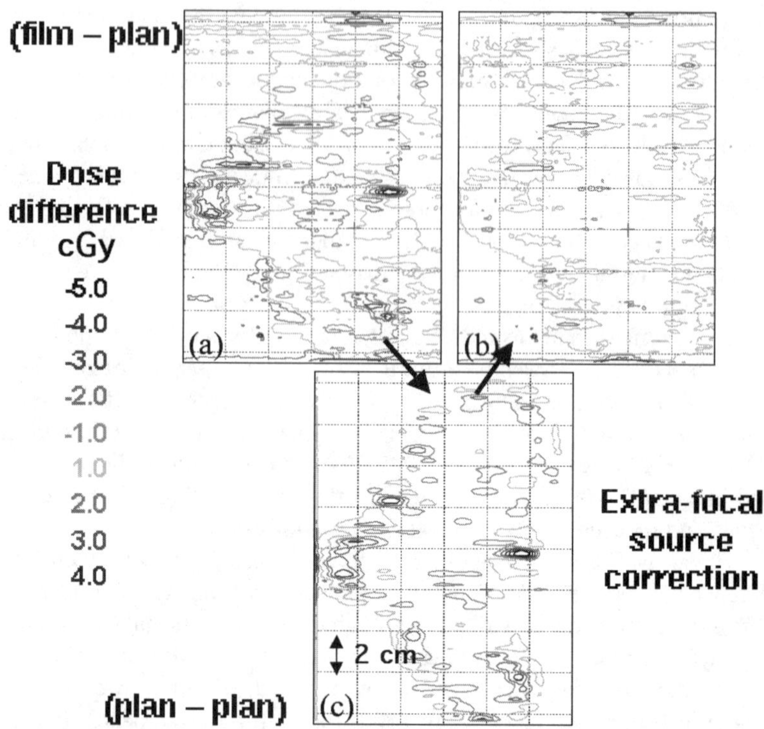


**Figure 8.** Comparison of dose differences (film-calculation) for the field in figure 6 using the (a) old source function and the (b) modified source function. The dose differences between the two calculations are shown in (c).

## Gap Width (DMLC Procedures – Varian Only)

### Narrow Sliding Window

If dynamic capabilities are supported, as for the Varian MLC, then alternate dosimetric methods with much greater precision are available in addition to the static methods described in the previous section. As these tests are more quantitative, they allow tracking of long-term stability. Given that the fluence (and consequently the dose measured) through a narrow gap is critically dependent on gap width, inversely, dosimetric measurements can be used as a sensitive monitor of gap width (Wang et al. 1996; LoSasso, Chui, and Ling 1998; Arnfield et al. 2000; LoSasso, Chui, and Ling 2001). For example, an output variation of 1%, which is easily measured, corresponds to a variation of ~0.05 mm for a 5.0 mm wide gap (with the round edge transmission not factored in). Based upon this relationship, we developed a number of dosimetric procedures utilizing an ion chamber or diode array.

## DMLC Output Vs. Static Field

The stability of the gap can be monitored utilizing an ionization chamber and a 5 mm sliding window beam delivery to measure the output. At the time of monthly x-ray beam output calibration, ion chamber readings for the narrow DMLC field are normalized to that measured in the static beam calibration field, using the same setup geometry to avoid uncertainties arising from changes in monitor chamber calibration; temperature and pressure corrections, and precise setup accuracy are also unnecessary. The long-term results, over a 4-year period from 1998–2002, for several treatment machines at MSKCC are displayed in figure 9. Here we plot the ratio of the DMLC output to static field output versus time. The variation in radiation output during this period is <1% for all three machines, and is less than that corresponding to the 0.2 mm tolerance on gap width (indicated by the vertical arrow marked 0.2 mm). Given the <1% output variation for the gap width of 5 mm used for the reference DMLC field, the variation would be even less (<0.3%) for typical clinical fields with a gap width of ~2 cm. The dashed lines in figure 9 indicate adjustments to the calibration parameters, which led to small changes in the DMLC outputs.

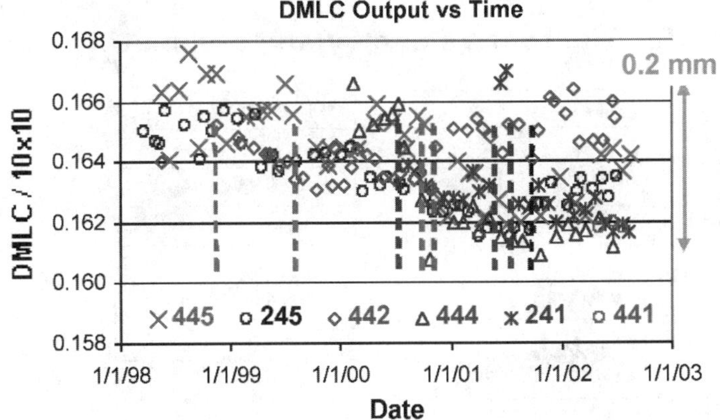


**Figure 9.** DMLC output stability over time. The ratios of the dynamic field to the reference field are plotted for six Varian MLCs. The 0.2 mm range in gap width corresponds to a 3% change in the ratio. The dashed lines indicate changes to the calibration parameters in the MLCXCAL files. [Reprinted from *A Practical Guide to Intensity-Modulated Radiation Therapy*, MSKCC staff. © 2003, with permission from Medical Physics Publishing.]

## DMLC Output Vs. Gantry And Collimator Angles

Leaf position variations imposed by the effects of gravity at different gantry angles should be documented periodically. Changes in leaf position between gantry angles are indicative of problems with leaf drive assemblies or carriage supports and can lead to significant dose errors. For SMLC these effects can only be observed with film techniques, using the doubly exposed film test described earlier or using the "picket fence" or similar pattern. Variation in fixed gaps at four orthogonal gantry angles should be observed. Scanning is advisable as the changes associated with skewness cannot be quantified visually. When DMLC is available, dosimetry is an option using ion chambers or diode arrays to measure output changes from narrow gaps at different points along the gap.

A standard monthly DMLC test for this purpose uses a cylindrical ion chamber (with appropriate buildup cap) at the isocenter; a fixed dose using the 5 mm sliding window field described above is delivered, and normalized to the dose from a fixed static field, at different gantry and collimator angles. The time trends of dose output for six combinations of gantry and collimator angles for four MLC are presented in figure 10. It is apparent that each MLC has a distinctive pattern. The horizontal dashed lines represent the output range that ±0.2 mm gap variation would impose. The vertical dashed lines are the adjustments to the calibration as in figure 9. These graphs show that for any specific set of gantry and collimator angles the clinical output is stable over time to within about 1%. Furthermore, since daily treatments are generally delivered with multiple gantry angles that compensate each other, the deviation due to carriage instability is usually much less than 1%.

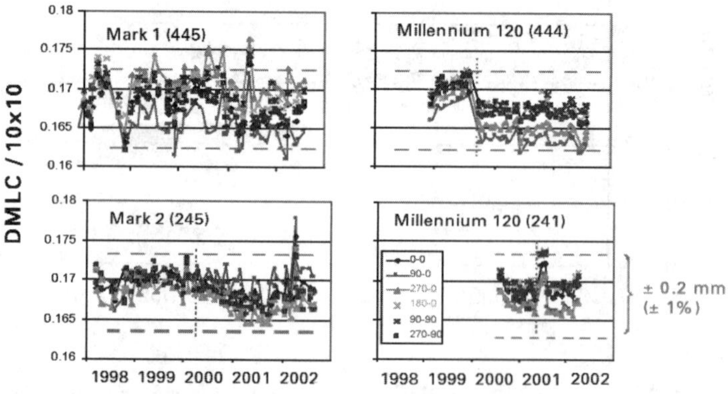



**Figure 10.** DMLC output stability vs. gantry and collimator angle for four MLCs over time. The DMLC outputs are normalized to the outputs for the static reference field at each angle. The dashed lines represent ±0.2 mm range in gap width (1% clinical dose variation).

## DMLC Output, Off-Axis Perpendicular To Leaf Motion

Off-axis dosimetry measurements indicate the relative skewness at a number of gantry and collimator angles. Data obtained with a linear diode array for a Varian MLC for gantry angles of 90° and 270° are shown in figure 11. The individual diode readings are normalized to the readings with both the gantry and collimator at 0°. The diodes see varying amounts of interleaf leakage. Fitting these data points to straight lines yields the dashed lines for gantry angles of 90° and 270° relative to the 0°-gantry position. Some backlash is unavoidable in mechanical systems. Fortunately, such variations, as observed here at 90° and 270°, tend to compensate each other during treatment. Nevertheless, output vs. gantry angle is variable among the MLC, and output changes over time may indicate mechanical problems.

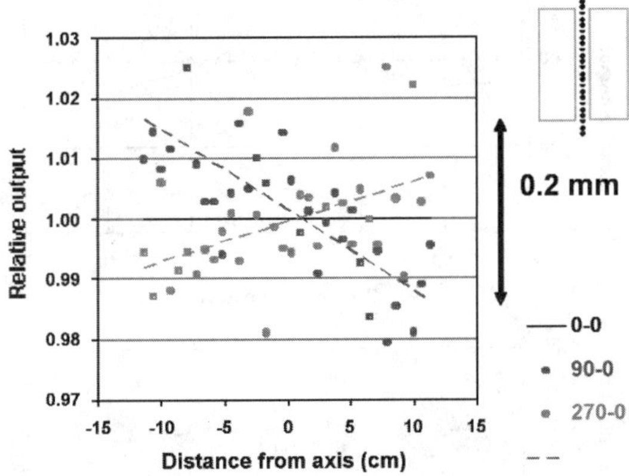


**Figure 11.** DMLC output stability vs. gantry angle measured with a linear diode array. The array is mounted in the blocking tray holder and aligned perpendicular to the direction of leaf motion. DMLC outputs are first normalized to the static reference field at each angle and then normalized to the output at 0°. [Reprinted from *A Practical Guide to Intensity-Modulated Radiation Therapy*, MSKCC staff. © 2003, with permission from Medical Physics Publishing.]

## DMLC Output, Off-Axis Parallel To Leaf Motion

A dynamic slit field can be used to verify the off-axis gap width accuracy dosimetrically. The method compares symmetry and flatness of relative dose profiles for an open field with that for a 1.0 cm wide dynamic field moving at a constant speed (cm/MU). Measurements may be obtained at arbitrary intervals with an ion chamber, a detector array, or film. Ideally, the normalized dose profile for the dynamic field should mimic that for the open static field.

The gap-width accuracy at off-axis positions verified with ionization measurements for one MLC is shown as relative dose profiles (i.e., normalized to the dose at the central axis) in figure 12a and 12b for 6 MV X-rays. Figure 12a shows the static field and DMLC field profiles and the ratios of these profiles for each of three fields, centered at the axis and at ±8 cm off-axis at a depth of 10 cm. Near the central axis, the open field and dynamic profiles agree within 0.5%; however, at 10 cm from the axis, the ratio of the profiles decreases by ~2%. This decrease is not due to changes in the gap-width, the measured transmission also decreases with increasing off-axis distance, to 92% of the central axis transmission at 10 cm off-axis. Figure 12b shows that the ratios of the profiles for the DMLC fields and the static fields are much flatter, once the transmitted component of the dose is removed from the DMLC readings. Thus, the width of the gap for this MLC is relatively constant across the field.

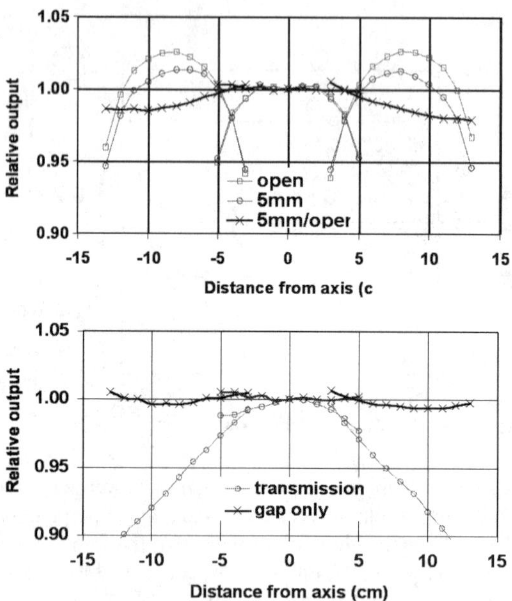


**Figure 12.** Measured dose profiles for a narrow, 0.5 cm, DMLC field are compared with those for an open static field. Due to the 15 cm field width limitation, fields are centered at the central axis and at ±8 cm off axis. (a) Ion chamber measurements at 1 cm intervals are normalized to the central axis. (b) The ratio of DMLC to open field is flat once the variation in off-axis transmission is measured and corrected for. [Reprinted from *A Practical Guide to Intensity-Modulated Radiation Therapy*, MSKCC staff. © 2003, with permission from Medical Physics Publishing.]

## Beam Characteristics For Small MUs

The delivery of IMRT using SMLC with Siemens and Elekta requires that the beam be cycled off and on (step and shoot). As the number of segments increases providing more control points, the monitor units (MUs) per segment will decrease. For complex intensity-modulated patterns with many subfields, large numbers of segments may be delivering small MU values, less than 2 MU (Ezzell and Chungbin 2001; Xia, Chuang, and Verhey 2002). For example, a 200 cGy prescribed daily fraction delivered with a

100 segment plan will average only 2 MU per segment. Since such small MU settings are outside the range of conventional treatments, the scope of acceptance testing and QA procedures do not normally address this issue.

Testing the accuracy of beam fidelity, i.e., dose output, symmetry, and flatness, for small MU can be done with an ion chamber positioned sequentially at the central axis and at four orthogonal off-axis points in a static field. At each point the dose for a fixed number of MU, X MU, is measured. At each point for X-1 MU segments the dose is also measured and then summed for comparison. Measurements may also be made with 2-D detector arrays or film. A summary of the experiences of small numbers of monitor units for several different machines concluded that individual centers need to make such measurements on their particular accelerator approximately monthly to ensure reliability (Webb 2001).

## Leaf Motor Issues

### Leaf Speed

Leaves have a maximum speed that is specified by the manufacturer. On occasion, leaf motors will not be able to maintain this speed during normal operation. Slowing is a symptom of excessive wear of the motor or other leaf assembly components. A buildup of dirt and grease migrating between the flat leaf surfaces from components of the drive mechanism may also tend to bind adjacent leaves; this possibility should be eliminated first. Variation in the maximum available leaf speed of individual leaves will influence treatment times since segments within an SMLC field will require longer leaf setup times.

For DMLC, which is only currently available with the Varian MLC, the reduction of the maximum leaf speed will have two possible effects. If a leaf is unable to maintain its programmed speed while the beam is on, then the MLC software will modulate the dose rate by increasing the number and duration of beam holdoffs during delivery, and thereby increase treatment times. More importantly, the delivered intensity profile may also differ from the prescribed profile if a leaf is lagging behind due to leaf speed issues, with or without beam holdoff indication. Thus, leaf speed is considered a more important QA issue for DMLC than for SMLC delivery, where the dose is unaffected. Detection of reduced leaf speed for an individual motor should be part of a QA program, so that the problem may be rectified by a service engineer.

The stability of leaf speed and the effects of leaf acceleration and deceleration on the delivered intensity profiles for DMLC have been recognized for several years (Chui, Spirou, and LoSasso 1996). To test the stability of leaf speed, specially designed leaf sequence files move pairs of leaves at constant speeds ranging from low to maximum speed. If the leaf speeds are constant across the field, then the measured dose profiles should be uniform. If leaf speeds are unstable, fluctuations would appear in the delivered profiles. Since leaf speeds are varied between programmed DMLC segments, the significance of acceleration and deceleration was also tested by intentionally interrupting the beam and then resuming the irradiation, which was judged not to be a concern.

Sub-par leaf speed can often be visually detected relative to other leaves when the leaves are moved at their maximum velocity during field setup or leaf retraction or by using a leaf exercise pattern designed for this purpose, which moves leaves in and out of the field. If the problem is subtle, it may only be noticeable during leaf movements at certain gantry angles when gravity is a compounding factor.

During a DMLC treatment with the Varian MLC, excessive beam hold-offs for one or more fields are an indication of such a problem. The therapists performing the treatments should have an ear open for these telltale signs and report them for servicing. A more objective approach is to evaluate DMLC leaf positions recorded by the Varian MLC controller in log files during delivery. The Dynalog File Viewer[3], a software tool for evaluating leaf positioning during IMRT delivery, tabulates leaf position errors [root mean square (rms) deviation of monitored and actual leaf positions for individual leaves] based upon their magnitude and frequency of occurrence during treatment. A test file which moves all the leaves in and out of the field in an alternating pattern at a speed close to the maximum can then be evaluated with the Dynalog File Viewer to identify errant leaf behavior. Individual leaves are suspect if their deviations appear significantly larger than the average for all the leaves. Performing such a leaf speed test at gantry angles of 90° and 270° may be best to incorporate the gravity factor as well.

## Motor Calibration Failures

Electromechanical components of the MLC may fail at any time. This may take the form of an abrupt failure, requiring immediate replacement of the part before treatment can resume, or, perhaps more troubling, it may be a gradual deterioration, requiring careful monitoring. Deterioration of motor speed has been described earlier. Another concern has to do with the long-term reliability of the primary encoders affixed to the Varian leaf motors; it is apparently related to the amount of usage of individual leaf motors. Chronic drift of the calibration of the leaf position encoder has been the principal symptoms of leaf motor failures for this MLC design until recently.

The data in figures 13 and 14 summarize the history of MLC leaf motor failures on three Varian MLC machines used primarily for DMLC treatments since 1996 at MSKCC. Approximately 80% of patients — ~30 patients/day, 5 fields/patient — on two machines, 245 and 445, have been IMRT prostate patients (prior to this time, 1992–1995, these MLC have been used primarily for static MLC treatments). In figure 13, the increased frequency of motor failure near the central axis, indicated by color, and multiple failure, indicated by numbers, is consistent with those leaves used for prostate fields. The solid lines in figure 14 graph the chronology of motor replacements. For each MLC, leaf motor failures became more frequent after the initiation of DMLC treatment. Leaf position errors, caused by calibration drift, were increas-

---

[3] "Dynalog File Viewer, Reference Guide," (2001) Varian Associates, Inc., Oncology Systems, Palo Alto, CA.

ingly detected during QA procedures and patient treatments. The frequency of MLC reinitialization was gradually increased during the treatment day. Eventually, beginning in 1998 the replacement of marginally performing motors became part of the QA program. With DMLC QA specifically targeting this problem, leaf drive motors were replaced at a steady rate between 1998 and 2001. Based on our QA records we have estimated what the MLC motor replacement rate would have been had we initiated this prophylactic motor replacement policy in 1995. These are shown as dashed lines in figure 13. It is postulated that the repeated abutment of opposing leaves especially during IMRT delivery caused many of these leaf motors to fail prematurely. New software developed by the manufacturer, with a 0.5 mm minimum gap criterion, was installed in June 2001, indicated by the vertical dashed line in figure 13. While it is too early to be definitive, the rate of motor replacement appears to have decreased at about the same time. Furthermore, the primary cause of leaf motor failure is no longer calibration drift.

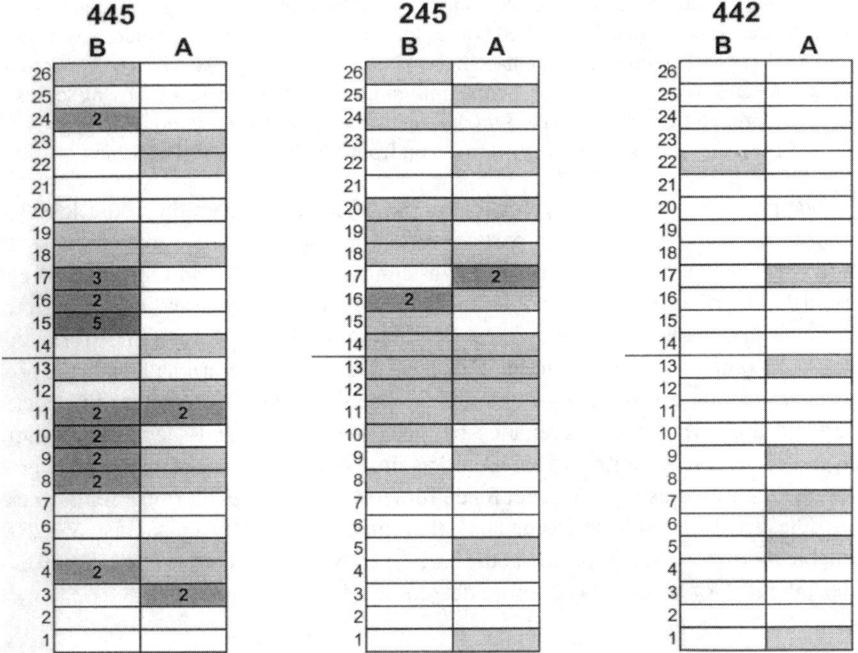


**Figure 13.** Leaf positions where motors have been replaced are shown in color for three MLC. Numbers indicate multiple motor replacements. The pattern of replacing centrally located motors for the MLCs in rooms 445 (left) and 245 (center) is consistent with the use of these MLCs almost exclusively for prostate treatments. [Reprinted from *A Practical Guide to Intensity-Modulated Radiation Therapy*, MSKCC staff. © 2003, with permission from Medical Physics Publishing.]

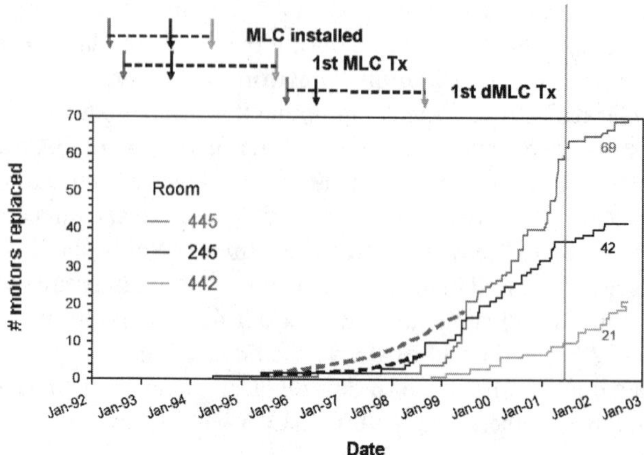


**Figure 14.** Cumulative motor replacements vs. time for three MLCs. The solid curves are the actual replacements. The dashed curves indicate that some motors would have been replaced earlier based upon the replacement criteria adopted in 1998. The vertical dotted line indicates the introduction of the 0.5 mm minimum gap criterion for moving leaves. [Reprinted from *A Practical Guide to Intensity-Modulated Radiation Therapy*, MSKCC staff. © 2003, with permission from Medical Physics Publishing.]

The problem just described for the Varian MLC stems from the count losses by the primary encoder, an integral part of the motor assembly. It becomes more severe during the course of the treatment day, assuming the MLC is initialized (self-calibrated) in the morning using its internal optical calibration system. On occasion that the count losses of a primary encoder become excessive, leaf position errors could exceed 0.5 mm at isocenter. Reinitializing the MLC will temporarily alleviate the problem, but position errors may go unnoticed since the secondary position interlock is triggered only when the discrepancy between the primary and secondary readouts reaches ~2 mm at isocenter. To safeguard against such errors, potential encoder problems are identified using the picket fence film test described earlier on a semi-weekly schedule. The film test is performed by a therapist, evaluated by a physicist, and questionable motors are then replaced at the earliest convenience. This condition may exist intermittently for several days before detection.

## Communication/Timing Errors

A number of studies have recently addressed the subject of communication delays, also referred to as timing errors, overshoot phenomenon, and latency issues, and the subsequent leaf position errors for the Varian MLC in dynamic mode. The concern arises due to the 55+ msec delay before the MLC control system can acknowledge and respond to the instruction for the next MU segment. In effect, the leaf lags behind its prescribed position, defined by the index, or fractional MU, in the leaf sequence file, at each moment of the delivery. It may appear as though the leaf speed is the issue, but rather the deviation in leaf position is caused by the communication delay.

For the SMLC mode, these errors mainly affect the delivered dose in the first and the last segment, which deliver slightly greater and less dose than planned, respectively. Intermediate segments also experience these delays; however, approximately the same "overshoot," i.e., the $\Delta$MU which is added to the end of each segment, is missing from the beginning of each segment. In this case two wrongs make it right; the intermediate segments generally receive the correct MU (Ezzell and Chungbin 2001; Xia, Chuang and Verhey 2002). This is demonstrated in figure 15, where the total MU per segment is varied from 0.25 to 25 at a delivery rate of 400 MU/min. For the smallest MU per segment such that the "overshoot" exceeds the planned MU for the segment, one or more of these intermediate segments may actually be skipped. The graphics in figure 16 illustrates this very clearly. In the upper diagram the planned segments are equal in MU per segment; the first segment delivers more dose and the last segment less than planned, while intermediate segments receive the correct dose. In the center diagram, a small intermediate segment, 3, is bypassed as a result of the overshoot. The lower diagram indicates the variable nature of the overshoot and the corresponding uncertainty this introduces to all delivered segments.

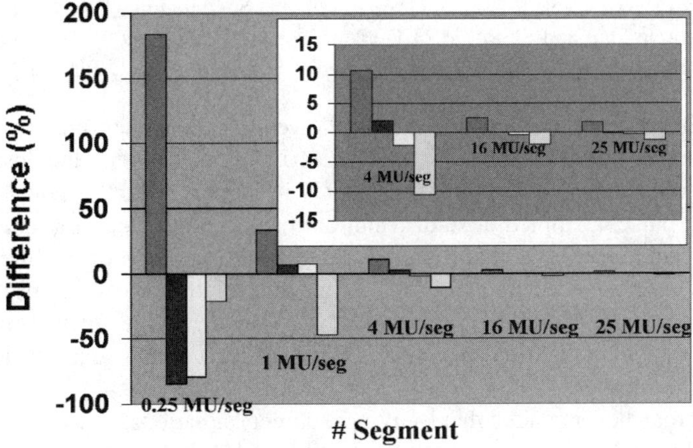


**Figure 15.** The relative dose variations among four segments as a function of MU per segment. The dose rate is 400 MU/min on a Varian 2300CD at 6 MV. [Courtesy of Ping Xia, UCSF.]

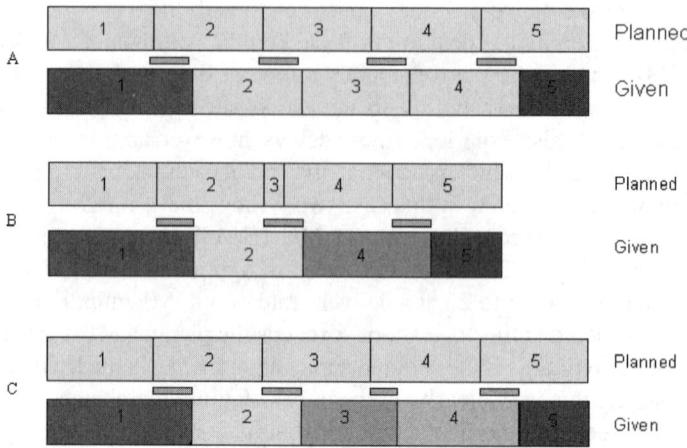


**Figure 16.** Schematic showing the effect of an overshoot in the MU delivery. (a) Overshoot is constant. Segment 1 is long, 5 is short, 2–4 are unaffected. (b) Overshoot exceeds the planned MU for segment 3, so it is skipped. (c) Overshoot is variable, so segment 3 is shorter than planned and segment 4 is longer. (Reprinted from *Journal of Applied Clinical Medical Physics*, vol. 2, issue 3, G. A. Ezzell, and S. Chungpin, "The Overshoot Phenomenon in Step-and-Shoot IMRT Delivery," pp. 138–128. © 2001, with permission from G. Ezzell and the *Journal of Applied Clinical Medical Physics*.]

In the DMLC mode, if leaf speeds are allowed to exceed their maximum values, dose rate modulation will result (Low et al. 2001). In this situation the dose is delivered in pulses as the beam holdoff is repeatedly invoked and the leaf deviation varies within each pulse; a rippled dose distribution results even though the intended leaf sequence is smooth. Another study offers a detailed description of the limitations of the delivery control system and proposes sequencing solutions to overcome these limitations (Litzenberg, Moran, and Fraass 2002b). However, the fluence modulation introduced by communication delays into DMLC delivery should also cancel for leading and trailing leaves.

Thus, it may be concluded that for typical clinical situations, i.e., when very small MU per field and MU per segment are avoided for SMLC and when appropriate leaf sequencing parameters (dose rate, leaf tolerance, and maximum leaf speed) are chosen for DMLC, timing errors will not lead to significant dose errors. There is some concern if these leaf sequences are used for QA purposes, where film and EPID may require shorter MU; the dose rate should be reduced in this case such that the maximum leaf speed is not exceeded.

## Log File Analysis (Varian Only)

Log files are generated by the Varian MLC control software after each IMRT field is delivered. These files contain the leaf positions as indicated by the primary leaf position encoder attached to each leaf motor. These monitored leaf positions and the prescribed leaf positions are recorded every 55 msec for each leaf. Analysis of these data can be a very useful QA tool, provided the information is properly interpreted. In this regard, it is important that the user understand that these are "monitored" leaf positions do not represent the "actual" positions of the leaves. They are the positions of the leaves from the perspective of the primary leaf position encoder attached to the leaf motor. Log files do not consider errors in the absolute leaf calibration, drift in the leaf calibration over time, or backlash in the leaf drive mechanism. Nevertheless, analysis of this data can provide information on the performance of MLC leaves individually.

Several applications of these log files have already been developed. During DMLC acceptance testing, log files were analyzed to study the impact of gantry and collimator rotations on leaf positioning (MSKCC 2003). The DMLC log files may also be converted to leaf sequence files which, with the prescribed MU and field size, permit the calculation of the "delivered" dose distributions (within the uncertainty due to leaf calibration and mechanical backlash) by the treatment planning system. The comparison of the delivered dose distributions with the planned dose distributions are useful to verify normal beam delivery and to study the effects of repeated beam holdoffs, invoked by gating signals, on IMRT dose delivery has been reported (LoSasso et al. 2001; Yorke et al. 2000). An example of such a comparison is shown as the dose overlay and difference in figure 17 for the posterior field of a 5-field DMLC prostate treatment. The dose difference distribution indicates discrepancies between the planned and delivered dose distributions of less than 1%.

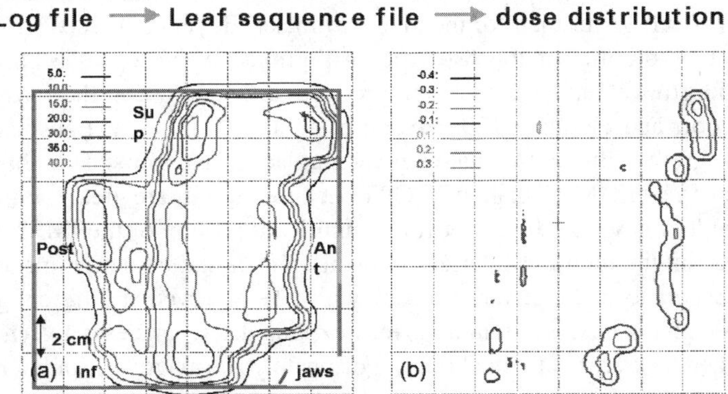


**Figure 17.** Comparison of a "delivered" dose distribution derived from a Dynalog file with the planned dose distribution. [Reprinted from *A Practical Guide to Intensity-Modulated Radiation Therapy*, MSKCC staff. © 2003, with permission from Medical Physics Publishing.]

Varian has provided a software package, the Dynalog File Viewer, to summarize the deviations of the leaves from their prescribed positions for leaves that were moving during the DMLC treatment. These treatment summaries currently only provide numerical scores, rms leaf position deviations, which are not directly correlated to dose delivery errors. However, they can be used to evaluate MLC in conjunction with appropriate test files to identify leaf motors that are not able to maintain their maximum speed.

A very detailed analysis of the Varian Dynalog files has been made to assess routine QA. (Litzenberg, Moran, and Fraass 2002a). In this study the authors derive, tabulate, and graphically display such quantities as leaf position and velocity deviations, gap deviations, and dose discrepancy profiles. They suggest that a routine of QA sequences be tested and analyzed daily to evaluate MLC performance. Although many of these features would overwhelm the average IMRT user, no doubt a modified version of this software, selecting specific parameters, targeting known problems would be a valuable QA and troubleshooting tool for the manufacturer to provide with each IMRT installation.

## Interleaf Transmission

All MLC are focused in the direction perpendicular to leaf motion. This requires that the leaves are divergent and that the sides of the leaves have an overlapping component, tongues and grooves or just a single step midway, to reduce the interleaf transmission through the narrow air spaces between the leaves. Variation in transmission for a specific MLC in the direction perpendicular to leaf motion is caused by differences between the midleaf thickness and the combined thickness of tongues and grooves, plus the transmission through the narrow air spaces, which is not completely blocked by the tongues and grooves. The overlap, which also adds stability, can take a number of shapes, but generally keeps the measured interleaf transmission to less than 3%, which is lower than for metal alloy blocks (Boyer et al. 2001).

Another by-product of the overlapping portions of the leaves is the so-called "tongue-and-groove" effect, which can produce an underdose in the interleaf space (van Santvoort and Heijmen 1996; Webb et al. 1997). Interleaf transmissions and tongue-and-groove effects fluctuate between adjacent leaf pairs. They have a more pronounced effect in IMRT than in 3DCRT because the MU are greater for IMRT and because the leaves shield the target for a significant portion of the IMRT treatment. For this reason, the range of interleaf transmission should be determined for all the leaves at acceptance testing; variations may also be observed at different gantry and collimator angles. Later, these findings may explain discrepancies between measured and calculated doses for individual fields. Fortunately, the magnitude of interleaf transmission and tongue-and-groove effects tend to negate each other as fields are combined in the composite plan.

Interleaf transmission is most easily quantified with film dosimetry using a tissue equivalent phantom and a high-resolution scanner. In general, the interleaf transmission exceeds the midleaf transmission for MLC as shown in figure 18 for Varian Mark 2 and Millennium MLC, where the transmission profiles for the blocked fields are normalized to that for the open field. As measured in phantom, the maximum interleaf transmission should not be more than twice the midleaf value. The full-width-half-maximum (FWHM) values are ~ 2.5 mm measured in phantom for 6 and 15 MV X-ray beams (LoSasso, Chui, and Ling 1998).

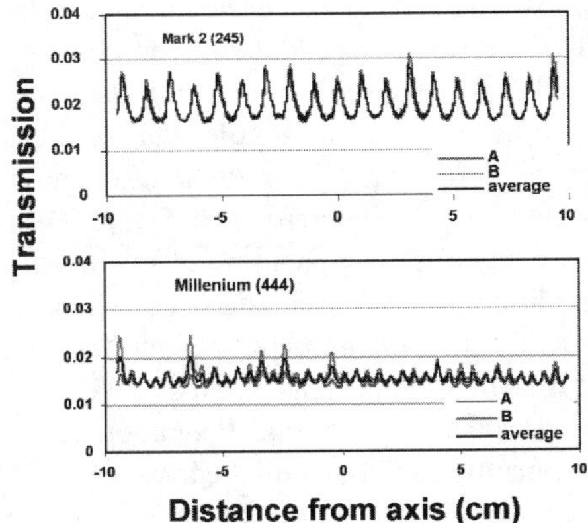



**Figure 18.** Interleaf and midleaf transmission profiles (A-side, B-side, and average) for the (a) Mark 2 and (b) Millennium™ 120 MLC. [Reprinted from *A Practical Guide to Intensity-Modulated Radiation Therapy*, MSKCC staff. © 2003, with permission from Medical Physics Publishing.]

## MLC Intercomparison

For centers with multiple MLC-equipped linacs, a diligent QA program will compare MLC parameters that affect the dose delivered. Values of parameters, such as midleaf and interleaf transmissions, variations in leaf position calibration, and output factors for small fields, are usually measured with static fields when commissioning the MLC; their comparison is straightforward.

A major concern for IMRT is the fluence through the leaf face. Each MLC design can be classified as either single- or double-focused. In the double-focused configuration (Siemens), the leaves move in an arc; the leaf face and the leaf sides nominally match the beam divergence. Single-focused leaves (Elekta and Varian) only have sides that are divergent. Since they move in a plane, they have rounded faces, allowing the leaves to maintain a constant penumbra width as the non-focused leaves move away from the central axis in a simple rectilinear motion. This is a complicating factor for dose calculation as the round leaf end transmits more of the primary beam than a flat leaf end, and the transmission is varying with distance from the edge. For the Varian and Elekta MLC, this added fluence will contribute a significant amount of the delivered dose within typical IMRT fields, perhaps 10% or more depending upon the degree of modulation in the plan. This transmission may vary somewhat with energy, MLC model, and distance from the central axis due to oblique path length through the leaf face and off-axis spectral changes. For the Siemens MLC, although the leaf faces are flat and focused to the source, even slight misalignment may introduce additional fluence.

Transmission through the leaf ends can be quantified with measurements of the effective gap offset (LoSasso, Chui, and Ling 1998; Arnfield et al. 2000; LoSasso,

Chui, and Ling 2001). An effective offset for a leaf can be thought of as the amount that a leaf would need to be retracted to add the same fluence as is transmitted through the leaf end. In one method film is used to measure integral dose in phantom for a set of nominal static gap widths including the smallest gap setting allowed with the leaves not touching. Leaf sequence files have been created for moving gaps with different fixed widths and constant leaf speed centered at 0, 5, and 10 cm from the central axis. An integrating ion chamber, either in a phantom or in air, serves the same purpose as film in the previous method. For each field, static or dynamic, the integrated reading is the sum of the fluence through the gap, the leaf end transmission, and the full leaf transmission. Full leaf transmission is measured using the same jaw setting and detector setup (note: measured transmission is dependent upon irradiation and geometry due to scatter and interleaf transmission), but with the leaves of the MLC blocking the field completely. The full leaf transmission varies for each gap field and must be subtracted from the measurement. This is derived from the average of the measured transmission for the two leaf banks with an adjustment for the spatial (film) or temporal (ion chamber) fraction that the detector is shielded by the leaves. The net ion chamber outputs, normalized to a static $10 \times 10$ cm$^2$ static field at the central axis and a depth of 10 cm for 6 MV and 15 MV beams, are displayed in figure 19. They are plotted against the nominal gap width and fit with straight lines. The intercept at zero dose yields the effective gap offset. Note that this measurement includes the effect from the uncertainty of the leaf gap calibration, the variations in attenuation due to energy and leaf design, and the limitations of the mechanical components of the MLC system.

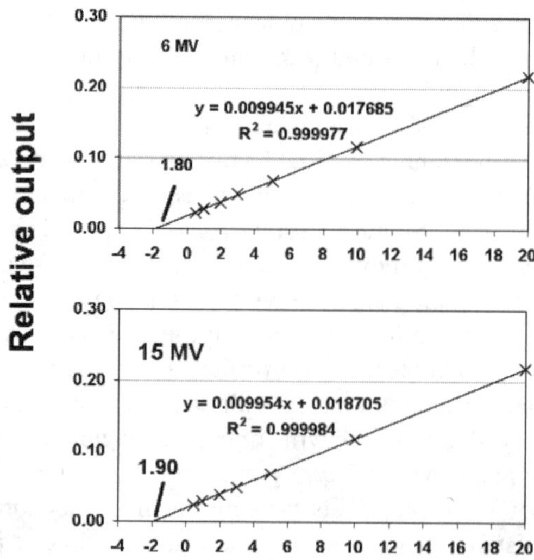


**Figure 19.** Output vs. DMLC gap width. The x-intercept is the effective gap offset due to the round leaf ends. [Reprinted from *A Practical Guide to Intensity-Modulated Radiation Therapy*, MSKCC staff. © 2003, with permission from Medical Physics Publishing.]

Effective gap offsets can then be compared for various rooms, MLC models, energies, and off-axis positions. Figure 20 summarizes measured offset values at the central axis, 5 cm, and 10 cm off-axis, parallel to leaf motion, for five Varian MLCs with three different leaf designs. For the same nominal energies, variation in the offset value was within ±0.15 mm at all positions. Except for the MLC in room 442, the variation in the offset value at the central axis is within ±0.05 mm. The lower offset for the MLC in room 442, in part, is due to the slightly lower beam energy observed for this 6 MV beam.

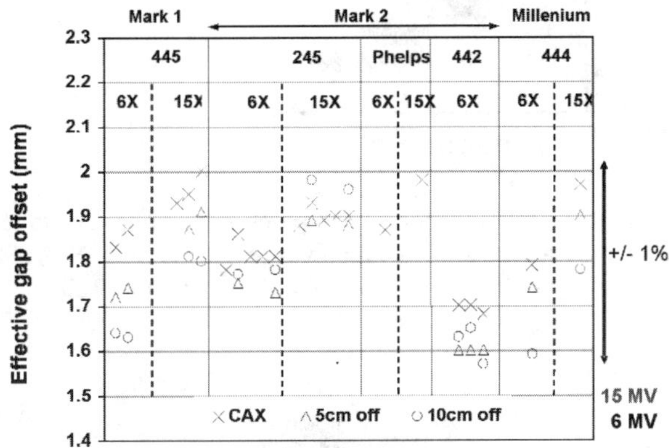


**Figure 20.** Comparison of measured effective offsets for five MLCs at the central axis and at 5 and 10 cm off-axis for 6 and 15 MV X-rays. [Reprinted from *A Practical Guide to Intensity-Modulated Radiation Therapy*, MSKCC staff. © 2003, with permission from Medical Physics Publishing.]

## Auxiliary Systems

Where the tumor and/or critical organs are potentially affected by respiratory motion, respiratory gating may be applied during simulation, scanning, and treatment to minimize movement. Gating during tumor localization will affect the apparent tumor size and location (Nehmeh et al. 2002). Gating during IMRT delivery has an added benefit, as intrafraction organ motion can distort the temporal and spatial dependent dose delivery. Figure 21 illustrates the cyclical motion of a point in the field, perpendicular and parallel to the leaf motion, caused by respiration. The impact on dose delivery of gating the accelerator beam with a respiratory monitoring system should be tested. This can be performed with film dosimetry techniques or by analyzing log files.

For large target volumes it is sometimes necessary to split fields into two subfields (figure 22) due to limitations in the field width used for IMRT. Dose distribution accuracy in the overlap region of split fields should be tested for clinical cases (Wu et al. 2000).

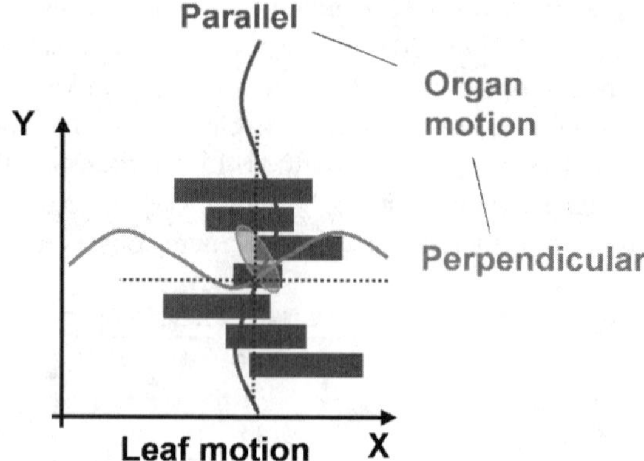


**Figure 21.** Diagram illustrating the motion of a point in the tumor due to respiratory motion relative to leaf motion for the sliding window type of treatment. Note: Step-and-shoot delivery is sensitive to respiratory motion as well.

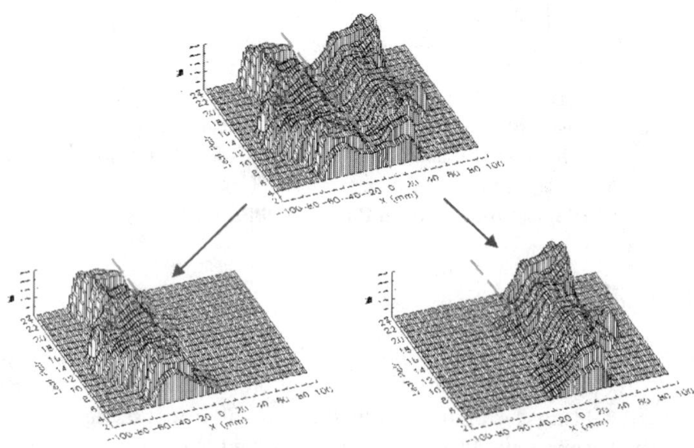

**Figure 22.** Diagram illustrating the splitting of large intensity pattern into two subfields.

## Frequency Of Checks

It is difficult to set a standard for frequency of performing QA. The frequency will vary with a number of factors including the type of delivery, i.e., SMLC or DMLC, the MLC design, the variety of tests used, the length and breadth of experiences of the individual institution, and the feedback of the composite experiences of all institutions with the MLC hardware and software. Ergonomic issues include the speed and simplicity of the tests, the stability of the parameters being tested for the individual MLC, and the significance of deviations on the delivered dose to the target and normal tissues.

Initially, the type and frequency of tests are performed on a schedule which reflects unfamiliarity with both the delivery problems and the clinical significance of apparent irregularities. Verification of all clinical fields for patient's plans, though labor intensive, is invaluable in the early stages of IMRT to evaluate the entire planning and delivery process. Gradually this heightened guard can be relaxed as understanding and confidence builds in the inherent safety features and a more efficient QA process.

Using MSKCC as an example, where thousands of patients have been treated with IMRT since 1995 and where the current rate is about 200 treatments per day on 14 MLC-equipped machines at the center and satellite facilities, routine QA requires less than 2 hours per month per MLC or about one-fifth of the daily and monthly QA for the linac. It is relatively rare that we verify clinical dose distributions for IMRT patients, currently less than 5% of patients have dose verification. Dosimetric evaluation of the entire field of each IM beam for each patient, using standard verification tools, would have overtaxed our medical physics resources and was judged not to be necessary. Individual patient dosimetry is currently relegated to new treatment sites, new MLC, or new software. Our current approach integrates existing methods, combining periodic QA and computer verification, to provide the necessary quality assurance in a safe and efficient manner (LoSasso, Chui, and Ling 2001). However, in the years surrounding the initiation of IMRT, QA with ion chamber and/or film dosimetry was performed for each field for hundreds of patients. This QA process has obviously evolved with time; it is likely that this program will be further refined in the future.

This startup intensity should be unnecessary considering the composite experiences of such institutions with these devices. Nevertheless, individual treatment centers should expect a learning curve for understanding novel treatment planning and QA issues. The urge to implement IMRT at individual therapy centers should be tempered while these issues come into focus and are addressed at each center.


## Summary

This chapter has addressed the quality assurance issues specific to IMRT delivery with an MLC, both for the SMLC and the DMLC modes. It does not address acquisition of commissioning parameters for the treatment planning system or the routine verification of treatments, which are discussed in other chapters.

One of the principal concerns for IMRT relative to conventional 3DCRT is the mechanical accuracy of the MLC. Leaf positioning and gap width are critical to the accuracy of the delivered dose in IMRT. Alignment of the MLC to the accelerator, direct and indirect measurements of leaf positions and gap widths, verification of reference static and dynamic fields, and analysis of feedback information provided by the MLC software are discussed. Procedures and results for a variety of mechanical, light field, and radiation field measurements using a feeler gauge, graph paper, film, and dosimeters have been presented.

# References


Arnfield, M. R., J. V. Siebers, J. O. Kim, Q. Wu, P. J. Keall, and R. Mohan. (2000). "A method for determining multileaf collimator transmission and scatter for dynamic intensity modulated radiotherapy." *Med. Phys.* 27: 2231–2241.

Boyer, A., P. Biggs, J. Galvin, E. Klein, T. LoSasso, D. Low, K. Mah, and C. Yu. *Basic Applications of Multileaf Collimators: Report of the AAPM Radiation Therapy Committee Task Group No. 50.* AAPM Report No. 72. Madison, WI: Medical Physics Publishing, 2001.

Budgell, G. J., J. H. L. Mott, P. C. Williams, and K. J. Brown. (2000). "Requirements for leaf position accuracy for dynamic multileaf collimation." *Phys. Med. Biol.* 45:1211–1227.

Chui, C. S., S. Spirou, and T. LoSasso. (1996). "Testing of dynamic multileaf collimation." *Med. Phys.* 23:635–641.

Ezzell, G. A., and S. Chungbin. (2001). "The overshoot phenomenon in step-and-shoot IMRT delivery." *J. Appl. Clin. Med. Phys.* 2:138–148.

Hounsell, A. R., and T. J. Jordan. (1997). "Quality control aspects of the Philips multileaf collimator." *Radiother. Oncol.* 45:225–233.

Ling, C. C., C. Burman, C. S. Chui, G. J. Kutcher, S. A. Leibel, T. LoSasso, R. M. Mohan, T. Bortfeld, L. Reinstein, S. Spirou, X. H. Wang, Q. Wu, M. Zelefsky, and Z. Fuks. (1996). "Conformal radiation treatment of prostate cancer using inversely planned intensity-modulated photon beams produced with dynamic multileaf collimation." *Int. J. Radiat. Oncol. Biol. Phys.* 35:721–730.

Litzenberg, D. W., J. M. Moran, and B. A. Fraass. (2002a). "Verification of dynamic and segmental IMRT delivery by dynamic log file analysis." *J. Appl. Clin. Med. Phys.* 3:63–72.

Litzenberg, D. W., J. M. Moran, and B. A. Fraass. (2002b). "Incorporation of realistic delivery limitations into dynamic MLC treatment delivery." *Med. Phys.* 29:810–820.

LoSasso, T., C. S. Chui, and C. C. Ling. (1998). "Physical and dosimetric aspects of a multileaf collimation system used in the dynamic mode for implementing intensity modulated radiotherapy." *Med. Phys.* 25:1919–1927.

LoSasso, T., C.-S. Chui, and C. C. Ling. (2001). "Comprehensive quality assurance for the delivery of intensity modulated radiotherapy with a multileaf collimator used in the dynamic mode." *Med. Phys.* 28: 2209–2219.

Low, D. A., J. W. Son, E. E. Klein, J. Markman, S. Mutic, and J. F. Dempsey. (2001). "Characterization of a commercial multileaf collimator used for intensity modulated radiation therapy." *Med. Phys.* 28:752–756.

MSKCC (Memorial Sloan-Kettering Cancer Center). *A Practical Guide to Intensity-Modulated Radiation Therapy.* Madison, WI: Medical Physics Publishing, 2003.

Mubata, C. D., P. Childs, and A. M. Bidmead. (1997). "A quality assurance procedure for the Varian multi-leaf collimator." *Phys. Med. Biol.* 42:423–431.

Nehmeh, S. A., Y. E. Erdi, C. C. Ling, K. E. Rosenzweig, E. D. Yorke, O. D. Squire, E. Ford, K. Sidhu, G. Mageras, L. E. Braban, S. M. Larson, J. L. Humm. (2002). "Effect of respiratory gating on reducing lung motion artifacts in PET imaging of lung cancer." *Med. Phys.* 29:366–371.

Van Esch, A., J. Bohsung, P. Sorvari, M. Tenhunen, M Paiusco, M. Iori, P. Engstrom, H. Nystrom, D. P. Huyskeens. (2002). "Acceptance tests and quality control (QC) procedures for the clinical implementation of intensity modulated radiotherapy (IMRT) using inverse planning and the sliding window technique: Experience from five radiotherapy departments." *Radiother. Oncol.* 65:53–70.

van Santvoort, J. P. C., and B. J. M. Heijmen. (1996). "Dynamic multileaf collimation without 'tongue and groove' underdosage effects." *Phys. Med. Biol.* 41:2091–2105.

Xia, P., C. F. Chuang, and L. J. Verhey. (2002). "Communication and sampling rate limitations in IMRT delivery with a dynamic multileaf collimator system." *Med. Phys.* 29:412–423.

Xing, L., B. Curran, R. Hill, T. Holmes, L. Ma, K. M. Forster, and A. L. Boyer. (1999). "Dosimetric verification of a commercial inverse treatment planning system." *Phys. Med. Biol.* 44:463–478.

Wang, X., S. Spirou, T. LoSasso, J. Stein, C.-S. Chui, and R. Mohan. (1996). "Dosimetric variation of intensity-modulated fields." *Med. Phys.* 23:317–327.

Webb, S. *Intensity-Modulated Radiation Therapy.* Bristol, UK: Institute of Physics Publishing, p. 180, 2001.

Webb, S., T. Bortfeld, J. Stein, and D. Convery. (1997). "The effect of stair-step leaf transmission on the 'tongue and groove problem in radiotherapy with a multileaf collimator." *Phys. Med. Biol.* 42:595–602.

Wu, Q., M. Arnfield, S. Tong, Y. Wu, and R. Mohan. (2000). "Dynamic splitting of large intensity-modulated fields." *Phys. Med. Biol.* 45:1731–1740.

Yorke, E., G. Mageras, T. LoSasso, H. Mostafavi, and C. Ling. (2000). "Respiratory Gating of Sliding Window IMRT." CD-ROM Proceedings of the World Congress on Medical Physics and Biomedical Engineering, July 23–28, 2000, Chicago, IL.

# Tolerance Limits And Action Levels For Planning And Delivery Of IMRT

**Jatinder R. Palta, Ph.D., Siyong Kim, Ph.D., Jonathan G. Li, Ph.D., and Chihray Liu, Ph.D.**
Department of Radiation Oncology
University of Florida, Gainesville, Florida



## Introduction

Intensity-modulated radiation therapy (IMRT) represents one of the most significant technical innovations of the modern day radiation therapy (IMRTCWG 2001; Leibel et al. 2002). It provides the ability for highly conformal dose distributions with sharp dose fall-off for complex target volumes that invaginate critical normal structures. This is accomplished with complex modulation of beam intensity of each IMRT field. Unlike conventional three-dimensional conformal radiation therapy (3DCRT), both the treatment planning and delivery of IMRT are more complex and less intuitive to the users. The intensity-modulated beams on linear accelerators with multileaf collimator (MLC) are generated with complex motion of the leaves. Each IMRT field includes many small, irregular, and asymmetric fields that completely obscure the relationship between monitor unit (MU) setting and radiation dose. The predominance of very small subfields in an intensity-modulated beam make the leaf positioning accuracy much more critical for IMRT as compared to 3DCRT. The proximity of critical normal tissues to target volumes in IMRT and the requirement for sharp dose gradients puts stringent demands on the accurate modeling of beam penumbra and dose outside the field in IMRT planning. Thus, IMRT requires much more diligence in understanding the whole planning and delivery process, associated quality assurance (QA) procedures, and QA tolerance limits with action levels over and beyond what is currently understood for 3DCRT using MLC.

IMRT is an emerging technology. The current IMRT planning and delivery systems can be classified as first generation systems. The published literature in terms of what is acceptable in IMRT planning and delivery accuracy is sparse (Budgell 1999; Budgell et al. 2000; LoSasso, Chui, and Ling 1998, 2001; Venselaar, Welleweerd, and Mijnheer 2001). This chapter provides an overview of what is currently understood as the requirements for QA tolerance limits and action levels for key components of the first generation IMRT planning and delivery systems using MLC. As the field matures, one can expect more formal recommendations and a code of practice for IMRT from the American Association of Physicists in Medicine (AAPM) in the near future.

## Importance Of Accuracy In Dose Planning And Delivery

It is well understood in radiation therapy that the dose-response curves are quite steep and there is clinical evidence that a small change (7% to 10%) in the dose to target volume can result in a change in the tumor control probability (ICRU 1976). Along the same argument, similar dose change may also result in a sharp change in the incidence and severity of radiation-induced morbidity, especially for serial critical structures such as spinal cord, optical chiasm, and brain stem. For IMRT, the accuracy in dose planning and delivery is even more important because a small displacement of the delivered dose distribution can easily change the topical dose that exceeds the threshold for undesirable clinical outcome. Based on clinical evidence on effective and excessive dose levels, the consensus in radiation therapy community is that the dose delivered to the tumor volume should be within 5% of the prescribed dose (Dische et al. 1993). Therefore, the guiding principle for establishing QA test procedures and tolerance limits for the performance of IMRT planning and delivery systems should be to minimize overall uncertainty (random and systematic) in delivered dose to less than 5%.

## Process Of IMRT Planning And Delivery

The process of IMRT from a QA perspective includes patient immobilization, 3-D imaging, inverse planning, leaf sequencing, plan verification, patient setup verification, and treatment delivery (IMRTCWG 2001). The requirements for accuracy in patient immobilization, 3-D imaging, and setup verification have been previously discussed in reference to conventional 3DCRT (Fraas et al. 1998). However, IMRT requires more stringent tolerance limits for patient immobilization than 3DCRT. This is because IMRT treatment delivery may take a longer time, thus increasing the potential for intrafraction patient motion. Moreover, the computer optimization process in inverse planning depends on the accurate delineation of target volume and critical structures and its spatial integrity relative to each other. In inverse planning, the clinical objectives are described mathematically and a computer optimization algorithm is used to determine optimal beam intensities that lead to the desired conformal dose distribution. These intensity distributions cannot be delivered directly by the delivery systems. They are first converted into an MLC leaf sequence. The leaf sequencing algorithms need to account for the mechanical limitations of the delivery system, beamlet size, leaf end leakage, leaf transmission, and leaf travel. Each one of these parameters has tolerance limits that impact the overall accuracy of the beam intensity delivery as planned. The complexity of the IMRT planning process and the nonintuitive nature of the beam intensity patterns makes it necessary to verify each IMRT treatment plan on a hybrid phantom as described herein by Xia (***Patient-Specific Quality Assurance In IMRT***). The sharp dose gradients in IMRT warrant much tighter tolerance limits in the verification of patient set up for treatment delivery. Finally, the accuracy of IMRT delivery as planned depends on the mechanical accuracy and integrity of the MLC system (LoSasso, Chui, and Ling 1998, 2001). IMRT places much greater mechanical demand on the MLC and can result in accelerated wear and tear of the system. Therefore, periodic QA test procedures with appropriate tolerance limits and action levels are crucial in the planning and delivery of IMRT.

## Sources Of Error In The IMRT Process

The IMRT process as described previously has multiple steps with a potential to incur small errors at each step along the way. Most of the treatment execution errors occur for each treatment fraction and are classified as *random* errors. There are other errors such as organ motion, that is, movement of the target with respect to the radiographic anatomy, that can occur both during imaging for treatment planning and treatment delivery, and the target delineation. The errors that occur only during treatment planning are classified as *systematic* errors. It should be noted that the systematic errors are the most significant in terms of undesirable clinical outcome in IMRT. It is generally believed that the total error in clinical practice of IMRT has normal distribution and that errors in each step can be added quadratically (van Herk et al. 2000). The total error can then be obtained by adding the standard deviations of each error in quadrature. It is quite obvious the overall error is dominated by the error in a step with the largest magnitude. Therefore, every attempt should be made to reduce that error. Errors cannot be eliminated completely and the only way to account for errors without compromising a positive clinical outcome is to select margins around clinical target volumes and organs at risk judiciously. It is critically important that the tolerance limits and action levels for the QA test procedures for the different steps in the IMRT process preserve the rationale used in the selection of margins for each disease site.

The error analysis should be done for each disease site specifically because as described earlier, the internal organ motion and target delineation uncertainties can vary from site to site and each one of these have much greater impact on the overall uncertainty (van Herk et al. 2000). As an example, we show uncertainty analyses for prostate, central nervous system (CNS), and head and neck patients treated with IMRT in our clinic with Segmental Multileaf Collimator (SMLC) technique shown in table 1. It is obvious from this table that for prostate patients, the largest spatial uncertainty of 7.35 mm in the patient setup dominates the overall uncertainty, which is 7.60 mm. This clearly shows that there is really no point in making the tolerance limits on other parameters of the planning and delivery system too stringent unless the set up uncertainty is minimized. The situation is a little different for CNS, head, and neck patients for whom the set up uncertainties are much smaller and are comparable to planning and delivery system uncertainties in our institution. One should use prudence in selecting the tolerance limits and action levels for QA test procedures for each step of the IMRT process. The impact of the spatial uncertainties on delivered dose to a patient depends strongly on the local dose gradients of isodose distributions. Therefore, it is fairly easy to convert spatial uncertainties into dose uncertainties.

One other parameter that can impact the overall uncertainty is the target and critical structure delineation, which is not included in the analysis shown in table 1. Several studies have shown the physician-to-physician variability in target delineation can also be very significant (Giraud et al. 2002; Leunens et al. 1993; Logue et al. 1998; Rasch et al. 1999; Tai et al. 2002). Having very explicit outlining protocols, adequate training, and frequent consultations with the diagnostic imaging experts can reduce the uncertainties in target and critical structure delineation.

## Overall Goal Of IMRT Quality Assurance Process

The overall goal of the IMRT QA process is to ensure that each patient treated with this modality receives the best possible long-term tumor control without significant morbidity. Compared to 3DCRT, certain components in the IMRT process are more complex and require much more diligence in establishing QA procedures. For example, the intensity-modulated beams require the positioning accuracy of MLC leaves to be much more precise than those used for 3DCRT and monitored more frequently. As mentioned before, the goal in any radiation therapy treatment is to deliver prescribed radiation dose with less than 5% overall uncertainty. This requires the set tolerance limits for the IMRT planning and delivery system be such that the overall uncertainty is within the acceptable limits. Therefore, the first logical step is to analyze uncertainties in the three major components of the IMRT process: IMRT treatment planning, IMRT delivery equipment, and patient specific QA.

**Table 1.** IMRT Process Uncertainty Analysis

| | Prostate | | | | | | | | Head and Neck/CNS | | | | | | | |
|---|---|---|---|---|---|---|---|---|---|---|---|---|---|---|---|---|
| | Voxel Size (mm) | | | Mean Displacement (mm) | | | Item Uncertainty (mm) | Process Uncertainty (mm) | Voxel Size (mm) | | | Mean Displacement (mm) | | | Item Uncertainty (mm) | Process Uncertainty (mm) |
| | X | Y | Z | X | Y | Z | | | X | Y | Z | X | Y | Z | | |
| **Imaging** **CT** | 0.94 | 0.94 | 3.00 | 0.47 | 0.47 | 1.50 | 0.87 | 0.87 | 0.94 | 0.94 | 1.50 | 0.47 | 0.47 | 0.75 | 0.55 | 0.55 |
| **Planning** **RTP** | | | | | | | | | | | | | | | | |
| *Data Input* | | | | | | | 1.00 | 1.22 | | | | | | | 1.00 | 1.22 |
| *Calculation* | | | | | | | 0.50 | | | | | | | | 0.50 | |
| *Non-dosimetric* | | | | | | | 0.50 | | | | | | | | 0.50 | |
| **Delivery** **Machine** | | | | | | | | | | | | | | | | |
| *Isocenter* | | | | 0.50 | 0.50 | 0.75 | 1.03 | 1.44 | | | | 0.50 | 0.50 | 0.75 | 1.03 | 1.44 |
| *MLC* | | | | | | | 1.00 | | | | | | | | 1.00 | |
| **Setup** *Inter-fraction* | | | | | | | 2.00 | 7.35 | | | | | | | 0.50 | 1.12 |
| *Intra-fraction* | | | | | | | 5.00 | | | | | | | | 1.00 | |
| *Organ motion* | | | | | | | 5.00 | | | | | | | | 0.00 | |
| | Overall Uncertainty (mm) | | | | | | | 7.60 | | | Overall Uncertainty (mm) | | | | | 2.85 |

## IMRT Treatment Planning QA

### What Is Different About IMRT Treatment Planning?

IMRT treatment planning is simply an advancement in the 3DCRT planning in which nonuniform instead of uniform radiation beam intensities are used to obtain the most conformal dose distribution for a given target volume. The nonuniform beam intensities in IMRT are often determined by various computer-based optimization techniques that are driven by clinically defined planning objectives and constraints. IMRT treatment planning is similar to 3DCRT treatment planning as it also uses targets and normal structures identified on multiple transverse images, field design based on beam's eye view projections, volumetric dose calculations, and volumetric plan evaluation tools such as dose-volume histograms (DVHs). The only difference is that IMRT seeks to provide a method of sparing normal critical structures that push into and are partially or fully surrounded by clinical target volume (CTV).

IMRT dose distribution is calculated by dividing each beam into smaller sections, called *beamlets* that can have varying intensities. Since these beamlets have a very small size, typically 1 cm × 1 cm, a small error in the size of the *beamlet* can result in a large change in the radiation output (LoSasso, Chui, and Ling 1998). Radiation parameters such as transmission through the collimators, penumbra, and dose outside the field affect the results at the edge of the field in 3DCRT, which has reduced clinical importance. However, in IMRT, variable beam intensities for the beamlets are obtained by moving the MLC leaves through the irradiated field; thus accurate modeling of penumbra and leaf transmission is crucial in IMRT planning

The computer optimization algorithm in the inverse planning system provides optimal intensity-modulated beams that meet the planning objectives. These modulated beams are then converted into delivery instructions for the MLC system. The accuracy with which the planned intensity distribution is reproduced on a delivery system depends on parameters such as collimator transmission, shape and size of the leaves, interleaf leakage, and mechanical limitations in the motion of the MLC. Idealized intensity patterns are almost never deliverable exactly.

### TG-40 And IMRT Treatment Planning

The AAPM Task Group 40 (TG-40) report on Comprehensive QA for Radiation Oncology recognized the treatment-planning computer is a crucial component of the treatment process (Kutcher et al. 1994). It discusses the importance of understanding the planning system documentation, initial and ongoing testing, detail outline of the treatment planning process, and treatment planning QA for individual patients. All these issues are equally important in the IMRT treatment planning system QA. The specific test procedures and the tolerance limits described in the TG-40 report for treatment planning are not directly applicable for IMRT application. IMRT treatment planning system QA includes but is not limited to: the integrity of imaging data for planning, the calculation of relative dose distribution for modulated beams, heterogeneity corrections, leaf sequencing, and MU calculation. Unfortunately, there is very little guidance available in this area in the literature at this time. New Task Group reports are needed that provide recommendations for the acceptance testing, commissioning, and establishment and implementation of QA programs for IMRT treatment planning systems. Each institution must develop its own QA program that suits the local environment, ensures patient safety, and enables treatment planning and delivery accuracy.

## TG-53 And IMRT Treatment Planning

AAPM TG-53 report on QA for clinical radiotherapy treatment planning provides guidance in developing and implementing a comprehensive QA program for 3DCRT treatment planning (Fraas et al. 1998). It encompasses image-based definition of patient anatomy, 3-D description of beam geometry, graphical user interface, 3-D dose calculation algorithms, and plan evaluation tools including DVHs. It provides the necessary framework for the task of creating a QA program that is customized to the needs of each institution. The acceptance testing, commissioning and QA procedures described in the TG-53 report are also applicable to IMRT treatment planning systems. Thus, the amount of effort required in clinically implementing and maintaining an IMRT planning system must not be underestimated. There are at least two aspects of IMRT that distinguish it from 3DCRT: first is the optimization process in the planning phase, and second is the use of modulated treatment beams in the delivery phase. The commissioning and testing of these two phases of IMRT have not yet been fully developed.

IMRT treatment planning systems are also different in that the commissioning and QA process must include the determination of the effect of the input parameters on the optimized dose distribution. There are currently no established criteria for testing the quality and acceptability of the dose distributions produced by automated optimization. These will evolve as each institution acquires more experience in IMRT. It is expected that a standard set of phantoms with defined geometries and planning objectives will enable meaningful comparison between different IMRT planning systems and development of criteria for acceptance testing, commissioning and QA.

## Achievable Accuracy In IMRT Treatment Planning

The IMRT treatment planning process includes patient positioning and immobilization, image acquisition, target and clinical structure delineation, beam arrangement, dose calculation and optimization, leaf sequencing, plan evaluation, and plan implementation. Most of these steps with the exception of plan optimization and leaf sequencing are analogous to 3DCRT treatment planning. Determining the required and achievable accuracy for IMRT treatment planning systems is very difficult, because what is achievable on one system may not be so with another system. Therefore, the onus is on each institution to establish limits of accuracy of their IMRT planning system in their own local environment and for each disease site. There are limited data on achievable accuracy in dose calculation that have started to emerge for IMRT planning systems, which can be used as general guidelines (Essers et al. 2001; Wang et al. 1996; Xing et al. 1999). The TG-53 report has also provided ranges of generally achievable tolerance limits for the 3-D radiotherapy planning (RTP) systems, which should be achieved by all IMRT planning systems. There are, however, two tolerance limits described in the TG-53 report that are very difficult to meet in IMRT treatment planning systems. These have to do with the agreement between calculated and measured dose in both high dose in a small dose gradient, and high dose in large dose gradient region.

IMRT treatment planning systems have difficulty in meeting the 2% tolerance limit in the high-dose region and 1 to 5 mm in the high-dose gradient region (Van Dyk et al. 1993). In IMRT, individual intensity-modulated beams that vary in complexity from beam to beam create these high-dose gradients. It is sometimes difficult to have agreement at all points in a 3-D dose distribution. A disagreement between measured and calculated dose values at a few points does not necessarily lead to a negative overall result if other comparable points are well within the established tolerance limits. Figure 1 shows a comparison between the measured and calculated cross-beam plot for an intensity-modulated beam. The agreement is generally very good except at a few points in the high gradient area that are displaced by almost 10 mm. But on the other hand, the statistical analysis of 330 points in the cross plot shows 322 points (97.5%) are within the acceptable tolerance limit of 3%. Venselaar et al. (Venselaar, Welleweerd, and Mijnheer 2001) introduced a similar concept that combines the influence of systematic and random deviations on a large number of data points. Similar to their recommendation, we define the confidence limit, $\Delta$ as:

$$\Delta = |\text{ Mean deviation }| + 1.96 \times \text{SD}.$$

The multiplicative factor of 1.96 implies that still 5% of the individual points exceed the tolerance for that particular situation. For a confidence probability $P = 0.065$, the multiplication factor is 1.5, which was arbitrarily chosen by Venselaar et al. to quantify the dose accuracy of photon beam calculations of 3-D treatment planning systems. We recommend a value of $P = 0.05$ for the IMRT planning systems.

## Recommended Limits And Action Levels

A typical IMRT treatment planning system validation procedure is done by comparing the measured and calculated dose distribution using well-defined criteria. As discussed earlier, Van Dyk et al. (1993) have published criteria for dose distribution comparisons that really do not work as well for IMRT treatment planning systems. Therefore, we have defined more appropriate criteria that allow meaningful validation of IMRT treatment plans. Table 2 summarizes the proposed values of the planning confidence limits and action levels for different regions in an IMRT treatment plan.

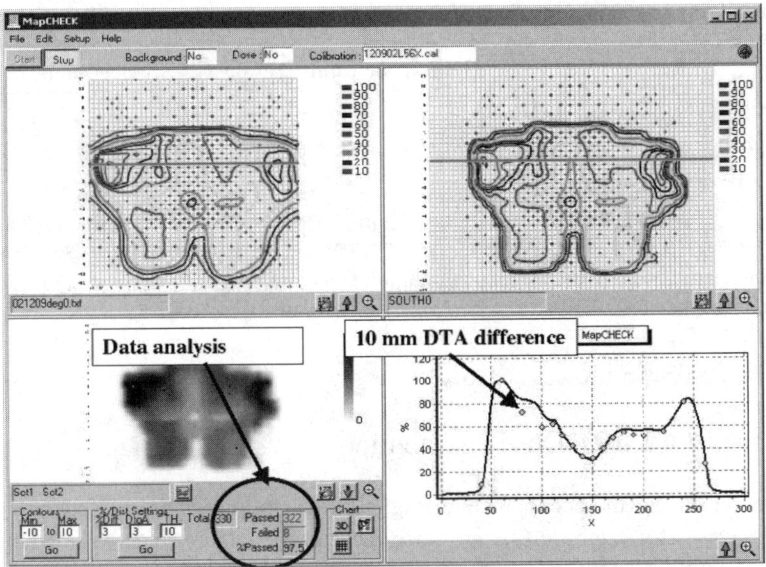

**Figure 1.** Comparison of a measured and calculated cross-plot (at 5 cm depth)
of an intensity modulated field incident on a flat phantom. A diode-array (*MapCheck;
Sun Nuclear Corp.*) was used for this comparison, which shows that 97.5% of the points
meet 3% criteria even though DTA (distance to agreement) for a few points is 10 mm.

These values were arrived at using the results of an IMRT questionnaire that was
mailed to 30 institutions that actively use IMRT. This questionnaire was designed to
collect data on how each institution views QA requirements and tolerance limits for
IMRT planning and delivery. There is recent literature that discusses patient-specific
point dose measurement for IMRT (Chen, Xing, and Nath 2002; Kung and Chen 2000;
Tsai et al. 1998). There is a developing consensus that the agreement between
measured and calculated dose points is of the order of 2% to 3%. We propose a confidence limit of 3% in high dose, small dose gradient region and a 10% in high dose,
and high gradient region. A large dose gradient is defined as being larger than 3% per
mm. The confidence limit for the low dose, small dose gradient is 4%. A larger limit
is used here because the dose calculations in the low dose region are inherently less
accurate. The action level values for each region are also included in table 2. The IMRT
treatment plan should not be used clinically if the measured dose difference is more
than the value given as the action level. The action level value serves as a pass-fail criterion. It should be noted that the mean deviation used in the calculation of confidence
limit $\Delta$, for all regions, is expressed as a percentage of the prescribed dose and not as
a percentage of the locally measured dose. The tolerance limits for the dose difference
in the high gradient region is also given in terms of distance to agreement. For each
measurement point, the calculated dose distribution is examined to determine the
distance between a measurement point and the nearest point in the calculated dose
distribution that has the same dose.

Jatinder Palta et al.

**Table 2.** Proposed Values of the Confidence Limits and Action Levels for IMRT Planning

| Region | Confidence Limit* (P=0.05) | Action level |
|---|---|---|
| $\delta_1$ (high dose, small dose gradient) | ±3% | ±5% |
| $\delta_2$ (high dose, large dose gradient) | 10% or 2 mm DTA$^\oplus$ | 15% or 3 mm DTA$^\oplus$ |
| $\delta_3$ (low dose, small dose gradient) | 4% | 7% |
| $\delta_{90-50\%}$ (dose fall off) | 2 mm DTA | 3 mm DTA |

* Mean deviation used in the calculation of confidence limit for all regions is expressed as a percentage of the prescribed does according to the formula,

$\delta_i = 100\% \; X \; (D_{calc.} - D_{meas.}/D_{\;prescribed})$

$^\oplus$Distance to agreement

## Validation Of IMRT Dose Distribution

An integral part of the acceptance testing, commissioning, and establishment of the baseline limits for ongoing QA are dose measurements and their comparison with IMRT planning system calculations. Dosimetric validation of an IMRT planning system should be conducted by first defining well-defined non-uniform beam intensities patterns and then applying them to a phantom so that the resulting dose distributions can be measured and validated unambiguously. Some examples of intensity patterns that can validate the input parameters of the dose calculation algorithms and determine its dosimetric accuracy are shown in figures 2 and 3. The strip, well, pyramid, and bar patterns shown in these figures (Ezzell, G. A., Private communication) can easily validate the input parameters of an IMRT dose calculation algorithm that include small field dosimetry, transmitted and leakage radiation, extra-focal radiation, and dose calculation resolution. Figure 4 shows a simple strip phantom can easily quantify the accuracy of dose calculation for varying intensities, which are a hallmark of an IMRT plan. The final step in the validation of the IMRT dose distribution is to plan and irradiate a geometric phantom that mimic the range of target volumes and critical structure geometries to be used clinically. The Radiological Physics Center (RPC) has designed several such phantoms to validate an IMRT treatment planning system for clinical use (Ibbott, G., Private communication). These phantoms are used by RPC to credential institutions for IMRT clinical protocols.

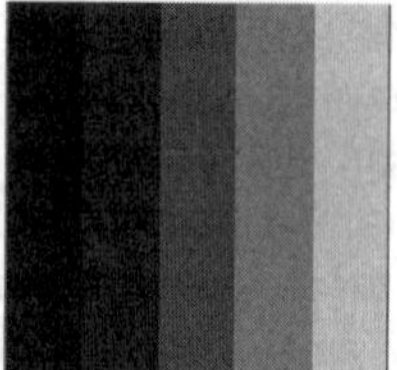 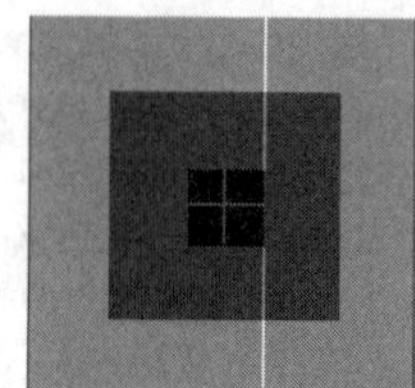 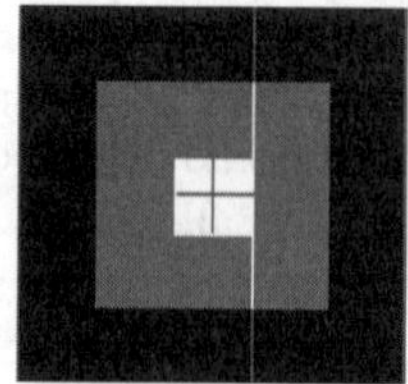

**Figure 2.** The intensity patterns used to validate the IMRT planning system. (a) A strip pattern, (b) a pyramid pattern, and (c) a well pattern.

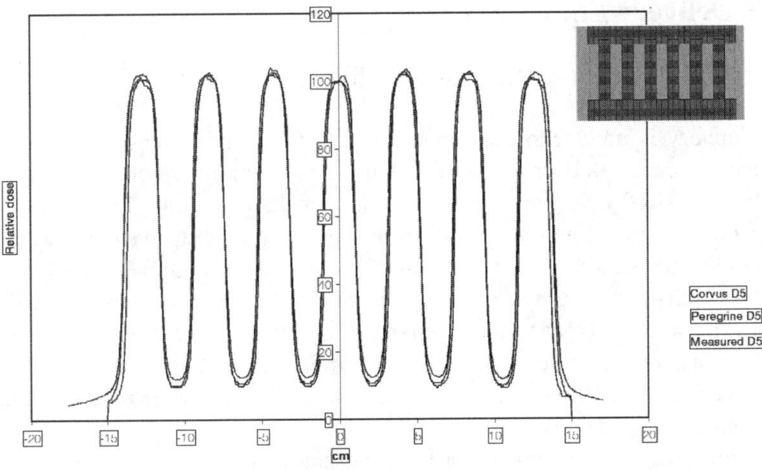



**Figure 3.** A bar pattern with 2-cm alternating strips. This type of a pattern can easily validate the input parameters of an IMRT dose calculation algorithm that include small field dosimetry, transmitted and leakage radiation, extra-focal radiation, and dose calculation resolution. For example, this validation test shows that the measured profile agrees well with the PEREGRINE® system calculation. The CORVUS® system overestimates the dose under the shielded area.

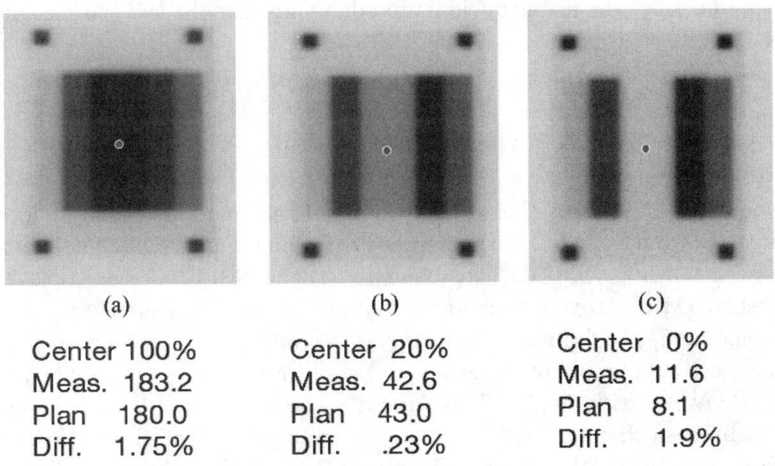



**Figure 4.** Comparison of calculated and measured dose for a strip intensity pattern with varying intensities (0% to 100%; theoretical) at the measurement point. The dose measured in frame (c) is from transmitted and scattered radiation under the blocked leaves. An acceptable agreement between the measured and calculated dose in all three frames indicates that the beam modeling in the IMRT planning system is adequate.

## IMRT Delivery Equipment QA

### Special Considerations In IMRT Delivery

IMRT delivery is much more complex than 3DCRT and it requires a much more precise and accurate delivery system. The three most important characteristics of the MLC-based IMRT delivery system include: mechanical integrity of the delivery system, precise spatial and temporal positioning of the MLC system, and radiation beam fidelity for small MUs. The mechanical demands on delivery system components, especially the MLC system, are on an order of magnitude more for IMRT than 3DCRT. The wear and tear of the mechanical system is also accelerated by the same magnitude. Therefore, special QA tests are required in addition to what is necessary for 3DCRT using MLC to ensure the delivery system continues to meet the functional performance specifications.

It is important to recognize that both the hardware and software control of the current IMRT delivery systems are relatively new and the potential for error is not completely understood at this time. Therefore, the testing of the IMRT delivery system needs to be more comprehensive and more frequent until it can be demonstrated with extended monitoring that a given parameter does not change over a period of time. The component of the IMRT delivery system requiring the most vigilance at this time is the MLC system (LoSasso, Chui, and Ling 2001). The MLC performance characteristics requiring continuous monitoring include the following: the leaf position accuracy and reproducibility, the leaf gap width reproducibility, and the leaf speed accuracy.

### IMRT Delivery Techniques And Delivery Equipment

IMRT delivery techniques fall into two distinct categories in which either the gantry is moving or fixed while the radiation beam is delivered (IMRTCWG 2001). Intensity-modulated arc therapy (IMAT) delivered with standard MLC and tomotherapy delivered with binary MLC are examples of dynamic gantry IMRT delivery techniques. Static MLC (SMLC) and dynamic MLC (DMLC) are examples of the fixed-gantry IMRT delivery techniques. Out of the dynamic gantry techniques, the serial tomotherapy with binary collimator is the only one that is in routine used to treat a significant number of patients with IMRT and discussed in detail by Curran (*IMRT Delivery Using Serial Tomotherapy*). The SMLC and DMLC methods of IMRT delivery techniques with fixed gantry are described by Boyer [Static MLC IMRT (Step And Shoot)] and Keall (Dynamic MLC IMRT) in the proceedings of this meeting. All the IMRT delivery techniques require a computer-controlled linear accelerator with a fast responding control system, which precisely synchronizes the motion of intensity modulation subsystem (MLC or binary collimator) and the radiation output from the accelerator. The functional requirements for a computer-controlled linear accelerator necessary for IMRT delivery are described by Waldron (*Functional Requirements For IMRT*).

## TG-40 And IMRT Delivery Equipment

AAPM TG-40 report on Comprehensive QA for Radiation Oncology provides a list of parameters and associated tolerance limits for a computer-controlled linear accelerator QA (Kutcher et al. 1994). The tolerance limits for QA tests described in the TG-40 report are not adequate for IMRT delivery system. Sharp dose gradients, which are typical of an IMRT delivery, mandate better mechanical accuracy of the delivery equipment to realize its full clinical potential. Therefore, the QA recommendations given in the TG-40 report are not exactly applicable to the delivery equipment used for IMRT. As suggested earlier, new Task Group reports are needed that provide recommendations for the acceptance testing, commissioning, and establishment and implementation of QA programs for IMRT delivery equipment. In the meantime, each institution must develop its own QA program that adequately monitors the functional performance characteristics of the IMRT delivery system for the chosen delivery technique to ensure patient safety and treatment delivery accuracy.

## MLC Characteristics That Impact IMRT Delivery Accuracy

Both the SMLC- and the DMLC-IMRT delivery techniques have relatively small gaps between opposed leaves while the radiation is delivered at each gantry position. LoSasso (*IMRT Delivery System QA*) has shown the radiation output for small gap widths is very sensitive to the size of the gap width, which changes the magnitude of the extra-focal radiation. In addition, leaves shield most regions most of the time during the radiation delivery. Therefore, the delivered dose is very sensitive to the transmission through the leaves and the rounded leaf ends. The requirements for MLC positional accuracy are more stringent for DMLC than SMLC because the gap between the opposing leaves tends to be much smaller for DMLC delivery. A variation of $\pm0.2$ mm in gap width for a 1.0 cm nominal gap can result in a dose variation of $\pm3\%$ for each DMLC field (LoSasso, Chui, and Ling 1998, 2001). Other factors impacting the accuracy of IMRT delivery with MLC include the following: leaf speed, dose rate of the linear accelerator, and the fidelity of the delivery control system for small MUs at high dose rates.

The accuracy of dose output and beam stability for small MUs cannot be overlooked in IMRT because a large fraction of the total MUs for each IMRT field is delivered with field segments that have very small MUs. An analysis of the first 100 head and neck patients treated with IMRT and planned with CORVUS® (NOMOS Corporation, Cranberry Township, PA) inverse planning at our institution shows that most sub-fields were treated with less than 5 MU as shown in figure 5. Recent investigations of IMRT beam delivery for small MUs show the delivered intensities can be very inaccurate, especially at higher dose rates (Ezzell and Chungbin 2001; Litzenberg, Moran, and Fraass 2002; Xia, Chuang, and Verhey 2002). Figure 6 shows some segments are completely dropped for a strip intensity pattern, and the MUs are redistributed at a high dose rate (600 MU/min) and a small MU for each subfield.

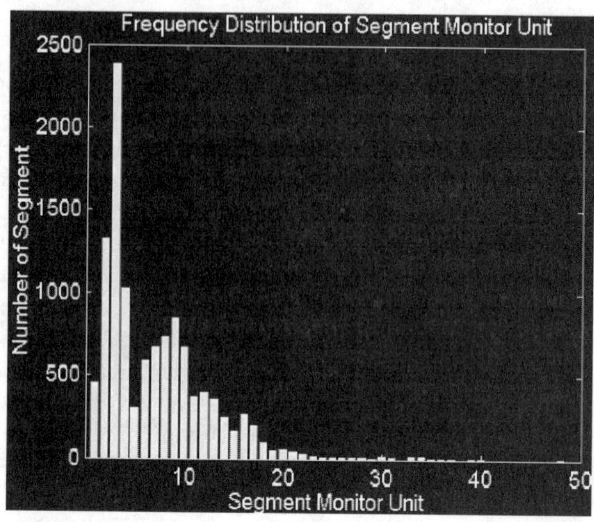


**Figure 5.** An analysis of first 100 head and neck patients treated with IMRT and planned with CORVUS inverse planning at the University of Florida. Most subfields have MUs less than 5.

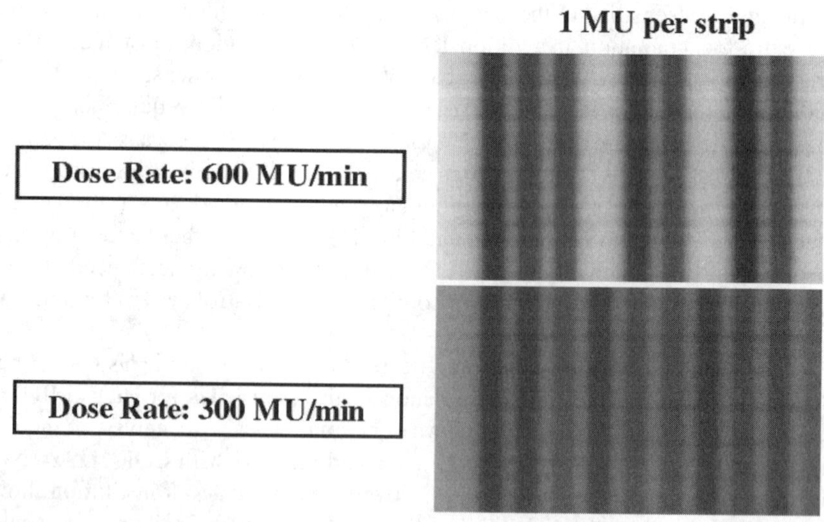


**Figure 6.** Film measurements of a 10-strip test pattern. The linac (Varian 2100 C/D) was instructed to deliver 1 MU per strip with the step-and-shoot IMRT delivery mode for a total of 10 MUs. The delivery sequence is from left to right. Some of the segments are completely dropped and the MUs are redistributed at high-dose rate (600 MU/min) and small MU for each subfield.

Another MLC characteristic impacting the accuracy of the IMRT delivery is the partial transmission through the rounded leaf ends on some MLC systems (Elekta and Varian). A film irradiation of contiguous abutting fields on these MLC systems will show thin lines of high dose at the field junctions. These lines cannot be avoided completely unless the leaf ends are focused (Siemens MLC system). The effect of leaf end transmission can be minimized only by intentionally introducing a constant offset in the leaf position setting. Figure 7 shows the impact of the leaf end transmission on abutting field and the minimization of this effect by introducing a leaf offset. The leaf end transmission has more of an impact on the accuracy of IMRT delivery with SMLC than the DMLC delivery technique. It is important to measure the leaf offset effect at different gantry and collimator angles to check the effect of gravity and MLC leaf carriage sag.

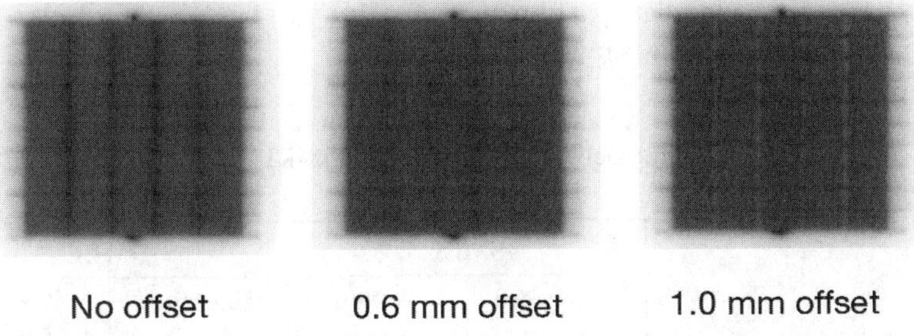



**Figure 7.** Films exposed with five abutting fields. A zero offset creates a high dose junction while 1 mm offset creates a cold spot. A compromise is an 0.6 mm constant offset. This test should be repeated at different gantry angles to rule out MLC carriage sag.

## Recommended Limits And Action Levels

The functional performance specifications of the MLC system for IMRT delivery need to be much tighter than for 3DCRT delivery. In 3DCRT, the MLC defines the outer aperture of the radiation field. A tolerance limit of up to 2 mm in leaf position may not have a consequential effect on the output. However, in IMRT the non-uniform fluence is obtained by adding several small subfields for which a small uncertainty in the field definition can result in a large discrepancy in the output of an intensity-modulated field. For this reason, the accuracy of leaf position must be maintained to a precision of better than a millimeter. As discussed earlier, the accuracy of the leaf position is much more important for DMLC than for SMLC. Furthermore, it is important to recognize that the overall accuracy of the delivered dose with an IMRT field depends on the reproducibility of the leaf position and the gap width. Another way to look at the leaf positioning accuracy and reproducibility is that the positioning inaccuracies of leaves spatially displace the modulated fields, whereas the lack of reproducibility results in a change in the fluence pattern. Thus, leaf-positioning inaccuracy increases systematic errors and the leaf position irreproducibility increases random errors in IMRT delivery.

The proposed values of tolerance limits and action levels for delivery systems used in IMRT are given in table 3. The action level for each parameter is typically set at a value twice the tolerance limit. We suggest the tolerance limit for the leaf positioning be 1 mm for SMLC and 0.5 mm for DMLC. This limit should provide spatial accuracy of intensity-modulated pattern to better than 1 pixel (0.3 to 0.94 mm) on a computed tomography (CT) image. The leaf position and gap width reproducibility are much more critical in IMRT delivery. Thus, the suggested tolerance limit value for these parameters is 0.2 mm to ensure a dose error less than 3% for any individual intensity-modulated field. The suggested tolerance limit for the leaf speed in DMLC delivery technique is ±0.1 mm/s. This should ensure a dose error of less than 3%. This is easily measured by irradiating a film with a fixed gap width and with pairs of leaves moving at different speed as shown in figure 8.

**Table 3.** Proposed Values of Tolerance Limits and Action Levels
for Delivery System Used in IMRT

| | SMLC | | DMLC | |
|---|---|---|---|---|
| | **Tolerance Limit** | **Action Limit** | **Tolerance Limit** | **Action Limit** |
| **MLC*** | | | | |
| Leaf position accuracy | 1 mm | 2 mm | 0.5 mm | 1.0 mm |
| Leaf Position reproducibility | 0.2 mm | 0.5 mm | 0.2 mm | 0.5 mm |
| Gap width reproducibility | 0.2 mm | 0.5 mm | 0.2 mm | 0.5 mm |
| Leaf speed‡ | N/A | N/A | +/− 0.1 mm/s | +/− 0.2 mm/s |
| **Gantry, MLC, and Table Isocenter** | 0.75 mm radius | 1.0 mm radius | 0.75 mm radius | 1.0 mm radius |
| **Beam Output Stability** | | | | |
| Low MU (<2 MU) | 2% | 3% | 3% | 5% |
| Low MU symmetry (<2 MU) | 2% | 3% | 2% | 3% |

*Measured at all four cardinal gantry angles.
‡Checked indirectly using a specially designed leaf sequence and film.

The suggested tolerance limit for the locus of gantry, collimator, and the table isocenters is a sphere of 0.75 mm radius. This is different from the recommendations given in the TG-40 report, where the tolerance limit for each individual isocenter is a sphere of 1 mm radius. We feel the IMRT delivery systems need to have tighter tolerance limits than the delivery system used for conventional radiation therapy.

We find it necessary to impose the tolerance limits on the output stability and beam symmetry for low MU delivery. Most intensity-modulated fields have many subfields with very small MUs. We suggest a tolerance limit of 2% both for beam output stability and beam symmetry at delivered MUs of 2 or less. The current QA devices such as diode array can easily and accurately measure output and beam stability for MUs less than 2. A fast film can also be used to measure the dose delivered at very high dose rates and for low MU in a dynamic delivery mode as shown in figure 6.

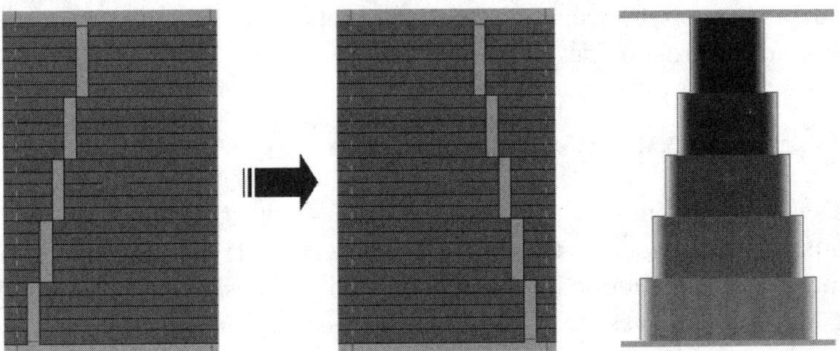

**Figure 8.** A "pyramid" test pattern to quantify the leaf speed accuracy of moving leaf pairs. The leaf pair speed increases from top to bottom in this example.

In summary, the IMRT delivery system QA should include the testing of all the parameters and with the frequency that are described in the TG-40 report. The scope of QA test procedures for the MLC system and the beam fidelity at low MUs need to be broadened. The tolerance limits and action levels for each parameter are delivery-technique dependent. In general, the DMLC delivery technique requires better accuracy of the sub components of the IMRT delivery system.

## Patient-Specific QA

The QA for 3DCRT planning and delivery typically relies on the performance evaluation of individual parameters of the system only. It is never necessary to perform patient-specific QA except when a clinical situation warrants the monitoring of dose to a specific area of interest with *in vivo* dosimeters. This is always with an assumption that once the system is properly commissioned, then the periodic QA checks of the subsystem will guarantee that all patients are treated with accuracy that is within the limits of established QA criteria.

For IMRT, the traditional QA is not sufficient. It is very difficult to anticipate all likely problems in IMRT. Often the intensity patterns are complex and non-intuitive. There is little correlation between the MUs and the delivered dose from each intensity-modulated field. Therefore, direct measurements are commonly made of a "hybrid plan" which is generated by applying the intensity-modulated field from a patient plan to a CT study of a geometric phantom. The computed dose distributions are then compared with the measured dose distributions with either a film or a diode array device. Often, an ion chamber is also used to measure the dose in a high dose, low gradient region in the phantom. We suggest that the patient-specific QA should have the same values of the confidence limits as described in table 2. There is no reason why the data from a phantom measurement should not have the same criteria of acceptability as the IMRT planning system. One must recognize that the patient-specific QA is only a total system check. It does not tell anything about the accuracy with which the patient receives an IMRT treatment. The accuracy of the patient treatment is strongly dependent on the accuracy of patient positioning, internal organ motion, and the presence of heterogeneities.

## Resource Requirements For IMRT QA

IMRT is a nascent technology and there are few QA metrics that are well established at this time. In order to ensure that IMRT services consistently meet the highest clinical standards, each institution must invest in a comprehensive QA program for IMRT planning and delivery. Besides a large initial investment in the IMRT hardware and software, adequate qualified personnel resources are necessary for the initial commissioning and ongoing QA of IMRT systems. Current estimates of additional resources necessary for the implementation and maintenance of an IMRT program (40 IMRT patients out of a total of 300 patients treated per year on a single machine) are 550 hours. This includes: 100 additional hours for machine QA, 50 additional hours for treatment planning QA, 200 hours for patient specific QA, and 200 additional hours for IMRT treatment planning. It should also be noted that IMRT decreases daily throughput on the machine. The maximum machine workload is expected to go down from 32 to 27 patients per day (8-hour shift). Also, the machine uptime is expected to go down from 99% to 95% due to more wear and tear of delivery equipment hardware and complexity of the control software.

## Summary

Current IMRT planning and delivery systems are first-generation systems. These systems are changing very rapidly and the peer-reviewed literature in IMRT is appearing at a very fast rate (over 600 publications in the last 5 years). We do not have a consensus on what is clinically acceptable in IMRT planning or delivery accuracy. Therefore, each facility offering IMRT must develop its own guidelines and criteria for the acceptance and QA of IMRT planning and delivery systems. We have proposed the tolerance limits and action levels for some important parameters in planning and delivery of IMRT. These recommendations are based on the results of a survey of facilities actively involved in IMRT. There is no doubt that the recommended values presented in this chapter will be discussed and debated over a period of time before a consensus is reached.

# References

Budgell, G. J. (1999). "Temporal resolution requirements for intensity modulated radiation therapy delivered by multileaf collimators." *Phys. Med. Biol.* 44:1581–1596.

Budgell, G. J., J. H. L. Mott, P. C. Williams, and K. J. Brown. (2000). "Requirements for leaf position accuracy for dynamic multileaf collimation." *Phys. Med. Biol.* 45:1211–1227.

Chen, Z., L. Xing, and R. Nath. (2002). "Independent monitor unit calculation for IMRT using MIMiC multileaf collimator." *Med. Phys.* 29:2041–2051.

Dische, S., M. I. Saunders, C. Williams, A. Hopkins, and E. Aird. (1993). "Precision in reporting the dose given in a course of radiotherapy." *Radiother. Oncol.* 29:287–293.

Essers, M., M. de Langen, M. L. Dirkx, and B. J. Heijmen. (2001). "Commissioning of a commercially available system for intensity-modulated radiotherapy dose delivery with dynamic multileaf collimation." *Radiother. Oncol.* 60:215–224.

Ezzell, G. A. Private communication, 2003.

Ezzell, G. A., and S. Chungbin. (2001). "The overshoot phenomenon in step-and-shoot IMRT delivery." *J. Appl. Clin. Med. Phys.* 2:138–148.

Fraass, B., K. Doppke, M. Hunt, G. Kutcher, G. Starkschall, R. Stern, and J. Van Dyk. (1998). "American Association of Physicists in Medicine Radiation Therapy Committee Task Group 53: Quality assurance for clinical radiotherapy treatment planning." *Med. Phys.* 25:1773–1829.

Giraud, P., S. Elles, S. Helfre, Y. De Rycke, V. Servois, M. F. Carette, C. Alzieu, P. Y. Bondiau, B. Dubray, E. Touboul, M. Housset, J. C. Rosenwald, and J. M. Cosset. (2002). "Conformal radiotherapy for lung cancer: different delineation of the gross tumor volume (GTV) by radiologists and radiation oncologists." *Radiother. Oncol.* 62:27–36.

Ibbott, G. Private communication, 2003.

ICRU Report 24. Determination of Absorbed Dose in Patient Irradiated by Beams of X-Gamma Rays in Radiotherapy Procedures. Washington DC: International Commission on Radiation Units and Measurements, 1976.

IMRTCWG (Intensity Modulated Radiation Therapy Collaborative Working Group). "Intensity-modulated radiotherapy: Current status and issues of interest." *Int. J. Radiat. Oncol. Biol. Phys.* 51:880–914.

Kung, J. H., and G. T. Chen. (2000). "Intensity modulated radiotherapy dose delivery error from radiation field offset inaccuracy." *Med. Phys.* 27:1617–1622.

Kutcher, G. J., L. Coia, M. Gillin, W. F. Hanson, S. Leibel, R. J. Morton, J. R. Palta, J. A. Purdy, L. E. Reinstein, G. K. Svensson, M. Weller, and L. Wingfield. (1994). "Comprehensive QA for radiation oncology: Report of AAPM Radiation Therapy Committee Task Group 40." *Med. Phys.* 21:581–618.

Leibel, S. A., Z. Fuks, M. J. Zelefsky, S. L. Wolden, K. E. Rosenzweig, K. M. Alektiar, M. A. Hunt, E. D. Yorke, L. X. Hong, H. I. Amols, C. M. Burman, A. Jackson, G. S. Mageras, T. LoSasso, L. Happersett, S. V. Spirou, C. S. Chui, and C. C. Ling. (2002). "Intensity modulated radiotherapy." *Cancer J.* 8:164–176.

Leunens, G., J. Menten, C. Weltens, J. Verstraete, and E. van der Schueren. (1993). "Quality assessment of medical decision making in radiation oncology: variability in target volume delineation for brain tumours." *Radiother. Oncol.* 29:169–175.

Litzenberg, D. W., J. M. Moran, and B. A. Fraass. (2002). "Verification of dynamic and segmental IMRT delivery by dynamic log file analysis." *J. Appl. Clin. Med. Phys.* 3:63–72.

Logue, J. P., C. L. Sharrock, R. A. Cowan, G. Read, J. Marrs, and D. Mott. (1998). "Clinical variability of target volume description in conformal radiotherapy planning." *Int. J. Radiat. Oncol. Biol. Phys.* 41:929–931.

LoSasso T., C.-S. Chui, and C. C. Ling. (1998). "Physical and dosimetric aspects of a multileaf collimation system used in the dynamic mode for implementing intensity modulated radiotherapy." *Med. Phys.* 25:1919–1927.

LoSasso, T., C. S. Chui, and C. C. Ling. (2001). "Comprehensive quality assurance for the delivery of intensity modulated radiotherapy with a multileaf collimator used in the dynamic mode." *Med. Phys.* 28(11):2209–2219.

Rasch, C., I. Barillot, P. Remeijer, A. Touw, M. van Herk, and J. V. Lebesque. (1999). "Definition of the prostate in CT and MRI: A multi-observer study." *Int. J. Radiat. Oncol. Biol. Phys.* 43:57–66.

Tai, P., J. Van Dyk, J. Battista, E. Yu, L. Stitt, J. Tonita, O. Agboola, J. Brierley, R. Dar, C. Leighton, S. Malone, B. Strang, P. Truong, G. Videtic, C. S. Wong, R. Wong, and Y. Youssef. (2002). "Improving the consistency in cervical esophageal target volume definition by special training." *Int. J. Radiat. Oncol. Biol. Phys.* 53:766–774.

Tsai, J. S., D. E. Wazer, M. N. Ling, J. K. Wu, M. Fagundes, T. DiPetrillo, B. Kramer, M. Koistinen, and M. J. Engler. (1998). "Dosimetric verification of the dynamic intensity-modulated radiation therapy of 92 patients." *Int. J. Radiat. Oncol. Biol. Phys.* 40:1213–1230.

Van Dyk, J., R. B. Barnett, J. E. Cygler, and P. C. Shragge. (1993). "Commissioning and quality assurance of treatment planning computers." *Int. J. Radiat. Oncol. Biol. Phys.* 26(2):261–273.

van Herk, M., P. Remeijer, C. Rasch, and J. V. Lebesque. (2000). "The probability of correct target dosage: dose-population histograms for deriving treatment margins in radiotherapy." *Int. J. Radiat. Oncol. Biol. Phys.* 47:1121–1135.

Venselaar, J., H. Welleweerd, and B. Mijnheer. (2001). "Tolerances for the accuracy of photon beam dose calculations of treatment planning systems." *Radiother. Oncol.* 60:191–201.

Wang, X., S. Spirou, T. LoSasso, J. Stein, C. Chui, and R. Mohan. (1996). "Dosimetric verification of intensity-modulated fields." *Med. Phys.* 23(3):317–327.

Xia, P., C. Chuang, and L. Verhey. (2002). "Communication and sampling rate limitations in IMRT delivery with a dynamic multileaf collimator system." *Med. Phys.* 29:412–423.

Xing, L., B. Curran, R. Hill, T. Holmes, L. Ma, K. M. Forster, and A. L. Boyer. (1999). "Dosimetric verification of a commercial inverse treatment planning system." *Phys. Med. Biol.* 44:463–478.

# Quality Assurance: When And What Is Enough For IMRT?

**Gary A. Ezzell, Ph.D.**
Mayo Clinic Scottsdale
Scottsdale, Arizona

This chapter serves as an introduction to a panel discussion at the Summer School on the topic of intensity-modulated radiation therapy (IMRT) quality assurance (QA). Its purpose is more to raise issues and provoke discussion than to provide an answer to the difficult question posed in the title. To be sure, this is a question worth discussing. Our QA practices should change as IMRT techniques evolve and we gain experience. We may take it as given that the QA we do now will not be what we do in the future, but we must make a conscious effort to develop processes that are efficient and effective. I will argue here that our current practices need to change because they are neither efficient nor effective.

Let us start with some observations, assertions, and caveats.

1.  We do not know what all the problems are. IMRT is so new and varied in its manifestations that the potential failure modes are not all understood and foreseen.

2.  Doing measurements for every patient in the manner we do now is very time-consuming and inherently inefficient.

3.  Doing such measurements is also not very effective. They can indicate that a problem exists, but not what the problem is or how to fix it. There are also many potential problems that such measurements will not detect.

4.  Billing constraints should not drive our QA practices. We need to assure the well-being of our patients and ourselves by being effective and efficient. Reimbursement is a consequence, not a cause. Ultimately, the market favors efficiency.

5.  Dosimetric QA, directed at ensuring the patient receives the dose prescribed, is necessary but insufficient. QA also includes evaluating the quality of the plan, and is directed at ensuring that the "inverse plan" has not become a "perverse plan." This discussion will concentrate on dosimetric QA, but the clinical physicist must not narrow his/her professional focus to that only.

6.  As a further caveat, this discussion is limited to ongoing QA and will not address the challenge of commissioning. The question of "when can I start treating" is important but mercifully beyond the scope of this chapter. However, I will argue below that commissioning does not stop when treatment starts.

Let us now examine some of these points in more detail.

### We do not know all the failure modes

Measurement is king. IMRT planning and delivery are so new that we do not know all the ways that they can go wrong. Planning can be inaccurate because of problems in dose calculation, linac/MLC modeling, or leaf sequencing. Delivery can be inaccurate because of information transfer or changes in linear accelerator/multileaf collimator (linac/MLC) performance. These are complex systems with interacting components, many of which are deeply imbedded and hidden from the operator. We are well advised to be careful and skeptical. Thankfully, we are not blind and helpless. The commissioning process should uncover any systematic defects that exist. Nevertheless, whenever beginning a new type of treatment, it is reasonable and prudent to include verification measurements for each patient during the initial phase. These are total system tests that should be considered part of the commissioning process, continued until the process is well established and stable, and re-instituted when the process changes.

### Per-patient measurements are time-consuming and inefficient

Measurement is king, but even kings are subject to greater laws. In this case, the issue is cost versus benefit. If measurement and analysis take hours, then physicists will need to look for faster alternatives that are also effective. If measurements can be quick and efficient, then they can be readily continued. The history of *in vivo* measurements for conventional beams is instructive. Such measurements only became common when diode systems evolved to the point that they were easy to use. It was not worthwhile to do TLD measurements for every patient, because using thermoluminescent dosimeters (TLDs) is laborious and the number of errors slipping through the existing QA mesh is small. For IMRT, the analogous technology may be electronic portal imaging device (EPID) dosimetry. But until an analogous technology is available, we should concentrate on creating a new QA mesh that includes per-patient calculations (to look for blunders in treatment preparation) and measurements of delivery accuracy (to look for consistency in machine performance.)

### Per-patient measurements are not very effective

Verification measurements do not sample the entire treated volume. Dosimetric errors caused by problems with a particular MLC leaf's motion may not be discovered by measurement to a single point or plane.

Furthermore, verification measurements are not done on the patient, but in a phantom to which the patient's plan has been applied. The results of the measurement are compared to the expectation generated by the planning system for that new geometry, and the new doses are not the same as the patient's doses. There are a number of possible planning blunders that would never be caught by this process, because the blunder would simply be transferred to the phantom. The measurement would confirm the new prediction but not flag that the prediction of the patient dose was wrong.

For example, the patient calculation might be in error because the CT couch was included in the patient's thickness. Or an inappropriate electron density correction might have caused effective depths to be scaled up by 20%. Or a software glitch might have associated the 6 MV beam name with the 15 MV data file. Applying that incorrect calculation to a phantom and then confirming the measurement in the phantom would not help the patient.

Finally, the phantom measurement may show that an error exists, without isolating the source of the error. It would then still be necessary to look for the cause in the planning, information transfer, or delivery processes.

Therefore, an effective and efficient QA system should include the following components.

1. Standardized tests of delivery system performance frequent enough to find problems before any patient's outcome is compromised. These would likely include daily, weekly, and monthly tests. These tests would look for problems/errors related to MLC/MU delivery control, e.g., errors in MLC positioning leading to output variations from small fields and/or hot/cold regions where beamlets should be abutting. For step-and-shoot IMRT delivery, films taken of sequential strips with abutting edges are very sensitive indicators of MLC accuracy. Such films can be quickly taken at different gantry angles at frequent intervals. For dynamic IMRT delivery, tests of leaf speed constancy need to be included as well.

2. For each patient:

   a. A visual check that plan data have been properly transferred from the planning system to the delivery system.

   b. An independent calculation of dose to target and critical normal tissues that is based on the leaf sequence used for treatment and measurements of source-to-surface distance (SSD) and depth that are independent of the planning system.

   c. Portal images that verify that the isocenter matches that used for planning and that field orientations are correct.

It should be emphasized that the independent calculation should be based on the patient treatment file that has been created in the computerized delivery system, not on the file that comes directly from the planning system. This is analogous to the plan check process we use for conventional treatments. As part of the plan check, the physicist inspects the patient's chart to see how the therapists have been instructed to treat the patient, and then does a dose calculation based on that information. In that way, if a wedge has been left out of the treatment instructions, the calculated dose will not match the expectation. To check an IMRT plan, the physicist should extract the treatment information from the computerized delivery system and input that into a calculation program. SSDs (and effective depths if density corrections are used) should be independently verified and entered into this program.

Commissioning the independent calculation method is, of course, a non-trivial exercise that will involve many measurements. But eventually, independent IMRT calculations should replace phantom measurements for every patient.

The question for this 2003 Summer School is: What should IMRT QA look like in 2004?

# IMRT For Prostate Cancer

**Alan Pollack, M.D., Ph.D. and Robert A. Price, Ph.D.**
Department of Radiation Oncology
Fox Chase Cancer Center, Philadelphia, Pennsylvania



## Rationale For IMRT

Essential to maximizing the control of prostate cancer is the delivery of radiation dose sufficient for tumor eradication. Dose escalation is at the forefront of prostate cancer radiotherapy-based trials. Several retrospective analyses have shown an improvement in freedom from biochemical failure (bNED), primarily in patients with intermediate-to-high risk features (Hanks et al. 1998; Lyons et al. 2000; Pollack, Smith, and von Eschenbach 2000). A prospective sequential dose escalation trial has been reported in a number of articles by the Memorial Sloan-Kettering group (Zelefsky et al. 1998, 2001, 2002). They have shown a significant gain in bNED over the years of the study, as dose was increased. The problem with the retrospective and sequential dose escalation analyses is that stage migration (Amling et al. 1998; Hankey et al. 1999; Jhaveri et al. 1999; Ung et al. 2002) and a shift in Gleason scoring (Schellhammer et al. 2000, 2002; Chism et al. 2002; Smith et al. 2002) have occurred during the time of these studies, that could influence bNED. Kupelian and colleagues (2002), as well as our own analyses (Pollack et al. 2002a, b), have demonstrated that year of treatment is a significant determinant of outcome in patients treated with radiotherapy for prostate cancer.

There is some radiobiological evidence for a lower than expected $\alpha/\beta$ ratio for prostate cancer. Fowler et al. (2002) and Brenner et al. (2002) have shown that $\alpha/\beta$ ratio may be as low as 1.5 to 3.0, which is similar to that of normal tissues. IMRT may offer a mechanism for the safe exploitation of hypofractionation for prostate cancer without harming neighboring normal tissue and lowering the overall cost of radiation therapy.

There are two randomized dose escalation trials that have reached maturity. Shipley et al. (1995) in a pre-PSA (prostate-specific antigen) trial of locally advanced patients found an improvement in local control for patients with Gleason 8-10 disease when dose was increased from 67.2 to 75.6 Gy with protons. In a more contemporary cohort, Pollack et al. (2002a) described a gain in bNED using a conformal boost technique when the isocenter dose was increased from 70 Gy to 78 Gy. This gain was most pronounced for intermediate to high-risk patients with a pretreatment PSA of >10 ng/ml (figure 1).

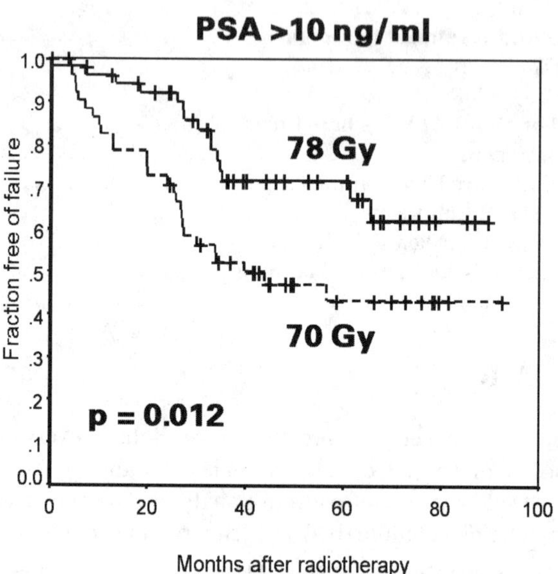


**Figure 1.** Kaplan-Meier freedom from biochemical failure curves for patients in the M.D. Anderson prostate cancer dose escalation trial who had a pretreatment PSA >10 ng/ml. The patients were randomized to treatment with 70 versus 78 Gy. [Reprinted from *International Journal of Radiation Oncology Biology Physics*, vol 53, A. Pollack, G. K. Zagars, G. Starkschall, J. A. Antolak, J. J. Lee, E. Huang, A. C. von Eschenbach, D. A. Kuban, and I. Rosen. "Prostate cancer radiation dose response: Results of the MD Anderson phase III randomized trial," pp. 1097–1105. © 2002, with permission from Elsevier.]

A number of studies have documented a dose-volume relationship for rectal complications, while that for bladder reactions is not well described. Grade 2 or higher rectal toxicity in the proton boost trial was 13% (Gardner et al. 2002). An appositional perineal field was used for the proton boost and a strong dose-volume histogram (DVH) relationship for the anterior rectal wall was identified (table 1). A significant increase in 5-year grade 2 or higher rectal complications was also found in the M.D. Anderson randomized trial (Pollack et al. 2002a). Figure 2 shows that the freedom from a grade 2 or higher rectal reaction was 26% in those who received 78 Gy, versus 12% for those who received 70 Gy. As depicted in table 1 (Pollack 2002), as dose is increased there is an increased risk of late rectal reactions. Table 2 (Pollack 2002) shows that as the volume of the rectum that receives a specified dose is increased, rectal toxicity is increased, similar to the pattern identified in the M.D. Anderson series (figure 2). The rectal outline method varied in the reports described, so it is important when adopting DVH constraints for planning that attention be paid to outlining features.

**Table 1.** Prostate Cancer Radiotherapy Dose and ≥ Grade 2 Rectal Reactions

| Author | Year | Dose | GI Toxicity (%) |
|---|---|---|---|
| Smit | 1990 | ≤70 Gy | 22 (2 yr Act) |
| | | >70–75 Gy | 20 |
| | | >75 Gy | 60 |
| Shipley | 1995 | 67.2 Gy | 12 (10 yr Act) |
| | | 75.6 CGE | 32 |
| Lee | 1996 | <72 Gy | 7 (18 mo Act) |
| | | 72–76 Gy | 16 |
| | | >76 Gy | 23 |
| Zelefsky | 1998 | ≤70.2 Gy | 6 (5 yr Act) |
| | | >75.6 Gy | 17 |
| Pollack | 2001 | 70 Gy | 12 (5 yr Act) |
| | | 78 Gy | 26 |

[Modified from Pollack, A. (2002), *Moss's Radiation Oncology: Rationale, Technique, and Results*, J. J. Cox and K. K. Ang (eds.). © 2002, Reprinted with permission from Mosby.]

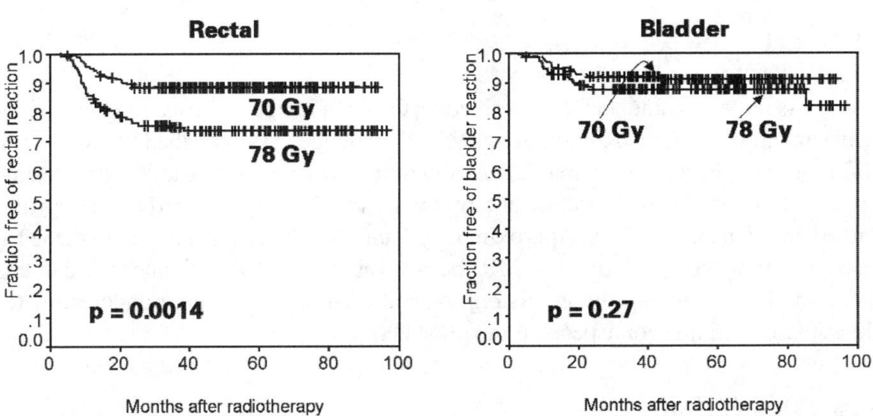


**Figure 2.** Kaplan-Meier curves for freedom from grade 2 or higher rectal toxicity (left) and bladder toxicity (right), as stratified by radiation dose administered in the M.D. Anderson Cancer Center Randomized trial. [Reprinted from *International Journal of Radiation Oncology Biology Physics*, vol 53, A. Pollack, G. K. Zagars, G. Starkschall, J. A. Antolak, J. J. Lee, E. Huang, A. C. von Eschenbach, D. A. Kuban, and I. Rosen. "Prostate cancer radiation dose response: Results of the MD Anderson phase III randomized trial," pp. 1097–1105. © 2002, with permission from Elsevier.]

**Table 2.** Prostate Cancer Radiotherapy: Rectal Volume Irradiated and ≥ Grade 2 Reactions

| Author | Year | Dose | Rectal Vol | GI Toxicity (%) |
|---|---|---|---|---|
| Benk | 1993 | 75 CGE | <40%ARW | 19 (40 mo Act)† |
| | | 75 CGE | ≥40%ARW | 71 |
| Lee | 1996 | 74–76 Gy | Rect Block | 10 (18 mo Act) |
| | | 74–76 Gy | No Block | 19 |
| Dearnaley | 1999 | 64 Gy | 3DCRT | 8 (5 yr Act) |
| | | 64 Gy | Conven-RT | 18 |
| Biersma | 1998 | 70 Gy | ≤30% | 0 (Crude)* |
| | | 70 Gy | >30% | 9 |
| Pollack | 2002 | 70 Gy | ≤25% | 16 (6 yr Act) |
| | | 70 Gy | >25% | 46 |

† Any rectal bleeding *Severe rectal bleeding ARW= anterior rectal wall
[Modified from Pollack, A. (2002), *Moss's Radiation Oncology: Rationale, Technique, and Results*, J. J. Cox and K. K. Ang (eds.). © 2002, Reprinted with permission from Mosby.]

The data from the M.D. Anderson randomized trial (Pollack et al. 2002a), combined with a more complete analysis by Huang et al. (2002a,b) that included clinical risk factors for rectal toxicity after radiation therapy (RT), resulted in the derivation of strict dose-volume constraints on the rectum (described below). Using intensity-modulated radiation therapy (IMRT) the rectal constraints have been met with more consistency than with conventional conformal radiotherapy (Dong et al. 2001).

## GTV/CTV Target Volumes

The gross target volume (GTV) is defined on CT-scan images or fused magnetic resonance imaging/computed tomography (MRI/CT) images. As described below, we use MRI routinely because of better delineation of the prostate base-bladder and prostate apex-rectum interfaces. The clinical target volume (CTV) is assumed to be approximately the same as the GTV. Approximately 6 mm (two slices) are added to the GTV at the prostatic apex as defined on MRI because about one-third of cancers are in this location, there is no capsule in this region, and CT-image averaging underestimates the superior and inferior aspects of the prostate.

## Prostate Motion

In the not too distant past, large volumes were used to treat the prostate and seminal vesicles, and for locally advanced disease the pelvic nodes were included for the first 45 to 50 Gy. Treatment volumes have been substantially reduced without full knowledge of the consequences. Even though prostate motion considerations have been largely ignored, the results have been encouraging. The question is whether outcome may be further improved by accounting for setup and target motion uncertainties.

Typical planning target volume (PTV) margins applied to the CTV in the treatment of prostate cancer with three-dimensional conformal radiation therapy (3DCRT) or IMRT are 1.0 cm in all dimensions, except posteriorly where the margin is 0.5 cm. These rather tight margins are necessary to minimize the rectal volume receiving high doses when the minimum PTV dose prescription is 75 Gy or above. Without consideration of the uncertainties in patient setup and interfraction prostate motion, such a posterior margin would result in a geometric miss in a significant proportion of treatments, especially since the disease often presents in the posterior aspect of the prostate capsule. Antolak et al. (1998) calculated, in a serial CT-scan study, that the PTV would have to be 1.1 cm in the anterior-posterior (AP) dimension in order to cover the CTV 95% of the time. More recently, Chandra and colleagues (Chandra et al. 2001) used BAT® (B-Mode acquisition and targeting system) ultrasound imaging (NOMOS Corporation, Cranberry Township, PA) on 147 patients that were undergoing IMRT for prostate cancer to measure the extent of the shifts implemented to center the prostate in the PTV. There were over 3500 interfraction shifts measured. The mean displacement of the BAT shift measurements was close to zero (0.5 mm in the AP dimension), indicating a near Gaussian distribution. In the AP dimension 25% to 30% of the shifts were over 5 mm, confirming that some form of adjustment for interfraction prostate motion is necessary.

Other methods for correcting interfraction prostate motion include the use of fiducial markers implanted in the prostate and daily electronic portal imaging (Litzenberg et al. 2002), and daily guidance such as CT-scanner in the linear accelerator treatment room (Hua et al. 2003), and cone beam CT-scanning (Jaffray et al. 2002), which will be available commercially in 1 to 2 years. Pretreatment CT-scan imaging has been used to adapt the PTV margin and hence dose (the smaller the margin permissible, the higher the PTV dose) (Martinez et al. 2001). CT-scan measurements performed at Memorial Sloan-Kettering Cancer Center (Hua et al. 2003) prior to treatment have documented that the PTV would be compromised over 25% of the time using standard bony landmark criteria without adjusting for prostate motion, which is remarkably similar to the conclusions based on BAT ultrasound studies (Chandra et al. 2001). Another approach is to immobilize the prostate with a rectal balloon (Teh et al. 2001). The ideal method may be to use a rectal balloon combined with pretreatment imaging, particularly if higher than conventional fractional doses are given.

Adjustments for interfraction motion are relatively straightforward compared to intrafraction motion. With IMRT treatments for prostate cancer approaching 20 to 25 minutes with imaging prior to treatment it is possible that rectal and/or bladder filling may change over this time period. Cine MRI studies (Padhani et al. 1999; Mah et al. 2002) have documented prostate positional changes over this time period, but in the majority the changes have been within a few millimeters and would not violate the PTV. Prostate intrafraction motion has also been measured by aligning the prostate to the planned CTV before treatment using the BAT system and repeating a BAT alignment after treatment (Huang et al. 2002b). An analysis of the recorded post-treatment BAT shifts revealed that only 1% required a readjustment after treatment of >5 mm in the AP dimension. Intrafraction motion has also been approximated by tracking fiducials in real time (Kitamura et al. 2002); these investigators found that patients treated supine had little intrafraction motion, while in those positioned prone intrafraction motion was considerable. It appears that intrafraction motion within a 20-minute time frame is relatively insignificant in the supine position as compared to interfraction motion.

Besides the facilitation of interfraction prostate alignment from imaging daily before treatment, imaging the prostate daily during RT allows one to monitor prostate size for patients receiving androgen deprivation (AD) and bladder filling. We have not quantified the extent of shrinkage during RT, but in some cases there appears to be a smaller prostate volume not completely filling the pretreatment CTV outline on the BAT ultrasound system. There also may be a discrepancy in the size of the prostate between ultrasound (smaller) versus CT. In these cases it is wise to set the posterior border at the prostate-rectal interface to avoid excessive rectum in the treatment field. The ability to visualize bladder volume daily on BAT ultrasound images is helpful in monitoring whether the desired amount of bladder filling is being achieved. In patients with significant urinary symptoms it is possible to differentiate between urinary retention and irritative effects that result in frequency and an empty bladder. Ultrasound imaging is very useful in selecting which patients should undergo post-void residual quantification and possible catheter placement.

## Risk Groups And Treatment Paradigms

### Favorable Risk

Nearly everyone agrees that favorable risk patients are those with a pretreatment PSA $\leq 10$ ng/ml, Gleason score of $\leq 6$, and $\leq$T2a disease (AJCC 2002 staging system). Recent data also suggest that if >50% of pretreatment biopsy cores are involved with cancer, such patients are better defined as intermediate risk (D'Amico et al. 2001). The CTV in favorable risk cases is considered to be nearly the same as the GTV, and mainly is comprised of the prostate as visualized on CT-scan and/or MRI. As depicted in figure 3, there is often a divot in the outline of the prostate where the seminal vesicles insert. On the couple of transverse images where the seminal vesicles insert, it is very difficult to know where the prostate ends and the seminal vesicles start. Therefore, we always include the most proximal 2 to 3 seminal vesicle cuts in the CTV and this area receives the full dose.

### Intermediate To High Risk

Intermediate risk includes any patient that is not classified as favorable or high risk. There are two main models that are used routinely in the clinic (D'Amico et al. 1998; Zelefsky et al. 1998; Pollack et al. 2003), although there are a host of other models. In the single factor high-risk model, either a PSA >20 ng/ml, Gleason score $\geq 8$ or T3 disease must be present. It should be noted that sometimes in the single factor high-risk model T2c disease is classified as high risk (D'Amico et al. 1998). In the two factor high-risk model, at least two of the following factors must be present: a PSA of >10 ng/ml, Gleason score of ≥7 or ≥T2b disease (Zelefsky et al. 1998).

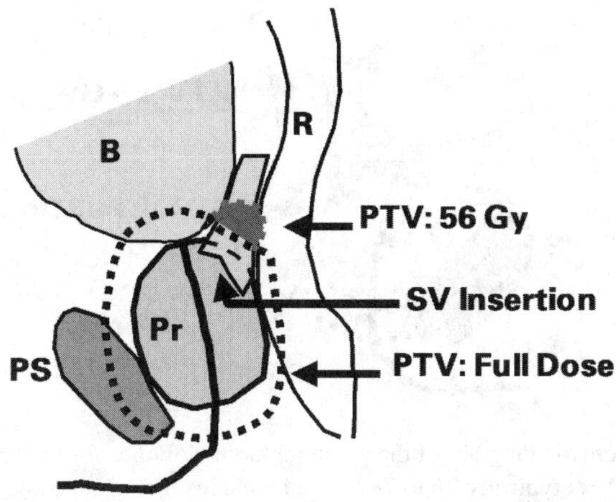


**Figure 3.** Schematic diagram of the insertion of the seminal vesicles (SVs) into the prostate and the planning target volumes for intermediate risk patients. There is uncertainty (poor definition combined with image averaging) in defining exactly what is prostate and what is SV. For these couple of 3 mm CT or MRI cuts, this region should be defined as prostate. This figure also shows how we include a second PTV for the proximal SVs in intermediate risk patients. The prescription for the second PTV is that the $D_{95}$ is 56 Gy (distributed over the total number of fractions of the treatment, e.g., 38 fractions for a primary PTV dose of 76 Gy).

The CTV for intermediate risk patients is essentially the same as that for low risk patients; however, at Fox Chase Cancer Center (FCCC) the proximal (<50%) seminal vesicles are treated to 56 Gy (figure 3). The CTV for high-risk patients includes the proximal seminal vesicles, covering approximately 50% or more (including all gross disease), which are treated to full dose and the distal seminal vesicles, which are treated to 56 Gy (figure 4). In addition, the periprostatic and periseminal vesicle lymph nodes are also treated to 56 Gy. With the results for Radiation Therapy Oncology Group (RTOG) protocol 94-13 (Roach, Lu, and Lawton 2001) there has been renewed interest in treating the whole pelvis to 45 Gy prior making a field reduction to the prostate and seminal vesicles. In this trial, the combination of neoadjuvant and concurrent androgen deprivation plus whole pelvic radiotherapy was superior to whole pelvic radiotherapy combined with adjuvant androgen deprivation (after RT) or prostate-only radiotherapy combined with either androgen deprivation sequencing regimen. Treatment of the pelvic lymph nodes with IMRT should reduce bowel and bladder toxicity (Nutting et al. 2000). In our experience, coverage of the external and internal iliac lymph nodes compromises the dose to the bladder and rectum, and will result in the need to reduce prostate dose or relax existing constraints. At the present time we are not treating these lymph node areas.

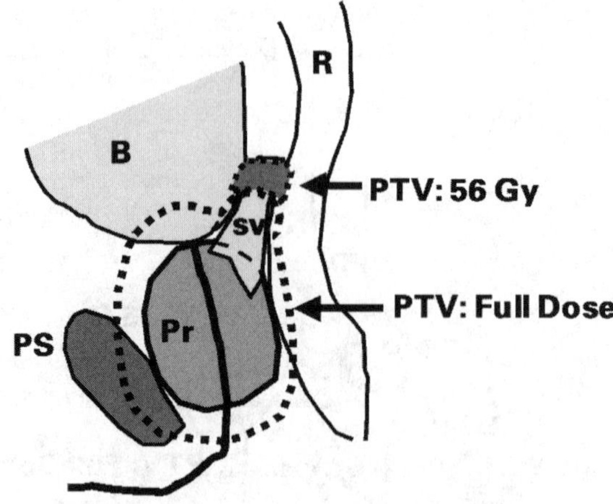


**Figure 4.** Schematic diagram of the planning target volumes for high risk patients. The primary PTV $D_{95}$ is typically 76 to 78 Gy and includes the prostate and proximal seminal vesicles. The secondary PTV $D_{95}$ is typically 56 Gy and includes the distal seminal vesicles.

## Simulation For IMRT At Fox Chase Cancer Center

Patients are simulated supine with a full bladder and an empty rectum, without a thermoplastic shell over the pelvis. An alpha cradle is used with a Plexiglas™ cradle for the feet. There appears to be less respiratory motion of the prostate in the supine position without a thermoplastic shell, as opposed to prone or supine with a thermoplastic shell (Malone et al. 2000a,b). The bladder should not be overly full at simulation because during treatment it is difficult for most patients to maintain a very distended bladder for the duration of treatment. An enema is administered prior to simulation to empty the rectum. As shown in figure 5, the filling status of the rectum will affect the calculation of the rectal constraint parameters. By performing CT-simulation with the rectum empty, the proportion of the rectum treated above the constraint threshold (e.g., 70 Gy) will be at the highest possible—a worst-case scenario. Since most patients have more frequent bowel movements, and consequently a reduced rectal volume after 2 weeks of radiotherapy (Antolak et al. 1998), this maneuver makes the simulation more representative of the extent of rectal filling during treatment.

MRI gives a much better image of the borders of the prostate at the base and the apex than CT-scan, and obviates the need for contrast (e.g., retrograde urethrogram). Indeed, the instillation of contrast in the bladder and rectum, or the use of retrograde urethrogram, may distort the anatomy (Malone et al. 2000b). A 0.23 Tesla MRI simulator (Philips Medical Systems, Bothell, WA) is used on a routine basis at FCCC to better define the prostate, and the images are then fused to the planning CT-scan. In the near future, routine CT-planning will be dropped and planning will be based entirely on MRI. The main problem with using MRI alone is the deformation at the edges of the field and this has been addressed.

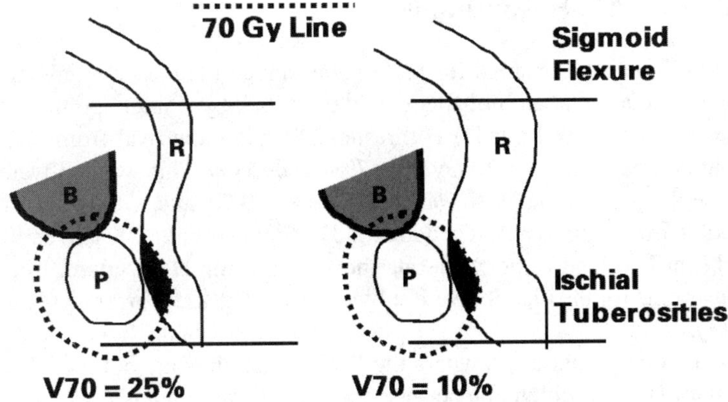


**Figure 5.** Schematic of the effect of the simulating and planning with an empty rectum (left) versus a full rectum (right). The V70 went from 25% (left) to 10% (right).

## Planning Constraints

The general planning approach that we use revolves around three sets of constraint parameters that are considered for plan approval. These are listed below.

### Absolute And Effective PTV Constraints

Perhaps the most important factor for plan acceptance is meeting the DVH constraints. PTV coverage is foremost. The absolute conditions used at FCCC include that 95% of the PTV and 100% of the CTV receive the prescription dose. The minimum dose to the PTV should be above 65 Gy (a small percentage, <1%, may fall below 65 Gy). The maximum dose to the PTV should not exceed 17% above the prescription dose. Newer software has reduced heterogeneity and adherence to the maximum dose constraint is much easier.

Our standard PTV margins on the CTV are 8 mm in all dimensions, except posteriorly at the rectum where a 5 mm margin is used. The effective PTV, which is defined here as the volume encompassed by the prescription line, is smaller or larger than the PTV desired. The effective PTV is influenced by three-dimensional changes in target shape. A typical range for the effective PTV margin on the CTV is 6 to 1.3 mm in all dimensions except posteriorly where the typical range is 3 to 7 mm. Attention is paid to these margins on a slice-by-slice basis. There may be a couple of CT-cuts (taken at a 3 mm spacing) in which the effective PTV margin on the CTV is less than the range desired; on these cuts attention is given to the location of the 90% line to ensure that CTV coverage is not significantly compromised.

## Normal Tissue DVH Constraints

The dose-volume relationships for rectal, and maybe bladder, complications are a continuous function and are not adequately described by a single point. As a consequence, we have reduced our DVH threshold for plan approval from ≤25% of the rectal volume treated to over 70 Gy to ≤17% over 65 Gy. This was motivated in part because the daily fractional dose was increased to 2.0 Gy and with IMRT this condition could be met regularly. A second rectal DVH constraint, ≤35% over 40 Gy, was rather arbitrarily added to better define the shape of the DVH curve. Likewise the DVH constraints for the bladder were subjectively set at ≤25% over 65 Gy and ≤50% over 40 Gy.

There are occasional cases where the DVH constraints are not met. The bladder in particular may be problematic because the patient was simulated when the bladder was not full. In these cases the patient is encouraged to have a full bladder during treatment and bladder filling is monitored with daily BAT ultrasound images. When the DVH criteria for the rectum are not met, it is often due to a short and/or very narrow rectum. In this setting a plan may be accepted if the DVH values are within 7% of the target limitations; this would bring the DVH maximums to ≤25% over 65 Gy and ≤42% over 40 Gy.

## Normal Tissue Dose Gradient Constraints

In plan evaluation the dose gradient across the surrounding normal tissues should be examined carefully. The goal is for abrupt fall-off to maximize normal tissue sparing. For prostate cancer the dose gradient across the rectum appears to be very important. Not only will a sharp gradient improve the DVH, but it may be an independent correlate of rectal complication risk. Skwarchuk et al. (2000) have shown that when the 50% line falls outside of the posterior aspect of the rectum, the complication risk is significantly elevated. Our criteria are similar. On examination of the isodose lines on a CT slice-by-slice basis, the 90% line should fall at less than half the width posteriorly and the 50% should fall at less than half the full width posteriorly.

## **Beam Arrangements And Inverse Planning**

At present, all prostate IMRT plans at this institution are generated using the CORVUS® inverse planning system (NOMOS Corporation, Cranberry Township, PA). Delivery is performed using the segmented multileaf collimation (SMLC) technique and Siemens Primus linear accelerators at 6, 10, and 18 MV. A precautionary age limit of ≥65 has been set for patients treated with 18 MV photons due to the increase in neutron production through photonuclear interactions. Even though inverse treatment planning is utilized, the entire process remains iterative. Aside from meeting the strict dose requirements for the target(s) as well as normal structures, plans are generated with delivery efficiency in mind.

Typically, six axial beam directions are used initially and increase to as many as nine with efforts to avoid parallel opposed beam arrangements. Efforts are also made to utilize avoidance techniques during the selection of beam directions minimizing the volume of critical structures being irradiated where possible. Additionally, the use of non-coplanar beam arrangements are often used in effort to meet the planning criteria (Price et al. 2002). We also define isocenter to coincide with fiducials and subsequent tattoos placed during the initial CT simulation process. Any subsequent shift is determined exclusively by daily localization (BAT ultrasound). All treatment plans utilize five intensity levels and result in an approximate range of 45 to 110 total segments and resulting treatment delivery times of approximately 10 to 25 minutes for 6 MV and 7 to 18 minutes for 10 and 18 MV. The initial input parameters are "templated" for ease of implementation and typically allow for only minor adjustments for each individual case. We have also improved the planning process through the addition of regions for dose constraint. By designating subsets of tissue as concentric regions around the target(s) and carefully defining each region's dose constraints, an increased measure of control over the dose gradient outside the target boundaries has been realized. This increased control manifests as two distinct endpoints that are beneficial to the IMRT process: increased dose conformity and decreased treatment time (Price, Murphy, and McNeeley 2003).

# References


Amling, C. L., M. L. Blute, S. E. Lerner, E. J. Bergstralh, D. G. Bostwick, and H. Zincke. (1998). "Influence of prostate-specific antigen testing on the spectrum of patients with prostate cancer undergoing radical prostatectomy at a large referral practice." *Mayo Clin. Proc.* 73:401–406.

Antolak, J., I. Rosen, C. Childress, G. K. Zagars, and A. Pollack. (1998). "Prostate target volume variations during a course of radiotherapy." *Int. J. Radiat. Oncol. Biol. Phys.* 42:661–672.

Chandra, A., L. Dong, E. Huang, L. O'Neil, I. Rosen, and A. Pollack. (2001). "Evaluation of ultrasound-based daily prostate localization during IMRT for prostate cancer." *Int. J. Radiat. Oncol. Biol. Phys.* 51:167–167.

Chism, D. B., A. L. Hanlon, P. Troncoso et al. (2002). "Impact on outcome of the Gleason score shift." *Int. J. Radiat. Oncol. Biol. Phys.* 54:265–266.

D'Amico, A., R. Whittington and S. Malkowicz, D. Schultz, K. Blank, G. A. Broderick, J. E. Tomaszewski, A. A. Renshaw, I. Kaplan, C. J. Beard, and A. Wein. (1998). "Biochemical outcome after radical prostatectomy, external beam radiation therapy, or interstitial radiation therapy for clinically localized prostate cancer." *JAMA* 280:969–974.

D'Amico, A. V., D. Schultz, B. Silver, L. Henry, M. Hurwitz, I. Kaplan, C. J. Beard, and A. A. Renshaw. (2001). "The clinical utility of the percent of positive prostate biopsies in predicting biochemical outcome following external-beam radiation therapy for patients with clinically localized prostate cancer." *Int. J. Radiat. Oncol. Biol. Phys.* 49:679–684.

Dong, L., J. C. O'Daniel, L. G. Smith, S. Bounds, I. Rosen, and A. Pollack. (2001). "Comparison of 3D conformal and intensity-modulated radiation therapy for early-stage prostate cancer." *Int. J. Radiat. Oncol. Biol. Phys.* 51:320–320.

Gardner, B. G., A. L. Zietman, W. U. Shipley, U. E. Skowronski, and P. McManus. (2002). "Late normal tissue sequelae in the second decade after high dose radiation therapy with combined photons and conformal protons for locally advanced prostate cancer." *J. Urol.* 167:123–126.

Hankey, B. F., E. J. Feuer, L. X. Clegg, R. B. Hayes, J. M. Legler, P. C. Prorok, L. A. Ries, R. M. Merrill, and R. S. Kaplan. (1999). "Cancer surveillance series: Interpreting trends in prostate cancer—part I: Evidence of the effects of screening in recent prostate cancer incidence, mortality, and survival rates." *J. Natl. Cancer Inst.* 91:1017–1024.

Hanks, G. E., A. L. Hanlon, T. E. Schultheiss, W. H. Pinover, B. Movsas, B. E. Epstein, and M. A. Hunt. (1998). "Dose escalation with 3D conformal treatment: Five year outcomes, treatment optimization and future directions." *Int. J. Radiat. Oncol. Biol. Phys.* 41:501–510.

Hua, C., M. Lovelock, G. S. Mageras, M. S. Katz, J. Mechalakos, E. P. Lief, T. Hollister, W. R. Lutz, M. J. Zelefsky, and C. C. Ling. (2003). "Development of a semi-automatic alignment tool for accelerated localization of the prostate." *Int. J. Radiat. Oncol. Biol. Phys.* 55: 811–824.

Huang, E., L. Dong, A. Chandra, D. A. Kuban, I. Rosen, A. Evans, and A. Pollack. (2002a). "Intrafraction prostate motion during IMRT for prostate cancer." *Int. J. Radiat. Oncol. Biol. Phys.* 53:261–268.

Huang, E. H., A. Pollack, L. Levy, G. Starkschall, L. Dong, I. Rosen, and D. A. Kuban. (2002b). "Late rectal toxicity: Dose-volume effects of conformal radiotherapy for prostate cancer." *Int. J. Radiat. Oncol. Biol. Phys.* 54:1314–1321.

Jaffray, D. A., J. H. Siewerdsen, J. W. Wong, and A. A. Martinez. (2002). "Flat-panel cone-beam computed tomography for image-guided radiation therapy." *Int. J. Radiat. Oncol. Biol. Phys.* 53:1337–1349.

Jhaveri, F. M., E. A. Klein, P. A. Kupelian, C. Zippe, and H. S. Levin. (1999). "Declining rates of extracapsular extension after radical prostatectomy: Evidence for continued stage migration." *J. Clin. Oncol.* 17:3167–72.

Kitamura, K., H. Shirato, Y. Seppenwoolde, R. Onimaru, M. oda, K. Fujita, S. Shimizu, N. Shinohara, T. Harabayashi, and K. Miyasaka. (2002). "Three-dimensional intrafractional movement of prostate measured during real-time tumor-tracking radiotherapy in supine and prone treatment positions." *Int. J. Radiat. Oncol. Biol. Phys.* 53:1117–1123.

Kupelian, P. A., J. C. Buchsbaum, C. Patel, M. elshaikh, C. A. Reddy, C. Zippe, and E. A. Klein. (2002). "Impact of biochemical failure on overall survival after radiation therapy for localized prostate cancer in the PSA era." *Int. J. Radiat. Oncol. Biol. Phys.* 52:704–711.

Litzenberg, D., L. A. Dawson, H. Sandler, M. G. Sanda, D. L. McShan, R. K. Ten Haken, K. L. Lam, K. K. Brock, and J. M. Balter. (2002). "Daily prostate targeting using implanted radiopaque markers." *Int. J. Radiat. Oncol. Biol. Phys.* 52:699–703.

Lyons, J. A., P. A. Kupelian, D. S. Mohan, C. A. Reddy, E. A. Klein. (2000). "Importance of high radiation doses (72 Gy or greater) in the treatment of stage T1-T3 adenocarcinoma of the prostate." *Urol.* 55:85–90.

Mah, D., G. Freedman, B. Milestone, A. Hanlon, E. Palacio, T. Richardson, B. Movsas, R. Mitra, E. Horwitz, and G. E. Hanks. (2002). "Measurement of intrafractional prostate motion using magnetic resonance imaging." *Int. J. Radiat. Oncol. Biol. Phys.* 54:568–575.

Malone, S., J. M. Crook, W. S. Kendal, and J. Szanto. (2000a). "Respiratory-induced prostate motion: quantification and characterization." *Int. J. Radiat. Oncol. Biol. Phys.* 48:105–109.

Malone, S., R. Donker, M. Broader, S. Dahrouge, J. Szanto, L. Gerig, G. Bociek, and J. Crook. (2000b). "Effects of urethrography on prostate position: Considerations for radiotherapy treatment planning of prostate carcinoma." *Int. J. Radiat. Oncol. Biol. Phys.* 46:89–93.

Martinez, A. A., D. Yan, D. Lockman, D. Brabbins, K. Kota, M. Sharpe, D. A. Jaffray, F. Vicini, and J. Wong. (2001). "Improvement in dose escalation using the process of adaptive radiotherapy combined with three-dimensional conformal or intensity-modulated beams for prostate cancer." *Int. J. Radiat. Oncol. Biol. Phys.* 50:1226–1234.

Nutting, C. M., D. J. Convery, V. P. Cosgrove, C. Rowbottom, A. R. Padhani, S. Webb, and D. P. Dearnaley. (2000). "Reduction of small and large bowel irradiation using an optimized intensity-modulated pelvic radiotherapy technique in patients with prostate cancer." *Int. J. Radiat. Oncol. Biol. Phys.* 48:649–656.

Padhani, A. R., V. S. Khoo, J. Suckling, J. E. Husband, M. O. Leach, and D. P. Dearnaley. (1999). "Evaluating the effect of rectal distension and rectal movement on prostate gland position using cine MRI." *Int. J. Radiat. Oncol. Biol. Phys.* 44:525–533.

Pollack, A. "The Prostate" in *Moss' Radiation Oncology, 8th Edition: Rationale, Technique, Results.* J. Cox and K. Ang (eds.). St. Louis, MO: Mosby, pp. 629–680, 2002.

Pollack, A., L. Smith, and A. von Eschenbach. (2000). "External beam radiotherapy dose-response characteristics of 1127 men with prostate cancer treated in the PSA era." *Int. J. Radiat. Oncol. Biol. Phys.* 48:507–512.

Pollack, A., G. K. Zagars, G. Starkschall, J. A. Antolak, J. J. Lee, E. Huang, A. C. von Eschenbach, D. A. Kuban, and I. Rosen. (2002a). "Prostate cancer radiation dose response: Results of the MD Anderson phase III randomized trial." *Int. J. Radiat. Oncol. Biol. Phys.* 53:1097–1105.

Pollack, A., A. L. Hanlon, B. Movsas et al. (2002b). "Correlates of distant metastasis and death in prostate cancer patients treated with radiotherapy." *Int. J. Radiat. Oncol. Biol. Phys.* 54:11–12.

Pollack, A., E. Horwitz, B. Movsas, et al. (2003). "Mindless or mindful? Radiation oncologists' perspective on the evolution of prostate cancer." *Urol. Clin. North Am.* In press.

Price, R., S. Murphy, and S. W. McNeeley (2003). "A method for increased dose conformity and segment reduction for SMLC delivered IMRT treatment of the prostate." *Int. J. Radiat. Oncol. Biol. Phys.* Submitted.

Price, R., G. E. Hanks, S. W. McNeeley, E. M. Horwitz, and W. H. Pinover. (2002). "Advantages of using noncoplanar vs. axial beam arrangements when treating prostate cancer with intensity-modulated radiation therapy and the step-and-shoot delivery method." *Int. J. Radiat. Oncol. Biol. Phys.* 53:236–243.

Roach III, M., J. Lu, and C. Lawton (2001). "A phase III trial comparing whole pelvis (WP) to prostate only (PO) radiotherapy and neoadjuvant to adjuvant total of androgen suppression (TAS): Preliminary analysis of RTOG 9413." *Int. J. Radiat. Oncol. Biol. Phys.* 51:3–3.

Schellhammer, P. F. (2002). "Re: Trends in Gleason score for prostate cancer diagnosed between 1983 and 1993." *J. Urol.* 168:2555–2556.

Schellhammer, P. F., R. Moriarty, D. Bostwick, and D. Kuban. (2000). "Fifteen-year minimum follow-up of a prostate brachytherapy series: comparing the past with the present." *Urol.* 56:436–439.

Shipley, W. U., L. J. Verhey, J. E. Munzenrider, H. D. Suit, M. M. Urie, P. L. McManus, R. H. Young, J. W. Shipley, A. L. Zietman, P. J. Riggs et al. (1995). "Advanced prostate cancer: The results of a randomized comparative trial of high dose irradiation boosting with conformal protons compared with conventional dose irradiation using photons alone." *Int. J. Radiat. Oncol. Biol. Phys.* 32:3–12.

Skwarchuk, M. W., A. Jackson, M. J. Zelefsky, E.S. Venkatraman, D. M. Cowen, S. levegrun, C. M. Burman, Z. Fuks, S. A. Leibel, and C. C. Ling. (2000). "Late rectal toxicity after conformal radiotherapy of prostate cancer (I): multivariate analysis and dose-response." *Int. J. Radiat. Oncol. Biol. Phys.* 47:103–113.

Smith, E. B., H. F. Frierson, Jr., S. E. Mills, J. C. Boyd, and D. Theodorescu. (2002). "Gleason scores of prostate biopsy and radical prostatectomy specimens over the past 10 years: Is there evidence for systematic upgrading?" *Cancer* 94:2282–2287.

Teh, B. S., W. Y. Mai, B. M. Uhl, M. E. Augspurger, W. H. Grant 3rd, H. H. Lu, S. Y. Woo, L. S. Carpenter, J. K. Chiu, and E. B. Butler. (2001). "Intensity-modulated radiation therapy (IMRT) for prostate cancer with the use of a rectal balloon for prostate immobilization: Acute toxicity and dose-volume analysis." *Int. J. Radiat. Oncol. Biol. Phys.* 49:705–712.

Ung, J. O., J. P. Richie, M. H. Chen, A. A. Renshaw, and A. V. D'Amico. (2002). "Evolution of the presentation and pathologic and biochemical outcomes after radical prostatectomy for patients with clinically localized prostate cancer diagnosed during the PSA era." *Urol.* 60:458–463.

Zelefsky, M., S. Leibel, P. Gaudin, G. J. Kutcher, N. E. Fleshner, E. S. Venkatraman, V. E. Reuter, W. R. Fair, C. C. Ling, and Z. Fuks. (1998). "Dose escalation with three-dimensional conformal radiation therapy affects the outcome in prostate cancer." *Int. J. Radiat. Oncol. Biol. Phys.* 41:491–500.

Zelefsky, M. J., Z. Fuks, M. Hunt, H. J. Lee, D. Lombardi, C. C. Ling, V. E. Reuter, E. S. Venkatraman, and S. A. Leibel. (2001). "High dose radiation delivered by intensity modulated conformal radiotherapy improves the outcome of localized prostate cancer." *J. Urol.* 166(3):876–881.

Zelefsky, M., Z. Fuks, M. Hunt, Y. Yamada, C. Marion, C. Ling, H. Amols, E. S. Venkatramen, and S. A. Leibel. (2002). "High-dose intensity modulated radiation therapy for prostate cancer: Early toxicity and biochemical outcome in 772 patients." *Int. J. Radiat. Oncol. Biol. Phys.* 53(5):1111–1116.

# Intensity-Modulated Radiation Therapy For Head And Neck Cancer

**K. S. Clifford Chao, M.D.[1] and Angel I. Blanco, M.D.[2]**
[1]Department of Radiation Oncology, The University of Texas,
M.D. Anderson Cancer Center, Houston, Texas
[2]Department of Radiation Oncology, Washington University
St. Louis, Missouri



## Introduction

Malignant tumors of the head and neck (H&N) are amenable to conformal radiotherapy for multiple reasons. Physical examination and radiographic evaluation with modern tools such as computed tomography (CT), magnetic resonance imaging (MRI), and, in some instances, fluorine-18 fluorodeoxyglucose positron emission tomography (FDG-PET) (Teknos et al. 2001; Kresnik et al. 2001) permit precise delineation of the primary tumor and involved lymph nodes. Critical structures lie in close anatomic proximity to regions at risk for primary tumor spread and lymphatic metastasis (Martinez-Monge et al. 1999). Intensity-modulated radiation therapy (IMRT) offers several theoretical advantages compared with standard three-dimensional conformal radiotherapy (3DCRT) (Low 2003). With IMRT, the fluence intensity at the target edges can be enhanced to partly compensate for the beam penumbra; with 3DCRT, the portal boundary must be extended beyond the target volume to increase the dose near the target periphery. Further, the 3DCRT dose distributions are generally convex, since all beams contribute to the prescription dose at the center (isocenter) of the radiation fields. IMRT dose distributions, in contrast, can have concave configurations (assuming a sufficient number of beams are used), allowing greater conformation than with 3DCRT. IMRT usually permits better avoidance of organs at risk (OARs). The dose gradients may potentially improve the therapeutic ratio by delivering tumoricidal doses to the target volumes while limiting radiation damage to critical structures (Brahme 2000).

Typical 3DCRT courses involve treatments to multiple target volumes delivered sequentially, each with different prescription doses. The dose per fraction is often the same for all subplans. The tolerance dose is often reached using a relatively high dose per fraction and subsequently a very low dose per fraction (scatter dose). Due to limitations of early commercial IMRT treatment planning systems, a single set of beams was initially used for treatment delivery (Zelefsky et al. 2001). Unique doses per fraction were prescribed to multiple target volumes to achieve different total doses in each target. The radiobiological consequences of the resulting range in fraction size required changes to the total target prescription doses relative to the classic, sequential dose prescriptions. This approach was implemented at Washington University (see table 1).

**Table 1.** IMRT Clinical Target Volume (CTV) and Normal Tissue Dose Specification with Biological Equivalent Dose (BED) Correction for Head and Neck Cancer— Washington University Guideline

| Target Volume | Conventional Technique | IMRT | | |
|---|---|---|---|---|
| | | Definitive (35 fractions) | High-risk Postoperative (33 fractions) | Intermediate-risk Postoperative (30 fractions) |
| CTV1 | 66-70 / 2 Gy | 70 / 2 Gy | 66 / 2 Gy | 60 / 2 Gy |
| CTV2 | 50-54 / 2 Gy | 56 / 1.66 Gy | 54 / 1.64 Gy | 52 / 1.73 Gy |

Normal Tissue Tolerance for IMRT prescription: Optic nerve and optic chiasm 55 Gy, Retina 45 Gy, Brain stem 50–55 Gy, Spinal cord 45–48 Gy, Parotid gland 20–30 Gy, Mandible 70 Gy

Adequate immobilization, an important factor influencing setup accuracy for the planning target volume (PTV) (ICRU 50, 1993), is achievable in the clinical setting in a cost-effective manner using thermoplastic masks, as demonstrated by Gilbeau et al. (2001) in an analysis of 915 portal images in 30 patients with brain or H&N tumors assigned to one of three different thermoplastic masks. For the whole population, total displacements reached a standard deviation (SD) of 0.22 cm at the level of the H&N.

IMRT is typically delivered using any of four approaches, including two that use conventional multi-leaf collimators (MLCs), called segmental MLC (SMLC) and dynamic MLC (DMLC), one that uses a dedicated IMRT MLC (tomotherapy), and physical modulators (compensators). The principal differentiation of SMLC and DMLC is that the leaves do not move while the linear accelerator beam is on in the former, while the leaves move during irradiation in the dynamic mode. Tomotherapy is a form of dynamic IMRT that uses a narrow multileaf collimator while the linear accelerator is rotated during beam-on. Finally, custom-designed physical modulators can also generate the complex, non-uniform fluence distributions characteristic of IMRT plans.

IMRT aims to improve the dose conformity through computerized, iterative treatment plan optimization and the use of intensity-modulated radiation beams (Hsiung et al. 2002). IMRT plan optimization, also described as inverse planning, may be defined as the process by which the intensity distribution of each beam employed in a plan is determined such that the resultant dose distribution can best meet the criteria specified by the planner (Chui and Spirou 2001). In the treatment of certain H&N tumors, IMRT confers a dosimetric advantage compared with traditional 3DCRT. Hsiung and colleagues compared IMRT versus 3DCRT for boost or salvage treatment in a series of 14 patients with nasopharyngeal carcinoma (NPC); 13 patients received an initial 45 Gy delivered via 2 bilateral portals covering the nasopharynx and upper neck and an anterior-posterior (AP) portal covering the lower neck. The neck lymphatics were boosted to 60 Gy using electron beams. Subsequently, a conformal boost was delivered to 25 Gy using 3DCRT. Five- and seven-portal IMRT plans were generated for each patient. Comparison of treatment plans revealed improved target dose homogeneity for the IMRT plans versus 3DCRT. The brainstem, spinal cord, and orbits received lower doses with IMRT. Overall, the study demonstrated superior results for 5-and 7-field IMRT plans compared with 5-field 3DCRT, as assessed by dose-volume histogram (DVH) (Drzymala et al. 1991).

The theoretical benefits of IMRT in the treatment of NPC were further established by Cheng, Chao, and Low (2001), who compared target volume coverage and normal tissue sparing of serial tomotherapy-based IMRT and fixed-field IMRT for NPC with those of conventional beam arrangements; 12 patients with NPC underwent CT simulation at Washington University. Conventional beam arrangements were designed following the guidelines of Intergroup NPC Study 0099 (Chao et al. 2001a). Similar dosimetric criteria were used to assess the target volume coverage capability of IMRT. Serial tomotherapy achieved equivalent target volume coverage as conventional techniques, while coverage for static-field IMRT was inferior. However, gross target volume (GTV) (LN) coverage at 70 Gy was significantly better with both IMRT techniques. Clinical target volume (CTV) coverage at 60 Gy was also significantly better with the IMRT techniques. The fixed-field IMRT technique exhibited the best parotid-sparing despite less desirable target coverage. The pituitary gland, mandible, spinal cord, and brain stem were also better spared by both IMRT techniques.

Xia and colleagues (Xia et al. 2000) also corroborated the dosimetric advantages of IMRT over 3DCRT in the treatment of NPC. A case of locally advanced NPC with intracranial extension was planned using two IMRT techniques. The IMRT plans achieved better sparing of normal critical structures. In addition, both IMRT plans delivered ≥95% of the prescription dose of 70 Gy to ≥95% of the GTV, while the 3DCRT plan delivered <89% of the prescribed dose to ≥95% of the GTV. The IMRT dose distributions conformed better to the target volumes compared with the 3DCRT plan while maintaining better sparing of critical structures.

IMRT technology confers dosimetric advantages over conventional therapy in other H&N tumor subsites. In an effort to preserve binocular vision and improve the dose distribution to the target volume, Claus and colleagues (Claus et al. 2001) have designed an IMRT protocol for the treatment of ethmoid sinus tumors. The study incorporated dose escalation, with initial tumor doses of 60 to 66 Gy and ultimate target prescription of 70 Gy in 2 Gy fractions. A class-solution approach for IMRT planning of ethmoid sinus cancer was proposed. Planning and dose delivery involved the use of an SMLC technique with seven beam incidences (20 to 37 segments). Longer followup is needed to assess the tumor control and late toxicities with this technique.

A dosimetric study by Bragg and colleagues (Bragg, Conway, and Robinson 2002) compared 3DCRT versus inverse-planning MLC-based IMRT in the treatment of parotid gland tumors in 10 IMRT beam arrangements calculated for nine patients. The target dose was comparable in the 3DCRT and IMRT plans, although improvements were seen when seven and nine IMRT fields were used. IMRT reduced the mean dose to the contralateral parotid gland and the maximum doses to the brain and the spinal cord, but increased the ipsilateral lens dose in some cases. A five-field setup was proposed as a class solution suitable for the majority of patients with parotid gland cancer.

## Tumor Control Of Head And Neck Cancer By IMRT

Quality assurance of IMRT plans is more complex than for traditional external beam therapy, necessitating additional physics support for successful implementation (Low et al. 1998). A study by Perez and colleagues (Perez, Kobeissi, and Chao 1999) estimated the average IMRT planning time at approximately 4 hours and the daily treatment time at 35 minutes, compared with 2 hours and 15 minutes for treatment planning and daily treatment time for conventional radiotherapy. There also exists some concern that IMRT treatment planning systems might achieve "too tight" dose distributions compromising tumor control with respect to conventional radiotherapy (Webb 2001); further, the technology is also complex and error-prone. A summary of the available IMRT data on tumor control is shown in table 2.

**Table 2.** Reported Outcomes of Select Published IMRT Series

| Author | N | Subsite | LC (%) | LRC (%) | OS (%) |
|---|---|---|---|---|---|
| Butler et al. (1999) | 20 | Multiple | N/A | 85* | N/A |
| Chao et al. (2003) | 126 | Multiple | N/A | 85 (2-y) | N/A |
| Dawson et al. (2000) | 58 | Multiple | N/A | 79 (2-y) 75 (5-y) | N/A |
| Lee et al. (2002) | 67 | NPC | 97 (4-y) | 98 (4-y) | 88 (4-y) |

Abbreviations: N = Number of patients, LC = Local control, LRC = Local-regional control, OS = Overall Survival, N/A = Not reported, NPC = Nasopharyngeal carcinoma

*Local-regional control includes 1 patient with persistent disease. Mean f/u in this series was 15.2months.

## Multiple Subsites

An initial publication by Chao and colleagues (Chao et al. 2000) demonstrated the feasibility of this approach in 17 H&N cancer patients. A system for determination and delineation of nodal target volumes and dose prescription which maximized the capabilities of the treatment planning system in use (PEACOCK®, NOMOS Corp., Cranberry Township, PA) was developed (Chao et al. 2002). The nomenclature defined CTV1 as the high dose target and encompassed the gross tumor and any clinically involved lymph nodes plus adjacent regions for definitive cases and the residual tumor, surrounding regions, surgical bed, and areas of extracapsular extension for postoperative cases. A second target, CTV2, was defined in selected definitive and postoperative cases and included prophylactically treated neck regions. Target doses were defined for high and intermediate risk categories defined according to institutional treatment guidelines. To minimize the possibility of underdosing the periparotid space, only the lateral lobe of each parotid was spared. The concept of biological equivalent dose (BED) (Dale 1985) was used to adjust daily target doses.

More recently, Chao and colleagues (Chao et al. 2003) examined the patterns of failure among 126 patients treated at Washington University with definitive (52 patients, 41%) or postoperative (74 patients, 59%) inverse-planning IMRT. Multiple H&N subsites were included. Thirty-five patients treated with definitive IMRT (67%) also received concurrent cisplatinum-based chemotherapy. IMRT was used in the upper neck to preserve salivary function; the lower neck was treated with a conventional AP portal abutted to the inferior IMRT dose distribution border. At a median follow-up of 26 months, 17 local-regional recurrences were identified. DVH analysis of those failures within the IMRT field revealed that the recurrent or persistent tumor volumes, defined as Vf, received comparable or superior dose coverage relative to the corresponding CTVs. To facilitate comparisons with the published literature, each Vf, was subclassified as "in-field," "marginal," or "out-field" using the University of Michigan definitions. For each recurrent patient, the radiographic image obtained at the time of failure was co-registered with the pre-RT CT dataset used in treatment planning. Among the failures, 9 (53%) were inside CTV1; 1 (6%) was marginal to CTV1 but included in CTV2; 1 failure (6%) occurred outside CTV1 but was included in CTV2; 1 failure (6%) was marginal to CTV2; 5 additional failures (30%) were found outside of the IMRT field and in the lower neck. The results showed the in-field failures are the most frequent.

A study by Dawson and colleagues (Dawson et al. 2000) examined the patterns of failure among 58 H&N cancer patients requiring bilateral neck irradiation treated at the University of Michigan in a parotid-sparing protocol. Multiple H&N tumor subsites were studied. Twenty-four patients (41%) were treated using a conformal technique; the remaining 34 (59%) received forward-planning segmental IMRT intended to provide adequate coverage of the primary target and lymph nodes at risk. No attempt was made to spare the parotid gland in the side of the neck containing the highest probability of metastasis. Strict criteria for target volume coverage required that the 95% isodose surface encompassed all planning target volumes (PTVs). Conventional fraction sizes, ranging from 1.8 to 2.0 Gy, were used. With a median follow-up of 27 months, 12 patients had developed a local-regional recurrence. For all recurrent patients, a recurrent tumor volume (Vrecur) was defined radiographically. Each recurrent tumor was classified as occurring locally or regionally, in the gross tumor, operative bed, or subclinical disease. Failures were characterized further as "in-field," "marginal," or "outside". Of 16 local and regional recurrences in 12 patients, 12 (75%) were in-field, 2 (13%) were marginal, and 2 (13%) were outside. The study demonstrated that in-field recurrences continue to be the predominant mode of failure following parotid-sparing conformal RT or static IMRT. This failure pattern is unchanged relative to that observed following classic two-dimensional radiotherapy (Piggott, Dische, and Saunders 1995).

## Fractionation Scheme

Extensive research efforts have been devoted to defining the optimal fractionation parameters for H&N tumors, especially after recognition of the strong correlation between overall treatment time and tumor control probability (Hansen et al. 1997). As demonstrated with altered fractionation schemes such as hyperfractionation (HF) (Parsons et al. 1988) and accelerated fractionation with concomitant boost (AF-C) (Ang and Peters 1992; Ang 1998; Ang et al. 2001; Horiot et al. 1992; Fu et al. 2000) among others, the local control of certain H&N cancers might improve with optimized fractionation schemes.

Mohan and colleagues (Mohan et al. 2000) examined IMRT fractionation strategies based on radiobiological considerations and defined the term "simultaneous integrated boost" (SIB) to describe IMRT treatments designed to synchronously deliver different dose levels to different tissues of the H&N region. The detailed pros and cons of various fractionation schemes will be discussed.

In general, an optimal fractionation scheme has not been conclusively defined for IMRT, and more clinical information is needed to address acute toxicities and late complications (i.e., soft tissue fibrosis, bone exposure, stricture of pharynx or esophagus).

## Oropharyngeal Carcinoma

Chao and colleagues (Chao et al. 2001b) evaluated 430 patients with oropharyngeal carcinoma treated at Washington University. Five patient groups were identified: Group I consisted of 153 patients who received preoperative chemoradiotherapy (CRT). Group II consisted of 142 patients treated with postoperative CRT. Group III consisted of 153 patients who received definitive CRT. Group IV was composed of 14 patients who received postoperative IMRT, and group V encompassed 12 patients treated definitively with IMRT. The results showed similar 2-year local-regional control among comparable groups (76% in group II vs. 100% in group IV, p = ns; and 68% in group III vs. 88% in group V, p = ns) (Ozyigit and Chao 2002). They also demonstrated that after IMRT treatment only 17% to 30% of the patients had late grade 2 xerostomia as compared with approximately 75% among those treated with CRT.

## Nasopharyngeal Carcinoma (NPC)

Definitive chemoradiotherapy has become the standard of care for advanced NPC in the United States following publication of Intergroup Study 0099 (IGS) (Al-Sarraf et al. 1998). Wolden and colleagues (Wolden et al. 2001) reported on 68 patients with NPC treated at Memorial Hospital using a 3D conformal boost technique to treat the tumor bed to a median dose of 70 Gy. The boost dose was prescribed to the isodose line that completely encompassed the PTV, resulting in a 13% higher mean dose compared to 2-D techniques for the same prescribed dose. Approximately one-half of patients (52%) received concurrent chemotherapy. With a median followup of 42 months, the actuarial local control at the primary site was 77%, the regional control in the neck was 97%, progression-free survival 56%, and overall survival 58%. All patients reported some degree of xerostomia. The overall incidence of late complications (Ang et al. 1990; Wang 1989) was thought comparable to that reported with 2-D techniques. In addition, the 5-year local control rate of 77% did not represent significant improvement over historical control rates with 2-D radiation (Hoppe, Goffinet, and Bagshaw 1976; Perez et al. 1992; Sanguineti 1997).

The Washington University experience with treatment of nasopharyngeal malignancies was recently presented (Chao et al. 2001a). The institutional results were compared with those of the Intergroup Study 0099 (IGS). One hundred and three patients were treated with conventional radiation therapy alone (MIR-RT). Twenty-two patients received conventional radiation with concomitant chemotherapy according to the IGS regimen. Among them, 13 patients were treated by conventional chemoradiotherapy (MIR-CRT), and 9 patients were treated with IMRT (MIR-CIMRT). The median followup was 4.9 years (range, 1–29 year). Results: Three-year progression-free survival for radiation therapy alone was 51% for MIR patients as compared with 24% in IGS ($p < 0.05$). Progression-free survival 3 years after chemoradiotherapy was 90% for MIR patients and 69% in IGS ($p < 0.05$). One year after radiation therapy, moderate to severe xerostomia (>RTOG grade 2) was significantly less in the IMRT patients.

The potential clinical benefit of the improved dose distributions for advanced NPC achievable using IMRT is best demonstrated in the large series from the University of California-San Francisco (Sultanen et al. 2000; Lee et al. 2002). Sixty-seven NPC patients were treated with IMRT using three different techniques. The gross tumor and positive lymph nodes were prescribed 65 to 70 Gy at 2.12 to 2.25 Gy per fraction. The CTV received 60 Gy at 1.8 Gy per fraction, and the prophylactically treated lymphatics 50 to 60 Gy at 1.8 to 2.0 Gy per fraction. In addition, 26 patients (39%) received an intracavitary high-dose rate (HDR) brachytherapy boost, given in 2 fractions 1 to 2 weeks after completion of external radiotherapy. The dose delivered was 5 to 7 Gy. Fifty patients (75%) received cisplatinum-based chemotherapy. The prescribed dose was chosen as the minimum dose that encompassed the target volume. Only 3% of the GTV and CTV volumes received <95% of the prescribed dose; rather, most voxels typically received more than 105% of prescription. The local and local-regional progression-free survival rates were considerably higher than reported with CRT techniques at 97% and 98%, respectively. Overall survival at 4 years was 88%. Only 1 patient failed in the upper neck. Toxicity was also acceptable with this regimen: The worst reported toxicity was Grade 1 in 20 patients (30%), Grade 2 in 15 (22%), Grade 3 in 7 (10%), and Grade 1 in 1 patient (1%). The authors also demonstrated the time-dependence of post-RT xerostomia. At 24 months post-RT, <10% of patients had RTOG grade 0-1 xerostomia.

## Head And Neck Lymphatics

Based on analysis of the patterns of nodal failure at a median follow-up of 26 months in 126 patients treated with IMRT at Washington University (Horiot et al. 1992, Chao and colleagues (Chao et al. 2002) developed guidelines for target volume determination and delineation of head and neck lymph nodes in patients receiving definitive or postoperative IMRT. Persistent or recurrent nodal disease was found in 6 of 52 (12%) patients receiving definitive IMRT; also, 7 of 74 (9%) patients receiving postoperative IMRT failed in the nodal region.

## Normal Tissue Protection

Among radiation therapy side effects, parotid gland damage is particularly significant since it typically produces xerostomia, leading to permanent alteration of speech and deglutition. In addition to being cited by head and neck cancer patients as a major cause of decreased quality of life (QOL) after irradiation, xerostomia also increases the risk of developing oral ulcers, fissures, dental cavities, infections, and secondary nutritional deficiencies (Beumer et al. 1979; Harrison et al. 1997). The early changes in salivary gland function during and following conventional radiotherapy indicate a rapid reduction in salivary flow rate (FR) ranging from 18% to 50% of the pretreatment FR one week after the initiation of radiotherapy (Leslie and Dische 1992; Shannon and Chauncey 1967; Dreizen et al. 1977; Shannon, Trodahl, and Starske 1978; Eneroth, Henriksson, and Jakobsson 1972; Mossman, Shatzman, and Chencharick 1981).

The potential for an improved therapeutic ratio with IMRT stems from the increased conformality of the resulting dose distributions, which provide an opportunity for increased sparing of normal tissues and, in particular, the salivary glands.

The University of Michigan experience with parotid-sparing 3-D conformal and IMRT was reported by Eisbruch et al. (1999) and included 88 patients. Normal tissue complication probability (NTCP) modeling revealed that parotid glands receiving a mean dose less than or equal to 24 Gy (unstimulated saliva) or 26 Gy (stimulated saliva) showed substantial functional sparing and recovery capacity. An update by Eisbruch and colleagues (Eisbruch et al. 2001) reviewed the functional outcomes among 132 patients; 84 (64%) received bilateral neck RT. Forty-eight patients (36%) of patients with well-lateralized tumors judged to be at low risk for contralateral lymphatic extension received unilateral neck RT. Contralateral parotid gland FRs declined in the initial post-RT period but rose thereafter in the bilateral group. FRs for bilateral patients declined initially after treatment but recovered and approached the pretreatment levels after 12 months. Contralateral parotid gland FRs were initially similar to pretreatment levels; during the second year post-RT, the flow rates increased and were significantly higher than pre-RT FRs (p = 0.006). Ipsilateral parotid glands received mean doses exceeding 30 Gy in both groups, and the corresponding FRs were very low. XQ analysis showed that, at 2 years, unilateral-irradiated patients had less discomfort than bilaterally treated patients. Among unilateral patients, the XQ scores rose initially post-RT but decreased close to baseline levels by 1 year. Scores in the bilateral group remained significantly higher than in the unilateral group at all measurement points. The mean dose to the oral cavity emerged as a significant predictor of the severity of xerostomia: Sparing of the uninvolved oral cavity in addition to the salivary glands should be an important objective in salivary-function sparing irradiation.

Chao and colleagues (Chao et al. 2001c; Deasy, Chao, and Markman 2001) reported the initial results of a prospective study of salivary function sparing in H&N cancer among 41 patients; 27 were treated with IMRT and 14 with forward-planning 3DCRT. Fourteen patients received concurrent chemotherapy. The patients underwent stimulated and unstimulated saliva collection and completed a five-question QOL questionnaire 1 week before RT and 6 months after completion of therapy. The relationship between salivary function and irradiated parotid dose and volume was investigated using two empirical models. The first, an "equivalent uniform dose" (EUD) model, assumes that each parotid gland contributes 50% of the post-RT FR. The resulting EUD parameter was nearly 1 (0.47), indicating that EUD is equivalent to mean dose. The second, "parallel-exponential" (PEX) model, assumes that each CT voxel corresponding to the parotid gland represents a parallel functional subunit and operates independently, with each voxel's saliva function decreasing exponentially as a function of quadratic polynomial in voxel dose. Results showed that mean parotid dose was lower in patients receiving IMRT versus 3DCRT. A correlation between mean parotid dose and the fractional reduction of stimulated saliva output at 6 months post-RT was observed. Both models examined (EUD and PEX) provided highly predictive fits, which shows the observed and (according to the EUD model) predicted FRs versus mean right and left parotid dose. The EUD model predicted that reduction in FRs will occur independently for each parotid gland at a exponential rate of 4% per Gy of mean parotid dose. Thus, xerostomia (<25% pre-RT FR) can be predicted for mean doses of 32 Gy or more, consistent with the findings reported by Eisbruch and colleagues (Eisbruch et al. 1999, 2001).

Ozygit and Chao (2002) have compared incidence of grade 2-3 acute skin toxicity and mucositis in oropharyngeal patients treated with postoperative CRT, definitive CRT, postoperative IMRT, and definitive IMRT. The side effect profiles appear comparable for the four studied groups.

## Conclusion

The emerging use of IMRT, either alone or in combination with cytotoxic chemotherapy or radioprotectors, will be discussed. By the strictest criteria, the data should be considered preliminary, as these results were not derived from prospective, randomized fashion. Two ongoing, prospective RTOG protocols within the RTOG aim to investigate the use of IMRT-based radiotherapy in a multi-institutional setting. The first, H-0022 (RTOG 2001), will assess the feasibility of adequate target coverage and major salivary gland sparing in patients with oropharyngeal cancer treated with IMRT techniques, determine the rate and pattern of locoregional tumor recurrence, and examine the nature and prevalence of acute and late side effects (using RTOG scales) and their relationship to local dose. The second protocol will study the feasibility and tumor control in nasopharyngeal cancer patients treated exclusively with IMRT. With obvious dosimetric advantages in target coverage and normal tissue sparing of IMRT over conventional techniques, a phase III randomized study to address whether IMRT is superior to CRT may not be conducted due to ethical concerns.

Despite this lack of prospective, randomized evidence, optimism remains based on the early IMRT results. Chao et al. (2001b) showed local tumor control of oropharyngeal lesions is at least equivalent to historical controls. In addition, the local-regional recurrence-free survival of 97% reported by Lee et al. (2002) surpasses that reported in any other large series. Further, this technology is amenable to substantial improvements with advance in inverse-planning and delivery methods, optimized fractionation schedules, better combinations of cytotoxic chemotherapy, radioprotectors and irradiation, and as functional imaging techniques permit a more precise delineation of microscopic tumor extensions (and thus clinical target volumes) and radioresistant hypoxic tumor sub-regions (Chao et al. 2001d).

## References

Al-Sarraf, M., M. LeBlanc, P. G. Giri, K. K. Fu, J. Cooper, T. Vuong, A. A. forastiere, G. Adams, W. A. Sakr, D. E. Schuller, and J. E. Ensley. (1998). "Chemoradiotherapy versus radiotherapy in patients with advanced nasopharyngeal cancer: Phase III randomized Intergroup study 0099." *J. Clin. Oncol.* 16:1310–1317.

Ang, K. (1998). "Altered fractionation in head and neck cancer." *Semin. Radiat. Oncol.* 8:230–236.

Ang, K. K., L. J. Peters, R. S. Weber, M. H. Maor, W. H. Morrison, C. D. Wendt, and B. W. Brown. (1990). "Concomitant boost radiotherapy schedules in the treatment of carcinoma of the oropharynx and nasopharynx." *Int. J. Radiat. Oncol. Biol. Phys.* 19:1339–1345.

Ang, K. K., and L. J. Peters. (1992). "Concomitant boost radiotherapy in the treatment of head and neck cancers." *Semin. Radiat. Oncol.* 2:31–33.

Ang, K. K., A. Trotti, B. B. Brown, A. S. Garden, R. L. Foote, W. H. Morrison, F. B. Geara, D. W. Klotch, H. Goepfert, and L. J. Peters. (2001). "Randomized trial assessing risk features and time factors of surgery plus radiotherapy in advanced head-and-neck cancer." *Int. J. Radiat. Oncol. Biol. Phys.* 51(3): 571–578.

Beumer 3rd, J., T. Curtis, and R. E. Harrison. (1979). "Radiation therapy of the oral cavity: Sequelae and management, part 1." *Head Neck Surg.* 1:301–312.

Bragg, C. M., J. Conway, and M. H. Robinson. (2002). "The role of intensity-modulated radiotherapy in the treatment of parotid tumors." *Int. J. Radiat. Oncol. Biol. Phys.* 52(3):729–738.

Brahme A. (2002). "Development of radiation therapy optimization." *Acta Oncol.* 39(5):579–595.

Butler, E. B., B. S. Teh, W. H. Grant 3rd, B. M. Uhl, R. B. Kuppersmith, J. K. Chiu, D. T. Donovan, and S. Y. Woo. (1999). "Smart (simultaneous modulated accelerated radiation therapy) boost: A new accelerated fractionation schedule for the treatment of head and neck cancer with intensity modulated radiotherapy." *Int. J. Radiat. Oncol. Biol. Phys.* 45(1):21–32.

Chao, K. S., D. A. Low, C. A. Perez, and J. A. Purdy. (2000). "Intensity-modulated radiation therapy in head and neck cancers: The Mallinckrodt experience." *Int. J. Cancer* 90:92–103.

Chao, C. .K., M. Cegniz, C.A. Perez, and M. Arquette. (2001a). "Superior Functional Outcome with IMRT in Locally Advanced Nasopharyngeal Carcinoma." Proceedings of the American Society of Clinical Oncology (ASCO). May 14, 2001, San Francisco.

Chao, K. S., N. Majhail, C. J. Huang, J. R. Simpson, C. A. Perez, B. Haughey, and G. Spector. (2001b). "Intensity-modulated radiation therapy reduces late salivary toxicity without compromising tumor control in patients with oropharyngeal carcinoma: A comparison with conventional techniques." *Radiother. Oncol.* 61:275–280.

Chao, K. S., J. O. Deasy, J. Markman, J. Hayne, C. A. Perez, J. A. Purdy, and D. A. Low. (2001c). "A prospective study of salivary function sparing in patients with head-and-neck cancers receiving intensity-modulated or three-dimensional radiation therapy: Initial results." *Int. J. Radiat. Oncol. Biol. Phys.* 49:907–916.

Chao, K. S., W. R. Bosch, S. Mutic, J. S. Lewis, F. Dehdashti, M. A. Mintun, J. F. Dempsey, C. A. Perez, J. A. Purdy, and M. J. Welch. (2001d). "A novel approach to overcome hypoxic tumor resistance: Cu-ATSM-guided intensity-modulated radiation therapy." *Int. J. Radiat. Oncol. Biol. Phys.* 49:1171–1182.

Chao, K. S., F. J. Wippold, G. Ozyigit, B. N. Tran, and J. F. Dempsey. (2002). "Determination and delineation of nodal target volumes for head-and-neck cancer based on patterns of failure in patients receiving definitive and postoperative IMRT." *Int. J. Radiat. Oncol. Biol. Phys.* 53(5):1174–1184.

Chao, K. S. C., G. Ozyigit, B. N. Tran, M. Cengiz, J. F. Dempsey, and D. A. Low. (2003). "Patterns of failure in patients receiving definitive and post-operative IMRT for head and neck cancer." *Int. J. Radiat. Oncol. Biol. Phys.* 55(2):312–321.

Cheng, J. C., K. S. Chao, and D. Low. (2001). "Comparison of intensity modulated radiation therapy (IMRT) treatment techniques for nasopharyngeal carcinoma." *Int. J. Cancer* 96(2):126–131.

Chui, C. S., and S. V. Spirou. (2001). "Inverse planning algorithms for external beam radiotherapy." *Med. Dosim.* 26:189–197.

Claus, F., W. De Gersem, C. De Wagter, R. Van Severen, I. Vanhoutte, W. Duthoy, V. Remouchamps, B. Van Duyse, L. Vakaet, M. Lemmerling, H. Vermeersch, and W. De Neve. (2001). "An implementation strategy for IMRT of ethmoid sinus cancer with bilateral sparing of the optic pathways." *Int. J. Radiat. Oncol. Biol. Phys.* 51(2):318–331.

Dale, R. G. (1985). "The application of the linear-quadratic dose-effect equation of fractionated and protracted radiotherapy." *Cancer* 75:2351–2355.

Dawson, L. A., Y. Anzai, L. Marsh, M. K. Martel, A. Paulino, J. A. Ship, and A. Eisbruch. (2000). "Patterns of local-regional recurrence following parotid-sparing conformal and segmental intensity-modulated radiotherapy for head and neck cancer." *Int. J. Radiat. Oncol. Biol. Phys.* 46(3):1117–1126.

Deasy, J. O., K. S. C. Chao, and J. Markman. (2001). "Uncertainties in model-based outcome predictions for treatment planning." *Int. J. Radiat. Oncol. Biol. Phys.* 51(5):1389–1399.

Dreizen, S., L. R. Brown, T. E. Daly, and J. B. Drane. (1977). "Prevention of xerostomia-related dental caries in irradiated cancer patients." *J. Dent. Res.* 56:99–104.

Drzymala, R. E., R. Mohan, L. Brewster, J. Chu, M. Goitein, W. Harms, and M. Urie. (1991). "Dose-volume histograms." *Int. J. Radiat. Oncol. Biol. Phys.* 21:71–78.

Eisbruch A., R. K. Ten Haken, H. M. Kim, L. H. Marsh, and J. A. Ship. (1999). "Dose, volume, and function relationships in parotid salivary glands following conformal and intensity-modulated irradiation of head and neck cancer." *Int. J. Radiat. Oncol. Biol. Phys.* 45:577–587.

Eisbruch, A., H. M. Kim, J. E. Terrell, L. H. Marsh, L. A. Dawson, and J. A. Ship. (2001). "Xerostomia and its predictors following parotid-sparing irradiation of head-and-neck cancer." *Int. J. Radiat. Oncol. Biol. Phys.* 50:695–704.

Eneroth, C. M., C. O. Henriksson, and P. A. Jakobsson. (1972). "Effect of fractionated radiotherapy on salivary gland function." *Cancer* 30:1147–1153.

Fu, K. K., T. F. Pajak, A. Trotti, C. U. Jones, S. A. Spencer, T. L. Phillips, A. S. Garden, J. A. Ridge, J. S. Cooper, and K. K. Ang. (2000). "A Radiation Therapy Oncology Group (RTOG) phase III randomized study to compare hyperfractionation and two variants of accelerated fractionation to standard fractionation radiotherapy for head and neck squamous cell carcinomas: First report of RTOG 9003." *Int. J. Radiat. Oncol. Biol. Phys.* 48:7–16.

Gilbeau, L., M. Octave-Prignot, T. Loncol, L, Renard, P. Scalliet, and V. Gregoire. (2001). "Comparison of setup accuracy of three different thermoplastic masks for the treatment of brain and head and neck tumors." *Radiother. Oncol.* 58:155–162.

Hansen, O., J. Overgaard, H. S. Hansen, M. Overgaard, M. Hoyer, K. E. Jorgensen, L. Bastholdt, and A. Berthelsen. (1997). "Importance of overall treatment time for outcome of radiotherapy of advanced head and neck carcinoma: Dependency on tumor differentiation." *Radiother. Oncol.* 43(1):47–51.

Harrison, L. B., M. J. Zelefsky, D. G. Pfitser, E. Carper, A. Raben, D. H. Krause, E. W. Strong, A. Rao, H. Thaler, T. Polyak, and R. Portenoy. (1997). "Detailed quality of life assessment in patients treated with primary radiotherapy for squamous cell cancer of the base of the tongue." *Head Neck* 19:169–175.

Hoppe, R. T., D. R. Goffinet, and M. A. Bagshaw. (1976). "Carcinoma of the nasopharynx. Eighteen years' experience with megavoltage radiation therapy." *Cancer* 37:2605–2612.

Horiot, J. C., R. LeFur, T. N'Guyen, C. Chenal, S. Schraub, G. Alfonsi, W. Gardini, W. Van den Bogaert, S. Danczak, M. Bolla, M. Van Glabbeke, and M. De Pauw. (1992). "Hyperfractionation versus conventional fractionation in oropharyngeal carcinoma: Final analysis of a randomized trial of the EORTC cooperative group of radiotherapy." *Radiother. Oncol.* 25: 231–241.

Hsiung, C. Y., E. D. Yorke, C. S. Chui, J. Hu, J. P. Xiong, M. A. Hunt, C. C. Ling, E. Y. Huang, C. C. Sung, Y. J. Huang, C. J. Wang, H. C. Chen, S. A. Yeh, H. C. Hsu, and H. I. Amols. (2002). "Intensity modulated radiation therapy versus conventional three-dimensional conformal radiotherapy for the boost or salvage treatment of nasopharyngeal carcinoma." *Int. J. Radiat. Oncol. Biol. Phys.* 53(3):638–647.

ICRU Report 50. Prescribing, Recording and Reporting Photon Beam Therapy. Washington, DC: International Commission on Radiation Units and Measurements, 1993.

Kresnik, E., P. Mikosch, H. J. Gallowitsch, D. Kogler, S. Wiesser, M. Heinisch, O. Unterweger, W. Raunik, G. Kumnig, I. Gomez, G. Grunbacher, and P. Lind. (2001). "Evaluation of head and neck cancer with 18-FDG PET: A comparison with conventional methods." *Eur. J. Nucl. Med.* 28(7):816–821.

Lee, N., P. Xia, J. M. Quivey, K. Sultanem, I. Poon, C. Akazawa, P. Akazawa, V. Weinberg, and K. K. Fu. (2002). "Intensity-modulated radiotherapy in the treatment of nasopharyngeal carcinoma: An update of the UCSF experience." *Int. J. Radiat. Oncol. Biol. Phys.* 53(1):12–22.

Leslie, M. D., and S. Dische. (1992). "Changes in serum and salivary amylase during radiotherapy for head and neck cancer – a comparison of conventionally fractionated treatment with CHART." *Radiother. Oncol.* 24:27–31.

Low, D. A. "Physics of Intensity Modulated Radiation Therapy for Head and Neck Cancer" in *Head and Neck IMRT* (1st edition). K. S. C. Chao and G. Ozyigit (eds.). Philadelphia: Lippincott Williams and Wilkins, 2003.

Low, D. A., K. S. C. Chao, S. Mutic, R. L. Gerber, C. A. Perez, and J. A. Purdy. (1998). "Quality assurance of serial tomotherapy for head and neck patient treatments." *Int. J. Radiat. Oncol. Biol. Phys.* 42(3):681–692.

Martinez-Monge, R., P. S. Fernandes, N. Gupta, and R. Gahbauer. (1999). "Cross-sectional nodal atlas: A tool for the definition of clinical target volumes in three-dimensional radiation therapy planning." *Radiol.* 211:815–828.

Mohan, R., Q. Wu, M. Manning, and R. Schmidt-Ullrich. (2000). "Radiobiological considerations in the design of fractionation strategies for intensity-modulated radiation therapy of head and neck cancers." *Int. J. Radiat. Oncol. Biol. Phys* 46(3):619–630.

Mossman, K. L., A. R. Shatzman, and J. D. Chencharick. (1981). "Effects of radiotherapy on human parotid saliva." *Radiat. Res.* 88:403–412.

Ozyigit, G., and K. S. C. Chao. (2002). "Clinical experience of head-and-neck cancer IMRT with serial tomotherapy." *Med. Dosim.* 27(2):91–98.

Parsons, J. T., W. M. Mendenhall, N. J. Cassisi, J. H. Isaacs Jr., and R. R. Million. (1988). "Hyperfractionation for head and neck cancer." *Int. J. Radiat. Oncol. Biol. Phys.* 14(4):649–658.

Perez, C. A., B. J. Kobeissi, and K. S. C. Chao. Cost Benefit of Three-Dimensional Conformal or Intensity Modulated Radiation Therapy. 3-D Conformal Radiation Therapy and Intensity Modulated Therapy in the New Millennium. Houston, TX: Baylor College of Medicine, Office of Continuing Medical Education: Section 10, 1999.

Perez, C. A., V. R. Devineni, V. Marcial-Vega, J. E. Marks, J. R. Simpson, and N. Kucik. (1992). "Carcinoma of the nasopharynx: Factors affecting prognosis." *Int. J. Radiat. Oncol. Biol. Phys.* 23:271–280.

Pigott, K., S. Dische, and M. I. Saunders. (1995). "Where exactly does failure occur after radiation in head and neck cancer?" *Radiother. Oncol.* 37:17–19.

Radiation Therapy Oncology Group (RTOG) H-0022. Phase I/II Study of Conformal and Intensity Modulated Irradiation for Oropharyngeal Cancer. Feb 2001 (Rev. 1-2, Jan 15, 2002). Available at rtog.org.

Sanguineti, G., F. B. Geara, A. S. Garden, S. L. Tucker, K. K. Ang, W. H. Morrison, and L. J. Peters. (1997). "Carcinoma of the nasopharynx treated by radiotherapy alone: Determinants of local and regional control." *Int. J. Radiat. Oncol. Biol. Phys.* 37:985–996.

Shannon, I., and H. Chauncey. (1967). "A parotid fluid collection device with improved stability characteristics." *J. Oral. Ther. Pharm.* 4:403–412.

Shannon, I. L., J. N. Trodahl, and E. N. Starcke. (1978), "Radiosensitivity of the human parotid gland." *Proc. Soc. Exp. Biol. Med.* 157:50–53.

Sultanem, K., H. K. Shu, P. Xia, C. Akazawa, J. M. Quivey, L. J. Verhey, and K. K. Fu. (2000). "Three-dimensional intensity-modulated radiotherapy in the treatment of nasopharyngeal carcinoma: The University of California-San Francisco experience." *Int. J. Radiat. Oncol. Biol. Phys.* 48:711–722.

Teknos, T. N., E. L. Rosenthal, D. Lee, R. Taylor, and C. S. Marn. (2001). "Positron emission tomography in the evaluation of stage III and IV head and neck cancer." *Head Neck* 23(12):1056–1060.

Wang, C. C. (1989). "Accelerated hyperfractionation radiation therapy for carcinoma of the nasopharynx. Techniques and results." *Cancer* 63:2461–2467.

Webb, S. (2001). *Intensity-Modulated Radiation Therapy.* Bristol: Institute of Physics (IOP) Publishing, 2001.

Wolden, S. L., M. J. Zelefsky, M. A. Hunt, K. E. Rosenzweig, L. M. Chong, D. H. Krause, D. G. Pfister, and S. A Leibel. (2001). "Failure of a 3D conformal boost to improve radiotherapy for nasopharyngeal carcinoma." *Int. J. Radiat. Oncol. Biol. Phys.* 49:1229–1234.

Xia, P., K. K. Fu, G. W. Wong, C. Akazawa, and L. J. Verhey. (2000). "Comparison of treatment plans involving intensity-modulated radiotherapy for nasopharyngeal carcinoma." *Int. J. Radiat. Oncol. Biol. Phys.* 48(2):329–337.

Zelefsky, M. J., Z. Fuks, M. Hunt, H. J. Lee, D. Lombardi, C. C. Ling, V. E. Reuter, E. S. Venkatraman, and S. A. Leibel. (2001). "High dose radiation delivered by intensity modulated conformal radiotherapy improves the outcome of localized prostate cancer." *J. Urol.* 166(3):876–881.

# Lung Cancer Radiotherapy

Craig W. Stevens, M.D., Ph.D.[1], Thomas Guerrero, M.D., Ph.D.[1],
and Kenneth M. Forster, Ph.D.[2]

[1]Department of Radiation Oncology, [2]Department of Radiation Physics
The University of Texas M.D. Anderson Cancer Center, Houston, Texas



More than 60% of lung cancer patients will receive radiotherapy at some point in their disease, 45% for initial treatment and 17% for palliation (Tyldesley et al. 2001). Since about 170,000 patients will develop lung cancer (Greenlee et al. 2002), there will be over 100,000 Americans irradiated for lung cancer this year. Therefore, it is critical that we aggressively implement the best of new technologies because, with such large patient numbers, even small advances can improve the lives of many patients. Experienced teams are required to manage patients optimally, particularly when combined modality therapy is used, with demonstrably better outcomes when patients are treated by experienced personnel (Bach et al. 2001; Lee et al. 2002).

Radiation therapy for lung cancer is rapidly changing. Our ability to define target volumes and avoid normal structures has been aided by advancements in computed tomography (CT) technology and in [18]FDG-PET (fluorodeoxyglucose radiolabeled with [18]F-positron emission tomography) scanning. It is also now possible to measure and account for individual variations in respiratory tumor motion. Treatment planning algorithms can account for tissue inhomogeneity, which can improve delivered dose distributions to target volumes. In fact, our way of thinking about lung cancer planning has changed to utilize International Commission on Radiation Units and Measurements (ICRU) report 62 definitions of volumes and doses so that true three-dimensional (3-D) conformal radiotherapy is routinely achieved. We look forward to the effective implementation of intensity-modulated radiation therapy (IMRT), and eventually the use of proton therapy. We also anticipate the rational integration of new biologic therapies into standard treatment.

## Radiation Treatment Planning

### Defining Treatment Volumes For Lung Cancer

The ICRU has defined several volumes that are important for the modern treatment of lung cancer: Gross tumor volume (GTV), which is the tumor that is visible by any imaging modality; clinical target volume (CTV), which is the volume that is likely to contain microscopic disease; and planning target volume (PTV), which includes the CTV with a margin to account for daily setup error and target motion. Another volume, the internal target volume (ITV), was defined in ICRU report 62 and is an expansion of the CTV in which target motion is explicitly measured and taken into account. The final PTV is then formed by adding a setup margin (to account for daily setup variations) to the ITV.

### Gross Target Volume (GTV)

Delineation of GTV is the subject of some controversy. Radiologists and radiation oncologists define GTVs somewhat differently, suggesting that radiation oncologists must be well trained in imaging (Giraud et al. 2001). The pulmonary extent of lung tumors must be delineated on pulmonary windows, and the mediastinal extent of tumors must be delineated using mediastinal windows. Improper windowing/leveling can result in GTVs that vary by several centimeters (figure 1). We have actively involved our diagnostic imaging physicians in the calibration of our CT simulators to ensure that the "lung" and "mediastinal" settings are similar in our departments. This makes it somewhat easier to compare diagnostic and treatment planning studies. We calibrate each of the monitors that access our CT simulator data sets to comply with a Society of Motion Picture and Television Engineers (SMPTE) test pattern. This ensures that the programmed window/level will be displayed in an identical way on each monitor.

Another important issue involves the contouring of spiculations. Data from the 1970's suggest that spiculations contain tumor cells more often with adenocarcinomas than with squamous carcinomas. No radiographic-histologic correlation studies have been done recently to explicitly address this problem. We generally assume that all spiculations contain tumor. It is important to differentiate spiculations from branching vessels (figure 1, arrows), and this can sometimes be easier with a contrast-enhanced scan.

Intravenous (IV) contrast has been used in our department in very selected cases (figure 2). In our experience, contrast can help with delineation of hilar and occasionally mediastinal lymph nodes. The procedure for the use of contrast initially involved the training of therapists, nurses and physicians about the management of contrast reactions. While the risk of reaction is low for non-ionic contrast, it is not zero. Clinical parameters for safe contrast administration should be cleared with your radiology department, as should the procedure for management of contrast reactions.

A non-contrast study is obtained first. The contrast is then infused according to a schema from our diagnostic radiology group, and the contrast-enhanced CT obtained. Contours are then drawn on the contrast study and transferred to the non-contrast study for treatment planning. This is important since planning should be done with heterogeneity corrections. The presence of IV contrast can result in dosimetric errors of 2% to 5% in regions [such as the anterior-posterior (AP) window] that are surrounded by vessels containing contrast.

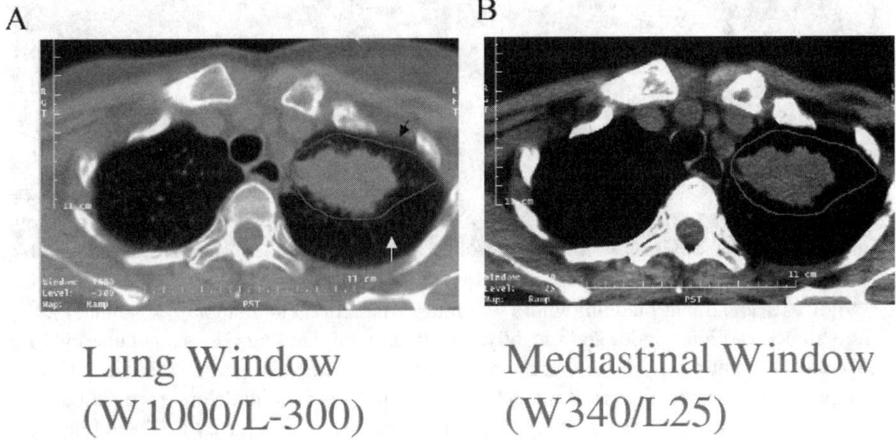



**Figure 1.** CT scans of a left upper lobe NSCLC using (a) lung and (b) mediastinal windows. Note that spiculations are poorly seen on mediastinal windows. Note too the branching of the vessels (white arrow) in contradistinction to the spiculation which do not branch (black arrow).

[18]F-FDG-PET scanning is another imaging modality that has become quite important for radiation treatment planning (Vanuytsel et al. 2000; Seltzer et al. 2002). It can reduce inter-observer differences in GTV contouring (Caldwell et al. 2001). It can help to categorize suspicious mediastinal/hilar lymph adenopathy as either benign or malignant, with higher standard uptake values (SUVs) being predictive of metastatic disease. It can also help to identify tumor within an atelectatic lobe, and thereby decrease the amount of normal lung irradiated. Finally, because FDG-PET scans detect distant metastases in about 30% of non-small-cell lung cancer (NSCLC) patients (particularly those with otherwise advanced disease), it can significantly help with patient triage (MacManus et al. 2001). In one study, use of FDG-PET scans for treatment planning altered the target volumes in 11/11 cases with seven volumes increased and four decreased (Erdi et al. 2002). It is not clear what impact the use of PET scanning will have on patterns of failure. One caveat is that FDG-PET scanning will make it difficult to compare results of PET-staged patients with earlier studies because of significant stage migration. A group at the Peter MacCallum Cancer Institute compared the survival of patients treated on two similar protocols, one of which required FDG-PET scanning

while the other was performed before PET scanning was available (MacManus et al. 2002). The median survival of PET staged patients was 31 months, compared with 16 months for conventionally staged patients.

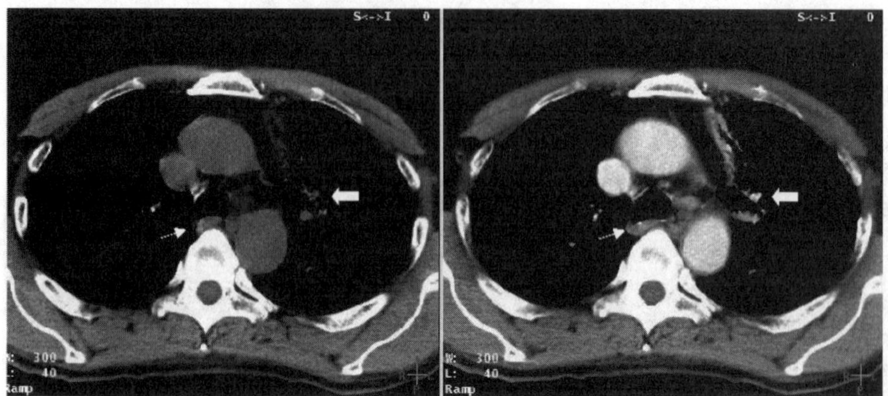

**Figure 2.** Treatment planning with IV contrast. Induction chemotherapy changed the lung tumor and hilar nodes significantly, so a treatment planning CT was obtained with IV contrast (right panel). Note that the hilar structures (large white arrow) enhanced, and so were not considered part of the GTV. One region in the contralateral mediastinum (small white arrow) did not enhance. The ~1 cm mass was positive by PET and biopsy. Without either the contrast or PET scan, this region could have been confused with the azygos vein and likely excluded from the high dose region.

Techniques for integrating PET scans into radiotherapy treatment planning are currently being developed. Several important technical points need to be made. First, it is desirable to minimize the time between the PET scan and treatment planning CT scan. This will lessen potential changes in tumor size or lung collapse that might make image registration difficult. Second, whenever possible, PET scans should be done on flat tables with patients immobilized in the treatment position. This will minimize systematic errors in soft tissue location (for example, the carina can move over 2 cm simply by changing arm position). Because the internal diameter of PET gantries, which are typically smaller than gantries of CT simulators (typically 50 to 60 cm), it may be necessary to check the physical size of patient immobilization devices before simulation to ensure clearance through the PET gantry. Third, PET and CT images should be registered using both surface fiducials and the spine. This reduces registration error. Most of these technical issues will be resolved when dedicated PET-CT units become more widely available (figure 3).

Contouring on the registered image sets can also be challenging. FDG-PET scanning is very poor at delineating tumor edges, particularly in areas of spiculation because the number of tumor cells per voxel may be rather low. Also, the time course of FDG-PET scanning (~5 minutes per bed position) is long relative to CT scanning (1 second or less per slice and falling). This causes a poorly characterized blurring of the edges along the axis of motion. Because of these edge effects, we found it best to contour suspected mediastinal/hilar lymph nodes using CT (with reference to the contrast-enhanced scans), and use the PET image data to confirm or reject nodal involvement. PET scanning is rarely useful for contouring of the primary tumor, but can sometimes identify hilar tumor in the setting of lobar/lung atelectasis. In this setting, one must be particularly careful to use CT to delineate the tumor edge.

A                                    B

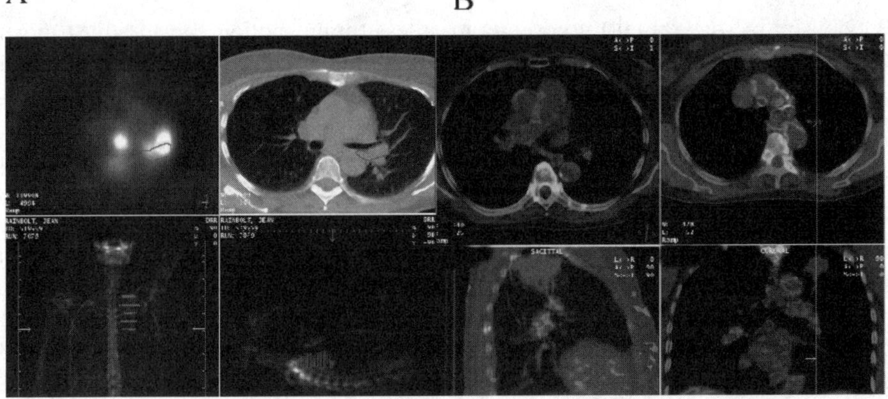

**Figure 3.** Comparison of sequential PET-CT with dedicated PET-CT. Sequential PET-CT images (a) demonstrate significant discrepancies between the regions of increased [18]F-FDG uptake and CT abnormalities. In contrast, a dedicated PET-CT (b) image of the same patient demonstrates that the [18]F-FDG-avid region and CT abnormality register quite well. Even in this case, note that the edge of the tumor seen in the bottom left panel of (b) shows poor [18]F-FDG uptake, despite these being clear spiculations.

## Clinical Target Volume (CTV)

It has historically been difficult to determine the extent of microscopic disease, both adjacent to the primary GTV and in the mediastinum. A radiographic-histopathologic comparison of lung tumor size was recently completed (Giraud et al. 2000). This study demonstrated that to include the tumor within the CTV with 95% accuracy requires GTV-to-CTV expansions of 6 mm for squamous cancers and 8 mm for adenocarcinomas. Expansions for other histologies have not been recently determined, but a conservative approach would be to use 8 mm. Generally, CTVs should not extend beyond anatomic boundaries unless there is evidence of invasion. For example, CTVs should not extend across interlobar fissures, into the chest wall or the mediastinum without CT/MR (magnetic resonance) evidence of invasion.

Appropriate CTVs for mediastinal lymph nodes have not been rigorously determined. We empirically use 8 to 10 mm expansions around involved nodes (either gross involvement or FDG-PET positivity). Obviously, these expansions should not necessarily be uniformly applied along all axes. In the absence of radiographic proof of invasion, CTVs for primary tumors should generally not extend into the chest wall or mediastinum. CTV expansions of lymph node disease should not extend into the major airways, vessels or lung.

## Tumor Motion And Internal Margin Volume (ITV)

Previously, we have used fluoroscopy to assess tumor motion and to adjust target volumes. However, it became apparent that two-dimensional measurement of tumor motion, such as might be done by fluoroscopy, was inadequate. Fluoroscopic detection of AP tumor motion was often quite poor because of the superposition of the mediastinal structures. We had also hoped that tumor motion might be predictable, but found that it was not (Stevens et al. 2001). Thus, we concluded that tumor motion was best assessed individually for each patient in three dimensions.

To understand the extent of the motion problem, at our institution we implemented a tumor motion protocol for our NSCLC patients. Twenty-three patients have been enrolled and evaluated. Entry criteria were that the patient should have a pathologically proven lung cancer, be able to be trained to use the spirometer, and have a planned treatment course of at least 6 weeks. Patients with more than segmental atelectasis were excluded. CT scans were obtained at normal inspiration and expiration. A SensorMedics Vmax22 computer-controlled occlusion spirometer and a Marconi PQ 5000 CT scanner were employed (figure 4a). Pulmonary function tests (PFTs) were performed primarily to assess the vital capacity (Vc) of the patient (figure 4b). Patients would hold their breath for 15 to 20 seconds. CT images over the entire lung volume were acquired at 100% tidal volume (normal inspiration) and at 0% tidal volume (end expiration). For each CT data set, the GTV was contoured and reviewed by two physicians. All CT image sets were registered, using the vertebral bodies, to the treatment planning CT for the assessment of tumor motion. Figure 5a demonstrates that lung motion is not uniform. For this case, the diaphragm moves anteriorly and inferiorly with inspiration, while the anterior chest wall moves slightly anteriorly. The carina can also move, in this case anteriorly and slightly inferiorly. The mediastinum generally narrows with inspiration, and the heart rotates. In this example, the upper lobe lung tumor moves about 6 mm anteriorly as well. In a second example (figure 5b), the geometric center of the tumor was identified on the inspiration and expiration CT. After registration, the motion of the geometric center for the GTV was determined. Figure 6 shows a scatter plot of the magnitude of tumor motion for 23 lung cancer patients. The magnitude of motion revealed that under normal respiration only 6 of the 23 patients had tumors that moved 3 to 5 mm, and no lesions moved less than 3 mm. The mean tumor displacement was 9.3 mm and the standard deviation was 4.3 mm. Most of the motion that was observed was in the superior-inferior (SI) and AP directions; while there was some right-left motion, it was typically smaller in magnitude. The mean magnitude of motion for a lower lobe lesion was 12.9 mm while for an upper lobe the mean was 7.8 mm. Tumor motion was not predicted by location, size, stage or pulmonary function (table 1).

A motion study was also repeated at the end of treatment in 10 patients. Tumor motion changed significantly over the course of treatment with both the direction and magnitude of tumor motion changing in all cases. Some tumors moved more, some moved less, and some changed direction! The motion of several tumors changed more than 1 cm during treatment. It was noted by spirometry that the amplitude and frequency of respiration changed with treatment, which was not surprising considering that the vital capacity could change by as much as 35%. The magnitude of motion change was surprising since no patient had large amounts of lung collapse. These data suggest that 3-D tumor motion should be assessed in each patient, and probably several times during treatment.

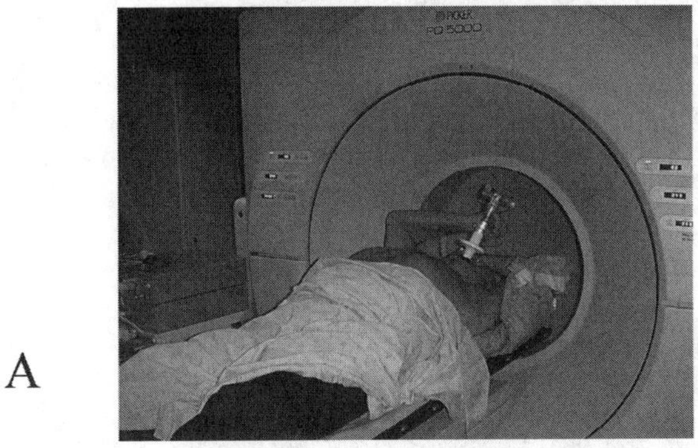

A

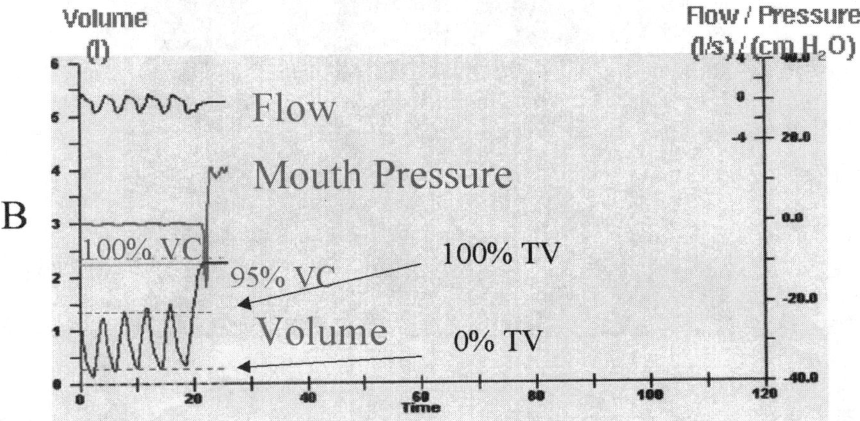



**Figure 4.** (a) Patient using spirometry-assisted breath hold for obtaining treatment planning CTs in various phases of the respiratory cycle. (b) A representative trace from the Sensor-Medics spirometer demonstrating flow, pressure, and lung volumes.

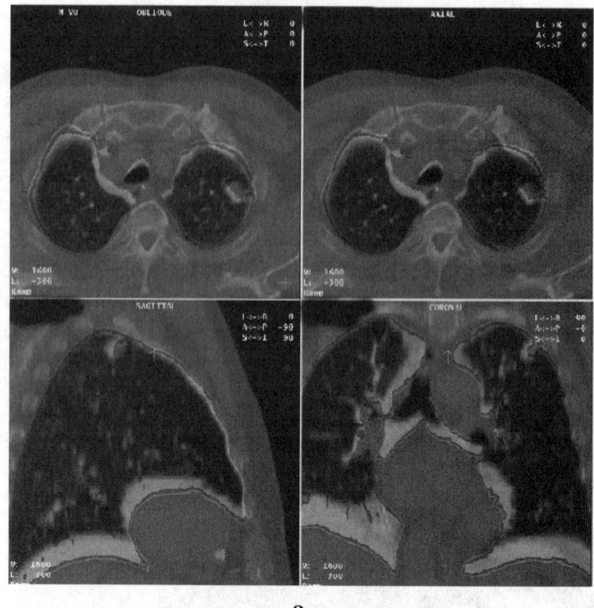

a.

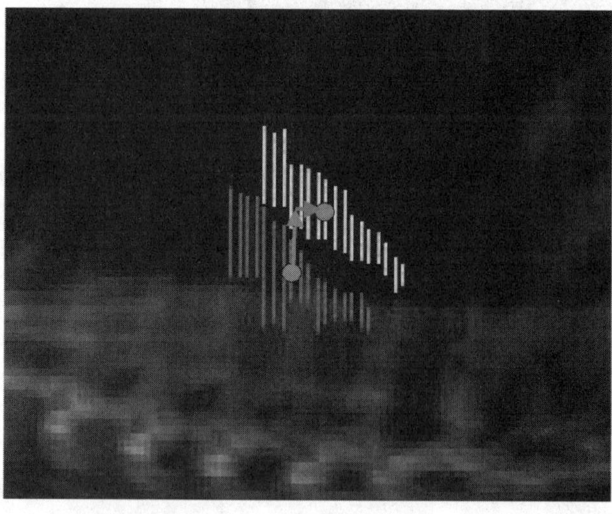

b.

**Figure 5.** Lung tumor motion. (a) The CTs were registered to the vertebral bodies in three dimensions. Note that motion is not uniform throughout the lung. In this example the diaphragm moves both anteriorly and inferiorly with inspiration, and the anterior chest wall moves anteriorly. The upper lobe tumor movement is essentially all AP during respiration. (b) In a second example, the tumor was contoured on the inspiration and expiration CT. The CTs were registered, and the motion of the center of mass is shown in one projection.

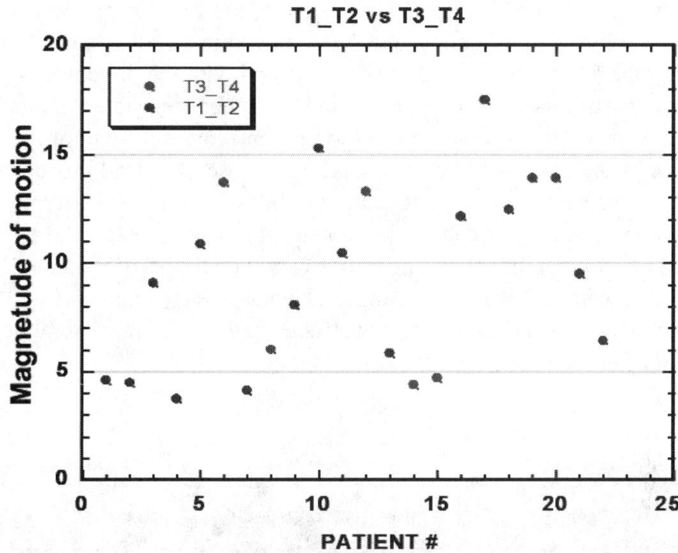


**Figure 6.** Again, CT scans were obtained during a breath hold at 100% tidal volume and 0% tidal volume and the center of mass motion determined in three dimensions. The total displacement of the tumor during quiet respiration is shown for each of 23 patients. Note that there is no obvious correlation between T-stage and the magnitude of tumor motion.

**Table 1.** Mean Magnitude Of Motion

| Mean | (mm) | STD |
| --- | --- | --- |
| T1/T2 | 9.5 | 4.2 |
| T3/T4 | 8.4 | 4.7 |
| Upper | 7.8 | 3.6 |
| Lower | 12.9 | 3.9 |
| Free | 12.4 | 3.4 |
| Attached | 7.8 | 3.9 |

Based on these studies, the application of a uniform margin to account for motion seems inappropriate since the tumor motion for our patients appears to be mainly in two directions. Following the guidelines of ICRU report 62 we have attempted to explicitly account for the tumor motion. The ITV represents the volume occupied by the CTV during normal quiet respiration. In order to determine this volume, CT image data sets at normal expiration (0% tidal volume) and at normal inspiration (100% tidal volume) as well as quiet-breathing image sets needed to be acquired. GTVs for each CT image set were delineated and expanded to form CTVs. Finally the two breath-hold data sets were registered to the quiet respiration data set and the envelope of the three CTVs represents the ITV. As can be seen in figure 7 and as previously discussed, lung tumors can move significantly, and often the motion is along the AP direction as well as along the SI axis. CT images were obtained with the patient in the treatment position during inspiration and expiration, and the images registered. Panel 7a demonstrates the expansion that would be used to take motion into account if only the AP view had been used (as would be typical with fluoroscopy). Had this been done, the tumor would have been outside of the target volume for part of the treatment, which would have resulted in significant under-dosing. If tumor motion is measured in three dimensions, as shown in panel 7b, the tumor would be properly irradiated. This technique also helps with choosing beam angles, because beam angles parallel to the axis of motion will usually irradiate less normal tissue. In this example, lateral fields or very oblique fields should be avoided.

## Fig 7A

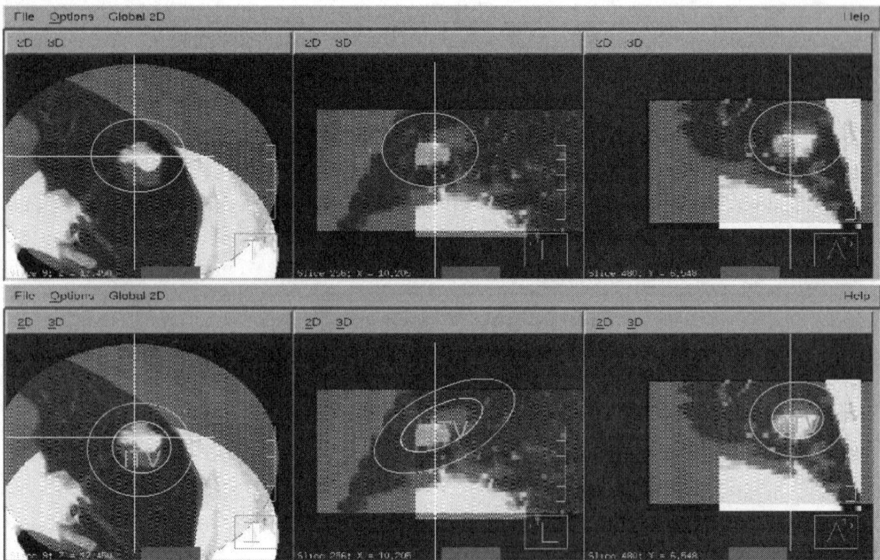

## Fig 7B

**Figure 7.** CT scans were obtained through the target volume on a representative patient at inspiration and expiration, and the images registered. If the target volume had been limited to the tumor motion seen on the AP projection (panel a), tumor would have been near the edge of the treatment field for any treatment with oblique fields. However, if an internal target volume had been drawn to include the tumor motion in three dimensions (panel b), such potential underdosing would have been avoided.

Our experience with 3-D measurement of lung tumor motion suggests that about one-third of lung tumors move less than 0.5 cm with respiration. For this third of patients, simple expansion along the axis motion is adequate. For the other two-thirds, the treatment machine can be gated with respiration, or the patient can use an assisted breath-hold technique, or an ITV-based approach can be used. A commercially available system can be used to gate the linear accelerator (linac) (Ramsey et al. 1999). This technique uses an externally placed fiducial which is tracked as the patient breathes. The beam can be triggered at a chosen point in the respiratory cycle, typically end-expiration because this is the longest, most reproducible portion of the respiratory cycle. This requires that patients be able to breath slowly in a regular pattern. Active breathing control (ABC) (Sixel et al. 2001) and deep inspiration breath hold (DIBH) (Rosenzweig et al. 2000) are two techniques that have been pioneered to help patients hold their breaths at reproducible points in the respiratory cycle. These two techniques limit patient respiratory excursion to fixed volumes. The radiation beam is then initiated. They limit diaphragm excursion to about 5 mm, instead of 10 to 15 mm (Ford et al. 2002). These techniques require very cooperative patients, who are able to hold their breath for at least 15 seconds. Unfortunately, patients with poor pulmonary function (who would most benefit from reduction in irradiated lung volumes) are the patients least able to comply with breath holding techniques. Thus, it is not clear which is the best method to temporally immobilize lung tumors. Our feeling is that, until gating techniques are improved, that an ITV-based approach offers the most reliable method of explicitly accounting for respiratory dependent lung tumor motion.

## Planning Target Volume (PTV)

PTV is designed to account for setup uncertainty (and motion if the ITV approach is not used). Because several respiratory cycles and associated motion typically occur during the treatment of a single fraction, the margin for motion and setup uncertainty should be combined linearly. Preliminary data at our institution have shown that, when immobilizing patients with a Vac-Loc bag and T-bar, an expansion along all axes of 7 mm will account for 95% of the day-to-day setup uncertainty. However, we have dozens of therapists, 3 CT simulators, and 12 linacs. Thus, our setup measurements may not be similar to those of a smaller clinic. Setup uncertainty is likely both technique-dependent and institution-dependent, and should be measured individually for each technique and in each department.

## Treatment Planning

## Heterogeneity Corrections

Traditionally, radiation treatment planning for thoracic tumors has assumed a homogeneous patient. In fact, the clinical trials using radiation therapy for lung cancer have almost all been based on dose planned in a homogeneous body (Orton et al. 1998).

Radiation Therapy Oncology Group (RTOG) protocols for thoracic tumors continue to require homogeneous treatment planning because of the fear of underdosing the primary tumor when correcting for heterogeneity and to allow comparison with previous results. Nevertheless, the need for lung heterogeneity correction has been debated for some time (Orton et al. 1984; Klein et al. 1997; Papanikolaou and Klein 2000), and dose calculations taking into account the presence of heterogeneity have become commercially available (Papanikolaou and Klein 2000). Even though some studies have indicated that heterogeneity correction may result in isocenter doses 6% to 18% greater than those calculated without correction (Klein et al. 1997), the use of heterogeneity correction in treatment planning systems warrants serious consideration. However, it is important that any method incorporating heterogeneity correction factors make use of the clinical knowledge already gained from traditional homogeneous treatment planning.

To address this issue, we have recently developed a heterogeneity-corrected dose-volume prescription method that allows prescription to an isodose that circumscribes and ensures coverage of at least 95% of the PTV. This prescription was combined with a dose calculation that incorporates heterogeneity corrections using the convolution/superposition algorithm. With our change in prescription technique using ICRU-defined parameters, we realized the potential for a significant change in the actual dose delivered to patients with lung cancer. We therefore studied the effect of this change on dose distributions and target volume coverage (Frank et al. 2003).

Thirty stage I/II NSCLC tumors were treated from 1998 to 2001 at our institution using heterogeneity-corrected plans. Treatment planning was performed using 6 MV beams in the clinically-used geometries. Three treatment plans were generated for each case. The first treatment plan was generated using the traditional homogeneous point-dose method in which each prescription delivered a dose of 60 to 66 Gy to the tumor isocenter. The dose distribution for this plan was re-calculated using heterogeneity corrections, while maintaining the same number of monitor units (MUs) per beam. This more accurately reflects the actual clinical dose received. The second treatment plan incorporated heterogeneity corrections into the dose calculations while ensuring 95% coverage of the PTV. For the third technique (which is that currently used in our clinic), beam weighting and MUs were allowed to vary so as to produce an acceptable plan.

Maximum CTV and PTV doses were not statistically different for these planning techniques (5% differences or greater were considered significant). Similarly, the doses to the isocenter and the normal structures (lung, heart, esophagus, spinal cord) that are normally included in the evaluation of treatment plans were not significantly different. However, there was a significant difference in the PTV coverage prescribed by our method and the traditional homogeneous method ($P = 0.05$) (figure 8 shows an example in which the delivered plan was calculated using heterogeneity corrections, middle panel). Most importantly, the dose prescribed by traditional treatment planning for 14 of 30 tumors covered less than 90% of the PTV when heterogeneity was taken into account. Analysis of these 14 cases revealed no trends in tumor location, beam geometry, or target volume. In several cases, the prescription dose covered less than 80% of the PTV. Monte Carlo modeling of these effects is currently underway.

These data demonstrate that changing prescription techniques from the isocenter of a homogeneous target to 95% of the PTV does not significantly change the dose delivered to the isocenter, but usually improves coverage of the PTV. It also essentially eliminated the use of higher energy beams, because underdosing at the lung-tumor interface can result from the build-up of high-energy photons and electronic disequilibrium at the tumor surface. This results in a tumor-sparing effect similar to the skin-sparing effect produced by high-energy photons at the air-skin interface (Klein et al. 1993). Our change in technique has also slightly increased the distance from the PTV to the block edge (previously ~5 mm to now ~8 to 10 mm, particularly near PTV edges that are surrounded by lung).

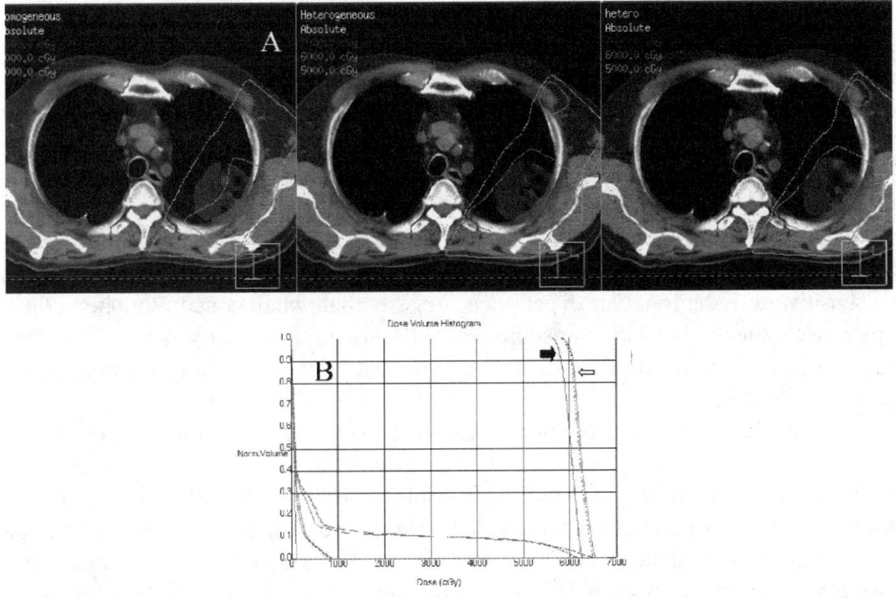


**Figure 8.** Treatment planning results using three different techniques: panel (a): prescribing dose to the isocenter of a homogeneous target; panel (b): using the monitor unit calculations from (a), but applying heterogeneity corrections; panel (c): prescribing to cover 95% of the PTV to the prescription dose.

Of course, it is too soon to know whether this change in prescription technique will improve local control. However, we recently reviewed our outcome for 83 patients with stage I NSCLC, and found that the only predictor of outcome was the margin from GTV to block edge. Tumor size, stage (IA vs. IB), location, and dose were not predictive of local control. While these patients were not planned using heterogeneity corrections, it is likely that larger margins resulted in better PTV coverage.

## Other Technical Issues

There has been much interest in developing techniques for intensity modulated treatment of lung cancers. There are several technical reasons to delay the widespread use of IMRT for lung cancer at this time. First is the issue of tumor motion. IMRT is not appropriate for mobile targets. Our recent data suggests that ~75% of lung tumors move more than 0.5 cm. Unless this motion can be predicted, or measured for each patient, IMRT may result in significant underdosing of tumor, while irradiating significant additional volumes of lung (which also moves!). IMRT plans are designed so that non-flat dose distributions from various beam geometries add up appropriately to achieve a very conformal dose distribution. Because of the nature of the dynamic delivery of IMRT, it is not clear how the doses will add when the target is also moving.

Secondly, there is still some uncertainty about the algorithms used to calculate beamlet doses in very inhomogeneous structures (Wang et al. 2002), although these problems can be minimized by the eventual use of Monte Carlo-based planning algorithms. The dose calculation algorithms used in most treatment planning systems are quite good at predicting the dose in heterogeneous structures (such as the lung) if the fields are large (figure 9a). However, as the field size falls, as it naturally does for IMRT, there can be significant dose calculation errors made (figure 9b). This is particularly problematic at tumor edges.

Thirdly, IMRT achieves highly conformal high dose regions by increasing volumes that receive relatively low doses. This may be a significant problem because lung is so sensitive to radiation. Our experience suggests that, when concurrent chemotherapy is used, the dose-volume most predictive of lung injury is not $V_{20}$, but ~$V_{14}$. Thus, for lung IMRT to be safe, the dose-volume constraints of the lung must be better defined and validated.

Clearly, there is still much work to be done before IMRT can be routinely applied to lung cancer outside of clinical trials. Our thoracic treatment planning group is currently exploring the use of IMRT for thoracic tumor types that minimize the above-mentioned problems. These include esophageal cancer, superior sulcus tumors, and mesothelioma (Amahad et al. 2003; Forster et al. 2003) after extrapleural pneumonectomy. Preliminary results (figure 10) demonstrate that IMRT may be quite useful in the treatment of lung cancer, but should not yet be used routinely outside of controlled clinical trials. In this case, the integral lung dose was actually less for the IMRT plan than for the conventional 3DCRT plan.

## Comparison of Dosimetry Algorithms: 6 MV Broad Beam Broad Target

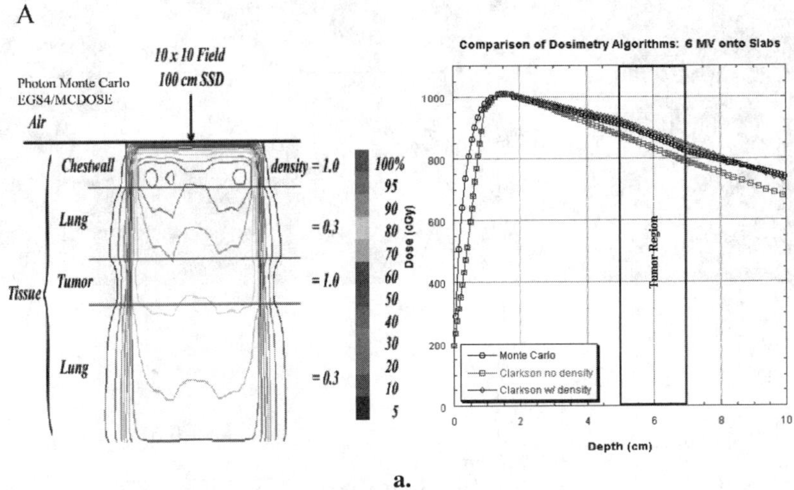



a.

## Comparison of Dosimetry Algorithms: 6 MV IMRT Beamlet Broad Target

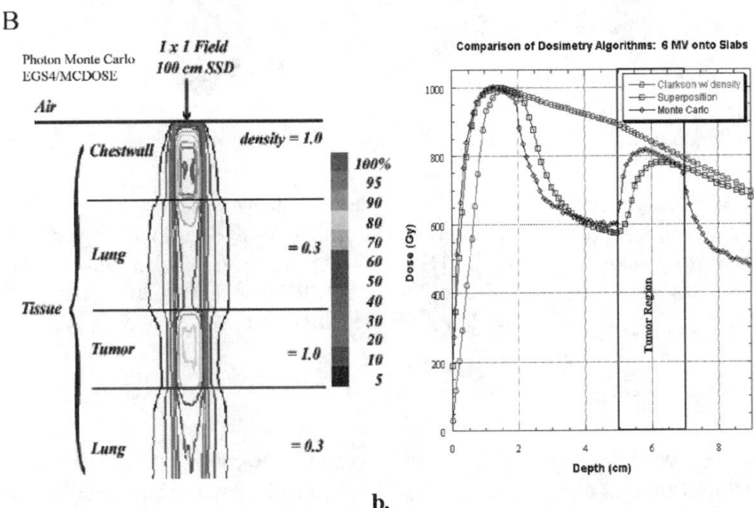



b.

**Figure 9.** Dose distributions in a heterogeneous target using (a) large field or (b) small fields. There is very good correlation between the three dose calculation algorithms when large fields are used, but Monte Carlo calculations suggest that there can be significant errors when these same algorithms are applied to very small inhomogeneous fields.

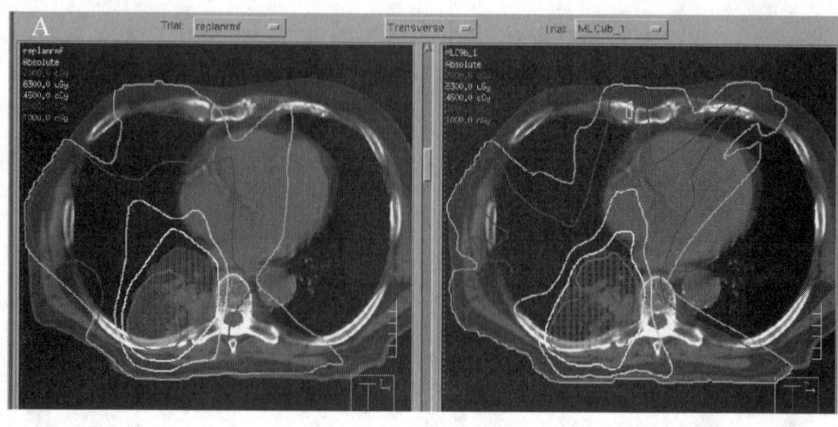

a.

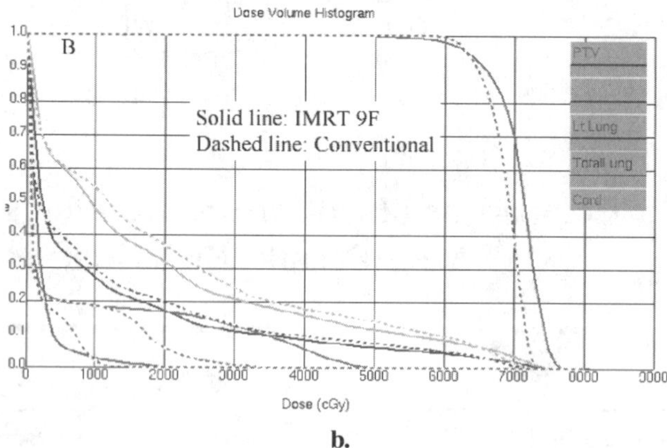


b.

**Figure 10.** Conventional vs IMRT. (a) The isodose distributions are compared for a four-field "conventional" plan and a nine-field IMRT plan for a lower lobe lung cancer case. (b) The dose-volume histogram (DVH) in this case demonstrated that the target volume coverage was slightly better for the 3DCRT plan, but the lung dose was lower for the IMRT plan.

## Acknowledgments

The authors would like to thank Drs. Lei Dong, George Starkschall, and Steven Frank for their input on this chapter, and Ms. Cora Bartholomew for her excellent administrative assistance in the preparation of this manuscript.

# References


Ahamad, A., C. W. Stevens, W. R. Smythe, A. A. Vaporcivan, R. Komaki, J. F. Kelly, Z. Liao, G. Starkschall, and K. M. Forster. (2003). "Intensity modulated radiation therapy: A novel approach to the management of malignant pleural mesothelioma." *Int. J. Radiat. Oncol. Biol. Phys.* 55:768–775.

Bach, P. B., L. D. Cramer, D. Schrag, R. J. Downey, S. E. Gelfand, and C. B. Begg. (2001). "The influence of hospital volume on survival after resection for lung cancer." *N. Engl. J. Med.* 345:181–188.

Caldwell, C. B., K. Mah, Y. C. Ung, C. E. Danjoux, J. M. Balogh, S. N. Ganguli, and L. E. Ehrlich. (2001). "Observer variation in contouring gross tumor volume in patients with poorly defined non-small-cell lung tumors on CT: The impact of $^{18}$FDG-hybrid PET fusion." *Int. J. Radiat. Oncol. Biol. Phys.* 51:923–931.

Erdi, Y. E., E. D. Yorke, A. K. Erdi, Y. C. Hu, L. E. Braban, H. M. Macapinlac, J. L. Humm, O. D. Squire, C. S. Chui, S. M. Larson, and K. Rosenzweig. (2002). "Radiotherapy treatment planning for patients with non-small cell lung cancer using positron emission tomography." *Radiother. Oncol.* 62:51–60.

Ford, E. C., G. S. Mageras, E. Yorke, K. E. Rosenzweig, R. Wagman, and C. C. Ling. (2002). "Evaluation of respiratory movement during gated radiotherapy using film and electronic portal imaging." *Int. J. Radiat. Oncol. Biol. Phys.* 52(2):522–531.

Forster, K. M., W. R. Smythe, G. Starkschall, Z. Liao, T. Takanaka, J. F. Kelly, A. Vaporicivan, A. Ahamad, L. Dong, M. Salehpour, and R. Komaki. (2003). "Intensity-modulated radiation therapy following extrapleural pneumonectomy for the treatment of malignant mesothelioma: Clinical implementation." *Int. J. Radiat. Oncol. Biol. Phys.* 55:606–616.

Frank, S. J., K. M. Forster, C. W. Stevens, J. D. Cox, R. Komaki, Z. Liao, S. Tucker, X. Wang, R. E. Steadham, C. Brooks, and G. Starkschall. (2003). "Treatment planning for lung cancer: Traditional homogeneous point-dose prescription compared with hetergeneity-corrected dose-volume prescription." *Int. J. Radiat. Oncol. Biol. Phys.* In Press.

Giraud, P., M. Antoine, A. Larrouy, B. Milleron, P. Callard, Y. De Rycke, M. F. Carette, J. C. Rosenwald, J. M. Cosset, M. Housset, and E. Touboul. (2001). "Evaluation of microscopic tumor extension in non-small-cell lung cancer for three-dimensional conformal radiotherapy planning." *Int. J. Radiat. Oncol. Biol. Phys.* 48:1015–1024.

Giraud, P., D. Grahek, F. Montravers, M. F. Carette, E. Deniaud-Alexandre, F. Julia, J. C. Rosenwald, J. M. Cosset, J. N. Talbot, M. Housset, and E. Touboul. (2001). "CT and (18)F-deoxyglucose (FDG) image fusion for optimization of conformal radiotherapy of lung cancers." *Int. J. Radiat. Oncol. Biol. Phys.* 49:1249–57.

Jemal, A., A. Thomas, T. Murray, and T. Thun. (2002). "Cancer statistics 2002." *CA Cancer J. Clin.* 52:23–47.

Klein, E. E., L. M. Chin, R. K. Rice, and B. J. Mijnheer. (1993). "The influence of air cavities on interface doses for photon beams." *Int. J. Radiat. Oncol. Biol. Phys.* 27:419–427.

Klein, E. E., A. Morrison, J. A. Purdy, M. V. Graham, and J. Matthews. (1997). "A volumetric study of measurements and calculations of lung density corrections for 6 and 18 MV photons." *Int. J. Radiat. Oncol. Biol. Phys.* 37:1163–1170.

Lee, J. S., C. B. Scott, R. Komaki, D. S. Ettinger, and W. T. Sause. (2002). "Impact of institutional experience on survival outcome of patients undergoing combined chemoradiation therapy for inoperable non-small-cell lung cancer." *Int. J. Radiat. Oncol. Biol. Phys.* 52:362–370.

MacManus, M. P., R. J. Hicks, J. P. Matthews, A. Hogg, A. F. McKenzie, A. Wirth, R. E. Ware, and D. L. Ball. (2001). "High rate of detection of unsuspected distant metastases by pet in apparent stage III non-small-cell lung cancer: Implications for radical radiation therapy. *Int. J. Radiat. Oncol. Biol. Phys.* 50:287–293.

MacManus, M. P., K. Wong, R. J. Hicks, J. P. Matthews, A. Wirth, and D. L. Ball. (2002). "Early mortality after radical radiotherapy for non-small-cell lung cancer: Comparison of PET-staged and conventionally staged cohorts treated at a large tertiary referral center." *Int. J. Radiat. Oncol. Biol. Phys.* 52:351–361.

Orton, C. G., P. M. Mondalek, J. T. Spicka, D. S. Herron, and L. I. Andres. (1984). "Lung corrections in photon beam treatment planning: Are we ready?" *Int. J. Radiat. Oncol. Biol. Phys.* 10:2191–2198.

Orton, C. G., S. Chungbin, E. E. Klein, M. T. Gillin, T. E. schultheiss, and W. T. Sause. (1998). "Study of lung density corrections in a clinical trial (RTOG 88-08)." *Int. J. Radiat. Oncol. Biol. Phys.* 41:787–794.

Papanikolaou, N., and E. E. Klein. (2000). "Point/Counterpoint: Heterogeneity corrections should be used in treatment planning for lung cancer." *Med. Phys.* 27:1702–1704.

Ramsey, C. R., D. Scaperoth, D. Arwood, and A. L. Oliver. (1999). "Clinical efficacy of respiratory gated conformal radiation therapy." *Med. Dosim.* 24:115–119.

Rosenzweig, K. E., J. Hanley, D. Mah, G. Mageras, M. Hunt, S. Toner, C. Burman, C. C. Ling, B. Mychalczak, Z. Fuks, and S. A. Leibel. (2000a). "The deep inspiration breath-hold technique in the treatment of inoperable non-small cell lung cancer." *Int. J. Radiat. Oncol. Biol. Phys.* 48(1):81–87.

Seltzer, M. A., C. S. Yap, D. H. Silverman, J. Meta, C. Schiepers, M. E. Phelps, S. S. Gambhir, J. Rao, P. E. Valk, and J. Czernin. (2002). "The impact of PET on the management of lung cancer: The referring physician's perspective." *J. Nucl. Med.* 43:752–756.

Sixel, K. E., M. C. Aznar, and Y. C. Ung. (2001). "Deep inspiration breath hold to reduce irradiated heart volume in breast cancer patients." *Int. J. Radiat. Oncol. Biol. Phys.* 49:199–204.

Stevens, C. W., R. F. Munden, K. M. Forster, J. F. Kelly, Z. Liao, G. Starkschall, S. Tucker, and R. Komaki. (2001). "Respiratory-driven lung tumor motion is independent of tumor size, tumor location, and pulmonary function." *Int. J. Radiat. Oncol. Biol. Phys.* 51:62–68.

Tyldesley, S., C. Boyd, K. Schulze, H. Walker, and W. J. Mackillop. (2001). "Estimating the need for radiotherapy for lung cancer: an evidence-based, epidemiologic approach." *Int. J. Radiat. Oncol. Biol. Phys.* 49:973–85.

Vanuytsel, L. J., J. F. Vansteenkiste, S. G. Stroobants, P. R. De Leyn, W. De Wever, E. K. Verbeken, G. G. Gatti, D. P. Huyskens, and G. J. Kutcher. (2000). "The impact of 18F- fluro-2-deoxy-D-glucose positron emission tomography (FDG-PET) lymph node staging on the radiation treatment volumes in patients with non-small cell lung cancer." *Radiother. Oncol.* 55:317–324.

Wang, L., E. Yorke, G. Desobry, and C. S. Chui. (2002). "Dosimetric advantage of using 6 MV over 15 MV photons in conformal therapy of lung cancer: Monte Carlo studies in patient geometries." *J. Appl. Clin. Med. Phys.* 3:51–59.

# Methods To Manage Respiratory Motion In Radiation Treatment

**John Wong, Ph.D.**
William Beaumont Hospital
Royal Oak, Michigan



## Introduction

Modern methods of radiation treatment, such as intensity-modulated radiation therapy (IMRT), have greatly enhanced our ability to deliver very high doses that conform tightly to the target, but which also drop steeply to avoid inflicting serious injury to the surrounding critical structures. The sharper dose gradient invites the use of tighter margin to achieve higher dose escalation. However, great care must be exercised to ensure that the reduced margin is adequate in accommodating the setup variation and organ motion that can occur during one (intra-) fraction, and between (inter-) fractions. With steep dose gradients, geometric misses would incur higher risk of serious complications. For tumors in the brain, head and neck, and lower abdominal regions, margin reduction is possible with, albeit sometimes invasive, patient immobilization. The judicious use of on-line or off-line image guidance methods can also be effective (Lattanzi et al. 1999; Martinez et al. 2001; Litzenberg et al. 2002). However, margin reduction remains challenging for treatment in the thoracic and upper abdominal regions. There, intrafraction respiratory motion is significant. Near the diaphragm, it is not uncommon to observe respiration motion with an amplitude of 2 cm. Given that a normal breathing cycle has a period of about 4 s, the tissue in that region is moving at a speed of roughly 1 cm per s. Table 1 lists the results from various studies on the range of tumor and organ motion associated with free-breathing.

**Table 1.** Summary of the Studies Reporting Free Breathing Tumor and Organ Motion [Courtesy of V. Remouchamps.]

| Author | Method | Object Analyzed | Location | Motion in mm Mean (SD) | Direction |
|---|---|---|---|---|---|
| Balter et al. 1996 | Fluoroscopy | Diaphragm | Diaphragm | 9.1 (2.4) | — |
| Davies et al. 1994 | Fluoroscopy | Diaphragm | Diaphragm | 12 (7) | — |
| Ekberg et al. 1998 | Fluoroscopy | — | — | 2.4 | Medio/Lat + AP/PA |
| | | | | 3.9 (0-12) | Cranio-caudal |
| Erridge et al. 2003 | Portal Images | Lung Tumors | More motion in the lower lobes | 7.3 (2.7) 12.5 (7.3) 9.4 (5.2) | Lateral Cranio-caudal Antero-posterior |
| Hanley et al. 1999 | Fluoroscopy | Diaphragm | Diaphragm | 26.4 | — |
| Korin et al. 1992 | MRI | Diaphragm | Diaphragm | 13 | — |
| Mah et al. 2000 | CT | Lung Tumors | — | 8 (5) | — |
| Ross et al. 1990 | Ultra Fast CT | Lung Tumors | Heart Aorta Diaphragm Chest Wall | 9.2 8.7 Out of view <3 | Lateral Lateral Cranio-caudal Unspecified |
| Seppenwoolde et al. 2002 | Fluoroscopy Gold Marker | Lung Tumors | Lower Lobes Attached to Aortic Arch | 12 (2) 2 (1) 1-4 | Cranio-caudal Lateral/AP-PA With Heart Beat |
| Shimizu et al. 2000 | Sequential CT at same Position | Lung Tumors | Inferior Lobes Superior Lobes | 39.4% in and out 0% in | — |
| Wade 1954 | Fluoroscopy | Diaphragm | Diaphragm | 17 (3) | — |
| Wagman et al. 2003 | Fluoroscopy, CT Port Films | Diaphragm, Liver, Spleen, Kidneys, GTV | Diaphragm/ Superior Abdomen | 22.7 12.8 | Diaphragm Other organs |
| Weiss, Baker, and Potchen 1972 | Fluoroscopy | Diaphragm | Diaphragm | 13 (5) | — |

## The Mechanics Of Breathing

It is useful to review briefly the basic mechanics and control of breathing that concern the development of methods to manage respiratory motion in radiation treatment. For more details, the reader can refer to standard physiology textbooks (West 1974; Nunn 1993).

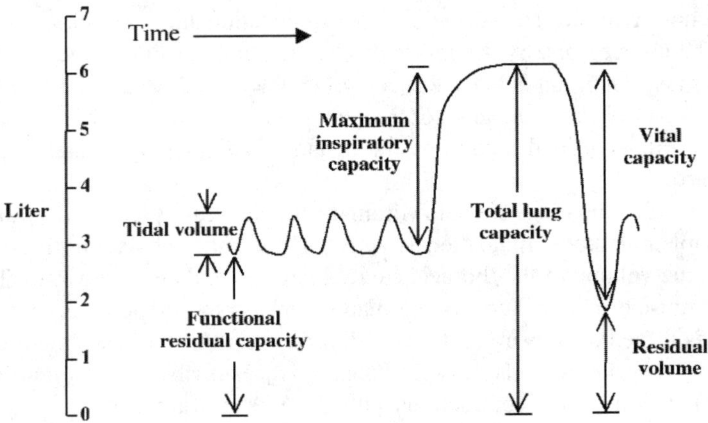


**Figure 1.** A schematic breathing trace of lung volumes that would be shown when a patient breathes through a spirometer. Note that residual volume and functional residual capacity cannot be measured with simple spirometry.

Figure 1 shows a schematic time trace of changing lung volumes that would be measured when a subject breathes through a spirometer. *Tidal volume* is the nominal gas volume that a person inhales and exhales during normal, quiet breathing. *Functional residual capacity* is the volume retained in the lungs at the end of normal exhalation. *Maximum inspiratory capacity* is the maximum gas volume that a person can breathe in with maximum inhalation effort. *Total lung capacity* is the maximum gas volume that the lungs can hold, and is equal to the sum of maximum inspiratory capacity and functional residual capacity. *Residual volume* is the volume retained after forced maximum exhalation. *Vital capacity* is the lung volume measured from maximum inhalation to maximum exhalation. Note that functional residual capacity and residual volume cannot be measured with simple spirometry. Instead, more involved methods of gas dilution or body plethysmograph need to be used.

The "static" lung volumes described in figure 1 can be highly variable between individuals. For a normal adult, tidal volume is roughly 500 ml, but can vary slightly from breath to breath because of the highly elastic nature of the lungs. About 150 ml of the tidal volumes are attributed to the dead space of the tracheo-bronchial tree that does not participate in gas exchanges. Tidal volume would increase if the dead space were artificially increased, such as when a patient is asked to breathe through a mouthpiece and tubing. For a normal adult, the vital capacity can range from 3 to 5 liters. The static lung volumes will vary noticeably with age, activities, and other physiological or disease status.

The primary function of the lung is to facilitate gas ($O_2$ and $CO_2$) exchange between blood and gas, thus maintaining normal levels of gas pressure, $P_{O_2}$ and $P_{CO_2}$, in the arterial blood. Respiration is an "involuntary" action; i.e., a person would continue to breathe despite being unconscious. Unlike cardiac motion, the respiratory motion is cyclic but not rhythmic. The periodic cycle of inhalation and exhalation is regulated, through chemoreceptors, by the levels of $CO_2$, $O_2$, and pH in the arterial blood. Of these, the most important is $P_{CO_2}$. Reducing $P_{CO_2}$, as would occur with hyperventilation, is a very effective means for reducing the urge to breathe, or sustaining breath-hold. Under normal conditions, the $O_2$ and pH stimuli play a small role in ventilation control.

Anatomically, the lungs are held within the thoracic cavity, encased by the liquid-filled intrapleural space. Inhalation is active. During the inhalation phase of quiet breathing, the volume of the thoracic cavity increases and air is drawn in. The most important muscle of inhalation is the diaphragm. As the diaphragm descends, the abdomen is forced downward and forward, increasing the vertical dimension of the chest cavity. The intercostals muscles connect adjacent ribs and also participate in normal inhalation. Their contractions pull the ribs upward and forward, thereby increasing both the lateral and anterior-posterior (AP) diameters of the thorax. Figures 2a and 2b show the schematic motions of the diaphragm and thorax during inhalation.

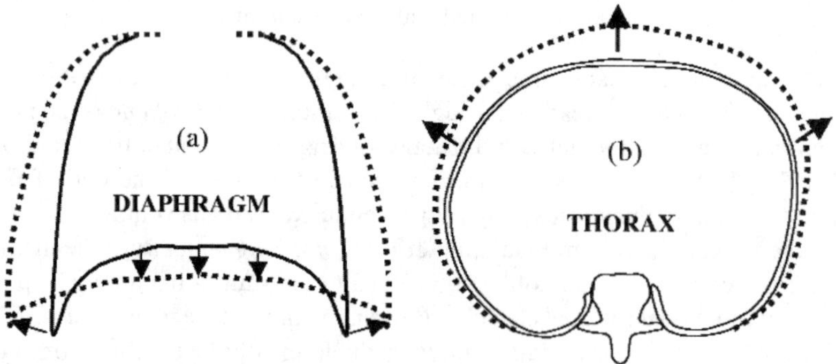


**Figure 2.** (a) On inhalation, the diaphragm contracts, the abdomen is forced down and forward, and the rib cage is lifted. (b) The intercostal muscles also contract to pull and rotate the ribs, resulting in increasing both the lateral and AP diameters of the thorax. [Reprinted from J. B. West, *Respiratory Physiology—The Essentials.* © 1974, with permission from Lippincott, Williams and Wilkins.]

Exhalation is passive for quiet breathing. The lung and chest wall are elastic and return passively to their pre-inhalation positions at the end of normal exhalation. Other ventilation muscles are involved only during active exhalation.

The normal pressure outside the lung is sub-atmospheric. The tendency of the lung to recoil to its deflated volume is opposed by the tendency of the chest cage to bow out. Indeed, the lung volume at the end of normal exhalation, i.e., functional residual capacity, is at equilibrium or the most relaxed state. Transpulmonary pressure, i.e., pressure around the lung, is lowered during inhalation, and recovered during exhalation. During normal breathing, the deflating lung volume is larger than the inflating volume at the same transpulmonary pressure. This is called "hysteresis," attributable to the complex respiratory pressure volume relationship of the lung and chest wall.

Few notable points can be made in regard to devising methods to manage breathing motion on radiation treatment. The lung is elastic and can be easily distended. As a result, tidal volume for each breath can vary. Diaphragmatic contraction is the major driving force for normal quiet inhalation. Intercostal muscles will also participate and may vary from breath to breath. At the end of normal exhalation, functional residual capacity represents the lung volume at its most neutral, thus reproducible, state. However, functional residual capacity may vary from day to day, depending on the physical and physiological conditions of the person. In so far that there is hysteresis in the inflating and deflating lung volumes, so would there be hysteresis in the positions of the chest wall, diaphragm, and thoracic contents during inhalation and exhalation. In active ventilation maneuvers, such as achieving maximum inhalation, all respiratory muscle groups will be recruited.

## Methods To Manage Respiratory Motion In Radiation Treatment

The traditional approach to accommodate the variation in target position associated with breathing is to examine its range of motion with fluoroscopy such that an adequate margin can be prescribed. The margin for breathing motion is typically more than 1 cm. When combined with the margin for setup error, the final margin is often 2 cm or more. In three-dimensions (3-D), the resultant planning target volume (PTV) would be expanded as the cube of the margin expansion, rendering significant irradiation of normal tissue volume.

Several methods are being developed to facilitate the reduction of margin for breathing motion. Inherently related to its acceptance by the treatment personnel and the patient, the accuracy and reproducibility of each procedure needs to be quantified. The problem needs to be studied in 3-D because breathing motion is non-uniform in 3-D. Figures 3a and 3b show the snapshots at end-exhalation and end-inhalation, respectively, from a cine-MRI (magnetic resonance imaging) study of quiet breathing in the coronal plane. Figure 3c shows the overlaid images where the regional difference in the lung outlines are shown in gray. Figures 4a, 4b, and 4c show the corresponding results from the cine-MRI study performed in the sagittal plane. For these selected image planes with the patient in the supine position, the lung expansion is more noticeable in the inferior and posterior directions of the diaphragm, than the expansion in the anterior and lateral directions of the chest wall.

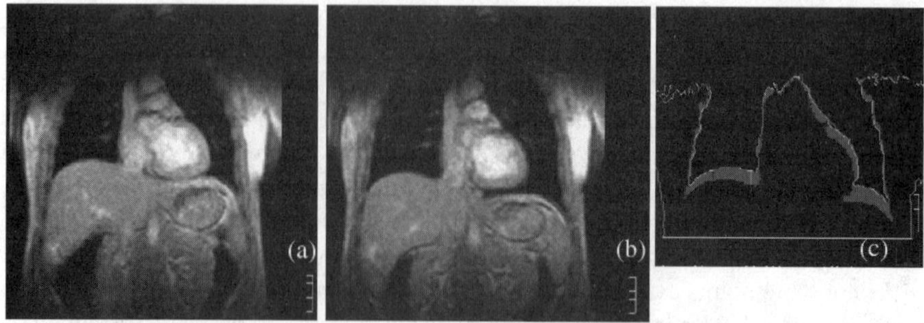

**Figure 3.** Snapshot images from a cine-MRI study of quiet breathing
in a coronal plane at (a) end exhalation and (b) end inhalation.
(c) The regional difference of the lung outlines is shown in gray shading.

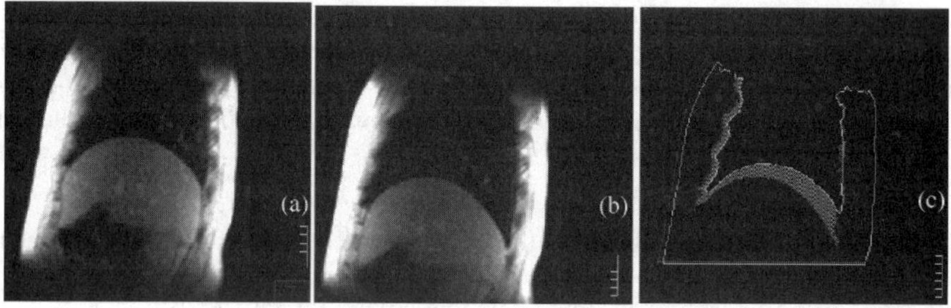

**Figure 4.** Snapshot images from a cine-MRI study of quiet breathing in a sagittal plane at
(a) end exhalation and (b) end inhalation. (c) The regional difference of the
lung outlines is shown in gray shading.

At present, there are two basic approaches to address the problem of breathing
motion in radiation treatment: (1) gating/tracking and (2) breath-hold maneuvers. Both
are active procedures that modify the operation of the treatment. In gating and tracking, the state of the treatment machine is adjusted in response to a signal that is
representative of a patient's breathing motion. With breath-holding, the lung volume
of the patient is directly immobilized prior to beam-on, and released after the beam is
off. Both approaches are similar to those techniques developed in the late 1980's for
x-ray computed tomography (CT) and MRI to minimize blurring of images due to
breathing motion (Korin et al. 1992; Jackson et al. 1993; Liu et al. 1993; Frohlich and
Dohring 1985; Jones 1982; Vock et al. 1990).

## Methods Of Gating And Tracking

For this chapter, the term "gating" pertains to turning the radiation beam on and off,
while tracking pertains to controlling the mechanical motion of the accelerator. Gating

and tracking are executed in response to a signal representative of the patient's respiration. These techniques allow the patient to breathe freely, and are considered more suitable for patients with compromised pulmonary status, such as those with lung cancers, who cannot sustain prolonged breath-hold.

The basic components of a gating or tracking system consist of a respiration sensor whose signal is processed and evaluated by a computer for suitability to trigger, or gate, the radiation. The earliest experience of applying respiratory-gated radiation therapy had come from Japan (Ohara et al. 1989; Osaka et al. 1997). In the United States Kubo reported the first technical feasibility study with a Varian 2100C accelerator in 1996 (Kubo and Hill 1996). A variety of respiration sensors were adapted in house in these earlier works, including strain gauge wrapped around the trunk, temperature sensor placed near the nose, spirometry (Kalender et al. 1990), and infrared light emitting diode [Osaka et al. 1997]. At present, a Real-time Position Management (RPM) system is commercially available from Varian Medical Systems (Palo Alto, CA) for automatic respiratory gating and has been employed by several investigators for evaluation and treatment (Mageras et al. 2001; Vedam et al. 2001).

*Respiratory Gating—Simulation*

The following material focuses primarily on the use of the Varian RPM system for respiratory gating and is largely the experience at Memorial Sloan-Kettering Cancer Center (MSKCC). The RPM system is based on the breathing synchronized radiation therapy camera-based system (Kubo et al. 2000), which tracks the motion of a small plastic block with a pair of reflective markers placed on the abdomen or chest of the patient (see figure 5). The positions of the corners of the marker block are tattooed on the skin for reproducible repositioning. A charge-coupled device (CCD) camera is used to capture the images of the markers illuminated by infrared emitting diodes. The software tracks the position of the top marker, while the separation between top and bottom markers provides a distance calibration. Figure 6 shows a graphical representation of the marker motion displayed on the workstation. An algorithm in the RPM system monitors the waveform and determines if it is regular. It also determines the phase of the breathing cycle, assigning phase = 0 to the waveform maximum.

In a combined immobilization and training session at a conventional simulator outfitted with the RPM system, fluoroscopy is recorded in synchrony with the external marker position. During simulation, the operator adjusts separately the phase for the start (beam enable) and end (beam disable) of the treatment gate, by inspecting the respiration waveform (see figure 6) and/or by viewing the resultant anatomic motion during the gate interval with fluoroscopic imaging.

When the RPM system is used with "normal" breathing (versus breath-hold), regular and reproducible breathing is important for efficient, accurate respiratory-gated simulation and treatment. The beam-enable or CT trigger signal is not issued with irregular breathing, which thus compromises the efficiency of the respiratory gating procedures. Worse, as shown in figure 7, an irregular breathing pattern can potentially result in image acquisition and/or beam delivery at the wrong phase of the breathing cycle.

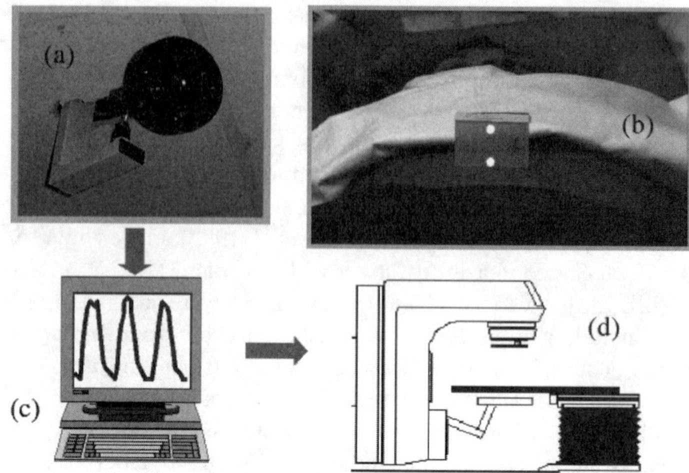

**Figure 5.** A pictorial schematic of the functioning of the Varian RPM system, consisting of (a) a wall-mounted infrared illuminator and CCD camera; (b) reflective external marker placed on a patient's abdomen or chest; (c) a workstation to process signals; and (d) generate trigger to the accelerator, simulator or CT scanner. The trigger can be based on amplitude or phase of the respiratory signal.

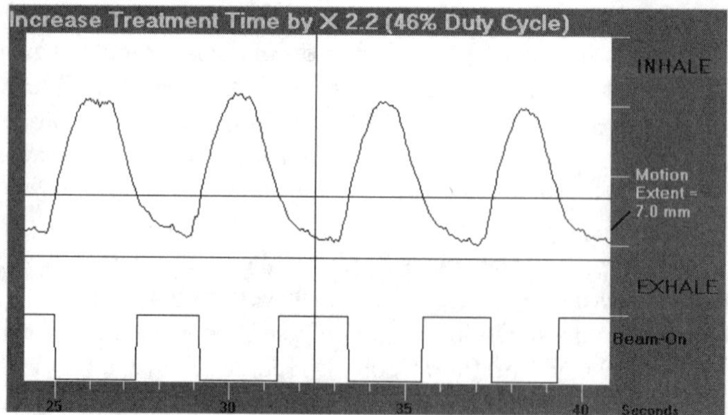


**Figure 6.** Example of a respiration trace from the RPM monitor screen for patient treated at end expiration. The horizontal lines specify the portion of the respiration trace within which the beam is enabled. The square-wave in the display indicates beam-enable status.

In order to reduce breathing irregularity, it is advisable to set the gating thresholds around end-exhalation, i.e., at functional residual capacity, for more stable lung volume and slower breathing motion. The longer quiescent period also provides a longer duty cycle. In addition, simple verbal coaching instructions ("breathe in…breathe out") have been shown to improve regularity (Mageras et al. 2001). Figure 8 shows that with verbal instructions, the patient can be coached to breathe with a higher and less variable tidal volume.

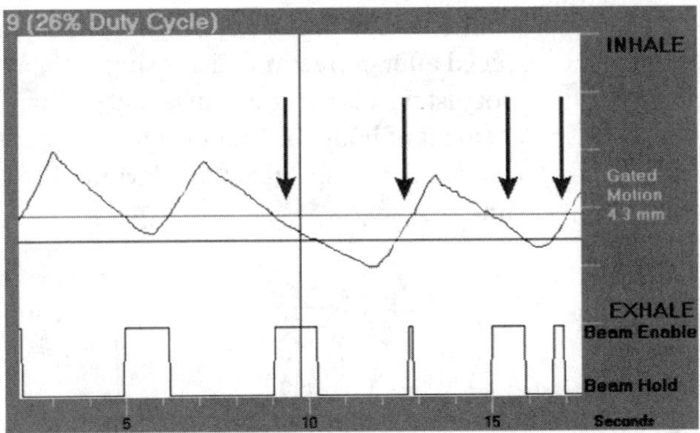



**Figure 7.** Irregular breathing can result in treatment or image acquisition at the wrong portion of the breathing cycle (arrows).

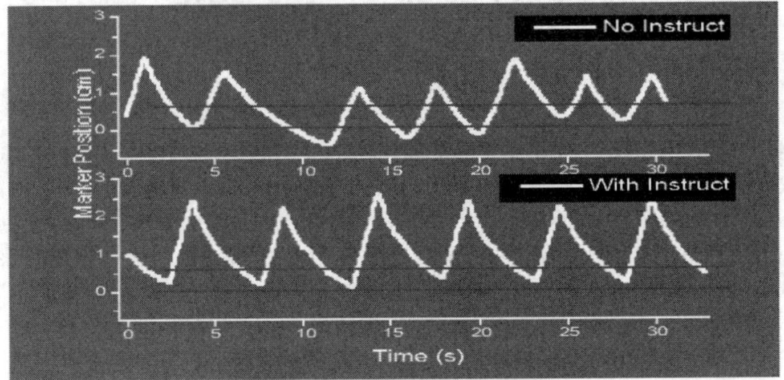



**Figure 8.** Comparison of the RPM traces : (top) for a free breathing sequence and (lower) one where the verbal instruction is given. Verbal instruction improves regularity of the breathing sequence. [Reprinted from *Journal of Applied Clinical Medical Physics*, vol 2, G. S. Mageras, E. Yorke, K. Rosenzweig, L. Braban, E. Keatley, E. Ford, S. A. Leibel, and C. C. Ling, "Fluoroscopic evaluation of diaphragmatic motion reduction with a respiratory gated radiotherapy system," pp. 191–200. © 2001, with permission from the American College of Medical Physics.]

It is important to note that, at present, clinical implementation of respiratory-gated radiation delivery using the RPM system requires considerable care and patient-specific quality assurance (QA). With any surrogate respiratory signal, it is assumed that there is a one-to-one correspondence between the signal (the motion of the markers on the patient's chest) and the patient's internal anatomy (tumor and critical normal tissues). Figure 9a shows the comparison of the trace of diaphragm position measured from the recorded fluoroscopic images with that of the RPM marker. There is an apparent lag of 0.7 s between them.

Figures 9b and c show the scatter-plot of the positions of diaphragm versus those of the markers before correction for a 0.7 s lag and after correction, respectively. The dispersion of the points is reduced after correction. The results indicate that for some patients, anatomical motion (not just the diaphragm) can be out of phase with the RPM marker trace. Given the involvement of both diaphragm and chest wall in ventilation, these observations are perhaps not surprising since the RPM marker block is placed only at one position on the trunk.

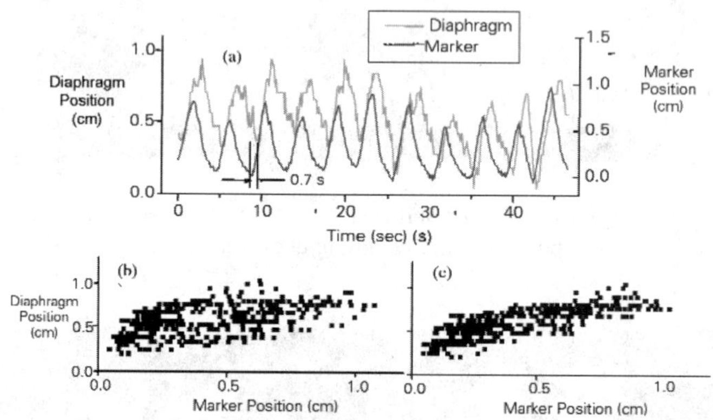


**Figure 9.** (a) Comparison of diaphragm positions measured from fluoroscopy with that of the RPM marker, showing a lag of 0.7 s. (b) Scatter-plot of the diaphragm positions versus those of the RPM marker before correction for a 0.7 s lag and (b) after correction. [Reprinted from *Journal of Applied Clinical Medical Physics*, vol 2, G. S. Mageras, E. Yorke, K. Rosenzweig, L. Braban, E. Keatley, E. Ford, S. A. Leibel, and C. C. Ling, "Fluoroscopic evaluation of diaphragmatic motion reduction with a respiratory gated radiotherapy system," pp. 191–200. © 2001, with permission from the American College of Medical Physics.]

*Respiratory Gating—CT Simulation And Studies*

The results of figure 9 indicate that with the respiratory gating, it is important to examine the relationship of the surrogate respiratory signal with the patient's internal anatomy. It follows that 3-D CT scans are needed at the intended treatment respiratory phase, not only for dose calculation purposes, but also in repeats for proper design of treatment margin.

**Respiratory-Triggered CT.** The initial method of Respiratory-triggered CT (RTCT) has been developed with the standard single slice helical CT scanner in mind. The methodology follows that of figure 5. The RPM system is mounted to move with the CT couch (see figure 10). The CT scanner is triggered by the RPM system. The projection data are acquired in the step-wise axial mode with 1 s gantry rotation. Even with regular breathing, respiration-triggered image acquisition will take longer than with free-breathing (FB) because only part of the breathing cycle is used. For example, if the breathing period is 5 s, acquiring a 60-slice study at the rate of one CT image per breathing cycle (e.g., only at end-expiration) on a single slice scanner requires 5 minutes under ideal conditions of regular breathing—compared to 1 min for helical, free-breathing acquisition at 1 slice/s.

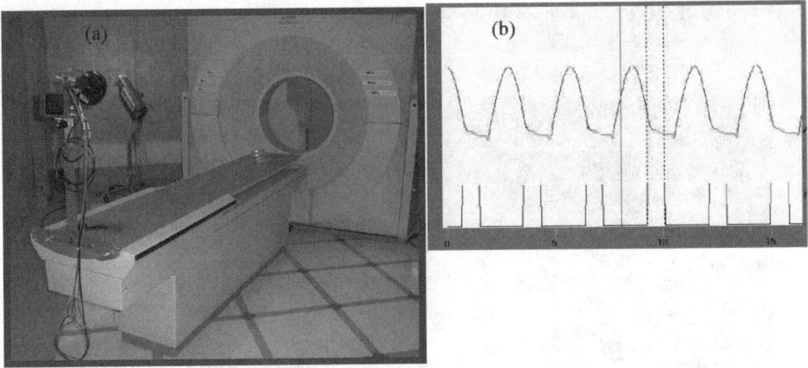

**Figure 10.** (a) A picture of the RPM system mounted on a CT scanner at MSKCC. (b) Display of the RPM trace that was used to trigger the 1 sec CT scan in the axial mode. [Courtesy of G. Mageras.]

Figures 11a and 11b show the sagittal view of the patient scan acquired in the standard helical mode; and one acquired with respiratory trigger, respectively. Motion artifacts at the diaphragmatic region are clearly visible in the former; but much reduced in the RTCT. However, despite vocal coaching, it is not uncommon for some irregular breathing to occur at CT simulation, causing out-of-phase slices and motion artifacts, as shown in figure 11c. At MSKCC, the "bad slices" during RTCT simulation are recorded for deletion if desired and reacquired when regular breathing resumes.

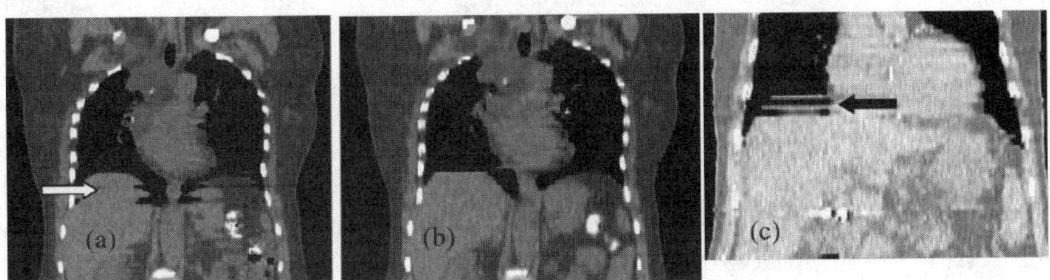

**Figure 11.** Sagittal views of (a) a helical scan acquired during free-breathing with motion artifacts (arrow); (b) a respiratory-triggered scan; (c) artifacts (arrow) can occur for RTCT if the patient's breathing is irregular.

Respiratory-triggered CT had been instrumental in demonstrating the potential gain of respiratory-gated treatment. In eight patients, end-exhalation (E) and end-inhalation (I) triggered scans were acquired. Shifts of the centroids of the liver, right and left kidneys, spleen, and gross target volume (GTV) were measured between the ends of the respiratory cycle (E-I), and also between repeat end-exhalation (E-E) scans. On average, the shift in the superior-to-inferior (SI) between E-I scans was 12.8 mm (range: 3.0 to 29.2 mm); and 2.0 mm (range: 0.0 to 6.4 mm) between repeat E-E scans. Figure 12 shows the results graphically. The larger variation observed for the spleen can be expected, given that this organ changes size with the cyclical wash-in and wash-out of blood.

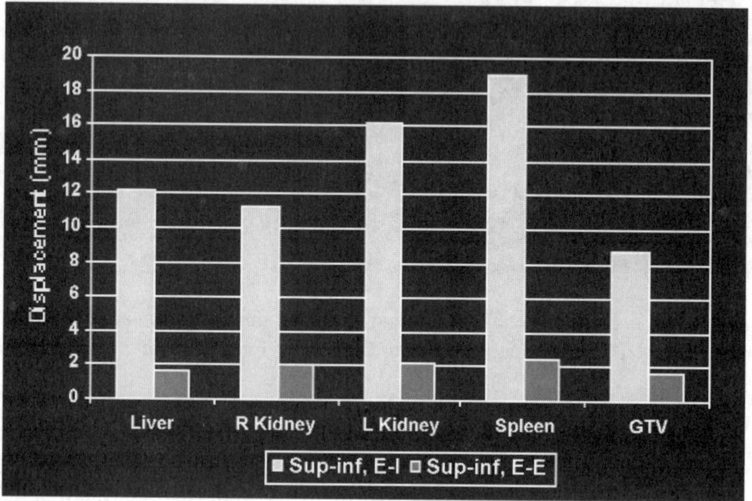



**Figure 12.** The displacements of the centroids of different organs measured using respiratory-triggered CT scans acquired at end-exhalation (E) and end-inhalation (I); and repeat end-exhalation scans. [Reprinted from *International Journal of Radiation Oncology Biology Physics*, vol 55, R. Wagman, E. Yorke, E. Ford, P. Giraud, G. Mageras, B. Minsky, and K. Rosenzweig, "Respiratory gating for liver tumors: use in dose escalation," pp. 659–668. © 2003, with permission from Elsevier.]

The RTCT technique, however, has two significant limitations. First, the CT sessions tend to be long. A study of reproducibility and margin design would require repeating multiple respiration-triggered scans. The long acquisition times increase the likelihood of patient movement and irregular breathing during the CT session. Second, with RTCT, the respiratory phase at which the slice acquisition is triggered must be decided before the scan is performed. The appropriate phase is usually chosen by inspecting the respiration waveform, or by examination of anatomic motion under fluoroscopy. There is no information about the variation of tumor and organ positions during breathing. Because of the 1 s scan time, there will be residual motion in each RTCT. A study of repeat CT scans at the same respiratory phase has found a mean variation in diaphragm position of 3 mm (Giraud et al. 2003) and would affect definition of the PTV. A more efficient approach than RTCT for acquiring CT scans at different phases is needed to provide important information in defining an appropriate PTV for respiratory-gated treatment.

**Respiration-Correlated Spiral CT**. Of significant importance to the study of respiratory motion with CT is the recent development of the Respiration-Correlated Spiral CT (RCCT) technique [Ford et al. 2003]. RCCT is an adaptation of the technique for cardiac imaging [Kachelriess, Ulzheimer, and Kalender 2000] which allows the acquisition of complete 3-D image data sets at multiple phases with a single spiral CT scan. The details of the method are published recently [Ford et al. 2003], and will only be described briefly in this chapter.

In the RCCT procedure, there is no triggering of the CT scanner by the RPM system. Instead, the x-ray ON signal and the corresponding spiral CT projection data are indexed with the respiration waveform from the RPM. The combined information is then used to retrospectively correlate CT slice with respiration phase. The principle of operation is illustrated in figure 13. By setting a small pitch, i.e., the ratio of table advance to the slice thickness acquired in one rotation, the table is moved slowly such that sufficient data can be acquired for CT image reconstruction over the entire respiratory cycle.

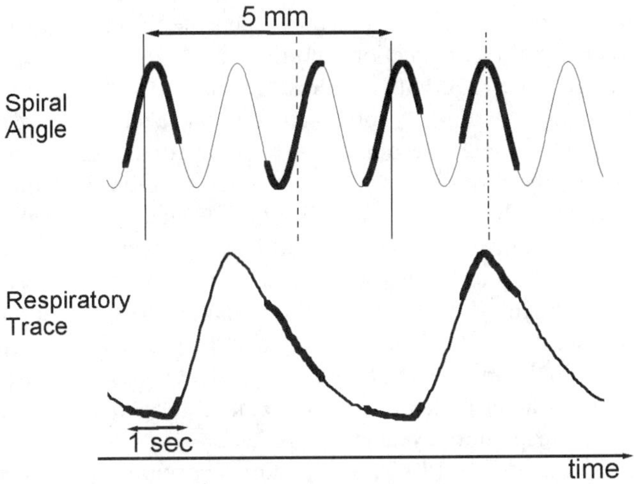


**Figure 13.** Schematic of the respiration-correlated CT (RCCT) technique. The respiratory waveform (lower part of figure, actual patient data) is acquired as the table is advanced in position and the spiral progresses (upper part of figure shows CT gantry angle vs. time). Vertical lines correspond to CT slices at end expiration (solid line), end inspiration (dot-dashed), and an intermediate respiratory phase (dashed). In this example, the data to reconstruct a slice span an interval of 230° or approximately 1 second (bold line segments), and the spacing between slices at the same respiratory phase is 5 mm. [Reprinted from *Medical Phys*ics, vol 30, E. C. Ford, G. S. Mageras, E. Yorke, and C. C. Ling, "Respiration-correlated spiral CT: A method of measuring respiratory-induced anatomic motion for radiation treatment planning," pp. 88–97. © 2003, with permission from AAPM].

Two quantities are important in acquiring an optimal RCCT data set. They are (1) the gap between slices from successive respiratory cycles, i.e., the region in which no CT data are acquired at a particular phase, and (2) the elapsed fraction of the respiratory period to acquire complete CT data for reconstructing one slice. For a 180° reconstruction algorithm and a fan beam CT geometry with the detector bank subtending an angle $\Phi$, the data for one complete slice are acquired with a gantry rotation of $\pi+\Phi$ (Ford et al. 2003).

Both the gap and elapsed respiratory fraction are dependent on the selection of the CT scan pitch and gantry rotation period. Minimizing the gap and fractional slice time would improve the quality of RCCT image. There are trade-offs. Depending on the pitch of the table, if the rotation period is short in comparison with the respiratory period, better temporal resolution is achieved but the gap is larger. Conversely, if the rotation period is long, the gap will be reduced, but the mixing of the temporal information will be increased. In general, using a smaller pitch is advantageous for reducing gaps. However, using a smaller pitch will increase the total time for a scan and will limit the length of the region that can be scanned before exceeding the x-ray tube heat capacity. The smallest pitch consistent with the requirements of the scan should be used. In addition, in order to achieve the best temporal resolution, one should also choose the smallest fraction of gantry rotation adequate for reconstructing one slice, such as selecting a 180° reconstruction algorithm.

The experience at MSKCC with a Philips/Marconi PQ5000 scanner indicates that for RCCT, a combination of gantry rotation of 1.5 s and a table pitch of 0.5 offers the best compromise for temporal resolution (~1 s per slice) and gap width. For a slice thickness of 3 mm, the resultant resolution in couch position (including slice thickness and gap width) is between 4 mm and 6 mm depending on respiratory period, comparable to the 5 mm slices acquired with RTCT. Depending on the respiratory period, a RCCT will produce CT data at different respiratory phases. Because the respiratory cycle and the gantry rotation are not coordinated, the CT data for some of the reconstructed phases are not unique, meaning that the projection data might be used in adjacent slices. In theory, the number of independent phases per breathing cycle is the ratio of the respiratory period and the time that it takes to acquire a slice. In the example where the respiratory cycle is 5 s, CT gantry rotation is 1.5 s, and only 0.64 of the rotation is needed for a 180° reconstruction algorithm, the number of independent phases is 5.

Phantom studies have been performed at MSKCC to determine the effectiveness of RCCT. Figure 14 shows the experimental setup. A motor driven rod is used to move a spherical plastic phantom in an elliptical (vertical and longitudinal) cycle. The RPM system is mounted at the end of the CT couch to track the waveform of the motion and to facilitate RCCT. The speed and amplitude of motion can be varied to simulate a wide range of respiratory motion.

Figure 15 shows "sagittal" image reconstructions, i.e., in the vertical plane through the center of the motion phantom with various scanning protocols. Panel A is a scan with the phantom stationary at the lowest vertical position, corresponding to end expiration. In the scans of panels B–D, the phantom was moving with a period of 5.0 s.

The vertical excursion was 2.3 cm and the longitudinal excursion 1.9 cm. Panel B is a conventional spiral scan. Scans in A and B had slice thickness of 5 mm. Panel C shows a respiration-triggered axial scan of the phantom at the lowest vertical position, with a slice thickness of 5 mm. Panel D shows a RCCT scan reconstructed at the lowest vertical position. The reconstructed slice thickness was 0.5 mm, with an effective spacing between slices at the same phase of 5 mm. The RCCT scan yields image quality similar to that of the respiration-triggered scan. The RTCT image shows somewhat sharper edges and better-defined inner cavities, owing to the better temporal resolution of 0.64 s per slice, compared to 0.96 s for RCCT. The slightly lower temporal resolution for the latter is a limitation of the available settings on the single-slice scanner, and is a compromise to maintain acceptable spatial resolution in the longitudinal direction.

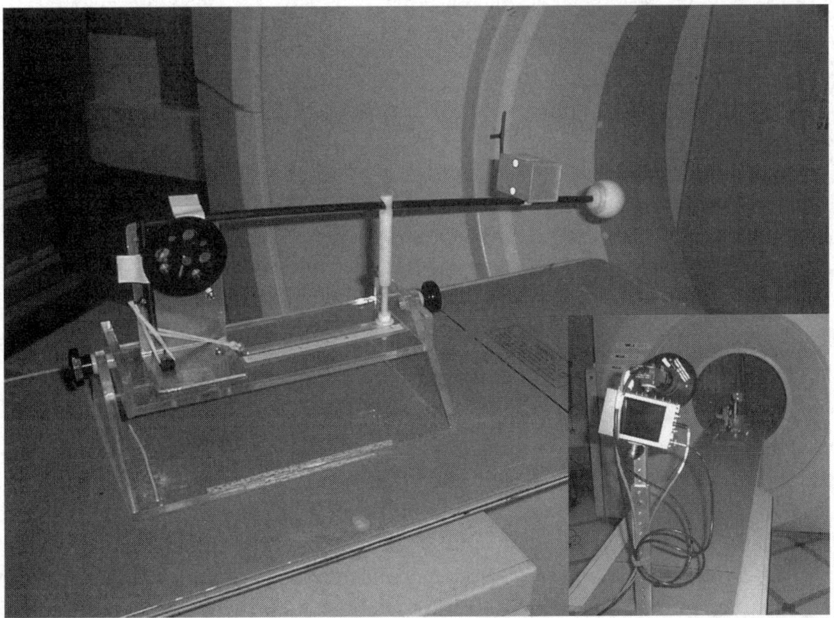

**Figure 14.** Motion phantom used for testing of the respiration-correlated CT technique. A plastic sphere, suspended on the end of the motor-driven rod, executes an elliptical motion in the vertical (anterior-posterior) and longitudinal (superior-inferior) directions. The speed is controlled remotely. The waveform of the marker block mounted on the rod is recorded by the RPM system. Inset shows the tracking camera of the RPM system mounted on the end of the CT couch. [Reprinted from *Medical Physics*, vol 30, E. C. Ford, G. S. Mageras, E. Yorke, and C. C. Ling, "Respiration-correlated spiral CT: A method of measuring respiratory-induced anatomic motion for radiation treatment planning," pp. 88–97. © 2003, with permission from AAPM].

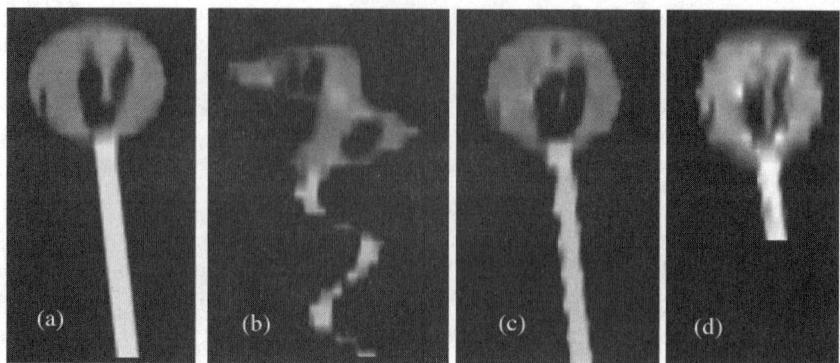



**Figure 15.** "Sagittal" section reconstructions from CT scans of the motion phantom at "end-expiration" (minimum of vertical motion) using various protocols. (a) Stationary phantom, standard spiral scan. (b) Moving phantom, standard spiral scan. (c) Moving phantom, respiration-triggered axial scan. (d) Moving phantom, respiration-correlated CT scan. The scans shown in panels (a) through (c) were acquired with 5 mm slice spacing and thickness. The phantom motion had a period of 5.0 seconds and excursions of 2.3 cm and 1.9 cm in the anterior-posterior (left-right) and superior-inferior (up-down) directions respectively. The dark regions within the plastic sphere are air cavities. [Reprinted from *Medical Physics*, vol 30, E. C. Ford, G. S. Mageras, E. Yorke, and C. C. Ling, "Respiration-correlated spiral CT: A method of measuring respiratory-induced anatomic motion for radiation treatment planning," pp. 88–97. © 2003, with permission from AAPM].

Figure 16 shows the sagittal views of the RCCT of the moving sphere at 10 different phases of the 5 s period. The centroid position of the sphere as a function of phase compares well to the expected position as measured with fluoroscopy. The mean difference is 1.1 mm in the AP direction (range: 0.1 to 4.0 mm), and 1.2 mm in the SI direction (range: 0.0 to 3.5 mm). Reconstructed volumes match those expected on the basis of stationary-phantom scans to within 5% in all cases. The surface distortions of the reconstructed sphere, as quantified by deviations from a mathematical reference sphere, are similar to those from a stationary phantom scan and are correlated with the speed of the phantom. The mean deviation is about 1 mm with the largest deviation of 3 mm occurring when the phantom is moving fastest.

RCCT is a major advance that will play an important role in the study of the effects of breathing motion on radiation treatment. It is significantly more convenient than RTCT. Multiple phases of respiration are imaged with RCCT in approximately the same scanning time required to image a single phase with a triggered axial scan. RCCT can be used in conjunction with respiratory-gated treatment to identify the patient-specific phase of minimum tumor motion, determine residual tumor motion within the gate interval, and compare treatment plans at different phases. The four-dimensional (4-D) temporal information is imperative in the development of tracking delivery method where the mechanical components of the accelerator tracks target motion associated with breathing. Equally important, RCCT provides a practical means for repeating important CT studies of the patient's breathing motion during the course of treatment, which, at present, is assumed to be maintained after the initial planning session.

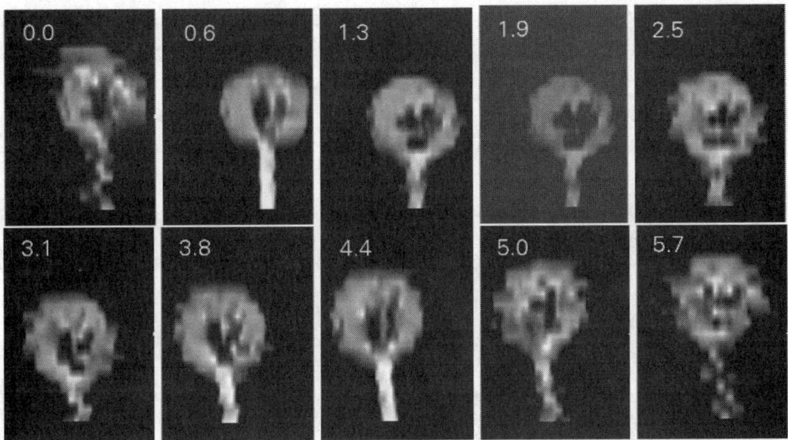

**Figure 16.** Sagittal reconstructions of the motion phantom from an RCCT scan from ten phases of the respiratory cycle. The respiratory phase of each image is shown in radians. The phantom motion had a period of 5.0 seconds and excursions of 2.3 cm and 1.9 cm in vertical and longitudinal directions respectively. [Reprinted from *Medical Phys*ics, vol 30, E. C. Ford, G. S. Mageras, E. Yorke, and C. C. Ling, "Respiration-correlated spiral CT: A method of measuring respiratory-induced anatomic motion for radiation treatment planning," pp. 88–97. © 2003, with permission from AAPM].

At present, the quality of RCCT scans, while acceptable, is inferior to breath-hold CT scans. It is limited by the temporal and spatial resolution of single slice helical scanner. X-ray tube heating also restricts the length of the scan region to 9 cm for typical RCCT settings. These limitations will be inconsequential with the advent of the multi-slice scanner. Figures 17a, 17b, and 17c show the transverse, coronal, and sagittal views, respectively, of a recent RCCT scan at the same respiratory phase (out of 10) acquired at MSKCC using a four-slice scanner (Discover QX/i, GE Medical Systems). The scan length spanned 30 cm, slice spacing was 2.5 mm and the scan period was 0.5 s. The improvement in resolution is impressive.

## Respiratory-Gated Treatment

At present, delivery of respiratory-gated treatment is under investigation at a few centers. The assumptions that (1) there is a one-to-one correspondence between the external respiratory signal and internal anatomy, and (2) this relationship is maintained over the entire course of treatment need to be validated before dissemination for general clinical use.

At MSKCC, the RPM system has been used for gated static and IMRT treatments of over 30 lung cancer and liver cancer patients (Wagman et al. 2003). RPM is well tolerated by patients and technical staff. Clinical implementation requires considerable care and patient-specific QA. Changes in breathing pattern can occur. They could be due to changes in the use of diaphragm and chest wall; or variation in the functional residual capacity from day to day. To promote breathing regularity, recorded voice instructions, customized for the individual patient, are played during treatments. Well-trained therapists are a vital component of RPM-gated treatments. They must watch the displayed motion trace and turn the beam off if they see serious irregularity or drift, then re-track the marker, and/or talk to the patient before proceeding.

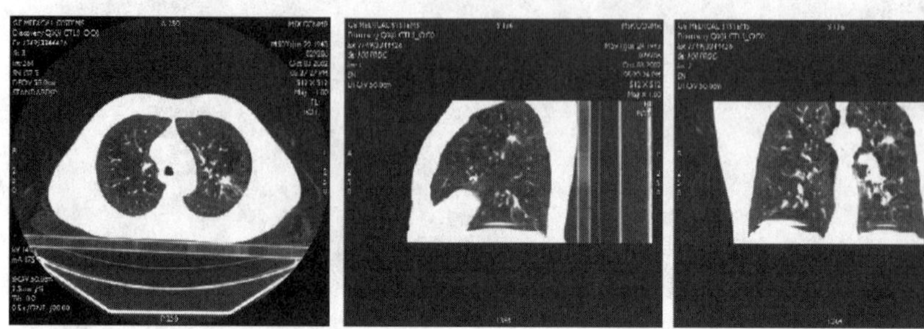

**Figure 17.** The (a) transverse, (b) coronal and (c) sagittal views at the same respiratory phase of a RCCT scan acquired at MSKCC using a 4-slice scanner. Ten phases were acquired at 0.5 s per slice, 2.5 cm slice spacing. [Courtesy of G. Mageras.]

Of necessity, gated beam delivery takes longer than conventional delivery. For example, if a patient breathes regularly with a 5 s period and the gate results in a 33% duty cycle, delivering 100 monitor units (MUs) on an accelerator operated at 300 MU/min takes 60 s (compared to 20 s without gating). Some time can be recovered by treating at maximum dose rate; of course, most of "treatment time" is spent on setup rather than beam delivery. Up to 10 min extra is allowed for gated treatment depending on patient compliance.

At MSKCC, megavoltage portal images have been used for treatment QA and to determine how well the RPM system controls internal anatomy. The diaphragm is the most visible surrogate for tumor motion and has been shown to correlate well for liver tumors (Dawson et al. 2001). For some lung cancer patients, there are also soft tissue features visible within the GTV. For each patient receiving gated treatment, AP or PA localization films (diaphragm films) showing the isocenter, diaphragm, and vertebral landmarks are taken in addition to the usual weekly double-exposed treatment port films. The distance between the diaphragm apex and a fixed bony landmark and the distance between the apex and isocenter are measured. The former distance reflects the gating system performance while the latter includes setup error and directly impacts the dose distribution in the patient. (see inset of figure 18).

Studies of fluoroscopic movies of the first eight patients treated with RPM at MSKCC [Ford et al. 2002] indicate that gated treatment is capable of reducing the patient-averaged standard deviation of the diaphragm position (i.e., intrafractional motion) from 6.9±2.1 mm (no gate) to 2.6±1.7 mm (gated). Anterior-posterior portal images (at least weekly) of these patients showed a mean deviation of the diaphragm position relative to bony anatomy (i.e., interfractional variation) of 2.8±1.0 mm. Figure 18 shows the results from the fluoroscopic studies and those from portal image analysis.

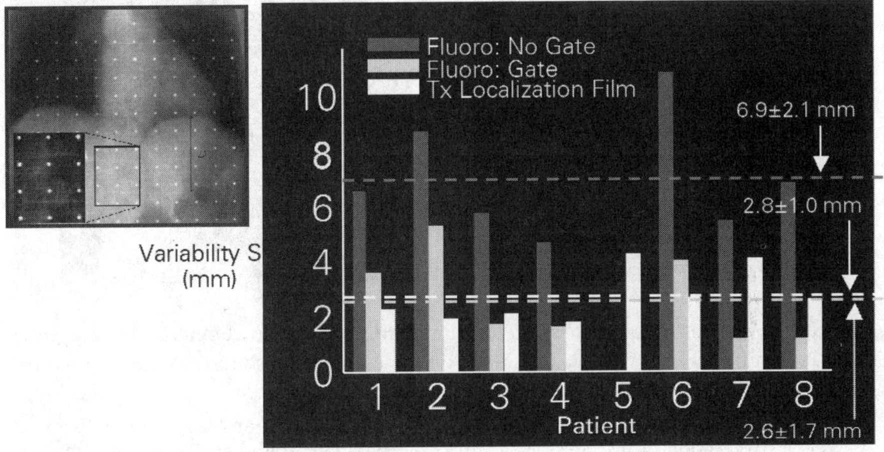


**Figure 18.** The comparison of diaphragm variability using gated fluoroscopy and gated localization film measurements, based on the landmark shown in the inset. [Reprinted from *International Journal of Radiation Oncology Biology Phys*ics, vol 52, E. C. Ford, G. S. Mageras, E. Yorke, K. E. Rosenzweig, R. Wagman, and C. C. Ling, "Evaluation of respiratory movement during gated radiotherapy using film and electronic portal imaging," pp. 522–531. © 2002, with permission from Elsevier.]

However, figures 19a and 19b show that for four of the eight patients, the diaphragm position on port films showed a systematic shift of more than 4 mm relative to its position on the digitally reconstructed radiograph (DRR) constructed from the planning CT simulation. Studies of subsequent patients confirm these initial findings, that systematic differences between the diaphragm position at simulation and at treatment occur for a significant fraction of patients. Care must be taken to detect and correct for such systematic shifts. At MSKCC, three diaphragm films are reviewed during each of the first 2 weeks of treatment. If no systematic differences are observed, the frequency of imaging is reduced, to bi-weekly then weekly. For systematic errors over 4 to 5 mm, the fields are adjusted according to the discretion of the physician. For the 30 patients treated with respiratory gating, field adjustments were made for 5 of the 30 patients. Techniques for convenient visualization of tumor location throughout the course of treatment, or to determine whether the diaphragm is a valid surrogate for lung tumor position would be a helpful adjunct to RPM gating—or any form of gating based on an external marker.

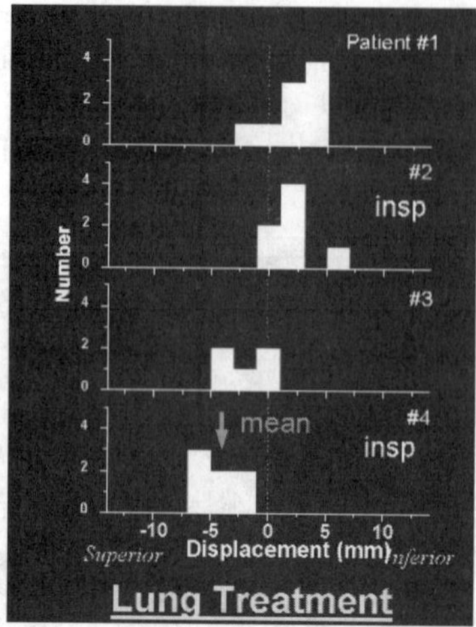


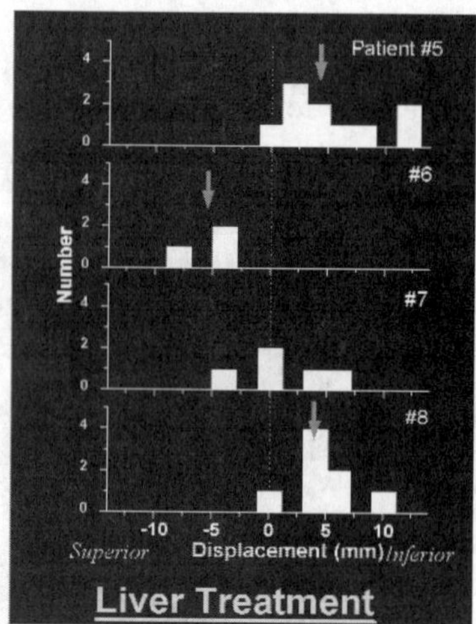


**Figure 19.** Analysis of the diaphragm position during the course of treatment using gated localization films. Four patients (arrows) exhibited systematic shifts of more than 4 mm relative to DRR. [Reprinted from *International Journal of Radiation Oncology Biology Physics*, vol 52, E. C. Ford, G. S. Mageras, E. Yorke, K. E. Rosenzweig, R. Wagman, and C. C. Ling, "Evaluation of respiratory movement during gated radiotherapy using film and electronic portal imaging," pp. 522–531. © 2002, with permission from Elsevier.]

Because of the uncertainty about the one-to-one correspondence between the external respiratory signal and internal anatomy with the RPM system, Shirato et al. (2000) has implemented a more direct approach of triggering radiation based on fluoroscopic images of a 2 mm gold marker implanted in the tumor or its vicinity. Figure 20 shows three of the four in-room mounted fluoroscopy units which, in pairs, allow continuous localization of the marker at 30 frames per sec (fps), regardless of gantry position. A pattern recognition software is used to detect when the marker is within a threshold window or "permitted dislocation" for triggering the radiation. Phantom studies with the marker have shown that a moving target can be irradiated with an accuracy of ±1 mm. The approach has merits, although the validity of the single marker as surrogate for 3D tumor motion needs to be validated. There are also concerns with the length of treatment and the corresponding increase of fluoroscopic dose to the patient.

*Methods Of Tracking*

An inherent limitation of respiratory-gated treatment is the shortened duty cycle. Respiratory tracking is a recent development that aims to alleviate the delivery inefficiency. Typically, the MLC is moved to conform to the moving target with the beam on continuously. The basic requirement is knowledge of the respiratory motion at all times, as provided by RCCT. A direct approach under development at Tohoku University in Japan (Takai et al. 2002) is to image and track the motion of a gold marker implanted in the tumor. Figures 21a and 21b show the accelerator-mounted dual fluoroscopy system

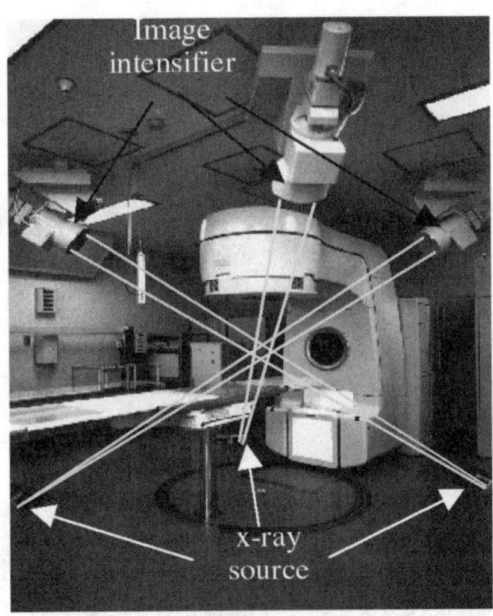



**Figure 20.** A picture of the in-room mounted fluoroscopy units to facilitate
real-time tracking of a gold marker in the tumor for triggering radiation. [Reprinted
from *International Journal of Radiation Oncology Biology Physics*, vol 48, H. Shirato,
S. Shimizu, K. Kitamura, T. Nishioka, K. Kagei, S. Hashimoto, A. Aoyama, T. Kuneida,
N. Shinohara, H. Dosaka-Akita, and K. Miyasaka, "Four-dimensional treatment planning
and fluoroscopic real-time tumor tracking radiotherapy for moving tumor,"
pp. 435–442. © 2000, with permission from Elsevier.]

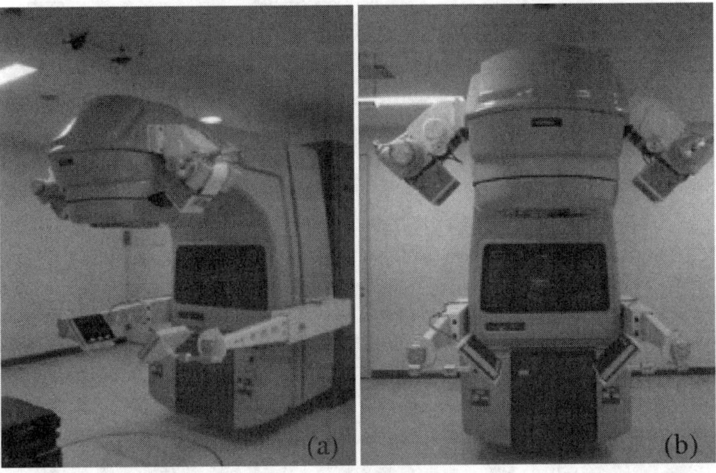



**Figure 21.** The side (a) and front (b) views of an accelerator-mounted dual fluoroscopic
imaging system with amorphous silicon flat panel detectors. Orthogonal images facilitate
continuous irradiation that tracks tumor motion (using gold marker). [Courtesy of Y. Takai.]

684                                    **John Wong**

using two amorphous silicon flat-panel detectors. Orthogonal fluoroscopic images are acquired of the markers during respiration as shown in figure 22. The (x,y,z) position of the marker is detected in real-time and the information is used to move the MLC for tracking, as shown in figure 23. Taking the tracking method one step further, it has been proposed that a robotic accelerator (Murphy et al. 2003) can be used to track tumor motion for delivering pencil beam irradiation from all orientations, taking advantage of its high degree of movement freedom. In-room fluoroscopic systems similar to that of figure 20 are used to provide the tracking signal. The pencil beam delivery approach readily accommodates complex intensity modulation. For robotic delivery, tracking tumor that moves due to respiration is a necessity given the long treatment time associated with the system (Murphy et al. 2002).

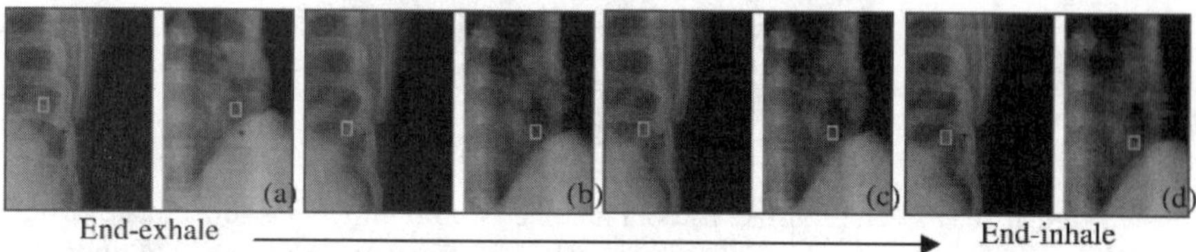


**Figure 22.** A sequence (a–d) of orthogonal pair images showing the gold seed motion with respiration, from end of normal exhalation to end of normal inhalation. The rectangles mark the region encompassing the implanted gold seed, which is analyzed in real-time for tracking (see figure 23). [Courtesy of Y. Takai.]

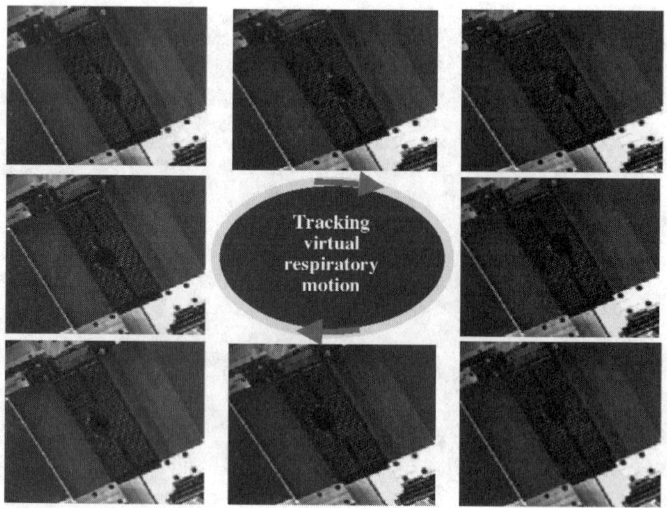


**Figure 23.** A sequence of pictures showing, as conceptual demon-stration, the use of the MLC to track the motion of the implanted gold seed during one cycle of respiration. [Courtesy of Y. Takai.]

Another interesting application of tracking delivery pertains to IMRT in the presence of breathing motion. Several publications (Ramsey, Cordrey, and Oliver 1999; Kubo and Wang 2000; Yorke et al. 2000) report negligible dosimetric effects of gated operation for both static and sliding window IMRT fields. The RPM system has been used for gated IMRT treatments in lung and liver cancer patients at MSKCC (Wagman et al. 2003). However, treatment time would increase. Combining the 50% duty cycle for IMRT delivery and 25% for gating, the duty cycle for gated IMRT can be as low as 12.5%. In order to overcome the inefficiency of respiratory-gated IMRT, Keall et al. (2001) have adapted the dynamic MLC segments to track the respiratory motion of the tumor. The external respiratory signal from the RPM system, correlated with the 4-D motion information from the RCCT, is used to drive the MLC segments. Film measurements with an oscillating sinusoidal motion phantom show that 4-D IMRT is feasible and its dosimetry is similar to the delivery of IMRT to a static target. The approach holds promise, although it is very much in the investigation stage.

It is important to note that with respiratory-gated or tracked delivery, great care must be exercised to establish sound correlation of the respiration signal and the internal target motion. This applies to external surrogate and also implanted internal markers. The validity of the surrogate signal in providing accurate translation and rotation motion information about the tumor needs to be established. Similarly, the degree of organ deformation that cannot be inferred from the surrogate signal must also be examined. It is therefore imperative that the breathing motion must be analyzed in 3-D in treatment planning. For a conventional course of fractionated treatment that might extend over a few weeks, it is equally important to monitor possible changes in the 4-D CT information and to derive a new plan if necessary. Information about breathing motion during course of treatment is currently unavailable. The use of RCCT to study and support respiratory-gated or tracked delivery is of paramount importance.

*Methods Of Breath-Hold*

Breath-hold methods minimize the effects of breathing motion on radiation treatment by means of immobilization. Breath-hold has long been used in diagnostic radiology to reduce the blurring of images. For radiation therapy, the requirement is to attain the same breath-hold position between beams delivered during a single treatment fraction, and also between treatment fractions. Reproducibility of the immobilization is based on the hypothesis that when the subject relaxes during breath-hold, the ventilation muscles would go to their predisposed positions associated with the given pulmonary volume or pressure. In principle, breath-hold delivery appears simpler to implement than respiratory-gated methods. Achieving immobilization seems less involved than determining the margin for residual motion in gated treatment. In practice, issues about reproducibility and patient compliance and comfort need to be addressed, particularly for those patients with compromised pulmonary status.

Because various ventilation muscles may or may not be involved in normal breathing, and the tidal volumes between breaths are variable, it is difficult for the patient to achieve reproducible breath-hold voluntarily during normal ventilation. Instead, breath-hold methods are typically applied at maximum or moderate deep inhalation (Hanley et al. 1999; Wong et al. 1999), or at the end of normal exhalation (Dawson et al. 2001), in hope of achieving better reproducibility. Deep inspiration actively recruits all ventilation muscles to expand the lungs, while the lung volume is at its most neutral state at the end of normal exhalation.

A breath-hold procedure typically involves applying a nose clip to the patient to prevent nose breathing (or leaking). A mouthpiece, connected to a digital flow-meter through tubing, is then given to the patient to breathe through. The flow-meter signal is converted to ventilation lung volume that can be displayed for visualization by the treatment personnel outside the room, or the patient for visual feedback purposes. A pre-defined lung volume is then used as the cue for applying breath-hold. Two approaches have been employed; voluntary deep inspiration breath-hold (DIBH), and breath-hold under active breathing control (ABC).

## Voluntary Deep Inspiration Breath-Hold (DIBH)

Voluntary DIBH was first implemented at MSKCC for radiation treatment of patients with lung cancer (Mah et al. 2000; Rosenzweig et al. 2000). (DIBH denotes breath-hold at *maximum* deep inspiration for the remaining text of this chapter). Each patient was instructed to first go through a few cycles of deep breathing (i.e., slow vital capacity maneuvers) to help decrease the volume of $CO_2$ in the lungs, and then coached to breathe in the largest lung volume possible and hold. Breath-holding at this level of maximum inspiration capacity is expected to be reproducible since the lungs could not expand any more. For the lung patients selected for treatment, the durations of breath-hold typically would allow a beam-on time of 10 s. The DIBH procedure would be repeated to complete delivery of a beam if necessary, or for another beam at a different gantry angle.

Figure 24a shows a subject in the voluntary DIBH treatment position. The reproducibility of the diaphragm position, in 1 standard deviation (SD), with respect to a bony landmark was examined with fluoroscopy during simulation, and also with port films acquired during the course of treatment. Figure 24b shows the results for seven patients. In general, the diaphragm position could be immobilized to within 2 mm during the same breath-hold; and 3 mm between breath-holds. The port film data show larger variability but include setup variation.

Over 20 lung patients were treated using DIBH at MSKCC since 1998 (Rosenzweig et al. 2000). As with respiratory-gated treatment which requires CT information at the intended phase for treatment, DIBH treatment requires CT and simulation information at DIBH. Because of the limited duration of breath-hold, DIBH CT scans of any extended length would need to be acquired piecemeal. Few advantages were noted. At large lung volume, the lung density would decrease and less lung mass would be irradiated. For some patients, as shown in figures 25a and 25b, deep inspiration would increase the separation of the target volume from a critical structure, such as the spinal cord, thereby making it easier to achieve normal tissue sparing. Even with keeping the same margin for free-breathing treatment, dose escalation was possible. Planning studies showed that on average, the target dose could be increased from 69.4 to 87.9 Gy, while keeping the lung NTCP at <25%. However, the most serious disadvantage of DIBH is patient compliance. The procedure requires significant effort and can tire the patient. At MSKCC, half the patients could not sustain DIBH for the duration of the treatment. Although it appears that DIBH would allow appreciable margin reduction of several millimeters, patients with lung cancer need to be screened for compliance before being selected for treatment at DIBH.

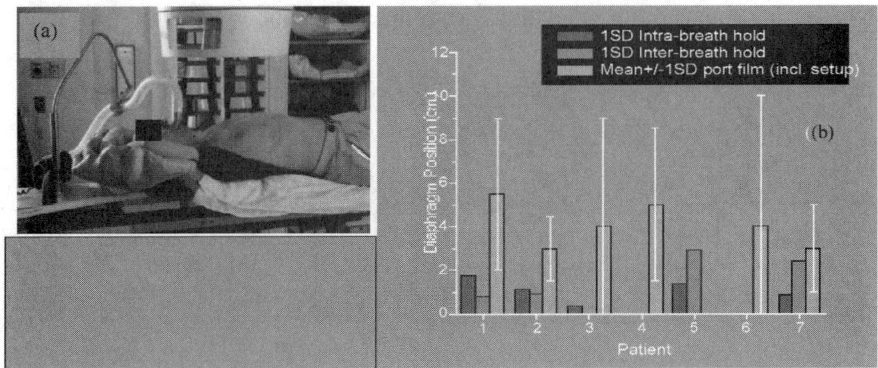


**Figure 24.** (a) A subject in the voluntary DIBH treatment position. (b) The variation of the diaphragm position with respect to a bony landmark measured using fluoroscopy during simulation and port films during the course of treatment. [Reprinted from *International Journal of Radiation Oncology Biology Phys*ics, vol 45, J. Hanley, M. M. Debois, D. Mah, G. S. Mageras, A. Raben, K. Rosenzweig, B. Mychalczak, L. H. Schwartz, P. J. Gloeggler, W. Lutz, C. C. Ling, S. A. Leibel, Z. Fuks, and G. J. Kutcher, "Deep inspiration breath-hold technique for lung tumors: The potential value of target immobilization and reduced lung density in dose escalation," pp. 603–611. © 1999, with permission from Elsevier.]

## Moderate Deep Inspiration Breath-Hold (mDIBH) With Active Breathing Control (ABC)

Active Breathing Control (ABC) is a method to facilitate reproducible breath-hold without requiring the patient to reach maximum inspiration capacity (Wong et al. 1999; Remouchamps et al. 2003a). The ABC method was developed at William Beaumont Hospital and is currently commercialized by Elekta Inc. (Norcross, GA) as the Active Breathing Coordinator. The ABC apparatus can be used to suspend breathing at any pre-determined position along the normal breathing cycle, or at active inspiration. The device consists of a digital spirometer to measure the respiratory trace, which is in turn connected to a balloon valve (see figure 26). In an ABC procedure, the patient breathes normally through the apparatus. When an operator "activates" the system, the lung volume and the phase (i.e., inhalation or exhalation) at which the balloon value will be closed are specified. The patient is then instructed to proceed to reach the specified lung volume, typically after taking two preparatory breaths. At this point, the valve is inflated with an air compressor for a pre-defined duration of time, thereby "holding" the patient's breath. The breath-hold duration is patient dependent, typically 15 to 30 seconds, and should be well tolerated to allow for repeated (after a brief rest period) breath-holds without causing undue patient distress. Figure 27 shows the display of the Elekta's ABC system, where the appearance of a green color shade (in this figure, the gray area above the waveform) serves to indicate both activation of the balloon valve and the lung volume at which it will close to maintain breath-hold. A timer display counts down remaining breath-hold duration in seconds.

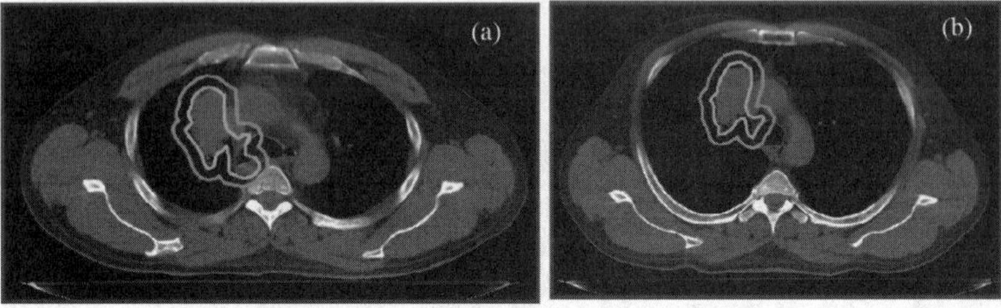


**Figure 25.** The separation between the PTV and the spinal cord in a (a) free-breathing plan is increased in the plan at (b) DIBH. [Courtesy of G. Mageras.]

## ABC Apparatus

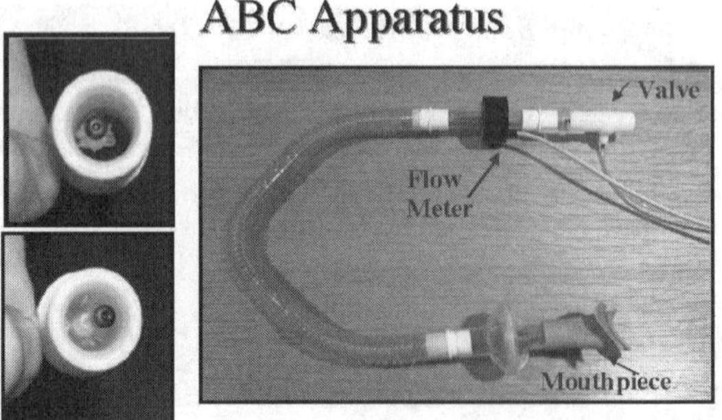


**Figure 26.** A photograph of the mouthpiece, digital flow meter, and balloon valve connection of the ABC apparatus. The insets on the left show the balloon valve in the open state (top) and in the closed state (bottom) as the balloon is inflated with an air compressor.

Our experience (Stromberg et al. 2000; Remouchamps et al. 2003a, 2003b) shows that a moderate deep inspiration breath hold (mDIBH) level set at 75% of the maximum inspiratory capacity achieves substantial and reproducible internal organ displacement while maintaining patient comfort. With the ABC system, the intended mDIBH position is calculated from the baseline at end of normal exhalation and set during an initial training session for each patient. Variation of the baseline between breaths is possible. In operation, verbal instructions are always given to help the patient achieve a steady breathing pattern. For each breathing cycle, the lung volume is intentionally re-normalized to a zero baseline each time zero flow is detected at the end of exhalation. Re-normalization occurs mostly at the beginning of a study. Once the patient achieves normal respiration in a relaxed manner, both the frequency and magnitude of the re-normalization becomes minimal. It is from this stable baseline that three measurements of the maximum inspiratory capacity are made. The mDIBH threshold is then set to approximately 75% of the average maximum inspiration capacity. The value is recorded and used for all subsequent sessions. Given the relatively large lung volume at mDIBH, the re-normalized baseline provides a sufficiently stable reference for achieving reproducible breath-holds.

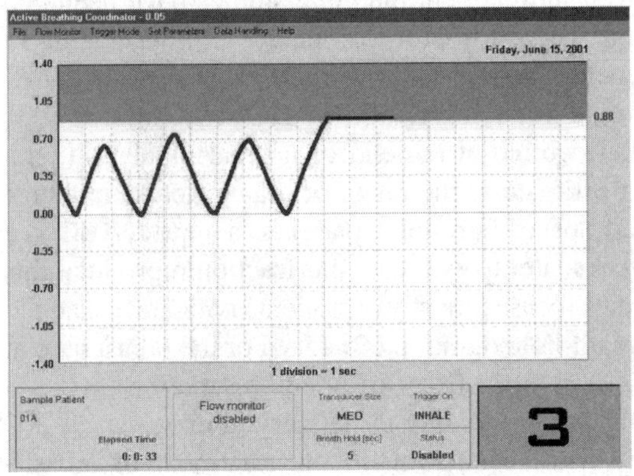


**Figure 27.** The screen display of the ABC system. The waveform is the ventilation signal converted from the digital flow-meter. The green shade (gray in this figure) indicates that the system is activated and also the lung volume for breath-hold. The bottom right display counts down the remaining duration of breath-hold in seconds. Note that this example does not show the large lung volume at moderate DIBH (mDIBH).

It is useful to discuss the stability of the respiration signal for methods of respiratory gating and breath-hold. For breath-hold methods, it seems logical to have a spirometer attachment since a valve is needed anyway. If the desire for respiratory-gating is to have the patient breathe freely without obstruction, then surface reflectors are employed instead of a spirometer. There have been some concerns as to the ability of these methods to provide robust respiration signals. The believers of the spirometry systems say that the surface reflector systems may not give an accurate portrayal of lung position because muscle relaxation can be out of phase with lung motion. This can be true. The involvement of the various muscles in normal breathing can result in variation between the surrogate signal and lung volume. The advocates for surface reflectors complain of signal drift with the spirometry systems. This can be true also. Some flow meters are more prone to non-linear variation with changing flow rates or with temperature changes. But first and foremost, it needs to be stressed that both surface markers and spirometers provide signals that are surrogates of tumor motion. Their applications must be validated by the users with fluoroscopic and CT imaging studies. For example, different surface marker positions will exhibit different sensitivity and relationship with breathing motion (Baroni et al. 2000). As for spirometry, if breath-hold is intended at the end of normal exhalation, then one should be aware that small variation in functional residual capacity is possible between breaths and potentially larger variation can occur between days.

## Reproducibility Of Breath-Hold With ABC

In order to develop the appropriate clinical procedures for treatment with ABC, extensive reproducibility and treatment planning studies have been performed at William Beaumont Hospital. The study protocol included the acquisition of a free-breathing CT scan for treatment planning and two mDIBH scans. The latter allowed examination of intrafraction reproducibility of the ABC procedure. In addition, a breath-hold CT scan each was acquired at the end of normal inhalation and exhalation. These provided an upper estimate of the range of organ motion in a breathing cycle, given the increased dead space. For some patients, a repeat ABC scan at mDIBH was acquired 1 to 4 weeks later to evaluate interfraction reproducibility.

The initial studies focused mostly on patients with breast and thoracic diseases who could tolerate a breath-hold duration of >15 s. For the breast patients, the CT data also allowed the study of (1) the effects of breathing motion on the dosimetry of whole breast IMRT using "step and shoot" delivery (Frazier et al. 2000), (2) the use of mDIBH to reduce heart irradiation in the treatment of left-sided breast patients (Remouchamps et al. 2003b), and (3) the use of mDIBH to facilitate loco-regional treatment with wide-tangents that included the inter-mammary nodes (Remouchamps et al. 2003a).

Figure 28a shows a patient being set up for an ABC CT study. The ABC display can be viewed by the patient on an auxiliary monitor. While all patients found verbal coaching imperative, less than half requested the visual information. During a CT study session, breath-hold procedures were repeated in order to facilitate the acquisition of piecemeal CT scans that spanned the entire thorax region. (As with RCCT, the inconvenience of piecemeal CT scans would not be a factor with the advent of multi-slice CT where a 40 cm scan length can be completed with a 10 s breath-hold). The analysis of breath-hold reproducibility involved removing the component of setup error by registering the two mDIBH scans with respect to the vertebrae. The lungs, the trachea and the first bifurcation were then contoured for each data set (see figure 28b). These contours were interpolated in 1 mm slice thickness from the original 5 mm slice thickness. Three-dimensional organ surfaces were formed for the contoured organs. An in-house algorithm was used to determine the closest distance-to-agreement (DTA) for each point between the two 3-D organ surfaces as a measure of reproducibility.

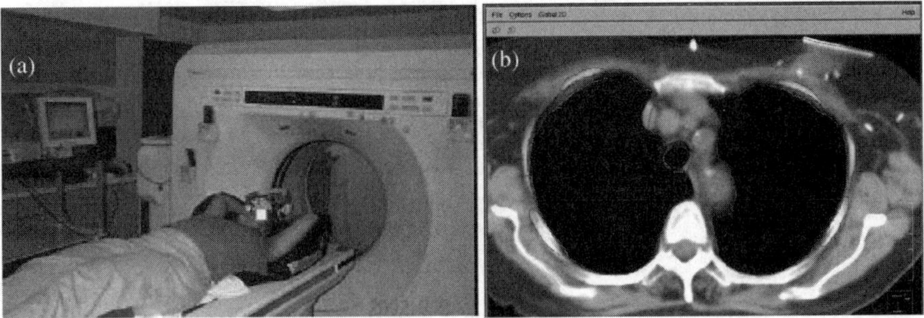

**Figure 28.** (a) A patient setup for an ABC CT study. (b) The contours of the lungs, ribs, and tracheas from two registered interfraction ABC scans at mDIBH are overlaid on one of the CT data. [Courtesy of V. Remouchamps.]

As shown in figure 29, the DTA surface map provides a measure of breath-hold reproducibility in 3-D. Data from 21 patients with breast cancer were analyzed and summarized in table 2 as mean and one standard deviation (SD) of the lung surface DTA distributions, divided into six regions. With the patient positioned in an Alpha cradle, the mean (and SD) intrafraction DTA is 1.1(1.2) mm for the left lung and 1.0(1.1) mm for the right lung. The corresponding values without the use of an Alpha cradle are significantly higher with 1.9(2.1) mm and 2.2(2.2) mm for the left and right lung, respectively ($p<0.005$ for the SD of the left lung and $p<0.0003$ for the SD of the right lung). The results confirm an earlier observation that the breath-hold reproducibility is inherently coupled with setup variation. Differences in setup position would impact on the participation of different ventilation muscles during breathing. The interfraction DTAs for the left and right lungs are 1.3(1.5) mm and 1.4(1.6) mm, respectively, similar to the intrafraction results. Immobilization with breath-hold can be effective if setup variation is minimized between treatment fractions.

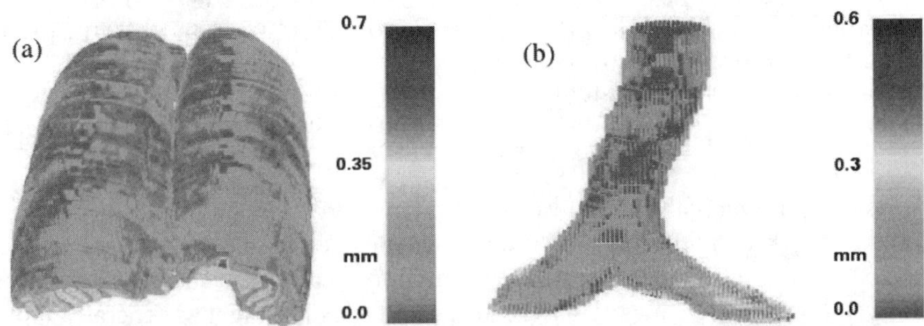

**Figure 29.** The DTA surface maps in millimeters (mm) for the (a) lungs and (b) carina of a patient study. [Courtesy of V. Remouchamps.]

**Table 2.** The Mean (1 standard Deviation) of DTA of 2 Lung Surfaces in Centimeters for Two Registered ABC Scans Acquired at mDIBH. The Figure in the Inset on the Right Shows the Division of the Lungs into Six Regions in the Analysis

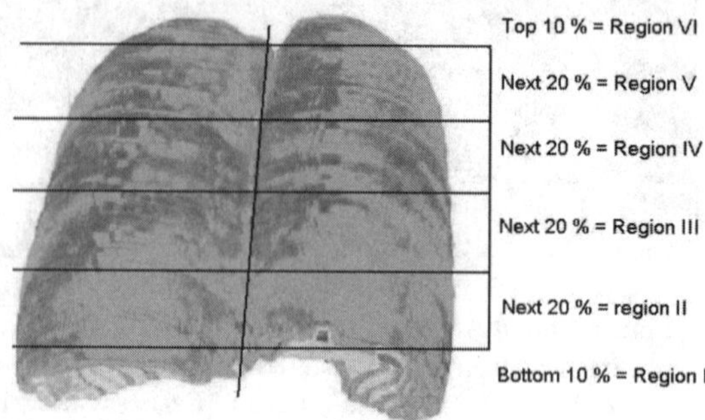


| | | Full Lung | Region I (Bottom | II (20%) | III (20%) | IV (20%) | V (20%) | Region VI (Top 10%) |
|---|---|---|---|---|---|---|---|---|
| No cradle *7 patients Intrafraction* | Left Lung | 0.19 (0.21) | 0.43 (0.34) | 0.25 (0.25) | 0.15 (0.12) | 0.14 (0.09) | 0.14 (0.09) | 0.14 (0.09) |
| | Right Lung | 0.22 (0.22) | 0.44 (0.32) | 0.35 (0.28) | 0.17 (0.11) | 0.14 (0.09) | 0.13 0.08 | (0.15) (0.12) |
| Alpha cradle Immobilization *14 patients Intrafraction* | Left Lung | 0.11 (0.12) | 0.17 (0.15) | 0.15 (0.14) | 0.10 (0.09) | 0.09 (0.08) | 0.08 (0.08) | 0.09 (0.07) |
| | Right Lung | 0.10 (0.11) | 0.10 (0.10) | 0.12 (0.13) | 0.09 (0.08) | 0.09 (0.08) | 0.08 (0.08) | 0.13 (0.09) |
| Alpha cradle *8 patients INTERFRACTION* (2-3 weeks later) | Left Lung | 0.13 (0.15) | 0.17 (0.15) | 0.17 (0.20) | 0.11 (0.12) | 0.09 (0.09) | 0.10 (0.09) | 0.15 (0.10) |
| | Right Lung | 0.14 (0.16) | 0.19 (0.18) | 0.17 (0.20) | 0.12 (0.09) | 0.11 (0.10) | 0.12 (0.11) | 0.16 (0.12) |

As a surface map, the DTA results for the lung are more pertinent for structures close to the chest wall. The DTA values obtained for the tracheal bifurcation are 0.9(0.8) mm for intrafraction and 1.4(1.0) mm for interfraction. The results for these more central structures suggest that the lung surface results might be generally applicable for the entire thorax. The speculation needs to be validated with further studies.

The regional analysis demonstrates that with ABC breath-hold at moderate deep inspiration, the upper two-thirds of the chest wall are better immobilized than the lower diaphragmatic region. With proper setup, a margin of 3 mm for breathing motion would suffice for ABC treatment at mDIBH in the upper two-thirds of the lung, and 5 mm for the lower third.

## Treatment At mDIBH With ABC

The reproducibility studies indicate that mDIBH with ABC can be a reproducible method to minimize the effect of breathing motion on radiation treatment in the thoracic regions, particularly for patients whose pulmonary functions are not compromised. Moderate DIBH also maintains the advantage of displacing critical structures from the radiation beam. For those patients with left-sided breast disease whose anatomies are predisposed to heart irradiation from tangential field arrangement, mDIBH with ABC can be applied to move the heart away from the fields (Sixel, Aznar, and Ung 2001; Sidhu et al. 2002; Remouchamps et al. 2003a). Figures 30a and 30b show the beam's eye views (BEVs) on DRRs at free breathing and mDIBH, respectively. The heart, shown in shaded contour, is displaced from the beam at mDIBH. Such observations have prompted the implementation of ABC treatment at mDIBH for those breast patients who would benefit.

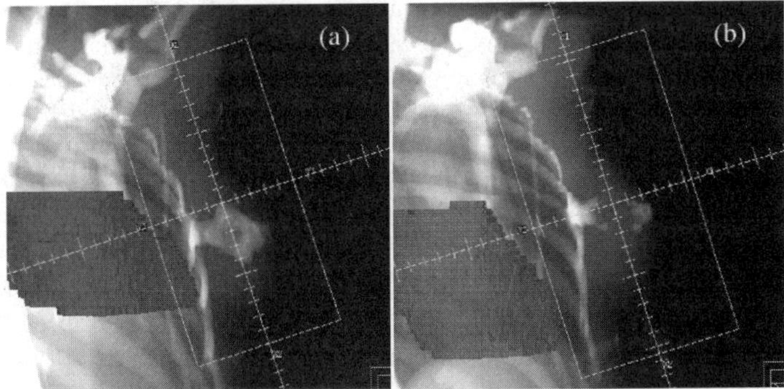


**Figure 30.** Beam's eye view displays showing, respectively, that (a) irradiation of a portion of the heart by the tangential field arrangement with the patient breathing freely, and (b) displacement of the heart from the field at mDIBH. [Reprinted from *International Journal of Radiation Oncology Biology Phys*ics, vol 55, V. M. Remouchamps, F. A. Vicini, M. B. Sharpe, L. L. Kestin, A. A. Martinez, and J. W. Wong, "Significant reductions in heart and lung doses using deep inspiration breath hold with active breathing control and intensity-modulated radiation therapy for patients treated with locoregional breast irradiation," pp. 392–406. © 2003, with permission from Elsevier.]

At present, 15 Beaumont patients have been treated at mDIBH with ABC. Twelve were patients with left-sided breast cancer treated with IMRT; one with right-sided breast cancer with a significant portion of her liver in the field; and two with lung cancers who could tolerate mDIBH for over 20 s. Figure 31a shows a breast patient in the treatment position with an electronic portal imaging device (EPID) deployed for treatment verification. Figure 31b shows the treatment personnel at the control station where a therapist (indicated by the box) is providing verbal instruction to the patient. Ideally, three therapists would man the treatment, although two had managed adequately in many occasions.

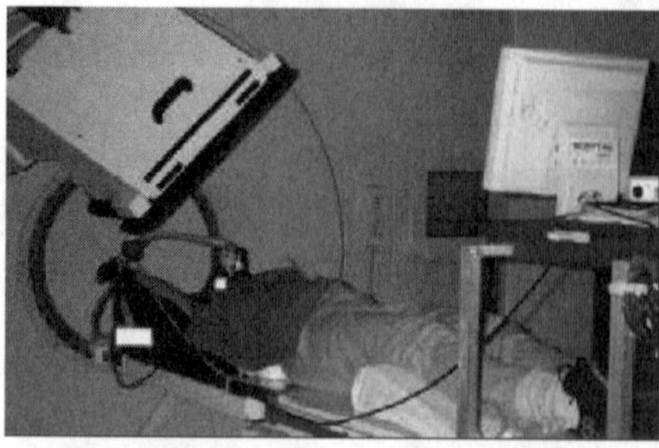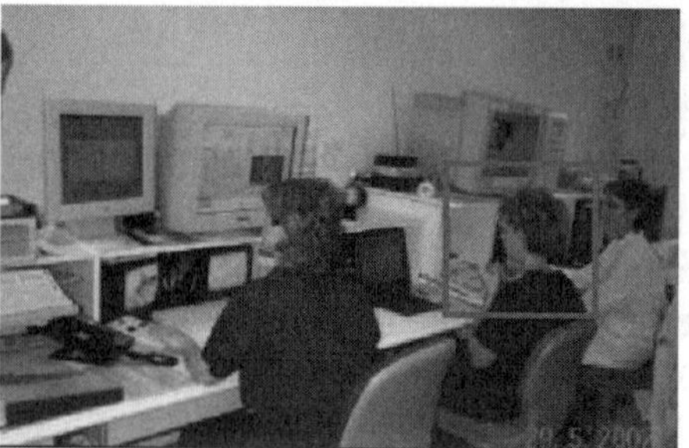

**Figure 31.** (a) A left-sided breast patient set up for treatment at mDIBH with the ABC system. A EPID was deployed for treatment verification. (b) Treatment therapists at the treatment counsel for ABC treatment. Verbal coaching was provided by a therapist using a dedicated audio system, rather than the intercom system. [Reprinted from *International Journal of Radiation Oncology Biology Phys*ics, vol 55, V. M. Remouchamps, F. A. Vicini, M. B. Sharpe, L. L. Kestin, A. A. Martinez, and J. W. Wong, "Significant reductions in heart and lung doses using deep inspiration breath hold with active breathing control and intensity-modulated radiation therapy for patients treated with locoregional breast irradiation," pp. 392–406. © 2003, with permission from Elsevier.]

The setup of ABC treatment with tangential fields requires special preparation and care. The details have been published (Remouchamps et al. 2003b). Briefly, free-breathing and mDIBH simulation and CT scanning are performed for the patient. Free-breathing information is used for marking the patient for setup, while the mDIBH information is needed for treatment planning and delivery. The source-to-surface distances (SSDs) are checked both at free breathing, and at mDIBH with a short 5 to 10 s duration. Companion PC components, such as keyboard and display, are found very useful for in-room operation of the ABC system. The IMRT delivery, the segments of each tangent are purposely divided into two or three separate deliveries to accommodate repeat breath-hold. Similarly, the open-field segment with a significant allocation of MUs is also split into two separate deliveries. Electronic portal images acquired of these open-field segments allow the examination of intra- and interfraction treatment variation that combine both breath-hold and setup. Figure 32 shows the dual window display from the electronic portal imaging system with (a) the reference DRR and (b) the portal image of the open-field segment.

Treatments at mDIBH with the ABC system were well tolerated by all selected patients and treatment personnel. Twenty minutes were allocated for breath-hold treatment. With the exception of the initial five patients, all ABC treatments were completed within 15 min. Figure 33 shows the time-trace of the lung volumes from a patient undergoing ABC treatment. There is an initial short breath-hold period for setup, followed by two 20 s breath-holds for the delivery of the medial beams, and two for the lateral beams. The level of mDIBH was set at 1.9 liters. With the slower response of the ABC system being used at William Beaumont Hospital, minor volume overshoot occurred when the patient breathed rapidly. However, the overshoot would result in minor positional variations due to already large lung volume at breath-hold.

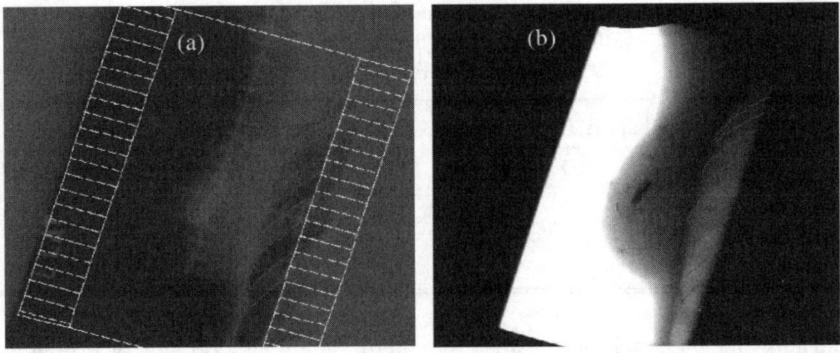


**Figure 32.** Dual window display from the electronic portal imaging system showing (a) the reference DRR and (b) portal image of the open field segment acquired during a delivery at mDIBH.

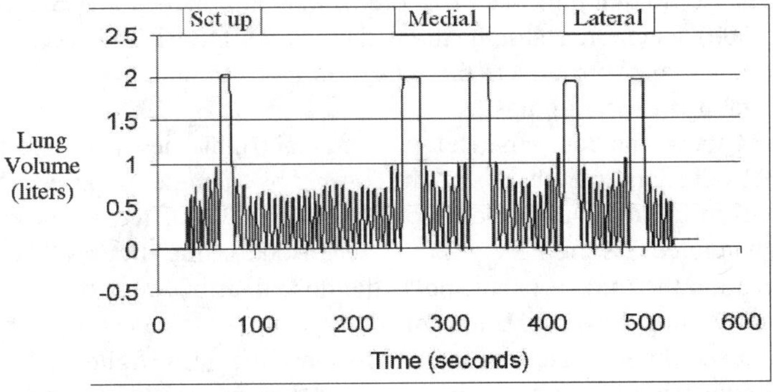


**Figure 33.** A time-trace of the lung volumes as recorded by the ABC system for a left-sided breast patient undergoing IMRT at mDIBH.

For the first five left-sided breast patients treated with breath-hold, daily electronic portal images were acquired of the open-field segments whenever possible. The variations of the chest wall from its reference DRR position were quantified using an in-house template alignment tool. The analysis combines setup error and breath-hold variation. The results for 509 electronic portal images are summarized in table 3. The magnitudes of the variations are small. The larger variation in the cranio-caudal direction is more indicative of setup error than breath-hold variation.

## Effects Of Lung Inhomogeneity On Dose Delivery At mDIBH

Results from the initial ABC treatments and reproducibility studies are very encouraging. They suggest that immobilization with breath-hold can be highly effective and

**Table 3.** Combined Variations of Setup and Breath-Hold (in mm) of Breast Tangent Treatments with ABC Measured from the 509 Daily Electronic Portal Images for the Five First Patients

| | Medial / BH1 | | Medial / BH2 | | Lateral / BH1 | | Lateral / BH2 | |
|---|---|---|---|---|---|---|---|---|
| | Mean | SD | Mean | SD | Mean | SD | Mean | SD |
| Transverse | 1.7 | 2.4 | 1.2 | 2.1 | 1.8 | 2.3 | 1.8 | 2.3 |
| Cranio-caudal | 2.0 | 3.2 | 2.1 | 3.1 | 3.4 | 3.1 | 3.2 | 3.3 |
| Rotation | 1.4 | 1.0 | 1.2 | 1.0 | 1.5 | 1.0 | 1.0 | 1.0 |

would allow the prescription of a small margin for breathing motion. However, it must be cautioned that for treatment in the lungs, the necessary beam aperture not only needs to encompass the PTV margins for setup error and breathing motion, but it must also be expanded to account for the width of the penumbra. For a lung density of 0.3 relative to water, significant broadening of the penumbra occurs as the range of the secondary electrons is extended. The width of the 95% to 50% isodose lines of a 6 MV beam increases from 6 mm in water to more than 10 mm in the lung (Sharpe, Miller, and Wong 2000), and more so for the inflated lungs at mDIBH. The necessary expansion of the beam aperture offsets the reduction in PTV margin made possible by respiratory gating or breath-hold.

Figure 34 shows the transverse (left) and sagittal (right) views of a treatment plan where the PTV (in dark gray shade) is to be covered by a parallel-opposed 6 MV beam arrangement. In the top panel, the dose distributions calculated for homogeneous water adequately covers the PTV with the 95% isodose line (figures 34a and 34b). Closer to reality, the middle panel shows the dose distributions corrected for lung inhomogeneity using the pencil beam convolution/superposition model. The penumbra broadens and the 95% isodose line shrinks into the PTV (figures 34c and 34d). Significant expansion of the beam aperture would be needed to compensate for the broadened penumbra. An alternative approach is to employ intensity modulation. The lower panel shows the recovery of the 95% isodose coverage of the PTV when the fluence at the 15 mm periphery of the beam aperture was increased by 15% (figures 34e and 34f).

## Summary And Conclusion

This chapter provides an updated report on the status of the different methods that are being developed to manage breathing motion in radiation treatment. Table 4 summarizes the results from investigations on the intra- and interfraction reproducibility of diaphragm positions using these methods. Significant progresses have been made in both respiratory-gated and breath-hold treatment delivery. Respiratory-gated delivery preserves the patient's comfort, at the expense of residual breathing motion within the intended gating window. Breath-hold with ABC effectively immobilizes the patient and allows substantial margin reduction. The procedure however, is not suitable for a

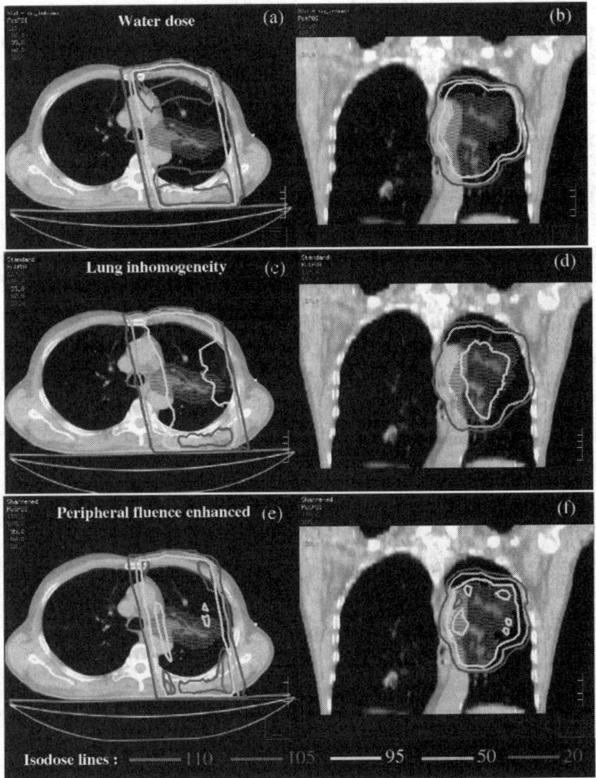


**Figure 34.** The transverse (left) and sagittal (right) views of a treatment plan where the PTV (in red shade) is to be covered by the 95% isodose lines from parallel-opposed 6 MV x-ray beams. Panels (a) and (b) on top show the dose distributions without lung corrections. Panels (c) and (d) in the middle show the dose distributions with lung corrections using a pencil beam convolution/superposition model. Panels (e) and (f) on the bottom show the dose distributions, corrected for lung inhomogeneity, that could be achieved when the fluence at a beam periphery of 15 mm was increased by 15%. [Reprinted from *Medical Physics*, vol 27, M. B. Sharpe, B. M. Miller, and J. W. Wong, "Compensation of x-ray beam penumbra in conformal radiotherapy," pp. 1739–1745. © 2000, with permission from AAPM.]

patient whose pulmonary health has been compromised by disease. It is important to note that these two approaches of managing breathing motion are not mutually exclusive. When the breath-hold signal is applied to automatically gate the machine, even for the short duration that can be maintained by the lung cancer patient, one may achieve the optimal combination of patient immobilization and efficient operation.

At present, both gating and breath-hold methods remain in the investigation stage. Although they are both commercially available and approved by the FDA, great care must be exercised when applied clinically. The validity of the external respiratory signal in inferring internal anatomic position needs further in-depth evaluation. Similarly, the potential for changes in breathing motion exists during the course of treatment, and must be investigated. The advent of multi-slice CT greatly enhances the in-depth studies of many of these issues. While clinical effectiveness of gating or breath-hold radiation treatments awaits long-term evaluations, the recent experience is encouraging and suggests that the many problems associated with breathing motion can be well managed.

**Table 4.** Summary of the Studies Reporting Breathing Immobilization or Gating Accuracy [Courtesy of V. Remouchamps.]

| Authors | Technique | Diaph Position Intrafraction Reproducibility Mean (SD) in mm | Diaph Position Interfraction Reproducibility Mean (SD) in mm | Estimated IM for Breath Hold Treatment (in mm) |
|---|---|---|---|---|
| Dawson et al. 2001 | BH at expiration with ABC device | — | 2.5 (range 1.8–3.7) | — |
| Hanley et al. 1999 | DIBH | 1 (0.9) | 2.5 (1.6) | 2-5 |
| Kim et al. 2001 | Voluntary self "gating" at Various Breath Hold positions | 2.6 (1.3) | <5 (SD 0.1-2.6) | — |
| Kubo et al. 2000 | Gating at Various Breath Hold positions with Varian system (infrared) | 2.6 (1.7) | 2.8 (1) * | — |
| Mah et al. 2000 | DIBH | — | 1 (4) * | — |
| Remouchamps et al. 2003c | mDIBH with ABC device | 1.4 (1.7) | 1.9 (2.2) | 3–4 upper two/thirds 6–7 lower third |
| Wagman et al. 2003 | Gating at expiration with Varian RPM | — | — 5.1 (2.1) Fluoro 2.2 CT scan (right) 3.8 CT Scan (left) | — |

SD = Standard deviation; IM = Internal Margin or organ motion margin for respiratory motion; BH = Breath Hold; Diaph = Diaphragm; *includes set up uncertainties.

## Acknowledgments

The author wishes to express his gratitude to Drs. G. Mageras and E. Yorke for their generous contribution of the information on the use of respiration-gated treatment at Memorial Sloan-Kettering Cancer Center. Dr. V. Remouchamp's provision of summary results from studies on breathing motion is also much appreciated.

# References


Balter, J. M., R. K. Ten Haken, T. S. Lawrence, K. L. Lam, and J. M. Robertson. (1996). "Uncertainties in CT-based radiation therapy treatment planning associated with patient breathing." *Int. J. Radiat. Oncol. Biol. Phys.* 36:167–174.

Baroni, G., G. Ferrigno, R. Orecchia, and A. Pedotti. (2000). "Real-time three-dimensional motion analysis for patient positioning verification." *Radiother. Oncol.* 54:21–27.

Davies, S. C., A. L. Hill, R. B. Holmes, M. Halliwell, and P. C. Jackson. (1994). "Ultrasound quantitation of respiratory organ motion in the upper abdomen." *Br. J. Radiol.* 67(803):1096–1102.

Dawson, L.A., K. K. Brock, S. Kazenjian, D. Fitch, C. J. McGinn, T. S. Lawrence, R. K. Ten Haken, and J. Balter. (2001). "The reproducibility of organ position using active breathing control (ABC) during liver radiotherapy." *Int. J. Radiat. Oncol. Biol. Phys.* 51(5):1410–1421.

Ekberg, L., O. Holmberg, L. Wittgren, G. Bjelkengren, and T. Landgerg. (1998). "What margins should be added to the clinical target volume in radiotherapy treatment planning for lung cancer?" *Radiother. Oncol.* 48(1): 71–77.

Erridge, S. C., Y. Seppenwoolde, S. H. Muller, M. van Herk, K. De Jaeger, J. S. Belderbos, I. J. Boersma, and J. V. Lebesque. (2003). "Portal imaging to assess set-up errors, tumor motion and tumor shrinkage during conformal radiotherapy of non-small cell lung cancer." *Radiother. Oncol.* 66(1):75–85.

Ford, E. C., G. S. Mageras, E. Yorke, K. E. Rosenzweig, R. Wagman, and C. C. Ling. (2002). "Evaluation of respiratory movement during gated radiotherapy using film and electronic portal imaging." *Int. J. Radiat. Oncol. Biol. Phys.* 52(2):522–531.

Ford, E. C., G. S. Mageras, E. Yorke, and C. C. Ling. (2003). "Respiration-correlated spiral CT: A method of measuring respiratory-induced anatomic motion for radiation treatment planning." *Med. Phys.* 30:88–97.

Frazier, R. C., F. A. Vicini, M. B. Sharpe, D. Yan, J. Fayad, K. L. Baglan, L. L. Kestin, A. A. Martinez, and J. W. Wong. (2000). "The impact of respiration on whole breast radiotherapy: A dosimetric analysis using active breathing control." (Abstract). *Int. J. Radiat. Oncol. Biol. Phys.* 48(Suppl. 1):200.

Frohlich, H., and W. Dohrin. (1985). "A simple device for breath-level monitoring during CT." *Radiol.* 156:235.

Giraud, P., E. C. Ford, K. E. Rosenzweig, E. Yorke, R. Wagman, K. Sidhu, M. A. Hunt, G. S. Mageras, H. Amols, C. C. Ling, and S. A. Leibel. (2003). "Reduction of organ motion in lung and liver tumors with respiratory gating." *Radiother. Oncol.* In press.

Hanley, J., M. M. Debois, D. Mah, G. S. Mageras, A. Raben, K. Rosenzweig, B. Mychalczak, L. H. Schwartz, P. J. Gloeggler, W. Lutz, C. C. Ling, S. A. Leibel, Z. Fuks, and G. J. Kutcher. (1999). "Deep inspiration breath-hold technique for lung tumors: The potential value of target immobilization and reduced lung density in dose escalation." *Int. J. Radiat. Oncol. Biol. Phys.* 45:603–611.

Jackson, P. C., S. C. Davies, F. V. Zananiri, J. P. Bean, D. H. Follett, M. Halliwell, and P. N. Wells. (1993). "The development of equipment for the technical assessment of respiratory motion induced artefacts in MRI." *Br. J. Radiol.* 66:132–139.

Jones, K. R. (1982). "A respiration monitor for use with CT body scanning and other imaging techniques." *Br. J. Radiol.* 55:530–533.

Kachelriess, M., S. Ulzheimer, and W. A. Kalender. (2000). "ECG-correlated imaging of the heart with subsecond multislice spiral CT." *IEEE Trans. Med. Imaging* 19:888–901.

Kalender, W. A., R. Rienmuller, W. Seissler, J. Behr, M. Welke, and H. Fichte. (1990). "Measurement of pulmonary parenchymal attenuation: use of spirometric gating with quantitative CT." *Radiol.* 175:265–268.

Keall, P. J., V. R. Kini, S. S. Vedam, and R. Mohan. (2001). "Motion adaptive x-ray therapy: A feasibility study." *Phys. Med. Biol.* 46:1–10.

Kim, D. J., B. R. Murray, R. Halperin, and W. H. Roa. (2001). "Held-breath self-gating technique for radiotherapy of non-small-cell lung cancer: A feasibility study." *Int. J. Radiat. Oncol. Biol. Phys.* 49(1):43–49.

Korin, H. W., R. L. Ehman, S. J. Riederer, J. P. Felmlee, and R. C. Grimm. (1992). "Respiratory kinematics of the upper abdominal organs: a quantitative study." *Magn. Reson. Med.* 23:172–178.

Kubo, H. D., and B. C. Hill. (1996). "Respiration gated radiotherapy treatment: A technical study." *Phys. Med. Biol.* 41:83–91.

Kubo, H. D., and L. Wang. (2000). "Compatibility of Varian 2100C gated operations with enhanced dynamic wedge and IMRT dose delivery." *Med. Phys.* 27(8):1732–1738.

Kubo, H. D., P. M. Len, S. Minohara, and H. Mostafavi. (2000). "Breathing-synchronized radiotherapy program at the University of California Davis Cancer Center." *Med. Phys.* 27:346–353.

Lattanzi, J., S. McNeeley, W. Pinover , E. Horwitz, I. Das, T. E. Schultheiss, and G. E. Hanks. (1999). "A comparison of daily CT localization to a daily ultrasound-based system in prostate cancer." *Int. J. Radiat. Oncol. Biol. Phys.* 43:719–725.

Litzenberg, D., L. A. Dawson, H. Sandler, M. G. Sanda, D. L. McShan, R. K. Ten Haken, K. L. Lam, K. K. Brock, and J. M. Balter. (2002). "Daily prostate targeting using implanted radiopaque markers." *Int. J. Radiat. Oncol. Biol. Phys.* 52(3):699–703.

Liu, Y. L., S. J. Riederer, P. J. Rossman, R. C. Grimm, J. P. Debbins, and R. L. Ehman. (1993). "A monitoring, feedback, and triggering system for reproducible breath-hold MR imaging." *Magn. Reson. Med.* 30:507–511.

Mageras, G. S., E. Yorke, K. Rosenzweig, L. Braban, E. Keatley, E. Ford, S. A. Leibel, and C. C. Ling. (2001). "Fluoroscopic evaluation of diaphragmatic motion reduction with a respiratory gated radiotherapy system." *J. Appl. Clin. Med. Phys.* 2(4):191–200.

Mah, D., J. Hanley, K. E. Rosenzweig, E. Yorke, L. Braban, C. C. Ling, S. A. Leibel, and G. Mageras. (2000). "Technical aspects of the deep inspiration breath-hold technique in the treatment of thoracic cancer." *Int. J. Radiat. Oncol. Biol. Phys.* 48:1175–1185.

Martinez, A. A., D. Yan, D. Lockman, D. Brabbins, K. Kota, M. Sharpe, D. A. Jaffray, F. Vicini, and J. Wong. (2001). "Improvement in dose escalation using the process of adaptive radiotherapy combined with three-dimensional conformal or intensity-modulated beams for prostate cancer." *Int. J. Radiat. Oncol. Biol. Phys.* 50:1226–1234.

Murphy, M. J., D. Martin, R. Whyte, J. Hai, C. Ozhasoglu, and Q. T. Le. (2002). "The effectiveness of breath-holding to stabilize lung and pancreas tumors during radiosurgery." *Int. J. Radiat. Oncol. Biol. Phys.* 2:475–482.

Murphy, M. J., S. D. Chang, I. C. Gibbs, Q. T. Le, J. Hai, D. Kim, D. P. Martin, and J. R. Adler. (2003). "Patterns of patient movement during frameless image-guided radiosurgery." *Int. J. Radiat. Oncol. Biol. Phys.* 55:1400–1408.

Nunn, J. F. *Nunn's Applied Respiratory Physiology, 4th ed.* Oxford: Butterworth-Heinemann, 1993.

Ohara, K., T. Okumura, M. Akisada, T. Inada, T. Mori, H. Yokota, and M. J. Calaguas. (1989). "Irradiation synchronized with respiration gate." *Int. J. Radiat. Oncol. Biol. Phys.* 17:853–857.

Osaka, Y., T. Kamada, Y. Matsuoka, S. Minohara, J.-E. Mizoe, H. Tomura, M. Endo, T. Kanai, and H. Tsujii. "Clinical Experience of Heavy Ion Irradiation Synchronous with Respiration" in *Proceedings of the XIIIth International Conference on the Use of Computers in Radiation Therapy.* D. D. Leavitt and G. Starkschall (eds.). May 27–30, 1997, Salt Lake City, Utah. Madison, WI: Medical Physics Publishing, pp. 176–177, 1997.

Ramsey, C. R., I. L. Cordrey, and A. L. Oliver. (1999). "A comparison of beam characteristics for gated and nongated clinical x-ray beams." *Med. Phys.* 26:2086–2091.

Remouchamps, V. M., F. A. Vicini, M. B. Sharpe, L. L. Kestin, A. A. Martinez, and J. W. Wong. (2003a). "Significant reductions in heart and lung doses using deep inspiration breath hold with active breathing control and intensity-modulated radiation therapy for patients treated with locoregional breast irradiation." *Int. J. Radiat. Oncol. Biol. Phys.* 55(2):392–406.

Remouchamps, V., N. Letts, F. Vicini, M. Sharpe, P. Chen, A. Martinez, and J. Wong. (2003b). "Initial clinical experience with deep inspiration breath hold using an active breathing control (ABC) device in the treatment of patients with left-sided breast cancer using external beam irradiation. *Int. J. Radiat. Oncol. Biol. Phys.* In press.

Remouchamps, V. M., N. Letts, D. Yan, F. A. Vicini, M. Moreau, J. A. Zielinski, J. Liang, L. L. Kestin, M. M. Martinez, and J. W. Wong. (2003c). "Three dimensional evaluation of intra- and inter-fraction reproducibility of lung and chest wall immobilization using active breathing control. *Int. J. Radiat. Oncol. Biol. Phys.* Submitted for publication.

Rosenzweig, K. E., J. Hanley, D. Mah, G. Mageras, M. Hunt, S. Toner, C. Burman, C. C. Ling, B. Mychalczak, Z. Fuks, and S. A. Leibel. (2000a). "The deep inspiration breath-hold technique in the treatment of inoperable non-small cell lung cancer." *Int. J. Radiat. Oncol. Biol. Phys.* 48(1):81–87.

Ross, C. S., D. H. Hussey, E. C. Pennington, W. Stanford, and J. F. Doornbos. (1990). "Analysis of movement of intrathoracic neoplasms using ultrafast computerized tomography." *Int. J. Radiat. Oncol. Biol. Phys.* 18(3): 671–677.

Seppenwoolde, Y., H. Shirato, K. Kitamura, S. Shimizu, M. van Herk, J. V. Lebesque, and K. Miyasaka. (2002). "Precise and real-time measurement of 3D tumor motion in lung due to breathing and heartbeat, measured during radiotherapy." *Int. J. Radiat. Oncol. Biol. Phys.* 53:822–834.

Sharpe, M. B., B. M. Miller, and J. W. Wong. (2000). "Compensation of x-ray beam penumbra in conformal radiotherapy." *Med. Phys.* 27:1739–1745.

Shimizu, S., H. Shirato, K. Kagei, T. Nishioka, X. Bo, H. Dosaka-Akita, S. Hashimoto, H. Aoyama, K. Tsuchiya, and M. Miyasaka. (2000b). "Impact of respiratory movement on the computed tomographic images of small lung tumors in three-dimensional (3D) radiotherapy." *Int. J. Radiat. Oncol. Biol. Phys.* 46(5):1127–1133.

Shirato, H., S. Shimizu, K. Kitamura, T. Nishioka, K. Kagei, S. Hashimoto, A. Aoyama, T. Kuneida, N. Shinohara, H. Dosaka-Akita, and K. Miyasaka. (2000). "Four-dimensional treatment planning and fluoroscopic real-time tumor tracking radiotherapy for moving tumor." *Int. J. Radiat. Oncol. Biol. Phys.* 48(2):435–442.

Sidhu, K., L. Hong, E. Yorke, G. Mageras, C. Chui, S. Spirou, K. Rosenzweig, C. Ling, and H. Amols. (2002). "Deep inspiration breath-hold technique and IMRT as methods to reduce volume of heart and liver in breast radiotherapy." *Int. J. Radiat. Oncol. Biol. Phys.* 54(Supplement 1):158–159.

Sixel, K. E., M. C. Aznar, and Y. C. Ung. (2001). "Deep inspiration breath hold to reduce irradiated heart volume in breast cancer patients." *Int. J. Radiat. Oncol. Biol. Phys.* 49:199–204.

Stromberg, J. S., M. B. Sharpe, L. H. Kim, V. R. Kini, D. A. Jaffray, A. A. Martinez, and J. W. Wong. (2000). "Active breathing control (ABC) for Hodgkin's disease: Reduction in normal tissue irradiation with deep inspiration and implications for treatment." *Int. J. Radiat. Oncol. Biol. Phys.* 48(3):797–806.

Takai, Y., M. Mitsuya, K. Nemoto, Y. Ogawa, H. Ariga, K. Takeda, C. Takahashi, H. Yamada, M. M. Mostafavi, C. Van Antwerp, and S. Manfield. (2002). "Development of real-time tumor tracking system with dMLC using dual x-ray fluoroscopy and amorphous silicon flat panel on the gantry of linear accelerator." *Int. J. Radiat. Oncol. Biol. Phys.* 54(Supplement):193–194.

Vedam, S. S., P. J. Keall, V. R. Kini, and R. Mohan. (2001). "Determining parameters for respiration-gated radiotherapy." *Med. Phys.* 28:2139–2146.

Vock, P., M. Soucek, M. Daepp, and W. A. Kalender. (1990). "Lung: Spiral volumetric CT with single-breath-hold technique." *Radiol.* 176:864–867.

Wade, O. L. (1954). "Movement of the thoracic cage and diaphragm in respiration." *J. Physiol.* 124:193–212.

Wagman, R., E. Yorke, E. Ford, P. Giraud, G. Mageras, B. Minsky, and K. Rosenzweig. (2003). "Respiratory gating for liver tumors: use in dose escalation." *Int. J. Radiat. Oncol. Biol. Phys.* 55(3):659–668.

Weiss, P. H., J. M. Baker, and E. J. Potchen. (1972). "Assessment of hepatic respiratory excursion." *J. Nucl. Med.* 13:758–759.

West, J. B. *Respiratory Physiology—The Essentials.* Baltimore, MD: Waverly Press, Inc., 1974.

Wong, J. W., M. B. Sharpe, D. A. Jaffray, V. R. Kini, J. M. Robertson, J. S. Stromberg, and A. A. Martinez. (1999. "The use of active breathing control (ABC) to reduce margin for breathing motion." *Int. J. Radiat. Oncol. Biol. Phys.* 44:911–919.

Yorke, E., G. Mageras, T. LoSasso, H. Mostafavi, and C. Ling. (2000). "Respiratory Gating of Sliding Window IMRT." CD-ROM Proceedings of the World Congress on Medical Physics and Biomedical Engineering, July 23–28, 2000, Chicago, IL.

# X-Ray–Guided IMRT


**David A. Jaffray, Ph.D.**
Department of Radiation Oncology
University of Toronto/Princess Margaret Hospital
Toronto, Ontario, Canada

## Overview Of The Challenges And Issues Surrounding Precise Radiation Field Placement In External Beam Radiation Therapy

Radiation therapy is a powerful localized therapeutic agent in the treatment of cancer. The nature of the biological action of therapeutic radiation with respect to diseased and normal structures supports the application of the total radiation dose over a number of treatment fractions. The technical challenges in accurately and precisely applying this localized agent to a well-defined target over the many (10 to 40) fractions of treatment are considerable. Advances in our capacity to generate conformal, patient-specific distributions of the radiation dose have highlighted the need for devices and methods of increasing the precision and accuracy with which this distribution can be placed within the human body. Over the past decade, there have been considerable advances in the development of x-ray based imaging systems that can be used during the treatment session to guide the placement of the radiation dose distribution. The goal of this chapter is to provide an overview of these developments; they will be discussed in relation to broad clinical practice including the topics of pre-treatment planning and preparation.

## Pretreatment Preparation And Fractionation In Radiation Therapy

Therapeutic intervention is a challenging task if it is to be performed with a high probability of success. More often than not, the therapeutic intervention must proceed without a complete description of all the relevant variables (state descriptors). State descriptors, here, are defined as dynamic constructs that contain all the known quantities relevant to patient treatment and the current estimate of their value. It is well understood that these values are estimates and are expected to deviate over the course of therapy. The refinement of the geometric components of this descriptor and schemes for intervention based upon these refined estimates is the topic of this chapter. A schematic representation of the state descriptor concept is shown in figure 1. These types of poorly described problems force the development of strategies that will make the solution robust regardless of "reasonable" variations in the state descriptors. Such concepts are used in many conditions in which the current and future states are not completely described by the measured quantities. Gospodarowicz and O'Sullivan (2001) have discussed such concepts in the coalescence of prognostic factors in cancer patients for the purpose of designing an appropriate treatment regimen. Failure to "freeze" the value of the variables at the current level of knowledge and make a decision would prevent intervention in an attempt to further increase the confidence in the planned course of therapy or in an attempt to consider alternate treatment schemes. This rather constrained approach is now being examined with the development of new information sources that would permit significant refinements to the values of the patient state descriptors.

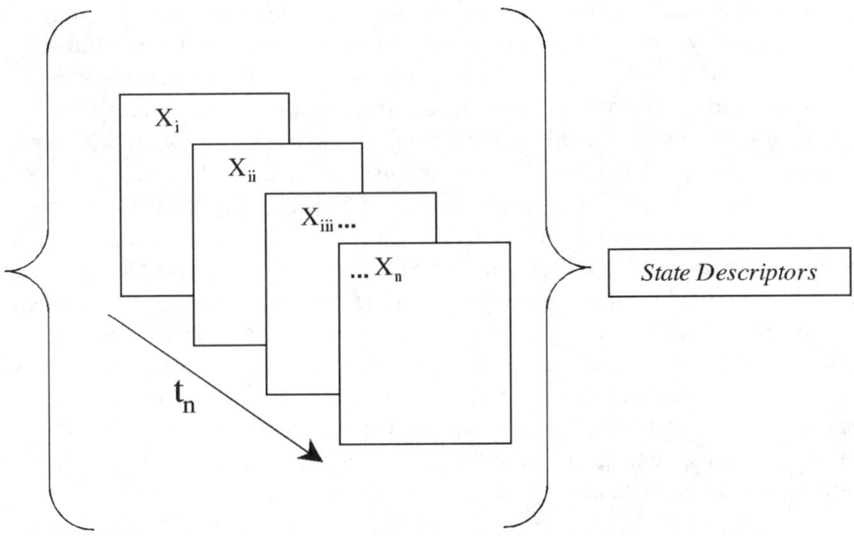


**Figure 1.** Schematic representation of the "state descriptor" concept. The need for image-guidance arises from the changes in state of the patient's anatomy or disease process through the course of time. The state descriptor contains all relevant variables and their values at a given point in time. The development of complex guidance systems is driven by the instability in the value of the state descriptor variables. This approach allows image-guidance for patient positioning, monitoring of disease response, and simple blood work to all be treated similarly in a generalized dynamic refinement model.

These state descriptors can take many forms ranging from status of disease and normal structures (extent/distribution of target structures, disease staging, patient performance status, etc.) to more geometric considerations (target location, correspondence between surrogate and target structures, repositioning skills, etc.). The development of imaging in the context of the treatment room permits the state descriptor values to be refined at a time closer to the moment of intervention, thereby, reducing the dependence on the strategic aspect of the planned intervention and increasing the confidence with which the therapeutic intervention will be executed. This is the essence of the "3-D hypothesis"—that increased geometric confidence permits the pursuit of dose escalation while maintaining tolerable levels of normal tissue complication.

The extension of these arguments to the remainder of the state descriptor opens the opportunity to embrace all updates to the state descriptor including biological descriptors derived from functional imaging sources, protein assays, physiological measures [i.e., tissue oxygen ($pO_2$) and interstitial fluid pressure (IFP)], or any number of clinical observations. Under this description, the development of image-guidance technologies is well positioned with respect to all other developments that will permit the pursuit of a full implementation of state descriptor refinement and response during the course of therapy.

One of the major challenges associated with state descriptor refinement over the course of therapy is the lack of prescription constructs that will permit refinement of the treatment without violation of the prescription. Currently, treatment prescriptions are constrained to dosimetric and geometric descriptors alone and, therefore, do not support refinements that would perturb the objectives over the course of radiation therapy. This is readily understood by considering a prescription to uniformly treat the clinical target volume (CTV) to a specified dose. In contouring the CTV, the geometric variables are fixed and reflect the CTV location and shape at the time at which the image set was acquired. It is highly unlikely that the CTV will present itself in exactly the same shape and form at another point in time, let alone at the moment of therapy. It is, therefore, highly unlikely that the prescription could ever be exactly carried out as specified. Similar challenges would also be raised by changes in other state variables being adjusted due to other changes in the state descriptor variables. For these reasons, the development of a more comprehensive prescription system needs to be developed that captures the intent of the prescription and makes it robust under minor perturbations in the state descriptor.

## Spatio-Temporal Instability Of Target And Normal Structures

The lack of robust positioning information at the time of treatment has long been accommodated by the use of enlarged treatment volumes to guarantee uniform dose coverage of the CTV over the course of therapy. There have been many investigations of the nature of spatio-temporal instability in the delivery of radiation therapy (Crook et al. 1995; de Boer and Heijmen 2001; Fontenla et al. 2001; Jaffray, Yan, and Wong 1999; Kaatee et al. 2002; Kitamura et al. 2002; Korin et al. 1992; Lebesque et al. 1992; Melian et al. 1997; Nuyttens et al. 2002; Roeske et al. 1995; Schewe et al. 1996; Stroom et al. 1999, 2000a; van Herk et al. 1995; Zelefsky et al. 1999). Some of the earlier investigations related the inability to accommodate these instabilities to local failure (Marks et al. 1974, 1976). These instabilities are accommodated by the irradiation of an increased volume of tissue. This increased volume is often described by a geometric margin that is applied to the CTV, resulting in the planning target volume (PTV). There are many recent publications on the appropriate development of this margin (Bedford et al. 1999; McKenzie, van Herk, and Mijnheer 2000; Remeijer et al. 2002) and additional publications that develop non-geometric descriptions for the accommodation of the geometric instabilities (Lockman, Yan, and Wong 2000; Yan and Lockman 2001). These methods avoid the geometric margin by evaluating dose coverage in the presence of geometric instability during the inverse planning stage.

## Sampling And Correcting For Apparent Discrepancies In Target Position

While the CTV to PTV margin accommodates the geometric uncertainties present in the delivery process, it is always advantageous to reduce the magnitude of the uncertainties such that smaller margins can be employed. This reduction permits the volume of normal tissue irradiated to be reduced and the prescription dose to be escalated. It is of paramount importance that the temporal nature of the instabilities be well understood if corrections are to be applied with confidence. This applies to both off-line and on-line correction strategies. Every effort must be made to characterize the temporal nature of the spatial instability over the time frame of the correction strategy.

## Simplification Of Geometric Uncertainties In Radiation Delivery: Systematic And Random Components

The general nature of the spatial instability can be described in many ways (Lof, Lind, and Brahme 1998). The development of probability density functions to describe the spatial instabilities offers an elegant description that covers most conditions. The use of probability density functions has been further simplified, such that these distributions are described by their first and second moments. The literature contains many descriptions of this simplification and relates them to clinical practice (Bel et al. 1994; Hurkmans et al. 2001; Kutcher, Mageras, and Leibel 1995; Lebesque et al. 1992; Shalev 1996; Yan et al. 1997a, 1997b). The description of geometric uncertainty is often separated into two components: systematic and random. Systematic components of the uncertainty are corrected through off-line strategies and random are corrected through on-line strategies. Investigators have developed schemes that use off-line approaches that refine their estimates of the random component for an individual patient and adjust the margins to accommodate the improved estimate (Yan et al. 1998, 2000). There are innumerous methods of implementation of these concepts with a variety of time frames for intervention whether they are in the form of patient-specific correction or patient-specific margin design. The key requirement is that the method is consistent in its utilization of correction and margin design such that the dose variation to the CTV falls within the prescribed limits. Finally, it is important to note that the use of a systematic and random component description applies well to geometric uncertainties but may not extend to the more general changes in the value of state descriptor variables.

## X-Ray Imaging Technologies For Guidance In The Radiation Therapy Setting

There is a rich history in the use of X-ray imaging technology to guide radiation therapy treatment. The majority of the developments have focused on the use of the megavoltage treatment source to generate a radiograph of the patient through the beam defining collimation assembly. This is referred to as "portal imaging"—images formed using the beam "port." The quality of portal films has traditionally been notoriously low when compared to the low-energy radiographs used in the simulation process. The development of electronic portal imaging systems have been responsible for substantial increases in image quality over the past 10 years with the development of amorphous silicon-based flat panel detectors.

## Portal Imaging Methods and Technologies

Portal imaging technology has undergone dramatic advances in the past 10 years. Portal film technology has also advanced in recent years with the introduction of Kodak's ECL series and the development of computed radiography (CR) systems. Munro (1999) provides an excellent review of electronic portal imaging devices in the clinical setting and identifies the current status of the commercially available devices. The quality of images generated with these new devices is acceptable at clinically acceptable imaging exposures (2 to 8 monitor units) and have sufficiently large field-of-view to cover most clinical fields. Images formed with these systems cannot only guide the treatment, but can also verify the shape and orientation of the treatment field (Bijhold et al. 1991; Creutzberg et al. 1993; Curtin-Savard and Podgorsak 1999; Mijnheer 1992; Partridge et al. 2000; Ploeger et al. 2002). The capacity to visualize a surrogate of target position and the edge of the treatment field in the same image has made the portal imaging approach extremely robust and relatively easy to integrate into clinical practice. Portal film can be used as a robust source of data for off-line correction schemes and many of the early feasibility studies on the implementation of off-line corrections strategies were tested on portal film based measurements. The development of the electronic portal imaging devices (EPIDs) has spurred the development of on-line strategies as well as provided a wealth of data for support of the off-line approach. While portal imaging technology has advanced substantially in recent years, the inherently low contrast in the megavoltage (MV) radiographs and restriction associated with imaging through the treatment port has spurred the development of kilovoltage (kV) imaging systems on the medical linear accelerator.

## Kilovoltage Radiography And Fluoroscopy For Bone And Implanted Surrogates.

There have been many embodiments of kV radiography and/or fluoroscopy integrated with the radiation therapy treatment device. Figure 2 illustrates a cobalt-60 treatment unit with an integrated kV x-ray tube for directing the treatment field. This type of direct integration of a kV x-ray source has been proposed by multiple investigators (Cho and Munro 2002; Nunan 1995). Others have proposed attaching a kV x-ray tube to the gantry and achieving MV and kV source coincidence by a gantry rotation or table translation (Biggs, Goitein, and Russell 1985; Jaffray et al. 1995; Pisani et al. 2000). There have also been developments in the construction of room-based kV imaging systems (Adler et al. 1997; Schewe et al. 1998; Shirato et al. 1999; Yin et al. 2002). Both approaches are designed to localize the bony anatomy or surrogate structures (markers, etc.) through acquisition of at least two radiographs. Typically, these are acquired at two distinct and known angles. In the gantry-based approach, a single imaging system is used in conjunction with the gantry rotation to generate the necessary images. Room-based systems typically include a minimum of two complete imaging systems (source and detector) and have been constructed with up to four separate systems. Shirato et al. (2000a) use four systems (shown in figure 3) to permit continuous stereo monitoring regardless of linear accelerator gantry angle. The types of detectors used in these systems range from conventional radiographic film, to image-intensifiers, to charge-coupled device (CCD)/phosphor screen-based systems, to large-area flat-panel detectors. The continued development of large-area, high-performance flat-panel detector technology can be expected to spur this technology in coming years. This is clearly demonstrated in the announcement of the Elekta Synergy System, the BrainLab Novalis unit, and Varian's robot mounted kV tube and detector device—all these technologies were demonstrated at the American Society of Therapeutic Radiation Oncology (ASTRO) 2002 exhibition in New Orleans, LA.

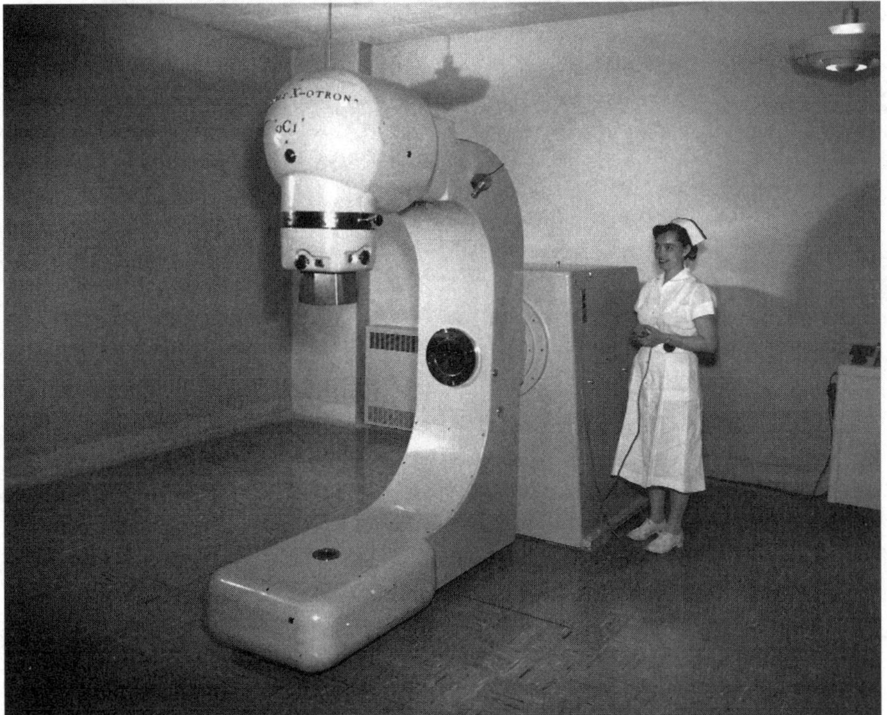


**Figure 2.** Photograph of the X-o-tron $^{60}$Co unit installed at Princess Margaret Hospital in the late 1950's. This unit was unique in that a kV x-ray tube was mounted above the source drawer of the $^{60}$Co source to allow kV radiographs to be acquired with appropriate shielding. The unit was in operation until 1983. [Courtesy of PMH Archives, Princess Margaret Hospital, Toronto, Canada]

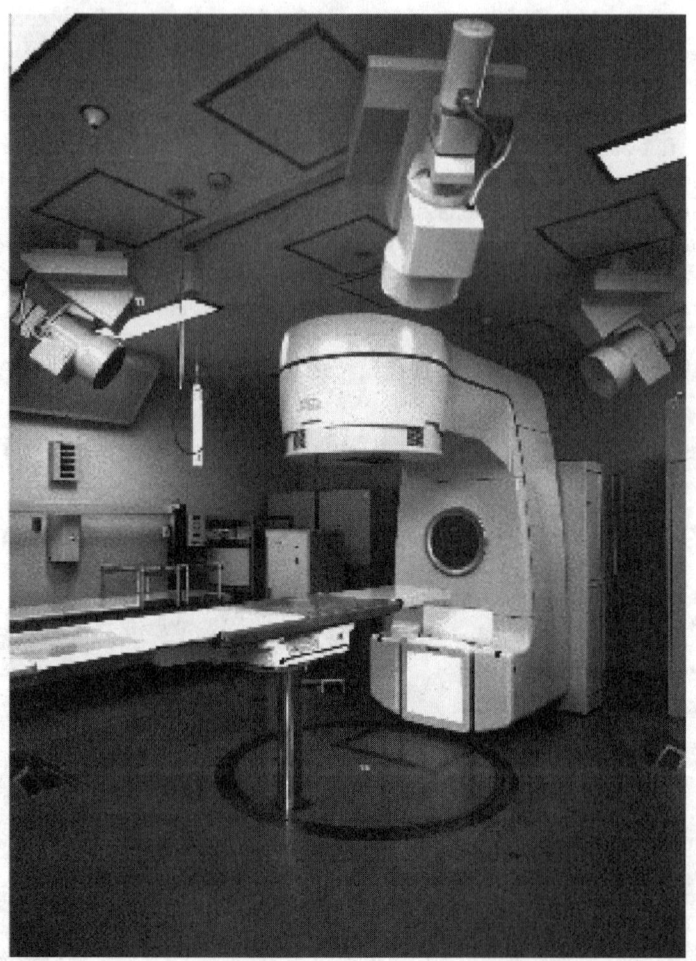

**Figure 3.** Real-time tumor-tracking system for gated radiotherapy highly integrated system (four x-ray tubes, four image intensifiers; temporal resolution: 30 fps; spatial targeting precision: 1.5 mm @ 40 mm/s). [Reprinted from *International Journal of Radiation Oncology Biology Physics,* vol. 48, H. Shirato, S. Shimizu, K. Kitamura, T Nishioka, K. Kagei, S. Hashimoto, H. Aoyama, T. Kunieda, N. Shinohara, H. Dosaka-Akita, and K. Miyasaka, "Four-dimensional treatment planning and fluoroscopic real-time tumor tracking radiotherapy for moving tumor," pp. 435–442. © 2000, with permission from Elsevier.]

## Kilovoltage Computed Tomography (kVCT)

The development of dedicated radiographic imaging systems in the treatment room promises to revolutionize radiation therapy practice by increasing the precision with which the patient's bony anatomy can be positioned with respect to the treatment beam. These systems also demonstrate great promise for increasing the precision of treatment for those sites in which fiducial markers can be placed directly in the targeted structures. However, this covers only a minority of the treatment sites and does not address the visibility of dose limiting normal structures. The advancement of a general solution for precision radiation therapy throughout the human body requires the capacity to visualize soft-tissue structures in the treatment context. There have been a number of volumetric imaging modalities proposed for this task, including, ultrasound (Holupka et al. 1996; Lattanzi et al. 2000), computed tomography (CT) (Brahme, Lind, and Nafstadius 1987; Jaffray, Yan, and Wong 1999; Mackie et al. 1993; Uematsu et al. 1996), and magnetic resonance (MR) imaging (J. Lagendijk, private communication). In this section, the development of CT as a method for guiding radiation therapy in the treatment room is reviewed.

*Conventional CT In The Treatment Room*

A straightforward approach to implementing CT-guided radiation therapy is to place a conventional CT scanner in the treatment room in a known geometric relationship to the medical linear accelerator's isocenter. Uematsu et al. (1998) have been developing this approach over the past 7 years (Kuriyama et al. 2003; Uematsu et al. 1996, 1998, 1999, 2001, 2002a). Currently, two manufacturers provide products of this type (Siemens' accelerator in combination with a Toshiba CT scanner; Mitsubishi's accelerator in combination with a General Electric CT scanner) (Kuriyama et al. 2003). Figure 4 illustrates the system reported by Kuriyama et al (2003). All systems are based upon a CT scanner placed in close proximity to the medical linear accelerator, allowing a single couch to be moved from an "imaging" position to the treatment position. These systems vary in the amount of motion and degrees of freedom required to move the patient from one position to the other. Both of the commercially available systems minimize the amount of couch movement by translating the CT scanner gantry during acquisition. This has the perceived importance of avoiding differences in couch deflection at different couch extensions (Kuriyama et al. 2003). While the installation of a second costly piece of equipment in the treatment room is perceived to be somewhat inelegant, it has a clear advantage in that it leverages all of the development that has been invested in conventional CT technology over the past 20 years—leading to unquestioned image quality and clinical robustness. In a recent article, Kuriyama et al. (2003) report a positional accuracy for the Mitsubishi-based system of under 0.5 mm. This accuracy in combination with excellent image quality promises excellent management of inter-fraction setup errors and organ-motion. The issues of motion between imaging and delivery remain and will have to be accommodated through the appropriate selection of PTV margin.

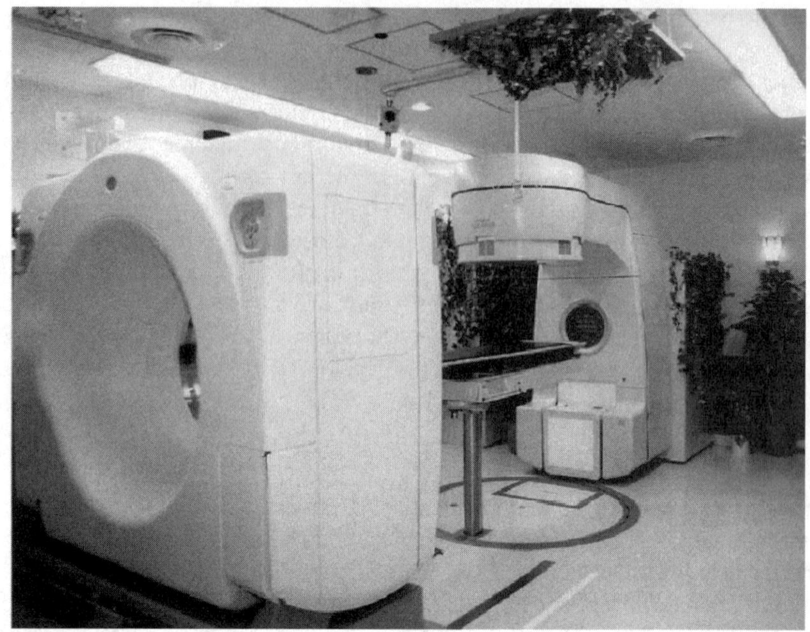

**Figure 4a.** A panoramic view of the integrated CT-linac irradiation system.
A linac gantry is placed on the opposite side of the CT gantry. Between these gantries
the common treatment couch is placed.

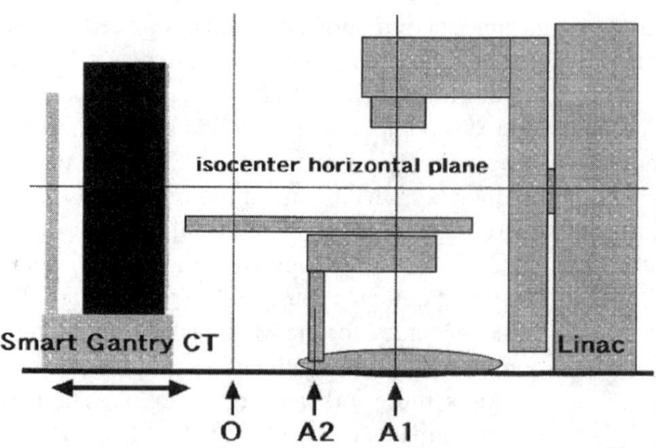


**Figure 4b.** Diagram of the integrated CT-linac irradiation system. The treatment couch
has two rotation axes; A1 is for isocentric rotation to make non-coplanar arcs, and A2 is
for rotation between CT and linac. The gantry axis of the linac is coaxial with that of the
CT scanner. A special self-driving device is equipped on the bottom of the conventional
CT gantry so that the gantry, not the couch, moves when scanning.

*Cone-Beam CT On The Medical Linear Accelerator*

An alternative approach for CT-based image guidance is to integrate the CT imaging system directly into the mechanics of the medical linear accelerator. Current medical linear accelerators are limited to approximately 360° of gantry rotation. This would limit a conventional CT approach on such a gantry to one slice per revolution. The International Electrotechnical Commission (IEC) limits on gantry rotation rate (~1 rpm) would make imaging with such a platform prohibitive. Recent advances in large area flat-panel detector technology offer the opportunity to implement cone-beam CT (Cho, Johnson, and Griffin 1995; Feldkamp, Davis, and Kress 1984), permitting a volumetric image to be acquired in a single revolution of the gantry structure (Jaffray 1999a; Jaffray et al. 2002; Jaffray and Siewerdsen 2000). Jaffray et al. (2002) have been exploring this approach over the past 7 years. Figure 5 contains a photograph of the cone-beam CT system mounted on an Elekta Precise™ accelerator and sample images generated with this technology. Advantages of such an approach are numerous, provided cone-beam CT image quality is sufficient to visualize soft-tissue structures of interest in the treatment context. This has been examined through numerous investigations (Siewerdsen and Jaffray 1999, 2000, 2001) and current flat-panel technology appears to provide a reasonable level of performance with continued performance enhancements anticipated. The cone-beam CT approach provides volumetric imaging in the treatment position and allows radiographic or fluoroscopic monitoring throughout the treatment procedure.

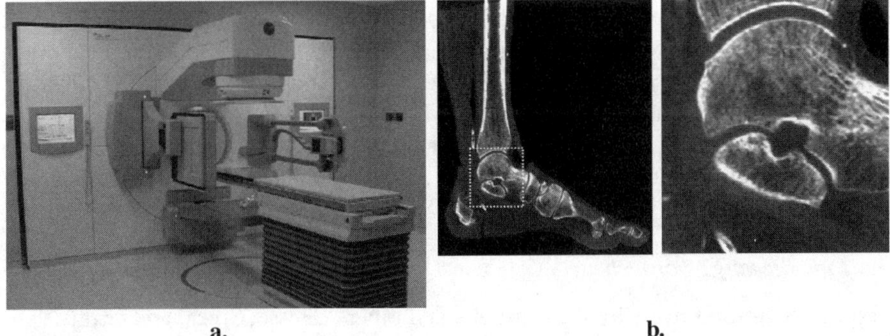

a.          b.

**Figure 5.** (a) Medical linear accelerator adapted to support kV cone-beam CT imaging. A conventional x-ray tube and flat-panel detector are mounted orthogonal to the treatment beam. (b) Sample cone-beam CT dataset acquired with a large area flat-panel detector and kilovoltage x-ray beam. [Courtesy of Princess Margaret Hospital, Toronto, Canada]

## Megavoltage Computed Tomography (MVCT)

The need for accurate electron density estimates for treatment planning was the initial rationale for developing MVCT imaging systems. Their use for patient and target structure localization was secondary. A number of investigators have been exploring the use of MV beams in CT imaging over the past 20 years.

*Single-Slice Techniques*

The initial development of an MVCT scanner for radiation therapy is attributed to Simpson et al. (1982). Their approach was based upon a 4 MV beam and a single linear array of detectors. Brahme, Lind, and Nafstadius (1987) proposed employing a 50 MV treatment beam for CT imaging in 1987. In their proposal, the high-energy beam would create contrasts comparable to a 300 keV due to the z-dependence of the pair production x-ray interaction process. Nakagawa et al. (2000) is the only group to have reported clinical experience in the direction of treatment based upon the MV CT images, using their single-slice system to treat 15 patients for metastatic and primary lung cancer. In this system, a single linear detector consisting of 75 cadmium tungstate crystals is mounted on the accelerator gantry and can be readily removed. The authors indicate that a spatial resolution of 0.5 mm and contrast resolution of 5% can be resolved with the system. Clinical imaging doses of 2.8 cGy were delivered during patient imaging.

*Cone-Beam MVCT On The Medical Linear Accelerator*

Limitations in gantry rotation have also spurred the development of cone-beam MVCT on a medical linear accelerator. With the exception of Mosleh-Shirazi et al. (1998), these developments have come as a by-product of advances in commercial portal imaging technology. Groh et al. (2002) have reported on the challenges associated with achieving high signal-to-noise performance at MV energies with low-efficiency flat-panel detector technology. Despite the low efficiency of these systems, the visibility of high contrast structures, such as air and bone, should be reasonable at clinically acceptable doses (~5 cGy). The MV cone-beam CT approach also suffers from the size of flat-panel detectors currently available in the market, limiting the field-of-view of such systems to roughly 25 cm in diameter and 25 cm in length.

*The Tomotherapy Approach*

Despite continued efforts by these groups and others (Hesse, Spies, and Groh 1998; Midgley, Millar, and Dudson et al. 1998; Mosleh-Shirazi, Swindell, and Evans 1998; Mosleh-Shirazi et al. 1998; Partridge, Evans, and Mosleh-Shirazi 1998; Spies et al. 2001), the development of a commercial system for MVCT imaging was not implemented until the development of tomotherapy (Mackie et al. 1999; Ruchala et al. 1999). The reader is referred to a number of references for a broad overview of the tomotherapy concept (Mackie et al. 1993; Olivera et al. 1999). In the original tomotherapy proposal, a kVCT scanner would be integrated into the treatment unit for localization of the target and normal structures. Ruchala et al. (1999) have investigated the use of a kVCT detector based upon pressurized xenon gas within a tungsten septa-filled housing for use with the MV beam. The detector has performed beyond expectations, largely due to the high cross section of the tungsten septa in the MV beam. The detector is estimated to have a detective quantum efficiency approaching 25%—almost 10 times higher than what can currently be achieved with MV flat-panel detectors. In addition, the tomotherapy approach employs a helical source and detector path to reduce slicing artifacts arising from the lack of noise correlations between adjacent slices.

## Clinical Procedures Employing X-ray Imaging Technologies

While there have been substantial developments in the field of imaging for therapy guidance over the past 10 years, it has only been in the past 2 years that integrated systems for imaging and correction have really begun to appear. In fact, the use of weekly portal films to verify field placement is still the predominant practice—this is somewhat surprising since the first commercial electronic portal imagers were released at the start of the 1990's. It is argued that this slow adoption is a by-product of the poor image quality in early systems and the lack of tools for clinical utilization. The AAPM Task Group #58 report provides recommendations for clinical implementation of electronic portal imaging devices and processes for their clinical utilization (Herman et al. 2001).

### Conventional Portal Film Practice

Portal film practice varies substantially from clinic to clinic with measurements occurring with varying frequency and a variety of correction protocols that range from regimented practice to clinician-specific interventions. Portal films have been employed in both off-line and on-line approaches. It is typical for portal films to be acquired on the first day of treatment with corrections applied to improve agreement between the films and reference simulator film or digitally reconstructed radiograph. Repeated portal films can be acquired on weekly intervals with review by the oncologist. The need for a correction in patient positioning or field shape/position is assessed by direct measurement from the film on a light box. This practice, while old, does describe a hybrid on-line and off-line approach to guiding radiation field placement and should not be discounted. Advancements in portal imaging technology have not been well accompanied by improvements in measurements and analysis tools until recently (Herman, Kruse, and Hagness 2000).

### Off-line Strategies Using Portal Imaging Technologies

The merits of image-guidance based upon portal films are substantial and significant gains in the accuracy of setup can be achieved using this technology to manage systematic errors. These gains require the development of robust clinical procedures for off-line analysis and decision-making. One of the first published articles on the topic was by Lebesque et al. (1992). This article described a methodology for systematic analysis for portal films to detect systematic errors. The development of an "action level" for on-line intervention was a natural hybrid of off-line and on-line methods (Bel et al. 1993). This approach has been furthered with the implementation of more elaborate approaches that address the workload issues (de Boer and Heijmen 2002). Yan et al. (1998) have proposed and implemented a generalized model for off-line correction of systematic errors and off-line accommodation of random errors. This approach is an excellent model of dynamic refinement addressing the issues of geometric positioning. These concepts can be readily extended to consider other surrogates for the position of anatomical targets. Wu et al. (2001) have employed an on-line portal imaging system and portal films for on-line correction of setup errors and off-line estimation of prostate marker displacement, respectively. Systematic correction for organ motion and setup error has a substantial impact on the margins required to guarantee CTV coverage. Systematic errors have a two to three times large impact on margin size than random errors for fractionated radiation therapy and the appropriate emphasis should be placed on their reduction (van Herk et al. 2000).

## On-line Strategies Using Portal Imaging Technologies

While off-line corrections can be implemented with minimal technological requirements, the simplicity of the on-line approach is attractive. On-line corrections require more work at the time of treatment, but reduce the need for off-line analysis and organized intervention. There have been many implementations and studies of the use of portal imaging for on-line re-positioning (Alasti et al. 2001; Balter et al. 1993; De Neve et al. 1992; Nederveen, Lagendijk, and Hofman 2001; Pisani et al. 2000; Stroom et al. 2000b). Figure 6 illustrates a typical on-line correction strategy. These strategies typically rely upon an estimate of the residual uncertainty in correction to define a threshold for intervention. A typical threshold for on-line intervention is 2 mm (Pisani et al. 2000), positioning errors below this value are not corrected. The magnitude of this residual uncertainty can be reduced through the development of robust positioning tables that support on-line correction (Brock, McShan, and Balter 2002).

## On-line Strategies Using kV Radiographic Technologies

There has been a dramatic increase in the number of radiation therapy delivery systems that are being equipped with integrated kV imaging systems. The capacity of these systems to generate images of the patient independent of the MV treatment beam has permitted their use in on-line correction and monitoring.

Pisani et al. (2000) report on a study of 14 patients that compares kV and MV radiographs generated with a single system. The authors conclude that the intra-observer variations in alignment were reduced for radiographs generated by the kV imaging system, although, these variations were small compared to the observed setup errors. The development of flat-panel kV and MV imaging detectors will affect these conclusions and further investigation is merited. Optimizing image quality will serve to provide higher quality data for semi- or fully automatic registration algorithms—a key requirement for efficient and robust on-line image guidance.

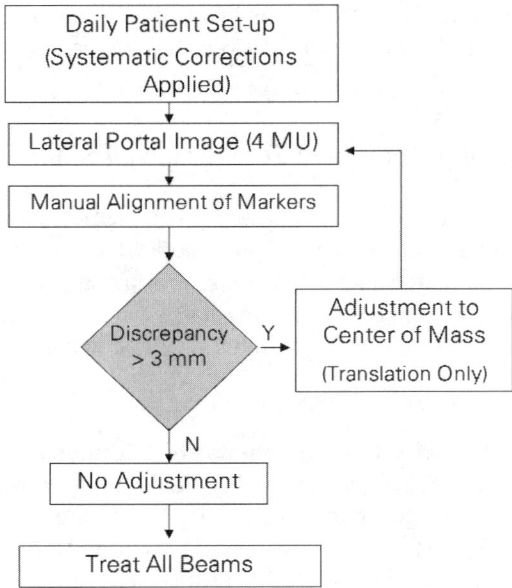


**Figure 6.** Daily on-line imaging and correction procedure for marker-based image-guided radiation therapy of the prostate. In this procedure, a single lateral portal image is taken to permit re-positioning in the anterior-posterior (AP) and superior-inferior (SI) directions. Intervention is required approximately 19% of the time. [Courtesy of T. Haycocks M.RT.(T), Princess Margaret Hospital, Toronto, Canada]

Shirato et al. (2000b) describe the development of a highly integrated, room-based kV radiography system and have employed it in numerous clinical investigations. The "real-time tumor tracking system" is capable of imaging at fluoroscopic rates and is interlocked with the treatment beam to suppress exposure when the targeted marker(s) are beyond geometric tolerances. This system has been employed in the treatment of numerous clinical sites (Shimizu et al. 2000, 2001; Shirato et al. 2000) and is of particular interest where intra-fraction motion is of concern. A similar design has been developed by BrainLab Inc. (Redwood City, CA). This system uses the room-based radiographic system for patient positioning only (Yin et al. 2002).

The on-line correction capacity of the Cyberknife (Adler et al. 1997) is another example of in-room kV radiography for on-line correction. In this system, however, the correction can be performed through the motion of the robotic support of the linear accelerator. The commercial source of this technology, Accuray Inc. (Sunnyvale, CA), has also been exploring the development of a system for dynamic tracking of internal structures affected by respiration. This is achieved through the use of an optical tracking system that measures the displacement of a marker whose motion has been correlated to the motion of internal structures.

The simplicity and speed of the radiographic approach offers an excellent platform for reducing setup errors. The introduction of a marker allows the systems to address inter- and intra-fraction organ motion. This is proving to be a powerful tool for many sites in the body.

## Methods Employing Computed Tomography Techniques

Limitations in the contrast resolution and lack of volumetric imaging information will ultimately limit radiographic methods to high contrast structures or structures in which surrogates can be easily implanted. The desire to provide non-invasive guidance of treatment and a volumetric record of the irradiated normal structures are driving the development of x-ray CT systems for guiding radiation therapy.

### Conventional CT For Off-line Correction

Yan et al. (2000a) have developed an innovative scheme that employs an off-line approach to characterize the spatial mobility of the prostate with respect to bony anatomy. In this scheme, a conventional CT scanner is employed for daily imaging of the prostate during the first 5 days of treatment. This information is used in combination with the initial treatment planning CT to estimate an organ occupancy volume that better represents the prostate position over the remaining fractions. This analysis is merged with a patient-specific estimate of setup error estimated from daily electronic portal images. The authors have demonstrated that their approach can be used to substantially reduce the PTV margin for the individual, thereby, permitting dose escalation (Martinez et al. 2001).

### On-line Methods With Conventional CT

The use of a conventional CT scanner in the treatment room for image-guided radiation therapy is being explored by a number of investigators and has resulted in two commercial offerings [PRIMATOM™, Siemens Medical Systems (Kuriyama et al. 2003)]. The clinical utilization of these devices has been largely restricted to Japanese centers. Uematsu et al. (1998, 2000, 2001, 2002b) have been exploring this approach for nearly a decade and have demonstrated its use in a variety of clinical sites. In their scheme, patients were transferred between a conventional simulator, a conventional CT scanner, and a conventional accelerator on a common couch top within the treatment room. In the treatment of lung cancer, respiratory motion is minimized through coaching under x-ray fluoroscopy, the target position is determined under CT, and, finally, the patient is transferred to the accelerator for treatment. This has been performed for 45 patients suffering from lung cancer with the number of fractions per patient ranging from 5 to 15. The overall accuracy of the system for rigid anatomical sites, such as stereotactic radiosurgery of the brain, is reported to be sub-millimeter. The FOCAL unit of Uematsu et al. (2000) demonstrates the merits of fluoroscopy and computed tomography in the treatment setting.

### Cone-Beam CT Approach For On-line Repositioning

Cone-beam CT approaches promise the combined advantages of fluoroscopic monitoring and volumetric imaging of the patient in the treatment position. Conceptually, such an approach would be a merger of the best of both worlds—providing the capacity for soft-tissue imaging in the treatment position and real-time radiographic monitoring during the treatment delivery. Jaffray et al. (2002) have been exploring the use of an independent kV imaging system for combined radiographic and tomographic imaging. Full utilization of this approach requires significant integration with the clinical treatment system if the treatment time is not to be significantly extended. To this end, comprehensive treatment processes have been proposed that focus on reducing the number of parameters to be extracted from the volumetric image sets (Jaffray et al. 2001). The use of megavoltage cone-beam CT for guiding radiation therapy is being explored, to date, no clinical treatment protocols have been pursued with this technology. Ford et al. (2002) have proposed the clinical implementation of this technology for verification of treatment targeting in lung lesions. The imaging would be performed during a rotational arc treatment delivery. As yet it is unclear how cone-beam CT technology will impact radiation therapy, however, the capacity for radiography, CT, and direct integration with the treatment unit will produce systems that can be employed in many ways.

### Other Megavoltage CT Approaches

Megavoltage CT has been used for on-line correction in the clinical setting since the mid-1990's (Nakagawa et al. 2000). The procedure used by Nakagawa and colleagues involves positioning the patient according to skin marks, collecting a single MVCT slice, evaluating and possibly adjusting the patient's position. This is repeated until a satisfactory match is achieved. The MV detector is also used during treatment to relate the beam geometry to the MVCT images. A visual inspection by the radiation therapists suffices for monitoring. To date, they have treated 15 lung cancer patients with this approach. The authors clearly indicate that the poor quality of these images restricts their use to lesions in the lung. While others have developed MVCT systems, there are no other groups that have actually treated patients with the systems.

### The Tomotherapy Approach—Megavoltage CT

The integration of an MVCT subsystem into the tomotherapy device has permitted the generation of images of the patient with soft-tissue contrast at clinically acceptable doses (2 to 5 cGy). While the tomotherapy process is broad and there are many potential approaches to utilizing the MVCT image sets, a simplified approach has been implemented in its current release (2002). The images generated with the system are registered to the planning CT dataset and shift and rotation estimates are derived. The patient position is corrected through lateral, longitudinal, and vertical couch movements.

## Summary

The developments surrounding the improved precision of radiation therapy are advancing at a remarkable pace. The capacity to detect and correct for geometric positioning errors is becoming readily available with the development of robust imaging systems and software tools to analyze the resulting images. The development of on-line volumetric imaging systems, such as integrated CT, cone-beam CT or MVCT offer much more than improved targeting. These systems will be capable of documenting the delivery of dose to diseased and normal structures at an unprecedented level.

## References

Adler, J. R., Jr., S. D. Chang, M. J. Murphy, J. Doty, P. Geis, and S. L. Hancock. (1997). "The Cyberknife: A frameless robotic system for radiosurgery." *Stereotact. Funct. Neurosurg.* 69:124–128.

Alasti, H., M. P. Petric, C. N. Catton, and P. R. Warde. (2001). "Portal imaging for evaluation of daily on-line setup errors and off-line organ motion during conformal irradiation of carcinoma of the prostate." *Int. J. Radiat. Oncol. Biol. Phys.* 49:869–884.

Balter, J. M., G. T. Chen, C. A. Pelizzari, S. Krishnasamy, S. Rubin, and S. Vijayakumar. (1993). "Online repositioning during treatment of the prostate: a study of potential limits and gains." *Int. J. Radiat. Oncol. Biol. Phys.* 27:137–143.

Bedford, J. L., V. S. Khoo, D. P. Dearnaley, and S. Webb. (1999). "Improved methods for adding transaxial two-dimensional margins to the superior and inferior regions of a clinical target volume." *Med. Dosim.* 24:169–175.

Bel, A., M. van Herk, H. Bartelink, and J. V. Lebesque. (1993). "A verification procedure to improve patient set-up accuracy using portal images." *Radiother. Oncol.* 29:253–260.

Bel, A., H. Bartelink, R. E. Vijlbrief, and J. V. Lebesque. (1994). "Transfer errors of planning CT to simulator: a possible source of setup inaccuracies?" *Radiother. Oncol.* 31:176–180.

Biggs, P. J., M. Goitein, and M. D. Russell. (1985). "A diagnostic X ray field verification device for a 10 MV linear accelerator." *Int. J. Radiat. Oncol. Biol. Phys.* 11:635–643.

Bijhold, J., M. van Herk, R. Vijlbrief, and J. V. Lebesque. (1991). "Fast evaluation of patient set-up during radiotherapy by aligning features in portal and simulator images." *Phys. Med. Biol.* 36:1665–1679.

Brahme, A., B. Lind, and P. Nafstadius. (1987). "Radiotherapeutic computed tomography with scanned photon beams." *Int. J. Radiat. Oncol. Biol. Phys.* 13:95–101.

Brock, K. K., D. L. McShan, and J. M. Balter. (2002). "A comparison of computer-controlled versus manual on-line patient setup adjustment." *J. Appl. Clin. Med. Phys.* 3:241–247.

Cho, P. S., R. H. Johnson, and T. W. Griffin. (1995). "Cone-beam CT for radiotherapy applications." *Phys. Med. Biol.* 40:1863–1883.

Cho, Y., and R. Munro. (2002). "Kilovision: Thermal modeling of a kilovoltage x-ray source integrated into a medical linear accelerator." *Med. Phys.* 29:2101–2108.

Creutzberg, C. L., V. G. Althof, H. Huizenga, A. G. Visser, and P. C. Levendag. (1993). "Quality assurance using portal imaging: The accuracy of patient positioning in irradiation of breast cancer." *Int. J. Radiat. Oncol. Biol. Phys.* 25:529–539.

Crook, J. M., Y. Raymond, D. Salhani, H. Yang, and B. Esche. (1995). "Prostate motion during standard radiotherapy as assessed by fiducial markers." *Radiother. Oncol.* 37:35–42.

Curtin-Savard, A. J. and E. B. Podgorsak. (1999). "Verification of segmented beam delivery using a commercial electronic portal imaging device." *Med. Phys.* 26:737–742.

de Boer, H. C. and B. J. Heijmen. (2001). "A protocol for the reduction of systematic patient setup errors with minimal portal imaging workload." *Int. J. Radiat. Oncol. Biol. Phys.* 50:1350–1365.

de Boer, J.C. and B. J. Heijmen. (2002). "A new approach to off-line setup corrections: Combining safety with minimum workload." *Med. Phys.* 29:1998–2012.

De Neve, W., F. Van den Heuvel, M. De Beukeleer, M. Coghe, L. Thon, P. De Roover, M. Van Lancker, and G. Storme. (1992). "Routine clinical on-line portal imaging followed by immediate field adjustment using a tele-controlled patient couch." *Radiother. Oncol.* 24:45–54.

Feldkamp, L., L. Davis, and J. Kress. (1984). "Practical Cone-beam Algorithm." *J. Opt. Soc. Am. A* 1:612–619.

Fontenla, E., C. A. Pelizzari, J. C. Roeske, and G. T. Chen. (2001). "Using serial imaging data to model variabilities in organ position and shape during radiotherapy." *Phys. Med. Biol.* 46:2317–2336.

Ford, E. C., J. Chang, K. Mueller, K. Sidhu, D. Todor, G. Mageras, E. Yorke, C. C. Ling, and H. Amols. (2002). "Cone-beam CT with megavoltage beams and an amorphous silicon electronic portal imaging device: Potential for verification of radiotherapy of lung cancer." *Med. Phys.* 29:2913–2924.

Gospodarowicz, M., and B. O'Sullivan. "Prognostic Factors: Principles and Application" in *Prognostic Factors in Cancer*, *2nd Ed.* M. K. Gospodarowicz, D. E. Henson, R. V. P. Hutter, B. O'Sullivan, L. H. Sobin, Ch. Wittekind (eds.). Chichester, West Sussex: John Wiley & Sons Ltd., pp. 17–35, 2001.

Groh, B. A., J. H. Siewerdsen, D. G. Drake, J. W. Wong, and D. A. Jaffray. (2002). "A performance comparison of flat-panel imager-based MV and kV cone-beam CT." *Med. Phys.* 29:967–975.

Herman, M. G., J. J. Kruse, and C. R. Hagness. (2000). "Guide to clinical use of electronic portal imaging." *J. Appl. Clin. Med. Phys.* 1:38–57.

Herman, M. G., J. M. Balter, D. A. Jaffray, K. P. McGee, P. Munro, S. Shalev, M. van Herk, and J. W. Wong. (2001). "Clinical use of electronic portal imaging: Report of AAPM Radiation Therapy Committee Task Group 58." *Med. Phys.* 28:712–737. Also available as AAPM Report No. 75, Clinical Use of Electronic Portal Imaging. Madison, WI: Medical Physics Publishing.

Hesse, B. M., L. Spies, and B. A. Groh. (1998). "Tomotherapeutic portal imaging for radiation treatment verification." *Phys. Med. Biol.* 43:3607–3616.

Holupka, E. J., I. D. Kaplan, E. C. Burdette, and G. K. Svensson. (1996). "Ultrasound image fusion for external beam radiotherapy for prostate cancer." *Int. J. Rad. Oncol. Biol. Phys.* 35:975–984.

Hurkmans, C. W., P. Remeijer, J. V. Lebesque, and B. J. Mijnheer. (2001). "Set-up verification using portal imaging; review of current clinical practice." *Radiother. Oncol.* 58:105–120.

Jaffray, D. A., and J. H. Siewerdsen. (2000). "Cone-beam computed tomography with a flat-panel imager: Initial performance characterization." *Med. Phys.* 27:1311–1323.

Jaffray, D. A., D. Yan, and J. W. Wong. (1999). "Managing geometric uncertainty in conformal intensity-modulated radiation therapy." *Semin. Radiat. Oncol.* 9:4–19.

Jaffray, D. A., K. Chawla, C. Yu, and J. W. Wong. (1995). "Dual-beam imaging for online verification of radiotherapy field placement." *Int. J. Rad. Oncol. Biol. Phys.* 33:1273–1280.

Jaffray, D. A., D. G. Drake, M. Moreau, A. A. Martinez, and J. W. Wong. (1999). "A radiographic and tomographic imaging system integrated into a medical linear accelerator for localization of bone and soft-tissue targets." *Int. J. Radiat. Oncol. Biol. Phys.* 45:773–789.

Jaffray, D., M. van Herk, J. Lebesque, and A. Martinez. "Image Guided Radiotherapy of the Prostate" in Proceedings of the Medical Imaging Computing and Computer-Assisted Intervention (MICCAI), pp. 1075–1080, 2001.

Jaffray, D. A., J. H. Siewerdsen, J. W. Wong, and A. A. Martinez. (2002). "Flat-panel cone-beam computed tomography for image-guided radiation therapy." *Int. J. Radiat. Oncol. Biol. Phys.* 53:1337–1349.

Kaatee, R. S., M. J. Olofsen, M. B. Verstraate, S. Quint, and B. J. Heijmen. (2002). "Detection of organ movement in cervix cancer patients using a fluoroscopic electronic portal imaging device and radiopaque markers." *Int. J. Rad. Oncol. Biol. Phys.* 54:576–583.

Kitamura, K., H. Shirato, Y. Seppenwoolde, R. Onimaru, M. Oda, K. Fujita, S. Shimizu, N. Shinohara, T. Harabayashi, and K. Miyasaka. (2002). "Three-dimensional intrafractional movement of prostate measured during real-time tumor-tracking radiotherapy in supine and prone treatment positions." *Int. J. Radiat. Oncol. Biol. Phys.* 53:1117–1123.

Korin, H. W., R. L. Ehman, S. J. Riederer, J. P. Felmlee, and R. C. Grimm. (1992). "Respiratory kinematics of the upper abdominal organs: a quantitative study." *Magn. Reson. Med.* 23:172–178.

Kuriyama, K., H. Onishi, N. Sano, T. Komiyama, Y. Aikawa, Y. Tateda, T. Araki, and M. Uematsu. (2003). "A new irradiation unit constructed of self-moving gantry-CT and linac." *Int. J. Radiat. Oncol. Biol. Phys.* 55:428–435.

Kutcher, G. J., G. S. Mageras, and S. A. Liebel. (1995). "Control, correction, and modeling of setup errors and organ motion." *Semin. Radiat. Oncol.* 5:134–145.

Lagendijk, J. Private communication.

Lattanzi, J., S. McNeeley, S. Donnelly, E. Palacio, A. Hanlon, T. E. Schultheiss, and G. E. Hanks. (2000). "Ultrasound-based stereotactic guidance in prostate cancer—quantification of organ motion and set-up errors in external beam radiation therapy." *Comput. Aided Surg.* 5:289–295.

Lebesque, J. V., A. Bel, J. Bijhold, and A. A. Hart. (1992). "Detection of systematic patient setup errors by portal film analysis." *Radiother. Oncol.* 23:198.

Lockman, D. M., D. Yan, and J. Wong. (2000). "Estimating the dose variation in a volume of interest with explicit consideration of patient geometric variation." *Med. Phys.* 27:2100–2108.

Lof, J., B. K. Lind, and A. Brahme. (1998). "An adaptive control algorithm for optimization of intensity modulated radiotherapy considering uncertainties in beam profiles, patient set-up and internal organ motion." *Phys. Med. Biol.* 43:1605–1628.

Mackie, T. R., T. Holmes, S. Swerdloff, P. Reckwerdt, J. O. Deasy, J. Yang, B. Paliwal, and T. Kinsella. (1993). "Tomotherapy: A new concept for the delivery of dynamic conformal radiotherapy." *Med. Phys.* 20:1709–1719.

Mackie, T. R., J. Balog, K. Ruchala, D. Shepard, S. Aldridge, E. Fitchard, P. Reckwerdt, G. Olivera, T. McNutt, and M. Mehta. (1999). "Tomotherapy." *Semin. Radiat. Oncol.* 9:108–117.

Marks, J. E., A. G. Haus, H. G. Sutton, and M. L. Griem. (1974). "Localization error in the radiotherapy of Hodgkin's disease and malignant lymphoma with extended mantle fields." *Cancer* 34:83–90.

Marks, J. E., A. G. Haus, H. G. Sutton, and M. L. Griem. (1976). "The value of frequent treatment verification films in reducing localization error in the irradiation of complex fields." *Cancer* 37:2755–2761.

Martinez, A. A., D. Yan, D. Lockman, D. Brabbins, K. Kota, M. Sharpe, D. A. Jaffray, F. Vicini, and J. Wong. (2001). "Improvement in dose escalation using the process of adaptive radiotherapy combined with three-dimensional conformal or intensity-modulated beams for prostate cancer." *Int. J. Radiat. Oncol. Biol. Phys.* 50:1226–1234.

McKenzie, A. L., M. van Herk, and B. Mijnheer. (2000). "The width of margins in radiotherapy treatment plans." *Phys. Med. Biol.* 45:3331–3342.

Melian, E., G. S. Mageras, Z. Fuks, S. A. Leibel, A. Niehaus, H. Lorant, M. Zelefsky, B. Baldwin, and G. J. Kutcher. (1997). "Variation in prostate position quantitation and implications for three-dimensional conformal treatment planning." *Int. J. Radiat. Oncol. Biol. Phys.* 38:73–81.

Midgley, S., R. M. Millar, and J. Dudson. (1998). "A feasibility study for megavoltage cone beam CT using a commercial EPID." *Phys. Med. Biol.* 43:155–169.

Mijnheer, B. J. (1992). "Quality assurance in radiotherapy: Physical and technical aspects." *Qual. Assur. Health Care* 4:9–18.

Mosleh-Shirazi, M. A., W. Swindell, and P. M. Evans. (1998). "Optimization of the scintillation detector in a combined 3D megavoltage CT scanner and portal imager." *Med. Phys.* 25:1880–1890.

Mosleh-Shirazi, M. A., P. M. Evans, W. Swindell, S. Webb, and M. Partridge. (1998). "A cone-beam megavoltage CT scanner for treatment verification in conformal radiotherapy." *Radiother. Oncol.* 48:319–328.

Munro, P. "Megavoltage Radiography for Treatment Verification" in *The Modern Technology of Radiation Oncology. A Compendium for Medical Physicists and Radiation Oncologists.* J. Van Dyk (ed.). Madison, WI: Medical Physics Publishing, pp. 481–508, 1999.

Nakagawa, K., Y. Aoki, M. Tago, A. Terahara, and K. Ohtomo. (2000). "Megavoltage CT-assisted stereotactic radiosurgery for thoracic tumors: Original research in the treatment of thoracic neoplasms." *Int. J. Radiat. Oncol. Biol. Phys.* 48:449–457.

Nederveen, A. J., J. J. Lagendijk, and P. Hofman. (2001). "Feasibility of automatic marker detection with an a-Si flat-panel imager." *Phys. Med. Biol.* 46:1219–1230.

Nunan, C. S. (1995). "Radiotherapy apparatus equipped with a low dose localizing and portal imaging x-ray source." U. S. Patent 5,471,516.

Nuyttens, J. J., J. M. Robertson, D. Yan, and A. Martinez. (2002). "The variability of the clinical target volume for rectal cancer due to internal organ motion during adjuvant treatment." *Int. J. Radiat. Oncol. Biol. Phys.* 53:497–503.

Olivera, G. H., D. M. Shepard, K. Ruchala, J. S. Aldridge, J. Kapatoes, E. E. Fitchard, P. J. Reckwerdt, G. Fang, J. Balog, J. Zachman, and T. R. Mackie. "Tomotherapy" in *The Modern Technology of Radiation Oncology. A Compendium for Medical Physicists and Radiation Oncologists.* J. Van Dyk (ed.). Madison, WI: Medical Physics Publishing, pp. 521–587, 1999.

Partridge, M., P. M. Evans, and M. A. Mosleh-Shirazi. (1998). "Linear accelerator output variations and their consequences for megavoltage imaging." *Med. Phys.* 25:1443–1452.

Partridge, M., J. R. Symonds-Tayler, and P. M. Evans. (2000). "IMRT verification with a camera-based electronic portal imaging system." *Phys. Med. Biol.* 45:N183–N196.

Pisani, L., D. Lockman, D. Jaffray, D. Yan, A. Martinez, and J. Wong. (2000). "Setup error in radiotherapy: on-line correction using electronic kilovoltage and megavoltage radiographs." *Int. J. Radiat. Oncol. Biol. Phys.* 47:825–839.

Ploeger, L. S., M. H. Smitsmans, K. G. Gilhuijs, and M. van Herk. (2002). "A method for geometrical verification of dynamic intensity modulated radiotherapy using a scanning electronic portal imaging device." *Med. Phys.* 29:1071–1079.

Remeijer, P., C. Rasch, J. V. Lebesque, and M. van Herk. (2002). "Margins for translational and rotational uncertainties: a probability-based approach." *Int. J. Radiat. Oncol. Biol. Phys.* 53:464–474.

Roeske, J. C., J. D. Forman, C. F. Mesina, T. He, C. A. Pelizzari, E. Fontenla, S. Vijayakumar, and G. T. Chen. (1995). "Evaluation of changes in the size and location of the prostate, seminal vesicles, bladder, and rectum during a course of external beam radiation therapy." *Int. J. Radiat. Oncol. Biol. Phys.* 33:1321–1329.

Ruchala, K. J., G. H. Olivera, E. A. Schloesser, and T. R. Mackie. (1999). "Megavoltage CT on a tomotherapy system." *Phys. Med. Biol.* 44:2597–2621.

Schewe, J. E., J. M. Balter, K. L. Lam, and R. K. Ten Haken. (1996). "Measurement of patient setup errors using port films and a computer-aided graphical alignment tool." *Med. Dosim.* 21:97–104.

Schewe, J. E., K. L. Lam, J. M. Balter, and R. K. Ten Haken. (1998). "A room-based diagnostic imaging system for measurement of patient setup." *Med. Phys.* 25:2385–2387.

Shalev, S. (1996). "On-line portal imaging: contributions and limitations in clinical practice." *Front. Radiat. Ther. Oncol.* 29:156–167.

Shimizu, S., H. Shirato, K. Kitamura, N. Shinohara, T. Harabayashi, T. Tsukamoto, T. Koyanagi, and K. Miyasaka. (2000). "Use of an implanted marker and real-time tracking of the marker for the positioning of prostate and bladder cancers." *Int. J. Radiat. Oncol. Biol. Phys.* 48:1591–1597.

Shimizu, S., H. Shirato, S. Ogura, H. Akita-Dosaka, K. Kitamura, T. Nishioka, K. Kagei, M. Nishimura, and K. Miyasaka. (2001). "Detection of lung tumor movement in real-time tumor-tracking radiotherapy." *Int. J. Radiat. Oncol. Biol. Phys.* 51:304–310.

Shirato, H., S. Shimizu, T. Shimizu, T. Nishioka, and K. Miyasaka. (1999). "Real-time tumour-tracking radiotherapy." *Lancet* 353:1331–1332.

Shirato, H., S. Shimizu, K. Kitamura, T. Nishioka, K. Kagei, S. Hashimoto, H. Aoyama, T. Kunieda, N. Shinohara, H. Dosaka-Akita, and K. Miyasaka. (2000a). "Four-dimensional treatment planning and fluoroscopic real-time tumor tracking radiotherapy for moving tumor." *Int. J. Radiat. Oncol. Biol. Phys.* 48:435–442.

Shirato, H., S. Shimizu, T. Kunieda, K. Kitamura, M. Van Herk, K. Kagei, T. Nishioka, S. Hashimoto, K. Fujita, H. Aoyama, K. Tsuchiya, K. Kudo, and K. Miyasaka. (2000b). "Physical aspects of a real-time tumor-tracking system for gated radiotherapy." *Int. J. Radiat. Oncol. Biol. Phys.* 48:1187–1195.

Siewerdsen, J. H., and D. A. Jaffray. (1999). "Cone-beam computed tomography with a flat-panel imager: effects of image lag." *Med. Phys.* 26:2635–2647.

Siewerdsen, J. H. and D. A. Jaffray. (2000). "Optimization of x-ray imaging geometry (with specific application to flat-panel cone-beam computed tomography)." *Med. Phys.* 27:1903–1914.

Siewerdsen, J. H. and D. A. Jaffray. (2001). "Cone-beam computed tomography with a flat-panel imager: magnitude and effects of x-ray scatter." *Med. Phys.* 28:220–231.

Simpson, R. G., C. T. Chen, E. A. Grubbs, and W. Swindell. (1982). "A 4-MV CT scanner for radiation therapy: the prototype system." *Med. Phys.* 9:574–579.

Spies, L., M. Ebert, B. A. Groh, B. M. Hesse, and T. Bortfeld. (2001). "Correction of scatter in megavoltage cone-beam CT." *Phys. Med. Biol.* 46:821–833.

Stroom, J. C., P. C. Koper, G. A. Korevaar, M. van Os, M. Janssen, H. C. de Boer, P. C. Levendag, and B. J. Heijmen. (1999). "Internal organ motion in prostate cancer patients treated in prone and supine treatment position." *Radiother. Oncol.* 51:237–248.

Stroom, J. C., M. Kroonwijk, K. L. Pasma, P. C. Koper, E. B. van Dieren, and B. J. Heijmen. (2000a). "Detection of internal organ movement in prostate cancer patients using portal images." *Med. Phys.* 27:452–461.

Stroom, J. C., M. J. Olofsen-van Acht, S. Quint, M. Seven, M. de Hoog, C. L. Creutzberg, H. C. de Boer, and A. G. Visser. (2000b). "On-line set-up corrections during radiotherapy of patients with gynecologic tumors." *Int. J. Radiat. Oncol. Biol. Phys.* 46:499–506.

Uematsu, M. (2002a). "[CT-guided stereotactic radiotherapy for early stage lung cancer]." *Nippon Rinsho* 60 *Suppl* 5:408–410.

Uematsu, M. (2002b). "[Stereotactic radiation therapy for non small cell lung cancer]." *Nippon Geka Gakkai Zasshi* 103:256–257.

Uematsu, M., T. Fukui, A. Shioda, H. Tokumitsu, K. Takai, T. Kojima, Y. Asai, and S. Kusano. (1996). "A dual computed tomography linear accelerator unit for stereotactic radiation therapy: A new approach without cranially fixated stereotactic frames." *Int. J. Radiat. Oncol. Biol. Phys.* 35:587–592.

Uematsu, M., A. Shioda, K. Tahara, T. Fukui, F. Yamamoto, G. Tsumatori, Y. Ozeki, T. Aoki, M. Watanabe, and S. Kusano. (1998). "Focal, high dose, and fractionated modified stereotactic radiation therapy for lung carcinoma patients: a preliminary experience." *Cancer* 82:1062–1070.

Uematsu, M., M. Sonderegger, A. Shioda, K. Tahara, T. Fukui, Y. Hama, T. Kojima, J. R. Wong, and S. Kusano. (1999). "Daily positioning accuracy of frameless stereotactic radiation therapy with a fusion of computed tomography and linear accelerator (focal) unit: evaluation of z-axis with a z-marker." *Radiother. Oncol.* 50:337–339.

Uematsu, M., A. Shioda, A. Suda, K. Tahara, T. Kojima, Y. Hama, M. Kono, J. R. Wong, T. Fukui, and S. Kusano. (2000). "Intrafractional tumor position stability during computed tomography (CT)-guided frameless stereotactic radiation therapy for lung or liver cancers with a fusion of CT and linear accelerator (FOCAL) unit." *Int. J. Radiat. Oncol. Biol. Phys.* 48:443–448.

Uematsu, M., A. Shioda, A. Suda, T. Fukui, Y. Ozeki, Y. Hama, J. R. Wong, and S. Kusano. (2001). "Computed tomography-guided frameless stereotactic radiotherapy for stage I non-small cell lung cancer: a 5-year experience." *Int. J. Radiat. Oncol. Biol. Phys.* 51:666–670.

van Herk, M., A. Bruce, A. P. Kroes, T. Shouman, A. Touw, and J. V. Lebesque. (1995). "Quantification of organ motion during conformal radiotherapy of the prostate by three dimensional image registration." *Int. J. Rad. Oncol. Biol. Phys.* 33:1311–1320.

van Herk, M., P. Remeijer, C. Rasch, and J. V. Lebesque. (2000). "The probability of correct target dosage: dose-population histograms for deriving treatment margins in radiotherapy." *Int. J. Radiat. Oncol. Biol. Phys.* 47:1121–1135.

Wu, J., T. Haycocks, H. Alasti, G. Ottewell, N. Middlemiss, M. Abdolell, P. Warde, A. Toi, and C. Catton. (2001). "Positioning errors and prostate motion during conformal prostate radiotherapy using on-line isocentre set-up verification and implanted prostate markers." *Radiother. Oncol.* 61:127–133.

Yan, D. and D. Lockman. (2001). "Organ/patient geometric variation in external beam radiotherapy and its effects." *Med. Phys.* 28:593–602.

Yan, D., F. A. Vicini, J. W. Wong, and A. A. Martinez. (1997a). "Adaptive radiation therapy." *Phys. Med. Biol.* 42:123–132.

Yan, D., J. Wong, F. Vicini, J. Michalski, C. Pan, A. Frazier, E. Horwitz, and A. Martinez. (1997b). "Adaptive modification of treatment planning to minimize the deleterious effects of treatment setup errors." *Int. J. Radiat. Oncol. Biol. Phys.* 38:197–206.

Yan, D., E. Ziaja, D. Jaffray, J. Wong, D. Brabbins, F. Vicini, and A. Martinez. (1998). "The use of adaptive radiation therapy to reduce setup error: a prospective clinical study." *Int. J. Radiat. Oncol. Biol. Phys.* 41:715–720.

Yan, D., D. Lockman, D. Brabbins, L. Tyburski, and A. A. Martinez. (2000). "An off-line strategy for constructing a patient-specific planning target volume in an adaptive treatment process for prostate cancer." *Int. J. Radiat. Oncol. Biol. Phys.* 48:289–302

Yin, F. F., S. Ryu, M. Ajlouni, J. Zhu, H. Yan, H. Guan, K. Faber, J. Rock, M. Abdalhak, L. Rogers, M. Rosenblum, and J. H. Kim. (2002). "A technique of intensity-modulated radiosurgery (IMRS) for spinal tumors." *Med. Phys.* 29:2815–2822.

Zelefsky, M. J., D. Crean, G. S. Mageras, O. Lyass, L. Happersett, C. C. Ling, S. A. Leibel, Z. Fuks, S. Bull, H. M. Kooy, M. van Herk, and G. J. Kutcher. (1999). "Quantification and predictors of prostate position variability in 50 patients evaluated with multiple CT scans during conformal radiotherapy." *Radiother. Oncol.* 50:225–234.

# Patient Positioning Using Optical And Ultrasound Techniques


Sanford L. Meeks, Ph.D.[1], Wolfgang A. Tomé, Ph.D.[2],
Lionel G. Bouchet, Ph.D.[3], A. Curtis Hass, M.D.[1],
John M. Buatti, M.D.[1], Francis J. Bova, Ph.D.[4]

[1]Department of Radiation Oncology, University of Iowa, Iowa City, Iowa
[2]Department of Human Oncology, University of Wisconsin Medical School,
Madison, Wisconsin, [3]ZMed Inc., Ashland, Massachusetts
[4]Department of Neurological Surgery, University of Florida, Gainesville, Florida




## Introduction

Over the last decade, virtual simulation has become the standard of care for planning the majority of external beam radiotherapy treatments. There are many obvious technical advantages of virtual simulation over conventional radiotherapy simulation. Target identification is more accurate, because the target may be identified directly on computer tomography (CT) and/or co-identified on magnetic resonance imaging (MRI), functional imaging scans, and positron emission tomography (PET) scans of the patient. Furthermore, the spatial relationship of the tumor to surrounding normal organs is more easily appreciated through direct target identification. This allows the treatment planner to more easily design beam orientations, sizes, and shapes that avoid these structures. The ability to iteratively alter the beam arrangement is also a major advance over conventional simulation. Virtual simulation allows trials of multiple beam entrances and exits without requiring patient participation. Furthermore, treatment with oblique angles is facilitated through virtual simulation, and the use of non-coplanar field arrangements has become practically achievable. Moreover, virtual simulation has provided the framework for three-dimensional (3-D) conformal therapy and intensity-modulated radiation therapy (IMRT).

While virtual simulation provides a significant improvement over conventional simulation techniques, the transfer of plan information from the virtual world to actual treatment has been limited by the accuracy of the fiducial systems traditionally chosen in radiation therapy. Optical and image-guided radiation therapy systems hold a great deal of promise for improving the precision of patient treatment by providing a more robust fiducial system. The ability to accurately position internal targets relative to the linear accelerator (linac) isocenter and to provide real-time patient tracking theoretically enables significant reductions in the amount of normal tissue included in the irradiated volume. Testing and implementation of these systems present new challenges for the clinical physicist, and it is important that the strengths and weaknesses of these systems are thoroughly understood. Our group has been active in the development and clinical application of non-invasive optical-guided techniques for both stereotactic radiosurgery and fractionated stereotactic radiotherapy. In addition, we have been active in extending the optical guidance paradigm to extracranial treatment sites. High-precision extracranial radiation delivery is challenging, however, because the target position can shift relative to bony anatomy between the time of image acquisition for virtual simulation and the time of treatment. Our group has recently investigated the use of optical-guided 3-D ultrasound for high-precision radiation delivery. The purpose of this chapter is to describe (1) optical and ultrasound guided radiotherapy techniques, (2) the underlying mathematics that drive image guidance, (3) quality assurance techniques, and (4) clinical implementation of optical- and ultrasound-guided patient positioning systems.

## Optical Tracking Systems

Tracking is the process of measuring the location of instruments, anatomical structures, and/or landmarks in three-dimensional space and in relation to each other. Systems for tracking and motion capture for interactive computer graphics have been explored for more than 30 years. Various technologies have been tested for determining an object's location, including mechanical, magnetic, acoustic, inertial, and optical position sensors. Most of these technologies have been tested for medical use in either image-guided surgery or image-guided tracking in radiation therapy. Description of technologies other than optical tracking is considered beyond this report, and can be found in more general works on tracking systems (Allen, Bishop, and Welch 2001).

Optical tracking systems use infrared light to determine an object's position. The object may either be an active or a passive marker. The most common active markers are infrared light emitting diodes (IRLEDs). Passive markers are generally spheres or disks coated with a highly reflective surface for passively reflecting infrared light from an external source. Various detectors can be used to determine the positions of an optical marker, but charge-coupled device (CCD) cameras are most often used. CCD cameras are simply a collection of light sensitive cells, or pixels, and these cells can be arranged in either a one- or two-dimensional (2-D) matrix. When light strikes a CCD cell, electrons are produced in proportion to the amount of light incident on the cell. The charge collected per cell provides a pixel luminance value; a 2-D CCD array thus provides a 2-D digital "image" of the target with brighter pixels corresponding to a higher light intensity incident on the cell and darker pixels corresponding to lower light intensity incident on the cell. This digital image can then be analyzed to determine the pixel with the highest intensity. Each camera in a 2-D CCD array determines a ray in 3-D. When an optical system uses two 2-D CCDs, the intersection of the 3-D rays from the cameras determines a point in space, and hence the 3-D marker location through a stereoscopic technique.

## Optical Tracking In Radiation Therapy

Several optical tracking systems have been developed and are commercially available for use in radiation therapy (Baroni, Ferrigno, and Pedotti 1998; Cardinale et al. 1999; Kai et al. 1998; Kubo et al. 2000; Menke et al. 1994; Rogus, Stern, and Kubo 1999; Wang et al. 2001). The theory of operation behind all the available systems is very similar; optical tracking of infrared markers (passive or active) attached to the patient is used to determine a patient's position relative to the linear accelerator. This real-time feedback can then be used to position the patient and/or gate the radiation beam. Our operational description will focus on the system that was originally developed at the University of Florida (Bova et al. 1997; Buatti et al. 1998; Meeks et al. 2000; Tomé et al. 2000, 2001; Ryken et al. 2001a) and is commercially available under the trade name RadioCameras™ (ZMed Inc., Ashland, MA). This system uses the Polaris position sensor unit (Northern Digital, Inc., Waterloo, Ontario) to optically track the position of either active or passive infrared markers arranged in an array to form a rigid body. Optical tracking systems have native coordinate systems that are most often located at the center of the detector. In the RadioCameras system, the Polaris is mounted in the ceiling above the linear accelerator (figure 1). Therefore, the origin for the camera system is located at the ceiling of the treatment room and the axes of the coordinate system are dependent upon the camera's orientation. The most logical origin for clinical use in radiotherapy is the machine isocenter, with the coordinate axes located parallel to the vertical, lateral, and longitudinal couch motions. A calibration procedure is required to transform the coordinate system from the Polaris' native coordinate system to the linear accelerator's coordinate system. This calibration utilizes a calibration apparatus that places passive markers at known coordinates relative to the machine isocenter (see figure 2). An optical measurement of the apparatus is obtained, thereby establishing a transformation matrix from camera coordinates to room coordinates. After this calibration, the position of any infrared marker in the room may be determined relative to the isocenter. Using this same calibration procedure, the origin and orthogonal reference system can be translated to any point. The system can therefore be adapted to any orthogonal reference system, making it compatible with most imaging systems, treatment delivery systems, or stereotactic frame systems.

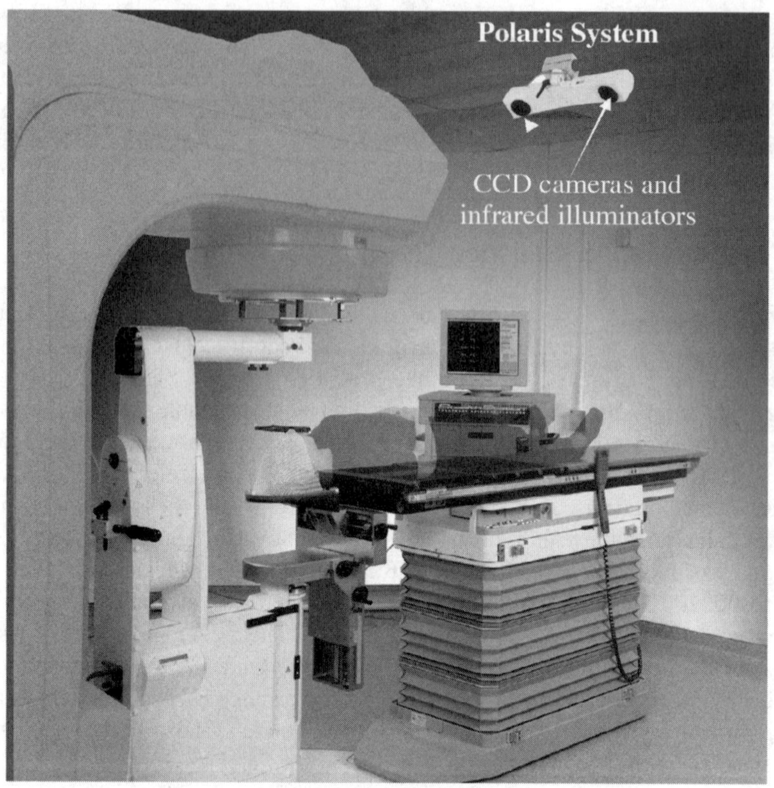


**Figure 1.** The setup for optical-guided radiotherapy includes a bite plate with six IRLEDs, a Polaris position sensor that images the position of the six IRLEDs, and a computer that determines the position of the IRLEDs relative to linac isocenter.

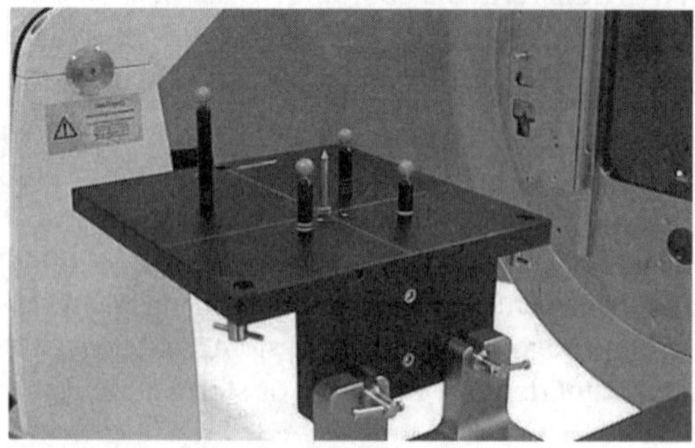

**Figure 2.** The optical calibration apparatus has four reflective spheres that can be placed at known positions relative to isocenter. After optically sampling their positions, a calibration matrix is established that transforms the position sensor unit from its native coordinate system to the room coordinate system.

Patient localization is accomplished through detection of an optical reference array containing four passive markers. This reference array is attached to a custom bite plate that links to the maxillary dentition of the patient to form a rigid system. The optically determined patient position is then compared to the desired patient position, as determined in the virtual simulation; the bite plate-reference array complex is kept in place during the virtual simulation CT scan (figure 3), and the image coordinates of the reflective markers are determined as part of the virtual simulation (figure 4).

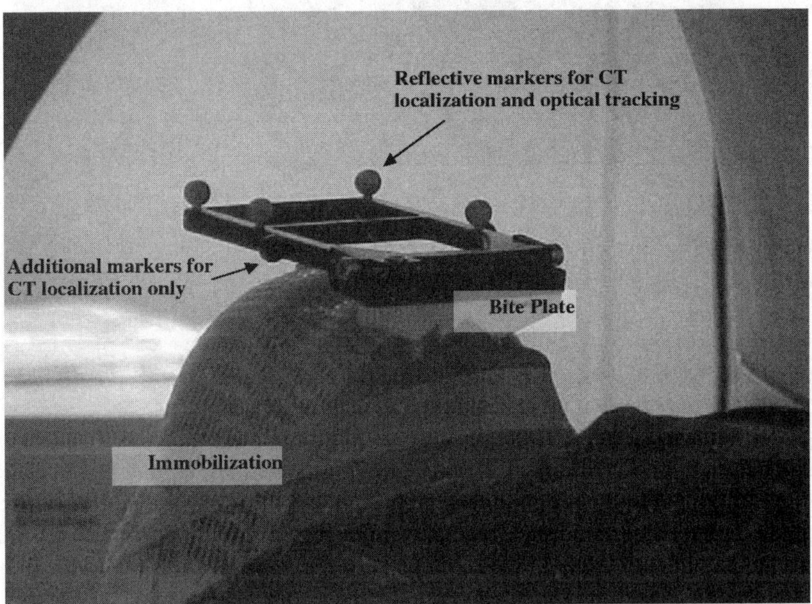


**Figure 3.** The optical reference array has six fiducials that can be localized in a CT scan. Four of these fiducials have a reflective surface that can be used for optical tracking. The reference array is attached to a bite plate. The custom bite plate is fabricated by placing dental impression material in an acrylic dental tray and allowing the impression material to form on the patient's maxillary dentition. Patients undergo CT scanning and treatment with the bite plate and reference array in position. Immobilization is accomplished using a custom pillow and facemask.

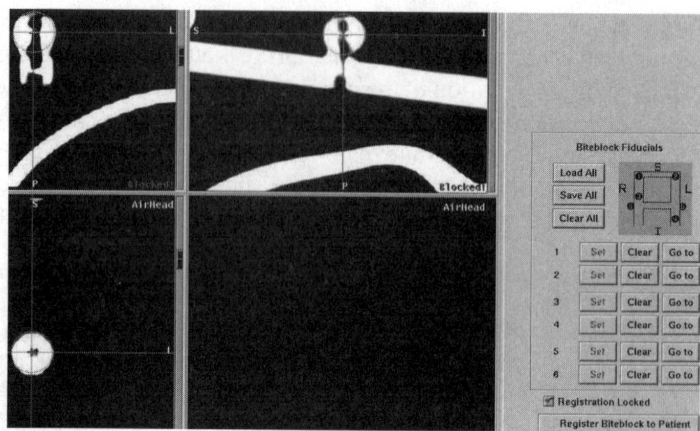


**Figure 4.** Image localization is accomplished by indicating the center of each spherical fiducial in the CT scan. Comparison of the image-localized positions of the sphere with the known fiducial array geometry provides the mean registration error.

## Mathematics Of Optical Tracking

In optical guidance for radiation therapy, we determine the image coordinates of the passive markers and the desired isocenter location from the virtual simulation CT scan, and we determine the room coordinates of the passive markers relative to the machine isocenter from optical tracking. The mathematics required for optical guidance simply entails the determination of the relationship between these two sets of points. Exhaustive details of the mathematics used in optical guidance can be found in the literature (Yang et al. 1999; Meeks et al. 2000; Bouchet et al. 2001; Tomé et al. 2002).

Since this is a minimization problem, iterative optimization algorithms can be used to find the best-fit rotation. Several different optimization algorithms have been used to solve the patient orientation problem in stereotactic radiotherapy, including simulated annealing and various downhill algorithms such as the downhill simplex and the Hooke and Jeeves pattern search algorithm (Yang et al. 1999; Shoup and Mistree 1987). The solution space for the stereotactic radiotherapy application has been shown to be relatively flat, and downhill methods have proven fast and effective for stereotactic radiotherapy (Yang et al. 1999).

## Commissioning And Quality Assurance For Optical Guidance

Optical-guided patient positioning systems present new challenges that must be thoroughly investigated prior to patient use. Testing procedures and expected tolerances can be found in the literature (Bova et al. 1997; Phillips et al. 2000; Meeks et al. 2002), and a basic review is presented here. For example, all infrared camera systems exhibit a spatial drift immediately after startup due to thermal changes. It is important to determine the magnitude and duration of this drift and ensure that it does not contribute to errors in the clinical process. This drift can be simply tested by rigidly fixing an optical reference array in the camera's field of view, and then optically sampling the position of the reference array at temporal intervals immediately following power on to the camera. Figure 5 graphically depicts the thermal drift that occurs when the camera is first switched on. Readings were taken at 10-minute intervals from the time of power on up to 100 minutes after the power was turned on. As can be seen in figure 5, the accuracy of the camera drifts more than 4 mm over the first 80 minutes that power is supplied to the camera. After this initial system warm-up, the reproducibility of the system can be evaluated by continuing to sample the position of the array at fixed temporal intervals. Figure 6 shows the results of repeat measurements taken at 10-minute intervals after the camera has stabilized. As can be seen graphically, the camera is extremely reproducible (within 0.04 mm) after the initial warm-up period. The results of these experiments indicate that the camera is extremely stable, but no camera calibration or clinical use should occur unless power has been supplied to the camera for a minimum of 90 minutes. The duration and magnitude of this initial instability is camera dependent, and should be tested independently at each site prior to clinical use.

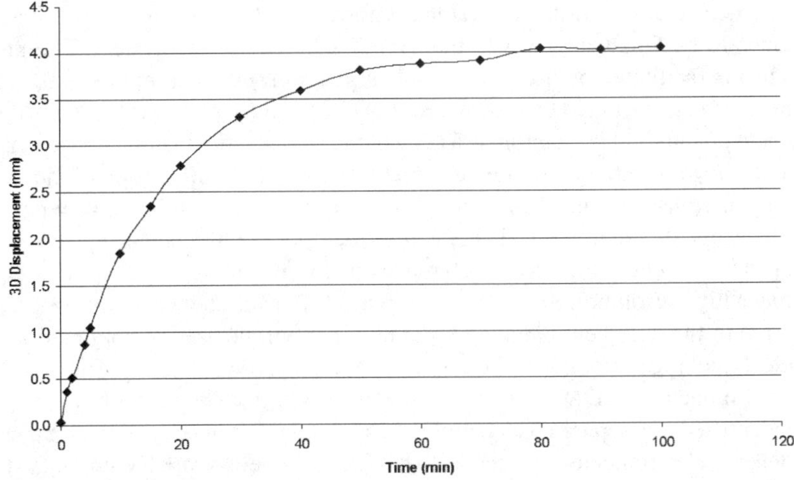

**Figure 5.** Thermal drift of the system as a function of time from time = 0 (power on to system) to time = 100 minutes.

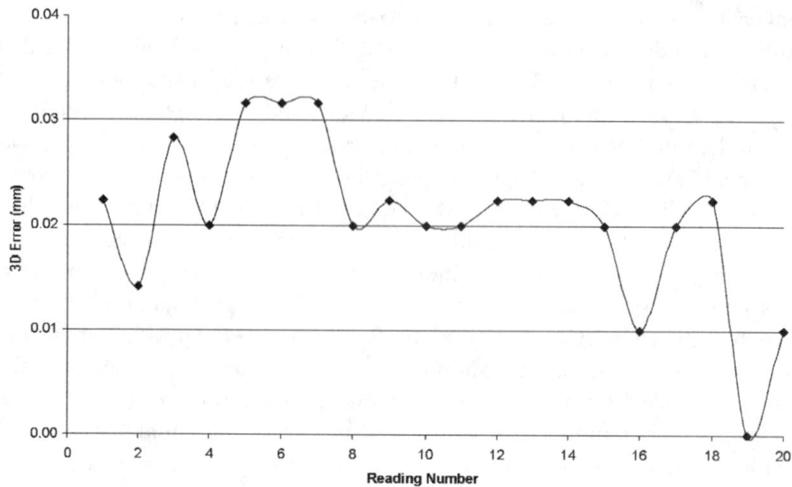

**Figure 6.** Reproducibility of the optical guided system after the camera has stabilized.

After system reproducibility is determined, acceptance tests should focus on the spatial accuracy of localizing known points in both the image coordinate system and the linear accelerator coordinate system. Known targets tests can be performed at acceptance to systematically verify the overall accuracy of the system. The known targets test is facilitated by use of an absolute phantom in which points in the phantom are precisely machined to known coordinates. We have previously designed such an absolute phantom; this phantom is a copy of the stereotactic ring that has six spheres at various known locations throughout stereotactic space. Being a copy of the stereotactic ring, the phantom attaches directly to any stereotactic localization devices, and also can accept stereotactic localizers and/or the optical reference array. Tests were performed by attaching the optical reference array to the absolute phantom, and then obtaining a high resolution ($0.7 \times 0.7 \times 1.0$ mm$^3$) CT scan. These CT images are then transferred to the treatment planning system(s) that will be used in conjunction with the optical tracking system; in our case, we use both FastPlan™ (ZMed Inc., Ashland, MA) and Pinnacle$^3$®(ADAC Laboratories, Milipitas, CA). The center of each sphere can be identified as a separate isocenter in the planning system(s), and the images and isocenters are electronically transferred to the RadioCameras workstation. In the treatment room, optical tracking is then utilized to place the center of each sphere at the isocenter of the treatment machine. Determining the sphere's true location can be performed with either conventional stereotactic positioning systems or film. For example, the absolute phantom can be attached to our stereotactic floor stand (Friedman and Bova 1989), as shown in figure 7. The RadioCameras station tracks the reference array and is used to move the center of each sphere to isocenter. The stereotactic coordinates are read from the floorstand. These experimentally determined coordinates are compared against the known values to determine the accuracy of image localization and optical guidance combined. On average, the six well-defined targets can be identified using FastPlan and optically localized in RadioCameras to within 0.6 mm total 3-D error. Similarly, on average, the six well-defined targets can be identified using Pinnacle and optically localized in RadioCameras to within 1.0 mm total 3-D error. The error with either system is within the image resolution, and indicates that the total error is dominated by the imaging and optical tracking actually contributes very little additional error to the overall process (Meeks et al. 2002).

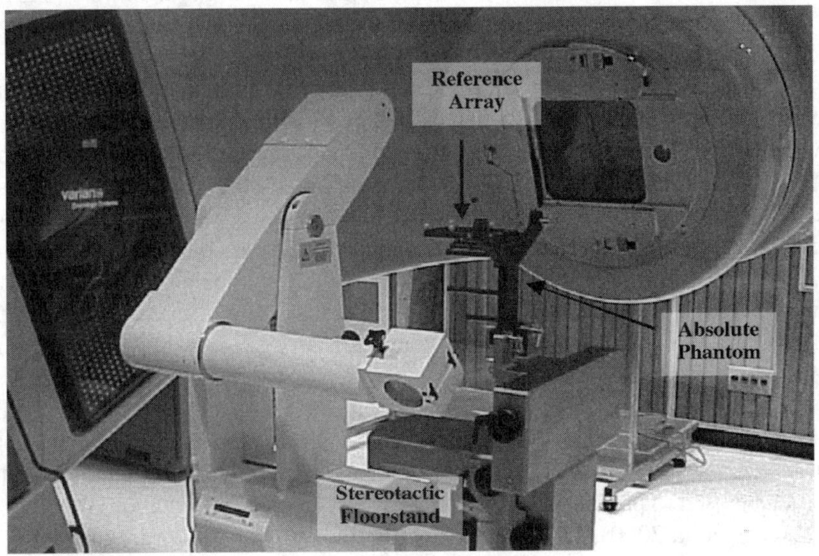


**Figure 7.** The accuracy of image localization and optical tracking can be determined using an absolute phantom. This shows the reference array attached to the absolute phantom, and the absolute phantom attached to the floorstand. Optical tracking is used to move the coordinate to experimentally determined coordinates, and these are then compared against absolute known coordinates.

The known targets test can alternatively be performed using spatial measurements of film as the standard experimental determination of each sphere's position. After CT scanning and treatment planning localization of each sphere, the aluminum spheres are replaced with tungsten spheres. Again, the phantom is optically tracked to place the center of each sphere at the machine isocenter. After the sphere is positioned, it is imaged using the linear accelerator's x-ray beam, and the sphere's deviation from machine isocenter is measured on radiographic film. Results using this technique are similar to those stated above, with average accuracy better than 1 mm. Regardless of the method used to commission an optical tracking system for radiotherapy, it is expected that the planning CT resolution will dominate the observed errors. The accuracy of well-manufactured optical tracking systems is so high that they should contribute very little additional error to the process.

## Clinical Implementation And Patient-Specific Quality Assurance

The entirely frameless process can be described as follows. Patients have their bite plate made the day of radiosurgery, and imaging is obtained with the bite plate fixed on the patient's maxillary dentition and the patient immobilized as shown previously in figure 3. During treatment planning the desired target, or isocenter, coordinates are determined in CT space. The centers of the spherical fiducial markers in the optical reference array are also localized in CT space, thus determining their positions relative to the treatment isocenter and defining a stereotactic coordinate system. After selecting the fiducials from the scan, the code determines the best fit between the image-defined coordinates of the reference array and the known geometry of the reference array. The residual error between the image localization of the markers and the known geometry after the best fit is obtained is called the *mean registration error*, and is calculated for each patient. The mean registration error provides quality assurance of the frameless localization system, as it ensures integrity of both the fiducial and imaging systems (Meeks et al. 2000). In phantom it has consistently been shown that the mean registration error is approximately 0.3 mm, due primarily to the finite CT voxel sizes used. In the vast majority of clinical situations, the mean registration error can be maintained below 0.5 mm. For a given image set, values larger than this are indicative of spatial CT inaccuracies, mechanical inaccuracy in the reference array, or patient motion during the CT scan. The mean registration error can then be projected to isocenter in order to predict the actual localization error at the point of treatment. It has been shown in both phantom and patient that the mean registration error can be used to predict the actual error at isocenter to within approximately 0.2 mm (Meeks et al. 2000), and this error prediction is a valid measure of the overall treatment accuracy.

In addition to validating the planning CT data set, it is important to verify the reproducibility of biteplate reseating. Bite plate reproducibility is determined by attaching a second reference array to the patient using an adjustable headband (figure 8). The patient is instructed to insert the bite plate, and the position of the reference array is determined relative to the headband reference array. The bite plate is removed and then reinserted, or reseated, and its position is re-sampled. The reproducibility value is determined by averaging the 3-D vector error in reseating the bite plate over 10 insertions. In the vast majority of clinical situations, including edentulous patients, this error is less than 0.3 mm (Bova et al. 1997; Buatti et al. 1998; Meeks et al. 2000; Tomé et al. 2001; Ryken et al. 2001a).

During patient setup, the RadioCameras system is used to determine the patient's position and to report the displacement from isocenter in real time. The system reports the translational misalignments along three orthogonal axes and reports the rotational misalignment about each of these axes. In addition, the system reports overall *vector* misalignment, which is the root mean square (rms) of the three translational misalignments, and hence, the 3-D displacement of the patient's target from isocenter. The patient's target is repositioned to the desired position in stereotactic space within 0.3

mm vector misalignment and 0.3 degrees of rotational misalignment about each axis. The patient is monitored in real time during treatment delivery. If patient motion resulted in a displacement of more than 0.5 mm from the planned isocenter, the treatment is interrupted until the patient's position is corrected. This process is repeated for each treatment field.

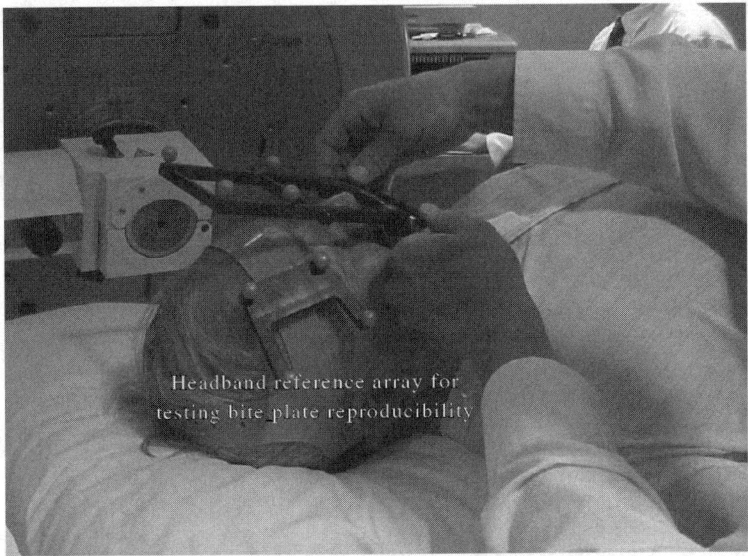


**Figure 8.** Bite plate reseating reproducibility can be tested on each patient by attaching an adjustable headband with reference array to the patient. The bite plate reference array is then dynamically tracked relative to this headband reference array.

## Optically Guided Ultrasound

While the initial system for optical-guided radiotherapy provides high localization accuracy, it has been limited to intracranial therapy. Outside of the cranium, soft-tissue targets can move relative to rigid fixation points (e.g., bone structures) between the times of image acquisition, treatment planning, and treatment delivery. Therefore, real-time imaging is required to establish extracranial stereotactic localization of the lesion at the time of treatment delivery. We have developed a system for 3-D ultrasound guidance (Bouchet et al. 2001, 2002; Ryken et al. 2001b; Meeks et al. 2003) that is commercially available under the trade name SonArray™ (ZMed Inc., Ashland, MA). Ultrasound was chosen because it is an inexpensive, yet flexible and high-resolution imaging modality that can easily be adapted for use in a radiation therapy treatment room. Systems have been developed that rely on 2-D ultrasound probes attached to mechanical tracking systems, and these have proven effective for improving the precision of patient localization for prostate radiotherapy (Troccaz et al. 1995; Lattanzi et al. 1999, 2000). The interpretation of 2-D ultrasound images is difficult, however, and can be highly dependent on the skill and expertise of the operator in manipulating the transducer and mentally transforming the 2-D images into a 3-D–tissue structure. Much of this difficulty results from using a spatially flexible 2-D imaging technique to view 3-D anatomy. Three-dimensional ultrasound reconstruction helps overcome this limitation. We generate 3-D ultrasound data sets through optical tracking of free-hand acquired 2-D ultrasound data. The operator holds the ultrasound probe and manipulates it over the anatomical region of interest. The raw 2-D data are transferred to a computer workstation using a standard video link. The position and angulation of the ultrasound probe in any arbitrary orientation is determined using an array of four IRLEDs attached to the probe (figure 9). Similar to our system for intracranial optical tracking, the Polaris camera system is used to determine the positions of the IRLEDs, and this information is input into the computer workstation. The position of each ultrasound pixel can therefore be determined using the IRLEDs, and an ultrasound volume can be reconstructed by coupling the position information with the raw ultrasound data (figure 10a and 10b).

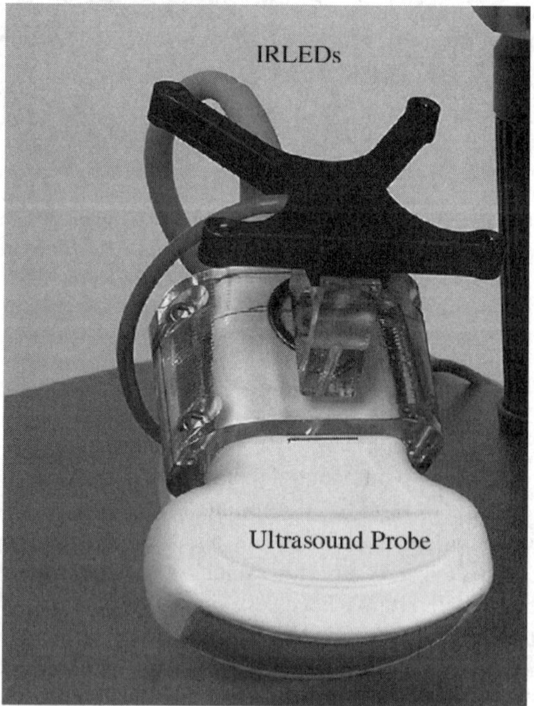


**Figure 9.** The ultrasound probe is tracked via an array of four IRLEDs rigidly attached to it. By tracking the probe, a 3-D ultrasound volume can be generated and tracked relative to the optical system's origin (typically isocenter).

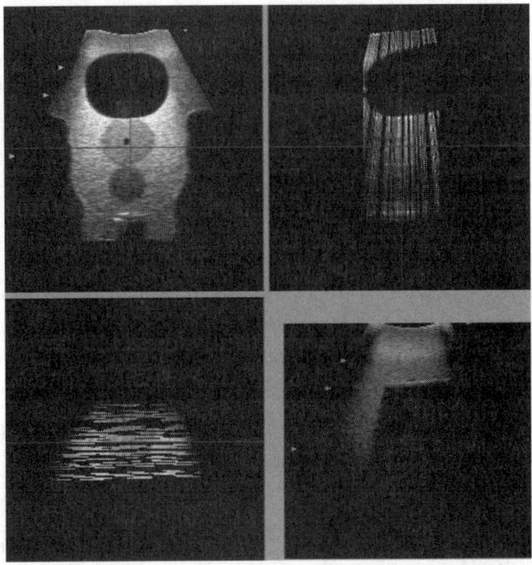

**Figure 10a.** Using freehand ultrasound acquisition, ultrasound data can be acquired at any orientation, and 2-D image planes are acquired until sufficient data are acquired to fill a cubic matrix. Orthogonal views through ultrasound images of a prostate phantom show that sufficient data are acquired to fill the matrix, but gaps may exist in the data due to the freehand acquisition.

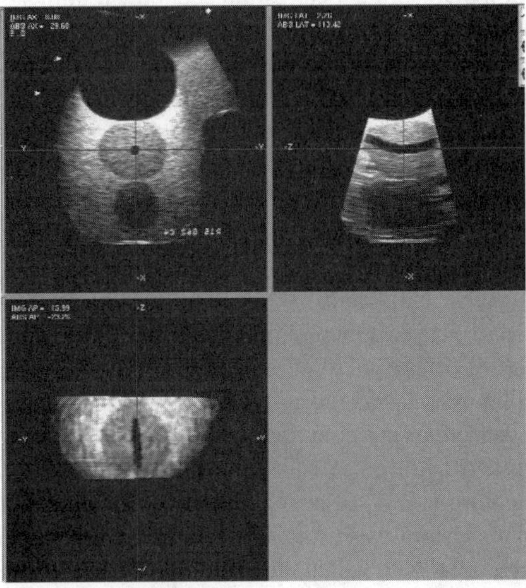

**Figure 10b.** Three orthogonal views of the images in figure 11a after linear interpolation has been used to complete the dataset and fill gaps in the data.

    

In addition to building the 3-D image volume, image optical guidance is used to determine the absolute position of the ultrasound volume in the treatment room coordinate system. Because the relative positions of the ultrasound volume and the ultrasound probe are fixed, the knowledge of the probe position in the treatment room coordinate system at the time of data acquisition is sufficient to determine the position of the image volume relative to the linac isocenter. The determination of the relative position of the image and probe corresponds to a calibration step that is performed at the time of system installation (Bouchet et al. 2001). This calibration procedure uses an optically tracked ultrasound phantom that contains echoic wires at 13 depths in an anechoic medium. Because the phantom is optically tracked, the room position of each wire is known very accurately. The ultrasound image coordinate of each wire is then determined by collecting multiple images of the phantom. It is then a simple mathematical procedure to determine the transformation matrix relating ultrasound image space to treatment room space.

## Commissioning And Quality Assurance For Ultrasound Guidance

To ensure accurate localization, all possible errors in the imaging, patient localization, and treatment delivery processes must be systematically analyzed (Bouchet et al. 2002; Tomé et al. 2002). Outlined below are test procedures necessary to meet the quality assurance challenges presented by an optically guided 3-D ultrasound system for real-time patient localization. While all tests were performed using the SonArray system, the general philosophy and procedures are applicable to all systems utilizing this technology. Determination of absolute localization accuracy requires the user to establish a consistent stereotactic, or 3-D, coordinate system in both the treatment planning system and the treatment vault. While we chose to establish this coordinate system through optical guidance, it can also be done using mechanical means, as in conventional stereotactic procedures, or other telemetry technologies that are commercially available. Regardless of the methodology utilized, it is imperative that acceptance tests are performed prior to clinical use of the system to ensure that the image-guided system allows for safe, controlled, and efficient delivery of both conventional and intensity-modulated radiotherapy.

For our testing, we used a specially designed ultrasound phantom (figure 11). This phantom consists of 12 echoic spheres imbedded in a tissue-equivalent non-echoic medium (with speed of sound 1470 m s$^{-1}$), with a passive infrared fiducial array attached to it. The spheres are arranged at five different nominal depths: one at 30 mm; two at 50 mm; and the remaining nine arranged in groups of three at nominal depths of 70 mm, 100 mm, and 130 mm. A CT scan ($0.49 \times 0.49 \times 2.0$ mm$^3$ resolution) of the phantom was acquired. Using the fiducial array for optical tracking, the same stereotactic coordinate system was established in the treatment planning system and in the treatment room, relative to which the positions of each sphere are known within imaging uncertainty. Each of the spheres was localized in the Pinnacle treatment planning system and its coordinates were transferred to the SonArray system as intended treatment isocenters. In order to reproduce the exact position of the ultrasound phantom at the time of the CT, a six-dimensional couch mount has been employed in the treatment room. This couch mount has three orthogonal translational degrees of freedom [anterior-posterior (AP), lateral, axial] and three orthogonal rotational axes (Couch, Spin, Tilt); this allows one to reproduce the position of the phantom to within a predefined error tolerance. Each target sphere was positioned at the treatment machine isocenter using the following method. First the isocenter corresponding to the target sphere chosen for ultrasound localization was selected on the control computer. The phantom was then moved using optical tracking and the couch controls until the rms error between actual and desired position of the target sphere was less than 0.2 mm. Once a target sphere had been positioned at the treatment machine isocenter using optical tracking, the ultrasound probe was fixed on top of the phantom. A 3-D ultrasound volume of each sphere was acquired using optical tracking as described above. The 3-D ultrasound-based position of the target sphere was determined by finding the center of the sphere in the axial, sagittal, and coronal planes using a circle tool placed on each of the three-orthogonal ultrasound views (figure 12). The target localization accuracy of the 3-D ultrasound optically guided system was thus determined by comparing the experimentally determined position of each sphere to its predicted position from the treatment planning system.

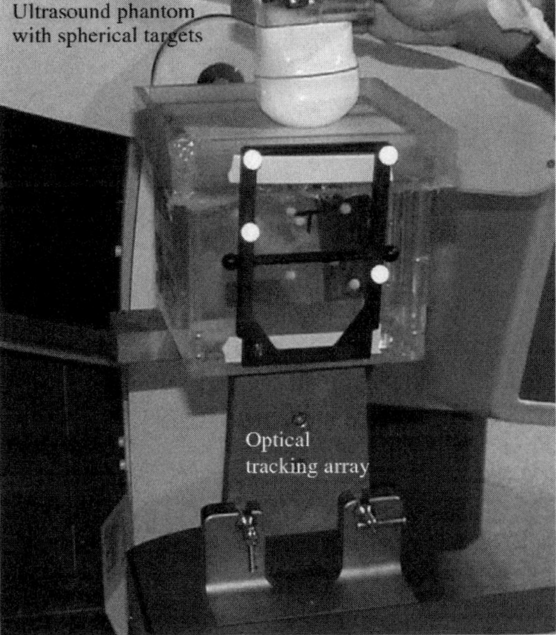


**Figure 11.** An ultrasound phantom was designed that has spherical targets in a non-echoic medium. The phantom may either be optically or mechanically tracked to determine the absolute coordinates of the spherical targets.

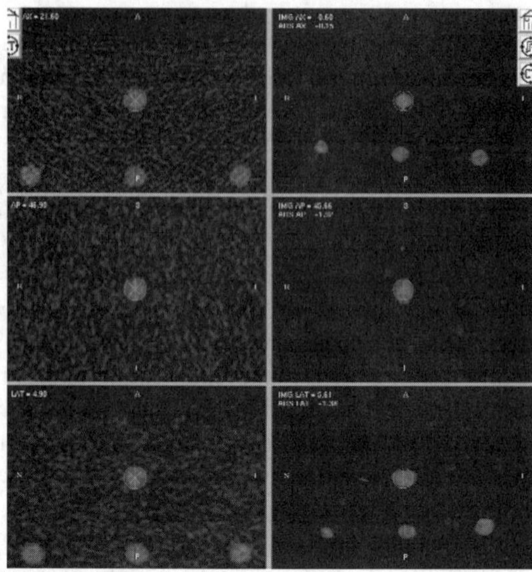

**Figure 12.** Orthogonal views of CT and 3-D ultrasound images of the ultrasound phantom used for determining the localization accuracy of an ultrasound guided system. A circle was positioned on all three orthogonal views to determine the position of the sphere centroids.

Our tests have indicated that the localization error does not depend on the target depth or the ultrasound focal depth used. Table 1 demonstrates representative values for such a test of optically guided 3-D ultrasound target localization for a 15 cm ultrasound probe format. Similar to optical guidance testing described previously, optically guided 3-D ultrasound localization should able to localize a well-defined internal target to within the inherent imaging uncertainty. However, localization errors in each of the spatial dimensions may exceed the predicted localization error due to finite image pixel size.

**Table 1.** Accuracy of Optically Guided 3-D Ultrasound as a Function of the Depth of the Target for a Focal Depth of 15 cm. Results are given in terms of the mean distance in the AP, lateral, and axial directions and the 95% confidence interval around that mean value.

| Depth (mm) | Anteroposterior Distance (mm) | Lateral Distance (mm) | Axial Distance (mm) |
|---|---|---|---|
| 30 | 0.8±0.6 | 0.5±0.3 | 1.0±1.7 |
| 50 | 0.1±0.7 | 0.6±0.8 | 1.3±1.6 |
| 70 | −0.2±0.6 | 1.0±0.9 | 0.1±1.5 |
| 100 | 0.2±0.8 | 1.2±0.9 | 0.3±1.8 |
| 130 | 0.3±0.6 | 1.1±1.0 | 0.2±1.5 |
| All depths | 0.2±0.7 | 0.9±0.6 | 0.6±1.0 |

Other experiments can be performed using anthropomorphic phantoms. We have previously described a sample test using a specially designed prostate phantom (Tomé et al. 2002), and performance of this test is outlined below. The phantom consists of three layers. The first layer contains the bladder, the second the prostate and urethra, and the third a model for the rectum in the form of a long cylinder. The bladder, prostate, urethra, rectum, and the background material are made of Zerdine with different echogenicity closely mimicking sound absorption and speed properties of the typical anatomy of a patient. A CT scan ($0.49 \times 0.49 \times 2.0$ mm$^3$ resolution) was acquired of the phantom with a passive infrared fiducial array attached. Using optical tracking as described previously, the positions of each segmented organ can be known in both CT image space and treatment room space within imaging uncertainty. The CT data set was segmented into four distinct regions of interest (ROIs): the bladder, the prostate, the urethra, and the rectum. A treatment isocenter was chosen in Pinnacle, and its position, along with the planning images and segmented ROIs, was transferred to the control computer of the SonArray system. The phantom was then set up on the treatment couch as shown in figure 13.

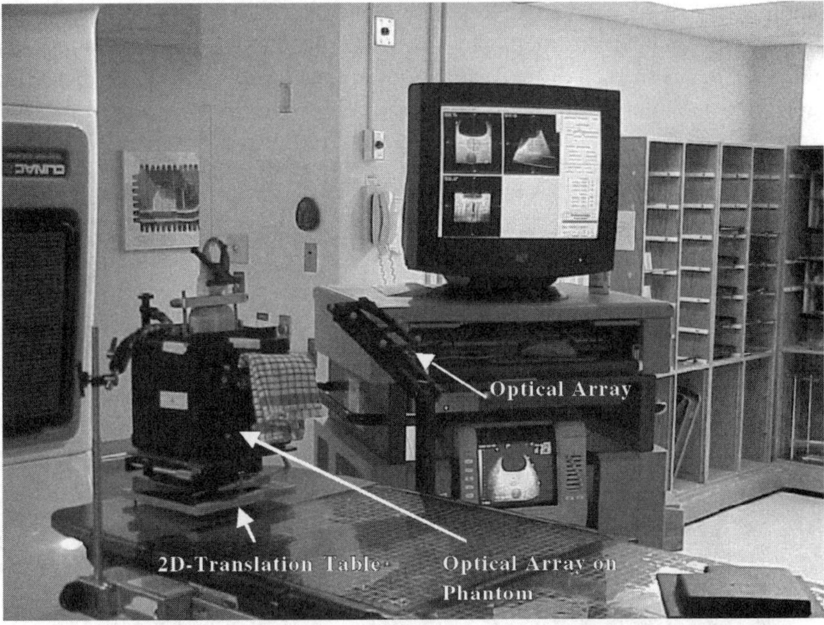


**Figure 13.** Experimental setup of the ultrasound guided system for determining known shifts in a target structure using 3-D ultrasound localization.

Optical tracking was again used to align the chosen treatment isocenter with the treatment machine isocenter within 0.2 mm rms error. The fiducial array attached to the phantom was then covered. A separate fiducial array was then attached to the treatment couch, and its position was recorded using SonArray. In this way we have established a fixed "bony anatomy" about which introduced internal organ motion can be studied. Next, internal organ motion with respect to the fixed bony anatomy was simulated. First the fiducial array attached to treatment couch was covered and the fiducial array attached to the phantom was uncovered. Then the phantom was shifted from its starting position ±5 mm in the lateral and superior/inferior directions using a 2-D translation table. These shifts were measured to within ±0.2 mm rms error using the optical positioning sensor system. Once the shifts had been made, the fiducial array attached to the phantom was again covered and the fiducial array attached to the treatment couch was uncovered. Since the treatment couch position remained fixed, the bony anatomy was not changed even though the phantom was physically moved. Hence, through the alternate use of two fiducial arrays we are able to introduce accurate apparent organ motion while maintaining a fixed bony anatomy in the control computer. This apparent organ motion can then be detected using the ultrasound localization system (figure 14). Once a shift had been measured using 3-D ultrasound localization, the phantom was shifted to a new position and a new 3-D ultrasound localization was performed. This procedure was followed until the required number of ultrasound localizations of each phantom shift had been obtained. Repeated performance of this test shows that one is able to localize an internal structure to within the inherent imaging uncertainty. Again, localization errors in each of the spatial dimensions may exceed the predicted localization error due to finite image pixel size.

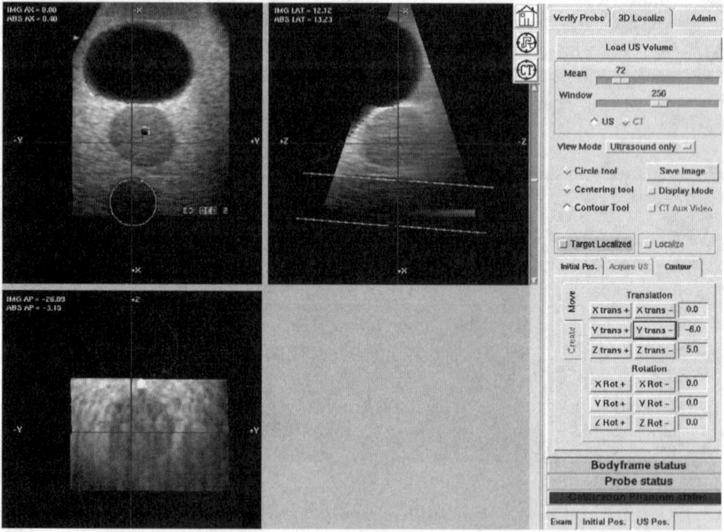

**Figure 14.** This depicts the graphical user interface that allows the user to register the treatment planning CT and 3-D ultrasound volumes. The contours obtained during treatment planning are overlaid on the 3-D ultrasound volume of the prostate phantom. In this case, simulated organ shifts were induced in the Y (lateral) and Z (axial) directions.

In the preceding paragraphs we have described two methods for quantitative testing of the accuracy of an image-guided system. While many qualitative tests exist for testing these systems, we believe that it is extremely important for the physicist to perform commissioning tests of the system that quantify the errors locally. As mentioned in the introductory paragraph of this section, this requires the user to establish some local standard coordinate system in the room. We have chosen to establish this through optical tracking, but the standard can be established using alternative mechanisms.

## Clinical Application

We have used ultrasound localization for conformal and intensity-modulated radiotherapy of prostate radiotherapy (Patel et al. 2003). In addition, the system has been used for patient localization for patients undergoing extracranial radiosurgery for a variety of abdominal, paraspinal, and pelvic lesions (Ryken et al. 2001b; Meeks et al. 2003). Clinical use of ultrasound image guidance proceeds as follows. Prior to CT scanning, the patient is immobilized using a custom vacuum cushion as is commonly used in radiation therapy (Vac-Loc™, Med-Tec, Inc., Orange City, IA). The CT is acquired with the patient immobilized in the same position that will be used during the radiotherapy treatment in order to maintain a generally consistent position of mobile anatomy. The CT images are transferred to our 3-D treatment planning system where the tumor volume and normal structures of interest are delineated. A treatment plan is then designed to conform the prescription dose closely to the planning target volume (PTV), while minimizing the dose to the nearby normal structures.

The day of the treatment, the patient is placed in the same immobilization cushion that was used during CT scanning. The patient is initially set up relative to isocenter using conventional laser alignment. A 3-D ultrasound volume is then acquired and reconstructed in the computer workstation. The target volume and critical structure outlines, as delineated on the planning CT scans, are overlaid on the acquired ultrasound volume in relation to isocenter. The contours determined from the CT scans are then manipulated until they align with the anatomic structures on the ultrasound images. The amount of movement required to align the contours with the ultrasound images determines the magnitude of the target mis-registration with isocenter based on conventional setup techniques. The target is then placed at the isocenter by tracking an infrared array attached to the treatment couch which allows precise translation from the initial position to the 3-D ultrasound determined position. Once all the setup information has been verified using repeat ultrasound acquisition and co-registration, treatment proceeds as planned.

While ultrasound localization provides high-precision target localization, it is important to note that ultrasound image interpretation requires training and skill from the end user. It is unlikely that end users with no ultrasound expertise will generate results that improve patient localization accuracy. As an example of this, a pilot study was run at the University of Iowa to determine the user variability of ultrasound localization of the prostate. Retrospective registration of 15 patient data sets was performed independently by nine different users. Four of these users had approximately 1 year of ultrasound localization experience, while the other five users had been trained with the ultrasound localization software but had no experience in ultrasound interpretation. Results of this study are tabulated in table 2, and indicate that the standard deviation among untrained users is unacceptably large; in fact, the standard deviation is nearly as large as the average required shift. Among those trained in ultrasound interpretation, however, the results are consistent, and indicate that significant increases can be obtained using daily ultrasound localization.

**Table 2.** User Variability in Prostate Localization Using Ultrasound Guidance

|  | AP (mm) | Lateral (mm) | Axial (mm) |
|---|---|---|---|
| **Average Shift** | 3.4 | 2.7 | 4.5 |
| **Standard Deviation (4 Trained Users)** | 1.2 | 0.9 | 1.4 |
| **Standard Deviation (5 Untrained Users)** | 3.6 | 1.5 | 2.9 |

# References


Allen, B. D., G. Bishop, and G. Welch. (2001). Tracking: Beyond 15 Minutes of Thought. Course 11, SIGGRAPH 2001.

Baroni, G., G. Ferrigno, and A. Pedotti. (1998). "Implementation and application of real-time motion analysis based on passive markers." *Med. Biol. Eng. Comput.* 36:693–703.

Bouchet, L. G., S. L. Meeks, G. Goodchild, F. J. Bova, J. M. Buatti, and W. A. Friedman. (2001). "Calibration of three-dimensional ultrasound images for image-guided radiation therapy." *Phys. Med. Biol.* 46:559–577.

Bouchet, L. G., S. L. Meeks, F. J. Bova, J. M. Buatti, and W. A. Friedman. (2002). "3D ultrasound image guidance for high precision extracranial radiosurgery and radiotherapy." *Radiosurg.* 4:262–278.

Bova, F. J., J. M. Buatti, W. A. Friedman, W. M. Mendenhall, C. C. Yang, and C. Liu. (1997). "The University of Florida frameless high-precision stereotactic radiotherapy system." *Int. J. Radiat. Oncol. Biol. Phys.* 38:875–882.

Buatti, J. M., F. J. Bova, W. A. Friedman, S. L. Meeks, R. B. Marcus Jr., J. P. Mickle, T. L. Ellis, and W. M. Mendenhall. (1998). "Preliminary experience with frameless stereotactic radiotherapy." *Int. J. Radiat. Oncol. Biol. Phys.* 42:591–599.

Cardinale, R. M., S. H. Benedict, E. A. Bump, B. D. Kavanaugh, and R. Mohan. (1999). "Automated target positioning for extracranial radiosurgery." *Int. J. Radiat. Oncol. Biol. Phys.* S45:206.

Friedman, W. A., and F. J. Bova. (1989). "The University of Florida Radiosurgery System." *Surg. Neurol.* 32(5):334–342.

Kai, J., H. Shiomi, T. Sasama, and Y. Sato. (1998). "Optical high-precision three-dimensional position measurement system suitable for head motion tracking in frameless stereotactic radiosurgery." *Comput. Aided Surg.* 3:257–263.

Kubo, H. D., P. M. Len, S. Minohara, and H. Mostafavi. (2000). "Breathing-synchronized radio-therapy program at the University of California Davis Cancer Center." *Med. Phys.* 27:346–353.

Lattanzi, J., S. McNeeley, W. Pinover , E. Horwitz, I. Das, T. E. Schultheiss, and G. E. Hanks. (1999). "A comparison of daily CT localization to a daily ultrasound-based system in prostate cancer." *Int. J. Radiat. Oncol. Biol. Phys.* 43:719–725.

Lattanzi, J., S. McNeeley, A. Hanlon, T. E. Schultheiss, and G. E. Hanks. (2000). "Ultrasound-based stereotactic guidance of precision conformal external beam radiation therapy in clinically localized prostate cancer." *Urol.* 55:73–78.

Meeks, S. L., F. J. Bova, T. H. Wagner, J. M. Buatti, W. A. Friedman, and K. D. Foote. (2000). "Image localization for frameless stereotactic radiotherapy." *Int. J. Radiat. Oncol. Biol. Phys.* 46:1291–1299.

Meeks, S. L., T. C. Ryken, E. C. Pennington, F. J. Bova, W. A. Friedman, and J. M. Buatti. (2002). "Testing and initial experience with an image-guided system for frameless stereo-tactic radiosurgery." *Radiosurg.* 4:251–261.

Meeks, S. L., J. M. Buatti, L. G. Bouchet et al. (2003). "Ultrasound guided extracranial radio-surgery: Technique and application." *Int. J. Radiat. Oncol. Biol. Phys.* In press.

Menke, M., F. Hirschfeld, T. Mack, O. Pastyr, V. Sturm, and W. Schlegel. (1994). "Photogram-metric accuracy measurements of head holder systems used for fractionated radiotherapy." *Int. J. Radiat. Oncol. Biol. Phys.* 29:1147–1155.

Patel, R. R., N. P. Orton, W. A. Tomé, R. Chappell, and M. A. Ritter. (2003). "Rectal dose-sparing with a balloon catheter and ultrasound localization in conformal radiation therapy for prostate cancer." *Radiother. Oncol.* In press.

Phillips, M. H., K. Singer, E. Miller, and K. Stelzer. (2000). "Commissioning an image-guided localization system for radiotherapy." *Int. J. Radiat. Oncol. Biol. Phys.* 48:267–276.

Rogus, R. D., R. L. Stern, and H. D. Kubo. (1999). "Accuracy of a photogrammetry-based patient positioning and monitoring system for radiation therapy." *Med. Phys.* 26:721–728.

Ryken, T. C., S. L. Meeks, E. C. Pennington, P. Hitchon, V. Traynelis, N. A. Mayr, F. J. Bova, W. A. Friedman, and J. M. Buatti. (2001a). "Initial clinical experience with frameless stereo-tactic radiosurgery: Analysis of accuracy and feasibility." *Int. J. Radiat. Oncol. Biol. Phys.* 51(4):1152–1158.

Ryken, T. C., S. L. Meeks, V. Traynelis, J. Haller, L. G. Bouchet, F. J. Bova, E. C. Pennington, and J, M. Buatti. (2001b). "Ultrasonographic guidance for spinal extracranial radiosurgery: technique and application for metastatic spinal lesions." *Neurosurg. Focus* 11(6):8.

Shoup, T. E., and F. Mistree. *Optimization Methods with Applications for Personal Computers.* Englewood Cliffs, NJ: Prentice-Hall, 1987.

Tomé, W. A., S. L. Meeks, J. M. Buatti, F. J. Bova, W. A. Friedman, and Z. Li. (2000). "A high-precision system for conformal intracranial radiotherapy." *Int. J. Radiat. Oncol. Biol. Phys.* 47:1137–1143.

Tomé, W. A., S. L. Meeks, T. R. McNutt, J. M. Buatti, F. J. Bova, W. A. Friedman, and M. Mehta. (2001). "Optically guided intensity modulated radiotherapy." *Radiother. Oncol.* 61:33–44.

Tomé, W. A., S. L. Meeks, N. P. Orton, L. G. Bouchet, and F. J. Bova. (2002). "Commission-ing and quality assurance of an optically guided three-dimensional ultrasound target localization system for radiotherapy." *Med. Phys.* 29(8):1781–1788.

Troccaz, J. N. Laieb, P. Vassal, Y. Menguy, P. Cinquin, M. Bolla, and J. Y. Giraud. (1995). "Patient setup optimization for external conformal radiotherapy." *J. Image Guid. Surg.* 191:113–120.

Wang, T., T. Solberg, P. Medin, and R. Boone. (2001). "Infrared patient positioning for stereotactic radiosurgery of extracranial tumors." *Comput. Biol. Med.* 31:101–111.

Yang, C. C., J. Y. Ting, A. Markoe, F. J. Bova, W. M. Mendenhall, and W. A. Friedman. (1999). "A comparison of 3-D data correlation methods for fractionated stereotactic radiotherapy." *Int. J. Radiat. Oncol. Biol. Phys.* 43:663–670

# Modulated Electron Therapy


Kenneth R. Hogstrom, Ph.D.[1], John A. Antolak, Ph.D.[1],
Rajat J. Kudchadker, Ph.D.[1], C.-M. Charlie Ma, Ph.D.[2],
and Dennis D. Leavitt, Ph.D.[3]
[1]Department of Radiation Physics
The University of Texas M.D. Anderson Cancer Center
Houston, Texas
[2]Department of Radiation Oncology
Fox Chase Cancer Center
Philadelphia, Pennsylvania
[3]Department of Radiation Oncology
University of Utah School of Medicine
Salt Lake City, Utah




## Introduction

Radiation therapy has recently progressed to the extent that the delivery of complex, computer-controlled therapy has become more acceptable in radiation oncology practice. Although such sophistication has been accepted for at least four decades for proton, pion, and heavy-ion therapy, the routine availability and utilization of conformal, intensity-modulated photon therapy has only recently occurred. Its acceptance has presented the opportunity to utilize modulated electron therapy (MET), which is capable of delivering highly conformal treatments to superficial targets. The high surface dose and minimal exit dose of electron therapy offers advantages over photon therapy for superficial targets. The rapid fall-off of the electron dose beyond the treatment volume can help reduce the dose to distal healthy tissues in the treatment of superficial tumors, such as those in the breast and head and neck regions.

The purpose of this chapter is to introduce the clinical medical physicist to the principles of modulated electron therapy, which undoubtedly will become an important tool for radiation therapy over the next decade.

Electron conformal therapy (ECT) is defined as the use of one or more electron beams for the following purposes: (1) containing the planning target volume (PTV) in the 90% (of given dose) dose surface; (2) achieving as homogeneous a dose as possible (e.g., 90% to 100%) or a prescribed heterogeneous dose distribution to the PTV; and (3) delivering a minimal dose to underlying critical structures and normal tissue. MET is defined as electron conformal therapy achieved through energy modulation and/or intensity modulation of the incident electron beam(s).

In MET, the energy and intensity of the incident electron beam are modulated in the plane perpendicular to the central axis of the electron beam. The beam intensity of an electron field can be modulated to improve the lateral dose conformity within the target volume, and different electron energies can be used to improve the dose conformity in the depth direction. Energy modulation can be achieved in either continuous or finite steps. Presently, there is no technology that allows the incident beam to have its energy spatially modulated in real time; therefore, electron energy is modulated by one of two methods. In the first method, energy modulation is achieved using electron bolus, which modulates the electron range in the patient by varying the bolus thickness across the beam. Because bolus thickness can be manufactured with 1 mm accuracy or better, the equivalent energy modulation is in steps of 0.2 MeV or less. In the second method, the patient is irradiated using multiple electron beams of differing energy. On conventional linear accelerators, energies are spaced at intervals ranging from approximately 1.5 to 4.0 MeV, corresponding to a 7- to 20-mm increment in beam penetration in unit density tissue. Beam intensity can be modulated using either a multileaf collimator (MLC) or multiple field cutouts. Three variations of energy and intensity modulation, namely, bolus ECT, segmented-field ECT, and intensity-modulated electron therapy (IMET), will be discussed in this chapter. The advantages and disadvantages of these variations will be discussed. Also, we will present how MET can be used to deliver electron arc therapy. Last, we will introduce the potential for mixed-beam therapy using MET. Our discussions will be limited to electron-beam energies currently available (6 to 25 MeV). MET for deep-seated tumors will not be discussed because it requires electron-beam energies substantially greater than 25 MeV, which are not commonly available.

MET has the same types of issues that intensity-modulated x-ray therapy (IMXT) does, namely, treatment planning, dose calculation, treatment delivery, quality assurance, and clinical utility. Each of these issues will be discussed for the various types of MET reviewed in this paper.

## Bolus Electron Conformal Therapy

Electron bolus has been defined as

> a specifically shaped material that is nearly tissue equivalent; it is normally placed either in direct contact with the patient's skin surface, close to the patient's surface, or inside a body cavity. This material is designed to provide extra scattering or energy degradation of the electron beam. Its purpose is to shape the dose distribution to conform to the target volume or to provide a more uniform dose inside the target volume.
>
> (Hogstrom 1992)

Bolus has been designed and used for many years to conform the fall-off of the electron beam dose distribution (e.g., the 90% dose surface) to the distal surface of the target volume. However, not until the work of Low et al. (1992) was the bolus designed to account for not only energy loss but also the effects of multiple Coulomb scattering of the electrons.

### Treatment Planning

Low et al. (1992) designed bolus along fan lines emanating from the virtual electron source. As shown in figure 1, the initial design of the bolus, referred to as "creation," determined the bolus thickness along each fan-line that fell within the uniform portion of the electron beam. The thickness was designed so that when added to the depth of the distal PTV surface, it equaled the therapeutic depth ($R_{90}$). The resulting dose distribution was calculated using the three-dimensional (3-D) implementation of the Hogstrom pencil-beam algorithm (Hogstrom, Mills, and Almond 1981; Starkschall et al. 1991b). Due to effects of multiple Coulomb scattering, the bolus shape required modification. This was accomplished by various operators that smoothed the bolus proximal surface to homogenize PTV dose and that added or subtracted bolus material to make small adjustments necessary to conform the 90% isodose surface to the PTV. During this process, the bolus was extended laterally to be sufficiently outside the beam aperture to intercept essentially all electrons in the penumbra. This forward planning approach was implemented into the The University of Texas M. D. Anderson Cancer Center treatment-planning system, COPPERPlan (Starkschall et al. 1991a, 1994).

### Treatment Delivery

Once the bolus is designed, the next step in the planning and delivery process is its fabrication. This was accomplished by milling a block of machineable wax using a tabletop milling machine (Antolak et al. 1994; Low et al. 1995). The machineable wax has a linear stopping and linear scattering power similar to that of polyethylene (Low and Hogstrom 1994). The distal and proximal surfaces of the bolus were milled to the dimensions for the bolus provided by the treatment planning system. The distal surface was milled to match the patient's skin surface, and the proximal surface was milled to provide the conformal dose distribution. Studies by Bawiec (1994) showed that the milling process was sufficiently accurate. Experience showed, however, that the milling process using a table-top milling machine took too much time to be practical as a long-term clinical solution. Larger milling machines better suited for this process are not likely to be available to most radiation oncology centers; therefore, the M. D. Anderson Cancer Center clinic presently uses a bolus milling service (.decimal, Sanford, FL), which receives an electronic file of the bolus, mills it, and provides it to the institution the next day via overnight mail. Figure 2 shows a bolus milled for use on a patient with head and neck cancer.

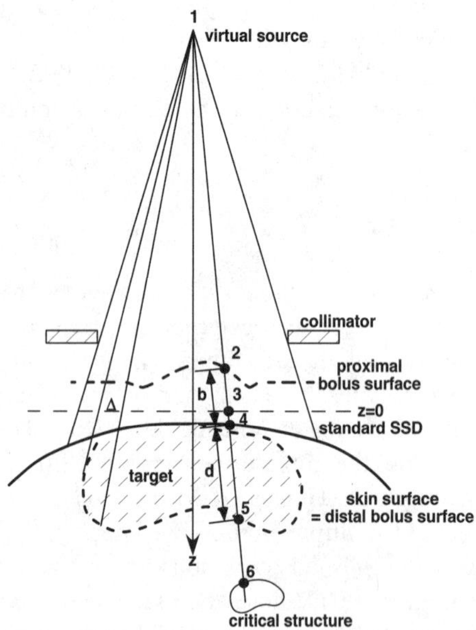


**Figure 1.** Sketch illustrating the fan geometry and design elements of the bolus design system. The design elements are illustrated through the representation of one fan line, on which points 1 through 6 are drawn. Point 1 represents the virtual electron source; points 2 through 6, the intersections of the fan line with the proximal bolus surface, the standard SSD plane, the proximal patient surface, the distal target volume surface, and the proximal critical structure surface, respectively. Bolus thickness, initially estimated by $b = R_{90}\text{-}d$, is modified to account for electron scatter and rate of energy loss in the bolus and patient. [Reprinted from *Medical Physics*, vol 19, D. A. Low, G. Starkschall, S. W. Bujnowski, L. L. Wang, and K. R. Hogstrom, "Electron bolus design for radiotherapy treatment planning: Bolus design algorithms," pp. 115–124. © 1992, with permission from AAPM.]

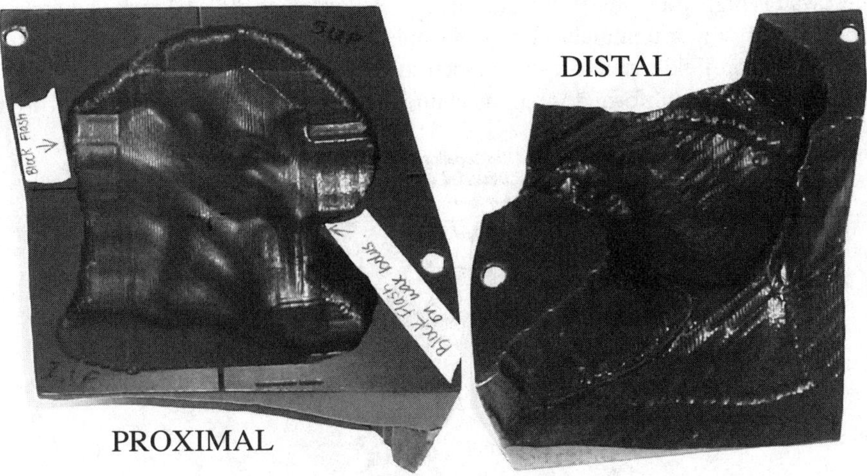


**Figure 2.** Custom electron bolus fabricated from machineable wax for head and neck treatment. The distal side is designed to match the patient's skin surface, and the proximal side is designed to modulate the penetration of the electron beam to match the PTV.

## Quality Assurance

Bolus quality assurance is required prior to the bolus use. The bolus manufacturer assures that the milling process was accurate, but this is inadequate to verify the proper positioning of the bolus on the patient and resulting dose to the patient. Positioning and dose are verified by placing the bolus on the patient, performing a planning computed tomography (CT) scan, calculating the dose with the bolus in place using the appropriate beam parameters, and verifying that the resulting dose distribution is consistent with that originally designed. Figure 3 demonstrates this in a case in which a patient was treated using an electron bolus for a posterior wall sarcoma (Low et al. 1995).

## Clinical Utility

The electron bolus has been clinically used primarily to treat postmastectomy chest wall and head and neck. In chest wall irradiation, the primary purpose of the electron bolus has been to minimize dose to the lung and heart. When treating the chest wall with electrons, surgical defects can often result in the chest wall thickness being highly irregular. Bolus can even the thickness, sparing considerable lung tissue. Alternatively, to spare lung, the chest wall is often irradiated using tangent photon beams that are abutted to an electron internal mammary chain (IMC) field. Such treatment is not as effective as bolus electron conformal therapy in cases in which disease at the IMC-chest wall field border is either known or highly likely or in which the anatomy of the chest wall is highly distorted owing to surgery (Perkins et al. 2001). Figure 4 compares a bolus plan with a treatment plan achievable by the conventional technique using tangent photon fields matched to an electron IMC field. The bolus plan produces a significantly more uniform dose in the abutted region where the cancer had recurred.

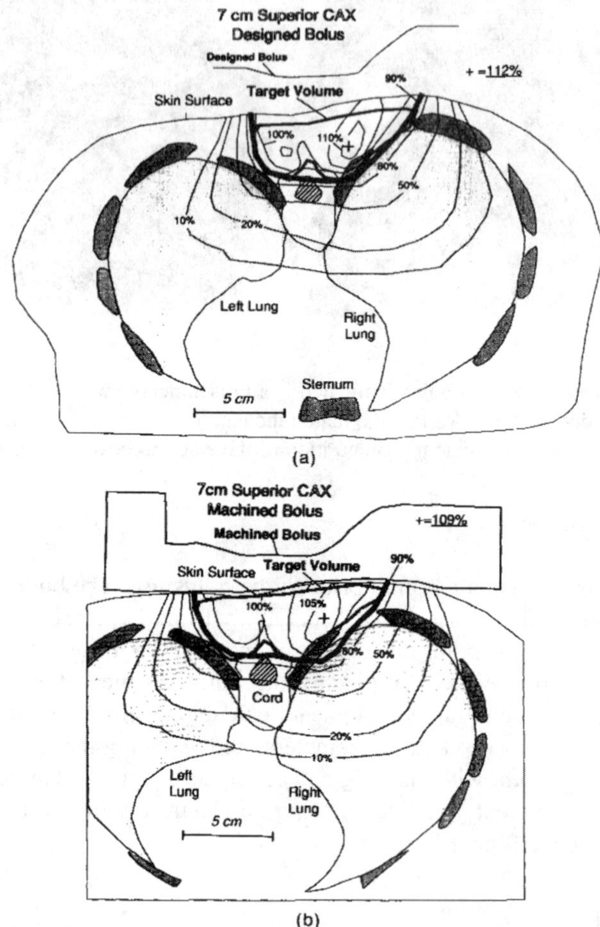


**Figure 3.** Example of quality assurance of bolus ECT for patient treatment of the paraspinal muscles. Anatomic structures, target volume, and the electron-beam isodose curves are superimposed on the transverse plane lying 7 cm superior to the central axis of the beam. (a) The treatment plan with the designed bolus. (b) The treatment plan for the CT scan with the bolus placed on the patient in treatment position. [Reprinted from *International Journal of Radiation Oncology Biology Physics*, vol 33, D. A. Low, G. Starkschall, N. E. Sherman, S. W. Bujnowski, J. R. Ewton, and K. R. Hogstrom, "Computer-aided design and fabrication of an electron bolus for treatment of the paraspinal muscles," pp. 1127–1138. © 1995, with permission from Elsevier.]

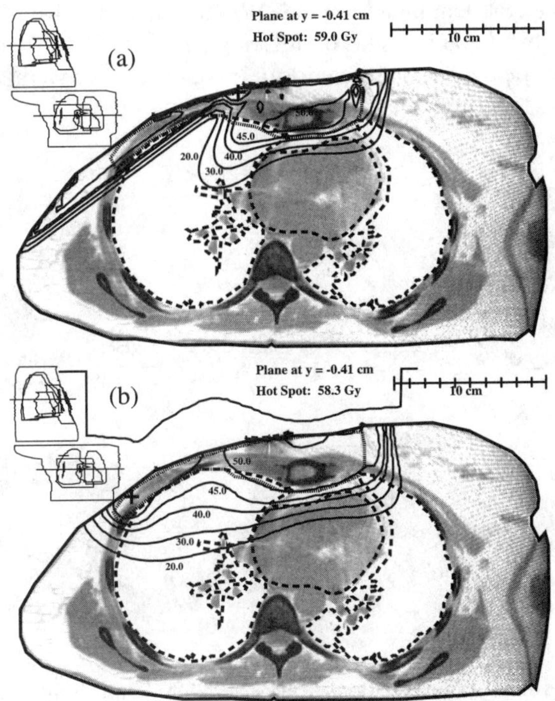



**Figure 4.** (a) Isodose curves (Gy) using standard tangent-IMC technique for a patient with a lesion in the right IMC area, with extension into the chest wall soft tissues. A dose of 50 Gy was prescribed to 100% of the given dose, using 12 MeV electrons for the IMC field, and the electron-field edge was matched to the medial tangent field edge on the patient's skin surface. The 45 Gy isodose line covers the target volume, except for the cold triangle directly beneath the junction line, an area of known disease. (b) Isodose curves (Gy) using the bolus ECT technique for the same patient. A dose of 50 Gy was prescribed to 100% of the given dose, using 16 MeV electrons, and the bolus was designed to deliver 90% of the given dose to the target volume. [Reprinted from *International Journal of Radiation Oncology Biology Physics*, vol 51, G. H. Perkins, M. D. McNeese, J. A. Antolak, T. A. Buchholz, E. A. Strom, and K. R. Hogstrom, "A custom three-dimensional electron bolus technique for optimization of postmastectomy irradiation," pp. 1142–1151. © 2001, with permission from Elsevier.]

Electron therapy in the head and neck is useful for sparing critical structures, such as the spinal cord, brain, and salivary glands. The use of electron beams in the head and neck can be further improved by using bolus conformal therapy. This is particularly true for PTVs that extend sufficiently inferiorly to overlay the spinal cord in the neck or superiorly to overlay brain tissue. The latter is exemplified in figure 5, which shows the PTV for a patient treated for a carcinoma of the left parotid gland. Figure 6 illustrates how the 90% dose surface conforms to the PTV in the same transverse planes as shown in figure 5. Figure 7 compares the dose-volume histogram (DVH) for the custom bolus treatment plan with the DVH for an alternative method of treating the patient using two separate fields of differing energy (a 20 MeV superior field and a 12 MeV inferior field). The bolus conformal plan improves coverage of the PTV and gives lower doses to the spine and brain.

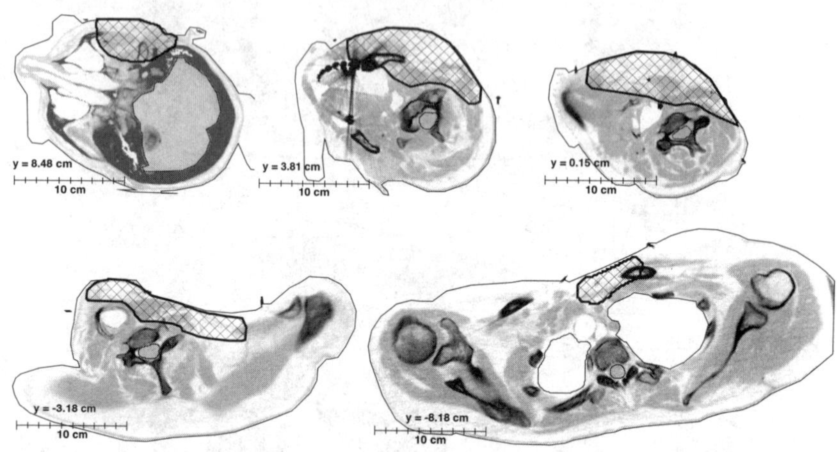

**Figure 5.** Transverse CT images (gray scale inverted for clarity) showing the location, depth, and shape of the parotid PTV (cross-hatched) at various levels. The maximum depth of the PTV is such that 20 MeV electrons were required for the bolus ECT treatment plan (Kudchadker et al. 2002a).

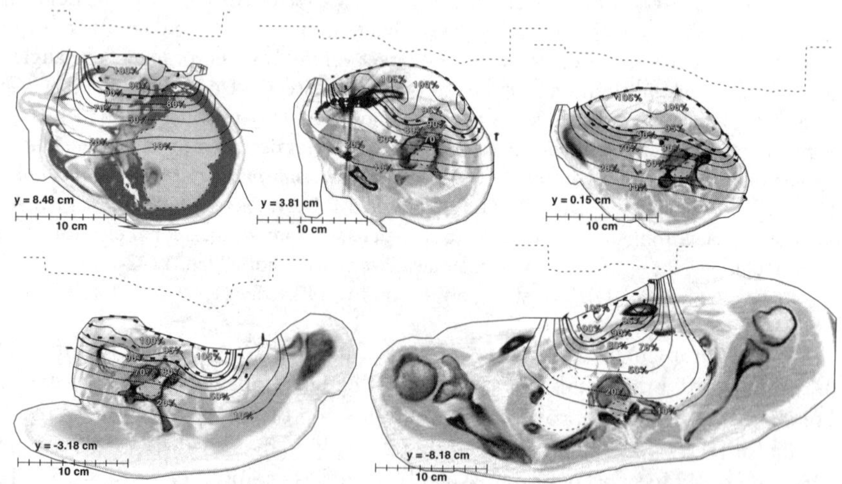

**Figure 6.** Dose distributions superimposed on transverse CT images from figure 5, illustrating how the bolus ECT treatment plan is able to conform the 90% isodose line to the PTV (dashed line) (Kudchadker et al. 2002a).

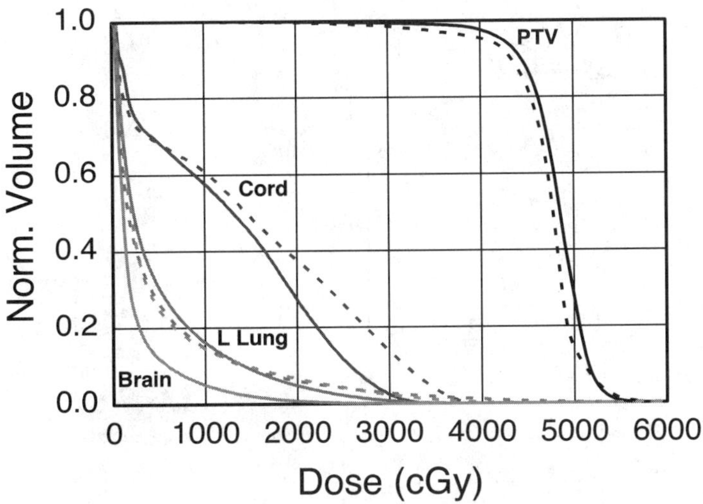


**Figure 7.** Dose-volume histograms for the PTV, spinal cord, left lung, and brain for the bolus ECT treatment plan shown in figure 6 (solid line) and a two-field plan with 20 MeV electrons superiorly and 12 MeV electrons inferiorly (dashed line) (Kudchadker et al. 2002a).

After planning bolus conformal therapy for many patients, Kudchadker et al. (2002b) observed that the irregular surface of the bolus increased the inhomogeneity of dose from a 10% variation (90% to 100%) in water (without bolus) to as much as a 20% variation (90% to 110%) in the patient (with bolus). This is illustrated in figure 8a, which shows the coronal plane dose distribution for a patient treated for carcinoma of the right buccal mucosa. Kudchadker et al. (2002b) showed that dose homogeneity could be restored by moderately modulating the intensity of the incident electron beam. Figure 8b shows the coronal dose distribution with intensity modulation, and the DVH comparison in figure 8c shows that the dose difference between 90% and 10% PTV coverage is reduced from 15% for the bolus plan to 9% for the bolus with the intensity-modulated plan. Figure 8d shows the relatively small amount of intensity modulation required for such a treatment.

The technique of bolus conformal therapy is relatively mature compared with the more recent MET techniques discussed below. Patients have been treated using bolus ECT technology for more than 10 years at M. D. Anderson, where its use has been demonstrated largely for breast and head and neck cancers. The treatment technique requires no modification to the electron treatment machine, and bolus fabrication with 1-day service is commercially available. A quality assurance process is well documented, and dose can be calculated using the pencil-beam dose algorithms presently available in 3-D treatment planning systems. The widespread use of bolus conformal therapy would require only the transfer of bolus design technology (Low et al. 1992) to commercial treatment planning systems.

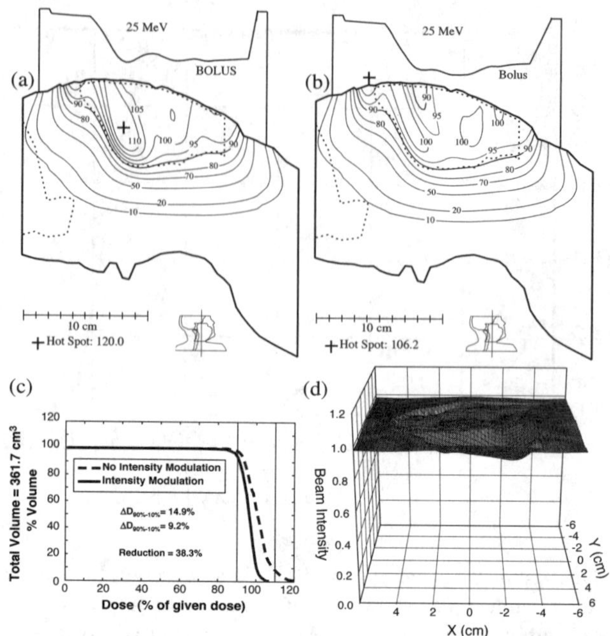



**Figure 8.** Bolus ECT dose distributions in a coronal plane are compared. Bolus ECT is planned with no intensity modulation (a), and with added intensity modulation (b). The treatment plans were designed to have the 90% isodose line cover the PTV (squamous cell carcinoma of the right buccal mucosa) and to deliver minimal dose to brain and other critical structures. The dotted lines demarcate the PTV and the base of brain. Note decrease in hot spot from 120% to 106%. (c) DVH for PTV comparing treatment plans with and without intensity modulation. (d) Beam intensity map required for the intensity-modulated bolus ECT plan. [Reprinted from *International Journal of Radiation Oncology Biology Physics*, vol 53, R. J. Kudchadker, K. R. Hogstrom, A. S. Garden, M. D. McNeese, R. A. Boyd, and J. A. Antolak, "Electron conformal radiotherapy using bolus and intensity modulation," pp. 1023–1037. © 2002, with permission from Elsevier.]

## Segmented-Field Electron Conformal Therapy

Segmented-field ECT is defined here as the utilization of multiple abutted electron fields, each having a common virtual source position but each having its own energy and weight, so as to conform the therapeutic dose surface (e.g., 90% of given dose) to the PTV. An example of segmented-field ECT (Zackrisson and Karlsson 1996) for postmastectomy chest wall irradiation is illustrated in figure 9. Segmented-field ECT can be applied to treatment of the parotid gland, improving upon the crude example in the previous section, where the superior segment (parotid) of the field was planned with a greater energy and the inferior segment (neck nodes) with a lesser energy so as to protect the spinal cord.

## Treatment Planning

Segmented-field ECT can be planned using existing technology, namely, using an appropriate 3-D treatment planning system. The 3-D treatment planning system needs a sufficiently accurate dose calculation (e.g., the Hogstrom pencil-beam algorithm) and the ability to model beam edges accurately. Unfortunately, manufacturers do not provide a key tool, a beam's eye view of PTV depth (Starkschall et al. 1994), which could be useful for manually segmenting the field. Figure 10 shows an example of such a tool and how it could be used to manually segment the field into smaller fields of differing energy and weights. It should be possible to automate this process by incorporating some basic rules of abutting electron fields into an algorithm.

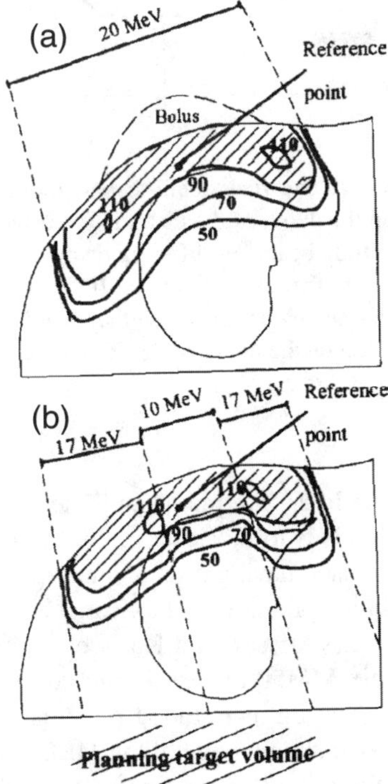


**Figure 9.** Comparison of bolus ECT with segmented-field ECT treatment plan for irradiation of the thoracic wall and the IMC after radical mastectomy. Dose distribution is shown in a transverse section for (a) the bolus ECT plan using 20 MeV electrons from a single portal and (b) the segmented-field ECT plan, which has three segments with a common isocenter. The segmented-field ECT plan uses 10 MeV electrons for the central segment and 17 MeV electrons for the medial and lateral segments. The reference point was used for dose normalization. [Reprinted from *Radiotherapy & Oncology*, vol 39, B. Zackrisson and M. Karlsson. "Matching of electron beams for conformal therapy of target volumes at moderate depths," pp. 261–270. © 1996, with permission from Elsevier.]

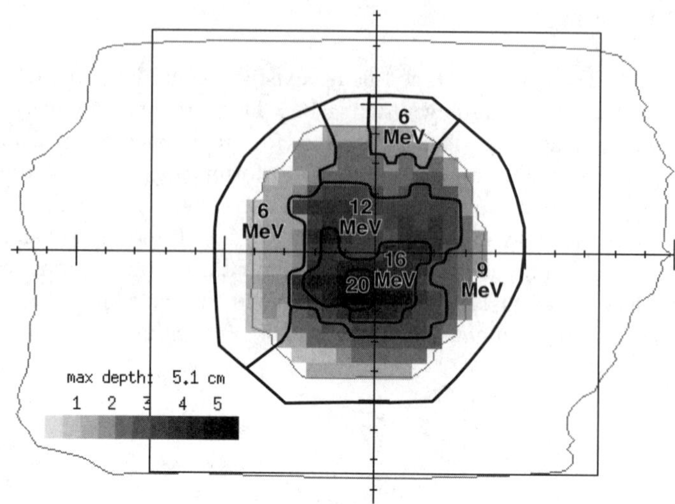



**Figure 10.** Potential of beam's eye view depth-display tool for segmented-field ECT. Gray levels are used to map the depth of the distal PTV surface. The depth map is used to segment the field into multiple beams of differing energy, selecting from the five beam energies available on the radiotherapy accelerator. In this example, for initial energy segmentation, the minimum beam energy whose therapeutic depth of the broad beam ($R_{90}$) exceeds the depth of the PTV is selected.

## Treatment Delivery

The delivery of segmented-field ECT remains an issue. Currently, the only practical way to deliver segmented fields is to fabricate multiple Cerrobend® inserts, one for each beam energy, with each insert having possibly multiple apertures. For this to work best, the Cerrobend edges should probably be fabricated with divergent edges. An alternative is to utilize an MLC. Zackrisson and Karlsson (1996) demonstrated that the x-ray MLC on a Scanditronix MM50 racetrack microtron can serve also as an electron MLC (eMLC). The electron penumbra remains sufficiently small for its utilization because (1) the downstream edge of the MLC is only 35 cm above isocenter, (2) the head of the machine is filled with helium, (3) the virtual source is small owing to the utilization of a scanned beam, and (4) the leaves are doubly focused. X-ray MLCs from other manufacturers are not sufficient to be used as eMLCs because (1) the downstream edges are too far from isocenter, (2) the heads of the machines are filled with air, and (3) the virtual sources are large because the beams are broadened by dual scattering foil systems. This is illustrated in figure 11, using data from Klein (1998). In this case, the penumbra from the Varian MLC was so great that it was not possible to segment beams in such a way as to track closely the sharp gradient in the distal edge of the anterior portion of the PTV for a parotid case. Potential solutions to this issue are to redesign the treatment head (Karlsson, Karlsson, and Ma 1999; Karlsson and Karlsson 2002) or to develop eMLCs that replace Cerrobend inserts (Lee, Jiang, and Ma 2000; Ma et al. 2000b) or the entire applicator system (Antolak, Boyd, and Hogstrom 2002; Boyd, Antolak, and Hogstrom 2002).

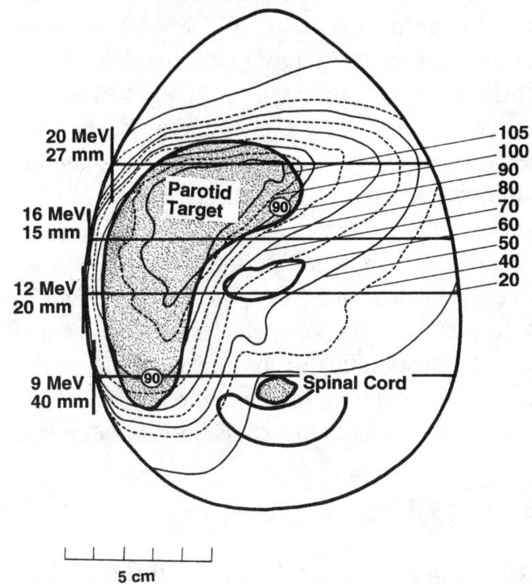


**Figure 11.** Dose distribution in a transverse plane through the parotid gland for a segmented-field ECT plan. The goal was coverage of the PTV by the 90% isodose contour while giving minimal dose to the spinal cord. [Reprinted from *Radiotherapy & Oncology*, vol 48, E. E. Klein, "Modulated electron beams using multi-segmented multileaf collimation," pp. 307–311. © 1998, with permission from Elsevier.]

## Quality Assurance

The issue of quality assurance for segmented-field ECT has not specifically been reported. However, it should be possible to verify delivery by using film to measure the dose in three orthogonal planes in a cubical solid-water phantom, two orthogonal planes containing the beam's central axis, and one perpendicular to the central axis (depth ≈1 to 3 cm). The measured dose could be compared to that calculated in a cubical solid-water phantom, using the patient-specific beams.

## Clinical Utility

Segmented-field ECT should be useful primarily in sites for which bolus ECT is useful (i.e., postmastectomy chest wall, parotid gland, and other head and neck sites that could benefit from ECT) to spare critical structures.

The major advantage of segmented-field ECT is that the dose fall-off beyond the 90% isodose surface distally is sharper than that with a bolus ECT treatment, as illustrated in figure 9. This is because bolus ECT requires that the maximum energy be used throughout the lateral extension of the field, and the $R_{90\text{-}10}$ is less for the lower energy electron beams that can be used for segmented-field ECT.

One disadvantage of segmented-field ECT results from the abutted fields not having matched penumbras, leading to dose inhomogeneity (hot and cold spots) in the abutment regions. This is evident in figure 9b, which shows hot spots of approximately 110% created just inside the edge of the higher energy beam. Varying the beam intensity near the beam edges to improve the matching of the penumbra could reduce or eliminate the dose inhomogeneity. Another disadvantage of segmented-field ECT is that the ability to conform the 90% dose surface might depend on the coarse energy resolution of existing radiotherapy accelerators; for example, the racetrack microtron has a rather coarse energy spacing of 5 MeV; the Varian Clinac 2100, an energy spacing of 3 to 4 MeV. Bolus, on the other hand, can be fabricated with a thickness accuracy of approximately 1 mm, corresponding to an energy spacing of 0.2 MeV. A final disadvantage arises if there are too many segmented fields; this leads to increased treatment time (or monitor units), which results in excess bremsstrahlung dose to the patient.

## Intensity-Modulated Electron Therapy

In contrast to bolus ECT and segmented-field ECT, IMET is defined as the utilization of multiple electron beams, each with its own energy and intensity pattern. IMET differs from bolus and segmented-field ECT in that IMET allows electrons of multiple energies at a single point within the beam. On the other hand, bolus ECT can more finely vary the beam energy, whereas IMET is limited to the available energies of the treatment machine. IMET has a lesser surface dose than bolus ECT does because no bolus is present.

IMET has garnered increasing interest in recent years, and significant progress has been made in researching IMET planning and delivery techniques (Hyödynmaa, Gustafsson, and Brahme 1996; Åsell et al. 1997; Ebert and Hoban 1997; Lee, Jiang, and Ma 2000; Lee et al. 2001; Ma et al. 2000b, 2003). Figure 12, an example by Åsell et al. (1997), illustrates how IMET might be used for chest wall irradiation. Multiple energy electron beams, ranging from 5 to 30 MeV, conform the dose distribution to the chest wall. However, this example also illustrates other key issues. Most significant, possible techniques for delivering intensity patterns with such sharp gradients are not apparent. This emphasizes the significance of having an integrated treatment planning and delivery system, which is the essence of the discussion about treatment and treatment planning below. Second, the 5 MeV energy spacing of the radiotherapy machine used in this study is likely too great and undoubtedly would often result in excessive lung irradiation; however, the closeness of energy spacing necessary for MET has not been studied. Third, the solution space may be so complex that it might be difficult to define cost functions that provide highly practical solutions and avoid needless irradiation of normal tissues to doses below tissue tolerances.

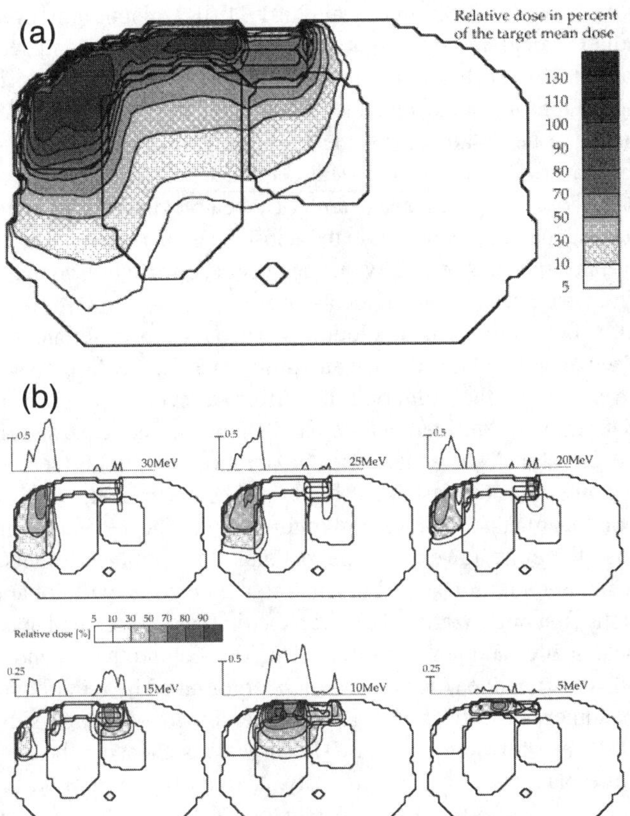



**Figure 12.** The potential of IMET is demonstrated by planning treatment of a chest wall phantom using a single beam portal in the anteroposterior (AP) direction. (a) The dose distribution resulting from six electron energies being used simultaneously is shown in a transverse plane. (b) The beam intensity versus position plot and the resulting dose distribution are plotted for each of the six electron beams, having energies ranging from 5 MeV to 30 MeV in 5 MeV steps. [Reprinted from *Physics in Medicine and Biology*, vol 42, M. Åsell, S. Hyödynmaa, A. Gustafsson, and A. Brahme, "Optimization of 3D conformal electron beam therapy in inhomogeneous media by concomitant fluence and energy modulation," pp. 2083–2100. © 1997, with permission from IOP Publishing.]

## Treatment Planning—Optimization

Treatment planning for IMET differs from that for bolus ECT and segmented-field ECT in that it requires an inverse planning approach. Many inverse planning algorithms have been developed to optimize intensity-modulated radiation therapy (IMRT) using either photon beams or electron beams (Brahme 1988; Webb 1989; Holmes and Mackie 1994; Ebert and Hoban 1997; Jiang et al. 2000; Jiang, Pawlicki, and Ma 2000; Ma et al. 2000b; Lee et al. 2001). IMRT planning is usually done by dividing a radiation field into small spatial elements, or beamlets, and determining the dose contribution from each beamlet as the first step in planning (ignoring leaf scatter and leakage). Optimizing the total dose distribution allows the weights or intensities for each beamlet to be obtained, and the resulting two-dimensional (2-D) intensity maps can be converted into an MLC leaf sequence for delivery. The optimization assumes that the dose computed on a beamlet-by-beamlet basis is the same as the dose delivered via the actual leaf sequence. In these instances, an additional adjustment must be applied to leaf sequences or simply during dose reconstruction so that planners can evaluate the true dose rather than an ideal dose.

Lee et al. (2001) proposed a solution to account for differences between the planned and actual MLC leaf sequence and differences in the dose between the planning and delivery stages; that solution is to perform a second optimization after a leaf sequence is determined. Considering a step-and-shoot leaf sequence algorithm, the leaf positions for each "shoot" segment define one or more small fields (segmented fields). Monte Carlo simulations of these MLC fields will be performed, which will be taken as a new set of "beamlets" in the second optimization. The second optimization will be fast because there are fewer segmented fields than initial beamlets, and thus it searches in a smaller solution space. In general, the outcome will not appear as optimal as that of the first optimization; however, the first optimization plan is nonrealistic without the leaf scatter and leakage effect. The idea behind the second optimization is that the leaf scatter and leakage effect can be minimized by reducing or increasing the weights of some segmented fields. This was demonstrated using a simple 2-D plan (Lee et al. 2001), as shown in figure 13. The target was chosen to be concave, with a critical structure placed within the concavity. A small region around the target was chosen to represent the normal tissue. The lateral extent of the target was approximately 20 cm. An array consisting of twenty 1-cm-wide beamlets was delivered into the phantom, covering the area from $x = -10$ to 10 cm. The resulting cumulative DVH is shown in figure 13. Idealized beamlets are optimized to give a dose distribution that agrees very well with the prescription, shown in figure 13 as a solid line. However, actual delivery of this plan adds the effect of the MLC leakage and scatter. The resulting DVH is right shifted and also has a change in the slope, suggesting poorer target coverage than was predicted by the idealized plan. However, once segment weights are re-optimized, the target coverage becomes very similar to that of the ideal beamlets, despite the non-idealities of the real collimator. The critical structure dose rises slightly with the addition of the leaves, owing to the leakage, but the final optimization reduces this effect somewhat. Figure 14 shows the intensity maps for different electron energies before and after the second optimization.

An alternative method to beamlet-based plan optimization is aperture-based plan optimization; for more information, the reader is referred to Jiang et al. (2000); Jiang, Pawlicki, and Ma (2000); and Deng, Lee, and Ma (2002).

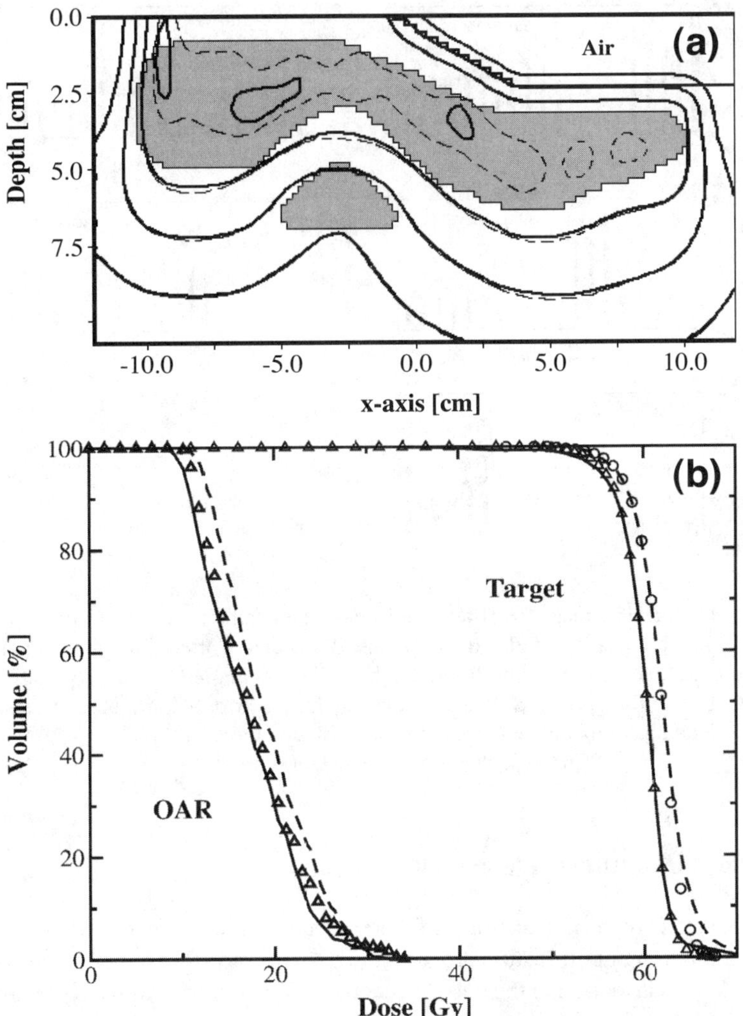



**Figure 13.** (a) Isodose plots for a 2-D homogeneous phantom. Shown are the simulated deliveries of plans generated accounting for leaf effects (solid) and ignoring leaf effects (dashed). Lines represent absolute dose: starting at the target moving outwards, 62.5, 50, 30, and 10 Gy. (b) DVHs for target and organ at risk (OAR): first optimization (solid), delivery of this plan with leaves in place without second optimization (dashed), and after second optimization (triangles). Also shown is the delivered target DVH (circles) for a plan in which a second optimization occurred, but in which segments only included leaf scatter, and not bremsstrahlung. [Reprinted from *Physics in Medicine and Biology*, vol 46, M. C. Lee, J. Deng, J. Li, S. B. Jiang, and C.-M. Ma, "Monte Carlo based treatment planning for modulated electron beam radiation therapy," pp. 2177–2199. © 2001, with permission from IOP Publishing.]

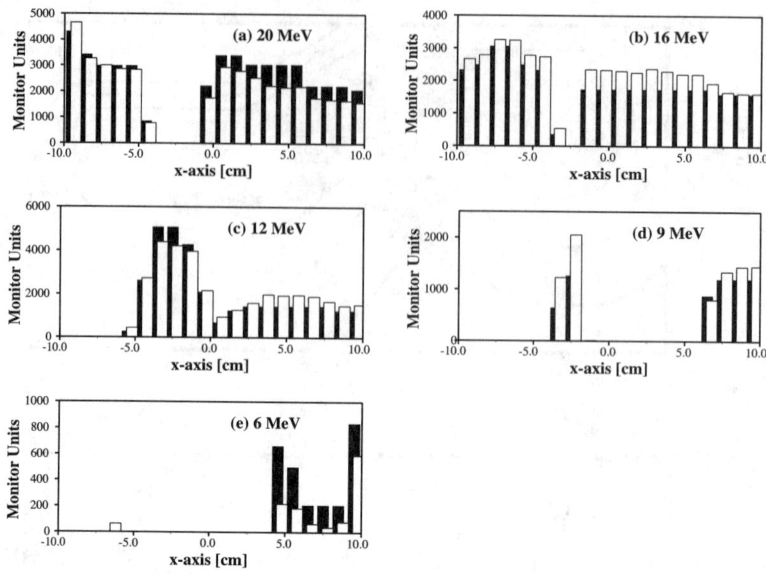

**Figure 14.** Intensity maps for different energies generated for the 2-D phantom plan of figure 13 by optimization of electron beamlets. Black bars = after first optimization; open bars = after second optimization. [Reprinted from *Physics in Medicine and Biology*, vol 46, M. C. Lee, J. Deng, J. Li, S. B. Jiang, and C.-M. Ma, "Monte Carlo based treatment planning for modulated electron beam radiation therapy," pp. 2177–2199. © 2001, with permission from IOP Publishing.]

## Treatment Planning—Dose Calculation

As emphasized above, the accuracy of dose calculation plays an important role in the treatment planning optimization process for intensity-modulated therapy because the beamlet dose distribution in the heterogeneous patient geometry must be accurate and the effect of MLC leaf leakage and scatter must be accounted for (Jeraj and Keall 1999; Ma et al. 1999b, 2000a; Pawlicki and Ma 2001; Siebers et al. 2002). This requirement is more stringent for electron beams than for photon beams owing to electron scattering in the treatment head, in the air between the treatment head and the patient, and inside the patient (Lee, Jiang, and Ma 2000; Ma et al. 2000b; Lee et al. 2001). Conventional pencil-beam dose algorithms appear insufficiently accurate for IMET owing to the inaccuracy for small fields, extended air gaps, and regions near material interfaces and inhomogeneities. Ma et al. (2000b) compared beamlet dose distributions computed using a 3-D pencil-beam algorithm, as implemented in the FOCUS treatment planning system (Computerized Medical Systems, St. Louis, MO), with those computed using a Monte Carlo algorithm. Figure 15 shows the dose distributions calculated using the Monte Carlo method (a, c) and the FOCUS 3-D pencil-beam algorithm (b, d) for a $1 \times 1$ cm², 12 MeV beamlet incident on a patient phantom built from CT data. For beamlets with normal incidence and a 10 cm air gap (figures 15a and 15b), the difference in the dose distributions in the heart was evident: the Monte Carlo calculated isodose lines varied with the heart contour, whereas the pencil-beam calculated isodose lines remained symmetrical despite the change in material densities. Figures 15c and 15d show the beamlet distributions for oblique incidence. The axis of the beamlet was intentionally placed to go through soft tissues and bones. The pencil-beam isodose lines seemed to stretch according to the beam axis path-length and showed no signs of electron build down near the lung.

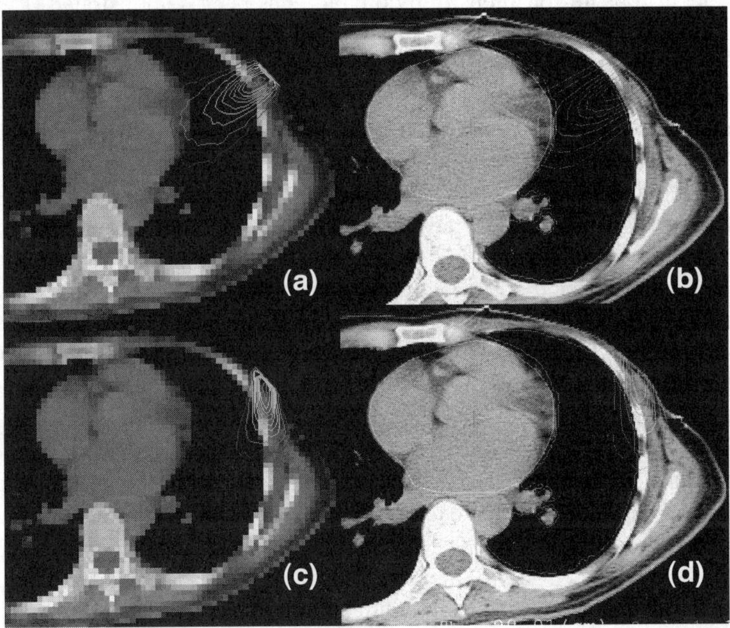

**Figure 15.** Comparison of dose distributions calculated using the Monte Carlo method (a,c) and the FOCUS 3-D pencil-beam algorithm (b,d) for a $1 \times 1$ cm², 12 MeV beamlet. The beamlet size is defined at 100 cm SSD. Two geometries are compared, normal incidence with 10 cm air gap (a,b) and oblique incidence (c,d). The isodose lines shown are 10, 20, 30, 40, 50, 60, 70, 80, and 90% of the maximum dose. [Reprinted from *Physics in Medicine and Biology*, vol 45, C.-M. Ma, T. Pawlicki, M. C. Lee, S. B. Jiang, J. S. Li, J. Deng, B. Yi, E. Mok, and A. L. Boyer, "Energy- and intensity-modulated electron beams for radiotherapy," pp. 2293–2311. © 2000, with permission from IOP Publishing.]

The results of Ma et al. (2000b) indicated that accurate dose calculation algorithms, such as Monte Carlo simulations (Mackie et al. 1994; Ma and Jiang 1999), are needed to compute electron beamlet distributions for the inverse planning process. Accurate dose calculation is also needed by IMET to account for the effect of bremsstrahlung leakage through the MLC leaves, electron scattering off the MLC leaf edges, and electron scattering in the air and inside the treatment head. Lee, Jiang, and Ma (2000) investigated the accuracy of Monte Carlo simulations and found good agreement with film measurement. Also, the Monte Carlo method has been found to be a useful tool for electron collimator design because of its ability to simulate electron transport accurately in complex geometry (Ma et al. 2000b).

## Treatment Delivery

Different techniques have been explored for IMET beam delivery. Utilization of a scanned electron beam for intensity modulation has been demonstrated (Lief, Larsson, and Humm 1996; Karlsson, Karlsson, and Zackrisson 1998); however, these applications were for lower gradients in the incident fluence than the gradient likely needed for IMET. At lower beam energies, the dose kernel width can become excessively large, making a scanned electron beam less attractive for IMET. Also, scanned beams are not available on commonly used clinical accelerators.

The most practical method for MET beam delivery might be the use of MLCs. X-ray MLCs are available but generally impractical for electron beams because of the large air gap between them and the patient; this results in inadequate lateral resolution of the pencil beams due to electron scatter in the air and scattering foil system (Brahme 1987; Zackrisson and Karlsson 1996; Janssen et al. 1997; Karlsson, Karlsson, and Ma 1999; Lee, Jiang, and Ma 2000; Ma et al. 2000b; McNeeley et al. 2001). One of the advantages of using an x-ray MLC is that x-ray and electron beams may be easily combined in the same plan. An essential requirement for matching an x-ray beam and an electron beam at different depths is that both beams share the same virtual source position. To accomplish this, several modifications to the design of a Varian Clinac 2300CD accelerator have been proposed (Karlsson, Karlsson, and Ma 1999). One proposed modification was to relocate the treatment head's dual scattering foil system to place the electron virtual source near that of the x-ray beam. Another was to replace the air in the treatment head with helium, which could significantly reduce the effect of electron scattering in the air on the beam penumbra. However, both of these proposed modifications require major changes to the existing treatment head design. Also, the beam properties deteriorate significantly for energies below 6 MeV, even for a helium-filled treatment head (Lee. Jiang, and Ma 2000).

Another alternative is to fabricate multiple electron cutouts. Although multiple electron cutouts are easy to fabricate and implement for small-scale clinical applications, their application to IMET would be too labor intensive and time consuming. To solve this problem, Ma et al. (2000b) investigated an alternative solution, a thin-leaf MLC at the electron cutout level to reduce the air scattering effect (figure 16a). The prototype eMLC consisted of 30 steel leaf pairs. Each leaf was 0.476 cm wide (0.5 cm projected to isocenter), 20 cm long, and 2.54 cm thick, with straight edges and ends. The leaves were mounted on a steel frame attached to the bottom scraper of a $25 \times 25$ $cm^2$ electron applicator on a Varian Clinac 2100C. The leaves slide in the steel frame, and the leaf positions are easily set using a precut cardboard for a beam segment. The largest radiation field available using the electron MLC was $15.7 \times 15.7$ cm$^2$, projected at 100 cm SSD (source-to-surface distance). A different eMLC design has been reported by McNeeley et al. (2001). Hogstrom and colleagues (Antolak, Boyd, and Hogstrom 2002; Boyd, Antolak, and Hogstrom 2002) designed a similar device for a Siemens PRIMUS accelerator (figure 16b); however, it was designed to be an applicator replacement and to be retractable. Their prototype utilized 3.0 cm thick brass leaves that had a 1 cm width projected to isocenter. The leaves could form a field up to $21 \times 20$ cm$^2$ and matched those of the PRIMUS x-ray MLC. Also, their design had diverging-leaf cross sections and rounded ends so that the electron scatter was minimal and penumbra independent of collimator position.

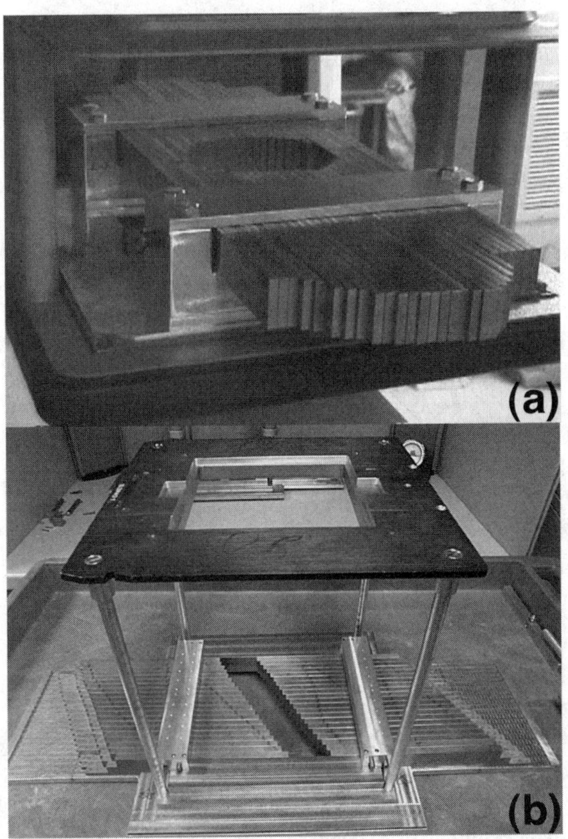


**Figure 16.** (a) Stanford prototype eMLC mounted in a $25 \times 25$ cm$^2$ applicator of a Varian 2100C accelerator. [(a) Reprinted from *Physics in Medicine and Biology*, vol 45, C.-M. Ma, T. Pawlicki, M. C. Lee, S. B. Jiang, J. S. Li, J. Deng, B. Yi, E. Mok, and A. L. Boyer, "Energy- and intensity-modulated electron beams for radiotherapy," pp. 2293–2311. © 2000, with permission from IOP Publishing.] (b) M. D. Anderson prototype eMLC designed for a Siemens Primus accelerator (Antolak, Boyd, and Hogstrom 2002).

Because of its thinner leaves and shorter distance to the patient surface, an eMLC can provide better dosimetric properties for small-field electron beams than an x-ray MLC can. Lee, Jiang, and Ma (2000) reported Monte Carlo and experimental investigations of multileaf collimated electron beams for IMET. They studied two proposed methods of electron-beam collimation: the use of existing x-ray MLC in a helium atmosphere to reduce in-air electron scatter, and an MLC specifically designed for electron-beam collimation. They concluded that an eMLC will have dosimetric characteristics similar to those of an x-ray MLC with focused leaf ends, but without the need to replace the air in the accelerator head with helium. The major disadvantage of the eMLC is its inablility to attenuate the contaminant bremsstrahlung dose in the electron beams. This effect is illustrated in figure 17, which shows Monte Carlo calculated dose distributions for a single $4 \times 4$ cm$^2$ electron field and a multiple abutting field of the same size formed by four $1 \times 4$ cm$^2$ electron fields. For a 20 MeV electron beam, the dose at the phantom surface for the abutting field shows about 4% fluctuation compared with that for a single electron field. This may result from the effect of leaf shape and extended source. The dose outside the field for the abutting field is about three times higher than it is for the single field; this effect is mainly caused by the leaf x-ray leakage. This is due to the longer beam-on time to deliver the four $1 \times 4$ cm$^2$ fields and electrons scattering off the leaf ends. This increased leakage is comparable to that for photon IMRT, where the beam-on time is generally 2.5 to 3.5 times longer than it is with a conventional photon treatment. The dose at a 3 cm depth shows little difference between the abutting field and the single field, except for the dose near the field edges and outside the field. For a 6 MeV electron beam, the dose at the phantom surface for the abutting field is almost the same as that for the single field (not shown). The effect of leaf leakage is very small for a 6 MeV beam, and the dose immediately outside the field is thought to be caused mainly by the effect of electron scattering in the air. It seems that field abutting with 1 cm beamlets collimated by an electron MLC can provide adequate beam characteristics for IMET for the beam energies investigated. However, the dose outside the field needs to be minimized through beam energy and leaf-sequence optimization.

## Clinical Utility

IMET should have the same clinical utility as the previously discussed MET techniques have. One potential untested application of IMET not previously discussed is treatment of intact breast. Figure 18 shows isodose plots, comparing 6 MV x-rays with IMET with 6, 9, 12, 16, and 20 MeV electrons (Ma et al. 1999a) in a left breast with a large target volume. Also, the x-ray plan included a 1.5 cm margin to account for breathing motion, whereas the IMET plan did not require this extra margin. The DVH curves shown in figure 18 demonstrate that with more energies to optimize, the lung dose can be significantly improved. The intermediate doses (25 to 50 Gy) were completely removed, and the lung volume that received a low dose (less than 3 Gy) was almost the same as that for the tangential photon beams, indicating that the bremsstrahlung effect was not significant with eMLC modulation. The improvement to the heart dose is equally significant with IMET. Further improvement in the target dose uniformity may be achieved through beam orientation optimization, i.e., by using more beam angles in the IMET optimization.

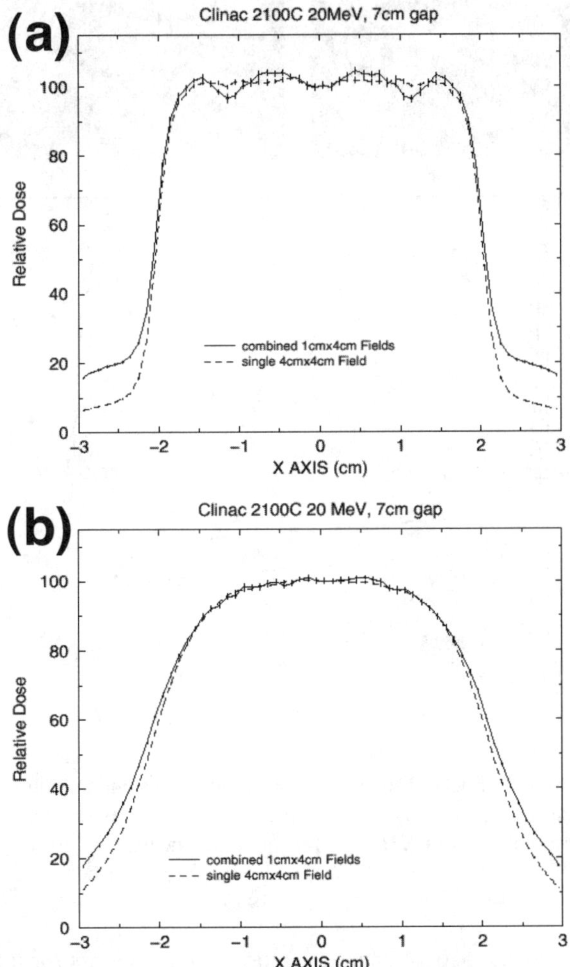


**Figure 17.** Demonstration of impact of x-ray leakage when using an eMLC for IMET. Monte Carlo calculated off-axis dose profiles in a water phantom for a 20 MeV electron beam collimated by an electron MLC of 1.5 cm thick tungsten leaves for a single $4 \times 4$ cm$^2$ electron field and for a $4 \times 4$ cm$^2$ field formed by four $1 \times 4$ cm$^2$ electron fields at depths of 0.5 cm (a) and 3 cm (b). [Reprinted from *Physics in Medicine and Biology*, vol 45, C.-M. Ma, T. Pawlicki, M. C. Lee, S. B. Jiang, J. S. Li, J. Deng, B. Yi, E. Mok, and A. L. Boyer. "Energy- and intensity-modulated electron beams for radiotherapy," pp. 2293–2311. © 2000, with permission from IOP Publishing.]

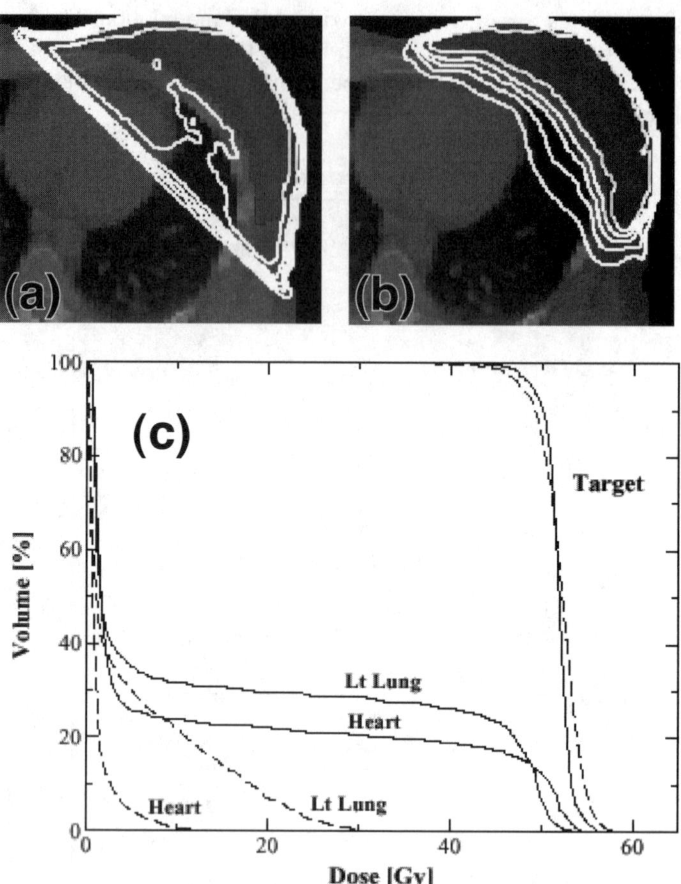



**Figure 18.** Comparison of dose distributions resulting from standard tangential 6 MV x-ray beams (a) with that from IMET (b) for intact breast irradiation. Isodose curves at 10, 20, 30, 40, and 50 Gy are plotted. (c) DVH plots for the target, heart, and left lung resulting from tangential 6 MV x-ray beams (solid lines) and from IMET (dashed lines) are compared (Ma et al. 1999).

Figure 19 shows the patient anatomy and isodose contours for intact breast irradiation; treatment was planned using intensity-modulated tangential beams, four-field IMXT, and eight-field IMET (Ma et al. 2003). The corresponding DVHs for the target, lung, and heart are shown in figure 20. This patient had a relatively thin breast and a flat chest-wall and therefore represented a more favorable case for tangential beams because less lung and heart would be exposed to the x-ray beams. However, conventional tangents usually result in higher doses in the thinnest regions of the breast (superior and inferior borders near the apex). These region-specific hot spots are most likely to manifest as clinical side effects, such as edema. Greater flexibility in intensity

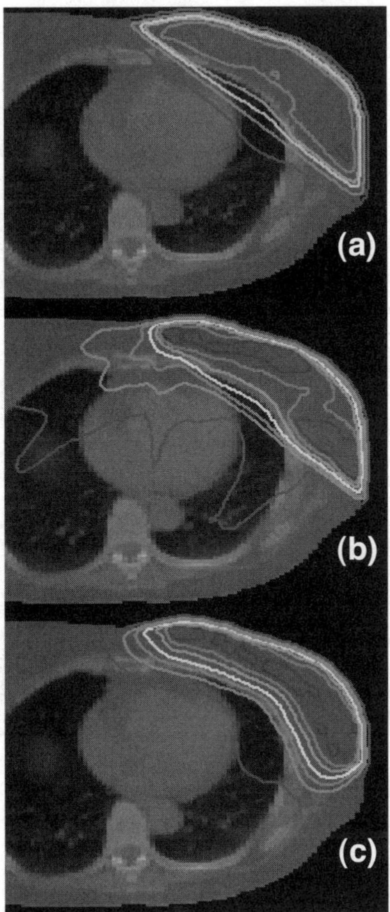

**Figure 19.** Isodose plots planned using two intensity-modulated tangential beams (a), four-field IMXT (b) and 8-field IMET (c) for a patient with breast cancer. The dose distributions are normalized to deliver 50 Gy to the 95% target volume. The 55, 52.5, 50, 45, 40, 25, 15, and 5 Gy isodose lines are shown. [Reprinted from *Physics in Medicine and Biology*, vol xx (submitted), C.-M. Ma, M. Ding, J. S. Li, M. C. Lee, T. Pawlicki, and J. Deng. (2003), "A comparative dosimetric study on tangential photon beams, IMRT and MERT for breast cancer treatment." © 2003, with permission from IOP Publishing.]

modulation allowed IMXT tangents to correct for this, though hotspots in entrance tissue may still occur especially in patients with large breasts. The dose heterogeneity in the target is greater with IMET (about 10%) than with IMXT tangents (about 5%), but it is better than with the four-field IMXT plan (about 15%). The lung and heart doses are much less than 20 Gy in the IMET plan. Unlike the x-ray plans, dose hotspots in the IMET plan were found to be more widely dispersed throughout the target region, not localized in specific geometric features. The multiple field IMXT technique was apparently inferior for breast treatment, with significant lung and heart volumes receiving low and medium doses (cf., figure 20a). It is also evident from the doses in healthy tissues (which represent everything inside the patient—external contour less the target volume) that multiple-field IMXT was inferior to intensity-modulated tangents and IMET. The volume of healthy tissues that received a 5 Gy dose was greater than 5000 cm$^3$ with four-field IMXT compared with less than 2000 cm$^3$ with intensity-modulated tangents and IMET (figure 20b). Because radiation-induced fatal risk is proportional to the integral dose (total energy deposited in the body), it is likely that IMET can be more beneficial than conventional tangents or IMXT in terms of late effects; however, more detailed studies are needed to make a general conclusion.

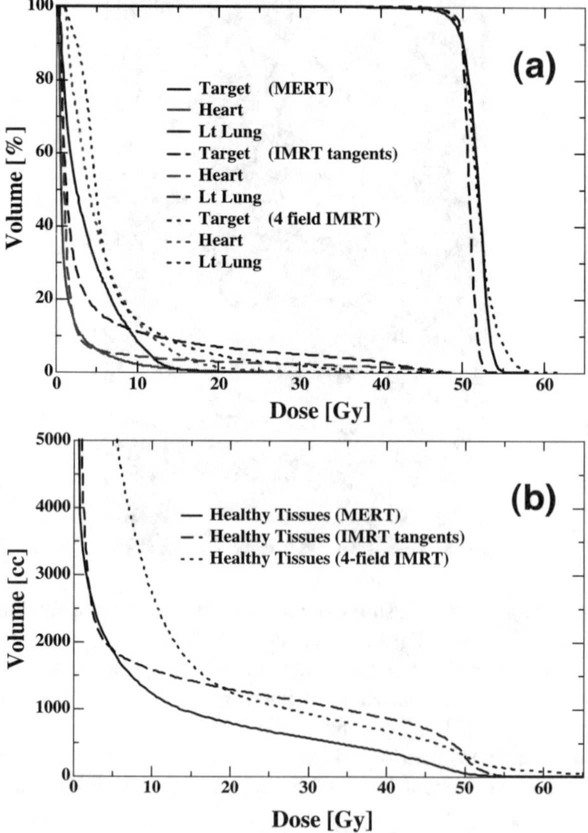



**Figure 20.** Dose-volume histograms for the target, lung, and heart (a) and healthy tissues, defined as all non-target volumes in the body (b), for the three intensity-modulated plans in figure 19. [Reprinted from *Physics in Medicine and Biology*, vol xx (submitted), C.-M. Ma, M. Ding, J. S. Li, M. C. Lee, T. Pawlicki, and J. Deng. (2003), "A comparative dosimetric study on tangential photon beams, IMRT and MERT for breast cancer treatment." © 2003, with permission from IOP Publishing.]

## Modulated Electron Arc Therapy

Modulated electron arc therapy (MEAT) is defined as the utilization of multiple arced beams of differing energies, with beam intensity varying with position along the arc and along the accelerator's isocentric axis. To achieve a uniform maximum dose ($D_{100}$) throughout the field, the electron beam fluence incident on the patient's surface has been varied by altering the width of the electron collimator (Hogstrom and Leavitt 1987). Present treatments utilize a fixed applicator, and the secondary collimator width is varied along the cephalo-caudal direction to account for variations in the patient's mean radius of curvature (i.e., distance from isocenter to patient surface along radial line) between transverse planes. Typically, the radius of curvature is less superiorly (lower neck) than inferiorly (lower chest). However, the radius of curvature within a single transverse plane can vary considerably, requiring that the secondary collimator width also vary with position along the arc. In other words, the secondary collimator width $W$ should vary with both position along the cephalo-caudal dimension ($Y$) and position along the angle of arc ($\theta$). Leavitt et al. (1989b) have demonstrated that this can be achieved by replacing the fixed secondary collimator with an eMLC whose shape varies with arc position [i.e., width $W = W(Y,\theta)$].

Electron arc therapy is used almost exclusively for treating postmastectomy, chest-wall cancer, where the PTV depth is the chest-wall thickness along rays emanating from isocenter. This is exemplified in figure 21, a typical patient treatment plan, in which one beam energy treats the internal mammary chain and another treats the chest wall, whose thickness is reasonably constant. However, the chest wall thickness might not always be constant. In some instances the postmastectomy chest wall has a highly variable thickness owing to excision of a significant portion of tissue. In such cases, custom bolus can be used to restore a constant thickness (Tobler and Leavitt 1996), much as that designed for fixed-beam bolus ECT and discussed above. Development of tools similar to those used for designing and constructing bolus for bolus ECT would enhance this process. An alternative technique would be to partition the beam energy in $Y$ as well as in $\theta$ [i.e., $E = E(Y,\theta)$], using techniques similar to those used for fixed-beam MET above, namely, segmented-field ECT or IMET. Because these techniques are just beginning to be investigated, we will discuss a general vision and needs for their future use.

### Treatment Planning

The area to be treated using arc therapy can be viewed in the same sense as the area to be treated with segmented-field ECT. The electron beam energies can be partitioned using a beam's eye view (i.e., viewing the patient anatomy from the virtual source of the electron beam). There is not a single virtual point source in MEAT, and although this does not create a problem, it does require a different way of thinking of the beam's eye view. In the plane of rotation, the mean directions of the electrons are focused toward isocenter. In a plane containing the central axis of the beam and the isocentric

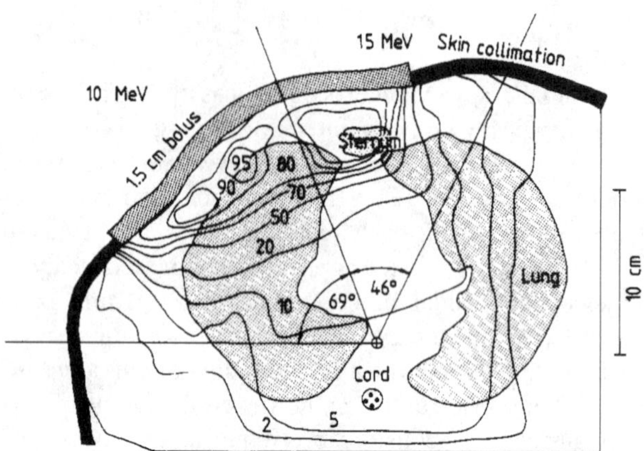


**Figure 21.** Typical arc electron treatment plan for a postmastectomy chest wall. Note that this patient required bolus to attain an adequate surface dose and to conform the 90% dose contour to the lung-chest wall interface. The plan required two beam energies, 15 MeV for the IMC and 10 MeV for the chest wall. Variation in chest-wall thickness in 3-D could require additional arced beams of different energies, similar to segmented-field ECT. Variation in the isocenter-to-patient-surface distance in 3-D could require methods for optimizing dose homogeneity, such as by varying secondary collimator width with angle of arc. [Reprinted from *Physics in Medicine and Biology*, vol 34, K. R. Hogstrom, R. G. Kurup, A. S. Shiu, and G. Starkschall, "A two-dimensional pencil-beam algorithm for calculation of arc electron dose distributions," pp. 315–341. © 1989, with permission from IOP Publishing.]

axis of the gantry, the virtual point source is the same as for a fixed beams (cf., figure 22; Hogstrom and Leavitt 1987). If a regular array of points is defined on the surface of a cylinder, the mean direction of electrons passing in the vicinity of each point is well defined and can be used to generate a PTV depth map. The beam energy can also be partitioned [$E = E(Y,\theta)$] so that the 90% dose surface encompasses the PTV, while conforming as closely as possible to its distal surface. Experience from 2-D–arc therapy planning shows that the boundary of the higher energy beams must extend adequately to account for electron penumbra. This can be appreciated from the two-energy plan previously shown for a single transverse plane (cf., figure 21).

Once the treatment is segmented for beam energy, $E(Y,\theta)$, it can be partitioned for collimator width, $W(Y,\theta)$, which controls dose uniformity. This can be calculated using the simple formula provided by Hogstrom and Leavitt (1987) and Leavitt et al. (1989b).

Because of the large air gap between the secondary collimator and the patient, the dose distribution at the end of an arc is large and its shape results largely from beam geometry (i.e., the collimator width). This provides broad matched penumbras, well suited for abutting arced beams of differing energy (Khan et al. 1991). A broad penumbra at the edges of the PTV can be made sharp by arcing 15° beyond the azimuthal extent of the PTV using skin collimation to restore the penumbra.

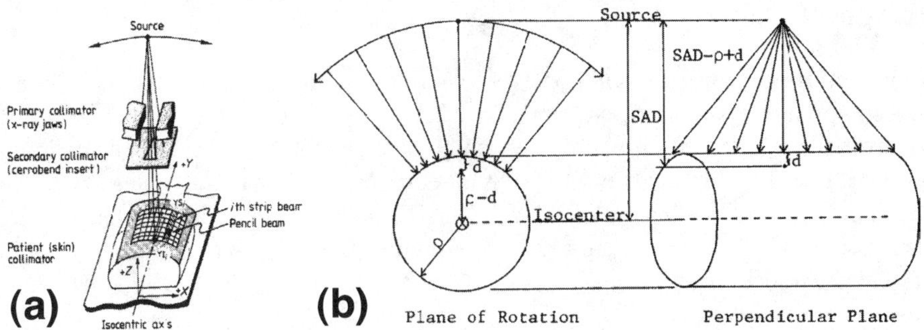


**Figure 22.** Geometry of arc therapy. (a) Illustration of the relationship between the x-ray collimator, secondary collimator (used to control dose homogeneity), and skin collimation on the patient. Note that the patient irradiated area can be partitioned into pixels for the purposes of treatment planning and dose calculation. [(a) Reprinted from *Physics in Medicine and Biology*, vol 34, K. R. Hogstrom, R. G. Kurup, A. S. Shiu, and G. Starkschall, "A two-dimensional pencil-beam algorithm for calculation of arc electron dose distributions," pp. 315–341. © 1989, with permission from IOP Publishing.] (b) Mean directions of electrons in plane of rotation are focused toward isocenter, and mean directions of electrons in plane perpendicular to isocenter show electrons emanating from a point source. [Reprinted from K. R. Hogstrom and D. D. Leavitt. "Dosimetry of Arc Electron Therapy" in *Radiation Oncology Physics–1986*, J. G. Kereiakes, H. R. Elson, and C. G. Born (eds.), pp. 265–295. © 1987, with permission from American Institute of Physics.]

Interestingly, for each beam, $E(Y,\theta)$ and $W(Y,\theta)$ are mostly independent of each other. Once specified, the dose distribution is calculated in 3-D. A first approximation to monitor units can be determined for each arc by prescribing to 90% of the maximum dose. Monitor units could be optimized to give the most uniform dose in the PTV while still conforming the 90% dose surface to the PTV. An alternative approach might be one similar to IMET, where beamlets are specified by beam energy ($E$), arc angle ($\theta$), eMLC leaf index ($Y$), and eMLC strip width ($W$).

Presently, treatment planning systems lack adequate capability for 3-D dose calculations for arc electron therapy. Dose calculation could likely utilize analytical or Monte Carlo methods. The algorithm could be configured to simulate an arced beam as (1) a collection of fixed beam dose calculations or (2) a two-step calculation. The latter transports electrons from the arced beam to the patient surface, where the skin surface is partitioned into pencil beams, and for each pencil beam the dose to the patient is calculated. This was the approach of Hogstrom et al. (1989) for multiplane, 2-D dose calculations, which could easily be extended to 3-D. However, with the ever-increasing speed of computers, it now seems more practical to simulate arc-beam dose distribution by summing fixed-beam dose calculations. Additionally, dose algorithms for arc electron therapy require the ability to model skin collimation and to accurately calculate x-ray dose.

In summary, treatment planning tools and dose-calculation tools must be developed and implemented into 3-D treatment planning systems before MEAT can be practical.

## Treatment Delivery

Treatment for this therapy will consist of an arced beam for each of the beam energies comprising a patient's treatment plan. Each arc will be specified by a range of arc rotation ($\theta_{start}, \theta_{stop}$), a number of monitor units to be delivered, and a variable collimator width $W(Y,\theta)$. Leavitt et al. (1989b) demonstrated that the latter could be accomplished by replacing the fixed, secondary collimator with a computer-controlled, dynamic MLC. Their prototype eMLC, pictured in figure 23, had a 4 cm leaf width projected to isocenter.

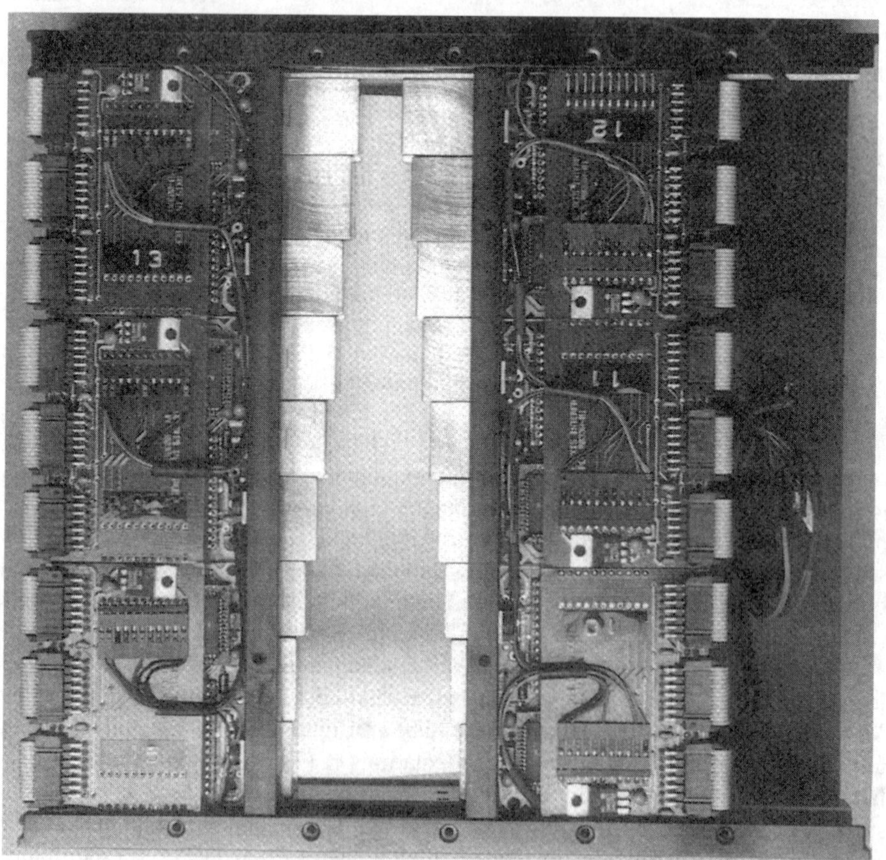

**Figure 23.** Beam's eye view of prototype eMLC for electron arc therapy. The leaf resolution (approximately 4 cm projected to isocenter) is coarse but could easily be improved.
[Reprinted from *International Journal of Radiation Oncology Biology Physics*, vol 17, D. D. Leavitt, J. R. Stewart, J. H. Moeller, W. L. Lee, and G. A. Takach, Jr., "Electron arc therapy: Design, implementation and evaluation of a dynamic multi-vane collimator system." pp. 1089–1094. © 1989, with permission from Elsevier.]

## Quality Assurance

Beam uniformity can be verified by *in vivo* dosimety on the chest wall surface using thermoluminescent dosimetry (TLD) or another appropriate dosimeter. Presently, methods have not been developed to verify the penetration of electron dose. However, a method similar to that standardly used for IMXT can be envisioned. Film could be used to measure the dose distribution in multiple transverse planes in a 30 cm diameter, cylindrical, solid-water phantom. The treatment planning system would calculate the dose in this phantom using patient-specific beam parameters, and those results would be compared to measurement for verification.

## Clinical Utility

The primary utility of MEAT will likely be postmastectomy chest wall therapy. The utility of intensity modulation to achieve dose uniformity was demonstrated by Leavitt et al. (1989a, c.f., figure 24). The patient's radius of curvature in the plane of rotation varied from approximately 12 cm to 19 cm, resulting in significant dose non-uniformity (approximately 70% to 110%) using a fixed collimator width. Allowing the field width to change 10 times over the approximately 190° arc improved the dose uniformity (to approximately 90% to 105%). This example utilized a single beam energy, although typically two energies are required, one for the chest wall and one for the internal mammary chain.

The radial depth dose in arc electron therapy shows considerably less surface dose (60% to 70%) than do fixed electron beams (cf., figure 25a). Leavitt, Stewart, and Earley (1990) have demonstrated the benefit of the superposition of multiple electron energies across an arc segment to achieve increased surface dose and improved radial depth dose uniformity (cf., figure 25b). Consequently, the benefit of an IMET-like technique for MEAT might be beneficial.

## Mixed-Beam Therapy

Mixed-beam therapy is defined as the combining of electron and photon beams for the purpose of achieving a more optimal patient dose distribution. Mixed-beam therapy includes both conventional and conformal therapy for the electron and photon beams.

The mixing of electron with x-ray therapy offers further benefits over either modality individually. Although the abutment of x-ray with electron fields offers significant treatment opportunities, mixed-beam therapy in the present context will be limited to the utilization of electron and x-ray beams to irradiate the same PTV. Historically, x-rays have been mixed with electrons to decrease surface dose, to increase therapeutic depth, and/or to increase dose homogeneity in the PTV (Fields and Hogstrom 1984). Such mixed-beam therapy has been utilized for irradiation of head and neck cancers and for irradiation of the IMC (Tapley 1976).

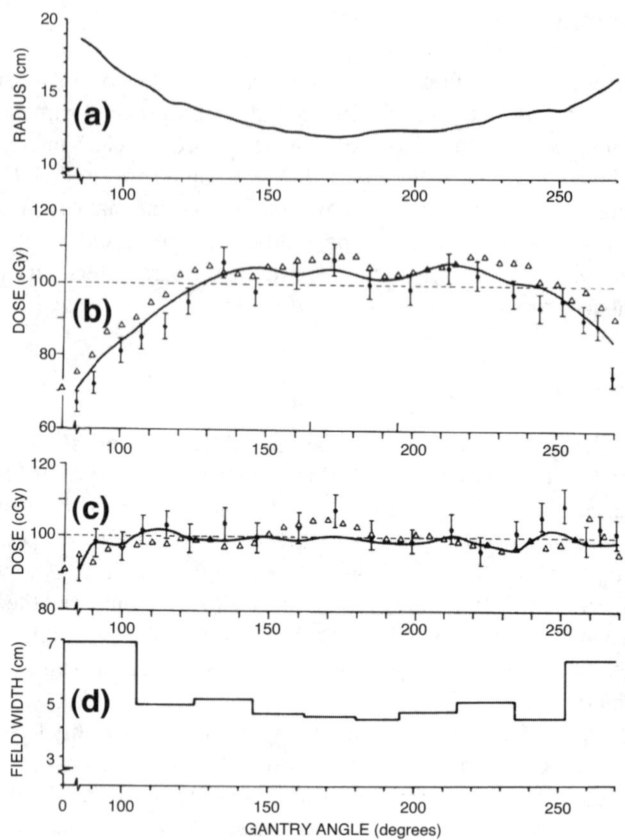



**Figure 24.** Utility of eMLC for bilateral arc therapy. (a) Radius of curvature versus arc position (gantry angle) varies significantly in superior transverse plane of patient. (b) Treatment with a constant-width secondary collimator produces significant dose inhomogeneity, as shown in plot of maximum depth dose versus arc position. (c) Treatment with a variable-width secondary collimator produces a uniform dose, as shown in the plot of maximum depth dose versus arc position. (d) Plot of secondary collimator width versus arc position required to achieve the dose in (c) above. [Reprinted from *International Journal of Radiation Oncology Biology Physics*, vol 16, D. D. Leavitt, J. R. Stewart, J. H. Moeller, and L. Earley, "Optimization of electron arc therapy doses by multi-vane collimator control," pp. 489–496. © 1989, with permission from Elsevier.]

IMXT and MET are at two ends of the treatment spectrum. Either can provide a conformal treatment to a superficial PTV, each having different strengths and weaknesses, as demonstrated above for irradiation of an intact breast. Using a similar technique, Li et al. (2000) found the mixed-beam IMRT to show improvement over the conventional tangential field technique, giving a reduced dose to the ipsilateral lung and heart.

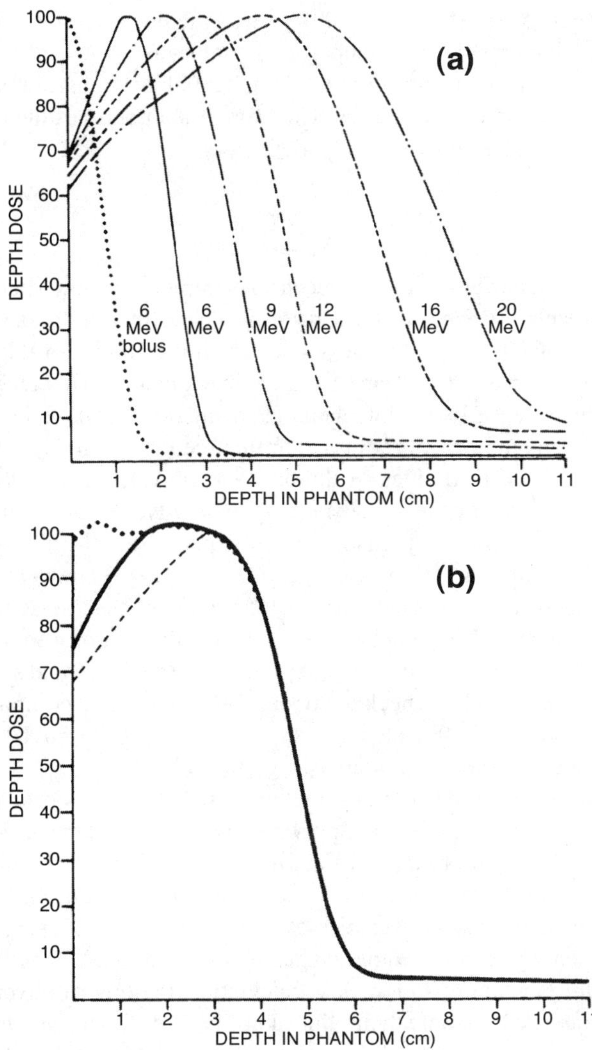


**Figure 25.** Utilization of energy modulation to achieve improved homogeneity of depth dose in MEAT. (a) Depth doses for an electron arc of 90° incident on a cylindrical phantom of 15 cm radius. Isocenter depth was set to 15 cm. Depth doses for 6, 9, 12, 16, and 20 MeV are shown, as well as the depth dose for a 6 MeV beam supplemented by 1.5 cm thick bolus. (b) Depth doses for a 12 MeV arced beam (dashed); addition of 6, 9, and 12 MeV arced beams (solid); and addition of 6, 9, 12 MeV, and "bolused" 6 MeV arced beams (dotted). [Reprinted from *International Journal of Radiation Oncology Biology Physics*, vol 19, D. D. Leavitt, J. R. Stewart, and L. Earley, "Improved dose homogeneity in electron arc therapy achieved by a multiple-energy technique," pp. 159–165. © 1990, with permission from Elsevier.]

Svatos, Rosenman, and Verhey (2000) showed the potential of mixed-beam therapy for reduced integral dose for superficial tumors (0 to 4 cm depth). Medical physicists at M. D. Anderson have seen similar potential in comparing bolus ECT with IMXT plans for head and neck cancers. Therefore, the mixture of the two modalities can be expected to find a future role in patient care.

## Conclusion

MET is a modality that offers improved electron therapy for patients, particularly those having disease near the surface and those having critical structures underlying the PTV. Methods for bolus ECT are well refined, and the clinical utility of this modality has been demonstrated for chest wall and head and neck cancer. This technology is not widely available because treatment planning manufacturers have not incorporated proven treatment planning methods into their treatment planning systems.

Segmented-field ECT provides an alternative to bolus ECT, and its utilization has also been demonstrated for the same sites; its main advantages are that it does not require fabrication of a bolus and that it has a sharper dose fall-off in depth from the PTV ($R_{90-10}$). This technology is not widely available, primarily owing to radiotherapy manufacturers not offering adequate MLCs and treatment head design.

IMET offers an inverse planning approach, which offers improved dose uniformity in the PTV. It is expected to provide an alternative to bolus ECT and segmented-field ECT in chest wall and head and neck treatments. Although more complicated than the previous two techniques, IMET also offers the potential for improved dose distributions and application in other major areas, e.g., intact breast.

These electron conformal therapy methods, with some modifications, can be applied to modulated arc electron therapy, which is most useful in the treatment of the postmastectomy chest wall. Finally, the ability to offer MET should allow its mixing with IMXT, providing treatment that is better than either modality alone, i.e., taking advantages of the strengths and weaknesses of each modality in a single treatment.

For these techniques to become available, research must continue to provide adequate tools for plan optimization, dose calculation, treatment delivery, and quality assurance and must demonstrate their clinical utility. Most important, unless the radiation oncology community can convince treatment planning system and radiotherapy accelerator manufacturers of its need, commercial availability and hence its widespread use will not be possible.

## References

Antolak, J. A., R. A. Boyd, and K. R. Hogstrom. (2002). "Evaluation of dosimetric issues related to IMET for a prototype EMLC." *Med. Phys.* 29:1285.

Antolak, J. A., G. Starkschall, E. R. Bawiec Jr., J. R. Ewton, and K. R. Hogstrom. "Implementation of an Automated Electron Bolus Fabrication System for Conformal Electron Radiotherapy" in *XIth International Conference on the Use of Computers in Radiation Therapy*. A. R. Hounsell, J. M. Wilkinson, and P. C. Williams (eds.). Manchester, UK: Christie Hospital NHS Trust, pp. 162–163, 1994.

Åsell, M., S. Hyödynmaa, A. Gustafsson, and A. Brahme. (1997). "Optimization of 3D conformal electron beam therapy in inhomogeneous media by concomitant fluence and energy modulation." *Phys. Med. Biol.* 42:2083–2100.

Bawiec Jr., E. R., (1994). The Effects of Accuracy in Milling of Electron Bolus on Dose Delivery. The University of Texas Health Science Center at Houston (M.Sc. thesis).

Boyd, R. A., J. A. Antolak, and K. R. Hogstrom. (2002). "Dosimetric characterization of a prototype EMLC for fixed beam therapy." *Med. Phys.* 29:1285.

Brahme, A. (1987). "Design principles and clinical possibilities with a new generation of radiation therapy equipment. A review." *Acta Oncol.* 26:403–412.

Brahme, A. (1988). "Optimisation of stationary and moving beam radiation therapy techniques." *Radiother. Oncol.* 12:129–140.

Deng, J., M. C. Lee, and C.-M. Ma. (2002). "A Monte Carlo investigation of fluence profiles collimated by an electron specific MLC during beam delivery for modulated electron radiation therapy." *Med. Phys.* 29:2472–2483.

Ebert, M. A., and P. W. Hoban. (1997). "Possibilities for tailoring dose distributions through the manipulation of electron beam characteristics." *Phys. Med. Biol.* 42:2065–2081.

Fields, R. S., and K. R. Hogstrom. "Optimization of Electron-Photon Mixed Beam Planning" in *Proceedings of the Eight International Conference on the Use of Computers in Radiation Therapy*. Silver Spring, MD: IEEE Computer Society Press, pp. 248–254, 1984.

Hogstrom, K. R. "Clinical Electron Beam Dosimetry: Basic Dosimetry Data" in *Advances in Radiation Oncology Physics: Dosimetry, Treatment Planning and Brachytherapy*. J. A. Purdy (ed.). AAPM medical Physics Monograph No. 19. Proceedings of the AAPM 1990 Summer School. New York, NY: American Institute of Physics, pp. 390–429, 1992.

Hogstrom, K. R., and D. D. Leavitt. "Dosimetry of Arc Electron Therapy" in *Radiation Oncology Physics–1986*. J. G. Kereiakes, H. R. Elson, and C. G. Born (eds.). AAPM Medical Physics Monograph No. 15. Proceedings of the AAPM 1986 Summer School. New York, NY: American Institute of Physics, pp. 265–295, 1987.

Hogstrom, K. R., M. D. Mills, and P. R. Almond. (1981). "Electron beam dose calculations." *Phys. Med. Biol.* 26:445–459.

Hogstrom, K. R., R. G. Kurup, A. S. Shiu, and G. Starkschall. (1989). "A two-dimensional pencil-beam algorithm for calculation of arc electron dose distributions." *Phys. Med. Biol.* 34:315–341.

Holmes, T., and T. R. Mackie. (1994). "A filtered backprojection dose calculation method for inverse treatment planning." *Med. Phys.* 21:303–313.

Hyödynmaa, S., A. Gustafsson, and A. Brahme. (1996). "Optimization of conformal electron beam therapy using energy- and fluence-modulated beams." *Med. Phys.* 23:659–666.

Janssen, J. J., E. W. Korevaar, P. R. Storchi, and H. Huizenga. (1997). "Numerical calculation of energy deposition by high-energy electron beams: III-B. Improvements to the 6D phase space evolution model." *Phys. Med. Biol.* 42:1441–1449.

Jeraj, R., and P. Keall. (1999). "Monte Carlo-based inverse treatment planning." *Phys. Med. Biol.* 44:1885–1896.

Jiang, S. B., T. Pawlicki, and C.-M. Ma. (2000). "An aperture-based inverse planning algorithm for modulated electron radiation therapy." CD-ROM Proceedings of the World Congress on Medical Physics and Biomedical Engineering, July 23–28, 2000, Chicago, IL.

Jiang, S. B., T. Pawlicki, F. Gracia, T. Guerrero, M. C. Lee, J. S. Li, J. Deng, D. R. Goffinet, A. L. Boyer, and C.-M. Ma. (2000). "Modulated electron radiation therapy: A new treatment modality." *Int. J. Radiat. Oncol. Biol. Phys.* 48(3 Suppl 1):218.

Karlsson, M. G., and M. Karlsson. (2002). "Electron beam collimation with focused and curved leaf end MLCs—experimental verification of Monte Carlo optimized designs." *Med. Phys.* 29:631–637.

Karlsson, M. G., M. Karlsson, and C.-M. Ma. (1999). "Treatment head design for multileaf collimated high-energy electrons." *Med. Phys.* 26:2161–2167.

Karlsson, M. G., M. Karlsson, and B. Zackrisson. (1998). "Intensity modulation with electrons: calculations, measurements and clinical applications." *Phys. Med. Biol.* 43:1159–1169.

Khan, F. M., K. P. Doppke, K. R. Hogstrom, G. J. Kutcher, R. Nath, S. C. Prasad, J. A. Purdy, M. Rozenfeld, and B. L. Werner. (1991). "Clinical electron-beam dosimetry: Report of AAPM Radiation Therapy Committee Task Group No. 25." *Med. Phys.* 18:73–109. (Also available as AAPM Report No. 32.)

Klein, E. E. (1998). "Modulated electron beams using multi-segmented multileaf collimation." *Radiother. Oncol.* 48:307–311.

Kudchadker, R., J. A. Antolak, W. H. Morrison, and K. R. Hogstrom. (2002a). "Conformal head and neck radiotherapy using custom electron bolus." *Med. Phys.* 29:1337.

Kudchadker, R. J., K. R. Hogstrom, A. S. Garden, M. D. McNeese, R. A. Boyd, and J. A. Antolak. (2002b). "Electron conformal radiotherapy using bolus and intensity modulation." *Int. J. Radiat. Oncol. Biol. Phys.* 53:1023–1037.

Leavitt, D. D., J. R. Stewart, and L. Earley. (1990). "Improved dose homogeneity in electron arc therapy achieved by a multiple-energy technique." *Int. J. Radiat. Oncol. Biol. Phys.* 19:159–165.

Leavitt, D. D., J. R. Stewart, J. H. Moeller, and L. Earley. (1989a). "Optimization of electron arc therapy doses by multi-vane collimator control." *Int. J. Radiat. Oncol. Biol. Phys.* 16:489–496.

Leavitt, D. D., J. R. Stewart, J. H. Moeller, W. L. Lee, and G. A. Takach, Jr. (1989b). "Electron arc therapy: Design, implementation and evaluation of a dynamic multi-vane collimator system." *Int. J. Radiat. Oncol. Biol. Phys.* 17:1089–1094.

Lee, M. C., S. B. Jiang, and C.-M. Ma. (2000). "Monte Carlo and experimental investigations of multileaf collimated electron beams for modulated electron radiation therapy." *Med. Phys.* 27:2708–2718.

Lee, M. C., J. Deng, J. Li, S. B. Jiang, and C.-M. Ma. (2001). "Monte Carlo based treatment planning for modulated electron beam radiation therapy." *Phys. Med. Biol.* 46:2177–2199.

Li, J. G., S. S. Williams, D. R. Goffinet, A. L. Boyer, and L. Xing. (2000). "Breast-conserving radiation therapy using combined electron and intensity-modulated radiotherapy technique." *Radiother. Oncol.* 56:65–71.

Lief, E. P., A. Larsson, and J. L. Humm. (1996). "Electron dose profile shaping by modulation of a scanning elementary beam." *Med. Phys.* 23:33–44.

Low, D. A., and K. R. Hogstrom. (1994). "Determination of the relative linear collision stopping and linear scattering powers of electron bolus material." *Phys. Med. Biol.* 39:1063–1068.

Low, D. A., G. Starkschall, S. W. Bujnowski, L. L. Wang, and K. R. Hogstrom. (1992). "Electron bolus design for radiotherapy treatment planning: Bolus design algorithms." *Med. Phys.* 19:115–124.

Low, D. A., G. Starkschall, N. E. Sherman, S. W. Bujnowski, J. R. Ewton, and K. R. Hogstrom. (1995). "Computer-aided design and fabrication of an electron bolus for treatment of the paraspinal muscles." *Int. J. Radiat. Oncol. Biol. Phys.* 33:1127–1138.

Ma, C.-M., and S. B. Jiang. (1999). "Monte Carlo modelling of electron beams from medical accelerators." *Phys. Med. Biol.* 44:R157–189.

Ma, C.-M., S. B. Jiang, T. Pawlicki, E. Mok, J. S. Li, J. Deng, A. Kapur, B. Yi, M. C. Lee, G. Luxton, and A. L. Boyer. (1999a). "Energy- and intensity-modulated electron beams for the treatment of breast cancer." *Int. J. Radiat. Oncol. Biol. Phys.* 45(3 Suppl 1):165–166.

Ma, C.-M., E. Mok, A. Kapur, T. Pawlicki, D. Findley, S. Brain, K. Forster, and A. L. Boyer. (1999b). "Clinical implementation of a Monte Carlo treatment planning system." *Med. Phys.* 26:2133–2143.

Ma, C.-M., T. Pawlicki, S. B. Jiang, J. S. Li, J. Deng, E. Mok, A. Kapur, L. Xing, L. Ma, and A. L. Boyer. (2000a). "Monte Carlo verification of IMRT dose distributions from a commercial treatment planning optimization system." *Phys. Med. Biol.* 45:2483–2495.

Ma, C.-M., T. Pawlicki, M. C. Lee, S. B. Jiang, J. S. Li, J. Deng, B. Yi, E. Mok, and A. L. Boyer. (2000b). "Energy- and intensity-modulated electron beams for radiotherapy." *Phys. Med. Biol.* 45:2293–2311.

Ma, C.-M., M. Ding, J. S. Li, M. C. Lee, T. Pawlicki, and J. Deng. (2003). "A comparative dosimetric study on tangential photon beams, IMRT and MERT for breast cancer treatment." *Phys. Med. Biol.* Submitted.

Mackie, T. R., P. J. Reckwerdt, C. M. Wells, J. N. Yang, J. O. Deasy, M. Podgorsak, M. A. Holmes, D. W. O. Rogers, G. X. Ding, B. A. Faddegon, C.-M. Ma, A. F. Bielajew, and J. Cygler. "The OMEGA project: Comparison among EGS4 electron beam simulations, Fermi-Eyges calculations and dose measurements." *XIth International Conference on the Use of Computers in Radiation Therapy.* A. R. Hounsell, J. M. Wilkinson, and P. C. Williams (eds.). Manchester, UK: Christie Hospital NHS Trust, pp. 152–153, 1994.

McNeeley, S., J. S. Li, R. A. Price, L. Chen, M. Ding, E. Fourkal, and C.-M. Ma. (2001). "An electron specific MLC for modulated electron radiation therapy." *Med. Phys.* 29:1286.

Pawlicki, T., and C.-M. Ma. (2001). "Monte Carlo simulation for MLC-based intensity-modulated radiotherapy." *Med. Dosim.* 26:157–168.

Perkins, G. H., M. D. McNeese, J. A. Antolak, T. A. Buchholz, E. A. Strom, and K. R. Hogstrom. (2001). "A custom three-dimensional electron bolus technique for optimization of postmastectomy irradiation." *Int. J. Radiat. Oncol. Biol. Phys.* 51:1142–1151.

Siebers, J. V., P. J. Keall, J. O. Kim, and R. Mohan. (2002). "A method for photon beam Monte Carlo multileaf collimator particle transport." *Phys. Med. Biol.* 47:3225–3249.

Starkschall, G., S. W. Bujnowski, J. A. Antolak, L.-H. Wang, and K. R. Hogstrom. "Tools for 3-D electron-beam treatment planning." *XIth International Conference on the Use of Computers in Radiation Therapy.* A. R. Hounsell, J. M. Wilkinson, and P. C. Williams (eds.). Manchester, UK: Christie Hospital NHS Trust, pp. 126–127, 1994.

Starkschall, G., S. W. Bujnowski, L. L. Wang, A. S. Shiu, A. L. Boyer, G. E. Desobry, N. H. Wells, A. L. Baker, and K. R. Hogstrom. (1991a). "A full three-dimensional radiotherapy treatment planning system." *Med. Phys.* 18:647.

Starkschall, G., A. S. Shiu, S. W. Bujnowski, L. L. Wang, D. A. Low, and K. R. Hogstrom. (1991b). "Effect of dimensionality of heterogeneity corrections on the implementation of a three-dimensional electron pencil-beam algorithm." *Phys. Med. Biol.* 36:207–227.

Svatos, M. M., J. G. Rosenman, and L. J. Verhey. (2000). "Effectiveness of mixing electrons with intensity modulated photons for reduction of integral dose for a variety of tumors sizes and depths." *Int. J. Radiat. Oncol. Biol. Phys.* 48(3 Suppl 1):140–141.

Tapley, N. D. (ed.). *Clinical Applications of the Electron Beam.* New York, NY: John Wiley & Sons, Inc., 1976.

Tobler, M., and D. D. Leavitt. (1996). "Design and production of wax compensators for electron treatments of the chest wall." *Med. Dosim.* 21:199–206.

Webb, S. (1989). "Optimisation of conformal radiotherapy dose distributions by simulated annealing." [Erratum appears in *Phys. Med. Biol.* 1990, 35(2):297]. *Phys. Med. Biol.* 34:1349–1370.

Zackrisson, B., and M. Karlsson. (1996). "Matching of electron beams for conformal therapy of target volumes at moderate depths." *Radiother. Oncol.* 39:261–270.

# Compensated And Intensity-Modulated Proton Therapy

**Tony Lomax, Ph.D.**
Paul Scherrer Institute
Villigen-PSI, Switzerland



## Introduction

The use of protons in radiotherapy, at least as an idea, is more than 50 years old. Robert Wilson first published his seminal paper on the subject in 1946 (Wilson 1946), and 8 years later the first patients were treated with protons at Berkeley. Since then, more than 32,000 patients have been treated worldwide at over 20 centers in 12 different countries (Sisterson 2002). As of July 2002, there were 21 centers around the world actively delivering clinical proton therapy, with more planned in the next few years. Historically, proton therapy has been the preserve of physics research laboratories. However, following the lead of Loma Linda University Hospital in California, who in 1990 began treatments with the world's first hospital-based proton therapy facility, and more recently Massachusetts General Hospital in Boston, the future for proton therapy clearly lies in the hospital.

It is the aim of this chapter to provide an overview of proton therapy from the point of view of physics, treatment delivery, clinical experience, and the potential of proton therapy to improve treatment outcome. The chapter is divided into the following sections:

Proton Interactions With Matter And Tissues

Sources Of Therapeutic Protons

Making Protons Useful I: Passive Scattering

Making Protons Useful II: Active Scanning

Intensity-Modulated Proton Therapy (IMPT)

Clinical Experience With Protons

When Are Protons Preferable?

Summary

## Proton Interactions With Matter And Tissue

### The Proton Depth-Dose Curve

As protons pass through a medium, they gradually lose energy, primarily through electromagnetic interactions with orbiting electrons. The resulting secondary electrons have a small range, and thus the energy lost through such interactions is deposited local to the original point of interaction. Mathematically, protons lose energy at a rate that is inversely proportional to the square of their velocity (see e.g., Bichsel 1972). Thus, as their energy decreases, the amount of deposited energy increases rapidly, resulting in the characteristic Bragg peak at the end of their range—i.e., where their velocity approaches zero (see figure 1). For purely mono-energetic protons, this Bragg peak would be extremely narrow, but is diluted in practice due to range-straggling effects— statistical fluctuations in energy loss—that result in energy-dependent fluctuations amounting to a few percent of the total range. Range straggling increases with increasing initial energy (greater penetration in matter), and thus higher energy beams will generally deliver broader Bragg peaks (see e.g., Berger 1993a). Further dilution of the Bragg peak results from the initial energy spectrum of the proton source, which for most therapeutic systems amounts to an additional 1% to 2% fluctuation of the nominal energy. In addition, protons can be completely lost from the beam due to interactions with atomic nuclei. Between entering the medium and the end of the proton range, about 20% of protons will be lost to such interactions. Although most of the proton energy from nuclear interactions is deposited locally (a little more than 50%), the rest is deposited in a "halo" of secondary particles, which remove the remaining energy away from the point of interaction with a fairly broad angular distribution (see e.g., Seltzer 1993 or Paganetti 2002).

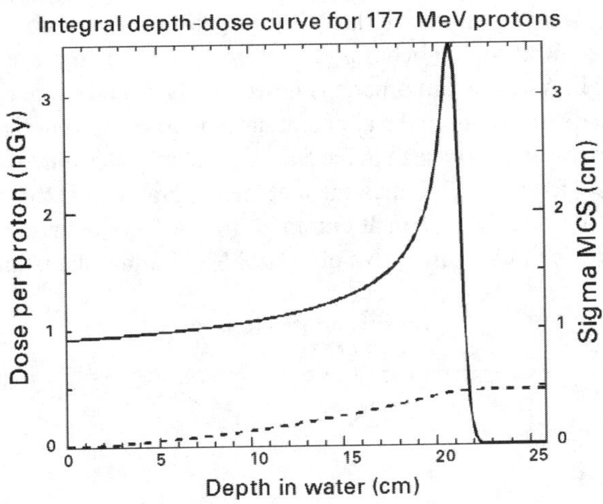


**Figure 1.** The integral depth dose curve for 177 MeV protons with a momentum band (energy spectrum) of 1.1% FWHM. The dotted line shows the lateral width of the beam due to multiple Coulomb scattering in the medium alone.

A depth-dose curve for 177 MeV protons is shown in figure 1. This shows the total dose deposited at any given depth, integrated over a plane perpendicular to the direction of propagation of the beam. This is the curve one would expect to observe if measuring at different depths in a broad beam source, or alternatively, in a narrow pencil beam when the diameter of the detector is very much larger than the beam width. The deposited dose increases slowly on entrance to the medium, gradually increasing as the protons lose energy and velocity, until the protons have little residual energy, and the deposited dose increases rapidly to the characteristic Bragg peak. Beyond this, the dose decreases to zero, typically in a few millimeters. Note, that proton beams demonstrate no skin sparing effect, a characteristic that can be problematic in some clinical circumstances.

## Multiple Coulomb Scattering

As protons lose energy, they are also deflected from their path through Coulomb scattering interactions. As each proton will experience many such deflections in a random manner, statistical considerations determine that Multiple Coulomb Scattering (MCS) of an infinitesimally small proton pencil beam will result in the beam having a Moliere distribution laterally, generally approximated as a Gaussian, whose width steadily increases with increasing penetration (see Moliere 1948; Preston and Koehler 1968; Berger 1993b; Scheib 1993). As an example, for 177 MeV protons, the width of the beam due to MCS alone at the Bragg peak is about 4 mm sigma, or about 9 mm FWHM (full width at half maximum) (figure 1). For such a pencil beam, the effects of MCS tend to remove increasing amounts of dose from the central axis as the depth of penetration increases. Figure 2 shows the *central axis* depth dose curve of a finite size pencil beam, with an initial width of 2.5 mm sigma. Where the effects of MCS are small near the entrance, the beam is still narrow, and the amplitude at the central axis relatively high. As the beam broadens however, more and more dose is removed from the central axis, resulting in the apparent drop of dose as a function of depth. The effects of MCS are most clearly seen in the Bragg peak, which is much less pronounced than for the integral Bragg peak, indicating that the integral dose at this depth, although about a factor of 4 higher here than at entrance (figure 1), is being distributed over a much larger area due to the cumulative effects of MCS along the beam's full range.

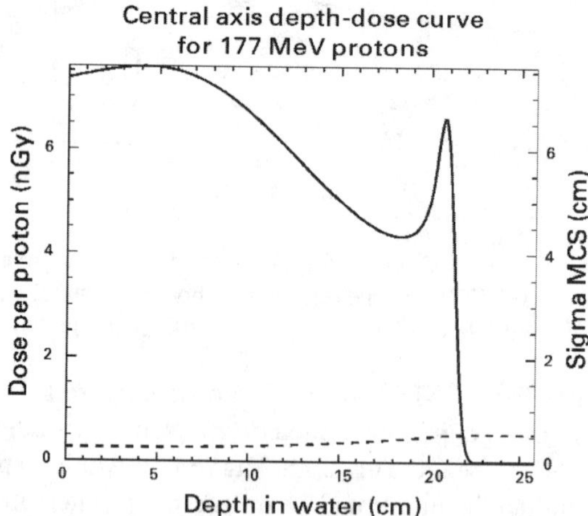


**Figure 2.** Central axis depth dose curve for 177 MeV protons for same parameters as figure 1. An initial width of the beam on entrance of 2.5 mm sigma has been assumed.

## Density Heterogeneities And Protons

The combined effects of the finite range of protons and the effects of MCS have some profound effects on the sensitivity of proton treatments to density heterogeneities within a patient. Although the fundamental physics of energy loss and scattering are well understood and robust mathematical models can predict their magnitudes with great precision in simple geometries (see e.g., Scheib 1993; Deasy 1998; Schaffner, Pedroni, and Lomax 1999; Szymanowski and Oelfke 2002), the complex density heterogeneities encountered by proton fields in patients bring special problems. Goitein first identified such effects for proton therapy in the early 1980's when he showed analytically the effects of thin slivers of bone on a clinical proton beam (Goitein 1978; Goitein et al. 1978). This work was expanded by the same group to model the degradation of the Bragg peak for a proton pencil beam passing along a bone/soft-tissue interface (Goitein and Sisterson 1978; Urie et al. 1986). The problem is relatively straightforward to understand, and is shown schematically in figures 3a and 3b. For a pencil beam passing parallel to an interface between two materials with different densities, some of the protons will pass through the higher density material, whilst some will pass through the lower density material. In addition, different protons will pass through different amounts of each material depending on how they are scattered, with some protons being scattered from the low-density material into the high, and vice versa. As the total energy loss depends on the path lengths the protons have taken through the two mediums, the proton beam beyond the interface has a significantly broadened spectrum. This has the effect of "diluting" the spectrum, and therefore the shape, of Bragg peaks that are delivered at depths beyond the interface (i.e., in figure 3, $\Delta R_{inhom} \gg \Delta R_{hom}$). For instance, in the situation shown in figure 3b, two distinct Bragg peaks could actually be formed behind the heterogeneity (see e.g., Schneider et al. 1998; Schaffner, Pedroni, and Lomax 1999).

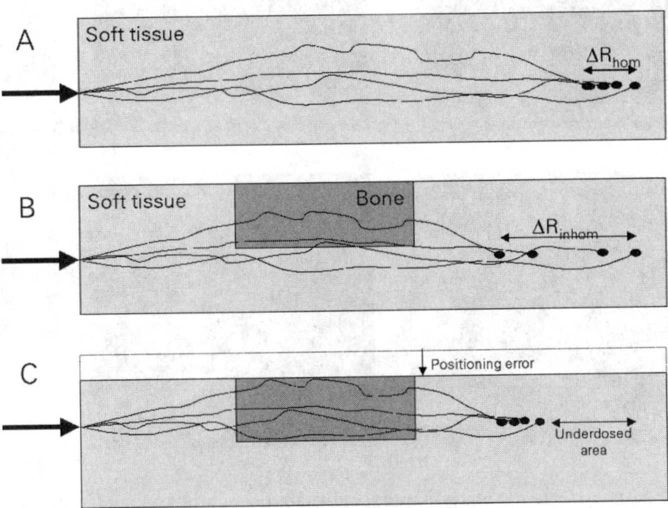


**Figure 3.** Schematic representation of density heterogeneity problems for protons. (a) Example of proton tracks through a homogenous medium. (b) The same tracks partially passing through a bone-soft tissue interface. Note the wider dispersion of Bragg peak ranges distal to the interface. (c) The same situation as (b), but with the interface shifted in relation to the beam. Note the change in shape and range of the Bragg peak due to this small positioning misalignment.

The example in figure 3 is for a relatively simple geometry, but density hetero-geneities encountered in patients are generally more complicated. This puts great demands on the dose calculation algorithms used for planning proton treatments. Although analytical dose calculations are very accurate in water or other homogenous mediums, there is a question mark over their effectiveness in the presence of gross heterogeneities. For this reason, some groups have developed Monte Carlo calcula-tion models that can be used in computer tomography (CT) planning geometries. Figure 4 shows a comparison of a Monte Carlo and analytical dose calculation from the proton treatment planning system of the Paul Scherrer Institute in Switzerland (Tourovsky, Pedroni, and Schneider 1993). Two fields are shown. For the top exam-ple (figure 4a and b), the field is passing through relatively homogenous anatomy, and there is very good visual agreement between the Monte Carlo and the analytical calcu-lations. A more quantative analysis showed that for this field, 99% of all calculation points agreed to better than ±5% between the two calculation methods. For the field at the bottom however, which is passing through more heterogeneous anatomy, only 89% of points agree to better than ±5%, and there are clear differences between the two dose distributions (figure 4c and d).

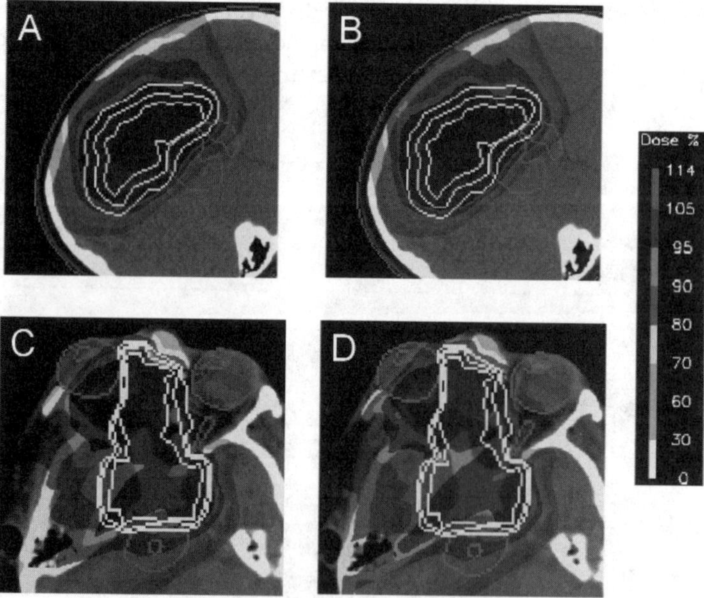


**Figure 4.** Monte Carlo vs. analytical dose distribution comparisons for two fields. (a) Analytical dose calculation for a field traversing relatively homogenous anatomy. (b) Monte Carlo calculation for the same geometry. (c) Analytical calculation for field traversing inhomogenous anatomy. (d) Monte Carlo calculation for same geometry.

Density heterogeneities do not only affect the accuracy of the dose calculation however. Even if a Monte Carlo calculation is used, there is another effect that simply cannot be avoided and must be taken into account when applying proton therapy clinically. That is the sensitivity of the delivered dose distribution to delivery errors such as patient positioning inaccuracies.

Figure 3c shows the situation if the geometry of figure 3b is shifted slightly in relation to the beam (i.e., the patient is poorly positioned in relation to the planning CT). Now, instead of having a diluted Bragg peak, the whole Bragg peak is shifted towards the entrance, as the bone has moved more into the beam. In the worst case, this could lead to significant underdosing (or conversely dose overshoot) distal to the Bragg peak purely due to a small misalignment of the patient with the beam. Although this example is a rather extreme case, it does illustrate that caution should be used when using protons in particularly heterogeneous geometries.

## Relative Biological Effectiveness (RBE)

The energy deposited by any radiation type is only a surrogate for biological effect, and this is particularly true for proton irradiation. The relationship between deposited energy and biological effect is a complex one, but can be related to the linear energy transfer (LET) of the irradiation (see e.g., Berger 1993a,b). In the Bragg peak, where the protons have very low energies and consequently lose a lot of energy to each interaction, the LET can be considerably higher than that seen for other radiation qualities like photons. This has lead to fears that the relative biological effectiveness (RBE) of protons could be considerably higher in this region. Cell experiments performed in the 1970's indicated that protons may well have a slightly higher RBE than photons and a standard factor of 1.1—indicating about 10% higher efficiency for protons than for photons—was adopted (Tepper et al. 1977; Urano et al. 1980, 1984). This standard has been adopted by all facilities now treating with protons.

It should be noted however, that from the many *in vitro* RBE studies performed, there are some fears that the RBE in the Bragg peak, and particularly in the distal fall-off region where the highest proportion of low-energy protons are, could be considerably higher. For example, in the comprehensive review of proton RBEs performed by Paganetti (Paganetti et al. 2002), RBE values as high as 2 have been found in some cell experiments in the distal end of a Spread Out Bragg Peak (SOBP) (e.g., Bettega et al. 2000). However, such high values are generally found, or predicted, in beams with narrow energy spectrums. When the spectrums are broader, then there is a greater mixture of low and higher energy protons in the Bragg peak, which somewhat "smears" out the higher RBE effects. In addition, there is some uncertainty as to how reliable cell experiments are in predicting RBE values in living tissue, and from the review of Paganetti, *in vivo* measurements have generally been found to yield lower RBE values than *in vitro* measurements, and closer to the accepted value of 1.1 currently used.

After 30 years of proton therapy, and more than 30,000 patients treated, there is no clinical evidence to indicate a higher RBE at the distal end of the beam, or to warrant a change from a global value of 1.1. Nevertheless, it is worth taking a cautious attitude regarding RBE, especially at the distal end of the beam.

In order to differentiate physical proton dose, expressed in Gray, and the biologically effective dose, proton doses delivered to patients are expressed in terms of Cobalt Gray Equivalent, or CGE. This is simply the physical dose (in Gy) multiplied by the RBE of 1.1. This CGE concept will be used throughout this article when discussing clinical doses delivered by proton plans.

## Sources Of Therapeutic Proton Beams

Unlike photons or electrons, the production of high-energy protons for the treatment of deep-seated tumors, where energies as high as 250 MeV may be required, requires large and specialized accelerators. This is mainly due to their mass (more than 1000 times the mass of an electron), which also has a consequence on the size of gantry required to deliver the therapy. In principle, any type of particle accelerator could be used as a proton source. Of the current operational facilities, both cyclotrons and synchrotrons are being used as sources, and a linear accelerator solution has been proposed for a facility in Italy. Each accelerator type, of course, has its champions and detractors. Broadly stated however, cyclotrons have the advantage of being able to generate relatively high proton currents in a direct current (DC) beam. In addition they are relatively compact, and are a mature and reliable technology. Almost all cyclotrons currently used for proton therapy use room temperature magnets, although a low-energy superconducting cyclotron has recently been installed in Sicily for the treatment of ocular tumors, and the German company Accel (RPTC, Munich) is building a 250 MeV superconducting cyclotron for a new facility at Paul Scherrer Institute (PSI) in Switzerland and a hospital-based facility in Bavaria (see figure 5). Both types of superconducting cyclotrons have been developed in collaboration with Michigan State University (Blosser et al. 1997).

On the down side, cyclotrons are inherently fixed energy machines. In order to vary energy, therefore, one needs additional mechanical energy degraders somewhere in the beam-line between accelerator and patient. As these energy degraders are nothing more than varying thicknesses of material inserted into the beam, the process of degrading a pristine proton beam to lower energies is a rather dirty affair from the point of view of beam utilization and activation. As an example, to degrade a 250 MeV primary beam down to 70 MeV—the energy typically used for treatments of ocular tumors—up to 99% of the protons emitted from the cyclotron may be lost simply through the degrading process and subsequent collimation.

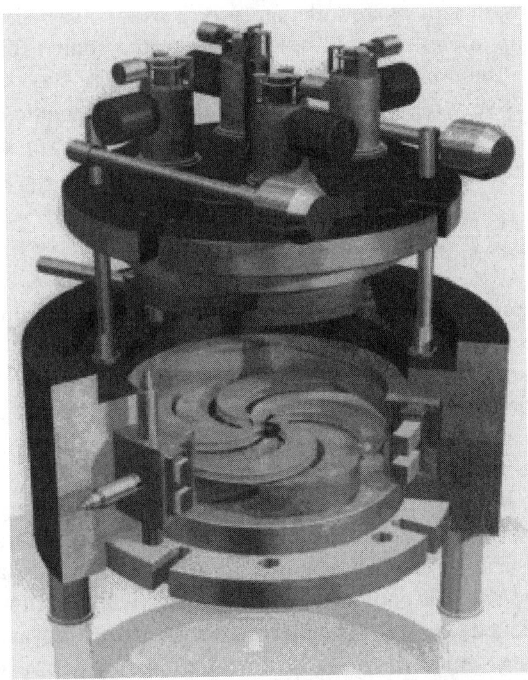

**Figure 5.** The Accel superconducting cyclotron.

Synchrotrons, on the other hand, are pulsed machines, capable of changing the delivered energy pulse-to-pulse. In principle, they provide improved beam utilization and a system in which the problem of activation can be substantially reduced in comparison to a cyclotron. However, the pulses tend to be short in duration and high in current, making precise control of the delivered dose within each pulse problematic. This can have consequences for some methods of delivering proton therapy, for example active scanning (see section below). A synchrotron was adopted as the proton source for the world's first hospital-based proton therapy facility at the Loma Linda University Hospital in Loma Linda, California, and a research synchrotron is being used for heavy ion therapy at GSI in Germany. For a full discussion of the different types of accelerators proposed and used for proton therapy, see the article by Mandrillon (1997).

One last method of generating protons should be mentioned. In theory, the use of very high power lasers (in the Petawatt region) applied to very thin metal targets can cause a short-lived plasma and very high electromagnetic fields in the region where the laser impinges on the target (see e.g., Bulanov and Khoroshkov 2002). The fields are so high, that protons released from the target can be accelerated to a 100 MeV or more in a few millimeters. A number of experiments and research centers have shown the feasibility of this approach and have suggested the potential of such systems for proton therapy. However, there are still many problems to solve before it can be demonstrated that such an approach could be a viable proton source for a proton therapy center. One of the main problems seems to be the energy spectrum of the protons produced, which is very broad, and anything but mono-energetic. Nevertheless, this remains a very interesting development, if a long way from being a practical solution for a clinical facility.

## Making Protons Useful I: Passive Scattering

The attraction of protons for radiotherapy has mainly been the finite range of these particles; with the potential that one uses protons of just sufficient range to reach the distal end of the target, thereby sparing all normal tissues beyond. However, the characteristics of single Bragg peaks, although fulfilling this potential admirably, are not very useful for treating anything but the smallest tumors. Simply put, the high dose region of a single Bragg-peak is too well defined in space to be able to deliver a homogenous dose to larger tumors. In order to produce a clinically useful field, one must first laterally broaden the narrow proton pencil beam produced by the proton accelerator. This is analogous to the shaping of the target in a linear accelerator (linac) to produce a broad and flat photon beam from a relatively narrow incident electron beam. Once broadened laterally, the delivered cross-sectional form of the broad beam can be shaped using similar methods as in photon therapy. However, in proton therapy, one is also faced with the problem of spreading out the dose in depth, usually to form a homogenous distribution through the target volume. A practical delivery system must therefore provide a mechanism for broadening the delivered dose distribution both laterally and in depth.

### Extending The Bragg Peak In Depth

The first solution to this problem was developed in the late 1950's, and has been successfully applied in almost all proton therapy facilities ever since. The method is called "passive scattering." The principle is rather simple, and is shown schematically in figure 6. A narrow proton pencil beam, emitted from the accelerator with a fixed energy, is first modulated in energy using a rapidly rotating and shaped wheel. As the energy of the proton beam is directly related to its range, this has the effect of superimposing many different Bragg peaks, each shifted by a small amount in depth, in the patient (Koehler, Schneider, and Sisterson 1975). With careful shaping of the range-shifter wheel, the weights of these depth-shifted Bragg peaks can be modulated such that a flat dose in depth, the SOBP can be delivered.

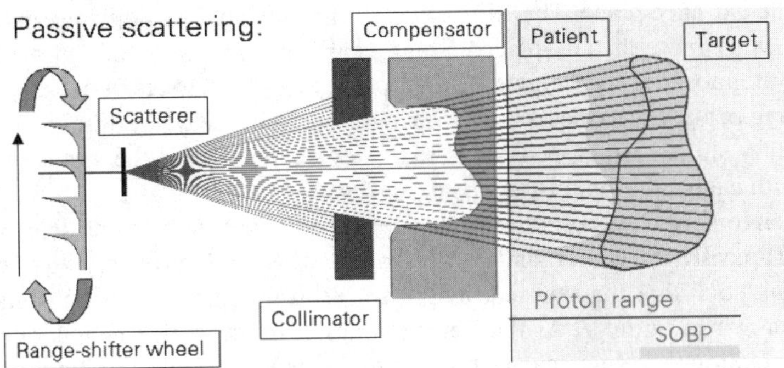


**Figure 6.** The principles and hardware of passive scattering proton therapy.

Figure 7 shows a typical SOBP. For comparison, the depth-dose curve for a 15 MV photon beam is also shown. Both curves are normalized such that the mean dose to the target region (between 15 cm and 5 cm in depth) is the same. The potential advantage of protons is clear, with a homogenous dose in the target and significantly reduced dose distal and proximal to the target. Only for the first few millimeters immediately after the entrance does the photon beam have an advantage, due to the lack of a skin sparing effect for proton beams.

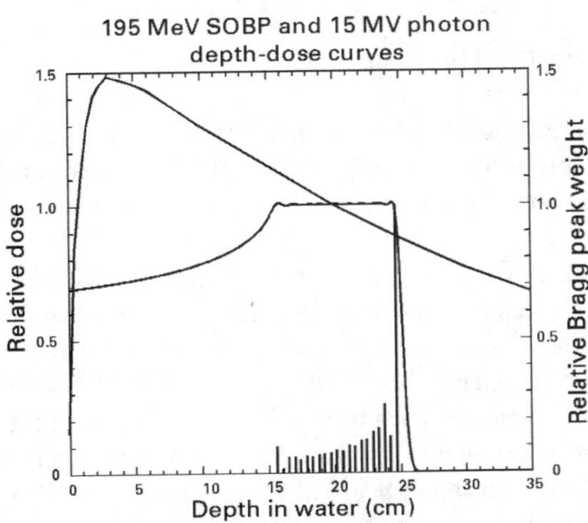


**Figure 7.** A proton SOBP in comparison to a 15 MV photon beam and the Bragg peak weights required to form the SOBP as a function of their depth. Bragg peak spacing is 5 mm is depth.

Figure 7 also shows the relative weights of each Bragg peak required to produce a flat SOBP for 177 MeV protons (incident on the range shifter wheel). One clearly sees how the weights of the Bragg peaks rapidly diminish as they are shifted back towards the entrance plane. This is an effect of the plateau dose delivered to the proximal tissues by more distally placed Bragg peaks. For instance, the most distal, and therefore the most highly weighted Bragg peak, already delivers about 20% to 25% of the Bragg peak dose to the tissues close to the surface (see figure 1). Given that each subsequently shifted Bragg peak adds to this dose, the dose at the surface increases rapidly with each additional Bragg peak.

The range shifter wheel design must reflect this very non-linear distribution of weights. Typically, different radial portions of the wheel will have varying thicknesses of material, such that the segment length for each thickness is proportional to the weights shown in figure 7. As the flat distribution in the SOBP is generated artificially, its position and length can be tailored to the treatment volume, and the therapist will have a number of range-shifter wheels to choose from when planning a patient's treatment. The rotation of the range-shifter wheel is rapid enough that to all intents and purposes, the SOBP can be considered to be a single entity when delivered to the patient.

Although the range-shifter wheel is the most widely used device for producing an SOBP, an alternative method is to use a ridge filter, whose multiple ridges are machined such that the protons of an incident pencil beam see many different thicknesses of degrading material. When shaped correctly, the "mix" of energies exiting from the filter are so weighted that the result is a flat SOBP delivered to the patient (see e.g., Petti et al. 1991).

## Lateral Broadening Of The Proton Pencil Beam

After the narrow pencil beam has been modulated in depth, it must also be broadened laterally in order to produce a clinically useful field size (figure 6). Again, there are a number of methods of doing this, the most common being single and double scattering.

In the first method, a single scatterer, such as a metal foil, is inserted into the beam. This has the effect of broadening the incident pencil beam through multiple Coulomb scattering. By having a sufficiently large drift space after the scatterer—in which the angular divergence of the beam introduced by the foil "amplifies" its lateral dimensions—clinically useful fields can be produced. The advantage of the single scatterer is that it is simple, is insensitive to its position in relation to the beam, and that the virtual source size for the divergent beam after scattering is small. When the broadened beam is subsequently collimated (see below), this reduces the apparent penumbra and provides a sharp lateral fall-off to the collimated beam. On the other hand, as a single foil produces a broadened beam with an essentially Gaussian profile, it is difficult to produce large fields with a satisfactory flatness, unless one has a large drift space between scatterer and patient. In addition, to achieve a uniformity of ±3% within the field, about 90% of the protons incident on the collimator will be lost, as these lie outside the flat region of the scattered beam. This also leads to a rather "dirty" and inefficient method, in that the majority of protons activate the surrounding metal structures rather than treat the patient.

To address the problems of limited field size and poor beam utilization inherent to the single scattering approach, double scattering systems have also been developed (Koehler, Schneider, and Sisterson 1977). In this method, a second scatterer is inserted into the beam after the initial metal foil. This is contoured, and consists of two materials of different atomic weights. The goal is to improve the efficiency of beam utilization, provide improved lateral dose uniformity for larger field sizes, while keeping the proton range constant, well defined and independent of radial position. On the down side, such scatterers are more complex to manufacture and the resulting virtual source size is considerably larger than for the single scatterer solution. This naturally leads to somewhat compromised lateral fall-off after collimation. In addition, to produce uniformly flat fields, the positioning of the second scatterer in relation to the beam is extremely critical, with even small misalignments resulting in observable asymmetries in the delivered lateral dose profile.

In practice, the use of single or double scattering systems can be seen as being complementary, with the single scattering method being used for the irradiation of smaller tumors where a sharp lateral fall-off is required (i.e., uveal melanomas), and double scattering being used when larger and/or more uniform fields are needed.


## Field Shaping For Passive Scattering

The result of depth modulation and lateral broadening is a field of some maximum useable size (determined by the acceptable range of flatness of the laterally spread beam) and an SOBP of user-defined position and extent in the patient. In principle, this is similar to a photon field from a linac, with the important exception of the form of the delivered dose in depth. Thus, the cross-sectional shape of the delivered field can be formed using identical methods as with photons, i.e., through the use of individually tailored and field-specific collimators which match to the projected shape of the target along the incident field direction. However, one also has the opportunity with protons to determine where exactly the distal fall-off of the SOBP is positioned in relation to the target. In the simplest approach, the maximum energy can be adjusted such that the most distal extent of the SOBP corresponds with the most distal portion of the target volume. More usefully, the position of the distal edge can be made to follow the distal surface of the target volume through the use of patient and field specific compensators. Such compensators are made of varying thickness material, where the thickness at any point inversely corresponds to the depth of the distal edge of the target volume when that point is projected along the incident beam direction. The result is a compensator that is thin where the distal end of the target is deep, and thick where the distal end is superficial (see e.g., figure 6).

## Passive Scattering In Practice

Through the use of passive scattering and field-specific collimators and compensators, a homogenous dose distribution, conformed both to the distal and lateral portions of the target volume, can be delivered from a single field direction. Figure 8a shows a single posterior field, as planned to a Ewing's sarcoma. As the extent of the SOBP is fixed across the field (the energy is modulated by the range shifter wheel *before* the beam is broadened by the scatterer), passively scattered fields provide no conformation of the high-dose region to the proximal side of the target volume. In practice therefore, multiple, angularly spaced fields are used, which radially "focus" the dose in the target volume (c.f., photons), thus improving the three-dimensional conformity of the dose to the target volume. An example of the three-field plan to the same case is shown in figure 8b.

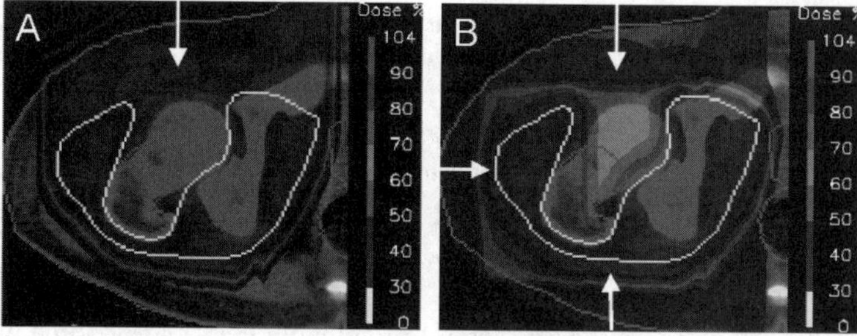


**Figure 8.** A single passively scattered field to a Ewing's carcinoma incident from the posterior (a) and a three-field plan to the same case (b). [Reprinted from *Physics Today*, September 2002, M. Goitein, A. J. Lomax, and E. S. Pedroni, "Treating Cancer With Protons," pp. 45–50. © 2002, with permission from American Institute of Physics.]

The majority of patients treated with protons have been treated using horizontal beam lines, such as that operational at the Harvard Cyclotron Laboratory until spring of 2002. However, to fully exploit the potential of proton therapy, it has been recognized that the clinician requires all the degrees of freedom typically available to a clinician working with a hospital linac. For this reason, a number of gantry-based proton systems have been developed over the past few years, the first being the hospital-based facility at Loma Linda in California. There are now a number world wide, including 4 in Japan and the new facility at Massachusetts General Hospital (MGH) in Boston, which became operational in November 2001. With these systems, the clinician has almost $4\pi$ access to the patient in order to optimally bring the dose on to the tumor.

However, the abrupt drop of dose beyond the SOBP can be exploited for more sophisticated delivery geometries. One such is the use of field-patching methods. This is a delivery approach that has been used widely at the Massachusetts General Hospital and Harvard Cyclotron Laboratory for the treatment of skull base tumors. In order to irradiate a tumor that partially surrounds a critical structure, such as the brain stem, a "Π" type dose distribution can be constructed around the structure, by abutting the distal end of two fields, one on the left side of the structure, the other on the right side, against the lateral edge of an orthogonal field passing above the structure. With such field-patching techniques, quite complex and conformal dose distributions can be constructed. Such a plan is shown in figure 9, in which a nasopharyngeal tumor wraps partially around the brain stem. Through the use of patched fields good dose conformation to the target can be achieved, whilst simultaneously avoiding the brain stem. It should be noted, however, that the planning of such treatments can be quite involved, and the delivery non-trivial, given the inevitable uncertainty of the actual position of the distal and lateral edges in the patient on any given day (Goitein 1985). For this reason, such treatments are usually delivered with "feathering," a method by which the range of the two distally abutting fields are varied a little day to day in order to smear out the potentially large hot and cold spots that can arise due to small misalignments along the patch lines. The excellent clinical results demonstrated for these tumors (see 'Clinical experience with protons' below) speak for the success of this approach.

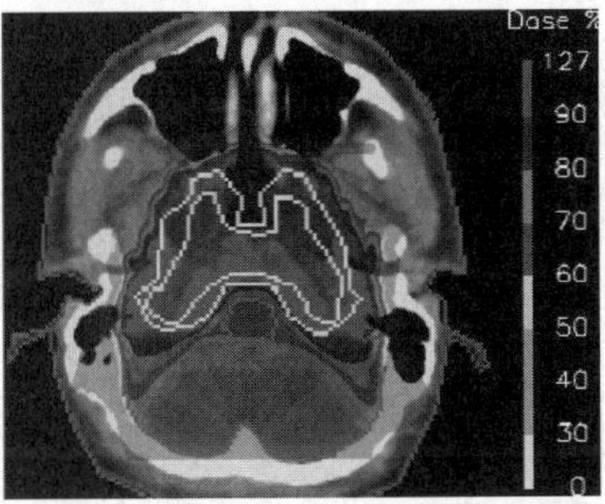

**Figure 9.** An example of a complex patched field proton plan to a nasopharynx tumor. Note the convex dose distribution around the brainstem and the sharp dose fall-offs laterally to the target.

An important exception to the use of multiple field directions is the irradiation of ocular lesions. These are small tumors located on the retina, which have been treated for nearly 30 years with protons. Typically, these are treated with a single, collimated field direction, but without the use of compensators other than simple wedges. For the eye treatment facility at PSI, the use of a low-energy proton accelerator (70 MeV) provides a sharp Bragg peak, which, together with the collimation, provides very sharp dose fall-offs distal and lateral to the tumor (Egger, Zografos, and Perret 1993). The principles of passive scattering then ensure that a homogenous dose can be delivered to the tumor, whilst critical structures such as the lens or optic nerves can be avoided.

## Passive Scattering: The Good And The Bad

Passive scattering is the most mature method for delivering proton therapy. Of the more than 30,000 patients treated with protons worldwide, all but a hundred or so have been treated with some variation of the passive scattering method outlined above. Thus, there is a wealth of experience, both clinical and practical, associated with the approach. It is also relatively simple and is, as the name implies, a passive method. That is, there is no dynamic component to the treatment (aside from the range shifter wheel, which rotates fast enough that it can be ignored). From this point of view, the use of passive scattered protons in areas of organ motion is no more questionable than the delivery of non-IMRT photons. Indeed, aside from the characteristics of protons, and the possibility of tailoring the position of the SOBP as a function of the distal edge of the target, many of the principles of its delivery are identical to that of conventional three-dimensional (3-D) photon therapy. The modulation of Bragg peaks in depth, however, provides both the possibility of delivering a homogenous and partially conformal dose from a single field direction, or of forming complex dose distributions through the use of field-patching methods.

Although passive scattering is the most widely used delivery method for proton therapy, its limitations are now being realized. As already mentioned, in many ways, passive scattered proton therapy is the proton analog to 3-D conventional photon therapy. Although there is undeniably a dynamic component to the delivery in the modulation of Bragg peak depth, this is only a tool for forming a clinically useful depth-dose curve, and the therapist has little or no control over this modulation, save for selecting range-shifter wheels for different positions and extents of the SOBP. Other than this, the delivery method is fixed and static. In addition, as the extent of the SOBP must be the same throughout the target volume, there is inevitably a large volume of normal tissue that receives the full target dose proximal to the target. Although this is not always clinically important, especially when performing multiple field treatments, this can mean that the full dose is deposited to the patient's skin, despite the fact that the target never extends to the surface at any point.

Such an example is shown in figure 10. This shows the same single field for the Ewing's sarcoma as in figure 8. Indicated is the maximum extent (10 cm) of the SOBP required to cover the widest portion of the target volume, as projected along the beam direction (solid white line). Note that the SOBP here does not extend to the patient's surface. However, at the lateral portions, the target is both thinner and its distal edge is less than 10 cm under the skin surface. Given that the extent of the SOBP must be the same here as for the widest part of the target (broken white lines), this means that the 100% dose extends from the tumor right back to the skin (and further if there was anything other than air) despite the fact that the tumor itself does not extend to the skin. Although the skin dose could be reduced through the use of multiple fields (see e.g., figure 8b), passive scattering inevitably delivers more dose to proximal tissues than is absolutely necessary.

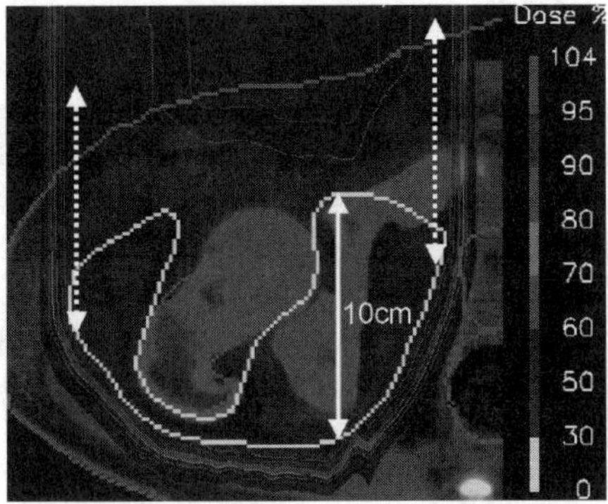


**Figure 10.** Fixed SOBP extents and skin dose. A SOBP of 10 cm extent is required to cover the widest part of the target volume (solid line). However, laterally, such a wide SOBP extends to and beyond the skin (broken lines), delivering full dose. [Reprinted from *Physics Today*, September 2002, M. Goitein, A. J. Lomax, and E. S. Pedroni, "Treating cancer with protons," pp. 45–50. © 2002, with permission from American Institute of Physics.]

## Making Protons Useful II: Active Scanning

Traditionally, delivering proton therapy has been looked upon as a problem of degrading a pristine Bragg peak and pencil beam such that it becomes a clinically useful broad field. However, a narrow pencil beam, with a near mono-energetic Bragg peak, can be viewed as a single "spot" of dose, well confined in three dimensions. If it were possible to dynamically position such Bragg peaks in three dimensions throughout the target volume, then it would be possible to use this dose spot to "paint" the dose to the target as required. This is the idea behind the active scanning approach to proton therapy, which is now gaining a certain amount of popularity within the proton therapy community (Kanai et al. 1980; Goitein and Chen 1983; Harberer et al. 1993; Pedroni et al. 1995; Marchand et al. 2000).

With active scanning techniques, the concept of an SOBP, a central component of the passive scattering approach, is abandoned. Instead, it relies on its ability to individually place and weight spots with full flexibility, and under computer control. From the treatment planning aspect, this requires algorithms for determining the optimal weight of each Bragg peak in three dimensions. Usually, this is performed using gradient-based optimization algorithms, very similar to the dose based optimization algorithms applied in IMRT (see e.g., Lomax et al. 1996). It should be noted, however, that for the majority of patients treated with discrete scanning, the sole constraint for the optimization is that each individual field applies a homogenous dose across the whole target. As such, this method on its own should *not* be directly compared to IMRT for photons, for reasons that will be discussed more thoroughly below.

## Discrete, Or Spot, Scanning

Active scanning can be accomplished by either mechanical or magnetic means, or a combination of the two. At the Paul Scherrer Institute in Switzerland, active scanning for proton therapy has been pioneered using the so-called "spot scanning approach" (Pedroni et al. 1995). A schematic representation of this approach is shown in figure 11. Discrete proton Bragg peaks are delivered on a 3-D grid throughout the target volume, typically with a spacing of about 5 mm in all directions (including in depth). At PSI, this is achieved through the combination of a magnetic deflection of the pencil beam, a mechanical motion of the patient table (in a direction orthogonal to the magnetic deflection), and the insertion of polyethylene plates into the beam line to quickly modulate the range in the patient. Through computer steering of these three elements, it is possible to position a Bragg peak anywhere in three dimensions within the target volume. In addition, it is also necessary to be able to individually modulate the dose delivered at each Bragg peak. As with most dynamic delivery systems, the dose at any given point is controlled by the length of time a spot dwells at each position, with the number of delivered protons being controlled by a fast monitor just before the patient. Once the desired number of monitor units has been delivered, then the beam at this point is switched-off using a fast magnetic deflection of the beam away from the treatment room. This fast switching of the beam is an important aspect of the spot scanning method, in that the beam is switched-off when the steering elements are being altered, and is only applied to the patient when all elements are stable. From this aspect, this method is analogous to the "step-and-shoot" approach for intensity-modulated radiation therapy (IMRT) (e.g., Bortfeld et al. 1994). It should be noted that although the PSI implementation includes a mechanical motion of the patient table as part of its scanning concept, this is not mandatory for a discrete scanning system, and there is no reason why this approach cannot also be delivered using a double magnetic scanning system.

The magnetic deflection of the beam is clearly the fastest motion, requiring about 5 ms to deflect the beam 5 mm. This is followed by the range-shifter plates, which require 50 ms to fall into the beam and finally the table motion, where about 1 second is required to move the table 5 mm. The beam can be switched-off in 50 μs once the desired monitor units have been reached for the spot. As delivery of the field is ordered with the magnetic deflection as fastest varying element, followed by the range shifter, the total dead times resulting from all the devices over the whole treatment are about equal (i.e., for a $10 \times 10 \times 10$ cm field, the beam is deflected 8000 times, a range shifter is inserted 400 times, but the table is only moved 20 times), and equate to about 50% to 60% of the total delivery time. With the current system at PSI, about 3000 Bragg peaks can be delivered each minute, enough to deliver 2 Gy to a target volume of about 300 ml. The whole spot scanning system outlined above has been implemented in a treatment gantry at PSI (figure 12), providing the clinician with similar degrees of freedom for bringing the beam into the patient as are available on a typical linac or commercial proton gantry.

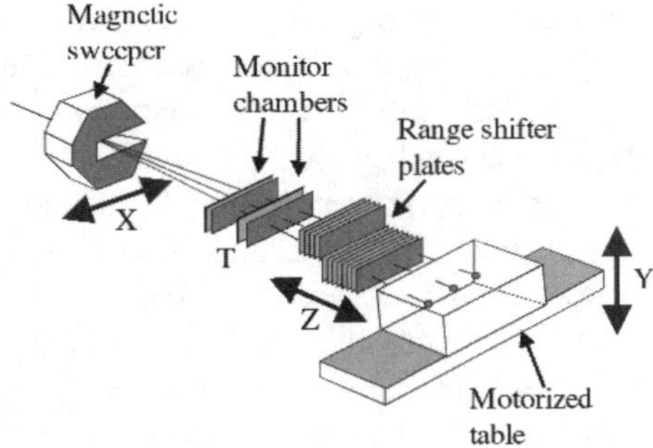



**Figure 11.** Schematic representation of spot-scanning hardware at PSI. With a magnetic sweeper, table motion, and variable number of range shifter plates in the beam, Bragg peaks can be delivered anywhere in three dimensions within the patient. Fast monitoring ensures that the dose at each Bragg peak position can also be precisely controlled.

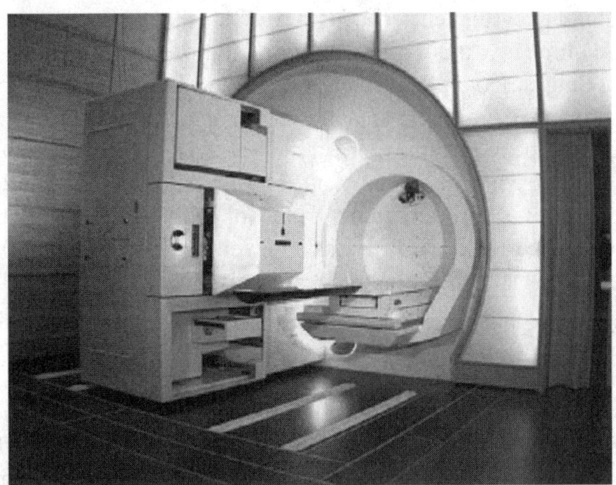

**Figure 12.** The PSI gantry treatment gantry. Using the steering hardware shown in figure 11, the gantry diameter can be reduced to about 3.5 m. The gantry can rotate ±180°, and the table ±120°, allowing for a similar flexibility as provided by a linac for photon therapy in the choice of incident field directions.

One interesting aspect of the PSI system is the Cartesian nature of its delivery geometry (Pedroni and Enge 1995). The beam optics of the gantry have been so designed that in the direction of the magnetic deflection, all pencil beams emitted from the gantry nozzle are parallel, regardless of the magnitude of their deflection away from the central axis. In other words, the system has an infinite source-to-skin distance, and therefore no divergence in its geometry. Aside from making the treatment planning algorithms considerably simpler, such geometry also brings other advantages. For instance, the patching of laterally displaced fields becomes relatively trivial. The PSI gantry allows for a magnetic deflection of ±10 cm. However, fields of more than 20 cm length in this direction can easily be treated by dividing the field into two or more subfields along the deflection axis. Between subfields, the table is moved in a direction parallel to the deflection and by the same amount as the width of the subfield. By this method, fields as large as 84 cm (see the section *Active Scanning In Practice* herein and figure 14 below) have been successfully delivered at PSI.

The main advantage of discrete scanning generally is that the manipulation of all steering elements is performed with "beam-off." This allows for the control system to set the elements and to check them (using functionally redundant systems) before the beam is applied to the patient. However, this approach leads to a relatively large dead time, as indicated above, leading to longer treatment times for the patient.

## Continuous, Or Raster, Scanning

The discrete scanning system currently used at PSI is the only proton scanning method currently in use clinically. It is not the only method of scanning, however. Ion Beam Applications, a Belgium manufacturer of proton therapy equipment, working together with MGH Boston are developing an active scanning system based on the continuous scanning of a proton pencil beam in a raster fashion through the target volume (Marchand et al. 2000). The concept here is that the treatment planning should provide a set of two-dimensional (2-D) proton fluence maps for each depth through the field, rather than a set of discrete Bragg peak positions and weights. These analog fluence patterns will then be delivered using a continuous scanning of the beam, with the proton fluence at each point being modulated by varying both beam intensity and scanning speed. Naturally, the different depth planes must still be delivered discretely, through the use of a stepped range-shifter wheel.

In comparison to discrete scanning, continuous scanning can provide a more efficient use of the accelerator, as the proton beam is continually switched on during the treatment, eliminating the dead time associated with discrete scanning. This will significantly reduce the time required to scan a field, consequently reducing the treatment time per patient. But perhaps more importantly, the increased efficiency can be utilized in other ways, such as allowing for multiple re-scannings of the field in clinically acceptable times. This could reduce the problems of organ motion to which active scanning approaches are prone (see below). However, controlling and checking the position, speed, and intensity of the beam continually poses some challenging problems for the control system, which will need to be considerably more complex than that required for discrete scanning.

## Hybrid Scanning

Discrete and continuous scanning represent the two possible extremes of scanning technology, and a number of groups are investigating the possibilities of hybrid solutions. At the German Heavy Ion research facility in Darmstadt, Germany, an active scanning system for the delivery of heavy ion therapy with carbon ions has been operational since 1997 (Harberer et al. 1993). This is truly a combination of continuous and discrete scanning, in that although the beam is not switched-off between spots, the steering elements move quickly between spot positions, where they remain until the desired dose is delivered. The dose delivered between spots (i.e., while the spot is being moved) is automatically compensated for in the delivery hardware.

For a second generation scanning gantry at PSI, a different type of hybrid system is being considered. In order to preserve the parallel delivery geometry of the current gantry system at PSI (see above), but to reduce dead-time and hence allow for fast re-scanning of the beam, a limited extent double scanning system is being investigated. Most anatomical organ motions are no more than 4 cm. Thus, it may not be necessary to rescan a whole field at one time. The proposal from PSI is to perform double scattering, but with the scattering in the transversal direction limited to 5 to 6 cm, with fields of larger size in this dimension being constructed with a mechanical table motion, as in their discrete scanning system. With this approach, fast re-scanning could be performed in each subfield (the 5 to 6 cm segments orthogonal to the main scanning axis), over a range larger than typical organ motions, whilst preserving the parallel delivery geometry and the advantages it brings.

## Active Scanning In Practice

A typical field for active scanning is shown in figure 13a, which can be directly compared to that for passive scattering shown in figure 8a. The flexibility introduced by scanning is clearly visible, in that not only is a homogenous dose delivered to the tumor, but also excellent conformation is achieved all around the target, including the proximal part. This is in stark contrast to the case for passive scattering. A three-field spot scanned plan for the same case is also shown (figure 13b), where a clear reduction of dose to all surrounding tissues through the use of scanning can be observed when compared to the same plan for passive scattering (figure 8b).

In many cases, reducing doses to proximal tissues is not an issue. However, for certain treatments, this can be important. Perhaps some of the most promising indications for proton therapy are pediatric tumors. One such, where protons could be close to ideal, is the irradiation of the cranio-spinal axis for tumor types such as medulloblastoma or primitive neuroectodermal tumor (PNET). Figure 14 shows a plan that was calculated and delivered for and to an Alderson/Rando phantom to demonstrate the feasibility of this approach using the spot scanning system of PSI. This consists of a single posterior field, 84 cm long, which irradiates the whole brain and spinal axis, whilst sparing the thorax, abdomen, and pelvis of the "child." From a clinical and practical point of view, a single posterior field would provide the best solution for such cases, however, only if the skin dose is not too high. In figure 14, it can be seen that through the use of scanning, the skin dose can be reduced, reducing the risk of acute skin reactions in comparison to passive scattering (c.f., figure 10).

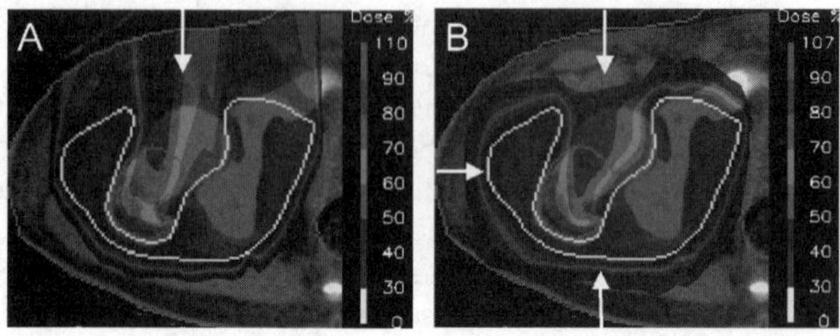

**Figure 13.** Single and multiple field spot-scanned plans to the Ewing's sarcoma. The improved dose distribution due to active scanning can be seen when comparing figure 13b to figure 8b for passive scattering. [Reprinted from *Physics Today*, September 2002, M. Goitein, A. J. Lomax, and E. S. Pedroni, "Treating cancer with protons," pp. 45–50. © 2002, with permission from American Institute of Physics.]

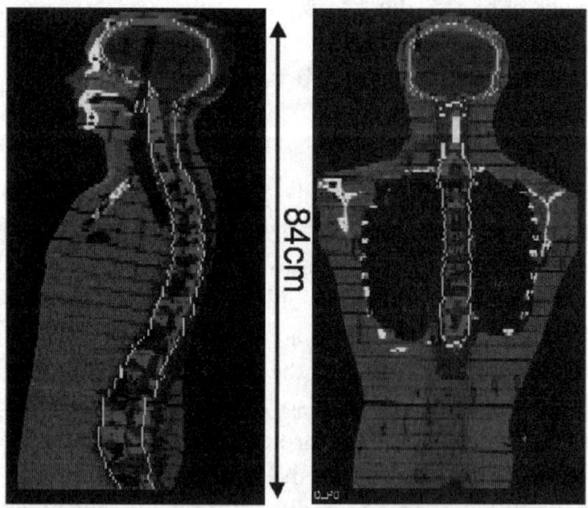


**Figure 14.** Phantom craniospinal irradiation planned using the spot scanning treatment-planning system at PSI. This was planned as a single field and automatically delivered as a set of five subfields in order to cover the 84 cm length. Film dosimetry showed a homogenous dose with no patch line artifacts and the field could be totally delivered in 15 minutes, fully automatically.

An interesting aspect of the plan shown in figure 14 is that this extremely long field was planned as a single treatment field using the PSI planning system. As the maximum range of magnetic scanning on the PSI gantry is 20 cm along the long axis of the patient, the field was actually delivered as a set of five, patched subfields, with a longitudinal table motion in between each subfield. However, as the PSI system has an infinite source to skin distance (i.e., all delivered pencil beams are parallel to each other) the subfields could be delivered one next to the other with no worries about matching divergent field edges. Film dosimetry of this field showed no patch line artifacts, and the whole field, including the whole brain irradiation, could be delivered from one control file in about 15 minutes.

## Active Scanning: The Good And The Bad

In principle, there are many potential advantages in using active scanning when compared to passive scattering, not least its potential for reducing the size of the treatment gantry. With passive scattering, a relatively large drift space is required between the scattering system and the patient in order to achieve clinically useful field sizes. This puts a lower limit on the size of the gantry required, and gantries with diameters of 10 to 12 meters are typical for such systems. However, one aspect of active scanning is that the broadening of a pencil beam through multiple Coulomb scattering is replaced by magnetic deflection of the beam. As the range of deflection, and hence field-size, is simply dependent on the strength of the scanning magnets, this can drastically reduce the diameter of the gantry. For instance, the PSI gantry has a diameter of only 3 meters, or a factor of 4 smaller than typical gantries designed for passive scattering. In addition, the patient and field specific collimators and compensators that are essential for passive scattering are no longer required with scanning. The computer-controlled selection of the relevant Bragg peaks to be delivered negates the need for such devices, and the optimization algorithm ensures that the resulting dose is homogenous. One advantage of this is that all protons exiting from the nozzle of the gantry are used to treat the patient—there is no need to cut away any of the beam with collimators before the patient—making active scanning a clean and efficient delivery system. In addition, multiple-field treatments can be delivered without the technologists having to enter the room, potentially improving patient throughput. On the other hand, there is no reason why collimators and compensators cannot be used with active scanning, and for certain cases (e.g., superficial lesions), the addition of collimators could bring some beneficial aspects.

However, perhaps the greatest potential for active scanning is its inherent ability to deliver intensity-modulated proton therapy (IMPT). This delivery technique will be discussed in more detail in the next section.

So what are the disadvantages of active scanning? Active scanning's great strength can also be considered its great weakness—the sequential application of individually modulated narrow pencil beams. When such a field is delivered in the presence of organ motion, there can be complex interplays between the dynamics of the delivery and the motion of the organs (Phillips et al. 1992). For instance, while a pencil beam is being delivered, a given point can either move away from the beam, resulting in a lower than desired dose, or remain within the beam as it moves. In the worst case, if the organ motion is in the same direction, and has the same speed, as the motion of the pencil beam, two consecutive pencil beams could be delivered to the same point within the patient. Of course, similar worries can be leveled at any dynamic delivery method, for instance IMRT or, to a lesser extent, dynamic wedges (see e.g., Yu, Jaffray, and Wong 1998; Pemler et al. 2001). However, for IMRT with dynamic multileaf collimators (DMLCs), the delivered field is made up of a set of open fields of varying shapes and sizes. Thus, well within each open field, organ motion will not be a problem (if the motion is smaller than the subfield), and the effects will only be seen at the edge of each subfield. For actively scanned protons on the other hand, the delivered sub-fields are very small—only the size of the incident pencil beam (typically 4 to 10 mm sigma)—and so organ motion effects can cause artifacts anywhere in the dose distribution. When treating in regions where organ motion could be a problem therefore, methods for reducing motion such as gating or active breathing are clearly desirable.

An alternative approach to dealing with motion artifacts, and one that is only realistic with active scanning, is to rapidly rescan many times for each field. Statistically, artifacts due to organ motion will be reduced by a factor equal to the square root of the number of re-scans, assuming that the motion is not correlated with the scanning pattern. Thus, rescanning a field 16 times, will reduce any motion artifacts within that field by about a factor of 4. If a double magnetic scanning system is used, then such a re-scan rate is not unrealistic, and this is the approach currently being developed by both IBA for raster scanning (Marchand et al. 2000), and for the second-generation scanning gantry at PSI (see above). Of course, if a four-field plan is applied, and each field homogenously covers the target, this can also be seen as a type of re-scanning, as can fractionation of the treatment over many treatment days. Recently, Bortfeld et al. (2002) have published the results of an interesting analysis on organ motion for both IMRT and scanned proton beams. Their analysis indicates that a three-times rescanning of an actively scanned proton field is sufficient to wash out motion artifacts over the duration of the treatment (i.e., when fractionation is also included). However, if faster re-scanning can be achieved, then it is clearly desirable to be able to deliver the calculated dose distribution per fraction as accurately as possible and methods for rapidly re-scanning the target will certainly be a part of any future active scanning devices.

One last potential weakness of active scanning should be mentioned. As typically field-specific collimators are not required, the lateral fall-off of an actively scanned field will be dependent on the size of the incident pencil beam. The smaller the spot size incident on the patient, the better the lateral fall-off that can be achieved. There are physical limits to what can be achieved, and a FWHM width of much less than 5 mm (before scattering in the patient) will be difficult to achieve due to scattering in the delivery equipment. For such a beam, and up to a depth of about 15 cm in the patient, the lateral fall-off for a proton field is comparable to that of a collimated photon beam. However, if a larger beam size is used, then the lateral fall-off will be compromised. Thus, the delivery hardware for active scanning beams must be carefully designed such that the beam width is close to this lower limit.

## Intensity-Modulated Proton Therapy (IMPT)

The introduction of IMRT into the clinic in the last few years has revolutionized radiotherapy. The development of software methods for calculating optimum fluence profiles for photon beams followed by the development of hardware for the realization of these profiles has led to impressive advances in the achievable level of dose conformation with photons. Indeed, at the 70% to 80% dose level, the dose conformation to even complex-shaped tumors is comparable between intensity-modulated (IM) photon plans and non-IM proton plans (see Lomax et al. 1999). However, the success of IMRT for photons can also show the way forward for proton therapy, where similar advances can be made. Indeed, the potential for intensity-modulated proton therapy (IMPT) is only just beginning to be explored.

## IMPT — What It Isn't And What It Is

Before looking into the methods and potential of IMPT, we must first define what it is. To do this, it is best to understand the real trick behind photon IMRT. Strictly speaking, the novelty of IMRT lies not in its ability to simply "modulate intensity." Firstly, as has been argued elsewhere (Webb and Lomax 2001), all commercially available methods of delivering IMRT actually modulate fluence. However, more importantly, the modulation of fluence is itself not the novel aspect of IMRT. The simple measure of inserting a collimator into a beam modulates fluence (if only in a binary way), as does the insertion of a wedge or any other compensating material. As such, various levels of fluence modulation have been used in radiotherapy for years. Thus, neither "intensity" nor "modulation" precisely identifies how IMRT differs from standard radiotherapy treatment methods. The key to the success of IMRT actually lies in a rather subtler difference from conventional delivery methods. That is, the novelty lies in its ability to calculate and deliver fields of *arbitrarily complex* fluence profiles, which combine in the target to provide a desired—usually homogenous—and highly conformal dose distribution around the target volume.

A common misconception is that any form of active scanning delivery is automatically IMPT. Whilst it is true that active scanning as a delivery method modulates individual pencil beam weights, and optimization is certainly a part of the treatment planning system, this does *not* mean that all treatments delivered using active scanning can be called IMPT. As stated above, current implementations of active scanning are calculated such that each individual field delivers a homogenous dose to the target volume. In this case, the optimization is simply being used to replace the use of fixed SOBPs to obtain a homogenous dose to the target.

So to deliver IMPT, we should employ the same "trick" as IMRT to proton therapy. That is, arbitrarily complex 3-D dose distributions should be delivered from different field directions, which when combined, produce the clinically required dose distribution. For active systems such as the spot scanning system at PSI, the move from standard delivery to IMPT simply involves moving from optimizing fields individually to optimizing pencil beams from all fields simultaneously (Lomax 1999).

This concept of IMPT is perhaps clearer with the aid of an example. Referring back to figure 13a, it is clear that discrete scanning delivers a homogenous dose across the whole target, with some sparing of the femoral head, which is proximal to, and deeply embedded in, the target volume. However, when we go to the three-field plan (figure 13b), apart from slightly improved sparing of the femoral head and a reduced skin dose for the posterior beam, no great improvement is seen in going from one to three fields.

Now take the same case calculated with IMPT. Figure 15 shows the same three-field plan calculated using IMPT methods (figure 15b). For this plan, the constraint that each field must deliver a homogenous dose has been relaxed, and free reign has been given to the optimization, with the algorithm being applied to all pencil beams from the three fields simultaneously. The result is a set of individually inhomogeneous fields (one of which is shown in figure 15a), which combine to form the final desired dose distribution. Although the spot scanned plan in figure 13b can successfully reduce the dose to the femoral head to about 60% to 70% dose level, IMPT allows one to get the dose even lower, in this case down below 30%. Thus, like its photon equivalent IMRT, IMPT provides the clinician with more flexibility in constructing the dose to complex targets than is possible with other proton delivery methods.

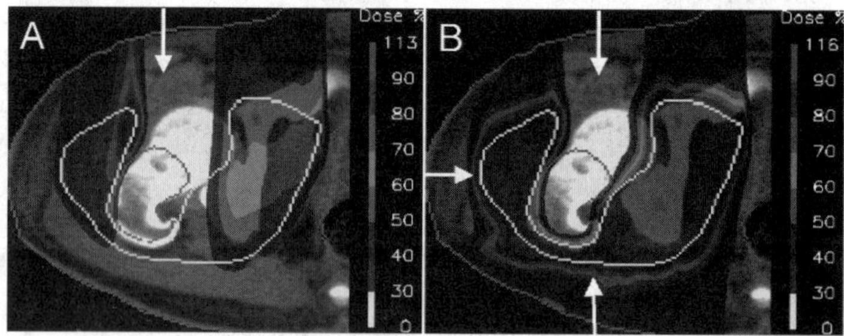

**Figure 15.** IMPT single field and three-field plan to the Ewing's sarcoma. The improved dose distribution resulting from IMPT can be seen when comparing figure 15b to figure 8b for passive scattering and figure 13b for discrete scanning. [Reprinted from *Physics Today*, September 2002, M. Goitein, A. J. Lomax, and E. S. Pedroni, "Treating cancer with protons," pp. 45–50. © 2002, with permission from American Institute of Physics.]

## 2-D, 3-D, And Distal Edge Tracking (DET) IMPT

In the above example, we have looked at one method of IMPT, which we call "3D-IMPT", as any given pencil beam distributed in three dimensions for any given field can be fully and independently modulated. Thus, 3D-IMPT can be considered the most general and flexible approach to IMPT. However, there are at least two other methods by which IMPT could be delivered, 2-D and Distal Edge Tracking (DET) (Lomax 1999).

2D-IMPT is a method that can be considered to be an almost exact analogy to photon IMRT. For photon IMRT, as the form of the depth dose curve for each beamlet of a field is identical, a field can only be modulated by varying the relative fluence of these beamlets across a plane perpendicular to the field direction. The situation is similar for passively scattered protons. Although the position of the SOBP can be modified through the use of a compensator, the extent and form of the SOBP is fixed across the incident field. Thus, a form of IMPT could also be delivered by simply varying the relative fluence of these SOBP beamlets using methods similar to those employed for photon IMRT. Although clearly not providing the degrees of freedom of 3D-IMPT, this approach has the advantage of being a method that could be applied to existing passive scattering systems in a relatively simple way.

Perhaps a more interesting method of IMPT that could be applied on conventional proton gantries is a method of IMPT first suggested by Deasy, Shepard, and Mackie (1997), which they callled "Distal Edge Tracking" ("DET"). In fact, this is very similar to 2D-IMPT, but instead of delivering beamlets in the form of SOBPs, single Bragg peak pencil beams are delivered with just enough energy to reach the distal end of the target. Through the application of multiple beam directions (four or more), and by modulating the fluence of each beamlet, it has been shown that this method can achieve excellent results for both conformation and dose homogeneity across the target. Indeed, it has been claimed that, at least for centrally positioned tumors, this method minimizes the total integral dose delivered to the patient and that a sharper lateral fall-off can be achieved than with 3D-IMPT (Oelfke and Bortfeld 2000). Although not clinically implemented yet, this method has the potential advantage of requiring many less pencil beams—if delivered using active scanning—or of providing a simple method of implementing IMPT on a passively scattered gantry.

Although DET is an interesting approach, it should be noted that this method is actually a special case of 3D-IMPT, and given a sophisticated enough optimization algorithm, the latter method should approach the DET solution if DET indeed is the optimum solution for any given case and delivery geometry.


## Delivering IMPT

Active scanning is currently the method of choice for delivering IMPT, either in practice or for future proton facilities, and can be easily configured to deliver any of the types of IMPT described above. Indeed, for active scanning, the method of IMPT to be used would only need to be defined at the treatment planning level, as the delivery method is flexible enough to deliver any set of 3-D or 2-D distributed sets of pencil beams that are requested.

What is perhaps not so obvious is that, at least theoretically, all methods can also be applied on passive scattering systems. Starting with the 2-D and DET approaches, these only differ in the form of the delivered beamlet. By adding a dynamic multileaf system to a passive scattering system, arbitrary cross-field fluences of either type of beamlet could be produced in exactly the same way as for IMRT with photons.

Although the collimators may need to be somewhat different—photon DMLCs would probably be thick enough to stop medium-energy protons, but the tongue-and-groove effect seen with DMLCs could lead to a significant proton leakage—such an approach is certainly practicable. In this case, 2-D and DET would only differ in the fact that the latter does not require the use of a range shifter wheel. Extending this further, a 3D-IMPT field is simply a set of depth-shifted 2-D fluence maps. Therefore, if a passive scattering delivery system could drive its range-shifter wheel in a stepped mode, the different fluence patterns at each depth could be equally well applied through the use of DMLCs, with a different DMLC sequence being applied at each range depth (Goitein 1997). Thus, even 3D-IMPT could in principle be applied on a passive scattering system, providing some additional hardware in the form of proton compatible DMLCs were available.

## IMPT In Practice

Currently, clinical IMPT is the preserve of the discrete scanning system of PSI in Switzerland. Five patients have now been treated with 3D-IMPT using the spot scanning approach, the first in 1999, and the method is slowly being integrated into the clinical routine. With the goal of IMPT being a major driving force, a number of proton facilities and manufacturers are developing active scanning systems, and in the next 4 to 5 years, IMPT will certainly become more prevalent. Interestingly, despite the apparent advantages of being able to deliver IMPT on existing passive scattering systems, as far as we are aware, no group is currently investigating the practicality, or otherwise, of this approach.

## Clinical Experience With Protons

### Passive Scattering

As of the summer 2002, more than 32,000 patients had been treated with protons worldwide. Although the majority of these patients have been treated at research facilities, the advent of hospital-based proton facilities, both in the United States and in Japan, means that the rate of increase of patient treatments is itself increasing rapidly (Sisterson 2002). Loma Linda University Hospital has already treated more than 7000 patients since 1990, and is currently treating more than 100 patients a day with their three-gantry facility, and since the start of treatments at MGH in November 2001, more than 100 patients have been treated, with about 20 patients a day being treated on a single gantry system. Up to three gantries are eventually planned at the MGH facility.

Still the most widely treated indication with protons is uveal melanoma, a rare tumor of the retina of the eye. For instance, more than 5000 patients with this indication have been treated at MGH and PSI alone, with about 200 to 250 patients a year currently being treated at PSI. Thus, there are good statistics and follow-up rates for these patients. Results are excellent, with local tumor control rates (LCR) of up to 98%

being achieved with proton therapy, together with a more than 90% eye retention rate (Egger et al. 2001). This latter figure is important, as the only alternative treatment to reach similar tumor control rates is surgical enucleation.

At the Harvard Cyclotron, some of the first tumors to be treated with protons were skull base sarcomas. These are relatively rare, bony lesions that are often directly in the neighborhood of the brainstem and optic structures, making surgery and conventional radiotherapy particularly difficult. In a series of more than 350 patients with either chondrosarcomas or chordomas, actuarial local control rates of 94% and 54% respectively have been achieved (Munzenrider and Liebsch 1999). Both figures are significantly better than comparable series with conventional photons, although the reason for the difference in local control between the two histologies is not currently known. Due to the proximity of a number of critical structures, patched field techniques have been routinely used in this series of patients, and no problems across the patch lines have been observed (see discussion above). In addition, these tumors are located in an anatomical area in which bone-tissue and bone-air interfaces are prevalent, traditionally problem areas for proton dose calculations. However, the excellent clinical results demonstrated in these tumor types, particularly for the chondrosarcomas, show that with careful planning methods, and a respect for the potential problems of density heterogeneities (i.e., beams pointing directly at critical structures are normally avoided), such problems can be minimized.

Since becoming operational in 1990, Loma Linda University Hospital has treated a series of more than 600 patients with prostate cancer to 74 to 75 CGE with protons. LCRs of between 100% and 53% have been achieved, depending on initial prostate specific antigen (PSA) activity (Slater et al. 1998), whereas for a subset of these patients with early stage tumors (T1-T2b), 5-year clinical and biochemical disease free survival was 97% and 88% respectively (Slater et al. 1999). In both sets of patients, very little in the way of treatment-related side effects were observed. Less successful was the prostate trial performed at MGH, where all patients were treated to 50.4 Gy with photons, but were then randomized into two arms, one of which received a boost of 16.8 Gy with photons, and the other which received a boost of 26.8 CGE using a single perineal proton field (Shipley et al. 1995). Although local recurrence-free survival was significantly improved in the proton arm for poorly differentiated tumors, overall survival was unchanged, and there was a trend towards higher rates of side effects (rectal bleeding and urethral stricture) in the proton arm. One should point out, however, that the proton plans delivered for this trial were severely restricted due to the hardware at the Harvard Cyclotron, where only a horizontal beam with 160 MeV (maximum range in water = 17 cm) was available, and thus a single, perineal field was the only option for delivering a proton boost to the prostate. An interesting potential area for proton therapy is in the treatment of lesions in the neighborhood of large, parallel organs such as the liver and lung, due to the reduced integral dose to the healthy portions of these organs resulting from their use. Initial clinical results in these areas are also encouraging. In Tsukuba, Japan, proton therapy has been used to treat hepatocellular carcinomas in over 120 patients, and local control rates of over 90% have been achieved. In a smaller series of lung patients treated at Loma Linda, local control rates of 86% have been achieved for the treatment of non-operable non-small-cell lung cancer (NSCLC) in 27 patients (Bush et al. 1999). Although these studies need to be followed up with randomized studies, the results nevertheless look promising.

The potential for protons has also been investigated in many smaller studies. Examples include paranasal sinus carcinomas (89% LCR at 3 years, Thornton et al. 1998), benign meningiomas (93% survival at 10 years, Suit and Goitein 2000), atypical and malignant meningiomas (80% LCR at 5 years, Suit and Goitein 2000) and sarcomas of the spine (between 100% and 54% LCR depending on the histology, Hug et al. 1995). In the latter cases, the finite range of protons when delivering dose to the spine from the posterior aspect has clear and obvious advantages in regard to sparing of the sensitive thoracic and abdominal organs when compared to conventional techniques. We will return to this theme later.

## Active Scanning

All the available clinical data for proton therapy are necessarily from passive scattering systems, as until very recently, this was the only method in clinical use. The first active scanning system at PSI in Switzerland came into use at the end of 1996, and by the end of 2002, 130 patients had been treated with this method, 5 of which had received 3D-IMPT plans as part of their treatment. As the facility has treated many different indications, it is too early yet to comment on the clinical outcomes, although the first curative patients treated with this approach are just reaching 5-year follow-up, and initial results for many indications look promising. For instance, of the 99 patients treated by the end of 2001, local control had been achieved in 82 with a median follow-up of 21 months. This figure includes 21 patients who were only treated with palliative intent, and the first IMPT patient, treated in 1999 for a chordoma in the thoracic spine (Lomax et al. 2001), who, more than 36 months post-treatment, is still locally controlled with no treatment-related morbidity. However, many more patients need to be treated before one can demonstrate a clinical advantage for active scanning or IMPT over passive scattering methods or conventional radiotherapy.

## When Are Photons Preferable?

## Clinical Comparisons Of Protons And Photons

Direct phase III clinical trials between protons and photons are sadly lacking, the prostate trial conducted at the Harvard Cyclotron and MGH being one of the few exceptions (Shipley et al. 1995). However, this example perhaps indicates some of the problems associated with such studies. Although the study was carried out in an exemplary way, and the results cannot be argued with, the fact that a very limiting treatment setup was used, restricting the possibilities for the proton part of the study, makes extrapolation to proton therapy generally as a tool for treating prostate cancer difficult—and for treating other sites, impossible. Indeed, the excellent results subsequently observed at Loma Linda in the treatment of prostate cancer (although sadly, not as part of a randomized clinical study), bear out this point (Slater et al. 1998, 1999).

In radiotherapy, the widespread introduction of new delivery techniques has not generally been the result of 'evidence' based on well-designed clinical trials. Thus, linear accelerators have been generally accepted as being superior to cobalt-60, 3-D conformal planning to 2-D and, more recently, IMRT to conventional therapy, without any formally conducted clinical trial to demonstrate these superiorities over a number of treatment sites and indications. Mainly, this is because such studies are extremely difficult to perform, and must run over such a long time-scale. Acquiring a few hundred eligible patients of a single indication in two separate arms can easily take a few years, even in the largest centers. Given that the follow-up for all the patients in the study should normally be at least 5 years, then even a relatively modest study can easily last 10 years or more. And there lies one of the problems. For example, consider what would have happened if a trial between proton and 3D-conformal photon therapies for skull base sarcomas had been started 10 years ago. The first solid results would just be appearing now. In the intervening time, however, there have been great advances in the delivery of photon radiotherapy, not least IMRT, and the results of this hypothetical trial would be, in all probability, already obsolete.

Due to these problems, the clinical acceptance of new methods has come about mainly through clinicians being persuaded that the improved dose distributions that can be achieved will bring clinical benefits. For example, IMRT is becoming widely disseminated, despite the fact that there is little evidence in the form of randomized clinical trials to demonstrate its superiority as of yet. Thus, together with pressure from the manufacturers, it is mainly the belief that improved dose distributions should bring clinical gain that is driving the current implementation of IMRT at many centers. Given this background, it is perhaps unsurprising that most of the arguments for proton therapy lie in the comparison of dose distributions, and their subsequent extrapolation to the clinical gains that may be expected from any observed differences.

## Comparative Treatment Planning Studies

Many treatment planning comparisons have been performed between protons and photons in the literature, and can be grouped into three main types; non-IM protons against non-IM photons, non-IM protons against IMRT and, more recently, IMPT against IMRT. For obvious reasons, all early papers comparing protons with photons fell into the first group. The results consistently showed better comformation with protons, including reduced dose to surrounding critical structures and significantly reduced integral doses to the patient, with some papers showing reductions of as much as a factor of 5 for some cases (Miralbell, Croweli, and Suit 1991; Slater, Slater, and Wahien 1992; Tatsuzaki, Urie, and Lingwood 1992; Tatsuzaki, Urie, and Willet 1992; Miralbell and Urie 1993; Lee et al. 1994; Isacsson et al. 1996; Miralbell, Lomax, and Russo 1997). However, given the recent advances in photon radiotherapy in recent years, many of these comparisons are now somewhat obsolete.

Although non-IMRT photons are still the standard of care in the majority of clinics and for the majority of indications, protons must be seen as a specialized technique, to be used primarily when standard methods are inadequate. As IMRT is becoming more accessible, and is also mainly seen in a similar role, then the potential efficacy of proton therapy should now primarily be gauged against this treatment modality. One of the first papers to directly compare non-IM protons with IMRT (and conventional photons) was the work of Lomax et al. (1999). A set of nine disparate cases were planned using both spot-scanned protons and IMRT. Although for the majority of cases, the doses to neighboring critical organs was reduced through the use of protons, the main differences were found below the 70% to 80% dose level, indicating that IMRT could provide a similar high dose conformation to the target volume, whilst protons better spared surrounding tissues in the mid-to-low dose region. Over all cases, the integral dose was found to be, on average, a factor of 2 lower for protons, although this was very case dependent and ranged from 1.0 to 4.5 over all the cases. A number of other papers can be found in the literature comparing non-IM protons with IMRT (e.g., Miralbell et al. 1997; Zurlo et al. 2000; Cozzi et al. 2001; Fogliata, Bolsi, and Cozzi 2002), and the results tend to be consistent over most tumor types, i.e., similar high dose conformation, and reduced dose to normal tissues below about the 70% level with protons.

One exception is the recent work on breast and regional node irradiations (Lomax et al. 2003), three plans of which are shown in figure 16. In this work, non-IM protons were compared to both conventional photons and IMRT, with interesting results. Although the IMRT methods (in this case calculated for nine equally spaced beams) could improve the dose homogeneity across the breast and regional node planning target volumes (PTVs) compared to the conventional approach, this could only be achieved at the cost of some additional dose to the heart, ipsilateral lung, contralateral breast, and contralateral lung (figure 16b). When the optimization criteria were changed in order to spare these organs, dose homogeneity was lost across the PTVs (see figure 16c). In addition, a literature review performed in this paper showed that the results of the study were consistent with other reported studies of IMRT for breast and regional nodes. In contrast, a two-field non-IM proton plan could provide both excellent dose homogeneity to all PTVs and excellent sparing of all the organs (figure 16a).

Perhaps the most currently relevant of the comparison studies are those dealing with comparisons of IMPT and IMRT. Given the limited number of centers that can calculate IMPT plans, the body of literature in this group is not so large, but nevertheless illuminating (Miralbell et al. 2000; Cella, Lomax, and Miralbell 2001; Lomax, Goitein, and Adams 2003). A number of sites have been investigated, from prostate to orbital lesions, and the results are nominally similar to those for other comparative studies concerning the level of high-dose conformity that can be achieved by both approaches. However, there is a point for any delivery method where the competing demands of the dose to critical organs and the target dose come into conflict, and an interesting question that can be asked when comparing the two methods is, to what extent can the normal tissues be spared whilst still applying an acceptable dose to the target volume? This question has been investigated for prostates, orbital tumors, and

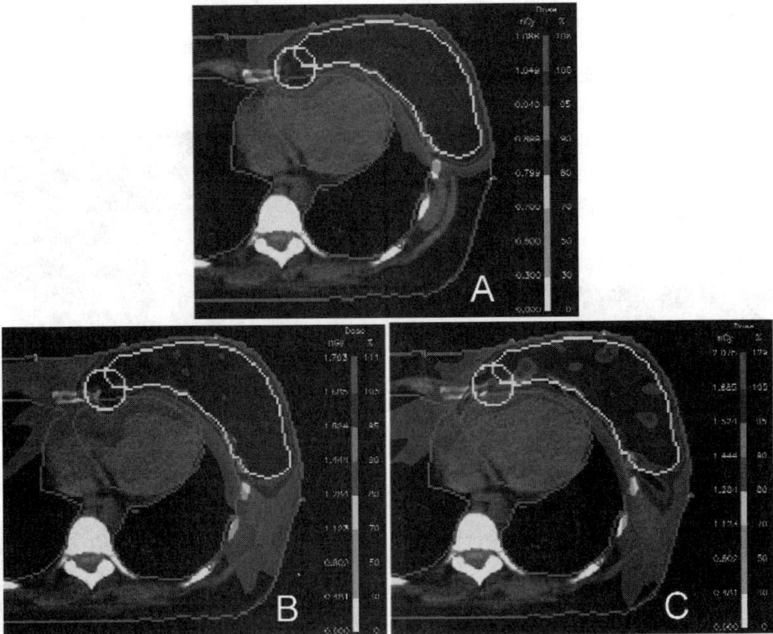

**Figure 16.** Proton and IMRT plans to the breast and regional nodes. (a) A two-field, discrete scanned proton field. (b) Nine-field IMRT with constraints set so as to preserve target dose homogeneity. (c) Nine-field IMRT plan with lower constraints on dose to heart and ipsilateral lung. Note the dramatic loss of homogeneity in PTV volumes. [Reprinted from *International Journal of Radiation Oncology Biology Physics*, vol. 55, issue 3, A. J. Lomax, L. Cella, D. Weber, J. M. Kurtz, and R. Miralbell, "Potential role of intensity-modulated photons and protons in the treatment of the breast and regional nodes," pp. 785–792. © 2003, with permission from Elsevier.]

paranasal sinus in the above papers. An additional example is included here to illustrate the typical results achieved.

Figure 17 shows three plans for the Ewing's carcinoma already considered elsewhere in this manuscript. On the left is the three-field IMPT plan already discussed. On the right are two IMRT plans. The top IMRT plan has been calculated such as to preserve dose conformation and homogeneity to the target. This nicely shows the typical results that one obtains from such comparisons. The dose conformations for the 70% to 80% dose level are very similar, but below this, there is a clear advantage for the protons, particularly in the femoral head region, and in the prostate and bladder (partially shown on the right of the images). However, in principle, the optimization criteria for the IMRT plan could be adjusted such that the mid-to-low doses to these organs are brought down to similar levels as for the proton plan. That is what has been done in the lower plan. From this, it is clear that the user, if he or she wishes, could force the IMRT plan to spare the femoral head to a greater extent, but only at the cost of a loss of high-dose conformation to the target volume. On the other hand, the proton plan has done this at the first time of asking, and with some more adjusting of the parameters, perhaps the doses to the normal tissues could even be reduced more.

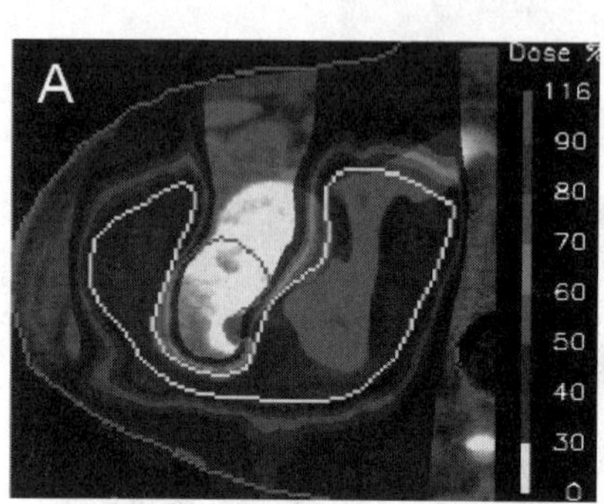
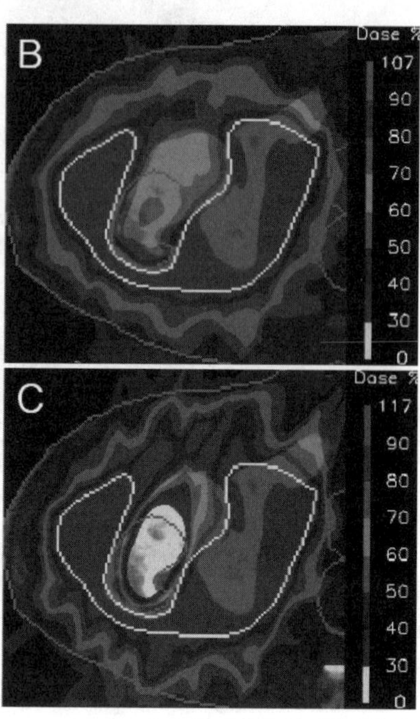

**Figure 17.** IMPT/IMRT comparison of the Ewing's sarcoma. (a) Three-field IMPT plan. (b) Nine-field IMRT plan with constraints set so as to preserve target dose homogeneity. (c) Nine-field IMRT with constraints to femoral head lowered so as to match dose delivered by IMPT plan. Note loss of conformity to PTV at the 80% to 90% dose level as result. Also note excellent sparing of bladder and prostate in the IMPT plan, partially seen on the right of each image. [Part (a) reprinted from *Physics Today*, September 2002, M. Goitein, A. J. Lomax, and E. S. Pedroni, "Treating cancer with protons," pp. 45–50. © 2002, with permission from American Institute of Physics.]

In summary, from comparative planning studies, protons generally provide an improved dose distribution, but it would seem that the main advantage of proton therapy lies in its ability to reduce the volume of normal tissues that receive mid-to-low doses, and in its flexibility in driving doses in selected normal tissues down to very low doses whilst still preserving target dose homogeneity.

## When Are Protons Preferable?

Given the above conclusions, for what type of cases and indications will protons have the most impact? As we have seen, a basic assumption in radiotherapy is that improved dose distributions will generally improve outcome, and there is no reason to think that this will not be the case with protons. On the other hand, proton therapy will certainly not replace photon therapy on a general basis, remaining a specialized treatment tool working as a complement to conventional radiotherapy. It is therefore necessary to identify those cases and indications where it will provide most benefit.

Perhaps the clearest indication is in pediatric radiotherapy. Pediatric radiotherapy generally is particularly successful from the point of view of local tumor control and overall survival. However, long-term treatment-related morbidity is known to be a problem, due to the irradiation of developing tissues and the long life expectancy of these patients. The advantage of protons in reducing overall dose to the pediatric patient has obvious advantages, as can be seen in figure 14 for the cranio-spinal axis irradiation (see also Miralbell et al. 1997; Miralbell, Lomax, and Russo 1997). Although there is little data on pediatric organ sensitivities, most clinicians would agree that tolerance doses, particularly to organs that are still developing, must be below those seen as acceptable for adults. Protons could therefore prove particularly advantageous for such treatments from the point of view of irradiation of the gonads, brain (see e.g., Miralbell et al. 1997) and bones (see e.g., dose to femoral head in Ewing's example in this script) to mention a few. In addition, there are compelling arguments to reduce the whole normal tissue dose to younger patients with good prospects of survival. For example, Schneider, Lomax, and Lombriser (2000) have used a case of a Hodgkin's lymphoma, a disease of predominantly young people, to estimate the risk of secondary malignancies as a result of radiotherapy with protons and IMRT. Unsurprisingly, it was found that the use of protons could reduce the risk of radiation-induced secondary cancer incidence by about a factor of 2, indicating the potential advantage of also reducing the overall integral dose to patients. Similar results have been predicted for other pediatric tumors (Miralbell et al. 2002).

Similar arguments for a probable decrease in tolerance dose to critical organs can be put forward for patients who are receiving concomitant therapies (e.g., chemotherapy), have been previously irradiated, or who have co-morbidity (e.g., patients who may have compromised organ functionality due to diseases other than their tumors). For instance, if a patient needs to be treated for a recurrence after previous radiotherapy in which the brainstem received 50 Gy, then there are clear reasons to want to reduce the dose to this organ as much as possible in subsequent salvage treatments.

Large and/or complex-shaped target volumes, particularly in the neighborhood of multiple or large critical organs, could also benefit from the use of protons. The Ewing's case discussed above is a good example of this, as are tumors in parallel organs such as the lung and liver. Alternatively, figure 18 shows an IMPT plan recently delivered at PSI to treat a completely resected chordoma of L5. The aim was to deliver 72 CGE to the PTV, whilst sparing the Cauda Equina to about 60 to 65 CGE, so as not to compromise the total dose in the PTV too much. A two-series treatment was used, of which figure 18a shows the plan for the second series. The plan consisted of two fields, separated by 20° (±10° from the posterior) and IMPT was used to selectively reduce the dose to the Cauda. An IMRT plan calculated for the same case and consisting of five equally spaced fields, optimized using exactly the same constraints, is shown for comparison.

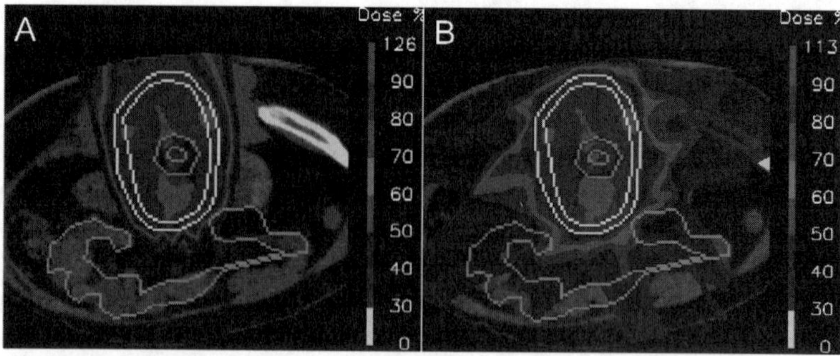

**Figure 18.** IMPT/IMRT comparison for a large sacral chordoma. (a) Two-field "narrow-angle" IMPT plan. The high maximum dose is a result of artifacts resulting from metal screws in the patient (who was treated post-operatively). The hot spots (>110%) were all found in the metal and GTV region. Note in particular, the selectively reduced dose around the Cauda Equina. (b) Five-field IMRT plan, optimized with exactly the same parameters as for the IMPT plan. The IMPT plan delivers 3.5 less integral dose to the patient than the IMRT plan.

What is interesting about this case is the ability of IMPT to selectively reduce doses to a critical structure in the middle of the PTV, despite the fact that only two, narrowly spaced angles have been applied. Through this narrow-angle approach, the target could be irradiated whilst delivering almost no dose to the intestine and other normal tissues distal and lateral to the PTV. Indeed, the total integral dose delivered to the non-target tissues for this patient would be 3.4 times higher with the IMRT plan than that delivered by the IMPT plan. Such almost surgical precision in the radiotherapy of larger target volumes is only possible with protons, and in particular with IMPT.

## Summary

Despite its relatively long history, proton therapy has, until recently, been mainly restricted to a few specialized centers in, or attached to, physics research laboratories. Although the clinical results are nevertheless promising, this has certainly restricted its spread and acceptance as a valid alternative to conventional therapy. This is now changing. In the United States there are now two hospital-based facilities (Loma Linda, CA, and MGH, Boston, MA) already operational, and more planned in the near future (the most mature projects being at M.D. Anderson in Houston, TX, and at the University of Florida in Jacksonville). In Japan, there are already four hospital-based facilities, with at least three more being planned, while in Europe, the first hospital-based facility should be operational in Bavaria in 2006. In addition, there are now a number of manufacturers offering proton therapy systems, Accel (Germany, active scanning), Hitachi (Japan, passive scattering), IBA (Belgium, passive with active scanning in development), and Optivus (United States, passive scattering). Thus, widespread availability of proton therapy is approaching. A critical question is the cost, and current estimates are that a proton facility is at least a factor of 3 more expensive than a comparable conventional facility. However, as the technology spreads, the costs are expected to reduce, and the running costs of a proton facility, which in the long term dominate the cost of treatment, are expected to be similar to conventional facility costs.

With the introduction of IMPT, proton therapy is being pushed to its physical limits, and only time will tell if the promise of protons translates into a real clinical benefit. With the advent of the hospital-based proton facility, we are beginning to have the tools to study this question, and challenging and fascinating times await us in the further development of radiotherapy.

# References

Berger, M. J. (1993a). Penetration of Proton Beams Through Water 1. Depth-Dose Distribution, Spectra and LET Distribution. NISTIR 5226, U. S. Department of Commerce, National Institute of Standards and Technology, Rockville, MD.

Berger, M. J. (1993b). "Penetration of Proton Beams Through Water 11. Three-Dimensional Absorbed Dose Distributions. NISTIR 5330, U. S. Department of Commerce, National Institute of Standards and Technology, Rockville, MD.

Bettega, D., P. Calzolari, P. Chauvel, A. Courdi, J. Herault, N. Ibarra, R. Marchesini, P. Massariello, G. L. Poli, and L. Tallone. (2000) "Radiobiological studies on the 65 MeV therapeutic beam at Nice using human tumour cells." *Int. J. Radiat. Biol.* 76:1297–1303.

Bichsel, H., "Passage of Charged Particles through Matter" in *American Institute of Physics Handbook.* 3$^{rd}$ Ed. D. E. Gray (ed.). New York: McGraw Hill, pp. 8-142–8-189, 1972.

Blosser, H., D. Johnson, D. Lawton, F. Marti, R. Ronningen, and J. Vincent. "A Compact Superconducting Cyclotron for the Production of High Intensity Protons" in *Proceedings of PAC97 (Particle Accelerator Conference).* Vancouver: IEEE Publishing, pp. 1054–1056, 1997.

Bortfeld, T., D. L. Kahler, T. J. Waldron, and A. L. Boyer. (1994). "X-ray field compensation with multileaf collimators." *Int. J. Radiat. Biol.* 28:723–730.

Bortfeld, T., K. Jokivarsi, M. Goitein, J. Kung, and S. B. Jiang. (2002). "Effects of intra-fraction motion on IMRT dose delivery: statistical analysis and simulation." *Phys. Med. Biol.* 47:2203–2220.

Bulanov, S. V., and V. S. Khoroshkov. (2002). "Feasibility of using laser ion accelerators in proton therapy." *Plasma Phys. Rep.* 28:5.

Bush, D. A., J. D. Slater, R. Bonnet, G. A. Cheek, R. D. Dunbar, M. Moyers, and J. M. Slater. (1999). "Proton-beam radiotherapy for early-stage lung cancer." *Chest* 116:1313–1319.

Cella, L., A. J. Lomax, and R. Miralbell. (2001). "Potential role of intensity modulated proton beams in prostate cancer radiotherapy." *Int. J. Radiat. Oncol. Biol. Phys.* 49:217–223.

Cozzi, L., A. Fogliata, A. J. Lomax, and A. Bolsi. (2001). "A treatment planning comparison of 3D conformal therapy, intensity modulated photon therapy and proton therapy for treatment of advanced head and neck tumours." *Radiother. Oncol.* 61:287–297.

Deasy, J. O. (1998) "A proton dose calculation algorithm for conformal therapy simulations based on Moliere theory of lateral deflections." *Med. Phys.* 25:476–483.

Deasy, J. O., D. M. Shepard, and T. R. Mackie. "Distal Edge Tracking: A Proposed Delivery Method for Conformal Proton Therapy Using Intensity Modulation." *XII International Conference on the Use of Computers in Radiation Therapy* (XIIth *ICCR*), Salt Lake City, Utah, May 27–30, 1997. D. D. Leavitt and G. S. Starkschall (ed.). Madison, WI: Medical Physics Publishing, pp. 406–409, 1997.

Egger, E., L. Zografos, and C. Perret. "Proton Beam Irradiation of Choroidal Melanoma's at PSI: Techniques and Results" in *Medical Radiology – Radiotherapy of Intraocular and Orbital Tumours*. Berlin: Springer Verlag, pp. 57–72, 1993.

Egger, E., A. Schalenbourg, L. Zografos, L. Bercher, T. Boehringer, L. Chamot, and G. Goitein. (2001). "Maximizing local tumour control and survival after proton beam radiotherapy of uveal melanoma." *Int. J. Radiat. Biol.* 51:138–147.

Fogliata, A., A. Bolsi, and L. Cozzi. (2002). "Critical appraisal of treatment techniques based on quasi-conventional, intensity modulated photon beams and proton beams for therapy of intact breast." *Radiother. Oncol.* 62:137–145.

Goitein, M. (1978) "A technique for calculating the influence of thin inhomogeneities on charged particle beams." *Med. Phys.* 5:258–264.

Goitein, M. (1985). "Calculation of uncertainty in the dose delivered during radiation therapy." *Med. Phys.* 12:608–612.

Goitein, M. (1997). "Ways to Implement Intensity Modulated Proton Beam Conformal Therapy." Presented at Proton Therapy Co-Operative Group (PTCOG) XXVII, November 17–19, 1997, Chiba, Japan.

Goitein, M., and G. T. Y. Chen. (1983). "Beam scanning for heavy charged particle radiotherapy." *Med. Phys.* 10:831–834.

Goitein, M., and J. M. Sisterson. (1978). "The influence of thick inhomogeneities on charged particle beams." *Radiat. Res.* 74:217–230.

Goitein, M., G. T. Y. Chen, R. J. Schneider, and J. M. Sisterson. (1978). "Measurements and calcultons of the influence of thin inhomogeneities on charged particle beams." *Med. Phys.* 5:265–273.

Harberer, T., W. Becher, D. Schardt, and G. Kraft. (1993) "Magnetic scanning system for heavy ion therapy." *Nucl. Instrum. Meth.* 330:296–305.

Hug, E. B., M. M. Fitzek, N. Liebsch, and J. E. Munzenrider. (1995). "Locally challenging osteo- and chondrogenic tumors of the axial skeleton: Results of combined proton and photon radiation therapy using three-dimensional treatment planning." *Int. J. Radiat. Oncol. Biol. Phys.* 31:467–476.

Isacsson, U., A. Montelius, B. Jung, and B. Glimelius. (1996). "Comparative treatment planning between proton and x-ray therapy in locally advanced rectal cancer." *Radiother. Oncol.* 41:263–272.

Kanai, T., K. Kanai, Y. Kumamoto, H. Ogawa, T. Yamada, and H. Matsuzawa. (1980). "Spot scanning system for radiotherapy." *Med. Phys.* 7:365–369.

Koehler, A. M., R. J. Schneider, and J. M. Sisterson. (1975). "Range modulators for protons and heavy ions." *Med. Phys.* 131:437–440.

Koehler, A. M., R. J. Schneider, and J. M. Sisterson. (1977) "Flattening of proton dose distributions for large fields." *Nucl. Instrum. Meth.* 4:297–301.

Lee, M., C. Wynne, S. Webb, A. E. Nahum, and D. A. Dearnaley. (1994). "Comparison of proton and mega-voltage X-ray treatment planning for prostate cancer." *Radiother. Oncol.* 33:239–253.

Lomax, A. J. (1999). "Intensity modulated methods for proton therapy." *Phys. Med. Biol.* 44:185–205.

Lomax, A. J., M. Goitein, and J. Adams. (2003). "Intensity modulation in radiotherapy: Photons versus protons in the paranasal sinus." *Radiother. Oncol.* 66:11–18.

Lomax, A. J., E. Pedroni, B. Schaffner, S. Scheib, U. Schneider, and A. Tourovsky. "3D Treatment Planning for Conformal Proton Therapy by Spot Scanning. Proc. 19th L H Gray Conference. London: BIR Publishing, pp. 67–71, 1996.

Lomax, A. J., T. Bortfeld, G. Goitein, J. Debus, C. Dysktra, P.-A. Tercier, P. A. Coucke, and R. O. Mirimanoff. (1999). "A treatment planning intercomparison of proton and intensity modulated photon radiotherapy." *Radiother. Oncol.* 51:257–271.

Lomax, A. J., T. Boehringer, A. Coray, E. Egger, G. Goitein, M. Grossmann, P. Juelke, S. Lin, E. Pedroni, B. Rohrer, W. Roser, B. Rossi, B. Siegenthaler, O. Stadelmann, H. Stauble, C. Vetter, and L. Wisser. (2001). "Intensity modulated proton therapy: A clinical example." *Med. Phys.* 28:317–324.

Lomax, A. J., L. Cella, D. Weber, J. Kurtz, and R. Miralbell. (2003). "Potential role of intensity-modulated photons and protons in the treatment of the breast and regional nodes." *Int. J. Radiat. Oncol. Biol. Phys.* 55:785–792.

Marchand, B., D. Prieels, B. Bauvir, R. Sepulchre, and M. Gerard. (2000) "IBA Proton Pencil Beam Scanning: An Innovative Solution for Cancer Treatment." Proc. 7th European particle Accelerator Conference (EPAC2000) Vienna, Austria.

Mandrillon, P. "Accelerators for Hadrontherapy" in *Advances in Hadrontherapy*. U. Amaldi, B. Larsson, and Y. Lemoigne (eds.). Amsterdam: Elsevier Science BV, pp. 160–180, 1997.

Miralbell, R., and M. M. Urie. (1993). "Potential improvement of three dimensional treatment planning and proton beams in fractionated radiotherapy of large cerebral arteriovenous malformations." *Int. J. Radiat. Oncol. Biol. Phys.* 25:353–358.

Miralbell, R., C. Croweli, and H. D. Suit. (1991). "Potential improvement of three dimensional treatment planning and proton therapy in the outcome of maxillary sinus cancer." *Int. J. Radiat. Oncol. Biol. Phys.* 22:305–310.

Miralbell, R., A. J. Lomax, and M. Russo. (1997). "Potential role of proton therapy in the treatment of paediatric medulloblastoma/primitive neuroectodermal tumors: Spinal theca irradiation." *Int. J. Radiat. Oncol. Biol. Phys.* 38:805–811.

Miralbell, R., A. J. Lomax, T. Bortfeld, M. Rouzaud, and C. Carrie. (1997). "Potential role of proton therapy in the treatment of paediatric medulloblastoma/primitive neuroectodermal tumors: Reduction of the supratentorial target volume." *Int. J. Radiat. Oncol. Biol. Phys.* 38:477–484.

Miralbell, R., L. Cella, D. Weber, and A. J. Lomax. (2000). "Optimizing radiotherapy of orbital and paraorbital tumors: Intensity modulated X-ray beams versus intensity modulated proton beams." *Int. J. Radiat. Oncol. Biol. Phys.* 47:1111–1119.

Miralbell, R., A. Lomax, L. Cella, and U. Schneider. (2002). "Potential reduction of the incidence of radiation-induced second cancers using proton beams in the treatment of pediatric tumors." *Int. J. Radiat. Oncol. Biol. Phys.* 54:824–829.

Moliere, G., (1948). "Theorie defrstreuung schneller geladener Teichen. II. Mehrfach-und Vielfachstreuung. Z. f. Naturforschung, 3a:78–97.

Munzenrider, J. E., and N. J. Liebsch. (1999). "Proton therapy for tumors of the skull base." *Strahlenther. Oncol.* 175:57–63.

Oelfke, U., and T. Bortfeld. (2000). "Intensity modulated radiotherapy with charged particle beams: Studies of inverse treatment planning for rotation therapy." *Med. Phys.* 27:1246–1257.

Paganetti, H. (2002). "Nuclear interactions in proton therapy: Dose and relative biological effect distributions originating from primary and secondary particles." *Phys. Med. Biol.* 47:747–764.

Paganetti, H., A. Niemierko, M. Ancukiewicz, L. E. Gerweck, M. Goitein, J. S. Loeffler, and H. D. Suit. (2002). "Relative biological effectiveness (RBE) values for proton beam therapy." *Int. J. Radiat. Biol.* 53:497–421.

Pedroni, E., and H. Enge. (1995). "Beam optics design of a compact gantry for proton therapy." *Med. Biol. Engr. Comput.* 33:271–277.

Pedroni, E., E. Bacher, H. Blattmann, T. Boehringer, A. Coray, A. J. Lomax, S. Lin, G. Munkel, S. Scheib, U. Schneider, and A. Tourovsky. (1995). "The 200 MeV proton therapy project at PSI: Conceptual design and practical realization." *Med. Phys.* 22:37–53.

Pemler, P., J. Besserer, N. Lombriser, R. Pescia, and U. Schneider. (2001). "Influence of respiration-induced organ motion on dose distributions in treatments using enhanced dynamic wedges." *Med. Phys.* 28:2234–2240.

Petti, P. L., J. T. Lyman, T. R. Renner, J. R. Castro, J. M. Collier, I. K. Daftari, and B. A. Ludewigt. (1991). "Design of beam-modulating devices for charged-particle therapy." *Med. Phys.* 18:513–518.

Phillips, M. H., E. Pedroni, H. Blattmann, T. Boehringer, A. Coray, and S. Scheib. (1992). "Effects of respiratory motion on dose uniformity with a charged particle scanning system." *Phys. Med. Biol.* 37:223–234.

Preston, W. M., and A. M. Koehler. (1968). The Effects of Scattering on Small Proton Beams. Harvard Cyclotron Internal Report.

Schaffner, B., E. Pedroni, and A. J. Lomax. (1999). "Dose calculation models for proton treatment planning using dynamic beam delivery system: An attempt to include density heterogeneity effects in the analytical dose calculation." *Phys. Med. Biol.* 44:27–41.

Scheib, S. (1993). "Spot-scanning mit protonen: Experimentelle resultate und therapieplanung." Technical High School (ETH), Zurich, Diss Nr. 10451.

Schneider U., A. J. Lomax, and N. Lombriser. (2000). "Comparatice risk assessment of secondary cancer incidence after treatment of Hodgkin's disease with photon and proton radiation." *Radiat. Res.* 154:382–388.

Schneider, U., B. Schaffner, A. J. Lomax, E. Pedroni, and A. Tourovsky. (1998). "A technique for calculating range spectra of charged particle beams distal to thick inhomogeneities." *Med. Phys.* 25:457–463.

Seltzer, S. M. (1993). An Assessment of the Role of Charged Secondaries from Non-Elastic Nuclear Interactions by Therapy Proton Beams in Water. NISTIR 5221, U.S. Department of Commerce, National Institute of Standards and Technology, Rockville, MD.

Shipley, W. U., L. J. Verhey, J. E. Munzenrider, H. D. Suit, M. M. Urie, P. L. McManus, R. H. Young, J. W. Shipley, A. L. Zeitman, P. J. Biggs et al. (1995). "Advanced prostate cancer: The results of a randomized comparative trial of high dose irradiation boosting with conformal protons compared with conventional dose irradiation using photons alone." *Int. J. Radiat. Oncol. Biol. Phys.* 32:3–12.

Sisterson, J., (2002). "World wide charged particle patient totals 2002." *Particles Newsletter.* 30.

Slater, J. D., J. M. Slater, and S. Wahien. (1992). "The potential of proton therapy in locally advanced carcinoma of the cervix." *Int. J. Radiat. Oncol. Biol. Phys.* 22:343–348.

Slater, J. D., L. T. Yonemoto, C. J. Rossi Jr., N. J. Reyes-Molyneaux, D. A. Bush, J. E. Antoine, L. N. Loredo, R. W. Schulte, S. L. Teichman, and J. M. Slater. (1998). "Conformal proton therapy for prostate carcinoma." *Int. J. Radiat. Oncol. Biol. Phys.* 42:299–304.

Slater, J. D., C. J. Rossi Jr., L. T. Yonemoto, N. J. Reyes-Molyneaux, D. A. Bush, J. E. Antoine, D. W. Miller, S. L. Teichman, and J. M. Slater. (1999). "Conformal proton therapy for early-stage prostate cancer." *Urology* 53:978–984.

Suit, H., and M. Goitein. (2000.) "Proton radiation therapy" ASTRO Refresher Course No. 202, ASTRO, Boston.

Szymanowski, H., and U. Oelfke. (2002). "Two-dimensional pencil-beam scaling: An improved proton dose algorithm for heterogeneous media." *Phys. Med. Biol.* 47:3313–3330.

Tatsuzaki, H., M. M. Urie, and R. Lingwood. (1992). "Comparative treatment planning: Proton versus X-ray beams against glioblastoma multiforme." *Int. J. Radiat. Oncol. Biol. Phys.* 22:265–274.

Tatsuzaki, H., M. M. Urie, and C. G. Willet. (1992). "3D comparative study of proton versus. X-ray radiation therapy for rectal cancer." *Int. J. Radiat. Oncol. Biol. Phys.* 22:369–374.

Tepper, J. E., L. J. Verhey, M. Goitein, H. Suit, and A. M. Koehler. (1977). "In vivo determination of RBE in a high energy modulated proton beam using normal tissue reactions and fractionated dose schedules." *Int. J. Radiat. Oncol. Biol. Phys.* 2:1115–1122.

Thornton, A. F., M. M. Fitzek, M. Vavares, and J. Adamset al. (1998). "Accelerated hyperfractionated proton/photon irradiation for advanced paranasal sinus cancer. Results of a prospective phase I-II study." *Int. J. Radiat. Oncol. Biol. Phys.* 42:222.

Tourovsky, T., E. Pedroni, and U. Schneider. (1993). "Monte Carlo codes for proton radiography and treatment planning." PSI Life Sciences Newsletter, Paul Scherrer Institute, 5232 Villigen, Switzerland, pp. 20–22.

Urano, M., M. Goitein, L. Verhey, O. Mendiondo, H. D. Suit, and A. Koehler. (1980). "Relative biological effectiveness of a high energy modulated proton beam using a spontaneous murine tumor in vivo." *Int. J. Radiat. Oncol. Biol. Phys.* 6:1187–1193.

Urano, M. L. J. Verhey, M. Goitein, J. E. Tepper, H. D. Suit, O. Mendiondo, E. S. Gragoudas, and A. Koehler. (1984). "Relative biological effectiveness of modulated proton beams in various murine tissues." *Int. J. Radiat. Oncol. Biol. Phys.* 10:509–514.

Urie, M. M., M. Goitein, W. R. Holley, and G. T. Y. Chen. (1986). "Degradation of the Bragg peak due to inhomogeneities." *Phys. Med. Biol.* 31:1–15.

Webb, S., and A. J. Lomax. (2001). "There is no IMRT?" *Phys. Med. Biol.* 46:L7.

Wilson, R. R. (1946). "Radiological use of fast protons." *Radiol.* 47:487–491.

Yu, C. X., D. A. Jaffray, and J. W.Wong. (1998). "The effects of intra-fraction organ motion on the delivery of dynamic intensity modulation." *Phys. Med. Biol.* 43:91–104.

Zurlo, A., A. J. Lomax A. Hoess, T. Bortfeld, M. Russo, G. Goitein, V. Valentini, L. Marucci, R. Capparella, and A. Loasses. (2000). "The role of proton therapy in the treatment of large irradiation volumes: A comparative planning study of pancreatic and biliary tumours." *Int. J. Radiat. Oncol. Biol. Phys.* 48:277–288.

# Socio-Economic Issues Of Intensity-Modulated Radiation Therapy

**Michael T. Gillin, Ph.D.**
Department of Radiation Physics
The University of Texas M.D. Anderson Cancer Center
Houston, Texas



## Introduction To Health Cost Issues

Cancer is a major public health issue in the United States. In 2001, it is estimated that there were 1,268,000 new cases of cancer diagnosed and 553,000 cancer deaths (American Cancer Society 2001). The National Cancer Institute estimated that in 1994 cancer care represented 5% of all health care costs, $41 billion (Brown, Hodgson, and Rice 1996), of the approximate $834 billion total costs. When the less malignant neoplasms, which include basal and squamous skin cancers and *in situ* carcinoma of the cervix, are excluded, the cost of cancer is still approximately 4% of direct health care expenditures. In 1995, Mr. Thomas Tucker, MPH, Associate Director for Cancer Control, University of Kentucky Markey Cancer Center, reported that cancer care costs break down to approximately 65% for hospital care, 24% for physician services, 4% for nursing home care, and 7% for drugs and other services (Tucker 1995). Mr. Tucker described a 1989 study, which was based on Medicare's Continuous Medical History sample file, which contains about 5% of all Medicare cases. This study includes all the expenditures related to care of patients who ultimately died of their diseases. This study sorted out direct expenditures into three parts, namely:

1.  The first three months of care.

2.  The monthly cost of continuing care.

3.  The terminal phase of care, i.e., the last 6 months of life.

The initial costs for patients with the same type of cancer varied substantially. The stage of disease and the initial treatment decisions were important variables. The cost of continuing care also varied, since it was a function of the number of months that the patient remained alive. The last 6 months of care for patients with the same initial diagnosis did not vary much.

Mr. Tucker used 1990 Medicare data to identify the five disease sites, which consumed more than two-thirds of the total cost of cancer care. These five sites, in order of expense, are: breast, colon, lung, prostate, and bladder. It was noted that breast cancer has a higher treatment cost than does lung cancer, because breast cancer patients live longer, which means that their continuing care cost is higher.

Brown et al., in 2001, published an article that examines the burden of cancer in terms of the economic cost and quality of life (Brown, Lipscomb, and Snyder 2001). They note that in 1997, four cancer sites (lung, prostate, breast, and colon/rectum) accounted for 52% of the estimated new cancers and 55% of the estimated cancer deaths. The relative 5-year survival rate varies greatly in these four sites, namely 93% for prostate cancer, 86% for breast cancer, 61% for colorectal cancer, and 14% for lung cancer. The economic burden of cancer is discussed in terms of cost-of-illness (COI) estimates. COI estimates include three main elements: direct cost, morbidity cost, and mortality cost. Direct cost is a measure of the expenditures for medical procedures and services associated with treatment and care of the disease entity. Morbidity cost is a measure of the lost income due to work disability and absenteeism associated with the disease entity. Mortality cost is a measure of the lost income associated with premature death. Table 6 of Brown et al., presents 1990 COI data from cancer. The largest component of this cost is the mortality cost (61.1%), which is followed by direct cost (28.6%), and morbidity cost (10.3%). The mortality-cost component has been criticized on a number of different grounds. It reflects economic cost to society only if the underlying assumptions, which are projected for several decades, are correct. Mortality cost is a good measure of loss of life years, expressed in monetary terms. When viewed from a cost-to-society perspective however, the message is very clear; namely, *expenditures for patient care that result in a cure are substantially less costly overall than expenditures for care that do not result in a cure.*

There is a small amount of literature that examines the cost of specific types of treatment for specific diseases. Warren et al. (2002) published an article reporting on the cost of treatment for elderly women with early stage breast cancer in fee-for-service settings. Their results indicate that the initial care costs for the first 6 months after diagnosis for women who underwent breast conserving surgery and radiation therapy were higher than for women who underwent modified radical mastectomy. However, the continuing care costs were significantly more expensive for the radical mastectomy patients. There was statistically no difference in the long-term costs. They conclude that individual preference should be the major factor in treatment option decisions.

The article by Brown et al. (2001) states that from 1963 to 1995, the cancer-related direct costs remained at approximately 5% of the total for all health care expenditures. Health care costs represent approximately 15% of the gross national product of the United States. The net result is that in the year 2000, the per capita cost of cancer care in the United States was more than $250, i.e., $250 for every man, woman, and child in the United States in the year 2000 was spent on cancer care. The American political system struggles to address specific issues related to health care, especially the future projective rise in costs as the population ages. There is a possibility that in the future cost-effectiveness may be important criteria in approving new procedures.

## Radiation Oncology Planning And Treatment Delivery Costs

Two of the major authorities on the estimates of the costs of radiation therapy are Perez (Perez et al. 1993) and Hayman (Hayman et al. 2000). In his comparison of two methods of estimating the technical costs of external beam radiation therapy, Hayman, using 1997 Medicare Cost-to-Charge ratios, provides estimates for the technical costs of four different radiation therapy treatments. Table 1 presents a summary of these estimates.

**Table 1.** Radiation Therapy Technical Costs

| Procedure | Estimated Technical Costs ($) |
|---|---|
| Palliative, simple, 10 fractions, no blocks | 1,285 |
| Palliative, complex, 10 fractions, blocks | 2,345 |
| Curative, breast cancer, 30 fractions, tangents plus Electron beam boost | 6,757 |
| Curative, prostate cancer, 35 fractions, 4 fields | 9,453 |

Hayman notes that the use of higher cost treatments will result in radiation therapy appearing less cost effective.

It is relatively easy to estimate the direct cost of providing radiation oncology treatment delivery and treatment planning costs. Table 2 assumes a 7-year depreciation for rooms and equipment, except for computers where a 3-year depreciation is assumed.

**Table 2.** Estimate of Direct Costs of Providing Radiation Oncology Treatment and Planning Services

| Item | Initial Cost ($) | Cost per Year ($) |
|---|---|---|
| Treatment Room, 600 sq. ft at $250/sq. ft | 150,000 | 25,000 |
| Accelerator | 2,000,000 | 300,000 |
| Maintenance | | 200,000 |
| Two Therapists | | 150,000 |
| 0.5 Physicist | | 62,500 |
| Approximate direct cost per hour for an accelerator room | | **350** |
| Planning room, 225 sq. ft at $200/sq. ft. | 45,000 | 6,500 |
| Planning System | 300,000 | 100,000 |
| Maintenance/Software Support | | 50,00 |
| Dosimetrist | | 100,000 |
| 0.5 Physicist | | 62,500 |
| Approximate direct cost per hour for a planning room | | **150** |

The actual direct cost for a specific service can easily be determined by knowing the amount of time required to provide that service. The direct technical costs for a course of treatment can also be easily calculated.

There are other direct costs for a radiation oncology clinic that are associated with the other functions in the clinic, e.g., nursing and clerical. Health care institutions also have indirect costs that cover a wide spectrum of costs from uncollected charges to salaries for the administrators (many institutions collect less than 50% of their charges). The amount of the indirect costs per procedure may be difficult for a medical physicist to obtain from any institution. The indirect costs charged to grants are common knowledge and are more than 50% of the direct costs.

Hospitals have been reporting their charge-to-cost ratios to the federal government for years. In fact, the dollar amounts associated with specific outpatient services as paid under the Hospital Outpatient Prospective Payment System is based, in part, as these hospital-reported values.

There is no universally accepted staffing model for radiation oncology. However, reasonably staffed clinics with moderate or high workloads generally have two therapists per accelerator, a dosimetrist, and a physicist. There are no criteria that recommend the number of dosimetrists or physicists per patient volume. Older criteria were developed before 3-D planning and delivery and before intensity-modulated radiation therapy (IMRT) [see for example, Table 1-11, Personnel Requirements for Clinical Radiation Therapy in Perez and Brady (1992)]. Those recommendations are inadequate to address modern planning and delivery needs. Depending upon the specific perspective (oncologist, physicist, dosimetrist, administrative) and the patient mix, the exact number of specialists per patient volume will vary.

It is a general approximation in radiation oncology that two-thirds of the costs are technical and one-third of the costs are professional. The professional fees are charged for individual patient-specific services. The exact charges are based upon a number of different considerations using a well-defined mechanism. An in-depth discussion of professional fees is beyond the scope of this work.

## IMRT Practice Costs

The planning and delivery of IMRT add additional professional and technical costs to radiation oncology, due to the added time and equipment required by this technique. The additional time includes time spent by the oncologist, the physicist, the dosimetrist, and the therapists. The exact amount of time required by each specialist will vary, depending upon the nature of the specific case, the experience of the individual, and the equipment being used. Table 3 contains a very rough estimate of the additional time required per IMRT case, assuming that all parties have a modest amount of experience with IMRT.

The current standard of practice for IMRT is that there be at least one measurement of the dose at a specific point and a measurement of the dose distribution pattern. The time required for this measurement and analysis is greater than the time required for the delivery of the treatment.

**Table 3.** Estimate of Additional Time Required by IMRT

| Specialist | Time Required per IMRT Case (Hours) | Percent Increase over 3-D (%) |
|---|---|---|
| Oncologist | 2 | 100 |
| Physicist | 4 | 200 |
| Dosimetrist | 8 | 200 |
| Therapist | 1 | 200 |

The initial planning experience with IMRT was based upon a planning system that only performed IMRT calculations. Currently, the standard 3-D planning systems offer IMRT modules, as an add-on for an additional price. Many larger institutions have more than one type of IMRT planning system. The initial treatment delivery experience with IMRT was based upon an IMRT-dedicated multileaf collimation (MLC) system. However, today IMRT is delivered using existing MLCs or other devices.

The modeling of the additional costs of IMRT is very dependent upon the initial assumptions. For the purposes of this discussion, assume the following:

1. An existing MLC is used in treatment delivery with additional wear and tear being the only added cost.

2. The treatment delivery time is doubled from 15 minutes to 30 minutes.

3. The treatment planning system cost is an additional $50/hour and that an additional 4 hours, over three-dimensional conformal radiation therapy (3DCRT), is required.

4. An additional two hours of physics time is required at a cost of approximately $60/hour.

Thus, the additional technical costs of an IMRT treatment over a 3DCRT treatment is approximately $100/treatment with the vast majority of this cost being the additional time required to deliver the treatment. If the time to deliver the treatment is doubled, then the cost of providing the treatment is at least doubled. The additional technical costs of IMRT planning over 3DCRT planning are on the order of $200 per plan, with labor being the primary component.

From the cost of a course of treatment perspective, treatment delivery is the highest costing technical charge. Progress in developing faster treatment delivery systems should reduce the overall cost of IMRT significantly.

## IMRT Benefits For Patients

Radiation oncology strives to obtain local control of the cancer being treated for curative purposes. Failure to obtain local control is a very ominous sign for the patient. Higher radiation doses have been known to increase cancer control in patients with adenocarcinoma of the prostate (Kuban, El-Mahdi, and Schellhammer 1987; Fuks et al. 1991). However, high radiation doses, which are delivered without conformal treatment planning, can lead to higher complication rates (Smit et al. 1990). Pollack et al. (2000) have reported a single institution randomized trial in which prostate cancer patients receiving 78 Gy to a reference point had a better biochemical disease-free survival (BNED) than patients receiving 70 Gy (79% to 69%, p = 0.058). The higher dose resulted in better outcomes for patients presenting with PSA >10 (prostate-specific antigen greater than 10), both in terms of higher BNED and lower rate of distant metastasis.

Dose is an important parameter in managing patients with non-small-cell lung cancer (NSCLC), despite the low long-term survival (8% to 14%) (Dillman et al. 1990; Sause et al. 1995). The Radiation Therapy Oncology Group (RTOG) protocol 83-01 was a prospective hyperfractionation trial in which patients were treated with 1.2 Gy, which was administered twice daily (Cox et al. 1990). The dose was escalated from 60 Gy, 64.8 Gy, 69.6 Gy, 74.4 Gy, to 79.2 Gy. A survival benefit was seen at 69.6 Gy among the favorable patients, but not at a higher dose level. There was a higher incidence of high-grade pneumonitis seen in the higher dose arms of the study. One interpretation of these results is that non-conformal dose escalation may have a negative effect on survival, given the known sensitivity of lung to radiation damage.

Malignant mesothelioma is a rare disease with a very poor prognosis. Recently, there have been reports of excellent local control with an acceptable rate of complications, using an IMRT treatment approach following extrapleural pneumonectomy. While the data still needs time to mature, this may represent an important clinical advance in the management of this disease (Ahamad et al. 2003; Forster et al. 2003).

Glioblastoma has also been shown to have a dose-response in the 50 to 60 Gy dose range, although the long-term survival is still abysmal, with less than 5% of the patients being expected to live more than 5 years (Mahley et al. 1989; Walker, Strike, and Sheline 1979). More than 20 years ago, the RTOG and the Eastern Cooperative Oncology Group (ECOG) conducted a dose escalation study which demonstrated no benefit in delivering 70 Gy as compared to 60 Gy. The lack of benefit may be related to increased toxicity. More than 15 years ago, Marks and Wong reported an 18% incidence of brain necrosis with doses higher than 64.8 Gy as compared to 0% with doses less than 57 Gy (Marks and Wong 1985).

Quality of life is an important endpoint for all cancer patients. Xerostomia is the most prevalent late side effect for patients receiving radiation for head and neck malignancies and is cited as the major cause of decreased quality of life (Harrison et al. 1997; Bjordal, Kaasa, and Mastekaasa 1994). The degree of xerostomia has been reported to depend on dose and volume of the salivary gland. Eisbruch et al. (1988) have reported the existence of dose and volume thresholds for the parotid salivary gland.

The RTOG has two different protocols designed to study major salivary gland sparing: one for patients with oropharyngeal cancer, H-0022, and the other is for patients with nasopharyngeal cancer, H-0225.

## IMRT Benefits For Institutions

There is a well-established system for coding physician services, the Physicians' Current Procedural Terminology (CPT), which is copyrighted by the American Medical Association (AMA). The content of the CPT is controlled by the CPT Editorial Panel, which consists of AMA-appointed physicians, representatives of the Centers for Medicare and Medicaid Services (CMS), and representatives of other insurance organizations. The CMS Common Procedure Coding System (HCPCS), which is used by both Medicare and Medicaid, is a uniform method for providers to report professional services, procedures, and supplies. The *ASTRO/ACR Joint Economics Committee's Radiation Oncology Coding User's Guide* presents a brief summary of how this system is designed to function (ASTRO/ACR 2002). It should be noted that on the professional side the pool of money used is fixed. Thus, when a code is established for one group of physicians, e.g., radiation oncologists for IMRT services, all other physicians receive less money for their services.

The Hospital Outpatient Prospective Payment System (HOPPS), which was implemented in August 2000, applies only to the technical component services for hospital outpatients. Under this system, services are grouped in Ambulatory Payment Classifications (APCs). APCs combine multiple CPTs that are clinically similar with respect to resource and include non-physician staff, supplies and equipment. Each APC is assigned a relative weight. There is an annual review of the APC groups, relative payment weights, wages and other adjustments. Table 4 is a partial listing of the 2003 Payments for Hospital Outpatient Procedures by APC (Federal Register 2002).

**Table 4.** 2003 Medicare Payments for Hospital Outpatient Procedures

| APC Title | CPT/HCPCS | Relative Weight | Payment Rate ($) |
|---|---|---|---|
| 0268 | US guidance, RT | 1.3856 | 72.26 |
| 0300 | Level I, RT | 1.5794 | 82.37 |
| 0301 | Level II, RT<br>RT delivery, IMRT* | 3.1588 | 164.73<br>400.00 |
| 0304 | Level I, RT Prep | 1.6182 | 84.39 |
| 0305 | Level II, RT Prep | 3.6530 | 190.51 |
| 0310 | Level III, RT Prep<br>RT Dose Plan, IMRT* | 13.6625 | 712.51<br>875.00 |

*The two IMRT APCs are included in the new technology section of the APCs and thus do not have relative weights assigned to them. They will be assigned to a specific APC after sufficient cost data have been reported by the hospitals and digested by CMS.

It is clear from the table that IMRT treatment delivery in 2003 provides hospitals with a substantial financial benefit over 3DCRT or any other treatment delivery approach. It should also be noted that this benefit may be adjusted in subsequent years.

## Socio-Economic Considerations

The 1997 Balanced Budget Act achieved some Medicare savings, but did not address the demographic problem in the United States; namely, the decline in the worker-to-beneficiary ratio from the current three-to-one to two-to-one by the time the last baby boomers retire. Rodger Doyle in the April 1999 issue of *Science and the Citizen* wrote an interesting article entitled "Health Care Costs" (Doyle 1999). He noted the following:

> Federal policy since World War II has emphasized medical technology and the widespread building of hospitals, even in rural areas. Other industrial countries, in contrast, followed the more cost-effective alternative of building up regional centers.

There are long-term consequences to having a substantially higher percentage of our gross national product being devoted to health care than our trading partners. These consequences will be seen both in terms of federal budget expenditures and in terms of our ability to compete in the world market. It will be very interesting to observe major economic forces using their political power to either control the rate of growth of spending on health care or to encourage further spending, as these issues are played out in the upcoming years.

The appropriate allocation of cancer care, which is based upon cost-effectiveness or efficacy, is a very challenging exercise. Eddy (1992) identified the four toughest problems; namely:

1.  Defining an understandable benefit, such as life-years saved.

2.  Dealing with inadequate information, e.g., finding that there is no evidence for efficacy of an accepted procedure.

3.  Measuring the costs of care.

4.  Defining the treatment efficacy outside of a clinical trial, i.e., results from a clinical trial may not transfer directly to the community setting.

Smith, Hillner, and Desch (1993) have proposed a decision-analysis model for oncology that contains eight elements. Decision analysis can be used as a method of deciding if society should fund a specific treatment approach (for example, is autologous bone marrow transfer in limited metastatic breast cancer too costly or a bargain?). These elements are:

1.  The natural history of the disease must be well described and quantifiable.

2.  Clinical trial data of efficacy must be used, or assumptions clearly specified.

3.  Costs, not charges, must be used.

4.  Utility values should be from the group in question, e.g., patients. Health care providers may be a suitable surrogate.

5.  A discount rate must be used and stated, with sensitivity analysis performed. (A discount rate of 5% for both time and money is commonly used.)

6.  The perspective must be clearly stated, i.e., the patient has a different perspective than does the insurance company.

7.  The level of application must be clearly stated.

8.  The sensitivity analysis must demonstrate robustness of the model in all clinically relevant alternative assumptions.

Using this decision analysis model, can IMRT be justified for prostate cancer patients with Gleason 7 and PSA <15? The natural history of the disease is well known. For surgical series, the 5-year PSA NED is on the order of 50%. For radiation series, the outcome depends upon the dose delivered. The results are approximately the same or worse than the surgical series, when the doses are less than 70 Gy. There is no prospective randomized clinical trial data that supports or does not support the use of IMRT. There is clinical trial data that does support conformal dose escalation. The increased actual costs for IMRT treatment depend upon the additional length of time that the treatment room is in use to deliver the IMRT treatment and may be doubled over 3-D conformal treatments. The informed consent process should provide the patient information upon which to make a judgment (prostate patients can present with a wide spectrum of medical conditions and may or may not be interested in taking risks relative to either their cure or possible toxicities). A discount rate of either time or money does not seem to be important for this analysis nor does the level of application. From the perspective of the insured patient, the risks associated with IMRT may be acceptable. From the perspective of the insurer, the lack of proven benefit of IMRT over 3DCRT and the possible toxicity would be emphasized. The sensitivity analysis permits setting the definition of thresholds, e.g., treatment efficacy or cost standards, before the cost-effectiveness can be judged. Thus, if the prostate patient is a healthy 60-year-old male, who has a full time job and is expecting to work for another 10 years, the added costs of treatment with an increase in local control may be justifiable from a socio-economic perspective, when reviewed against the possible mortality and morbidity costs. The same argument could not be made for a 75-year-old male.

A more challenging socio-economic IMRT question relates to the justification of the added cost of IMRT to prevent xerostomia. Assuming equal local control from

3DCRT treatment and IMRT treatments for a specific site stage of head and neck cancer, the continuing care costs and/or the morbidity costs must be considered. The added care costs per year to treat xerostomia will be greater than $1,000, assuming that medication is used. If there are additional medical care costs, the total additional costs due to this toxicity may be several thousands of dollars per year. The time required to reach a break-even point can be easily calculated. It should be appreciated, however, that individual patients may or may not develop this complication, independent of what treatment technique is used.

The potential economic gains from any new, effective cancer therapy, including IMRT, are substantial. Assume that a new treatment technique is able to cure 2% of the 500,000 cancer deaths per year, which equals 10,000 patients. Assume that the cost of care for these patients as their disease progresses through end of life care is $100,000, if the patient was not cured. Then the total cost savings for such patients would be $1 billion, which is 1/75 of the total cost of all cancer care in 2000. This simple approach provides an understanding of the potential effect from the socio-economic perspective of a new effective cancer therapy. This economic approach ignores the human impact of lives saved and the total cost in terms of productivity lost. The currently unanswered IMRT socio-economic question is how many additional cancer cures will result from this new treatment approach.

Currently, the free enterprise aspects of the American health care delivery system are running rampant. Hospitals understand the financial benefits to be gained by offering IMRT treatment for all tumor types. The concept of delivering higher doses to the target and lower doses to normal tissue is very attractive, even if there is very limited proof that higher cure rates and lower toxicity rates will result. Offering the patient hope is one important aspect of health care.

Medical physicists have an interesting role to play in the socio-economic evaluation of IMRT. One important contribution is the identification of the costs of treatment planning and treatment delivery. Hospitals are reporting costs to CMS. The reported costs should reflect the actual costs. The definition of IMRT, which is used for billing purposes, will be broadened over time as experience with other systems is reported. Other systems, e.g., physical modulators, may offer distinct advantages over the current treatment delivery approaches. Many institutions are having difficulties treating their patient load, given the longer treatment times required by IMRT. Medical physicists are exploring methods to make the treatment delivery process more efficient, which will lower the costs of IMRT.

IMRT offers potential surpassing some of the historical limitations of radiation oncology. For example, the 2 Gy per fraction standard can possibly be changed with IMRT to deliver a higher dose per fraction to the target while maintaining the current dose per fraction to the normal tissue. There are substantial socio-economic consequences to decreasing the number of fractions required to treat a specific disease. Such a change is possible if high-quality IMRT plans are developed and delivered.

The success of radiation as a cancer treatment modality is due in part to the high quality and safety of the entire process. As a new modality, such as IMRT, is introduced, medical physicists have a significant role in understanding the physical and clinical aspects of this modality and in serving as consultants to the oncologists in the application of this process. IMRT is an interesting evolution in making radiation more conformal. While there is still substantial progress to be made in both the IMRT treatment planning and treatment delivery processes, intensity-modulated X-ray therapy is just the beginning. It will soon be followed by energy and intensity-modulated electron therapy and energy and intensity-modulated proton therapy.

One fundamental economic fact perseveres in cancer management, namely that an expensive cure is far less costly in the long run than a treatment failure. Clearly, high technology medicine cannot cure all cancer patients. However, new technologies offer the possibility of making additional progress. At this point, society is not demanding that medical technology prove its cost-effectiveness or its efficiency prior to its mass utilization. This absence of proof does not, however, relieve medical professionals from the obligation of using new technology in a manner that serves the best needs of cancer patients.

# References


Ahamad, A., C. W. Stevens, W. R. Smythe, A. A. Vaporcivan, R. Komaki, J. F. Kelly, Z. Liao, G. Starkschall, and K. M. Forster. (2003). "Intensity modulated radiation therapy: A novel approach to the management of malignant pleural mesothelioma." *Int. J. Radiat. Oncol. Biol. Phys.* 55:768–775.

American Cancer Society, 2001. www.cancer.org.

*ASTRO/ACR Joint Economics Committee Radiation Oncology Coding User's Guide 2002.* Fairfax, Virginia: American Society of Therapeutic Radiology and Oncology, 2002.

Bjordal, K., S. Kaasa, and A. Mastekaasa. (1994). "Quality of life in patients treated for head and neck cancer: A follow-up study 7 to 11 years after radiotherapy." *Int. J. Radiat. Oncol. Biol. Phys.* 28(4):847–856.

Brown, M. L., T. A Hodgson, and D. R. Rice. "Economic Impact of Cancer in the United States" in *Cancer Epidemiology and Prevention*, Second Ed., D. Schottenfeld and J. F. Fraumeni Jr. (eds.). New York: Oxford University Press, pp. 255–266, 1996.

Brown, M. L., J. Lipscomb, and C. Snyder. (2001). "The burden of illness of cancer: Economic cost and quality of life." *Ann. Rev. Public Health* 22:91–113.

Cox, J. D., N. Azarnia, R. W. Byhardt, K. H. Shin, B. Emami, and T. F. Pajak. (1990). "A randomized phase I/II trial of hyperfractionated radiation therapy with total doses of 60.0 Gy to 79.2 Gy. Possible survival benefit with >69.6 Gy in favorable patients with Radiation Therapy Oncology Group stage III non-small cell lung carcinoma: Report of Radiation Therapy Oncology Group 83-11." *J. Clin. Oncol.* 8:1543–1555.

Dillman, R. O., S. L. Seagren, K. J. Propert, J. Guerra, W. L. Eaton, M. C. Perry, R. W. Carey, E. F. Frei 3rd, and M. R. Green. (1990). "A randomized trial of induction chemotherapy plus high-dose radiation versus radiation alone in stage III non-small-cell lung cancer." *N. Engl. J. Med.* 323(14):940–945.

Doyle, R. (1999). "Health care costs." *Science and the Citizen*. www.sciam.com.

Eddy, D. M. (1992). "Cost-effectiveness analysis. Is it up to the task?" *JAMA* 267:3342–3348.

Eisbruch A., R. K. Ten Haken, H. M. Kim, L. H. Marsh, and J. A. Ship. (1999). "Dose, volume, and function relationships in parotid salivary glands following conformal and intensity-modulated irradiation of head and neck cancer." *Int. J. Radiat. Oncol. Biol. Phys.* 45:577–587.

Federal Register, November 1, 2002.

Forster, K. M., W. R. Smythe, G. Starkschall, Z. Liao, T. Takanaka, J. F. Kelly, A. Vaporcivan, A. Ahamad, L. Dong. M. Salehpour, and R. Komaki. (2003). "Intensity-modulated radiation therapy following extrapleural pneumonectomy for the treatment of malignant mesothelioma: Clinical implementation." *Int. J. Radiat. Oncol. Biol. Phys.* 55:606–616.

Fuks, Z., S. A. Leibel, K. E. Wallner, C. E. Begg, W. R. Fair, A. Raben, L. L. Anderson, B. S. Hilaris, and W. F. Whitmore. (1991). "The effect of local control on metastatic dissemination in carcinoma of the prostate: Long-term results in patients treated with $^{125}$I implantation." *Int. J. Radiat. Oncol. Biol. Phys.* 21:537–547.

Harrison, L. B., M. J. Zelefsky, D. G. Pfitser, E. Carper, A. Raben, D. H. Krause, E. W. Strong, A. Rao, H. Thaler, T. Polyak, and R. Portenoy. (1997). "Detailed quality of life assessment in patients treated with primary radiotherapy for squamous cell cancer of the base of the tongue." *Head Neck* 19:169–175.

Hayman, J.A., K. A. Lash, M. L. Tao, and M. A. Halman. (2000). "A comparison of two methods for estimating the technical costs of external beam radiation therapy." *Int. J. Radiat. Oncol. Biol. Phys.* 47:461–467.

Kuban D., A. El-Mahdi, and P. Schellhammer. (1987). "Effect of local tumor control on distant metastasis and survival in prostatic adenocarcinoma." *Urol.* 30(5):420–425.

Mahaley, Jr., M. S., C. Mettlin, N. Natarajan. E. R. Laws Jr., and B. B. Pearce. (1989) "National survey of patterns of care for brain-tumor patients." *J. Neurosurg.* 71:826–836.

Marks, J. E., and J. Wong (1985). "The risk of cerebral radionecrosis in relation to dose, time, and fractionation." *Prog. Exp. Tumor Res.* 29:210–218.

Perez, C. A., and L.W. Brady. *Principles and Practice of Radiation Oncology.* Philadephia: Lea & Febiger, 1992.

Perez, C. A., B. Kobeissi, B. D. Smith, S. Fox, P. W. Grigsby, J. A. Purdy, H.D. Procter, and T. H. Wasserman. (1993). "Cost accounting in radiation oncology: A computer-based model for reimbursement." *Int. J. Radiat. Oncol. Biol. Phys.* 25:895–906.

Pollack, A., G. K. Zagars, L. G. Smith, J. J. Lee, A. C. von Aschenbach, J. A. Antolak, G. Starkschall, and I. Rosen. (2000). "Preliminary results of a randomized radiotherapy dose-escalation study comparing 70 Gy with 78 Gy for prostate cancer." *J. Clin. Oncol.* 18(23):3904–3911.

Radiation Therapy Oncology Group (RTOG) H-0022. Phase I/II Study of Conformal and Intensity Modulated Irradiation for Oropharyngeal Cancer, Feb 2001 (Rev. 1-2, Jan 15, 2002). Available at rtog.org.

Radiation Therapy Oncology Group (RTOG) H-0225. Nasopharyngeal Cancer. Available at rtog.org.

Sause, W. T., C. Scott, S. Taylor, D. Johnson, R. Livingston, R. Komaki, B. Emami, W. J. Curran, R. W. Byhardt, A. T. Turisi et al. (1995). "Radiation Therapy Oncology Group (RTOG) 88-08 and Eastern Cooperative Oncology Group (ECOG) 4588: Preliminary results of a phase III trial in regionally advanced, unresectable non-small-cell lung cancer." *J. Natl. Cancer Inst.* 87:198–205.

Smit, W. G., P. A. Helle, W. L. van Putten, A. J. Wijnmaalen, J. J. Seldenrath, and B. H. van der Werf-Messing. (1990). "Late radiation damage in prostate cancer patients treated by high dose external radiotherapy in relation to rectal dose." *Int. J. Radiat. Oncol. Biol. Phys.* 18:23–29.

Smith, T. J., B. E. Hillner, and C. E. Desch. (1993). "Efficacy and cost-effectiveness of cancer treatment: Rational allocation of resources based on decision analysis." *J. Natl. Cancer Inst.* 85(18):1460–1474.

Tucker, T. C. (1995). "Cancer care accounts for 5% of direct U.S. health expenditures." *Oncol. News Int.* 4:7.

Walker, M. D., T. A. Strike, G. E. Sheline. (1979). "An analysis of dose-effect relationship in the radiotherapy of malignant gliomas." *Int. J. Radiat. Oncol. Biol. Phys.* 5:1725–1731.

Warren, J. L., M. L. Brown, M. P. Fay, N. Schussler, A. L. Potosky, and G. F. Riley. (2002). "Costs of treatment for elderly women with early-stage breast cancer in fee-for-service settings." *J. Clin. Oncol.* 20:307–316.

# The Future Of IMRT

**Jerry J. Battista, Ph.D., and Glenn S. Bauman, Ph.D.**
London Regional Cancer Centre
London, Ontario, Canada



## Introduction

### The Rationale And Niche For IMRT

During this Summer School and in the preceding chapters, the focus has been on the hardware, software, procedures, and resources required to implement intensity-modulated radiation therapy (IMRT) clinically (IMRTCWG 2001). In this concluding chapter, we present a more philosophic overview, turning our attention to the principles behind IMRT and forecasting its role in the future of radiation oncology. *The underlying hypothesis is that loco-regional control of cancer remains a significant barrier to cancer cure for many common cancers* (Leibel et al. 2002; Tepper 2002). Through improved loco-regional control and minimal treatment complications, IMRT could potentially improve the outlook for many cancer patients (Teh et al. 2002). IMRT is undoubtedly a technical improvement over three-dimensional conformal radiotherapy (3DCRT). Better dose distributions are expected to translate into better clinical outcomes in accordance with the "Suit Credo" (Suit 1982, 2002; Suit and DuBois 1991; Suit and Miralbell 1989; Suit and Westgate 1986). The basic strategy is sketched in figure 1. Differential dose effects can be achieved between tumor and normal tissue, using stronger *dose gradients*.

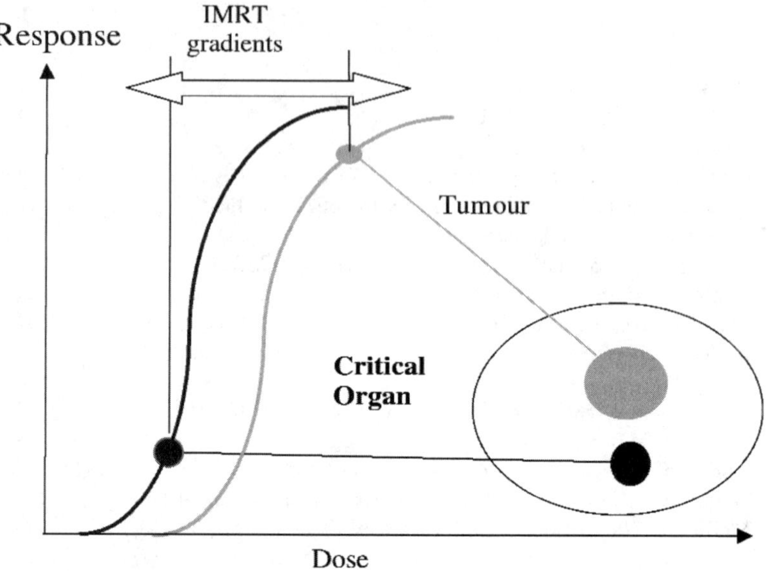


**Figure 1.** Dose gradients achieved with IMRT allow a greater differential in dose to be achieved between the target and normal tissues, assuming they are geographically separated. The inset shows a solid tumor overlaying a critical organ, with a gap.

This approach does, however, rely on the premise that the target and critical volumes can be segmented into geographically distinct regions. On a macroscopic scale, solid tumors are contoured from digital images and assumed to contain mostly tumorigenic cells, distinguishable from nearby critical organs. Radiosurgery, 3DCRT, and IMRT techniques are most readily applied to these situations, depending on the target volume size. For multiple lesions that are much more distributed within a predominantly healthy tissue matrix (e.g., regional lymph nodes), large coverage irradiation has been used with success (e.g., mantle techniques). To date, IMRT has not generally been applied to these situations except in an exploratory way to reduce toxicity through conformal avoidance of discrete critical structures within the region to be broadly irradiated (e.g., parotid sparing for head and neck treatment). For microscopic "liquid cancers," abnormal cells co-exist alongside normal cells in the blood stream or lymphatic channels; systemic treatment with cell-specific cytotoxic or radio-labeled agents seems more appropriate. However, local therapies may still be needed to deal with bulky regional disease (e.g., field of radiation added to chemotherapy for lymphomas). Clearly, IMRT will ultimately be used in combination with complementary therapies, to various degrees depending on the type of lesion: local, regional, or systemic.

The emphasis to date in the application of IMRT has been on treating solid local tumors, such as the prostate, to higher doses. We would like to draw attention to the potential for different roles of IMRT at tumor sites where current survival rates are poor: brain and lung. The treatment of brain metastases is an example where all three components of local, regional, or systemic approaches must be combined. Treatment of extracranial metastases is achieved through systemic therapy, irradiation of the brain in regions at risk of subclinical metastases, boosted by radiosurgery for intracranial solid lesions. To date, the modest benefits seen with aggressive radiotherapy of whole brain and radiosurgery are due mainly to progressive systemic disease. This is evidenced in patients with solitary brain metastases (with no extracranial metastases), where surgical resection or radiosurgery plus whole brain radiotherapy improves survival over radiotherapy alone. If one omits whole brain radiotherapy from either surgery or radiosurgery, there is a higher risk of intracranial recurrence and death from progressive neurological disease. Thus, in this case, all three components need to be at play: local, regional, and systemic, but currently systemic treatment is the "weakest link." With better systemic agents becoming available in the future, loco-regional control will gain in importance and IMRT will become even more critically important in years ahead. A second example relates to the treatment of lung disease where survival rates remain poor. The current trend is towards dose escalation in the radiographically evident tumor alone, combined with systemic therapy. Once the rate of local control and distant disease progression is seen to improve, it may then be necessary to revisit loco-regional radiation to treat potentially involved nodes. Focused beam delivery techniques will be necessary to keep the morbidity of this combination (high-dose local radiotherapy, chemotherapy, and regional radiotherapy) to acceptable tolerance levels. In summary, the role of IMRT will change in time and it will add great flexibility in "juggling" the concerted combinations of local, regional, and systemic therapies for better outcomes.

## The Evolution Towards IMRT

IMRT is sometimes viewed as a revolutionary breakthrough in cancer treatment, particularly by overly enthusiastic researchers and equipment manufacturers. In reality, it is the culmination of several decades of progress in convergent technologies, stemming from the imaging and radiotherapy worlds. IMRT is developing in the same way that conventional radiosurgery evolved based on available technology of the time. In fact, radiosurgery dates back to the 1950's with indications and sophistication evolving over the years to incorporate improvements in related fields, particularly imaging. Initially it was introduced as a simple predictable way to deliver highly focused dose distributions with circular collimators. Geometric rather than dosimetric treatment planning was used but this evolved quickly to take advantage of better targeting with angiography and computed tomography (CT) imaging, coupled with better immobilization frames, and treatment planning software. Multi-modality imaging continues to help improve the delineation of target volumes and critical structures. Multileaf collimators (MLCs) enable beam modification "on demand," replacing the fabrication and placement of mechanical blocks, wedges, and compensators. Thus, IMRT has become possible as a result of many ideas and technologies from diagnostic and therapeutic medical physics, engineering, and medicine. It is in fact a process refinement, likely to survive beyond the span of a contemporary "fad." Clinical IMRT will indeed force the further integration, automation, and streamlining of imaging, treatment planning, and treatment delivery. An example of this type of progression in radiotherapy includes the replacement of the physical wedge by a "virtual" dynamic wedge.

In some cases, a new technology may cause a fairly sudden "inversion" of the current approach rather than a "progression." Inversion is alternatively designated as a "shift in paradigm." An example is inverse treatment planning which is based on the "first principles" of radiotherapy and would have been the intuitive starting point, were it not for computer limitations of the past era. A non-medical example might help further illustrate this phenomenon. If the Internet capability had been established early in the late 1700's, would an international network of post offices have ever been formed? The reverse occurred but it did not prevent the development of alternative information delivery systems such as the telegraph, phone, fax machine, and Internet (using phone lines !).

In this chapter, we will refer to "IMRT" loosely, not only as a method of shaping dose distributions, but also including ancillary imaging methods for tumor targeting, tumor tracking, and beam verification. In fact, we expect that it will become progressively more difficult to distinguish the clinical impacts of improved dose delivery from those of better imaging and dose optimization schemes.

## Cost-Benefit Analysis

In industry and business, the cost-benefit ratio is usually a good prognostic factor for the longevity of a new product, process, or service. It is much more difficult to apply this methodology objectively to medical procedures because the "costs" and "benefits" are often less tangible and difficult to quantify. How do we quantify the addition of "n" years of good quality living to a cancer survivor? What is the gain in convenience and to society from a patient undergoing an abbreviated hypofractionated treatment schedule with an earlier return to productive work? What is the value of avoiding work-related injuries in staff using MLCs instead of repetitively moving shielding blocks? What is the "cost" of risk associated with using new technology that may induce long-term secondary cancers in a longer surviving cancer patient? What is the net benefit to society resulting from decreased side effects of treatment, and earlier return to work?

Figure 2 illustrates a qualitative ranking of various technologies and techniques, including IMRT, versus the technical complexity and cost required for implementation. Historically, external beam radiotherapy was applied using single kilovoltage fields, hand-shaped to conform to visible skin lesions. The introduction of megavoltage energy in the 1950's entailed a significant complexity in beam collimation because of the greater shielding mass required, but skin-sparing also paved the way to treating "deep" lesions, with less normal tissue damage. Three-dimensional imaging was triggered by the advent of X-ray CT scanning in the 1970's and extended consideration to the entire irradiated volume during computerized treatment planning. Rotational or arc therapy was used at the start of megavoltage radiotherapy but was discouraged by concerns over the large integral dose. It has undergone a renaissance with radiosurgery, intensity-modulated arc therapy (Wong, Chen, and Greenland 2002; MacKenzie and Robinson 2002; Yu et al. 2002) and tomotherapy (Mackie et al. 1999). High-LET (linear energy transfer) radiation beams (see the section *Cones, Fans, and Robots*) offer radiobiological advantages [relative biological effectiveness (RBE) and oxygen enhancement ratio (OER) differentials], while their physical advantages are now being challenged by multi-field X-ray IMRT (see *Accelerators: Light Electrons Or Heavy Charged Particles*).

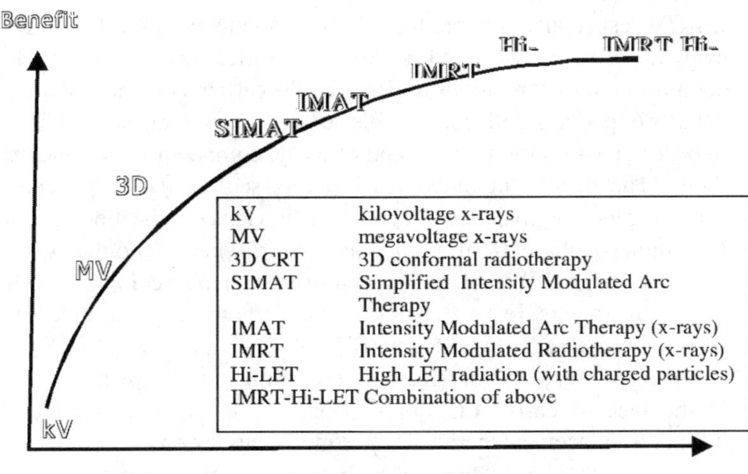


**Figure 2.** Schematic of the gains achieved with different major advances in radiotherapy.

The vertical axis in figure 2 is intended to be generic. It could apply to the treated populations of patients (see B below), reflecting tumor control probability (TCP), or the probability of *not* inducing a normal tissue complication $(1 - NTCP)$, or some combination $[TCP \times (1 - NTCP)]$. At the population level (see C below), it could represent "Person-years of life saved." The horizontal axis is the "cost" parameter and it can include amortized capital costs, operating costs, both primary and hidden secondary resource costs. The slope of the curve is inversely related to the cost-benefit ratio, and it is often expected to decrease as the methods mature to their fullest potential.

*Defining The Costs And Benefits On Different Scales*

In debating the pros and cons of any new technology, arguments have been voiced from a variety of perspectives at a different scale of concern:

(A)  Individual Patient
At this level, the outcome in terms of treatment success is essentially binary. The patient asks "Will I be one of the 70% who should survive or one of the 30% who will fail?" "Will I be one of the 5% to suffer severe side effects or not?" This cost-benefit analysis is done privately and interactively, with the advice of the oncologist and family. For an individual patient, IMRT improves the "odds" of achieving a complication-free survival, but there are no guarantees.

(B)  Cohorts of Patients
IMRT is especially suitable for selected patients with localized disease, no evidence of metastases, and where the historical level of success has been compromised by limitations imposed by the earlier technology. On this scale, cohorts of patients with comparable staging undergo phase I/II clinical trials in order to assess the toxicity and efficacy, compared with standard procedures. The benefit in outcomes is expressed as "% of patients treated achieving loco-regional control" or "% achieving complication-free survival." Randomized phase III trials are developed when a promising technique passes the phase I/II levels and is mature enough to be compared with a alternative treatments [e.g., 3DCRT versus cryotherapy, or 3DCRT versus non-conformal radiation therapy (RT)]. As with any new medical treatment, there are pressures to implement a new promising therapy as the "standard" in the face of early compelling phase I/II evidence. Examples include hormone replacement therapy for postmenopausal women, bypass techniques for carotid atherosclerotic disease: both are examples where the new "standard" failed to improve outcomes (or was associated with worse outcomes) compared to conventional therapy. Thus, there is a need for randomized clinical trails of IMRT, like any other form of new treatment. Such comparisons can be based on anticipated differences in side effects or changes in tumor control. Such comparisons can unveil changes in tumor control or side effects. In some clinical studies only equivalency is established between homologous technologies (e.g., GammaKnife versus linac radiosurgery, tomotherapy versus linac IMRT with cone-beam CT). In such cases, only differences in efficiencies or implementation gains may be revealed.

(C)  Populations
A "government's eye view" is useful when assessing the socio-economic benefits of a new technology. This "big picture" approach weighs the benefits to a society against financial investments in the context of alternative

cancer control or prevention strategies, or competing disease burdens such as heart disease versus cancer. Primary (prevention), secondary (early detection), and tertiary (treatment of established disease) care are other types of competing priorities at the societal level. This type of analysis is sometimes used to limit the rapid diffusion of new "unproven" technology. The disadvantage of this global approach is that it, by definition, does not consider an individual patient (A) or cohorts of patients (B). It may delay or deprive eligible individuals from having a better chance at a cancer cure, "for the good of the whole" population.

Much of the debate about the value of IMRT can be classified according to the different levels of scale identified above. Apparently opposed views may indeed be reconcilable, when corrected for different "magnifications" of the viewpoint. On an individual patient basis (level A), today's well-informed patients may request state-of-the-art techniques and thereby drive the market need for IMRT, based on a projected benefit. Better odds of treatment success and less morbidity will be potent forces, and this may ultimately overshadow any clinical trials results and cost–benefit analyses we do "on paper." Clinical researchers (level B) generally conclude that there is mounting evidence to support the 3DCRT and IMRT hypotheses. The techniques are feasible, produce less acute toxicity, and yield improved survival especially when coupled with dose escalation (Pollak et al. 2002; Purdy and Michalski 2001; Perez et al. 1997, 2001). A critical appraisal of the literature (Levitt and Kahn 2001; Cho, Khan, and Levitt 1999) in search of evidence "that IMRT is better" concluded that there may have been a "rush to judgment." This study was subsequently reviewed by Purdy and Michalski (2001) who added the Radiation Therapy Oncology Group (RTOG) trials experience and the debate continues (Levitt and Kahn 2002). Glatstein (2002) has summarized the pros and cons of IMRT, and highlights the non-physical reasons for failures of treatment and the potential for long-term carcinogenesis due to enhanced whole body integral dose (see *Long-Term Carginogenesis—The Hidden Cost of IMRT* below). Schulz (1999) and Schultz and Kagan (2002) based their opinions on the societal viewpoint (level C), arguing that gains in survival due to costly "fine tuning" of radiotherapy will be small. This null hypothesis did not go unchallenged (Mohan, Cardinale, and Hagen 1999) and the debate continued (Schulz 2001).

Multiplication of small gains by large populations yields a large number of individual patients who will benefit. Also, widespread development and implementation of a technique yields efficiencies and lower costs and can justify smaller incremental benefits across a larger patient population base. For instance, if IMRT technology and techniques could be developed to be reliable, economical, auto quality-assured, and exportable to the developing countries such as a cobalt tomotherapy machine (Schreiner 2001), the benefits would be enormous in terms of the absolute number of lives improved or saved by radiation therapy on a worldwide scale.

     **Jerry J. Battista and Glenn S. Bauman**

*How Many Patients Can Potentially Benefit From IMRT?*

In the population of 287 million in the United States, approximately 1.28 million will be diagnosed with cancer, and over 555,000 patients will succumb to their disease this year. The percentage of cancer patients who could potentially benefit from technological advances can be estimated based on those for whom loco-regional control and a "cure" is achievable, but whose present chances have been foiled by poor targeting, poor dose distribution, or insufficient dose. Figure 3 shows a "triage" of such cases, normalized (100%) to the number of diagnosis, and showing which failed patients could be "rescued" by technological innovation.

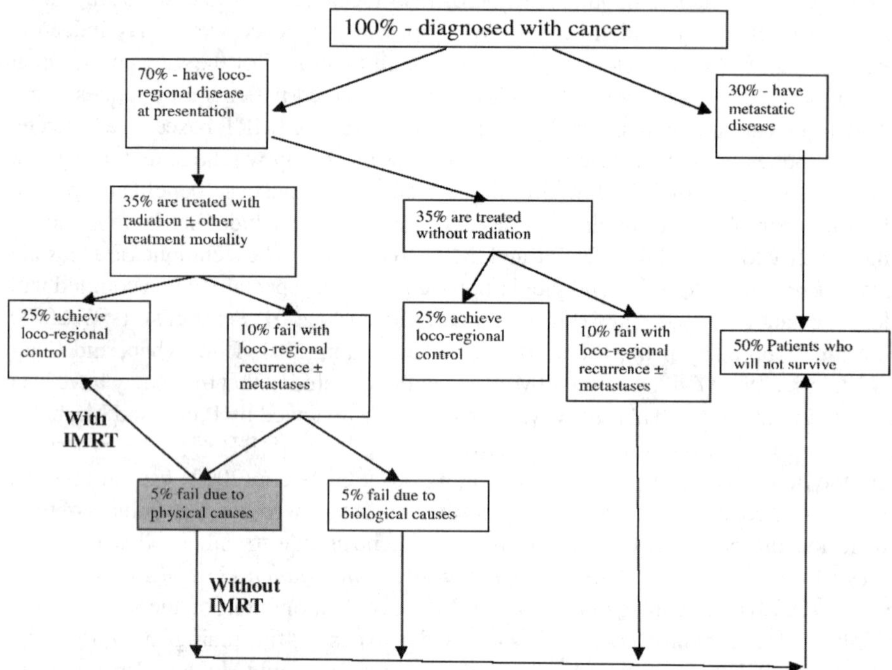


**Figure 3.** A triage of patients, normalized to the cancer incidence (100%).

The generic triage values in figure 3 are average values estimated from data for all tumors (Leibel et al. 1991) with assumptions on utilization of radiotherapy, surgery, and chemotherapy. Our goal here is to introduce the model and methodology rather than defend the input data. Mortality was forced to total up to 50% of the diagnosed cases (i.e., incidence). In this model, up to 5% of all diagnosed patients could benefit from technological advances in radiotherapy if all had access to IMRT. In the United States alone, this would correspond to 64,000 patients potentially benefiting—annually. Real gains could be lower if more failures are due to biological rather than poor dose distribution or underdosage. Clearly this type of analysis should be repeated on a tumor site-by-site basis, with more evidence-based triage numbers.

Such simplistic modeling also does not account for the cases where, currently, systemic progression due to inadequate drug therapies may be the main cause of failure, as discussed previously. For example, in extensive small-cell lung cancer, the incremental benefit of thoracic and prophylactic cranial radiotherapy is negated by systemic progression. Loco-regional control will become more important as systemic therapies improve; this is becoming apparent in limited stage small-cell lung cancer where thoracic radiotherapy and effective chemotherapy have been shown to be of benefit. Another example is lymphoma patients who benefit from combined chemotherapy and radiotherapy, at lower doses from each modality with less combined toxicity. Similarly, high-risk breast patients with positive nodes have been shown to benefit from adjuvant chemotherapy or hormones, with loco-regional chest wall radiotherapy starting to demonstrate an incremental survival benefit. This benefit has only become evident in recent years as technology and treatment techniques have improved and different bottlenecks to success are re-evaluated and cleared. New beam arrangements avoid large dose per fraction to normal tissues and *en-face* cobalt fields to treat internal mammary nodes. Historically, these have led to increased cardiac toxicity and deaths, overshadowing the anti-cancer benefit that may now advance into the foreground.

There are many promising agents that are aimed at controlling systemic disease. Adjuvant therapeutic agents of the future will possibly include novel biologic agents such as growth factor inhibitors, anti-angiogenesis agents, and tumor invasion inhibitors. These will address the microscopic systemic disease, leaving behind loco-regional tumor deposits that can be approached effectively with radiation, IMRT, and with less combined toxicity. All the numbers assumed in figure 3 need to be refreshed every 5 years to account for shifts in the combination of adjuvant therapies and their revised outcomes.

*Purely Dollars And Sense*

When CT scanners were first introduced to improve targeting and dose calculations in radiotherapy, Goitein (1980) showed that even a small improvement in local tumor control proved cost-effective. The offset costs were due to the large differential between the costs of initially successful radiotherapy ($12,000 in 1978 U.S. dollars) and that of a failed treatment ($36,000). A similar methodology can be applied to justify IMRT-related procedures, if it also reduces the rates of costly sequelae of treatment failures. In the period of 1992–1995, Perez et al. (1997) monitored the reimbursements of successful standard radiotherapy (average $10,900) and 3DCRT (average $13,800). Thus the incremental cost of implementing 3DCRT of the prostate was approximately $3,000. More notable in the original study was the major difference in cost between successful 3-D radiotherapy and failed radiotherapy followed by long-term use of hormonal therapy (total of $40,800). In the period of 1992–1997, Perez et al. (2001) extended their financial study to include IMRT. The technical costs were $7,100 for 3DCRT of the prostate, $9,200 for IMRT of the head and neck, and $6,000 for standard radiotherapy of the prostate. These translate to a 50% increase for IMRT over regular radiotherapy, but only a 20% change over 3-D radiotherapy. Actual net revenues (collected) for technical and professional aspects of the procedures were $15,600, $18,100, and $10,800, respectively. These translate to a 16% differential between IMRT and 3-D radiotherapy, as paid by patients and their insurance companies. Gillin (2002) recently suggested that the main additional costs of IMRT are attributable to treatment planning and this component would increase by only 25% on an hourly basis (from 3DCRT to IMRT).

It is relatively easy to predict the improvement in TCP that is needed in order to justify the extra costs of any new procedure. Assume N patients are eligible for either standard treatment or IMRT. Then,

Case 1: Standard Treatment (SRT) is used

N patients treated at @cost $$C_{SRT}$ per case　　　$C_{SRT}$ N$

If $TCP_{SRT}$ is achieved by SRT, then

Failures $= (1 - TCP_{SRT}) \times N$

Failures cost extra $\$\Delta F$ per case　　　$\Delta F (1 - TCP_{SRT}) N$

Total　　　$[C_{SRT} + \Delta F (1 - TCP_{SRT})] N$　　　(1)

Case 2: IMRT is used instead

N treated by IMRT with extra cost $\Delta C$　　　$(C_{SRT} + \Delta C) N$

$TCP_{IMRT}$ improves by $\Delta TCP$

Failures $= (1 - TCP_{IMRT}) \times N$

$= [1 - (TCP_{SRT} + \Delta TCP)]N$

Failures costs $\$F$ per case　　　$\Delta F (1 - (TCP_{SRT} + \Delta TCP)) N$

Total Cost　　　$[(C_{SRT} + \Delta C) + \Delta F(1 - (TCP_{SRT} + \Delta TCP))] N$　　　(2)

Equating (1) and (2) to obtain the "break even" equilibrium condition yields:

$$\Delta C = \Delta TCP \times \Delta F$$

Thus the extra costs ($\Delta C$) are exactly balanced by the expectation value of the savings ($\Delta TCP \times \Delta F$). Alternatively, the break-even point occurs when the absolute increase in TCP ($\Delta TCP$) equals the ratio of the extra costs for failure to the extra costs of IMRT:

$$\Delta TCP = \Delta C / \Delta F$$

In this simple model, the equilibrium point does *not* depend on the starting TCP value or the baseline cost of the standard treatment ($C_{SRT}$) and the number of cases treated (N); in reality, a larger number of treated cases may lead to economies of scale and thereby reduce the unit incremental cost ($\Delta C$). Using numbers from Perez et al. (1997), $\Delta F = \$27,000$ and $\Delta C = \$3,000$. Thus, the gain in TCP ($\Delta TCP$) required for IMRT to break even is $\$3,000/\$27,000 = 0.11$. If the $TCP_{SRT}$ of standard treatment were 80%, then IMRT would have to achieve a TCP of 91% to become "cost neutral."

Comparable gains in TCP values have been demonstrated in some 3DCRT and IMRT clinical trials when dose escalation is applied to prostate cases.

The key to purely financial cost effectiveness is therefore selection of patients most likely to benefit from the change in technology and avoidance of costly re-treatments. The above simple analysis, however, did not account for other cost savings that may result from implementing IMRT:

- Avoiding medications and procedures for treatment complications

- "Learning curve" overhead that will decrease when the equipment and procedures become better streamlined for IMRT

- Delegation to specialized technical staff (e.g., from physicist to dosimetrist), as procedures become robust and documented

- Efficiency gains in patient setup and delivery with arc therapy *versus* multi-field setups, and possible hypofractionation

- Cost avoidance due to lower supplies costs (e.g., shielding block fabrication *versus* MLC) and the reduced frequency of "lifting" injuries in staff

As a spin-off benefit, IMRT developments will spark creativity, generating new products or avenues for novel treatment design. Most of our thinking about radiation prescriptions (dose per day, total dose) has been constrained by technology that necessitated larger volumes of normal tissue irradiation. By having a tool to sculpt any dose-volume shape, the "solution space" is expanded, leading to the opportunity to optimize fraction size as well as total dose and overall treatment time. For example, hypo-fractionation may become possible for some tumors with favorable radiobiological characteristics (Fowler 2001). This might consume fewer machine resources, take less overall treatment time, and make it more convenient for patients. However, the need for extra quality assurance in such cases (e.g., more frequent portal imaging) may offset such potential cost savings.

In the short term, the newer methods are inevitably more costly or cumbersome to use. In time, these hurdles are overcome. Widespread development and implementation of a technique yields efficiencies and lower costs and can also justify smaller incremental benefits across a larger patient population base. Most of the economic arguments against IMRT will fade if we accept that a concerted drive to achieve efficiency will eventually lead to lower costs, aided by economy of scale.

*Long-Term Carcinogenesis—The Hidden Cost Of IMRT?*

One of the most compelling arguments to "go slow" with IMRT implementation may be the integral dose argument. This stems from the irony that improved radiotherapy will allow patients to survive longer, running a greater risk of manifesting a secondary radiation-induced neoplasm. Conventional radiotherapy increases the risk of secondary cancers for patients treated for Hodgkins disease and cervix and prostate cancer. For Hodgkin's disease, a study of approximately 1500 survivors (Cellai et al. 2001) revealed an increased lifetime risk of leukemia, non-Hodgkin's lymphoma, lung, and breast disease in females. The lifetime risk of developing these cancers with prior radiotherapy (alone) was 10%, and 16% after latency periods of 15 and 20 years, respectively. These represent a doubling in risk, relative to the general comparable population. Similarly, large studies are discussed by Hall (2000). These studies link the subsequent development of breast cancers in female patients to prior radiotherapy, with a risk enhancement ratio of 2.24. A study of 51,000 patients treated for prostate cancer with radiation alone, revealed an increase of 34% in risk for developing secondary solid tumors (e.g., bladder, rectum, and lung), after a latency period of 10 years or more. The increase in risk for developing sarcomas within or near the treatment fields was much higher. The enhanced risk of lung tumors is noteworthy since the lungs were well "out-of-field" and received much less dose (e.g., <1% of target dose). However, confounding factors such as lifestyle (i.e., smoking) and predisposition for lung cancer cannot be ruled out.

In view of these findings of the past decades, what new additional risks will IMRT introduce? The potential for a "backfire effect" with IMRT is due to three factors: greater X-ray leakage through MLCs, more beam time to produce intensity modulation, and dose escalation. Table 1 summarizes these issues for standard radiotherapy, 3DCRT, and IMRT. Let us first consider "in field" effects of carcinogenesis. We define this region as that for which a dose distribution is calculated. The deterministic radiation effects are the main consideration in critical organ sparing, keeping dose levels below tolerance values. Any "extra" dose due to elevated MLC transmission (effect C), for example, could be accounted for during the dose calculations. The stochastic carcinogenic effect is of concern in the lower dose regimen. This includes generic tissues in the dose "spillage" regions of the dose distribution where there is potential survival of potentially transformed cells. This background "fog" of dose can be assessed through dose-volume histograms (e.g., bone DVH for sarcomas) or integral dose. From this viewpoint, any increase in collimator leakage could become part of a dose optimization penalty and adjusted to keep these lower dose levels to historical levels or even lower in or near the treatment zone.

Let us now consider the "out of field" regions that receive potentially carcinogenic whole-body low-dose levels. These peripheral doses are deemed important in transforming actively dividing cells that survive a more moderate radiation insult. Regulations require that the primary collimator limit the dose in far zones (outside of a field with 25 cm radius) to be less than 0.1% of central dose. This component is, however, generally small when compared with contributions from field-shaping collimators and in-patient scattering at intermediate distances. IMRT will increase the leakage dose due to MLC transmission and side-scattering, but this will be compensated for by reduced in-patient scatter using smaller fields.

The synchronized movements include: continuous gantry rotation with rapid opening and closing of tungsten shutters and linear movement of the patient couch into the gantry aperture. Image guidance systems, essential to the precision of IMRT, are also integrated into the designs of figure 4. These images can be taken on treatment day to enable re-targeting and, in the case of CT imaging capability (a and b), reconstruction of the "*in vivo* 3-D dose distribution of the day." In the C-arm gantry system (a), CT imaging is done in the cone-beam geometry.

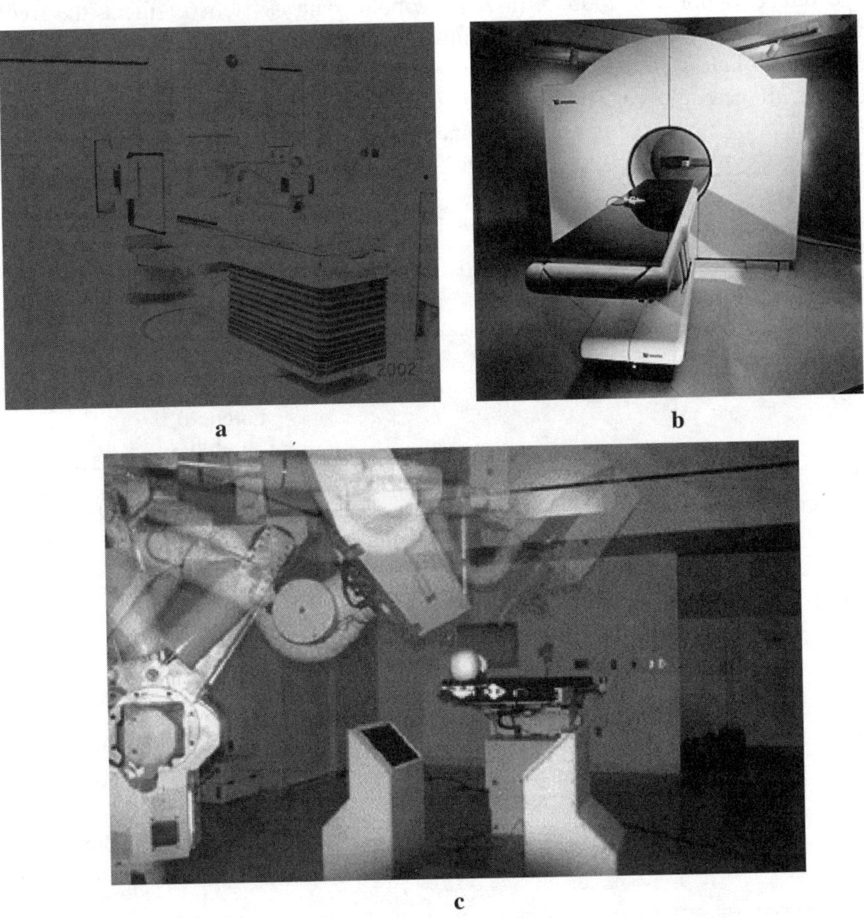

**Figure 4.** Three 3-D X-ray strategies using a broad cone beam (a), a thin fan beam (b), and (c) an articulated pencil beam. Image guidance is achieved with kilovoltage cone beam CT (a), megavoltage spiral CT (b), and radiography (c). Graphics courtesy of Dr. D. Jaffray and Elekta (a), Dr. T. R. Mackie and TomoTherapy Inc.(b), and Accuray's CyberKnife® (Newport Beach, CA).

 **Jerry J. Battista and Glenn S. Bauman**

A kilovoltage x-ray tube and flat panel detector are added to the C-arm, orthogonal to the 6 MV source and portal imaging system. Using fluoroscopy rather than radiography, some progress has been made in respiratory gating of the radiotherapy beam. The beam is triggered when the target, marked with internal high contrast beeds, is "in sight." In the future, a compact kilovoltage x-ray needle source (Cho and Munro 2002) may be added within the standard linac head, obviating the need for an extra x-ray tube. Ideally, this approach could use a dual-mode CT detector for kilovoltage and megavoltage (Seppi et al. 2003) X-rays. The robotic gantry system (c) directs the accelerator beam, and an independently mounted x-ray tube is used to perform biplanar radiography. This system is essentially a whole body radiosurgery system with radiographic image guidance used rather than CT or a mechanical guidance frame. IMRT may be achievable by using multiple pencil beams of different intensity aimed non-isocentrically to shape the dose distribution. Table 2 summarizes the various approaches.

**Table 2.** Different IMRT Gantry Designs, Irradiation Geometries, and Image Guidance Systems for the Systems Shown in Figure 4

| | Beam Geometry | Gantry Design | Degrees of Freedom | Beam Gating Potential Capability | Imaging |
|---|---|---|---|---|---|
| (a) Traditional Linac | Cone beam | C-arm | Non-coplanar | Breath-Hold or Beam Trigger | Fluoroscopy Kilovoltage CT |
| (b) Helical Tomo-therapy | Fan beam Continuous Helical Scan | Circular | Co-Planar without junctions | Breath-Hold with Interlaced Helices | Megavoltage CT |
| (a+b) Serial Tomotherapy | Fan beam Sequential Linear Steps | C-Arm | Co-Planar | Breath-Hold during Single Slice | Portal Imaging |
| (c) Robotic Linac | Pencil beam | Robotic Arm | Non-coplanar | Gated Beam | Biplanar Radiography |

It is our expectation that the treatment machines of the future will be distinguished more on the basis of their imaging and gating capability than their irradiation prowess! We predict the gradual replacement of portal radiographic imaging with on-board CT imaging or auxiliary ultrasound imaging. This is an essential change in the paradigm of verification imaging because soft tissues can be made visible nearer to the time of treatment—a crucial requirement to daily retargeting. We foresee a "David and

Goliath" competition between the C-arm gantry systems favored by traditional linac manufacturers (e.g., Elekta, Varian) and the ring gantry system more recently introduced by a startup company (TomoTherapy Inc). Multi-slice tomotherapy with a revolutionary new collimation system could be the next level of evolution, reducing treatment and imaging times, and possibly peripheral leakage dose. Clinical experience will begin to build on helical tomotherapy. The Madison unit was used to treat a patient for the first time in the summer of 2002 and the two first commercial units are been installed in Canada during 2003. The trade-offs in terms of degrees of freedom during dose optimization, CT imaging quality and convenience, leakage radiation characteristics, and respiratory gating capability will be evaluated relative to present linac designs.

## Accelerators: Light Electrons Or Heavy Charged Particles?

IMRT-like dose distributions have been produced for many years using "heavy charged particles" such as protons, $\pi^-$ mesons or heavier ions having a higher LET. There are over 30 mega-accelerators and the worldwide caseload treated thus far has been 35,000 patients (Particle Therapy Cooperative Group, Massachusetts General Hospital, Boston, MA). Over 85% of the treatments have been performed with proton beams, most often used to treat small lesions at the back of the eye. The high costs of the accelerators are such that these facilities are normally time-shared with basic scientific applications, with few exceptions (e.g., Boston, MA, and Loma Linda, CA). The "holy trinity" of this form of radiotherapy is as follows: (A) depth-dose characteristics featuring Bragg or "star" peaks at a well-defined depth; (B) relative biological effectiveness (RBE) that accentuates at the target depth; (C) reduced dependence on the oxygenation status of the tumor (i.e., lower OER than for X-rays) near the end of range. The RBE and OER are less applicable to proton beams, the most commonly used charged particle. Textbook comparisons between particle beams and X-ray beams have emphasized single-beam characteristics for monoenergetic particles. The depth-dose advantage is clear for "thin" lesions (protons are ideal for ocular lesions) but the depth-dose profile is degraded for modified beams that cover thicker lesions. The intrinsic "radiobiological gradient in RBE" along the beam path can produce a "turbo boost" of radiation damage in the peak region, particularly for the heavier charged particles. High-LET beams also produce more "direct" DNA damage in comparison with indirect chemical action, and therefore cell killing is less dependent on the level of hypoxia in tumors. This is a clear advantage over x-ray beam therapy but this is not in play for the most common applications using protons.

In many radiotherapy cases treated with x-rays, multi-field dose distributions are now used. For larger target volumes, conformal x-ray dose distributions can begin to compete with those of particle dose distributions, albeit using more fields (Lomax, Goitein, and Adams 2003). For smaller volumes, particle beams produce stronger dose gradients and less spillage dose into normal tissues, but the advantage has been narrowed with x-ray IMRT capability. Proton proponents argue that IMRT protons will always be better than IMRT photons "on paper" (Goitein 1992). The key question is whether this *in vitro* advantage translates into clinical benefit *in vivo*. While the intrinsic radiobiological advantages for treating hypoxic tumors remains with high-LET radiation, further advances in "high-resolution" MLC technology may allow "radiobiological compensators" to be designed to deliver higher doses specifically to hypoxic sub-regions of the tumor, if these zones can be imaged (see *Targets And Non-Targets: Functional Imaging In 3-D And 4-D*). Thus the general need for heavy particle radiotherapy, beyond "niche" tumor sites such as ocular lesions, is now debatable (Mackie and Smith 1999). With intense evolution and competition from X-ray IMRT, high-LET facilities are more likely to have a persistent, unique role in basic radiobiology research rather than mainstream radiotherapy. While it may be possible to also improve the conditioning of high-LET beams with IMRT, this does not appear to be an evolutionary pathway that will yield enough further advantage at reasonable cost. The step from IMRT to high-LET radiotherapy may have stepped into the realm of diminishing returns (figure 2). In this instance the ALATA principle (As Long As it is Technologically Achievable) may give way to the *ACARA principle* (As Conformal As is Reasonably Achievable).

## The Role of Brachytherapy

Brachytherapy was the first method to achieve "conformal radiotherapy," well before the advent of external beam therapy. There are clear advantages to implanting the radiation directly into the tumor bed, provided this placement can be verified during the implant procedure. The renaissance in $^{125}$I prostate implants is a prime example of the impact of image guidance on therapy. "Free hand" prostate implants showed inferior results to external beam radiotherapy, driving practice away from $^{125}$I implants until ultrasound guidance resurrected it. Clinical results are now essentially equivalent with those of external beam therapy (D'Amico et al. 1998; Zelefsky et al. 1999). In fact, this equivalence has allowed an estimate to be made of the radiobiological parameter $\alpha/\beta$ *in vivo*. The lower-than-expected value of $\alpha/\beta$ opened up new possibilities for hypofractionation using conformal external beams (Fowler 2001). There is clear synergy across the various forms of radiation delivery.

The next level of improved technique in brachytherapy lies in better control of the implant needle placement and seed deposition process. There is also opportunity to reduce morbidity using different "entry" approaches. For example, prostate implants are now done transperineally rather than suprapubically with a surgically open approach. This has reduced the recovery time for patients to the point that this is now an out-patient procedure with minimal hospital stay, resulting in significant cost and time savings, and freeing up machine resources.

In addition to imaging improvements such as 3-D ultrasound, the introduction of robotics may improve the precise execution and optimization of entry ports for the implant needles (a miniature variant of figure 4c). The robot may be used to reproducibly deposit seeds at predetermined coordinates in the patient coordinate space, using "smart" surgical navigation software that could also anticipate and avoid "collisions," such as pubic arch interference. Robotic techniques are not new to brachytherapy (i.e., remote afterloaders) but image-based navigation tools may add new flexibility and precision. This will potentially reduce the impact of the human "learning curve" on implant quality and outcomes. Peering further into the future of minimally- invasive procedures, robotics may allow telesurgery, an implant done under remote supervision and control by an expert in a major center.

The advantage of brachytherapy over teletherapy is that the treatment course duration appears shorter, although the sources remain active for several months, inactivating tumor cells with a continuous dose rate. The drawbacks are that the patient must be a reasonably good surgical candidate and that controls must be in place to assure radiation protection of the staff, patients, and their family. Brachytherapy also places more emphasis on operator skill in terms of ensuring the sources are placed in the planned matrix (D'Amico and Vogelzang 1999). Due to post-implant imaging of the seed matrix, and computation of the *delivered* dose distribution, one can readily quantify implant quality. It may be argued that it is easier to ensure a good quality of external beam treatments across a large number of physicians than a good quality implant. However, there is no hard evidence that "operator independence" prevails for external beam delivery, although this is more likely. Until we can image IMRT dose distributions *in vivo*, "less operator dependence" of external beam radiotherapy may be an illusion.

Will brachytherapy therefore still be used a few decades from now? IMRT dose distributions can be shaped more readily and offer more uniformity in dose at the target. Brachytherapy is less flexible because of limited access ports, and the straight-line needle trajectories for seed placements. There are several trends and forces that oppose brachytherapy evolution. In the surgical world, the trend is towards minimally invasive procedures. While brachytherapy may already qualify as being minimally invasive, external beam therapy is non-invasive! In the world of radiation protection and the ALARA (As Low As Reasonably Achievable) principle, the current mood is to steer away from the use, distribution, and storage of radioactive materials. To counteract these forces, brachytherapy may have intrinsic radiobiological "dose rate" advantages, and the dose distributions produce less "leakage dose" to neighboring tissues.

Our expectation is that brachytherapy will continue to evolve and play a significant role, but in a smaller subset of patients, unless robotics with vision and tactile functions transforms the procedures radically. The possibility of combining IMRT treatments with brachytherapy dose in different "boost" combinations is, however, tantalizing. It certainly is not an original approach, having been used for decades in cervical cancer but it may open up new possibilities. It has been suggested that tomotherapy be used to "top up" brachytherapy implants of inferior quality or dose level. Another instance may be when the diseased patient anatomy does not permit brachytherapy to be performed at all. An example includes locally advanced cervical cancer with destruction of tissue that precludes placement of the intrauterine stem.

When external beam therapy is used alone in this instance, clinical results are inferior to those obtained with intracavitary brachytherapy. If IMRT could be used to produce a substituted pseudo-intracavitary dose distribution, then good clinical results could be restored. Another possibility is to overtly combine brachytherapy with IMRT of regional lymph nodes using the conformal avoidance strategy. While taking full advantage of extremely steep dose gradients of brachytherapy, this may reduce morbidity due to broader regional node irradiation and enable dose escalation.

## Companion Technology And Competing Forces

### Targets And Non-Targets: Functional Imaging In 3-D And 4-D

Image guidance and image verification will become the *sine qua non* for IMRT of the future. Since dose volumes of any size and shape can be sculpted, two issues leap to the forefront as potential bottlenecks to progress: target volume definition and target volume tracking. This also applies to the localization of critical structures that must be regularly "missed" during treatment. Table 3 shows the various imaging techniques in a matrix of contributions to radiation oncology, with new and expanding roles of functional diagnostic imaging (Tepper 2001; Chapman et al. 2003), verification imaging, and dosimetric imaging.

Ling et al. (2000) proposed the concept of a "Biological Target Volume (BTV)." The current trend is towards "fusing" the target features extracted by each specialized imaging modality with its unique specificity and sensitivity. Combination gantries [e.g., tomotherapy with CT, positron emission therapy-computed tomography (PET-CT) scanners] facilitate direct image registration. PET-CT fusion in hardware or software enables functional PET information to be overlaid onto CT-delineated anatomy. Early clinical experience with PET-CT is showing great promise in avoiding "geographic misses" of metabolically active lung tumors, invisible to CT scanning alone. In the future, PET imaging will also identify poorly oxygenated sub-targets in human tumors. PET-CT simulation may be the next natural development. MR simulation is here already.

Future molecular imaging is important because it will hopefully generate sufficient "tumor signal" from voxels imaged by today's techniques. Indeed, this has been the traditional strength of nuclear medicine images, in which sub-voxel changes in uptake can be detected with more sensitivity than gross morphological change. With further advances in contrast and spatial resolution of imaging techniques, it may become possible to confirm that all tumor clonogens are 'covered' by the IMRT high dose volume. This will not be an easy accomplishment since there are potentially $\sim 10^6$ tumor cells per cubic mm (voxel) of tissue.

**Table 3.** Multi-Modality Imaging. Bracketed (x) Denote "Under Development"

| Feature | Simu-lator | CT | MRI | MRS | SPECT PET | Ultra-sound | Portal Imaging |
|---|---|---|---|---|---|---|---|
| Open Gantry | x | (x) | | | (x) | | x |
| Projection | x | x | (x) | | | | x |
| Tomography | | x | x | | x | x | |
| Beam's Eye View | x | x | (x) | | | | x |
| Fluoroscopy | x | | | | | x | (x) |
| Surface Contours | x | x | x | | | x | |
| Tissue Electron Densities | | x | | | | | |
| Vasculature | x | x | x | | | x | |
| Gross Target Volume | x | x | x | | x | x | (x) |
| Organs at Risk | x | x | x | | x | x | (x) |
| Clinical Target Volume | | | x | x | | | |
| Planning Target Volume | x | x | | | | | (x) |
| Biological Target Volume | | | x | x | x | | |
| Verification | | x | | | | x | x |
| 3-D Dosimetry | | x | x | (x) | | | |

In addition to identifying small numbers of tumorigenic cells, there is the difficulty of assuring that the imaged volume is stable in time. The old adage "If you can't see it, you can't hit it; if you can't hit it, you can't cure it" (attributed to H. E. Johns or W. Powers) takes on a timely corollary: "If it's moving, you can't hit it; if you can't hit it, you can't cure it." This "Heisenberg principle" may foil the best of attempts at precision treatment planning based on pre-treatment conditions. During the past decades, planning has emphasized 3-D anatomical images for better tumor targeting, but the plans are generated using an anatomical "snapshot" often taken weeks before start of treatment. However, the patient anatomy changes daily as organs fill (e.g., bladder, lung) and tissues deform and displace. These changes are evident from fluoroscopy on a traditional simulator. With greater emphasis on beam-shaping technology and tighter tumor margins, the issue of moving targets and critical structures becomes far more important. Strategies have evolved for accurate beam delivery in the thorax, where videometry, spirometry, or fluoroscopy (Shirato et al. 2000) are used to monitor the respiratory cycle. The patient either breathes normally and the radiation therapy beam can be "time-gated" (Keall et al. 2001) to activate only when the lung lesion is "in sight." Alternatively, the patient is trained to breath-hold reproducibly (Stromberg et al. 2000) so that the lesion is held stationary in space when the beam is delivered. While originally intended to target lung lesions, these methods may also enable the displacement of critical normal organs out of the beam paths (Hanley et al. 1999). These approaches will be implemented with variable degrees of ease for patients and beam efficiency on the various treatment delivery platforms (figure 4). The migration of imaging systems, such as CT and ultrasound, into the treatment rooms appears inevitable for "live" verification of the space-time coordinates of lesions and critical organs. Registration of these images with those gated during treatment planning (including biological imaging) will enable adaptive radiotherapy to proceed with confidence and credibility. Current experience suggests that non-linear registration (i.e., image warping) is required to account for the complex deformations and movements of the anatomy as a function of time. In the ultimate implementation of 4-D IMRT, target and non-target regions will be positioned and monitored within a virtual patient, incorporating changes based on the biomechanical properties of various tissue compartments.

## Modifying The Radiobiological Response

The basic strategy of developing biological modulators of radiobiological response is shown in figure 5, in contrast with the strategy depicted in figure 1. This approach separates the curves rather than separates the dose, shifting the tumor curve to the left and the normal tissue curve to the right.

This crossover has been the "holy grail" of radiobiology. Possible mechanisms may include promotion or suppression of DNA damage and repair, growth factors, apoptosis, or angiogenesis. If it were achieved, this would trigger the question: What then would be the role of IMRT, if any? Indeed, if an agent made tumors hypersensitive to radiation, relative to surrounding normal tissues, then uniform irradiation of a larger volume (e.g., with a parallel-opposed pair of beams) might be quite acceptable. Past decades of radiobiological research has resulted in agents that can sensitize hypoxic tumor cells by a factor of 3 at most (e.g., OER ~3 for X-rays), or desensitize some normal cells by a factor of less than 2 (e.g., amiphostine or WR2721), with most results being achieved *in vitro*. If both could hypothetically be used simultaneously *in vivo*, and *all* tumor and *all* surrounding normal cells were affected, one could hope for an effective therapeutic gain of less than 6. This six-fold differential is comparable with the dose gradients achievable today by IMRT without radiobiological modification (figure 1). However, many new developments are underway in molecular genetic manipulation (Bartelink 2001; Coleman 2001, 2002; Coleman and Cumberlin 2001), some including radio-activation of genes. With the human genome being mapped in detail, advances in molecular biology may uncover new targeting mechanisms (Brown 2001) that modify dose response. Highly conformal low dose distributions would still be needed to trigger the genetic reactions.

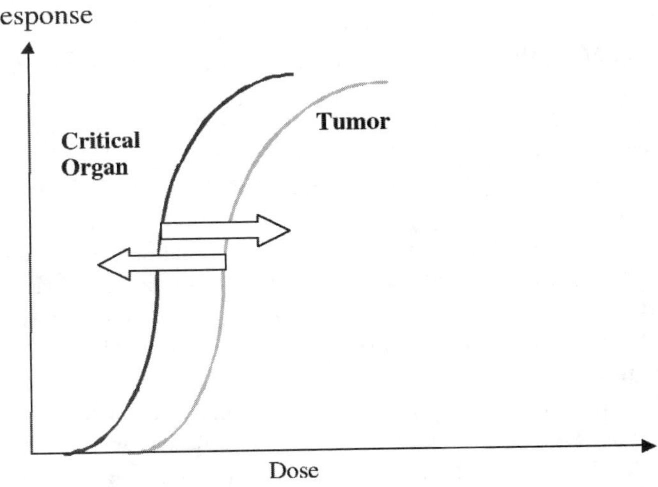


**Figure 5.** The strategy of "crossover," separating the dose response curves using radiobiological response modifiers.

In the past, there has been great difficulty in designing effective drug combinations that would work well *in vivo*, and are delivered specifically to the desired cell populations, without being systemically toxic. The expanding use of micro-array technology in biology labs will improve the search efficiency for relevant genes and proteins that are expressed only under certain cellular micro-environments, such as hypoxic stress. Better drug concentrations through specific delivery and absorption would certainly advance both chemotherapy and radiotherapy, including radio-immunotherapy. Approaches that rely on enhancing the absorption of external radiation, such as neutron capture therapy or photon activation therapy could be revisited with higher achievable molar concentrations.

Our expectation is that molecular therapy advances will come in time increments of decades rather than years. Initially, these advances will likely be more helpful in diagnostics and imaging of tumor cells rather than treating them. Indeed any agents that show promise will first be evaluated for *in vivo* distribution and specificity. This progression has historical precedents. The search for hypoxic cell sensitizers has resulted in new PET imaging agents rather than a therapeutically useful agent. Of course, such agents would then play a vital role in identifying the elusive biological target volume (BTV) for IMRT.

In summary, we can anticipate imaging benefits from the advances being made in designing new radiobiological modifiers and molecular markers. Combined with progress in new functional imaging techniques (functional CT and MRI), IMRT will benefit from the improved identification of targets and subtargets using blood flow measurements and molecular markers of key genetic and micro-environmental factors.

## Non-Radiation Modalities: Drugs, Lasers, And Thermal Energy

Alternatives to radiation have been developed and useful for specific tumor sites. The prostate as a localized, tumor-bearing structure that can be targeted is an attractive site for any number of local energy modalities: permanent implant ($^{125}$I, $^{103}$Pd), temporary high dose rate (HDR) brachytherapy, protons, implant microwave therapy, cryotherapy, photodynamic therapy with fibre optics, or combinations of the above. The comparison of these techniques and their future potential relative to IMRT must be based on their dosimetry, "invasiveness," effectiveness, toxicity, cost, convenience for the patient, and clinical outcomes. Hyperthermia is an example of a modality that is complementary to radiotherapy but problems in delivery and dosimetry have plagued its implementation on a wide scale. Some trials are in progress comparing the "mature" approaches such as external beam therapy, brachytherapy, surgery, and cryotherapy. However, many of the newer techniques are at a much earlier stage of development, particularly in the dosimetric and treatment planning aspects, and outcome measurements are preliminary. Successful treatment paradigms often combine therapies to improve the therapeutic ratio through a number of independent mechanisms. The complementary roles and synergy between radiotherapy, chemotherapy, and surgery have evolved over decades of clinical experience. These modalities have not been combined by accident but rather because these satisfy criteria such as synergy, low cross reactivity (toxicity), and "spatial cooperation."

## Conclusions

- Radiotherapy is a proven "curative" agent, that can approach its full potential through ongoing developments of IMRT, including tomotherapy.

- Radiotherapy is essentially non-invasive; toxicity can be reduced further using IMRT techniques

- Long-term carcinogenic effects are a concern for IMRT especially with higher energy x-ray beams (e.g., >10 MV X-rays). Lower energy IMRT with novel delivery and collimation systems will reduce the peripheral dose to historical levels or lower. The added risks of IMRT must be weighed against the survival benefits, within the perspective of background incidence of natural lifetime carcinogenesis.

- Efficiency and cost-effectiveness of IMRT will naturally evolve as this form of treatment becomes more widely adopted as the new future standard of precision radiotherapy.

- Ultimate advances in IMRT will hinge strongly upon better imaging of the biological target volume (BTV) to be treated effectively in space and in time.

- Clinical trials are showing early advantages for IMRT in terms of tumor control by dose escalation and reduced toxicity. The positive results are not universally accepted yet by the entire radiation oncology community but consensus is expected to build positively during this decade.

- IMRT will be complementary to many new forms of "avant garde" therapies, including those based on molecular targeting. It will continue to play a unique role as an agent that is especially efficient at killing tumor cells that find refuge in body regions that are not approachable through systemic channels.

- IMRT will produce an exciting technological milieu that enhances the retention and recruitment of a future generation of radiation specialists in our evolving field.

## Acknowledgments

We acknowledge fruitful discussions on the future of radiation oncology with all of our colleagues at the London Regional Centre, particularly Jake Van Dyk, Tomas Kron, Kevin Jordan, Eugene Wong, and Rashid Dar.

## References

Bartelink, H. (2001). "From translational research to improved local control and survival." Gilbert Fletcher Award Lecture, ICTR 2000, Lugano, March 2000. *Int. J. Radiat. Oncol. Biol. Phys.* 49:311–318.

Brown, J. M. (2001). "Therapeutic targets in radiotherapy." Keynote Lecture 2000, International conference on Translational Research and preclinical Strategies in Radio-Oncology (ICTR). *Int. J. Radiat. Oncol. Biol. Phys.* 49:319–326.

Carol, M., W. H. Grant 3rd, D. Pavord, P. Eddy, H. S. Targovnik, B. Butler, S. Woo, J. Figura, V. Onufrey, R. Grossman, and R. Selkar. (1996). "Initial clinical experience with the Peacock intensity modulation of a 3-D conformal radiation therapy system." *Stereotact. Funct. Neurosurg.* 66:30–34.

Cellai, E., S. M. Magrini, G. Masala, R. Alterini, A. S. Costantini, L. Rigacci, L. Olmastroni, M. G. Papi, M. A. Spediacci, F. Innocenti, G. Bellesi, P. R. Ferrini, and G. Biti. (2001). "The risk of second malignant tumors and its consequences for the overall survival of Hodgkin's disease patients and for the choice of their treatment at presentation: analysis of a series of 1524 cases consecutively treated at the Florence University Hospital." *Int. J. Radiat. Oncol. Biol. Phys.* 49:1327–1337.

Chapman, J. D., J. D. Bradley, J. F. Eary, R. Haubner, S. M. Larson, J. M. Michalski, P. G. Okunieff, H. W. Strauss, Y. C. Ung, and M. J. Welch. (2003). "Molecular (functional) imaging for radiotherapy applications: An RTOG symposium." *Int. J. Radiat. Oncol. Biol. Phys.* 55:294–301.

Cho, K. H., F. M. Khan, and S. H. Levitt. (1999). "Cost-benefit analysis of 3D conformal radiation therapy—treatment of prostate cancer as a model." *Acta Oncol.* 38, 603–611.

Cho, Y., and R. Munro. (2002). "Kilovision: Thermal modeling of a kilovoltage x-ray source integrated into a medical linear accelerator." *Med. Phys.* 29:2101–2108.

Coleman, C. N. (2001). "Investing in our future: Listening to those who will take us where we need to go." Young Investigators Workshop—Radiation Oncology Sciences Program. National Cancer Institute, National Institutes of Health, Aug 1–2, 2000. *Int. J. Radiat. Oncol. Biol. Phys.* 49:1505–1516.

Coleman, C. N. (2002). "Radiation oncology—linking technology and biology in the treatment of cancer." *Acta Oncol.* 41:6–13.

Coleman, C. N., and R. L. Cumberlin. (2001). "Translational research in radiation oncology." NCI Radiation Research Program Meeting Report. *Int. J. Radiat. Oncol. Biol. Phys.* 49:885–890.

D'Amico, A. V., and N. J. Vogelzang. (1999). "Prostate brachytherapy: Increasing demand for the procedure despite the lack of standardized quality assurance and long term outcome data." *Cancer* 86:1632–1634.

D'Amico, A. V., R. Whittington, S. B. Malkowicz, D. Schultz, K. Blank, G. A. Broderick, J. E. Tomaszewski, A. A. Renshaw, I. Kaplan, C. J. Beard, and A. Wein. (1998). "Biochemical outcome after radical prostatectomy, external beam radiation therapy, or interstitial radiation therapy for clinically localized prostate cancer." *JAMA* 280:969–974.

Fowler, J. F. (2001). "Biological factors influencing optimum fractionation in radiation therapy." *Acta Oncol.* 40:712–717.

Followill, D., P. Geis, and A. Boyer. (1997). "Estimates of whole-body dose equivalent produced by beam intensity modulated conformal therapy." *Int. J. Radiat. Oncol. Biol. Phys.* 38:667–672. [Published erratum appears in *Int. J. Radiat. Oncol. Biol. Phys.* 39(3):783].

Gillin, M. T. (2002). "Comments on 'On the role of intensity-modulated radiation therapy in radiation oncology'." *Med. Phys.* 29:2962–2963.

Glatstein, E. (2002). "Intensity-modulated radiation therapy: Ihe inverse, the converse, and the perverse." *Semin. Radiat. Oncol.* 12:272–281.

Goitein, M. U. (1980). "Benefits and cost of computerized tomography in radiation therapy." *JAMA* 244:1347–1350.

Goitein, M. U. (1992). "The comparison of treatment plans." *Semin. Radiat. Oncol.* 2:246–256.

Hall, E. J. *Radiobiology for the Radiologist.* Fifth Ed. Philadelphia: Lippincott Williams & Wilkins, 2000.

Hanley, J., M. M. Debois, D. Mah, G. S. Mageras, A. Raben, K. Rosenzweig, B. Mychalczak, L. H. Schwartz, P. J. Gloeggler, W. Lutz, C. C. Ling, S. A. Leibel, Z. Fuks, and G. J. Kutcher. (1999). "Deep inspiration breath-hold technique for lung tumors: The potential value of target immobilization and reduced lung density in dose escalation." *Int. J. Radiat. Oncol. Biol. Phys.* 45:603–611.

IMRTCWG (Intensity Modulated Radiation Therapy Collaborative Working Group). "Intensity-modulated radiotherapy: Current status and issues of interest." *Int. J. Radiat. Oncol. Biol. Phys.* 51:880–914.

Jaffray, D. A., J. H. Siewerdsen, J. W. Wong, and A. A. Martinez. (2002). "Flat-panel cone-beam computed tomography for image-guided radiation therapy." *Int. J. Radiat. Oncol. Biol. Phys.* 53:1337–1349.

Keall, P. J., V. R. Kini, S. S. Vedam, and R. Mohan. (2001). "Motion adaptive x-ray therapy: A feasibility study." *Phys. Med. Biol.* 46:1–10.

Leibel, S. A., Z. Fuks, M. J. Zelefsky, S. L. Wolden, K. E. Rosenzweig, K. M. Alektiar, M. A. Hunt, E. D. Yorke, L. X. Hong, H. I. Amols, C. M. Burman, A. Jackson, G. S. Mageras, T. LoSasso, L. Happersett, S. V. Spirou, C. S. Chui, and C. C. Ling. (2002). "Intensity modulated radiotherapy." *Cancer J.* 8:164–176.

Leibel, S. A., C. C. Ling, G. J. Kutcher, R. Mohan, C. Cordon-Cordo, and Z. Fuks. (1991). "The biological basis for conformal three-dimensional radiation therapy." *Int. J. Radiat. Oncol. Biol. Phys.* 21:805–811.

Levitt, S. H., and F. M. Khan. (2001). "The rush to judgment: Does the evidence support the enthusiasm over three-dimensional conformal radiation therapy and dose escalation in the treatment of prostate cancer?" *Int. J. Radiat. Oncol. Biol. Phys.* 51:871–879.

Levitt, S. H., and F. M. Khan. (2002). "In response to Purdy, J.A., and J. M. Michalski 'Does the evidence support the enthusiasm over 3D conformal radiation therapy and dose escalation in the treatment of prostate cancer?' *Int. J. Radiat. Oncol. Biol. Phys.* 51:867–870." *Int. J. Radiat. Oncol. Biol. Phys.* 53:1085–1086.

Lillicrap, S. C., H. M. Morgan, and J. T. Shakeshaft. (2000). "X-ray leakage during radiotherapy." *Br. J. Radiol* .73:793–794.

Ling, C. C., J. Humm, S. Larson, H. Amols, Z. Fuks, S. Leibel, and J. A. Koutcher. (2000). "Towards multidimensional radiotherapy (MD-CRT): Biological imaging and biological conformality." *Int. J. Radiat. Oncol. Biol. Phys.* 47:551–560.

Lomax, A. J., M. Goitein, and J. Adams. (2003). "Intensity modulation in radiotherapy: Photons versus protons in the paranasal sinuses." *Radiother. Oncol.* 66:11–18.

MacKenzie, M. A., and D. M. Robinson. (2002). "Intensity modulated arc deliveries approximated by a large number of fixed gantry position sliding window dynamic multileaf collimator fields." *Med. Phys.* 29:2359–2365.

Mackie, T. R., and A. R. Smith. (1999). "Intensity-modulated conformal radiation therapy and 3-dimensional treatment planning will significantly reduce the need for therapeutic approaches with particles such as protons." *Med. Phys.* 26:1185–1187.

Mackie, T. R., J. Balog, K. Ruchala, D. Shepard, S. Aldridge, E. Fitchard, P. Reckwerdt, G. Olivera, T. McNutt, and M. Mehta. (1999). "Tomotherapy." *Semin. Radiat. Oncol.* 9(1):108–117.

Mohan, R., R. Cardinale, and M. Hagen. (1999). "Comments on 'Further improvements in dose distributions are unlikely to affect cure rates'." *Med. Phys.* 26:2701–2705.

Mutic, S., and E. E. Klein. (1999). "A reduction in the AAPM TG-36 reported peripheral dose distributions with tertiary multileaf collimation." *Int. J. Radiat. Oncol. Biol. Phys.* 44:947–953.

Mutic, S., and D. A. Low. (1998). "Whole-body dose from tomotherapy delivery." *Int. J. Radiat. Oncol. Biol. Phys.* 42:229–232.

National Cancer Institute. (2003). Surveillance Epidemiology and End Results (SEER):1973-1999. Internet Communication. SUTP://seer.cancer.gov/csr/1973_1999/overview.pdf.

Perez, C. A., J. M. Michalski, S. Ballard, R. Dryzmala, B. J. Kobeissi, M. A. Locket, and T. H. Wasserman. (1997). "Cost-benefit of emerging technology in localized carcinoma of the prostate." *Int. J. Radiat. Oncol. Biol. Phys.* 39:875–883.

Perez, C. A., B. J. Kobeissi, K. S. C. Chao, J. M. Michalski, D. A. Low, M. Gupta, N. Dupoch, and T. H. Wasserman. "Cost-Benefit of 3D-CRT/IMRT" in *3-D Conformal and IMRT: Physics and Clinical Applications*. J. A. Purdy, W. H. Grant III, J. R. Palta, E. B. Butler, and C. A. Perez. Madison, WI: Advanced Medical Publishing Inc., pp. 589–601, 2001.

Pollack, A., G. K. Zagars, G. Starkschall, J. A. Antolak, J. J. Lee, E. Huang, A. C. von Eschenbach, D. A. Kuban, and I. Rosen. (2002). "Prosate cancer radiation dose response: Results of the MD Anderson phase III randomized trial." *Int. J. Radiat. Oncol. Biol. Phys.* 53:1097–1105.

Purdy, J. A., and J. M. Michalski. (2001). "Does the evidence support the enthusiasm over 3D conformal radiation therapy and dose escalation in the treatment of prostate cancer?" *Int. J. Radiat. Oncol. Biol. Phys.* 51:867–870.

Rogers, D. W., B. A. Faddegon, G. X. Ding, C.-M. Ma, J. We, and T. R. Mackie. (1995). "BEAM: A Monte Carlo code to simulate radiotherapy treatment units." *Med. Phys.* 22(5):503–524.

Schreiner, L. J. "The Potential for Modern Radiotherapy Using Cobalt 60" in MDS Symposium "Advances in Radiation Therapy" 50th Anniversary Celebrations of Cobalt-60 in Canada. London Regional Cancer Centre, London, Ontario, October 2001.

Schulz, R. J. (1999). "Further improvements in dose distributions are unlikely to affect cure rates." *Med. Phys.* 26:1007–1009.

Schulz, R. J. (2001). "Through the preoccupation with new technical developments, physicists have lost sight of the realities of cancer care and statistics. For the proposition." *Med. Phys.* 28:2185–2187.

Schulz, R. J., and A. R. Kagan. (2002). "On the role of intensity-modulated radiation therapy in radiation oncology." *Med. Phys.* 29:1473–1482.

Seppi, E. J., P. Munro, S. W. Johnsen, E. G. Shapiro, C. Tognina, D. Jones, J. M. Pavkovich, C. Webb, I. Mollov, L. D. Partain, and R. E. Colbeth. (2003). "Megavoltage cone-beam computed tomography using a high-efficiency image receptor." *Int. J. Radiat. Oncol. Biol. Phys.* 55:793–803.

Shirato, H., S. Shimizu, T. Kunieda, K. Kitamura, M. van Herk, K. Kagei, T, Nishioka, S. Hashimoto, K. Fujita, H. Aoyama, K. Tsuchiya, K. Kudo, and K. Miyasaka. (2000). "Physical aspects of a real-time tumor-tracking system for gated radiotherapy." *Int. J. Radiat. Oncol. Biol. Phys.* 48(4):1187–1195.

Stromberg, J. S., M. B. Sharpe, L. H. Kim, V. R. Kini, D. A. Jaffray, A. A. Martinez, and J. W. Wong. (2000). "Active breathing control (ABC) for Hodgkin's disease: Reduction in normal tissue irradiation with deep inspiration and implications for treatment." *Int. J. Radiat. Oncol. Biol. Phys.* 48(3):797–806.

Suit, H. (1982). "Potential for improving survival rates for the cancer patient by increasing the efficacy of treatment of the primary lesion." The American Society of Therapeutic Radiologists Presidential Address. October 1981. *Cancer* 50:1227–1234.

Suit, H. (2002). "The Gray Lecture 2001: Coming technical advances in radiation oncology." *Int. J. Radiat. Oncol. Biol. Phys.* 53:798–809.

Suit, H., and W. DuBois. (1991). "The importance of optimal treatment planning in radiation therapy." *Int. J. Radiat. Oncol. Biol. Phys.* 21:1471–1478.

Suit, H., and R. Miralbell. (1989). "Potential impact of improvements in radiation therapy on quality of life and survival." *Int. J. Radiat. Oncol. Biol. Phys.* 16:891–895.

Suit, H., and S. Westgate. (1986). "Impact of improved local control on survival." *Int. J. Radiat. Oncol. Biol. Phys.* 12:453–458.

Suit, H.D., J. Becht, J. Leong, M. Stracher, W. C. Wood, L. Verhey, and M. Goitein. (1988). "Potential for improvement in radiation therapy." *Int. J. Radiat. Oncol. Biol. Phys.* 14:777–786.

Teh, B., W. Y. Mai, W. H. Grant 3ʳᵈ, J. K. Chiu, H. H. Lu, L. S. Carpenter, S. Y. Woo, and E. B. Butler. (2002)."Intensity modulated radiotherapy (IMRT) decreases treatment-related morbidity and potentially enhances tumor control." *Cancer Invest.* 20:437–451.

Tepper, J. (ed.). (2001). "Functional imaging and its applications to radiation oncology." *Semin. Radiat. Oncol.* 11(1):no page number.

Tepper, J. (ed.). (2002). "Intensity modulated radiotherapy: A clinical perspective." *Semin. Radiat. Oncol.* 12(3):no page number.

Van Dyk, J., and J. A. Purdy. "Clinical Implementation of Technology and the Quality Assurance Process" in *The Modern Technology of Radiation Oncology.* J. Van Dyk (ed.). Madison, WI: Medical Physics Publishing, pp. 19–51, 1999.

Webb, S. (2000). "Regarding x-ray leakage during radiotherapy." *Br. J. Radiol.* 73:1339.

Williams, P. O., and A. R. Hounsell. (2001.) "X-ray leakage considerations for IMRT." *Br. J. Radiol.* 74:98–100.

Wong, E., J. Z. Chen, and J. Greenland. (2002). "Intensity-modulated arc therapy simplified." *Int. J. Radiat. Oncol. Biol. Phys.* 53:222–235.

Yu, C. X., X. A. Li, L. Ma, D. Chen, S. Naqvi, D. Shepard, M. Sarfaraz, T. W. Holmes, M. Suntharalingam, and C. M. Mansfield. (2002). "Clinical implementation of intensity-modulated arc therapy." *Int. J. Radiat. Oncol. Biol. Phys.* 53:453–463.

Zelefsky, M. J., K. E. Wallner, C. C. Ling, A. Raben, T. Hollister, T. Wolfe, A. Grann, P. Gaudin, Z. Fuks, and S. A. Leibel. (1999). "Comparison of the 5-year outcome and morbidity of three-dimensional conformal radiotherapy versus transperineal permanent iodine-125 implantation for early-stage prostatic cancer." *J. Clin. Oncol.* 17:517–522.

# Novel Uses And Applications Of IMRT

James S. Welsh, M.S., M.D.[1], Gustavo H. Olivera, Ph.D.[2],
and T. Rockwell Mackie, Ph.D.[2]
[1]Department of Human Oncology
University of Wisconsin Medical School, Madison, Wisconsin
[2]Department of Medical Physics, University of Wisconsin
and TomoTherapy Inc., Madison, Wisconsin



## Introduction

Intensity-modulated radiation therapy (IMRT) represents one of the greatest technological advances in modern radiation oncology. Helical tomotherapy exemplifies one
of the latest steps in the evolution of IMRT. Helical tomotherapy integrates a novel
radiotherapy unit with an innovative means of delivering IMRT (Mackie et al. 1999).
Physically, the helical tomotherapy unit can be considered a helical computed tomography (CT) scanner that harbors not a diagnostic x-ray tube, but rather a compact 6
MV linear accelerator capable of providing intensity modulated radiation therapy. The
intensity modulation is provided by an array of 64 leaves which function on a simple
binary (in or out) fashion. The patient is translated through the 85 cm bore, which
rotates about the patient, delivering therapy in a continuous helical fashion. The gantry
can rotate about the patient at various rates, ranging from 1 to 6 revolutions per minute.
In addition to its unique means of delivering IMRT, helical tomotherapy has the distinctive potential for adaptive radiotherapy conferred by its CT imaging component.
Housed within the gantry, opposite the accelerator is a xenon detector, which allows
megavoltage CT (MVCT) images to be generated. These MVCT images will replace
the conventional port films used in standard linac-based radiotherapy. They also
provide anatomical detail unprecedented in radiotherapy. Preliminary investigation
demonstrates that MVCT can provide excellent visualization of parenchymal lung
tumors and appears satisfactory for the purpose of tumor targeting in helical
tomotherapy (figure 1). Such image-guidance allows the potential for adaptive radiotherapy using helical tomotherapy. This is essentially the reconstruction of the actually
delivered dose (as opposed to the planned dose) followed by modifications in subsequent dose delivery and/or patient position, so that the entire course of radiotherapy
is more likely to achieve the desired radiation dose distribution.

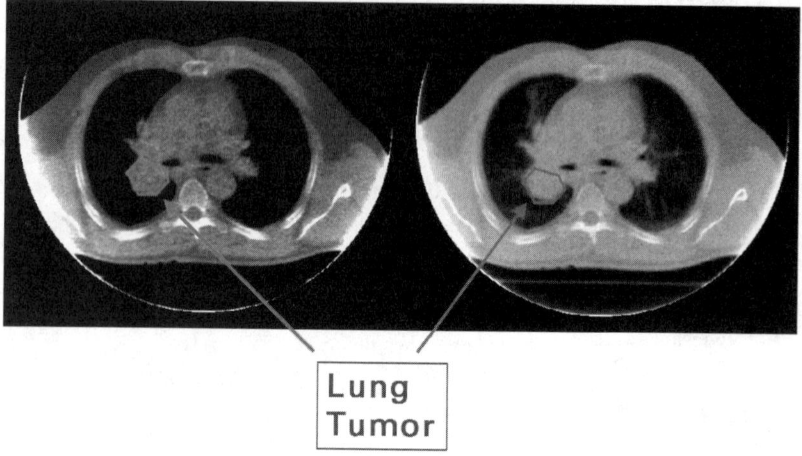


**Figure 1.** A transverse MVCT image of a patient with non-small-cell lung cancer, clearly illustrating the tumor mass. The absorbed radiation dose from the scan was 30 mGy.

Preliminary work at the University of Wisconsin suggests that helical tomotherapy appears to be particularly well suited for the specific avoidance of normal structures during treatments (Welsh et al. 2002). This strategy, known as "conformal avoidance" (Aldridge and Mackie 1998), aims to minimize radiation dose to sensitive normal organs/tissues rather than attempting to specifically target gross tumors and areas suspected of harboring occult disease. Conformal avoidance is thus the complement to conformal radiotherapy. In practice, it may be much easier to implement conformal avoidance than conformal therapy since normal sensitive structures such as lungs, liver, salivary glands, rectum, etc., are typically more readily visualized during treatment planning using conventional CT than complicated tumor volumes and nodal areas suspected of harboring micrometastases. Conformal avoidance radiotherapy through helical tomotherapy therefore opens up a vast array of possible applications of IMRT that heretofore have been considered impractical or impossible. In this chapter we look at several such unique applications that are currently under investigation at the University of Wisconsin.

## A New Mantle

The successful application of radiation therapy in the management of patients with Hodgkin's disease represented a milestone in the history of oncology. Prior to the routine use of radiation therapy for Hodgkin's disease, this disease was considered incurable and uniformly fatal. Early pioneers in the application of radiotherapy for Hodgkin's disease such as Gilbert and Peters paved the way for future clinical investigators to develop strategies using radiation therapy alone or in conjunction with chemotherapy to cure the vast majority of patients with early stage Hodgkin's disease. An integral component of radiation therapy for Hodgkin's disease has been the "mantle" field for disease above the diaphragm and the "inverted-Y" for disease below the diaphragm. While clinically proven to be effective, the mantle and to a lesser extent the inverted-Y have been implicated in a host of treatment-related complications. The mantle, with its simple AP/PA opposed fields, exposes relatively large volumes of normal lung, spinal cord, heart, thyroid, and larynx to unnecessary radiation. Although doses used for Hodgkin's disease are now modest, patients still experience occasional complications including radiation pneumonitis, Lhermitte's syndrome, hypothyroidism, and cardiac complications. Young children may experience growth abnormalities and women under the age of 30, especially in their teenage years may be particularly susceptible to breast cancer following treatment.

Using the strategy of conformal avoidance, we can now specifically aim to avoid unnecessary radiation of the key normal structures including thyroid, larynx, humeral heads, spinal cord, lungs, and heart yet, still provide full dose to the nodal regions at risk. Covering the nodal regions adequately is of paramount importance in any such strategy. This is because of the decades of clinical experience using the mantle and its various modifications, which have documented the importance of providing adequate dose to the nodal regions in the neck, mediastinum and supraclavicular, infraclavicular, and axillary regions. Attempting to implement conformal therapy to these regions can be difficult or impractical, as many clinicians who have attempted to contour such nodal chains can vouch for. Although grossly involved nodes are clearly visible and occasionally small lymph nodes can provide some indication of where the nodal chain is, the bulk of the lymph node chains are practically invisible to CT imaging. A common strategy used for conformal therapy to these regions is to contour the clearly visible vessels, such as the subclavian and axillary arteries and veins, and assuming that the nodal chain lies adjacent to these vessels. Such a strategy is risky since nodal anatomy may occasionally be aberrant and microscopically involved nodes could lie distant from the visible vessels and therefore not be targeted during conformal radiation therapy. Additionally, conformal targeting of these vessels and the (presumed) associated nodes is a much more limited field of radiation and thus differs from the time-tested and proven mantle fields. In our conformal avoidance approach we do not target the visible vessels, but rather target the entire "regions at risk" including the axillary, supraclavicular, infraclavicular, mediastinal, and neck regions while simultaneously conformally avoiding dose to normal structures which do not harbor disease, such as lungs, humeral heads, spinal cord, heart, thyroid, and larynx. Preliminary inverse treatment planning has yielded impressive radiation dose distributions and excellent dose-volume histograms (DVHs) (figure 2) (Welsh et al. 2003). Clinical implementation of this new mantle equivalent should begin in the near future.

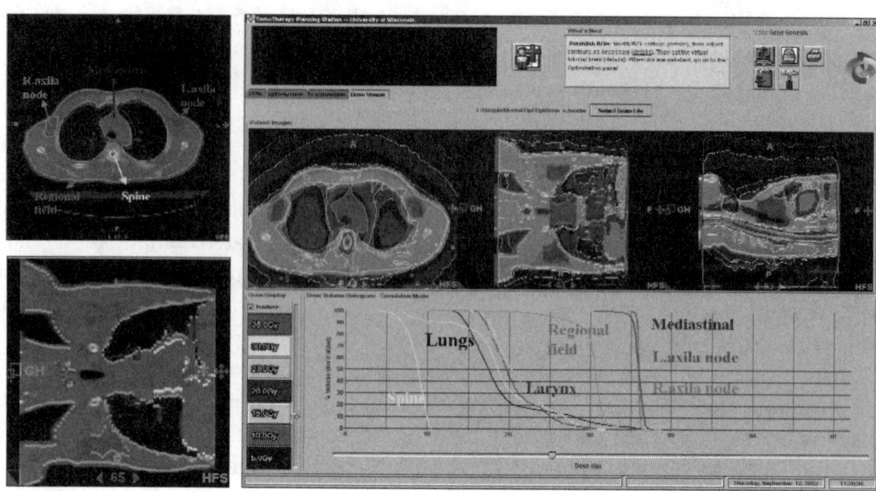



**Figure 2.** Effective sparing of key normal structures including spinal cord, lungs, and humeral head are evident in this helical tomotherapy-generated equivalent of a "mini-mantle" field.

## Brain-Sparing Total Scalp Irradiation/Scalp-Sparing Total Brain Irradiation

Although not commonly encountered, there are certain disease entities that involve the scalp alone and are amenable to total scalp irradiation with either curative or palliative intent. Such diseases include angiosarcoma, melanoma, non-Hodgkin's lymphoma, and benign diseases including dissecting cellulitis of the scalp. In such circumstances, a variety of different radiotherapeutic techniques have been employed, including multiple matched *en face* electron fields, combinations of photons and electrons, serial tomotherapy and most recently helical tomotherapy. The goal of all these approaches is to provide adequate dose to the scalp skin while minimizing radiation exposure to the underlying normal brain. Brain irradiation has been associated with a number of complications including cognitive deficits and induction of second malignancies including meningioma. Some of the techniques currently in use such as the combination of *en face* lateral electron fields to cover the lateral aspects of the scalp matched with opposed lateral proton fields to cover the sagittal strip of scalp skin appear to work quite well. A study from Mallinckrodt Institute (Locke et al. 2002) using IMRT by a serial tomotherapy found essentially no advantage to IMRT compared to their conventional technique. In our experience we have similarly found the electron-photon combination to be dosimetrically quite satisfactory, but in clinical practice a number of deficiencies can arise. This is because of the dosimetric uncertainties in the match-line region in the abutting electron and photon fields. In order to minimize hot spots or cold spots along this match line, one common approach is to "feather" the junction by moving the match line superior or inferior several millimeters every few days. While this reduces dosimetric uncertainties, daily patient setup can prove challenging and time-consuming for the radiation therapists. Again, employing the strategy of conformal avoidance and helical tomotherapy, we have been able to obtain surprisingly good dose distributions and DVHs. This unique application of IMRT via helical tomotherapy should prove to be far faster to deliver than the conventional electron/proton approach, yet provide equivalent or better brain sparing and tumor targeting.

Far more common in standard radiation therapy practice than total scalp irradiation is whole brain irradiation. Patients with limited brain metastases and controlled disease outside the central nervous system now have median survivals that are far longer thanks to the use of stereotactic radiosurgery and neurosurgical resection in conjunction with whole brain radiotherapy. Previously, when survival was typically measured in weeks to a few months, cosmetic outcome was of little concern. Now, however, with median survivals measuring a year or more in a number of patients, cosmesis obtains more relevance. This preservation of hair by conformal avoidance of the scalp during whole brain radiotherapy represents yet another potential application of IMRT that awaits formal investigation.

## Mesothelioma

Although a rare form of cancer, mesothelioma presents a particularly vexing challenge to radiation oncologists and medical physicists. In situations where the pleura cannot be surgically resected, radiation therapy remains the only hope of providing disease control. However, with the anatomical arrangement of the disease-ridden pleura wrapped around the entire lung, providing meaningful doses to the pleura without simultaneously irradiating large volumes of lung tissue to high doses has been practically impossible. Recently, the group from M. D. Anderson Cancer Center has come up with a strategy of using IMRT to provide dose to the pleura while minimizing normal lung parenchymal dose. A dosimetric analysis of their technique (Ahamad et al. 2003) has yielded surprisingly good radiation dose-distributions. Clinical implementation of this unique application of IMRT is currently underway at M. D. Anderson and preliminary results have been recently published (Forster et al. 2003). Other investigators have been successfully exploring intensity-modulated arc therapy (IMAT) for mesothelioma (Tobler, Watson, and Leavitt 2002). Helical tomotherapy, with its rotational method of radiation delivery, seems ideally suited for tangentially irradiating this complex volume in an efficient manner (figure 3).

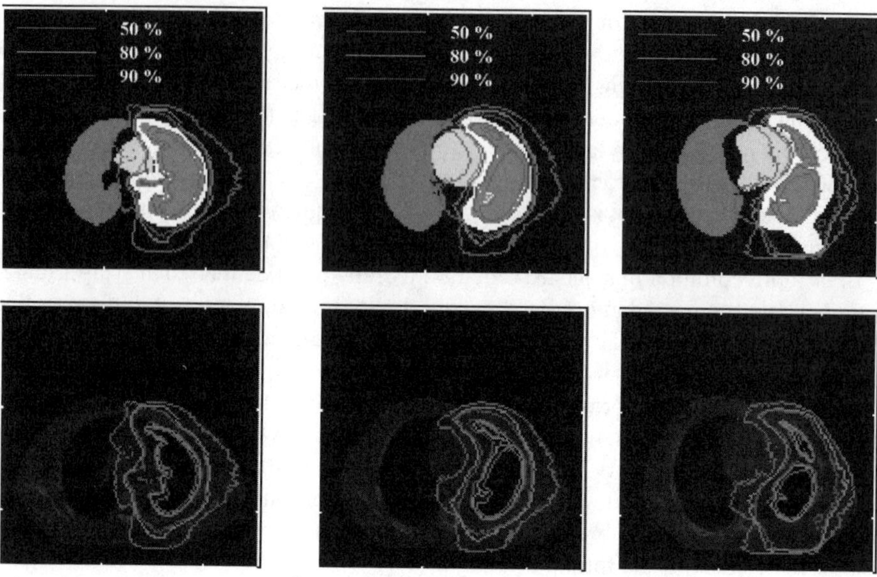


**Figure 3.** Radiation dose-distributions resulting from helical tomotherapy inverse treatment planning for mesothelioma.

## Total Body Irradiation (TBI)

Total Body Irradiation or TBI has been part of the preparative regimens for both autologous and allogeneic stem cell transplants for a variety of hematologic malignancies. Despite the fact that total doses are relatively low and treatment is often hyperfractionated, complications can and do occur. Among the more commonly encountered complications of TBI are radiation pneumonitis, liver injury, kidney injury, and cataracts. The currently popular approaches to TBI often involve some degree of lung-blocking, hyperfractionation, and low dose-rate of the administered treatment. While the low dose-rate is primarily a function of the distance away from the linac gantry required to cover the patient from head to toe, it secondarily has the presumably beneficial effect of reducing complications. Most centers do not attempt to specifically block the liver, kidneys, or lenses of the eye except in rare circumstances. Although not yet clinically tested, it is possible that TBI with a conformal avoidance strategy represents another potential new application of IMRT and plans are currently underway at the University of Wisconsin for a helical tomotherapy-based approach to TBI. It is worth mentioning that caution should be exercised with this or any other IMRT-based TBI technique because of the unknown effects of the altered dose-rate as well as the sparing of tissues normally included in conventional TBI protocols.

## Applications For Metastatic Disease

Patients with widespread metastatic disease, who are in need of palliation, represent a sizable fraction of most radiation oncology practices. On occasion, these cases can prove quite challenging such as when multiple sites are in need of palliation simultaneously. In such situations the current approach is to treat individual sites separately with conventional therapy, which can take up a fair amount of machine time. It also can be problematic in a patient who has been previously irradiated or if the areas that are in need of treatment require fields that will overlap in sensitive normal structures. In such situations IMRT may be of value. In our preliminary investigation of complex cases involving multiple sites that require treatment simultaneously, we found that linac-based IMRT and helical tomotherapy proved superior to conventional treatment planning and 3-D conformal therapy in terms of DVHs. Although the DVHs for linac-based IMRT and helical tomotherapy were essentially equal in terms of sparing of normal structures and providing full dose to the target, we found that in some situations the linac-based IMRT plan required several isocenters and over a dozen individual fields to achieve this same dose distribution. This would amount to an individual patient's treatment taking over an hour to administer and thus is impractical in most radiotherapy clinics. The helical tomotherapy plan would be able to treat the patient in an estimated 6 minutes and therefore represents a far more realistic solution to such complicated tumor volumes (Welsh et al. 2002).

This later observation generates a very interesting hypothesis about potential treatment of patients with widespread metastatic disease. Patients with metastatic disease are generally considered incurable and the role of radiation therapy is limited to palliation. In situations where metastatic deposits can be surgically resected, patient survival can occasionally be prolonged (e.g., limited liver metastases from colorectal cancer). Similarly, if metastatic disease can be controlled with radiation therapy, survival may be enhanced. In a prospective randomized clinical trial, patients with hormone-refractory prostate cancer were given combination chemotherapy followed by consolidation chemotherapy with or without [89]Sr (Tu et al. 2001). In this study, patients who received the consolidation with [89]Sr had significantly improved survival over the cohort who did not. This finding supports the hypothesis that chemotherapy can take care of micrometastatic disease while radiation therapy can attack the macroscopic deposits (in this case areas positive on bone scan). Following this logic, it remains possible that an approach could be developed in which disease visualized on CT/PET (positron emission tomogtaphy) would be tackled by radiation therapy while chemotherapy would eradicate the invisible microscopic disease. Future investigations employing helical tomotherapy or other IMRT techniques may make this formerly unthinkable scenario a reality for some patients with metastatic, currently incurable cancer.

# References


Ahamad, A., C. W. Stevens, W. R. Smythe, A. A. Vaporcivan, R. Komaki, J. F. Kelly, Z. Liao, G. Starkschall, and K. M. Forster. (2003). "Intensity modulated radiation therapy: A novel approach to the management of malignant pleural mesothelioma." *Int. J. Radiat. Oncol. Biol. Phys.* 55:768–775.

Aldridge, J. S., and T. R. Mackie. (1998). "Conformal avoidance radiation therapy." *Radiother. Oncol.* 48:S76.

Forster, K. M., W. R. Smythe, G. Starkschall, Z. Liao, T. Takanaka, J. F. Kelly, A. Vaporcivan, A. Ahamad, L. Dong, M. Salehpour, and R. Komaki. (2003). "Intensity-modulated radiation therapy following extrapleural pneumonectomy for the treatment of malignant mesothelioma: Clinical implementation." *Int. J. Radiat. Oncol. Biol. Phys.* 55:606–616.

Locke, J., D. A. Low, T. Grigireit, and K. S. Chao. (2002). "Potential of tomotherapy for total scalp treatment." *Int. J. Radiat. Oncol. Biol. Phys.* 52:553–559.

Mackie, T. R., J. Balog, K. Ruchala, D. Shepard, S. Aldridge, E. Fitchard, P. Reckwerdt, G. Olivera, T. McNutt, and M. Mehta. (1999). "Tomotherapy." *Semin. Radiat. Oncol.* 9(1):108–117.

Ruchala, K., G. Olivera, L. Forrest, M. Mehta, J. Kapatoes, J. Welsh, and T. Mackie. (2002). "Megavoltage CT for image-guided radiotherapy." *Radiother. Oncol.* 64(suppl 1):S12.

Tobler, M., G. Watson, and D. D. Leavitt. (2002). "Intensity-modulated photon arc therapy for treatment of pleural mesothelioma." *Med. Dosim.* 27:255–259.

Tu, S. M., R. E. Millikan, B. Mengistu, E. S. Delpassand, R. J. Amato, L. C. Pagliaro, D. Daliani, C. N. Papandreou, T. L. Smith, J. Kim, D. A. Podoloff, and C. J. Logothetis. (2001). "Bone-targeted therapy for advanced androgen-independent carcinoma of the prostate: A randomised phase II trial." *Lancet* 357:336–341.

Welsh, J., G. Olivera, S. Hui, D. Henderson, A. Forouzannia, W. Tomé, J. Kapatoes, K. Ruchala, W. Lu, P. Reckwerdt, M. Ritter, and T. R. Mackie. (2002). "Helical tomotherapy with conformal avoidance appears superior to 3-D CRT and IMRT for treatment of complex tumor volumes." *Radiol.* 225(P):360.

Welsh, J. S., S. Tannehill, G. Olivera, K. Bradley, M. Lock, S. Hui, J. Kapatoes, B. Kahl, S. P. Howard, and T. R. Mackie. (2003). "Conformal avoidance radiotherapy with helical tomotherapy for lymphoid malignancies: A new mantle." *J. Clin. Oncol.* In press.

# List Of Acronyms

| | |
|---|---|
| AAPM | American Association of Physicists in Medicine |
| ABC | Active breathing control |
| ABST | Anatomy-based segmentation tool |
| ACARA | As Conformal As is Reasonably Achievable |
| AD | Analog-to-digital |
| AD | Androgen deprivation |
| ALARA | As Low As Reasonably Achievable |
| ALATA | As Long As it is Technologically Achievable |
| AMA | American Medical Association |
| AMFPD | Amorphous silicon flat panel detector |
| AP/PA | Anterior-posterior/posterior-anterior |
| APC | Ambulatory Payment Classification |
| ART | Adaptive radiation therapy |
| ART | Adaptive radiotherapy |
| ART | Algebraic Reconstruction Technique |
| ASTM | American Society for Testing and Materials |
| ASTRO | American Society for Therapeutic Radiology and Oncology |
| BAT® | B-mode Acquisition and Targeting system |
| BED | Biologically effective dose |
| BEV | Beam's eye view |
| BIP | Block-iterative projections |
| BIS | Beam Imaging System |
| BNED | Biochemical disease-free survival |
| BOLD | Blood oxygenation level-dependent |
| BOT | Beam-on-time |
| BTV | Biological target volume |
| BUdR | Bromodeoxyuridine |
| CCD | Charge-Coupled Device |
| CDDP | Cisplatin |
| CF | Calibration factor |
| CFRT | Conformal Radiation Therapy |
| CGE | Cobalt Gray equivalent |
| CMS | Centers for Medicare and Medicaid Services |
| CNS | Central nervous system |
| COI | Cost-of-illness |
| COMM | Communications |
| CPT | (Physician's) Current Procedural Terminology |
| CSF | Cerebrospinal fluid |
| CSF | Collimator scatter factor |
| CR | Computed Radiography |
| CRT | Chemoradiotherapy |
| CT | Computed Tomography |
| CTV | Clinical target volume |

| | |
|---|---|
| CXRT | Conformal External Beam Radiotherapy |
| DA | Digital to analog |
| DAO | Direct aperture optimization |
| DAS | Data Acquisition System |
| DC | Direct current |
| DI | Deep inspiration |
| DIBH | Deep inspiration breath-hold |
| DICOM | Digital Imaging and Communication in Medicine |
| DICOM-RT | Digital Imaging and Communication in Medicine-Radiotherapy |
| DIE | Digital Input Encoder |
| DMF | Dynamic modulation factor |
| DMLC | Dynamic multileaf collimator |
| DRR | Digitally-reconstructed radiograph |
| DRS | Data Receiver Server |
| DTA | Distance to agreement |
| DTPA | Diethyletriammepentaacetate |
| DVA | Leaf sequence file |
| DVH | Dose-volume histogram |
| E-E | End-expiration |
| E-I | End-inspiration |
| ECOG | Eastern Cooperative Oncology Group |
| ECT | Electron conformal therapy |
| EDR | Enhanced dynamic range |
| EMI | Electromagnetic interference |
| eMLC | Electron multileaf collimator |
| EPID | Electronic Portal Imaging Device |
| EPR | Electron paramagnetic resonance |
| EPRI | Electron paramagnetic resonance imaging |
| EUD | Equivalent uniform dose |
| 4-D | Four-dimensional |
| F2T | Fluence to leaf trajectories |
| FB | Free-breathing |
| FC | Function Controller |
| FCCC | Fox Chase Cancer Center (Philadelphia, PA) |
| FDA | Food and Drug Administration |
| FDG | Fluorodeoxyglucose |
| $^{18}$F-FDG-PET | Fluorodeoxyglucose radiolabbeled with fluorine-18 positron emission tomography |
| fMRI | Functional magnetic resonance imaging |
| FPLA | Field-Programmable Logic Array |
| fps | Frames per second |
| FR | Flow rate |
| FSPB | Finite-size pencil beam |
| FSU | Functional sub-unit |
| FTP | File transfer protocol |

| | |
|---|---|
| FUdR | Floxuridine |
| FWHM | Full-width-half-maximum |
| GEMS | General Electric Medical Systems |
| GTV | Gross tumor volume |
| H&D | Hurter & Driffield (curve) |
| H&N | Head and neck |
| HCPCS | Hospital Common Procedure Coding System |
| HDR | High dose rate |
| HF | Hypoxic fraction |
| HMPAO | Hexamethylpropyleneamine oxime |
| HOPPS | Hospital Outpatient Prospective Payment System |
| HTCA | High Tension and Radio Frequency Control Area |
| HV | High voltage |
| HVL | Half-value layer |
| HVT | Half-value thickness |
| I/O | Input/Output |
| ICCA | Interface Cabinet Control Area |
| ICCR | International Conference on the use of Computers in Radiation therapy |
| ICRU | International Commission on Radiation Units and Measurements |
| IEC | International Electrotechnical Commission |
| IFP | Interstitial fluid pressure |
| IGS | Intergroup Study 0099 |
| IM | Intensity modulated |
| IM-WPRT | Intensity-Modulated Whole Pelvic Radiotherapy |
| IMAT | Intensity-Modulated Arc Therapy |
| IMC | Internal mammary chain |
| IMCO | Inverse Monte Carlo optimization |
| IMET | Intensity-Modulated Electron Therapy |
| IMPT | Intensity-Modulated Proton Therapy |
| IMRT | Intensity-Modulated Radiation Therapy |
| IMRTCWG | IMRT Collaborative Working Group |
| IMXT | Intensity-Modulated X-Ray Therapy |
| IOD | Information object definition |
| IRLED | Infrared light-emitting diode |
| IS | Information systems |
| ITV | Internal target volume |
| IV | Intravenous |
| LCR | Local tumor control rates |
| LET | Linear energy transfer |
| LGO | Lipschitz (continuous) Global Optimizer |
| LIF | Least-intensity feasible |
| linac | Linear accelerator |
| LMP | Linear multicriteria programming |
| LQ | Linear quadratic |

| MAA | Macro aggregated albumen |
| MASK | Medical Anatomy Segmentation Kit (project) |
| MC | Monte Carlo |
| MCDM | Multiple Criteria Decision Making (International society) |
| MCNP | Monte Carlo N-Particle |
| MCS | Multiple Coulomb scattering |
| mDIBH | Moderate deep inspiration breath-hold |
| MDP | Methylene diphosphonate |
| MEAT | Modulated Electron Arc Therapy |
| MET | Modulated Electron Therapy |
| MGH | Massachusetts General Hospital (Boston, MA) |
| MI | Mutual information |
| MIMiC® | Multileaf Intensity Modulating Collimator |
| MIP | Mixed integer programming |
| MLC | Multileaf collimator |
| MOSFET | Metal Oxide Semiconductors Field Effect Transistor |
| MR | Magnetic resonance |
| MRI | Magnetic Resonance Imaging |
| MRSI | Magnetic Resonance Spectroscopic Imaging |
| MSE | Mean square error |
| MSF | Multiple static field |
| MSKCC | Memorial Sloan-Kettering Cancer Center (New York, NY) |
| MTU | Multiplexer Terminal Unit |
| MU | Monitor unit |
| MVCT | Megavoltage Computed Tomography |
| NAA | N-acetylaspartate |
| NAL | No action level |
| NCI | National Cancer Institute |
| NCP | Nasopharyngeal carcinoma |
| NED | Disease-free survival |
| NEMA | National Electrical Manufacturers Association |
| NEOS | Network Enabled Optimization System |
| NKI | Netherlands Cancer Institute |
| NLP | Non-linear programming |
| NMR | Nuclear magnetic resonance |
| NSCLC | Non-small-cell lung cancer |
| NSF | National Science Foundation |
| NTCP | Normal tissue complication probability |
| 1-D | One-dimensional |
| OAR | Organ-at-risk |
| OBC | On-Board Computer |
| OEM | Original equipment manufacturer |
| OER | Oxygen enhancement ratio |
| OR | Organ at risk |
| PA | Posterior-anterior |

| PACS | Picture Archiving and Communication System |
| PB | Pencil beam |
| PC | Personal computer |
| PCB | Printed Circuit Board |
| PDD | Percent depth dose |
| PET | Positron emission tomography |
| PEX | Parallel exponential |
| PFS | Progression-free survival |
| PNET | Primitive neuroectodermal tumor |
| PO | Prostate only |
| POCS | Projection(s) onto convex sets (algorithm) |
| POI | Point of interest |
| pO2 | Tissue oxygen |
| pps | Pulse per second |
| PRF | Pulse repetition frequency |
| PRV | Planning organ at risk volume |
| PSA | Prostate-specific antigen |
| PSI | Paul Scherrer Institute (Switzerland) |
| PSU | Power Supply Unit |
| PSV | Planning structure volume |
| PTV | Planning target volume |
| QA | Quality assurance |
| QOL | Quality of life |
| R&V | Record and verify (system) |
| RAM | Random access memory |
| RBE | Relative biological effectiveness |
| RCCT | Respiration-correlated spiral computed tomography |
| RF | Radiofrequency |
| RHCA | Radiation head Control Area |
| RILD | Radiation-induced liver disease |
| RL | Right lateral |
| rms | Root mean square |
| ROI | Region of interest |
| RPM | Real-time position management (system) |
| RT | Radiation therapy |
| RT | Radiotherapy |
| RTCT | Respiration-triggered computed tomography |
| RTOG | Radiation Therapy Oncology Group |
| RTP | Radiation treatment planning |
| RTP | Radiotherapy treatment planning |
| RTTP | Radiation therapy treatment planning |
| RTU | Remote Terminal Unit |
| SA | Simulated annealing |
| SAD | Source-axis distance |
| SAL | Shrinking action level |

| Sc | Collimator scatter factor |
| SC | Secondary capture |
| SC | Superposition-convolution |
| SCC | Signal Conditioning Card |
| SCD | Source-to-collimator distance |
| SCP | Service class provider |
| SCU | Service class user |
| SD | Standard deviation |
| SF | Surviving fraction |
| SFD | Source-to-film distance |
| SI | Superior-inferior |
| SIB | Simultaneous integrated boost |
| SIP | Serial I/O Processor |
| SMLC | Segmented (segmental) multileaf collimation (step and shoot) |
| SMLC | Static multileaf collimation |
| SMLC | Step-and-shoot multileaf collimation |
| SOBP | Spread out Bragg peak |
| SOP | Service-object pair |
| SPECT | Single photon emission computed tomography |
| SRS | Stereotactic radiosurgery |
| SRT | Stereotactic radiotherapy |
| SSD | Source-surface distance |
| STC | Stationary Computer |
| SUV | Standard uptake value |
| SV | Seminal vesicle |
| SVD | Singular value decomposition |
| SWOG | Southwest Oncology Group |
| 2-D | Two-dimensional |
| 3-D | Three-dimensional |
| 3D-IMPT | Three-dimensional intensity-modulated proton therapy |
| 3DCRT | Three-dimensional conformal radiation therapy |
| T&G | Tongue and groove |
| T2F | Leaf trajectories to fluence |
| TAR | Tissue-air ratio |
| $TCD_{50}$ | Dose required to achieve a TCP at 50% |
| TCP | Tumor control probability |
| TD | Tumor dose |
| TG | Task Group |
| TLD | Thermoluminescent dosimeter |
| TMR | Tissue-maximum ratio |
| TV | Target volume |
| TVL | Tenth-value layer |
| UCSF | University of California at San Francisco |
| US | Ultrasound |
| VCU | Virginia Commonwealth University |